Rebhun's Diseases of Dairy Cattle

Third Edition

Simon F. Peek, BVSc, MRCVS, PhD, Dipl ACVIM

Clinical Professor
Large Animal Internal Medicine, Theriogenology, and Infectious Diseases
School of Veterinary Medicine
University of Wisconsin
Madison, Wisconsin

Thomas J. Divers, DVM, Dipl ACVIM, ACVECC

Steffen Professor of Veterinary Medicine
Large Animal Medicine
Department of Clinical Sciences
College of Veterinary Medicine
Cornell University
Ithaca, New York

ELSEVIER

ELSEVIER

3251 Riverport Lane
St. Louis, Missouri 63043

Notices

Practitioners and researchers must always rely on their own experience and knowledge in evaluating and using any information, methods, compounds or experiments described herein. Because of rapid advances in the medical sciences, in particular, independent verification of diagnoses and drug dosages should be made. To the fullest extent of the law, no responsibility is assumed by Elsevier, authors, editors or contributors for any injury and/or damage to persons or property as a matter of products liability, negligence or otherwise, or from any use or operation of any methods, products, instructions, or ideas contained in the material herein.

Library of Congress Cataloging-in-Publication Data

Names: Peek, Simon Francis, author. | Divers, Thomas J., author.
Title: Rebhun's diseases of dairy cattle / Simon F. Peek, BVSc, MRCVS, PhD,
   Dipl ACVIM, Clinical Professor, Large Animal Internal Medicine,
   Theriogenology, and Infectious Diseases, School of Veterinary Medicine,
   University of Wisconsin, Madison, Wisconsin, Thomas J. Divers, DVM, Dipl
   ACVIM, ACVECC, Steffen Professor of Veterinary Medicine, Large Animal Medicine,
   Department of Clinical Sciences, College of Veterinary Medicine, Cornell University, Ithaca,
   New York.
Description: Third edition. | St. Louis, Missouri : Elsevier, [2018]
Identifiers: LCCN 2017019322| ISBN 9780323390552 | ISBN 9780323396622 (ebook)
Subjects: LCSH: Dairy cattle--Diseases.
Classification: LCC SF961 .R43 2018 | DDC 636.2/142--dc23 LC record
available at https://lccn.loc.gov/2017019322

Senior Content Strategist: Jennifer Flynn-Briggs
Publishing Services Manager: Deepthi Unni
Project Manager: Nadhiya Sekar
Design Direction: Ryan Cook

Working together
to grow libraries in
developing countries

www.elsevier.com • www.bookaid.org

Contributors

John A. Angelos, DVM, PhD, Dipl. ACVIM
Professor
Department of Medicine and Epidemiology
School of Veterinary Medicine
University of California
Davis, California

Sebastien Buczinski DrVet, DES, MSc, Dipl ACVIM
Professor agrégé
Sciences cliniques
Faculté de médecine vétérinaire
Université de Montréal
Saint-Hyacinthe
Québec
Canada

Kevin J. Cummings, DVM, PhD
Associate Professor
Department of Population Medicine and Diagnostic
    Sciences
College of Veterinary Medicine
Cornell University
Ithaca, New York

Thomas J. Divers, DVM, Dipl ACVIM, ACVECC
Steffen Professor of Veterinary Medicine
Large Animal Medicine
Department of Clinical Sciences
College of Veterinary Medicine
Cornell University
Ithaca, New York

Alexander de Lahunta, DVM, PhD, Dipl ACVIM, ACVP
James Law Professor of Anatomy at Cornell
    University - Emeritus
Rye, New Hampshire

Norm G. Ducharme, DMV, MSc, Dipl ACVS
James Law Professor of Large Animal Surgery
Department of Clinical Sciences
College of Veterinary Medicine
Cornell University
Ithaca, New York

Gilles Fecteau, DVM, Dipl ACVIM
Professor titulaire
Sciences cliniques
Faculté de médecine vétérinaire
Université de Montréal
Saint-Hyacinthe
Québec
Canada

Susan L. Fubini, DVM, Dipl ACVS
Professor
Large Animal Surgery
Department of Clinical Sciences
College of Veterinary Medicine
Cornell University
Ithaca, New York

Robert O. Gilbert, BVSc, MRCVS, Dlp ACT
Professor and Head, Department of Clinical Sciences
Ross University School of Veterinary Medicine
(Professor Emeritus, Cornell University)

Anthony E. Good, DVM
Chief Veterinarian
Select Sires, Inc.
Plain City, Ohio

Erin L. Goodrich, DVM
Extension Associate
Veterinary Support Services Veterinarian
Animal Health Diagnostic Center
Department of Population Medicine and Diagnostic
    Sciences
College of Veterinary Medicine
Cornell University
Ithaca, New York

Charles L. Guard, DVM, PhD
Associate Professor
Department of Population Medicine and Diagnostic
    Sciences
College of Veterinary Medicine
Cornell University
Ithaca, New York

Nita L. Irby, DVM, Dipl ACVO
Ruttenberg Senior Lecturer
Department of Clinical Sciences
College of Veterinary Medicine
Cornell University
Ithaca, New York

Elizabeth A. Lahmers, DVM
Associate Veterinarian
Select Sires, Inc.
Plain City, Ohio

Jessica A.A. McArt, DVM, PhD
Assistant Professor
Ambulatory and Production Medicine
Department of Population Medicine and Diagnostic
  Sciences
College of Veterinary Medicine
Cornell University
Ithaca, New York

Sheila M. McGuirk, DVM, PhD, Dipl ACVIM
Professor Emerita
University of Wisconsin-Madison
3720 County Road M,
Dodgeville, Wisconsin

Donald R. Monke, DVM, MBA
Vice President
Production Operations
Select Sires, Inc.
Plain City, Ohio

Paolo Moroni, DVM, PhD
Director of Regional Ithaca Laboratory
College of Veterinary Medicine
Cornell University
Ithaca, New York

Daryl V. Nydam, DVM, PhD
Academic Director
Animal Health Diagnostic Center
Department of Population Medicine and Diagnostic
  Sciences
College of Veterinary Medicine
Cornell University
Ithaca, New York

Theresa L. Ollivett, DVM, PhD, Dipl ACVIM
Assistant Professor
Medical Sciences
School of Veterinary Medicine
University of Wisconsin
Madison, Wisconsin

Paula A. Ospina, DVM, PhD
Extension Associate
Animal Health Diagnostic Center
Department of Population Medicine and Diagnostic
  Sciences
College of Veterinary Medicine
Cornell University
Ithaca, New York

Simon F. Peek, BVSc, MRCVS, PhD, Dipl ACVIM
Clinical Professor
Large Animal Internal Medicine, Theriogenology, and
  Infectious Diseases
School of Veterinary Medicine
University of Wisconsin
Madison, Wisconsin

Jessica C. Scillieri-Smith, DVM
Senior Extension Associate
Animal Health Diagnostic Center
Department of Population Medicine and Diagnostic
  Sciences
College of Veterinary Medicine
Cornell University
Ithaca, New York

Danny W. Scott, DVM, Dipl ACVD, ACVP(Hon)
Professor of Medicine
Department of Clinical Sciences
College of Veterinary Medicine
Cornell University
Ithaca, New York

Raymond W. Sweeney, VMD, Dipl ACVIM
Professor of Medicine
School of Veterinary Medicine
University of Pennsylvania
Philadelphia, Pennsylvania

Justin L. Tank, DVM
Associate Veterinarian
Select Sires, Inc.
Plain City, Ohio

Belinda S. Thompson, DVM
Assistant Clinical Professor
Director of Veterinary Support Services
Animal Health Diagnostic Center
College of Veterinary Medicine
Cornell University
Ithaca, New York

Paul D. Virkler, DVM
Senior Extension Associate
Animal Health Diagnostic Center
Department of Population Medicine and Diagnostic
    Sciences
College of Veterinary Medicine
Cornell University
Ithaca, New York

Rick D. Watters, PhD
Senior Extension Associate
Animal Health Diagnostic Center
Department of Population Medicine and Diagnostic
    Sciences
College of Veterinary Medicine
Cornell University
Ithaca, New York

Francis L. Welcome, DVM, Dipl ACT, ABVP
Senior Extension Associate
Animal Health Diagnostic Center
Department of Population Medicine and Diagnostic
    Sciences
College of Veterinary Medicine
Cornell University
Ithaca, New York

Amy E. Yeager, DVM, Dipl ACVR
Hospital Staff Veterinarian
Imaging
College of Veterinary Medicine
Cornell University
Ithaca, New York

Michael J. Zurakowski, DVM
Senior Extension Veterinarian
Department of Population Medicine and Diagnostic
    Sciences
College of Veterinary Medicine
Cornell University
Ithaca, New York

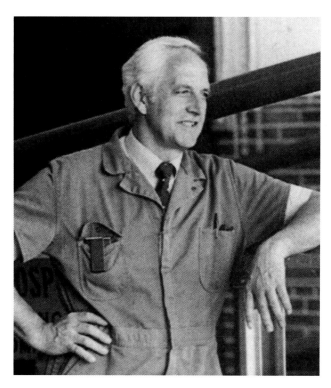

The third edition of *Rebhun's Diseases of Dairy Cattle* is dedicated to Dr. Robert Hillman, DVM, ACT, for his long and continuing contributions to teaching and practicing large animal medicine. Dr. Hillman (Bob)* may be best known professionally as a renowned large animal theriogenologist, with expertise in all large animal species but especially cattle and horses. Dr. Hillman also taught neonatology, lameness, and general medicine for horses and cattle and other large animal species during his career and is generally considered one of the best large animal veterinarians to ever practice and teach at Cornell University. Dr. Hillman taught mostly by example as he routinely performed his diagnostic and therapeutic magic in all areas of large animal medicine and

surgery. There is no doubt that the several thousand students that had the honor of working with him witnessed both state-of-the-art large animal practice and exemplary professional standards. Dr. Rebhun was one of the students of Dr. Hillman, and he often remarked that Dr. Hillman was probably the most skilled clinician he had ever met. Bob provided veterinary care for the local bull stud (Eastern, Federated Genetics, and Genex) from 1978 to 2015. It, therefore, seemed appropriate that we include a chapter on *Diseases of the Dairy Bull* in this third edition of *Rebhun's Diseases of Dairy Cattle,* and we thank Dr. Don Monke and his colleagues at Select Sire for writing this chapter in honor of Dr. Hillman.

Dr. Hillman is more than a respected clinician; he is also a gentleman in the truest sense—always polite, always willing to help with any endeavor, and always friendly. When greeted with a "Hi, Bob. How are you?" he always had the same response: "Fantastic." Dr. Hillman is currently retired (he actually has retired three times in the past but each time was hired back to fill a need in the Section of Theriogenology), but he can still be found at the veterinary college most mornings at 6 AM and is still occasionally asked to help with a difficult calving or foaling, examine a bull, provide acupuncture treatment, or perform treatment on the foot of a large cow. It is truly amazing to watch him almost effortlessly deliver a calf or foal or pare out a foot abscess in a 2400-pound bull.

We are certain the dedication of this book to Dr. Hillman for his tremendous contribution to veterinary medicine would be loudly applauded by Dr. Rebhun. Bob, we are so honored to have worked with you and learned from you, and we thank you for your numerous contributions to our veterinary profession!

Simon Peek
Thomas Divers

---

*Also commonly known as Uncle Bob because he frequently said to his patients, "Whoa, love. It's just your Uncle Bob who loves you like a brother."

Preface

Writing the preface to a book is conventionally an afterthought, something to be undertaken when the long and arduous tasks of writing and editing the text are nearly complete. Critically acclaimed authors and those with gravitas and standing often have the preface to their work written by a famous individual or public figure: Tom and I are writing our own. On the basis that those people who purchase this third edition are rather more interested in substance than literary style, we shall be brief. This book represents the collective work of multiple authors, the majority of whom still have some connection to Bill. In the elapsed time since publication of the second edition, three close colleagues and friends of Bill have passed away; the world, let alone the veterinary profession, is a poorer place for the passing of Drs. Francis Fox, John King, and Bud Tennant. Each of them defined excellence in their chosen fields and had contributed to the first two editions of this book with content, comment, images, and inspiration. Anyone with knowledge of Drs. Rebhun and Fox will be unable to avoid a smile, likely a chuckle, at the prospect of the two of them being reunited in some way. Bill would have been the first to say that his approach to veterinary medicine was strongly fashioned from the teachings of Dr. Fox, and as the latter said in his dedication to the second edition, Bill was the best he ever taught. It is in that spirit of striving for excellence that we assembled the contributor list for this third edition, and we are immensely grateful for their time, effort, and expertise; their outstanding contributions comprise the real substance of this latest edition. Undoubtedly, our goal has been to bring the most up-to-date information on diseases of dairy cattle together in one resource, adding a new chapter on diseases of dairy bulls and increasing the number of images and video clips that are available through web links. There are still substantial portions of the text that remain unchanged from when Bill wrote the first edition, on stacks of legal pads, patiently typed and collated by his secretary Mrs. Carolyn Richards, another who is no longer here to thank in person. Transcribing and editing a book has changed somewhat since the mid-1990s, but that does not lessen the debt of thanks that Tom and I owe to Penny Rudolph, Jolynn Gower, and the editorial team at Elsevier; their patience and forbearance have been sorely tested and found to be seemingly limitless. The video web page is a new feature of this edition, and we thank Cindy DeCloux and Julie Powell at Cornell for organizing and maintaining the site.

In the 20 years since the first edition was published the dairy industry in the United States has undergone change, most noticeably a move toward a smaller number of larger farms. With this consolidation has come a change in emphasis for veterinarians; within one generation, population medicine and herd-based approaches to cattle health have assumed greater importance than ever before. Consequently, veterinarians who work with dairy cattle must balance both individual animal knowledge with aspects of population medicine, applicable to the farms on which they work. We feel strongly that one follows from the other and hope that readers of this text will find the material applicable and still relevant. Bill was as strong an advocate of individual animal diagnostics and treatment as anyone who ever took the Veterinarian's Oath, but he would have championed a continued and pivotal role for veterinarians within dairy practice whatever twists and turns the industry took. For Bill, what was never acceptable was a lack of compassion for the patient or the failure to commit relentless attention to the pursuit of those clinical skills that distinguish veterinarians from all others in the industry. If nothing more, this book is meant to foster and reinforce those priorities.

Writing and editing this book have occupied the better part of almost 24 months, and in addition to thanking those listed previously, we would both like to express our gratitude to our families for their understanding and support. For Simon, mere words cannot express the love and thanks he feels toward his parents, Bill and Lorna; his children Emma, Michael, and Alexander; and his wife, Laurie, whose exceptional artistic talent now graces the front cover of this edition. For Tom, he sincerely thanks his wonderful family, Nita, Shannon, Bob, and Reuben, for tolerating his crazy work schedule and time spent away from the family. He especially thanks his ophthalmologist wife Nita for writing Chapter 14 and giving advice on this text and other veterinary and life issues that seem to arise almost daily.

Contents

PART I

Examination and Assessment

1

The Clinical Examination

THOMAS J. DIVERS AND SIMON F. PEEK

The clinical examination consists of three parts: (1) obtaining a meaningful history; (2) performing a thorough physical examination, including observations of the environment; and (3) selecting appropriate ancillary tests when necessary.

The goal of the clinical examination is to determine the organ systems involved; differential diagnoses; and, ideally, a diagnosis. In most cases, an accurate diagnosis will be reached by an experienced clinician. In difficult cases, the clinician, even when experienced, may formulate only a differential diagnosis that requires further information before an accurate diagnosis can be made.

The clinical examination is an art, not a science. The basic structure of the clinical examination can be taught, but the actual performance and interpretation involved require practice and experience. Clinicians who are lazy, who are poor observers, or who fail to interact well with clients will never develop good clinical skills.

The clinical examination is a search for clues in an attempt to solve the mystery of a patient's illness. These clues are found usually in the form of "signs" that are demonstrated to the examiner through inspection, palpation, percussion, and auscultation. Signs are the veterinary counterpart to the symptoms possessed by human patients. Stedman's Medical Dictionary defines a symptom as "any morbid phenomenon or departure from the normal in function, appearance, or sensation experienced by the patient and indicative of a disease." A sign is defined in the same source as "any abnormality indicative of disease, discoverable by the physician during the examination of the patient." Although somewhat pedantic, the veterinary interpretation of these terms has evolved to connote that animals cannot have symptoms, only signs. We cannot help but believe that sick cattle "experience" departures from normal and indicate it to experienced clinical examiners. However, we shall evade this pedantry and use the idiomatic "sign" throughout this text.

Signs are not the only clues that contribute to a diagnosis. Knowledge of the normal behavior of cattle, an accurate assessment of the patient's environment, the possible relationship of that environment to the patient's problems, and ancillary tests or data all may figure into the final diagnosis. A "tentative" diagnosis may be reached after the history is taken and physical examination is performed, but ancillary data are often required to translate the "tentative" into the "final" diagnosis.

The major stumbling block for neophytic clinicians remains the integration of information and signs into a diagnosis or differential diagnosis. An inexperienced clinician often focuses so hard on a single sign or a piece of historical data that the clinician "loses the forest for the trees." These same "trainees" in medicine are frustrated when a cow has two or more concurrent diseases. In such situations, the signs fail to add up to a textbook description of either disease, and the examiner becomes frustrated. A cow with severe metritis and a left abomasal displacement (LDA), for example, may have fever and complete anorexia. Such signs are not typical for LDA, so the inexperienced clinician may want to rule out LDA. The clinician must recognize that concurrent disease may additively or exponentially affect the clinical signs present. The clinical signs may cancel each other out, as may be seen in a recumbent hypocalcemic (subnormal temperature) cow affected with coliform mastitis (fever) that has a normal body temperature at the time of clinical examination.

Another stumbling block for even experienced veterinarians is that we may not take time to perform a thorough examination and miss a valuable piece of diagnostic information; we simply forget to look!! For experienced veterinarians, pattern recognition becomes increasingly important in arriving at a diagnosis but should not replace a thoroughly performed clinical examination. The two should be complementary. If pattern recognition becomes the predominant method of reaching a diagnosis without performing a complete examination or giving thought to pathophysiologic explanations for the clinical signs, diagnostic accuracy will decline. Much is made of "problems" possessed by sick animals and people. These problems constitute the basis of the problem-oriented medical record (POMR). We do not disagree with this thought process, but in fact it adds nothing to the skill or integrative ability of a good diagnostician. It is longhand logic that allows other clinicians or students to follow the thought processes of the clinician writing the POMR. Therefore, it may be valuable in communications among clinicians concerning a patient or as a means of evaluating a student or trainee in the early part of their clinical career. However, the major "problem" with the problem-oriented approach is that it does not make a bad diagnostician a good one. A clinician who cannot integrate data or recognize signs cannot recognize problems and will not formulate accurate plans. Therefore, the problem-oriented approach is not a panacea and in fact is merely an offshoot of the thought processes that a skilled diagnostician practices on a regular basis.

History

Obtaining an accurate and meaningful history or anamnesis is an essential aid to diagnosis. History may be accurate but not meaningful or may be misleading in some instances. The clinician must work to ask questions that do not verbally bias the owner's or caretaker's answers. When obtaining the history, the clinician also has the opportunity to display knowledge or ignorance regarding the specific patient's breed, age, use, and conformation. When the clinician appears knowledgeable concerning the patient, the owner is favorably impressed and often will volunteer more historical information. When the clinician appears ignorant of the patient and dairy husbandry in general, the owner often withdraws, answers questions tersely, and loses faith in the clinician's ability to diagnose the cause of the cow's illness. Therefore, part of the art of history taking is to communicate as well as possible with each owner. Bear in mind that owners are proud of their cattle, care for them, and have large economic investments in them. The clinician enhances credibility with dairy farmers by displaying knowledge and concern regarding the sick cow, the herd, and the dairy economy.

Where should a history begin? Usually the owner has called the veterinarian to attend to a specific problem, and the problem may be easily definable, or it may be vague. For example, a chief complaint of mastitis is specific as to location of the problem but not specific as to the cause, but a complaint of a cow "off feed" is very vague and requires a much more detailed history. For dairy cattle, several key questions usually need to be answered by an accurate history. In some instances, however, some of these questions may be omitted when the clinician can answer the question by observation. The following are examples of typical questions that should be asked while obtaining a history of an adult dairy cow.

1. When did the cow freshen? Or where in her lactation is she?
2. When did she first appear ill, what was the first clinical sign and what has transpired since that time? Did you take her temperature?
3. What have you treated her with? Has there been any response to treatment?
4. Has she had other illnesses this lactation or in past lactations?
5. What and how much does she eat now?
6. How much milk was she producing before she became ill, and what is she producing now?
7. What has her manure been like?
8. Is she ruminating normally?
9. Do you know if she received a reticular magnet?
10. What other unusual things have you noticed?
11. Have any other cows (calves) had similar problems? If so, what has been the end result?

Other information may be necessary. In most instances, an experienced clinician already will know breed, sex, approximate age, use, and other husbandry information. However, in some instances, specific age information may be necessary. The clinician can appear very observant by asking question three regarding treatments by the owner when it is obvious that the cow has had injections. Question ten is open ended and may yield valuable information from an observant owner or totally useless information from an unobservant owner. The clinician should be as complete as necessary in obtaining information but should avoid asking meaningless questions because they may annoy or confuse the owner. Frequently, when students are first gaining experience, they ask impertinent questions of owners; imagine a concerned owner, whose cow has an obvious dystocia, being asked what he feeds the cow. In such instances, the inexperienced clinician or student is trying to be thorough but has upset the owner, who usually will reply, "What difference does that make? She's trying to have a calf!"

Another important aspect of the history is to determine the duration of the disease. The general terms used to distinguish duration include peracute, acute, subacute, and chronic, although various experts disagree on the exact length of illness to define each category. Rosenberger suggests the following:

Peracute = 0 to 2 days
Acute = 3 to 14 days
Subacute = 14 to 28 days
Chronic ≥ 28 days

These durations are somewhat longer than those commonly used in the United States, and in general we suggest:

Peracute = 0 to 24 hours
Acute = 24 to 96 hours
Subacute = 4 to 14 days
Chronic ≥ 14 days

The interpersonal skills necessary for effective history taking and "bedside manner" in a veterinarian are similar to those used by physicians. The veterinary clinician, however, has to establish a doctor–client relationship, but the physician must foster a more direct doctor–patient relationship. A good relationship, together with the skills and interactions that create a good one, is the secret to acceptance by the human client just as for a human patient.

Experienced clinicians adjust to the owner's personality. Highly knowledgeable and educated clients require a much different use of language and grammar than do poorly educated clients who may be confused by or misunderstand scientific terms and excessive vocabulary.

The history also should clarify any questions regarding the signalment that the clinician cannot ascertain by inspection alone. Because we are concerned with the bovine species only, the use (dairy), sex, color, breed, size, and often age of the animal are apparent by inspection. It may be important to determine whether valuable cattle would be retained only for reproductive use if production should decrease drastically. The various components of the signalment are important to recognize because certain diseases occur more commonly in one sex and in some breeds, colors, and ages than in others.

Physical Examination

The physical examination begins as soon as the bovine patient comes into the clinician's view.

General Examination

A general examination consisting of inspection and observation is performed. The experienced clinician often makes this general examination quickly and sometimes while simultaneously obtaining verbal history from the owner. The general examination may be as short as 30 seconds or as long as 5 minutes if further observation is necessary. As part of the general examination, the clinician needs to establish the habitus—the attitude, condition, conformation, and temperament—of the sick animal. When the request for veterinary attention is a legitimate emergency or at least perceived as such by the client, then this initial inspection and observation will need to be brief. Inexperienced veterinarians must try hard to avoid rushing through this period of observation in their understandable hurry to commence the physical examination.

Attitude

The attitude or posture may suggest a specific diagnosis or a specific system disorder. The clinician must have basic knowledge of the normal attitude of dairy cattle, calves, and bulls before interpreting abnormal attitudes. The arched stance and reluctance of the animal to move as observed in peritonitis may indicate hardware disease, perforating abomasal ulcers, or merely a musculoskeletal injury to the back. A cow observed to be constantly leaning into her stanchion may have either nervous ketosis or listeriosis. A cow standing with her head extended, eyes partially closed, and exhibiting marked depression could have encephalitis or frontal sinusitis. A bull lying down with a stargazing attitude may have a pituitary abscess. A periparturient recumbent cow with an "S" curve in her neck is probably hypocalcemic. All of these attitudes are abnormal and indicative of disease. Many attitudes are not specific, however. A cow affected with hypocalcemia, for example, will often open her mouth and stick out her tongue when stimulated or approached, but some nervous cattle assume this attitude even when healthy. An arched stance with tenesmus may be observed in simple vaginitis, coccidiosis, or rectal irritation

but also may be observed occasionally with liver disease, diarrhea due to bovine viral diarrhea virus, and rabies.

Cattle stand by first elevating their rear quarters while resting on their carpal areas and then rising to their forelegs with a slight forward lunge. It is unusual for cattle to get up on their front legs first as do horses, but some cattle, especially Brown Swiss cows, cows with front limb lameness, or late pregnant cattle, do this normally. Therefore, again, it is important to be familiar with normal variations. It is impossible to enumerate all the possible abnormal attitudes assumed by cattle, but Table 1.1 is a partial list.

Condition

The condition of the animal is another component of the habitus that is assessed during the general examination. Condition is judged both subjectively and experientially in most instances. The clinician may assess the condition of a calf or an adult cow in comparison with the animal's herdmates, as well as with the bovine population in general. Excessively fat cattle are predisposed to metabolic diseases during the periparturient period and, when sustaining musculoskeletal injuries, may become recumbent more easily than leaner cattle.

Cattle may be thin yet perfectly healthy. When a cow loses weight and is thin because of illness, she generally appears much different than her herdmates. Healthy, thin cattle have normal hair coats and hydration status, appear bright, and possess normal appetites. Emaciated cattle that have lost weight because of chronic illness have coarse, dry hair coats and leathery dehydrated skin and appear dull. The clinician must remember that severe acute disease may cause weight loss of 50 lb or more per day. The condition of the animal correlates largely with the duration of the illness. Extreme emaciation is associated with chronic problems such as parasitism, chronic abscessation, chronic musculoskeletal pain, Johne's disease, advanced neoplasia, and malnutrition.

The body score of dairy cattle is a system designed to add some objectivity to the subjective determination of condition. Body score is used in herd management to assess the nutritional plane of the cattle and to correlate this to milk production, relative energy intake, and stage of lactation. Body score is arrived at subjectively by observation and palpation of the cow's loin, transverse processes of the lumbar vertebrae, and tail head area from the rear of the animal. Scores are recorded in half point gradations from 0 to 5 with 0 being very poor and 5 being grossly fat. Ideal scores have been suggested as 3.5 for calving cows, 2.0 to 2.5 for first service, and 3.0 for drying off (see Chapter 15).

Conformation

The conformation of the animal is the third component of the habitus to be assessed during the general examination. Familiarity with normal conformation is an obvious asset when observing conformational defects that may predispose

TABLE 1.1 Some Examples of Abnormal Attitudes Assumed by Cattle

Arched back, anorexia, abducted elbows ("painful stance")	Peritonitis, pleuritis
Arched back, anorexia, limbs placed farther under body than normal, reluctance to stand	Polyarthritis
Arched back, normal appetite, legs placed farther ahead (front) and behind (back) body than normal	Musculoskeletal back injury
Bloat, elevated tail head, weather vane head and neck, legs placed farther ahead (front) and behind (back) body than normal, anxious expression, ears erect, nictitans protruding	Tetanus
Recumbent with forelegs extended	Musculoskeletal injury to forelegs—usually carpus
Lateral recumbency but alert and responsive	Occasionally normal for brief time
Usually indicative of musculoskeletal pain causing reluctance to flex one or more limbs
Ventral abdominal pain caused by udder swelling, udder hematoma, ventral abdominal hernia, or cellulitis
Recumbency with "S" curve neck, depressed, or comatose	Hypocalcemia
Lateral recumbency, opisthotonos, depression	
Calves	Polioencephalomalacia or other CNS disease
Cows	Occasional hypomagnesemia or other CNS disease
Recumbency, hyperexcitability	Hypomagnesemia, occasional hypocalcemia
Grinding teeth, blindness with intact pupillary responses, depression	Lead poisoning, polioencephalomalacia
Grinding teeth, pushing nose against objects	Chronic abdominal pain, sinusitis, musculoskeletal pain
Colic	Indigestion with small intestinal gas and fluid accumulation, small intestinal obstruction, pyelonephritis or other urinary tract abnormality, cecal distention or volvulus and uterine torsion
"Praying position" with rear raised but resting on carpi	Laminitis
Tenesmus	Vaginitis, rectal irritation, coccidiosis, rabies, hepatic failure, BVDV
Dog-sitting position	May be normal before raising rear quarters in some Brown Swiss and occasionally in other late pregnant cattle, some lamenesses
If cow or bull cannot raise rear quarters but can raise front end, it may indicate a thoracolumbar spinal cord lesion
Hind feet under body, forefeet in front of body, reluctance to stand or move	Acute laminitis or severe forelimb lameness
Hind feet standing on edge of platform with heels non–weight bearing	Sore heels, overgrowth of claws, sole ulcers, heel warts
Hind feet in gutter with rear legs extended behind body	Spastic syndrome, too short a platform for cow, heel pain
Hind feet in gutter with rear legs extended behind body and lordosis	Chronic renal pain, chronic pyelonephritis, other causes of colic
Forelimbs crossed, reluctance to move	Bilateral lameness of medial claws, laminitis
Chewing on objects, biting water cup, licking pipes, licking and chewing skin, aggressive behavior, collapse	Nervous ketosis or organic CNS disease

BVDV, bovine viral diarrhea virus; *CNS,* central nervous system.

to or indicate specific diseases. For example, udder conformation in the dairy cow is extremely important, and cattle with suspensory ligament laxity are prone to teat injuries and mastitis. Calves with kyphosis may have vertebral abnormalities such as hemivertebrae. Splayed toes may predispose to interdigital fibromas, and weak pasterns often lead to chronic foot problems. A crushed tail head allows chronic fecal contamination of the perineum and vulva, with the potential for reproductive failure or ascending urinary tract infection. Chronic cystic ovaries may change the conformational appearance of many cows so that they display thickened necks, prominent tail head, relaxed sacrosciatic ligaments, and a flaccid perineum.

Temperament

Temperament is the fourth component of habitus and should be evaluated from a distance in addition to when the animal is approached during general examination. From practical and medicolegal standpoints, it is imperative that the clinician anticipates unpredictable or aggressive patient behavior whenever possible, lest caretakers, the clinician, or the animal itself be injured. Dairy bulls should never be trusted, even when they appear docile. Dairy cattle with newborn calves should be approached cautiously because people have been injured or killed by apparently quiet cows that suddenly became aggressive to protect a calf. Rarely, individual dairy cattle may be wild and vicious. They should be approached with extreme care or restrained in a chute if possible. Fortunately, most dairy cattle are rather docile and, unless startled or approached without warning, may be examined thoroughly without substantial restraint.

As a general rule, free-stall cattle are wilder than cattle housed in tie-stall barns, but there are exceptions. The manners and nature of the owner (or herdsperson) are directly reflected in the contentment or lack thereof observed in the herd. Some herds consist of truly quiet and contented cows, but in other herds, all cattle will act apprehensive and jumpy and fear all human contact. These latter herds, without exception, are handled roughly and loudly and frequently are mistreated. The veterinarian will quickly learn to adjust to the variable husbandry of herds within the practice. The increase in size of herds coupled with the impersonal nature of free-stall housing has decreased the prevalence of husbandry skills that facilitated human–cow contact. A worthy piece of advice, to which all those who work with dairy cattle should aspire, was provided by WD Hoard, founder of Hoard's Dairyman, circa 1885:

> *NOTICE TO THE HELP*
> *THE RULE to be observed in this stable at all times, toward the cattle, young and old, is that of patience and kindness. A man's usefulness in a herd ceases at once when he loses his temper and bestows rough usage. Men must be patient. Cattle are not reasoning beings. Remember that this is the Home of Mothers. Treat each cow as a Mother should be treated. The giving of milk is a function of Motherhood; rough treatment lessens the flow. That injures me as well as the cow. Always keep these ideas in mind in dealing with my cattle.*

Occasionally, cows that are transported or moved from familiar to unfamiliar surroundings will go wild and become extremely apprehensive or aggressive. These cattle may act as if affected by nervous ketosis but frequently are not.

The clinician should question the owner as to perceived changes in the temperament of the patient. Docile animals that become aggressive warrant consideration of nervous ketosis, rabies, and other neurologic diseases. Vicious cows that become docile again should be thought of as either very ill or perhaps affected with organic or metabolic central nervous system disease.

People unfamiliar with dairy cattle anticipate kicking as the major risk in handling cattle. It is true that cattle can "cow kick" with a forward-lateral-backward kick, but some cows also kick straight back with amazing accuracy. Not discounting the dangers of being kicked, clinicians should be aware that a cow's head may be her most dangerous weapon. Anyone who has been maliciously butted or repeatedly smashed by a cow's head understands the inherent dangers. Similarly, a mature bull's head is a potentially lethal weapon.

Entire herds of cattle or large groups of cattle within a herd that suddenly become agitated, apprehensive, or vocal or refuse to let milk down signal to the clinician the possibility of stray electrical voltage. Occasional spontaneous demonstrations of anxiety or agitation in cattle may also be associated with ectoparasitism.

Hands-on Examination

After the general examination and history are complete, the hands-on part of the physical examination should begin and proceed uninterrupted. It is important that the clinician is allowed to initiate and complete the hands-on examination in the absence of interference by others and during a period when other environmental interference (e.g., feeding, movement of cattle in the immediate vicinity) is kept to a minimum. A "group" approach to physical examination or one that is performed within a distracting environment only serves to minimize the reliability of physical diagnostics and will challenge even the best diagnostician.

Because dairy cattle are less apprehensive when approached from the rear, the physical examination starts at the rear of the animal. Adult dairy cattle are accustomed to people working around the udder, and their reproductive examinations or inseminations are frequent enough such that their overall anxiety is less when the examination starts at the hindquarters. Approaching the head or forequarters causes the cow to become more excitable, and this alters baseline parameters such as heart rate and respiratory rate.

The examination begins with insertion of a rectal thermometer—preferably a 6-inch large-animal thermometer—to obtain the rectal temperature. The thermometer should be left in place for 2 minutes (except for digital thermometers that provide rapid readings), during which time the animal's pulse rate is determined by palpation of the coccygeal artery (6 to 12 inches from the base of the tail) and a respiratory rate is recorded by observation of thoracic excursions. The clinician should use this 2-minute period to further observe the patient and its environment and to determine the habitus. The rear udder should be palpated, as well as the supramammary lymph nodes, during the time the temperature is taken. Enlargement of the supramammary lymph nodes necessitates consideration of mastitis, lymphosarcoma, and other diseases capable of causing local or general lymphadenopathy. Lymphosarcoma can cause both generalized, symmetric lymphadenopathy, or occasionally, marked asymmetric enlargement. However, the majority of cases of lymphosarcoma do not result in obvious peripheral lymphadenopathy. The mucous membranes of the vulva may also be inspected to detect anemia, jaundice, or hyperemia, as well as observed to detect any vulvar discharges. The veterinarian's sense of smell is also used during this time. The distinct, fetid odor of septic metritis, necrotic vaginitis, or retained fetal membranes; the necrotic odor of udder dermatitis; the sweetish odor of melena; or the "septic tank" odor of Salmonella diarrhea may be apparent to a trained clinician. If manure stains the tail, is passed during the examination, or has accumulated in the gutter behind the cow, the veterinarian should assess the consistency and volume of the manure visually as compared with herdmates on the same diet. Extreme pallor of the teats and udder may suggest anemia in cattle such as Holsteins that often have fully or partially nonpigmented teat skin. Inspection from the rear also may suggest a "sprung rib cage" on the left or right side, suggestive of an abomasal displacement. Bilateral abdominal distention when viewed from behind might be associated with the "papple" appearance of chronic bloat or vagal indigestion or, on extremely rare occasions, ascites or a dropsical pregnancy.

Body Temperature

The normal body temperature range for a dairy cow is 100.4° to 102.5°F (38°–39.17°C). Other authors allow the upper limit to reach 103.1°F, but this is above normal for the average dairy cow in temperate climate ranges. Calves, excitable cattle, or cattle exposed to high environmental heat or humidity may have temperatures of 103.1°F or higher, but this should not be considered normal for the average cow unless these qualifications exist. True hypothermia may occur as a result of hypocalcemia when ambient temperature is less than body temperature, exposure in extreme winter weather, and hypovolemic or septic shock. False hypothermia may occur when pneumorectum exists or the rectal thermometer has not been left in place long enough. Hyperthermia may be of endogenous origin (fever) or exogenous (heat exhaustion, sunstroke). Usually exogenous causes of hyperthermia can be explained readily based on the general examination and assessment of the environment. Under conditions of high ambient temperature and humidity, one should bear in mind the possibility of exogenous, environmental explanations for elevated rectal temperature even in housed cattle. If a clinician examines an animal under such environmental conditions and discovers an elevated temperature but cannot find an explanation from the remainder of the physical examination, then it can be highly informative to obtain rectal temperatures from herdmates nearby. It is often tempting to assign a diagnosis of respiratory disease, even pneumonia, to such cattle because they are frequently hyperpneic and tachypneic, but the absence of other evidence of respiratory illness (cough, nasal discharge, upper airway noise or adventitious sounds) is key and can alert the clinician to the fact that the increased respiratory rate is a normal physiologic response in a hyperthermic animal. It should be noted that hypocalcemic cows or recumbent cows—especially if they are darker colored rather than predominantly white—can become hyperthermic when unable to move out of the sun or when ambient temperatures are greater than their body temperature. The fine distinction between 103.1° and 102.5°F as the upper limit of normal temperature has resulted from our observation of scores of hospitalized cattle with confirmed chronic peritonitis but which maintain daily body temperatures between 102.5° and 103.1°F (39.2° and 39.5°C). Therefore, unless exogenous hyperthermia is suspected, rectal temperatures above 102.5°F should alert the clinician to inflammatory diseases. However, a normal body temperature does not rule out all inflammatory infectious diseases! At least 50% of the patients with confirmed traumatic reticuloperitonitis in our clinics, for example, register normal body temperatures. This phenomenon also has been observed by other authors.

Fever may be continuous, remittent, intermittent, or recurrent. Remittent fevers go up and down but never drop into the normal range. Intermittent fevers fall into the normal range of body temperature at some time during the day. Recurrent fever is characterized by several days of fever alternating with 1 or more days of normal body temperature.

It must be emphasized that true fever is a protective physiologic response to sepsis, toxemia, or pyrogens. It represents the body's response to infectious organisms or the systemic response to inflammation. As such, it is a normal protective defense mechanism. Fever in cattle should not be masked by antiinflammatory or antipyretic medications nor should their use be a knee-jerk response to the presence of an elevated temperature. Cattle do not have the tendency for laminitis secondary to fever that is observed in some horses. Therefore, the primary disease—not the fever—should be treated. Fever provides an excellent means of assessing the clinical response of the cow or calf to appropriate therapy of the primary disease.

Pulse Rate

The normal pulse rate for adult average-sized cattle is 60 to 84 beats/min. Larger cows that are healthy and quiet tend to be closer to 60 beats/min and sometimes lower, while smaller cows such as Jerseys are often toward the upper normal range. Calves have a normal pulse rate of 72 to 100 beats/min. Various authors disagree on the normal pulse rates of cattle, but these figures constitute an average for a nonexcited animal. Interpretation of extraneous factors affecting the pulse rate must be left to the clinician who is performing the examination and taking environmental factors and habitus into consideration.

Tachycardia is an elevated heart rate (pulse rate) and is present when the patient is excited or has any of a number of organic diseases. Tachycardia, although abnormal, is not system specific and may exist in infectious, metabolic, cardiac, respiratory, neoplastic, or toxemic conditions. Tachycardia also is present in painful diseases, including musculoskeletal pain. With musculoskeletal pain of the appendicular skeleton, a large difference in pulse rate will be found between when the animal is recumbent (lower) and when it stands.

Bradycardia is a lower-than-normal heart rate (pulse rate) and is present in very few conditions in cattle. Pituitary abscesses, vagus indigestion, and botulism are the major diseases considered to result in bradycardia in cattle. Not all cattle with these conditions have bradycardia, however. It has been initially reported also by Dr. Shelia McGuirk that normal cattle deprived of feed and water for several hours frequently develop bradycardia. We frequently find this in cattle that are not systemically ill but are held off feed in preparation for anesthesia and elective surgery. Except for an occasional cow with ketosis, we have only rarely observed development of bradycardia in sick cattle that have been off feed for a prolonged time. It may be that veterinarians seldom see normal cattle off feed for long periods because we are only called to examine sick cattle. One exception is the "broken drinking cup" phenomenon in confined cattle, in which the animal does not eat because she has had no water for 1 or more days. Hypoglycemic or hyperkalemic calves also may have bradycardia.

Pulse deficits or arrhythmias encountered when obtaining the pulse rate may dictate further consideration of both cardiac and metabolic disease.

Respiratory Rate

The normal respiratory rate for a dairy cow at rest ranges from 18 to 28 breaths/min according to Gibbons and 15 to 35 breaths/min according to Rosenberger. The frequency, depth, and character of respiration should be assessed. Depth is increased by excitement, exertion, dyspnea, and anoxia. Calves at rest breathe 20 to 40 times per minute. Some calves with pneumonia have normal respiratory rates when standing but elevated rates when lying down. Metabolic acidosis results in both increased depth and rate of respiration. High environmental temperatures and humidity also increase the rate and depth of respiration. Depth of respiration is decreased by painful conditions involving the chest, diaphragm, or cranial abdomen. The depth and rate of respiration are also decreased in severe metabolic alkalosis as the cow compensates to preserve CO_2.

The character of respiration may be normal costoabdominal, thoracic, or abdominal. Thoracic breathing occurs in those with peritonitis and abdominal distention in which either pain or pressure on the diaphragm, respectively, interferes with the abdominal component of respiration. Abdominal breathing is noted when cattle are affected with painful pleuritis or fibrinous bronchopneumonia or have severe dyspnea caused by pulmonary conditions such as bullous emphysema, pulmonary edema, acute bovine pulmonary emphysema, proliferative pneumonia, and other conditions that result in reduced tidal volume of the lower airway.

Dyspnea is synonymous with difficult or labored breathing, but many veterinarians also use the term to describe an increased rate of breathing (i.e., simple dyspnea). Polypnea and tachypnea are perhaps better words to describe an abnormal elevation of respiratory rate. Hyperpnea implies an increased depth of respiration. The examiner should note whether the maximal dyspnea occurs with inspiration (inspiratory dyspnea), expiration (expiratory dyspnea), or equally during inspiration and expiration (mixed dyspnea). Classically, whereas inspiratory dyspnea tends to originate from the upper airway, expiratory dyspnea usually incriminates the lower airway. Mixed dyspnea occurs in many conditions such as anoxia, severe pneumonia, and narrowing of the lower tracheal lumen. Audible respiratory noise, mostly on inspiration, is characteristic of an upper respiratory obstruction. The head and neck are often abnormally extended in cattle with respiratory dysfunction, and when pneumonia is present, the cattle often cough after rising.

Left Side

After the initial portion of the hands-on physical examination is completed at the rear of the animal, the examiner moves to the left side of the cow.

Auscultation of the Heart and Lungs

Auscultation of the heart on the left side should be completed at the three sites that correspond to the pulmonic valve, aortic valve, and mitral valve (see Chapter 3). If the animal is excited by the presence of the examiner near her forelimb, the heart rate may be higher than the pulse rate previously obtained. Heart rate, rhythm, and intensity of heart sounds should be assessed during auscultation of the heart. The heart rate or frequency of contraction should fall within the normal limits as described for pulse rate. The rhythm should be regular, and the intensity or amplitude of cardiac sounds should be even and commensurate with the depth of the thoracic wall. For example, the heart sounds are relatively louder in a calf than a fat dairy cow. The clinician must auscultate many calves and adult cattle to learn the normal intensity or amplitude of the cardiac sounds. A "pounding" heart with increased amplitude of heart sounds is heard in extreme anemia, after exertion, and in some cases of endocarditis.

Relative increased amplitude is observed in extremely thin animals and cattle with consolidated ventral lung fields. Decreased intensity of heart sounds may be associated with shock, endotoxemia, severe dehydration, or an extremely thick chest wall, as in adult bulls or fat cattle.

Extremely decreased or "muffled" heart sounds occur bilaterally in those with pericarditis, pneumomediastinum, and diffuse myocardial or pericardial infiltration caused by lymphosarcoma. Decreased or muffled heart sounds unilaterally may occur with unilateral thoracic abscesses, diaphragmatic hernias, thoracic neoplasia including lymphosarcoma, or tuberculosis.

The first heart sound, or systolic sound, occurs during the start of ventricular systole and usually is thought to be associated with closure of the atrioventricular (AV) valves and contraction of the ventricles. The second heart sound, or diastolic sound, occurs at the start of diastole and is thought to be caused by closure of the aortic and pulmonic valves. Many dairy cattle have a split first heart sound that results in a gallop rhythm (e.g., bah-bah-boop, bah-bah-boop). This split first heart sound is attributed to asynchronous closure of the AV valves or asynchronous onset of contracture of the ventricles and should be considered in most cases a normal variant. The third heart sound can be heard in some excited cattle with mild tachycardia, and the fourth heart sound may be heard in some cows with bradycardia.

Heart murmurs, or bruits, may be abnormal and should be assessed as to valvular site of maximal intensity, relation to systole and diastole, and loudness or intensity. Grading systems such as those used in small animals may be applicable when describing bovine heart murmurs (e.g., a grade II/VI holosystolic murmur), but in cattle, this is a very subjective evaluation because few practitioners will encounter enough cattle with heart murmurs to be objective about the intensity of the murmur. Heart murmurs occur in those with congenital cardiac anomalies, acquired valvular insufficiencies, endocarditis, anemia, and some cardiac neoplasms and may occur as a result of dynamic or positional influences in cattle in lateral recumbency. Cattle receiving a rapid infusion of high-volume intravenous fluid may have a transient murmur associated with fluid administration. Low-intensity (grade I or II) systolic murmurs are audible in some healthy cattle.

The heart sounds may radiate over a wider anatomic area than the normal cardiac location when conducted through fluid (pleural effusion) or solid (consolidated lung tissue) media. Such radiation of sound should be considered abnormal. In sick adult cattle, heart sounds also may radiate through an extremely dry rumen, becoming audible in the left paralumbar fossa. This has been classically described in cattle with primary ketosis, but the phenomenon is not limited to this disease.

Splashing sounds associated with the heart beat usually suggest a pericardial effusion, most commonly associated with traumatic or idiopathic pericarditis. Thoracic or lung abscesses located adjacent but external to the pericardium also occasionally may give rise to splashing sounds should liquid pus in the abscess have been set in motion by the beating heart. These splashing sounds would most likely be unilateral, as opposed to bilateral splashing sounds coupled with muffling of the heart sounds present in pericarditis patients.

Atrial fibrillation is the most common cardiac arrhythmia in dairy cattle and is most often associated with hypochloremic, hypokalemic metabolic alkalosis. Hypocalcemia also may be contributory, but hypokalemia seems to be the most consistent finding in cattle affected with atrial fibrillation. Some clinicians have found atrial fibrillation in a small percentage of cattle with endotoxemia secondary to gram-negative mastitis. A rapid (88–140 beats/min) erratic heart rate of varying intensity and a pulse deficit characterize the physical findings in atrial fibrillation. When atrial fibrillation is suspected, simultaneous auscultation of the heart and palpation of the facial artery or median artery are indicated to determine a pulse deficit. Cardiac arrhythmias other than atrial fibrillation are rare in adult dairy cattle. Calves affected with white muscle disease and calves that are hyperkalemic may have cardiac arrhythmias including bradycardia in calves with hyperkalemia.

After auscultation of the heart, auscultation of the left lung field should begin. The entire lung field should be auscultated and subsequently the trachea auscultated to rule out referred sounds from the upper airway. The caudal border of the lung field extends approximately from the 6th costochondral junction ventrally to the 11th intercostal space dorsally. If auscultation detects any abnormalities, thoracic percussion and thoracic ultrasonography should be performed to further aid diagnosis. The anterior ventral portion of the lung that lies under the shoulder should be carefully auscultated by forcing the stethoscope under the shoulder and triceps muscles. A comparison of sounds between both sides and different locations on the chest should be emphasized. Cattle with severe pneumonia often do not have crackles and wheezes, but auscultation of a tracheal or "sucking soup sound" in the thorax is indicative of lung consolidation. It is also helpful to have the owner hold the cow's mouth and nose shut for 15 to 45 seconds to force the cow to take a deep breath. Alternatively, increased respiratory effort, thereby exaggerating abnormal lung sounds, can also be achieved by holding a plastic bag over the cow's muzzle, forcing her to inspire an ever-increasing fraction of CO_2 and diminishing fraction of O_2 over a 1- to 2-minute period. In addition to enhancing adventitious lung sounds, other signs of lower airway disease may include a rapid intolerance of the procedure and development of dyspnea or the initiation of spontaneous and frequent coughing during the rebreathing period. Calves can be backed into a corner, and the examiner can hold the nose and mouth shut to auscultate the lungs without additional help. As awareness of the clinical relevance of respiratory disease in dairy calves has grown, increased efforts have been made to reach a diagnosis of pneumonia in a more timely manner. Such is the value of thoracic ultrasonography or the above described deep breathing techniques in calves in particular, that one might consider them part of the routine examination. Dorsal lung sounds should be heard during labored breathing, and absence of lung sounds on one or both sides may indicate pneumothorax or bullous emphysema.

During auscultation of the heart and lungs in the left hemithorax, the examiner may also palpate the jugular and mammary (superficial abdominal) veins for relative degrees of tension, pulsation, or thrombosis. In addition, the superficial cervical lymph node, peripheral skin temperature (ear and lower limbs), and skin turgor may be evaluated at this time. When the clinician suspects cardiac disease to be present based on initial physical examination, it is prudent to subsequently evaluate jugular and mammary vein character and fill as a means of corroborating the presence or severity of cardiac disease. Do not forget, however, the normal, significant, distention of the mammary veins in a high-producing dairy cow such that mammary vein distention and turgor must be interpreted in light of stage of lactation and recent production. More precise evaluation of cardiac function can be pursued through echocardiography (see Chapter 3).

Assessment of the Rumen and Left Abdomen

The examination proceeds to the left abdomen and begins with assessment of the rumen. Palpation and auscultation of the rumen should be performed. Auscultation in the left paralumbar fossa for a minimum of 1 minute will quantitate and qualitate rumen contractions. Palpation of the left lower quadrant and paralumbar fossa may aid this evaluation and is a better means of determining the relative consistency of rumen contents. Healthy cattle have one or two primary rumen contractions per minute. Hypomotility suggests stasis caused by endotoxemia, peritonitis, hypocalcemia, or other causes. Hypermotility may suggest vagal indigestion and ruminal distention. During auscultation of the rumen, the left superficial inguinal lymph node should be palpated, and the hair coat and skin may be further assessed.

The examination continues with simultaneous auscultation and percussion of the left abdomen to detect resonant areas (pings) indicative of gaseous or gas/fluid distention of viscera in the left abdomen. In descending order of frequency of occurrence, these include left displacement of the abomasum, rumen gas cap, pneumoperitoneum, rumen collapse, and abdominal abscesses secondary to rumen trocharization (see Chapter 5). It is very important to "ping" the entire left side of the abdomen because many LDAs may be located ventral to the typical location in the mid to upper abdomen at the 10th to 13th rib spaces. In calves, LDAs commonly ping more ventral and caudal than in adult cattle. When pings are identified, simultaneous ballottement and auscultation should be performed to determine the relative amount of fluid present. LDAs have inconsistent "splashy" sounds in comparison to RDAs due to a comparatively decreased fluid accumulation in LDAs. In the recent era of increased drenching of cattle with large volumes of fluid on farm, it is common to identify "splashy" rumens when a veterinarian auscultates and succusses the rumen of a cow with a static, low-fiber-content rumen within a few hours of orogastric fluid administration. These cows do not ping in the typical manner of a LDA, but "toilet"-like sounds may be heard coincident with weak and insignificant rumen contractions or ballottement. Careful questioning of the owner or herdsperson about treatment history will typically reveal that the cow has been drenched with several gallons of fluid within the previous few hours.

Right Side

The right thorax is evaluated next.

Auscultation of the Heart and Lungs

Auscultation of the right heart and lung fields is similar to that performed on the left side. In general, the heart sounds on the right side are slightly less audible than those on the left side because the majority of the heart lies in the left hemithorax. Auscultation of the right heart requires the examiner to force the head of the stethoscope as far as possible cranially under the right elbow of the cow. Murmurs originating from the right AV valve are best heard on the right side around the third intercostal space at the level of the elbow. Similarly, the loud, holosystolic murmur associated with a ventricular septal defect is loudest over the right hemithorax but can be heard on the left as well. Although the right lung is larger than the left, the auscultable basal border of the lung remains clinically identical to that found on the left side. Again, during auscultation of the right hemithorax, the examiner should assess the ipsilateral jugular vein, mammary vein, superficial cervical lymph node, skin turgor, peripheral skin temperature, hair, and skin. Suspicious areas discovered during auscultation of the right hemithorax may be evaluated further by percussion or ultrasound.

Assessment of the Right Abdomen

Evaluation of the right abdomen begins with simultaneous percussion and auscultation of the entire abdominal area. Many viscera and conditions in the right abdomen may give rise to pings (see Chapter 5). Simultaneous ballottement and auscultation will allow a relative assessment of the quantity of fluid present in a distended viscus when pings have been identified. Large amounts of fluid are commonly detected by succussion in cattle with RDA, cecal dilatation or volvulus and small intestinal distension. The best anatomical area for detecting excessive fluid in the small intestine of cattle is the caudal lower right abdomen. The fingertips should be used for determination of localized abdominal pain in the right abdomen. Deep pressure is exerted in the intercostal regions, paralumbar fossa, and right lower quadrant. This same technique may be used to palpate an enlarged liver that protrudes caudal to the 13th rib.

Ventral Abdomen

The next step in the physical examination is the determination of localized abdominal pain in the ventral abdomen.

Several means have been suggested for this determination. We prefer the examiner to be positioned in a kneeling position near the right fore udder attachment. A closed fist is rested on the examiner's left knee, and gentle but deep pressure is applied intermittently to specific areas to the left and right of midline as the examiner moves forward until the xiphoid area is reached. The cow should be allowed 2 to 5 seconds between compressions of each area to allow her to relax before pressure is applied to the next area. An average of 8 to 10 deep pressure applications is used while the examiner observes the patient's head, neck, and elbows for signs indicative of pain. When a painful area is identified, the cow usually will lift her abdomen off the examiner's fist and then tighten her neck musculature and show an anxious expression. She may also close her eyelids, open her eyelids widely, groan audibly, guard her abdomen, or abduct her elbows excessively. The examiner does not need to watch the abdomen because one will feel the cow's abdomen lift away. Subtle or chronic peritonitis cases may demonstrate only tightening of the neck musculature or show facial expressions indicative of pain. Peracute cases may show more violent reactions, and the patient may either move away from the examiner or kick, especially if the patient is a nervous cow. Other examiners prefer the withers pinch technique, in which firm pressure is applied to the withers area with one or both hands by grasping the withers and pinching. A normal cow should lower the withers to avoid this contact. A cow with peritonitis may be reluctant to lower her withers and thereby "push" against the painful peritoneal surface. This technique requires more subjective analysis because many nervous cows are reluctant to respond to the withers pinch. If simultaneous pressure is applied upward from the xiphoid region while the withers pinch is applied, some cattle with peritonitis may also audibly grunt. Although these examination procedures are routine in cattle with suspected peritonitis, the sensitivity and specificity of the test may not be as high as older textbooks suggest. Ultrasound examination, if possible, should be used to supplement these examination procedures.

In young calves, the umbilicus should be routinely palpated to determine if there is an abdominal hernia and if the umbilical remnants are normal. The umbilicus and remnants can be palpated best by placing the calf in lateral recumbency to perform deep palpation of the abdomen and the umbilical vein coursing rostral toward the liver. In a normal calf, the umbilical arteries and urachus cannot be manually palpated or identified on ultrasound examination of the umbilical stump beyond a few days of life. The umbilical stump can also be palpated in the standing calf to determine if a hernia is present and if intestinal loops are in the hernia.

Mammary Gland

Evaluation of the mammary gland is then conducted by palpation and examination of mammary secretions in all quarters. The conformation and any suspensory weaknesses may be evaluated but have been noted by observation, usually during the general examination. Dry cows are assessed first by palpation, and secretion is examined only if palpation detects firmness or heat suggestive of mastitis in one or more quarters. Milking cows routinely require a strip plate evaluation of the secretion from each quarter. The strip plate should have a black plate to highlight abnormalities, and a normal secretion from one quarter is left as a pool on the strip plate so that potential abnormal secretions can be milked into it. Other tests such as the California mastitis test or pH strips may follow the use of the strip plate (see Chapter 8 for further details). Generalized edema and focal areas of induration, abscessation, edema, or fibrosis detected by palpation of the udder should be recorded. The teats should be examined individually for teat end abnormalities, obstruction to milk flow, condition of the skin, inflammatory or neoplastic conditions, frostbite, photosensitization, edema, or evidence of previous injury.

At the Head

After the udder and teats have been examined, the cow's head is examined. Because examination of the head leads to the most patient apprehension, this part of the examination is left to next to last and followed by rectal examination. The head should be assessed for symmetry, nasal discharges, relative air flow from each nostril, cranial nerve deficits, and relative enophthalmos or exophthalmos. The eyes will be sunken as a result of dehydration or extreme emaciation. Specific examination may include ophthalmic examination and inspection of mucous membranes for hemorrhages, icterus, anemia, erosions, or ulcerations. The frontal and maxillary sinuses should be evaluated by percussion. Lymph nodes should be palpated. If previous physical findings suggest the possible diagnosis of rabies, then examination of the head should be performed with great caution, and examination of the oral cavity should be performed with gloved hands. The jaws and tongue should be manipulated to evaluate their strength and the teeth inspected for excessive or uneven wear, fractures, or loss. The age of the cow may be estimated by examination of the teeth. Calves have three or four incisors on each side of the mandible at birth, and these are replaced by permanent teeth at approximately 20 months for the central incisor, 30 months for the medial incisor, 40 months for the lateral incisor, and 48 months for the corner incisor. The six permanent premolars on each side (three on top and three on the bottom) erupt between 24 and 36 months. The six permanent molars on each side erupt between 6 and 30 months.

The palate and oral mucous membranes should be examined with the aid of a focal light for erosions or ulceration. The odor of the breath and oral cavity should be noted. Examiners who can smell ketones on the cow's breath may be able to evaluate this parameter. A manual oral examination is performed if foreign bodies, inflammatory lesions, or masses are suspected in the oral cavity or pharynx, larynx, or proximal esophagus. The muzzle should be examined for the degree and symmetry of moisture present, because Horner's syndrome may result in ipsilateral dryness of the affected side of the muzzle and nares as the most apparent clinical sign. Motor and sensory function of the facial musculature and skin should be assessed if cranial nerve lesions are suspected; this is especially important if listeriosis or otitis interna or media are possible diagnoses. The throat latch area and proximal jugular furrow can also be included in the examination of the head, although it is also appropriate to include jugular vein palpation as part of the cardiovascular evaluation of the right and left hemithoraces. Even docile cattle resent palpation of the retropharyngeal or throat latch area, and if there is any obvious external swelling, head and neck extension, or other indication that there may be a clinically relevant problem in this region, it is wise to have a halter on and the animal restrained. The area immediately caudal to the vertical rami of the mandibles and the proximal jugular furrow should be palpated carefully and bilaterally for swelling, pain, and asymmetric enlargement. When swelling is present, it is usually diffuse and most often the result of pharyngeal trauma or retropharyngeal infection, so one can anticipate significant resentment to the examination. The mandibular lymph nodes should always be palpated in the intermandibular space. Although there is some normal variation in size, clearly enlarged nodes may suggest lymphoma or infection of the mandibular or pharyngeal area. On rare occasions, the mandibular salivary gland may be enlarged and easily palpated. The mandibular salivary gland is multilobed, allowing it to be distinguished from the smooth lymph node. Although most dairy cattle have been dehorned, those with horns should have the horns palpated to detect horn fractures or fractures of the skull at the cornual base of the horn.

A few comments on clinical evaluation of hydration status are pertinent at this point of the examination because examination of the head and neck is key in detecting dehydration. Dehydration can be estimated by pinching the skin of the neck or eyelids, occluding the jugular vein near the thoracic inlet and looking for speed of jugular distention, and examining the mucus of the mouth for viscosity, the nose for wetness, and the position of the eyes in the orbit. All of these should be quickly performed because none of them alone has a high sensitivity and specificity for dehydration (sunken eyes may occur from severe weight loss alone, and skin turgor is an inconsistent indicator of dehydration in calves). The ears can be palpated for temperature because cold ears may indicate poor perfusion from septic shock or milk fever.

Rectal Examination

Before completing the physical examination, a rectal examination is mandatory in appropriately-sized cattle. Rectal examination allows evaluation of the reproductive tract,

palpation of the dorsal and ventral sacs of the rumen, left kidney, iliac and deep inguinal lymph nodes, urinary bladder, proximal colon, pelvic bones, and ventral aspect of the lumbar and sacral vertebrae. The rectal examination may confirm many causes of abdominal distention suspected by the external examination, including cecal distention with or without volvulus, small intestinal distention, ruminal enlargements, rumen collapse, pneumoperitoneum, right-sided abomasal displacements with volvulus, some abdominal or pelvic abscesses, fat necrosis, dropsical pregnancy, and occasional neoplastic lesions. Caudal abdominal or pelvic adhesions and rectal tears also may be confirmed by palpation examination. When reproductive abnormalities such as metritis, dystocia, uterine torsion, or retained placenta are detected or suspected, a manual vaginal examination is indicated after cleansing and preparation of the vulva and perineum. Vaginal examination is also indicated if pyelonephritis is suspected because palpation of unilateral or bilateral ureteral enlargement is better performed via vaginal rather than rectal examination. After the rectal or vaginal examination, cattle with pelvic pain should be observed for persistent tenesmus, and if present, epidural administration may be required. In recumbent cattle for whom partial or complete coxofemoral luxation is a possibility, the rectal examination also provides an opportunity to identify referred crepitus in the pelvis. In cases of caudoventral dislocation, the head of the femur may be palpated within the obturator foramen. This may require an assistant to manipulate the affected limb in multiple directions while the veterinarian is performing the rectal examination.

Obtaining Urine for Analysis

Urine should be obtained, ideally before rectal examination, by repeated stroking of the cow's escutcheon and vulva using the flat of one's hand, straw, or hay to stimulate urination. Urine obtained in this manner should be tested with multiple-reagent test strips or tablets for urinary ketones, specific gravity, and other abnormal constituents that might suggest further evaluation via a catheterized urine sample.

Additional Evaluations

If lameness or musculoskeletal abnormalities are suspected, specific examination of the limbs, feet, or additional observation of the cow may be indicated. These procedures are discussed in Chapter 12. If neurologic abnormalities are suspected, examination of this system should be performed (see Chapter 13).

Ancillary Tests

At the completion of the physical examination, the examiner may have arrived at a specific diagnosis or may have formulated a differential diagnosis requiring ancillary tests or special system evaluation to arrive at a final diagnosis. Some ancillary procedures are available immediately, but others require laboratory evaluation or special equipment that may require economic decisions before undertaking.

Ultrasonography

If an ultrasound machine with a sector probe is available, then an ultrasound examination is often the most useful ancillary test that will provide immediate information in many sick cattle. Pneumonia, endocarditis, pleural and pericardial effusion, intestinal distenion, thickened intestinal wall, abdominal abscessation, and many other abnormalities can be immediately determined by ultrasound examination. With time, onsite ultrasound examination of sick cattle is becoming a more common occurrence. A great deal of diagnostically useful information can be acquired with just two ultrasound probes and a modern, well-maintained machine. Medium- to high-frequency (6–10 MHz) linear probes are useful for rectal examination of the reproductive tract, pelvis, and caudal abdominal structures. Such probes can also be used for evaluation of pleural and peripheral pulmonary lesions (see Chapter 4). A medium-frequency sector or convex (3.5–7 MHz) probe is most useful for the evaluation of the abdomen and in many cases can provide cardiac images of diagnostic quality for structural lesions (congenital defects, valvular disease, pericardial disease). A specific 2-5 MHz probe with more extensive software is needed for "state-of-the-art" echocardiographic examination and measurements of cardiac function and valvular competence (see Chapter 3).

Abdominal Paracentesis

Abdominal paracentesis is indicated when peritonitis is suspected or exfoliative cytology may be helpful to diagnosis. The procedure is performed best in the ventral abdomen to the right of midline but medial to the right mammary vein. The left abdomen and midline are contraindicated because the rumen visceral peritoneum lies in direct apposition to the parietal peritoneum and usually results in a contaminated tap. If the right ventral abdomen fails to produce fluid, paracentesis may be attempted lateral to the right fore udder in an area devoid of obvious mammary vessels. In either event, the selected area should be clipped and surgically prepared before abdominal paracentesis. The tap is performed with a 3.75-cm, 18-gauge needle with the needle advanced carefully to avoid gut contamination. Alternatively, a blunt teat canula can be used, but it requires local anesthetic in the skin and subcutis before a small stab incision is made to facilitate passage of the canula (see Chapter 2). It is much more difficult to obtain abdominal fluid in cattle than it is in horses, but the procedure can be an extremely useful aid to confirm peritonitis in questionable cases. Normal values for bovine abdominal fluid vary, but in general, total protein should be no greater than 3.0 g/dL, and the total white blood cell (WBC) count should not exceed 5000 to 6000 cells/μL. One author also implies that neutrophils making up greater than 40% of the WBC and less than 10% eosinophils are more important indicators of peritonitis than are the aforementioned protein and total WBC values.

Thoracocentesis and Pericardiocentesis

Thoracocentesis and pericardiocentesis may be indicated for pleural fluid accumulation, suspected thoracic abscesses or neoplasms, and pericardial transudates or exudates. These procedures are performed after surgical preparation of the specific area (usually the lower third, fourth, or fifth intercostal space) and use of an 8.75-cm, 18-gauge spinal needle, advanced as far as necessary. Obviously, the relative risk of this diagnostic step needs to be discussed with the owner before the procedure, but concurrent ultrasound examination can make this a much less risky procedure than was previously the case.

Arthrocentesis

Arthrocentesis is indicated for cytologic and culture study when septic arthritis or degenerative joint disease is suspected. This procedure requires surgical preparation and uses needles of various lengths, depending on the exact joint involved.

Aspiration

Aspiration may be required to diagnose fluid-filled masses occurring anywhere on the cow's body. In most instances, aspiration will differentiate abscesses, hematomas, and seromas. The procedure is contraindicated if physical examination and anamnesis make acute hematoma (proximity to a major vessel or anemia) the most likely diagnosis. Therefore, on a practical basis, aspiration is used to differentiate seromas that do not require drainage from abscesses that subsequently require surgical drainage. Experience suggests that even aseptic preparation of an aspiration site is no guarantee that an apparently sterile seroma will not become an abscess over the subsequent days to weeks. It can never be certain whether the aspiration procedure, hematogenous spread, or external access via damaged or bruised skin is the definitive cause when a seroma becomes an abscess, but the likelihood of this happening should impress on veterinarians the advisability of sterile technique and a pragmatic conversation with the owner prior to the procedure. Ultrasonography can be of value when attempting to differentiate among a seroma, hematoma, or abscess. Seromas tend to have a uniformly anechoic (black) appearance, but because of the prevalence of gas-producing anaerobes in pyogenic infections in cattle, an abscess often gives images with mixed echogenicity and gas (white) shadowing, especially when mature. Hematomas do not have any gas within them as they transition from peracute anechoic blood through various stages of clot formation and resolution with a mixed echogenicity. Frequently, hematomas have a septate or honeycombed appearance in the subacute stages and a more solid appearance chronically.

Aspiration of tracheal secretions (tracheal wash) for cytologic examination and culture can provide valuable information about cause and treatment of respiratory diseases. The procedure can be performed by clipping the midneck region directly over the trachea. After proper scrubbing and local infusion of lidocaine, a small cut is made through the skin on the midline and directly over the trachea. A 14-gauge needle is placed into the trachea, and a 16-gauge catheter is introduced. When the catheter is in the trachea, 20 to 30 mL of sterile preservative-free saline is flushed into the trachea and aspirated back. The procedure is most easily performed if two halters (with one lead on the right side and one on the left side) are placed on the cow and, just before making the tracheal puncture, the cow's head is elevated and tied on both sides. In calves, the head can be elevated manually. Due to the smaller trachea and narrow space between tracheal rings in calves the procedure has higher difficulty than in cows. After collection of the sputum, it is important that the fluid be placed in appropriate transport vials for delivery to the laboratory.

Biopsy

Biopsy may be required for solid masses, such as neoplasms, granulomas, and fat necrosis, or for specific organ histopathology, such as the liver, kidneys, mammary glands, and lungs. Tru-Cut (Baxter Healthcare Corp., Valencia, CA) biopsy needles are the most versatile instrument for this purpose and are applicable to most lesions and organs listed. Lesions in the upper or lower respiratory tract may require special biopsy devices, which are used through the channel of an endoscope. Again, surgical preparation of the site and scalpel puncture of the prepared skin before percutaneous biopsy of organs or tissues are required. Intraoperative biopsy of abdominal organs via laparotomy is a legitimate alternative to percutaneous sampling.

Urinary Catheterization

Urinary catheterization (see Chapter 11, Fig. 11.1) may be required to obtain urine if exogenous contamination of voided urine is anticipated or urine culture is required. A Chambers catheter works well for this procedure, and bovine practitioners need to become practiced in catheterization, lest the suburethral diverticulum confound proper catheterization.

TABLE 1.2	Normal Complete Blood Count Values	
Parameter	**Reference Range**
Hematocrit (Hct)	22%–33%
Hemoglobin (Hgb)	8.5–12.2 g/dL
Red blood cell (RBC)	5.1–7.6 million/µL
Mean cell volume (MCV)	38–50 fl
Mean corpuscular hemoglobin (MCH)	14–18 pg
Mean corpuscular hemoglobin concentration (MCHC)	36–39 g/dL
Red blood cell distribution width (RDW)	15.5%–19.7%
White blood cells (WBCs)	4.9–12.0 thousands/µL
Segment neutrophils (N)	1.8–6.3 thousands/µL
Band N	Rare
Lymphocyte (L)	1.6–5.6 thousands/µL
Monocytes	0–0.8 thousands/µL
Eosin	0–0.9 thousands/µL
Basophils	0–0.30 thousands/µL
N:L ratio	0.4–2.34
Platelets	193–637 thousands/µL
Mean platelet volume	4.5–7.5 fl
Total solids—refractometer	5.9–8.1 g/dL

Special Consideration in the Interpretation of Hematology Profiles in Calves: Calves have higher red blood cell count but progressively lower mean cell volume during the first 4 weeks of life.
Calf neutrophil count is often higher than lymphocyte count during the first week of life.
Calf lymphocyte count is similar to adult values during the first 2 months and then transiently increases above adult values between months 2 and 7.

Milk Sampling

Examination of the milk and the California mastitis test are part of the routine examination for all lactating dairy cattle, and this is further discussed under the section on mastitis (see Chapter 8).

Hematology and Serum Chemistry

Blood collection for laboratory analyses may be required for many different reasons. Routine complete blood count and chemistry panels are most valuable in assessing sick cows that have no obvious problem on physical examination. Specific laboratory data are presented in each chapter for specific diseases. Normal values used at our clinics for adult cattle are listed in Tables 1.2 and 1.3.

TABLE 1.3 Hitachi (917) Reference Ranges—Cornell University

Parameter	Reference Range	Parameter	Reference Range
Na	134–145 mEq/L	Total bilirubin	0–0.1 mg/dL
K	3.9–5.3 mEq/L	Direct bilirubin	0–0 mg/dL
Cl	94–105 mEq/L	Cholesterol	73–280 mg/dL
Total CO$_2$ (venous)	25–35 mEq/L	Creatine kinase	77–265 IU/L
Anion gap	17–24 mEq/L	Lactate dehydrogenase	659–1231 IU/L
Blood urea nitrogen	10–25 mg/dL	Magnesium	1.7–2.2 mg/dL
Creatinine	0.4–1.0 mg/dL	Triglyceride	7–25 mg/dL
Glucose	31–77 mg/dL	Bile acids	9–455 Too variable to be of use in dairy cattle
Alkaline phosphatase	23–78 IU/L		
Aspartate aminotransferase	53–162 IU/L	Glutathione peroxidase	≥60 Eu/g of hemoglobin (whole blood)
Iron	113–226 mg/dL		
TIBC	362–533 mg/dL	Heparin blood pH (venous)	7.35–7.50
γ-Glutamyltransferase	11–39 IU/L	PCO$_2$ (venous)	41–50 mm Hg
Calcium total	8.3–10.4 mg/dL	Bicarbonate	24–34 mEq/L
Calcium ionized	1.06–1.33 mmol/L	Osmolality	270–300 mOsmol/kg
Phosphorus	4.2–7.7 mg/dL	Osmolar gap	0–15 mOsmol/kg
Total protein	7.2–9.0 g/dL	Colloid oncotic pressure	21-25 mm Hg (adults) 17-23 mm Hg (calves)
Albumin	3.2–4.2 g/dL		
Globulin	3.5–5.8 g/dL		

TIBC, Total iron-binding capacity.
Nonesterified free fatty acids (NEFFAs): greater than 0.4 mEq/L in a late pregnant cow (2 weeks to 2 days before freshening) suggests excessive negative energy balance.
Beta hydroxybutyrate (BHBA): 1400 µmol/L (or 14.4 mg/dL) suggests threefold increased risk for ketosis (subclinical or clinical); cows with clinical ketosis often have BHBA >3000 µmol/L or >26 mg/dL.
Special Consideration in the Interpretation of Biochemistry Profiles in Calves:
Biochemistry values in milk-fed calves can vary from the adult reference range listed above and in summary:
  Calf glucose value is normally 80–90 mg/dL.
  Calf gamma-glutamyl transferase is >200 IU/L the first week of life because of colostral absorption and remains above adult cow values for 2 weeks.
  Calf aspartate transaminase is below adult cow values for at least the first 3 months of life.
  Calf globulins and total protein values are below the adult cow reference range.
  Calf creatinine, creatine kinase, and packed cell volume are greater than those of adult cows for the first 1–3 days of life.

Summary for Clinical Examination

As our clinical experience increases, pattern recognition becomes an increasingly important armamentarium for arriving at an accurate diagnosis. Enhanced pattern recognition can both improve diagnostic accuracy and lower the number of diagnostic tests required. However, it has been our experience that if pattern recognition becomes the predominant means of reaching a diagnosis without completing a thorough clinical examination or seeking to understand a probable pathophysiologic explanation for the clinical signs, diagnostic clinical accuracy will then actually decline (Fig. 1.1). Experienced practitioners should use pattern recognition to improve the accuracy of the clinical examination but guard against excessive reliance on it.

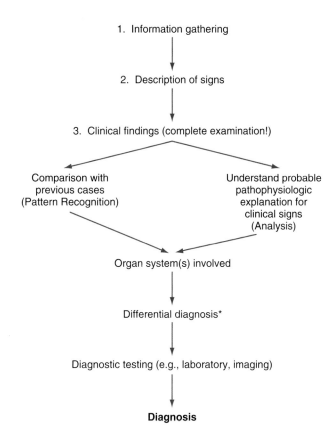

1. Information gathering

2. Description of signs

3. Clinical findings (complete examination!)

Comparison with previous cases (Pattern Recognition)

Understand probable pathophysiologic explanation for clinical signs (Analysis)

Organ system(s) involved

Differential diagnosis*

Diagnostic testing (e.g., laboratory, imaging)

Diagnosis

*A list of differential diagnoses for each clinical sign can be found at http://www.vet.cornell.edu/consultant/consult.asp

• **Fig. 1.1** Summary of steps in establishing an accurate diagnosis.

Suggested Readings

Brun-Hansen, H. C., Kampen, A. H., & Lund, A. (2006). Hematologic values in calves. *Vet Clin Path, 35,* 182–187.

Eddy, R. G., & Pinsent, P. J. N. (2004). In A. Andrews, R. H. Blowey, H. Boyd, et al. (Eds.), *Bovine medicine* (2nd ed.) (pp. 135–138). Oxford, UK: Blackwell.

George, J. W., Snipes, J., & Michael Lane, V. (2010). Comparison of bovine hematology reference intervals from 1957 to 2006. *Vet Clin Path, 39,* 138–148.

Gibbons, W. J. (1966). *Clinical diagnosis of diseases of large animals.* Philadelphia: Lea and Febiger.

Pérez-Santos, M., Castillo, C., Hernández, J., et al. (2015). Biochemical variables from Holstein-Fresian calves older than one week are comparable to those obtained from adult animals of stable metabolic status on the same farm. *Vet Clin Path, 44,* 145–151.

Perkins, G. A. (2004). Examination of the surgical patient. In S. L. Fubini, & N. G. Ducharme (Eds.), *Farm animal surgery* (2nd ed.) (pp. 3–14). St. Louis: WB Saunders.

Radostits, O. M., Gay, C. C., Blood, D. C., et al. (2000). *Veterinary medicine* (9th ed.) (pp. 3–40). Philadelphia: WB Saunders.

Rosenberger, G. (1979). Clinical examination of cattle. In Dirksen G, Gründer H-D, Grunert E, et al, collaborators, and Mack R, translator. Berlin: Verlag Paul Parey.

Terra, R. L. (2002). In B. P. Smith (Ed.), *Large animal internal medicine* (3rd ed.) (pp. 1–14). St. Louis: Mosby.

Wilson, J. H. (1992). The art of physical diagnosis. *Vet Clin North Am Food Anim Pract, 8*(2), 169–176.

2

Therapeutics and Routine Procedures

THOMAS J. DIVERS AND SIMON F. PEEK

Venipuncture

The jugular vein is the major vein used to administer most intravenous (IV) medications and large volumes of IV fluids in dairy cattle. The middle caudal vein ("tail vein") is used for collection of blood samples and for administration of small volumes (<5.0 mL) of medications. If the tail vein or artery is used for drug administration, only aqueous agents that will be nonirritating (if they leak perivascularly) should be used because it is harder to avoid some degree of leakage at this location than when a well-seated needle is used in the jugular vein. The mammary vein should not be used for either blood sampling or drug administration because complications of mammary venipuncture may have disastrous results, such as mammary vein thrombosis or phlebitis (see Figs. 3.47 and 3.48), persistent unilateral mammary edema, and endocarditis. In general, it is contraindicated to use the mammary vein therapeutically unless the cow has a life-threatening illness and is in a compromised position, such that the jugular vein is inaccessible. Cattle with bilateral jugular vein thrombosis also may necessitate the risk of mammary vein venipuncture. In severely dehydrated calves, it is necessary occasionally to use a cephalic or dorsal metatarsal vein in case the jugular veins become thrombosed during repeated fluid administration. Before any venipuncture, the overlying skin and hair should be moistened and smoothed down with alcohol or a chlorhexidine solution. The vein should be "held off" by applying digital pressure proximal to the heart from the site of venipuncture (Fig. 2.1).

Neophytes seldom apply pressure of sufficient magnitude or duration before venipuncture and consequently have difficulty palpating or viewing the distended vein. Experienced clinicians are very patient and allow the vein adequate time to fill with blood, making venipuncture easier. Choke ropes or chains seldom are necessary in routine jugular venipuncture but may be helpful in extremely dehydrated patients. Using gravity by allowing the head to hang over the side of a raised platform or table or even by hanging the calf over a stall divider or gate can distend the jugular vein significantly to facilitate venous access in very dehydrated calves. Commercial instruments such as Witte's neck chain and Schecker's vein clamp are available aids used in Europe.

Jugular venipuncture may be performed with a variety of needles, but the needle must be suited to the drug's viscosity and volume and the duration of time anticipated for delivery. Stainless steel 14-gauge needles that are 5.0 to 7.5 cm in length are favored for most fluid infusions that do not exceed 2 L and that are to be administered promptly. Although many practitioners use disposable 14-gauge needles that are 3.75 cm in length, these needles are too short and so sharp that, with minimal patient struggling, such complications as laceration of the intima of the vein or perivascular administration of medications may occur. These shorter, disposable needles are acceptable for recumbent or extremely well-restrained cattle only. In general, venous complications such as thrombosis and perivascular leakage are more common with the shorter needles. The longer 5.0- to 7.5-cm stainless steel needles are long enough to remain well positioned within the vein and are less sharp and therefore less likely to lacerate the intima of the vein and thus tend to cause less frustration to the practitioner faced with an unruly patient. The disadvantage of stainless steel 14-gauge needles is that they require cleaning, sterilization between uses, and periodic sharpening with an Arkansas stone. Cleaning and sterilization between uses are extremely important in preventing spread of bovine leukemia virus (BLV) and bacterial infections. Although most practitioners prefer 14-gauge needles, some practitioners successfully use 12-gauge, 5.0- to 7.5-cm stainless steel needles to allow an even more rapid administration of solutions such as dextrose and balanced electrolytes through the jugular vein. Careful pressure over the venipuncture site after removal of the needle is important in preventing hematoma formation, which may contribute to venous thrombosis.

When an indwelling IV catheter is to be placed in the jugular vein, a selected area in the cranial third of the jugular furrow should be clipped and prepared surgically before inserting the catheter. Catheters may be secured by skin sutures, adhesive tape, cyanoacrylate to the skin, or combinations of these techniques. Catheter placement is similar to placement of stainless steel needles, but a much greater length of catheter must be threaded into the vein. It is imperative that the vein distal to the site of placement remains compressed during the procedure. Because cattle,

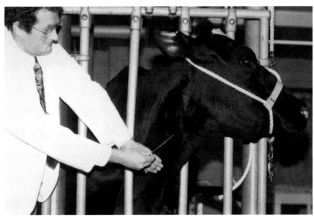

• **Fig. 2.1** Jugular venipuncture. The cow is restrained forward in the stanchion and has her head tightly secured by a rope halter tied with a quick-release halter tie. The jugular region has been swabbed with alcohol, and the vein is held off by pressure on the heart side of the venipuncture site. A pointer indicates the distended vein.

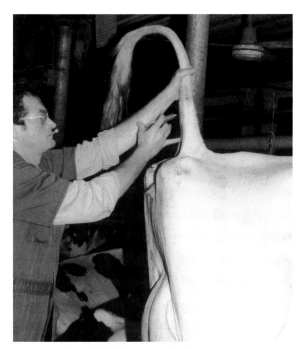

• **Fig. 2.2** Middle caudal (tail) venipuncture.

and especially dehydrated cattle, have an extremely thick hide, skin puncture with a no. 15 scalpel blade aids greatly in the placement of IV catheters in dehydrated cattle or young calves.

Catheter materials have improved considerably over the past decade or two, and their use need not be confined to university teaching hospitals. Less thrombogenic catheter materials such as those made with polyurethane rather than Teflon or silicone are now commonly used and even antimicrobial impregnated catheters (usually with chlorhexidine or silver sulfadiazine) can be used for hospitalized adult and neonatal patients at risk for thrombosis and septic thrombophlebitis. More traditional Teflon catheters are often perfectly fine for short-term IV fluid and drug administration in both adults and calves. Jugular catheters in adults should always be at least 16 gauge in diameter and typically 14 gauge and 13 cm in length to ensure proper seating. In calves, it is also commonplace to use IV catheters of up to 13 cm in length in the jugular vein, and 14 gauge, 16 gauge, and 18 gauge varieties are often used. Clipping and aseptic site preparation are always recommended.

Venipuncture of the middle caudal vein ("tail vein") is performed by inserting a needle on the ventral midline of the proximal tail. The exact distance from the anus may vary depending on the animal's size, but the site is usually 10.0 to 20.0 cm distal to the base of the tail. The vein and artery are thought to run side by side as far as the fourth caudal vertebrae; the artery then usually runs ventral to the vein. However, this anatomy often varies. It is rarely important to distinguish if the needle puncture and blood collection or drug administration has occurred in the coccygeal vein or artery. After removing the needle, a spurt of blood or hematoma formation would suggest the artery has been punctured. When performing tail vein venipuncture, the clinician must provide restraint by elevating the tail perpendicular to the top line. Forgetting to do this may result in a painful lesson in restraint. The tail is raised with the clinician's less adroit hand, and the venipuncture is performed

with the preferred hand (Fig. 2.2). Needles already should be connected to the syringe that holds the drug or with a Vacutainer (Becton Dickinson, Franklin Lakes, NJ) partially inserted so that the entire procedure can be done with one hand. Needles should be 18 or 20 gauge and 2.5 to 3.75 cm in length. The needle is inserted on the ventral midline perpendicular to the longitudinal axis of the tail and advanced until it gently strikes bone. Aspiration of blood is then attempted. If successful, the drug is administered or blood collected. If unsuccessful, the needle is gently backed off the bone 1 to 5 mm, and aspiration is attempted again. Use of the middle caudal vein for administration of small volumes (<5.0 mL) of medications and blood collection has largely replaced jugular venipuncture for these procedures in dairy cattle. Tail bleeding is far less stressful to the patient, avoids bellowing and excessive restraint, and is quicker because one person performs both restraint and venipuncture. Although primarily valuable for blood collection in adult dairy cattle, the tail vein may be used for blood collection in cattle of 300 kg or more. The procedure is more difficult in heifers and young bulls of this size, however, frequently because of behavioral responses to the needle placement combined with the smaller vessel diameter. Tail bleeding should not be attempted in young calves, lest permanent damage to caudal vessels occur.

Selection of appropriate needles for intramuscular (IM) injections in cattle requires consideration of density or viscosity of the drug to be administered, size of the patient, and desired depth of injection. Needles of too narrow bore prolong the time necessary for injection, often causing increased patient apprehension, struggling, or kicking. Needles too large of bore allow leakage of the administered drug from the site and cause more bleeding. Whereas

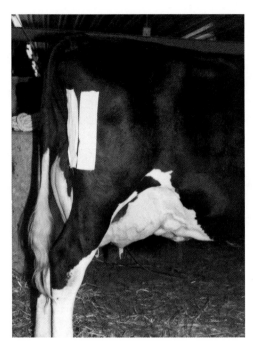

• **Fig. 2.3** Caudal and caudolateral (white tape) thigh sites for intramuscular injections.

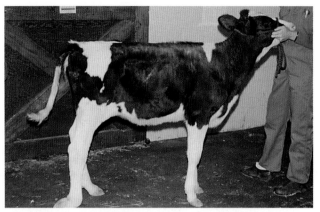

• **Fig. 2.4** Sciatic nerve injury secondary to intramuscular injection in the gluteal region of a Holstein calf.

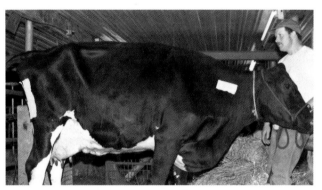

• **Fig. 2.5** Site (white tape) for intramuscular injection of small volumes in the cervical musculature. Be sure to inject dorsal to the cervical vertebral region if this site is chosen.

most aqueous-based drugs can be administered IM via an 18-gauge, 3.75-cm needle in adult cattle, injection of oil-based or more viscous drugs (e.g., penicillin, oxytetracycline HCl) is facilitated by a 16-gauge, 3.75-cm needle. Most practitioners use disposable needles for IM injections to avoid the bothersome task of cleaning and sterilizing used needles. Increasing concerns regarding carcass spoilage as a result of the IM administration of therapeutic and biologic agents in grade dairy cattle have prompted a move toward subcutaneous (SC) administration of many products (antibiotics, hormones) that were previously given IM. Subcutaneous administration may require additional milk withdrawal due to slower rate of absorption in comparison to IM administration. Carcass trimming with subsequent lost revenue from meat is a relevant issue because the slaughter value of a culled dairy cow represents a significant revenue stream for many modern producers.

In dairy calves younger than 2 months of age, a 20- or 18-gauge, 2.5-cm needle may be better for IM injections. In all instances, judgment is essential because the difference between a 1-week-old Jersey calf and an adult Holstein bull dictates selection of a needle based on the individual patient.

The primary site for IM injections in cattle is the caudal thigh musculature, especially the semimembranosus and semitendinosus. Occasionally, the caudal biceps femoris is used as well (Fig. 2.3). The gluteal region should not be used for IM injections in calves or adult dairy cattle because of the relative lack of musculature in a "dairy-type" animal. Injections in this area risk temporary or permanent injury to the sciatic nerve branches traversing the gluteal region when repeated IM injections or an IM injection of irritating drugs is necessary. Gluteal injections are especially contraindicated in dairy calves (Fig. 2.4). Although many textbooks and

publications advocate IM injections in the gluteal region, this procedure should be avoided in dairy cattle.

Other available sites for IM injections include the triceps brachia (triceps) and the caudal cervical muscles (Fig. 2.5). From a practical standpoint, dairy cattle generally are more excited by injections in their front end than by injections in their hind end. If a cow is well restrained with a halter, IM injections can be made safely in the caudal cervical or triceps region. In poorly restrained cattle, these injection sites frequently cause wild and aggressive behavior. Most dairy cows tolerate IM injections in the caudal thigh muscles without kicking. However, unnecessary prolongation of the injection because of improper needle selection, multiple IM injections, or failure to prepare the patient for the "shot" all may lead to violent behavior. In addition, some dairy cattle are dangerous and require additional restraint before IM injections to avoid injury to themselves or their handlers.

The caudal cervical muscles in a calf provide an easily accessible site for IM injections of less than 5.0 mL of non-irritating solutions. The clinician can restrain the calf by straddling its neck and bending the calf's head to one side while the injection is made (Fig. 2.6). A similar restraint technique can be used for IV injection or blood sampling in calves.

Selecting a clean site (free of manure and moisture) and swabbing it with 70% alcohol or chlorhexidine solution

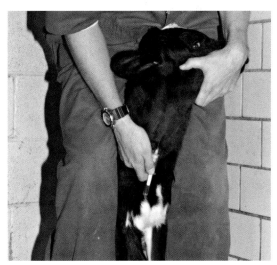

• **Fig. 2.6** Restraint and positioning of a young calf for jugular venipuncture. An intramuscular injection in the caudal cervical musculature or subcutaneous injection in this region can also be performed in a similar manner.

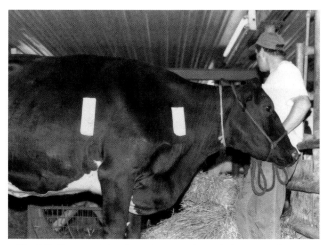

• **Fig. 2.7** Sites cranial and caudal to the forelimb (white tape) for subcutaneous injections.

should precede IM injections. The needle is held by the hub between the thumb and forefinger, and the cow is slapped repeatedly with the back of the clinician's hand near the site of the injection. Quickly rotating the hand, the clinician then slaps the needle into the selected IM site. The needle must be submerged all the way to its hub. A visual inspection for blood coming from the needle is made, and if none is seen, the syringe of medication is quickly attached to the needle.

Aspiration on the syringe plunger will detect needles placed within vessels. If blood is aspirated, the injection is aborted, and the needle should be placed at a different site. If no blood is observed, the injection is made as quickly as possible. Up to 20 mL of drug may be deposited at an IM site in an adult cow, but probably no more than 5 mL should be placed at any one site in a young calf. Consideration of the drug's irritability to tissue may also influence specific volumes deposited at IM sites.

For cattle restrained in stanchions, usually little additional restraint is necessary. For cattle in free stalls or cows that appear apprehensive, haltering and tail restraint by an assistant may be necessary.

Subcutaneous injections are indicated for certain antibiotics and calcium preparations in adult cattle. In calves, balanced fluid solutions and certain antibiotics are administered. The recommended sites for SC injections in dairy cattle are (1) caudal to the forelimb at the level of the midthorax where loose skin can be grasped easily and (2) cranial to the forelimb in the caudal cervical region where loose skin can be grasped easily (Fig. 2.7). Care must be taken to avoid hitting the scapula with the needle!

It is important to avoid injury or irritation to the forelimbs when injections at these sites are made, and irritating drugs or excessive volumes should be avoided, lest the animal experience pain associated with forelimb motion. To speed the administration, a large-gauge needle, such

as a 14-gauge needle, should be used for adult cattle, and a 16-gauge needle should be used for calves. A disposable 3.75-cm needle is sufficiently long for this purpose. Whereas a 500-mL bottle of calcium borogluconate usually is divided into three or four sites (e.g., left and right side front of forelimbs, left and right side caudal to forelimb), an antibiotic injection may be made at one site in the morning, another in the evening, and yet another site the following day. Calves requiring SC balanced fluid solutions may receive 250 to 1000 mL at a single site, depending on the size of the patient. During the injection, the bleb of fluids should be gently compressed and spread out by the clinician to distribute the fluids, improve absorption, and decrease leakage following withdrawal of the needle. SC injections of irritating drugs or dextrose-containing solutions must be avoided. SC injections at the base of the ear are common due to the widespread use of a crystalline free acid suspension of sodium ceftiofur. This is a relatively easy injection to perform and needs only basic restraint. Approximately 1 in 1000 injections with this product at this site results in acute death of the cow, most likely due to inadvertently administering the treatment intraarterially. Therefore, the value of the cow might be considered when performing this treatment.

Intraperitoneal injections seldom are performed in dairy cattle, with the exception of calcium solutions administered to hypocalcemic cows by laypeople untrained in venipuncture. Some over-the-counter calcium–dextrose solutions come complete with instructions recommending intraperitoneal injections through the right paralumbar fossa. Although this technique may be lifesaving for severely hypocalcemic cows, it also is dangerous for the following reasons:

1. Depending on the position of the cow and length of the needle used, the solution may enter SC, IM, intraperitoneally, or into a viscus such as the proximal colon.
2. Chemical peritonitis occurs if dextrose is present in the calcium solution.
3. Large intestinal adhesions are possible complications.

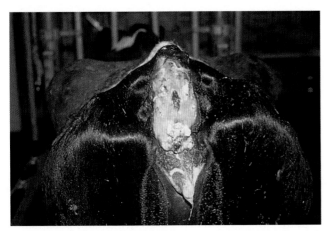

• **Fig. 2.8** Complete sloughing of the tail in a Holstein cow after perivascular injection of phenylbutazone.

In adult dairy cattle, a needle at least 5.0 cm in length would be necessary for intraperitoneal injection, and risks of damage to viscera are minimized by rolling a recumbent cow to her left side before puncturing the right paralumbar fossa.

Complications of jugular IV injections include hematoma formation, thrombosis, thrombophlebitis, tissue sloughing caused by perivascular injections of irritating drugs, endocarditis, and Horner's syndrome (see Figs. 3.46 and 14.11). The most irritating drugs commonly administered IV in cattle are 40% to 50% dextrose, 20% sodium iodide, and calcium. Avoiding perivascular deposition of these three drugs is extremely important. Good technique and adequate restraint are the keys to avoiding complications from IV injections. Similar advice regarding restraint and proper training for venipuncture technique currently must apply to the administration of flunixin meglumine to dairy cattle. Federal regulations in the United States require that this drug be administered IV. Because of its capacity for tissue irritation, combined with increased surveillance for violative drug residues in the carcass of cull cows, it has become extremely important that not only is the drug administered in the vein but that careful attention is paid to the avoidance of perivascular leakage.

Complications of tail vein injections include hematoma formation, thrombosis, thrombophlebitis, and rarely sloughing of the tail (Fig. 2.8).

Complications of IM injections include tissue necrosis with subsequent lameness; peripheral nerve injury, especially sciatic nerve branches in the gluteal region or tibial branches in the caudal thigh muscles of calves; clostridial myositis; severe pain following injection and procaine reactions. Peripheral nerve injury can be prevented best by avoiding the gluteal region when performing IM injections. In calves, palpation of the groove separating the biceps femoris and semitendinosus proximal to the stifle and injecting medial or lateral to this groove will help avoid sciatic nerve injury. Clostridial myositis is always a risk when injecting irritating drugs that may create a focal area of tissue necrosis and a subsequent anaerobic environment in the IM site. Although *Clostridium chauvoei* (blackleg) spores may lie dormant in tissue locations already, most clostridial myositis cases secondary to IM

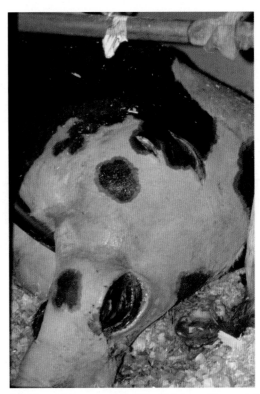

• **Fig. 2.9** Clostridial myonecrosis (*Clostridium perfringens* infection) associated with prostaglandin injection in the lateral thigh musculature.

injections are caused by *Clostridium perfringens* or *Clostridium septicum* (Fig. 2.9). Currently, prostaglandin solutions are the most commonly incriminated solutions to result in clostridial myositis (see also Fig. 16.1). Using sterile syringes and sterile needles and avoiding contamination of multidose drug vials are important preventive measures. In addition, IM injections should not be made through skin covered by dirt or manure without first cleaning the site.

Procaine reactions occur when procaine penicillin preparations inadvertently enter a vein. Subsequent hyperexcitability, propulsive tendencies, shaking, collapse, or other neurologic signs may develop within 60 seconds of the injection. Clinicians or veterinary students who have made IM injections resulting in procaine reaction adamantly say that they "checked for blood by syringe aspiration before injection and definitely were not in a vessel!" Indeed, these clinicians probably were not in a vessel at the start of the injection, but by pushing to force the thick procaine penicillin out of the syringe through an 18-gauge or smaller needle, they inadvertently forced the needle tip into a vessel. This is more likely to happen when multiple injections have already been given causing an increased vascularity to the area. Entering a vessel can happen to anyone, but it can be best avoided by using needles that are big enough to both detect blood when aspirating before injection and to deliver the drug quickly IM without undue force on the syringe. When a procaine reaction does occur, leave the patient alone—do not try to restrain the animal and keep people away from the animal to avoid human injury. Procaine reactions seldom are fatal in cattle unless a large amount of drug enters the bloodstream. It is common for laypeople or inexperienced

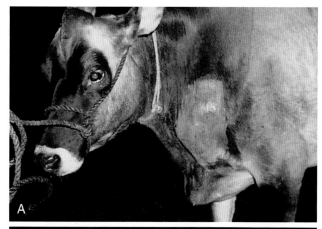

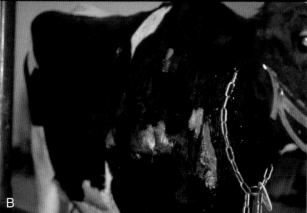

• **Fig. 2.10** Painful cellulitis and abscessation of the caudal cervical region secondary to subcutaneous calcium-dextrose solution administration in a Jersey cow (**A**). Similar outcome in a Holstein heifer with abscessation and cellulitis secondary to subcutaneous administration of a 50% dextrose solution (**B**). (Photo (B) courtesy of Dr. Gary Oetzel.)

clinicians to mistake the classic procaine reaction for a penicillin "allergy" or hypersensitivity; the latter generally has more obvious signs of vasoactive amine release with systemic or cutaneous evidence of anaphylaxis. However, distinguishing the two is important because a procaine reaction does not necessitate cessation of penicillin therapy, merely more careful attention to injection technique.

Complications of SC injections include chemical and infectious inflammation. Chemical inflammation with eventual tissue necrosis and sterile abscessation is common if dextrose or calcium dextrose combinations are injected SC. Infectious inflammation, phlegmon, and eventual abscessation may result from poor skin-site preparation or technique. Common signs include painful, diffuse swellings that gravitate ventrally from the SC injection site, lameness and stiff gait caused by pain associated with forelimb movements, fever, and depression (Fig. 2.10). Treatment consists of hydrotherapy, warm compresses, analgesics, and eventual drainage.

Various cannulas and commercial mastitis tubes are available for intramammary infusions. Individual sterile plastic cannulas (2-cm) with syringe adapters are used most commonly for infusion of noncommercial mastitis products, and stainless steel 14-gauge, 5.0 to 10-cm blunt-tip teat cannulas are sometimes used to facilitate milk-out from injured teats or for diagnostic probing of obstructed teats.

In all instances and regardless of the cannula used, the teat and teat end should be prepared aseptically before insertion of the cannula through the streak canal. After cleaning the teat thoroughly, the teat end should be swabbed repeatedly with alcohol before the cannula is inserted and again after the cannula is removed (see also Chapter 8). Large-volume infusions (>100 mL) may be administered via gravity flow with the aid of simplex tubing and a sterile teat cannula.

Instruments used to deliver medications to the pharynx, esophagus, or rumen require passage through the oral cavity; the only exception is nasoruminal intubation. Balling guns, oral specula and stomach tubes, a variety of dose syringes, and drenching devices are available for use in cattle. These instruments have tremendous potential to cause injury to cattle when used improperly or in a rough manner. Veterinarians should train laypeople in the proper use of instruments intended for oral delivery of medications to cattle because most injuries to the pharynx, soft palate, or esophagus of cattle are iatrogenic and caused by laypeople.

Balling Guns

Balling guns are available as single- or multiple-bolus instruments. Single-bolus instruments require two people for administration unless the person holding the cow's head releases the head each time a bolus is administered. Obviously, the patient becomes harder to catch each time the head is released. Multiple bolus magazines have become popular because they avoid the need for "reloading."

Both types of balling guns are safe when used properly, and both are lethal weapons if used improperly. Before passing a balling gun into the patient's oral cavity, a quick assessment of the patient's size is mandatory. The administrator of the bolus using a balling gun should ask themselves the following questions: Where is the pharynx in this patient? How much of the instrument should be advanced into the oral cavity? Balling guns passed too far caudally abut the soft palate or dorsal pharyngeal wall, thereby allowing pharyngeal injury when forceful expulsion of a bolus or multiple boluses occurs. In adult Holstein cattle, commercial balling guns are in correct position when the holding finger rings (not the plunger finger ring) are resting against the commissure of the patient's lips (Fig. 2.11). However, this same position in a Jersey cow or a yearling Holstein places the bolus too far caudally in the oral cavity, thereby risking pharyngeal injury when the bolus is forcibly discharged. Balling guns can be dangerous when used in recumbent cattle. Particular care with all oral medication is necessary with any patient demonstrating signs of hypocalcemia because normal swallowing and protective upper airway reflexes may be depressed.

Adult cattle balling guns should not be used in calves or young stock without extreme care or else splitting of the soft palate may occur. Smaller balling guns are available for calves and are preferable. Multiple-dose balling guns with sharp ends should be avoided. Gentle introduction and lubrication of balling guns, as with most instruments used in the oral cavity, will limit iatrogenic injuries. Balling guns should be of single-piece construction to avoid accidental

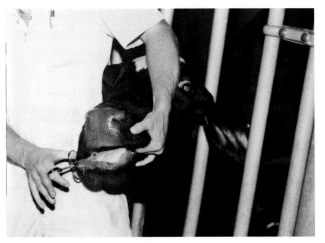

• **Fig. 2.11** Proper position for delivery of medication using a standard balling gun in an adult Holstein cow. Note that the operator's opposite hand is used to restrain the head and exert gentle fingertip pressure on the patient's hard palate such that the cow opens her mouth. In smaller cattle, the depth of insertion of the balling gun into the oral cavity needs to be adjusted to avoid pharyngeal injury.

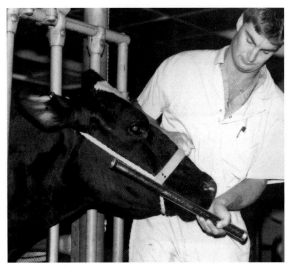

• **Fig. 2.12** Determining the length of a Fricke speculum to be advanced into the oral cavity of the patient before stomach tubing.

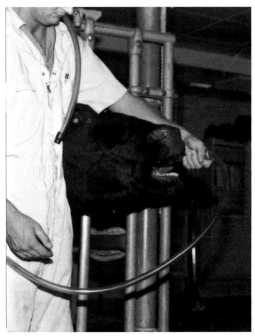

• **Fig. 2.13** Passing a stomach tube with the aid of a Fricke speculum. Note that the veterinarian uses his left arm to both restrain the head tightly to his body and to hold the speculum. The right hand is used to advance the tube. The patient's head should be held straight, not pulled to either side because this makes passage of the tube difficult and potentially injurious to the patient's pharynx.

loss of the magazine portion of the instrument into the rumen (which may occur with two-piece instruments!).

Stomach Tubes

Before passage of a stomach tube through the oral cavity of a cow, a speculum or gag must be used to guard the tube. Both the tube and some types of specula have the potential to cause iatrogenic injury. Stomach tubes should have smooth, tapered ends; appropriate flexibility; and measurement markers. A variety of gags are used to prevent cattle from chewing on or "eating" the stomach tube. Properly used gags present little potential for patient injury. However, a pipe and Fricke speculum are the oral specula used most commonly in dairy cattle and are potentially dangerous instruments. The length of a Fricke speculum exceeds the length of a cow's oral cavity so that the operator can safely hold a portion of the speculum external to the patient's mouth. Introducing a Fricke speculum too far caudally into the patient's oral cavity causes repeated gagging and coughing and interferes with passage of the stomach tube because the tube repeatedly contacts the pharyngeal wall rather than the pharyngeal cavity when advanced.

Overzealous forcing of the tube in this incorrect position results in injury to the patient. Before a Fricke speculum is used, the patient should be "sized up" to determine how much of the speculum should be advanced into the oral cavity (Fig. 2.12). The speculum should be continually grasped during the procedure or the cow may swallow the speculum. Any metallic speculum should be periodically checked for sharp or irregular ends or edges because natural wear and tear can lead to damaged metal that can induce significant trauma. A speculum appropriately sized for adult cattle should not be used in young stock, or splitting of the soft palate may occur. Cows that repeatedly regurgitate when placing a speculum and passing an oral stomach tube can be tubed through the nasal cavity, although a smaller diameter tube must be used.

A variety of stomach tubes are available. For cattle, a tube should have some flexibility, and the flexibility should be adjustable by temperature so that either warm or cold water can be used to add flexibility or add rigidity, respectively. Whereas tubes that are too soft and flexible will double back during passage, tubes that are completely inflexible risk iatrogenic injury to the pharynx, soft palate, or esophagus. Stomach tubes for adult cattle should have at least a ¾-inch (1.88-cm) outside diameter to speed delivery of medications or evacuation of gas (Fig. 2.13). Tubes of smaller diameter plug with rumen digesta too easily. Larger tubes, up to the

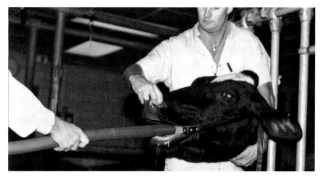

• **Fig. 2.14** Passage of a Kingman tube with the aid of a cut-out wooden gag attached by a head strap. It is imperative that the patient's head and neck be held straight and that the head not be elevated. This position facilitates passage of the well-lubricated tube and minimizes the chances of inhalation should regurgitation occur.

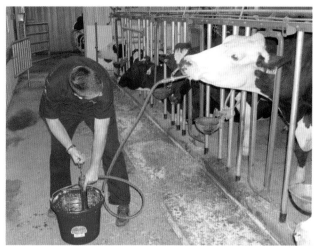

• **Fig. 2.15** McGrath pump. The pump is passed into the esophagus and verified by palpation to be in the correct location before the nose tongs are used to secure the device in place. Fluids can then be administered by bilge pump by just one person.

"ultimate tube" (the Kingman), require excellent patient restraint, an appropriate gag or speculum, lubrication of the tube, and appropriate head position of the patient (Fig. 2.14).

The Kingman tube is used to evacuate abnormal rumen contents or for rumen lavage. It may be used in cases of selected frothy bloats, lactic acidosis, and extreme fluid overload of the rumen. When passing a Kingman or other large-diameter stomach tube, the cow's head must be held straight forward and not pulled to the side because these tubes cannot be passed around a "corner." The cow's head should not be held higher than horizontal or the normal postural position during passage of the tube in case regurgitation around the tube (a frequent complication) occurs. This technique will help to avoid inhalation of regurgitated rumen contents.

The increasingly common practice of routine or therapeutic drenching of periparturient and postparturient cattle has led to the widespread use of the McGrath pump (Fig. 2.15) in modern dairies. This apparatus has the advantage of only requiring one person to position and then administer

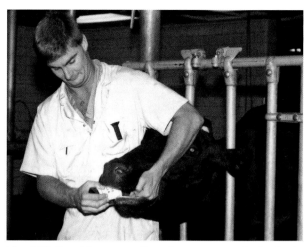

• **Fig. 2.16** Drenching a cow. Fingertip pressure on the hard palate with the off-hand facilitates introduction of the drench bottle. The cow's head is held horizontally, straight ahead, and close to the operator's ribs.

the fluids because it is maintained in place by a built-in set of nose tongs. Veterinarians should not hesitate to train laypeople in proper restraint, positioning, and administration techniques when using this or any other stomach tube or oral drenching device because inadvertent aspiration and drowning are tragic but occasional consequences of their use by unqualified or poorly trained personnel.

Common sense, lots of lubrication, and gentle technique are minimal requirements for veterinarians using large-bore stomach tubes.

Dose Syringe and Drench Bottles

Oral medicaments such as rumenotorics and propylene glycol often are administered by oral drenching or dosing. These techniques are less likely to injure the oral cavity or pharynx physically but do risk inhalation pneumonia when performed inappropriately.

After the cow's head is restrained, the drench bottle or syringe is introduced into the oral cavity at the commissure of the lips on the same side as the operator. Introduction is facilitated by finger pressure directed on the patient's hard palate by the operator's hand that is holding the patient's head (Fig. 2.16). The cow's muzzle should be held so that the head from pole to muzzle is horizontal to the ground or slightly higher. Holding the head too high or twisting the head to the side interferes with swallowing and risks inhalation of irritating chemicals. Allowances for spillage should be made when calculating the drug volumes to be administered.

Esophageal Feeders

Popular for delivery of colostrum or electrolyte solutions to newborn or young calves, esophageal feeder devices are potentially dangerous when used by impatient or poorly trained laypeople or when worn or brittle. Pharyngeal and esophageal lacerations are all too common iatrogenic

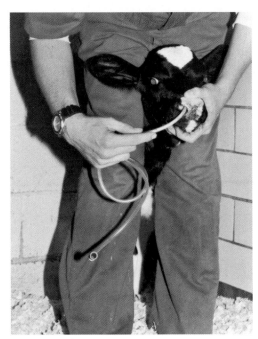

• **Fig. 2.17** Introducing a soft rubber stomach tube into the ventral meatus of a calf.

complications, and inhalation pneumonia is a less common complication. Laypeople should only be allowed to use these devices after training by a veterinarian. Proper disinfection of esophageal feeders that have been used to administer colostrum, milk replacer, or electrolyte solution is an important preventive measure in the control of infectious enteric disease in calves. In cold, northern climates, the plastic of these feeders can become weakened when "scored" heavily by teeth because of repeated use, making them brittle and prone to breakage as moisture freezes and thaws repeatedly within the damaged plastic. It is much more economical to replace these periodically than to have veterinarians attempt to retrieve parts of the device endoscopically or at surgery when swallowed (Video Clip 2.01). Even in young calves, soft plastic stomach tubes should not be passed orally without a calf speculum for fear of being bitten off and swallowed.

Magnet Retrievers and Other Instruments Designed to Retrieve Hardware from the Reticulum

All of these instruments are extremely dangerous to patients. Although some clinicians have had success with these instruments, they cannot be recommended because of an extremely high complication rate associated with their use. Iatrogenic pharyngeal lacerations are the most common complications encountered.

Oral Calcium Gels or Pastes

Tubes similar to those used to hold caulking compound have been marketed with various calcium and ketosis preparations

for oral administration to dairy cattle. Although most of the nozzles have been shortened, some tubes may still have extremely pointed and sharp delivery tips that can result in soft palate or pharyngeal laceration when advanced roughly or in an overzealous manner into the oral cavity of patients. Products with sharp or elongated tips should have the tips cut off before introduction into the cow's mouth. Commercially available balling guns, custom made for specific boluses (Bovicalc, Boehringer-Ingelheim), are available and generally safe when used appropriately and according to instructions.

Nasogastric Intubation

Nasogastric intubation with soft rubber tubing is the preferred method for tube feeding neonatal calves. A soft rubber stallion urinary catheter is passed through the ventral meatus into the esophagus (Fig. 2.17). Verification of the tube's placement within the rumen is made by blowing through the end while ausculting the rumen through the left paralumbar fossa. The tube can also be felt in the esophagus when palpating the proximal cervical area next to the trachea. This intubation technique is easy to perform; easy on the patient; avoids injury to the oral cavity, pharynx, and esophagus by mechanical devices used in oral tubing; and can be done by one person.

The stallion urinary catheter should be flexible and made of either rubber or soft polyethylene. After the catheter is in place, colostrum, milk, or fluids may be administered by attaching a funnel, or dose syringe, to the end of the tube. A catheter that fits tightly into the nasal cavity allows more rapid administration, particularly of more viscus fluids such as colostrum. The tube may be taped in place if ongoing fluid needs are anticipated, but patients usually are more comfortable without indwelling nasogastric tubes. Larger nasogastric tubes may be used for larger young stock or adult cattle and are preferred by some practitioners to oral intubation. Nasogastric tubes may be used to force-feed cows that persistently regurgitate during oral-pharyngeal tubing.

General Principles for Administration of Oral Medications

Restraint is best provided by a stanchion or head gate that limits the patient's mobility and allows the operator to grasp the head without being thrown about or injured. When a cow is approached from the front, she tends to back away and lower her head. Cows that have received oral medications or have been subjected to nose lead restraint in the past will lower their muzzles to the ground to make it difficult to grasp. Cows that are in tie stalls are more difficult to restrain for oral medications and may require use of a halter to minimize bidirectional movement.

The cow's head is grasped with the operator's less adroit hand and the head held tightly to the operator's body (Fig. 2.18). Holding the head tightly allows the operator to move with the cow and also prevents butting injuries that can break human ribs or cause other injuries. The operator is

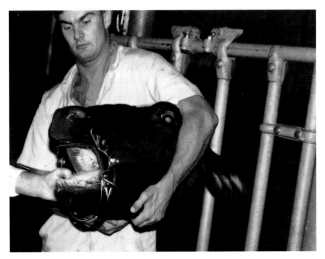

• **Fig. 2.18** The cow's head is held tightly to the operator's body, and the head is restrained in a horizontal, straight-ahead position while examination of the oral cavity is performed with the aid of a Weingart bovine mouth speculum.

braced by standing with feet placed at least shoulder width apart and with the upper body holding the patient firmly. When a stanchion or head gate is available, the operator also may rest against these objects to further prevent movement.

When securely positioned, the operator exerts pressure on the patient's hard palate using the hand that is holding the cow. This gentle pressure causes the patient's mouth to open and allows medications or devices to be positioned. Common errors to be avoided during oral medication procedures include:

1. Use of a halter: A cow cannot open her mouth if it is held tightly shut by a fastened halter. The halter must be removed or loosened or a nose lead used for restraint rather than a halter.
2. Keep the head straight forward: Excessive twisting or pulling the head to the side makes swallowing difficult for the patient and may increase the likelihood of pharyngeal injury when stomach tubes are used. Never attempt to pass a large-bore stomach tube with the patient's head twisted to the side.
3. Do not hold the head too high: Holding the head such that the muzzle is higher than the poll increases the likelihood of inhalation pneumonia, allows stomach tubes to enter the trachea more easily rather than the esophagus, and makes swallowing difficult.
4. Lack of lubrication: Always lubricate, even if just with water, any instruments being introduced in the oral cavity. This helps avoid iatrogenic injury.

Vaginal Examinations

Vaginal examinations are performed to evaluate or medicate the postpartum reproductive tract, to monitor or assist parturition, to palpate the ureters in patients suspected of having pyelonephritis, to allow urinary catheterization, and for various other procedures. Before vaginal examination, the tail should be tied to the patient or held by an assistant.

A thorough cleaning of the entire perineum should then be performed with mild soap and clean, warm water. Iodophor soaps, Ivory soap, or tincture of green soap are acceptable soaps for this preparation. Sterile lubricant or mild soap should be used to minimize vulvar or vaginal trauma when the sleeved hand and arm of the examiner are introduced into the reproductive tract.

After the vaginal examination, all soap and vaginal discharges should be washed away from the perineum, escutcheon, and rear udder and the area dried. If discharges have reached the teat ends, these should be cleaned and dipped in teat dip. This latter step emphasizes regard for overall cleanliness and udder health specifically.

Rectal Examinations

Although the procedure of rectal examination is simple, the skills necessary for rectal palpation of the reproductive tract and viscera are complex and require thousands of repetitions. We believe that neophytes should be required to wear latex rubber gloves and sleeves when performing rectal examinations on cattle. These gloves not only allow more sensitive touch but help protect the patient from inevitable rectal irritation associated with neophytic palpators and plastic sleeves. Adequate lubrication of glove and sleeve, backraking and removal of excessive manure in the rectum, patience, and gentle manipulations are critical to obtaining diagnostic information from the patient during a rectal examination.

Urinary Catheterization

Before urinary catheterization, the patient's tail is restrained, and the perineum is cleaned and scrubbed as described for the vaginal examination. Sterile gloves and lubricant should be used. A sterile Chambers catheter or catheter as depicted in Figure 11.1 is ideal for the urinary catheterization of cows. One gloved hand is introduced into the vestibule and used to identify the suburethral diverticulum. This is less than one hand's length from the lips of the vulva in most cattle and lies on the ventral floor of the vestibule. The urethra's external opening is a slit in the cranial edge of the vaginal origin of the diverticulum. The urethra is tightly compressed by smooth muscle tone and is much less obvious than the suburethral diverticulum. Therefore, it is best to loosely fill the diverticulum with a single finger and introduce the sterile, lubricated catheter dorsal to that finger so as to avoid diversion of the catheter into the diverticulum. Gentle, patient manipulation will allow the catheter to enter the urethra along the cranial edge of the diverticulum's juncture with the vaginal wall. After the urethra is entered, gentle pressure easily advances the catheter into the urinary bladder. Sterile technique is extremely important because urinary tract infections can be induced easily by dirty or traumatic catheterization, as frequently happened when dairy cows were catheterized routinely to obtain urine for ketone evaluations. *Corynebacterium renale* and other normal inhabitants of the caudal reproductive tract, as well as contaminants, can be introduced to the urinary tract by poor catheterization techniques.

Caudal Epidural Anesthesia

Caudal epidural anesthesia is required in cattle for both medical and surgical reasons, such as:
1. Relieve straining and tenesmus during dystocia
2. Relieve straining and tenesmus when replacing a uterine or vaginal prolapse
3. Relieve tenesmus secondary to colitis, rectal irritation, or vaginal irritation
4. Provide anesthesia for surgical procedures involving the perineum (e.g., Caslick's surgery)

The site of caudal epidural anesthesia is the space between the first and second caudal (CA1-CA2) vertebrae. Usually this space is identifiable as the first movable joint caudal to the sacrum. Lifting the tail up and down allows palpation to identify this movement. Crushed tail heads or previous sacrocaudal trauma may make identification of the CA1 to CA2 space difficult. After the space is identified, the area should be surgically prepared and an 18-gauge, 3.75-cm sterile needle used to deliver the anesthetic. Very large (>800 kg) cattle or adult bulls may require a longer 18-gauge needle. The cow's tail is moved up and down gently to allow the CA1 to CA2 space to be palpated, and the needle is inserted on the dorsal midline over the space. The needle then is gently and carefully advanced in a ventral direction until the resistance to advancement suddenly stops or a negative pressure "sucking" sound is heard, indicating that the needle has entered the epidural space. The sensation as one advances the needle into the epidural space has been referred to as "popping into the space" and is identical to that experienced during cerebrospinal fluid (CSF) collection. After the needle has been positioned, the selected anesthetic may be injected. Resistance to flow should be minimal to nonexistent if the tip of the needle is in fact positioned in the epidural space. Many clinicians attempt to confirm proper needle placement by dropping one or two drops of anesthetic from the syringe tip into the needle hub. If the needle is properly placed, then these drops quickly flow from the needle hub into the epidural space. If the needle is improperly positioned, then tissue resistance will prevent the drops from leaving the needle hub. After the needle is placed and the sucking sound of air is heard, the injection should be given promptly; if air is allowed to enter the needle for a prolonged period, then air emboli may occur, causing the cow to develop a rapid respiratory rate with abdominal lift.

The volume of anesthetic (most commonly 2% lidocaine) injected during caudal epidural anesthesia should be as little as possible to avoid ascending anesthesia that could affect locomotion or hind limb function. In most instances, 3 to 6 mL of 2% lidocaine is sufficient to establish anesthesia, relieve tenesmus, and so on in an adult cow. Other drug combinations have been used for epidural anesthesia, an example being combinations of 2% lidocaine and xylazine (4 mL of 2% lidocaine and 1 mL of 20 mg/mL

xylazine) in fractious cattle. A combination of 0.22 mg/kg, 2% lidocaine, and 1 mL of 10% sterile magnesium sulfate has been examined experimentally and found to provide a longer duration of action than 2% lidocaine alone. Whichever drug combination is selected, the animal should be standing or in sternal recumbency and should not have its front end lower than the hind, lest anesthetic too easily ascend the epidural space. Animals that develop any degree of limb paralysis or weakness after caudal epidural anesthesia should be confined to an area with good footing and hobbled loosely to prevent musculoskeletal injury until the anesthetic wears off. One of the major postoperative complications of true spinal (lumbar) anesthesia in cattle is musculoskeletal injury during the recovery period as the patient repeatedly attempts to rise despite its neurologic deficits. Lumbar anesthesia seldom is used in our hospitals because of fear of this aforementioned complication.

After the anesthetic is delivered to the epidural space, the needle should be removed. Needles left in place because of anticipated repeat dosing (e.g., prolonged dystocia) can lacerate the spinal nerves inadvertently, resulting in permanent neurologic deficits.

Longer-acting anesthetics than lidocaine should be considered only as a final option for a patient requiring repeated epidural anesthesia because these drugs may create irreversible complications and prolonged anesthesia. If repeated administration of anesthetics is expected, an epidural catheter (commercially prepared kits can be purchased or one can use sterile Silastic tubing that will fit through a 14-gauge needle) can be placed in the epidural space. A sterile gauze should be glued over the site following placement of the catheter to maintain sterility. We have also used epidural catheters for daily or twice-daily administration of preservative-free morphine (0.3 mg/kg) in treating cattle with severe hind limb or pelvic pain.

Blood Transfusions

Blood transfusions may be lifesaving for patients with extreme anemia, acute blood loss, thrombocytopenia, and other coagulation defects that result in hemorrhage, as well as for neonatal calves that failed to receive adequate passive transfer of immunoglobulins. Despite these and other well-known indications, whole blood transfusions are performed with reluctance (and sometimes not at all) by many veterinarians, primarily because of concern over improper collection or administration techniques that result in inefficient or prolonged procedures. Cross-matching is unnecessary in cattle unless the cow has received a prior transfusion. Therefore, blood transfusion must be simple, rapid, and easy on the donor, recipient, and veterinarian for the technique to be practiced. The following blood transfusion technique outlined is simple and rapid and has evolved through many years as we have sought to minimize frustration and wasted time associated with earlier techniques.

The donor cow should be a large healthy cow, preferably known to be BLV negative and free of persistent bovine viral diarrhea virus (BVDV) infection. The stage of lactation or gestation is flexible, but an open cow destined for culling

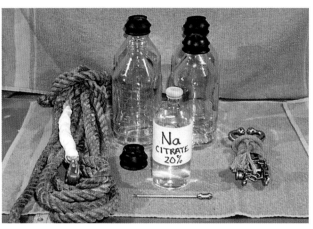

• **Fig. 2.19** Equipment necessary for blood collection from a sedated donor cow includes a choke rope; four or more wide-mouth 1-L glass bottles; 20% sodium citrate solution (35 mL/L as an anticoagulant); halter or nose leads; and a 15-cm, 8-gauge trochar.

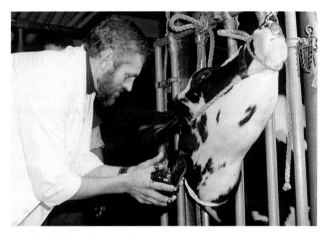

• **Fig. 2.20** Collection of blood from a well-restrained donor cow.

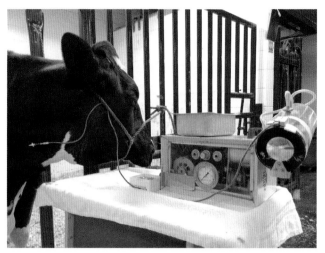

• **Fig. 2.21** Alternative, "closed," sterile system for obtaining whole blood from a well-restrained donor cow using a vacuum system.

after her current lactation is ideal. Blood typing is seldom necessary because cattle have a large number of blood types. However, if major and minor cow matching is available (as for a hospital patient), blood typing procedures minimize the potential for incompatibility if the cow requires multiple transfusions several days apart. The collective experience of the authors would place a risk of a clinically significant transfusion reaction in cattle at less than 1%. Six liters of whole blood may be taken from large (≥700 kg) healthy cows without risk. The donor cow should be sedated with 15 to 25 mg of xylazine IV, a jugular site clipped and prepped, and the animal confined to a stanchion or head gate in which her head can be restrained tightly by a halter or nose lead. A choke rope is placed around the caudal one third of the cervical area, and a 15-cm, 8-gauge trochar is placed in the jugular vein. Blood can be collected into wide-mouth 1- to 2-L bottles that contain 35.0 mL of 20% sodium citrate/L as an anticoagulant (Figs 2.19 and 2.20). The blood is then caught in the collection bottles by free flow while the administrator gently swirls the bottles to ensure an adequate mixture of blood and anticoagulant (Fig. 2.20). This technique allows collection of 6 L of whole blood in less than 15 minutes. After collection of the desired quantity of blood, the choke rope is released, the trochar

withdrawn, and external pressure applied to the jugular collection site for 2 minutes. Commercial transfusion needles, lines, and bags may also be used and would have less risk of bacterial contamination, but the collection process is slower. Careful catheter or trochar placement by experienced individuals, alongside aseptic technique under sedation, will allow a donor cow to be used monthly for several years.

An alternative method allows for vacuum-assisted blood collection through a 14-gauge catheter into commercial sterile blood collection bags; the disadvantage is slower collection speeds and the requirement for greater equipment (Fig. 2.21). Two-liter Baxter evacuated glass containers allow for a rapid collection; make sure the vacuum is not lost when adding the citrate.

The recipient is prepared for jugular catheterization, and a 14-gauge IV catheter is placed. The collected blood is administered at a slow to moderate rate through a blood administration set with in-line filter (Travenol Infuser; Travenol Laboratories, Deerfield, IL). Although rapid administration may be necessary in selected emergency situations, too-rapid administration may result in tachycardia, tachypnea, or collapse. Administration time varies from 30 to 120 minutes in most cases.

Sedation and adequate restraint of the donor coupled with rapid collection via the large trochar and choke rope alleviate donor and veterinarian frustration and apprehension that are often associated with alternative means of blood collection on farm. Incompatibility, although uncommon, will be manifested in the recipient by signs of urticaria or anaphylaxis. Urticaria, edema of mucocutaneous junctions, tachycardia, and tachypnea observed in the recipient dictate that blood transfusion cease and appropriate treatment (most commonly antihistamines) of the allergic reaction be provided. Cross-matching or random selection of another donor must then follow. Slow administration for the first few minutes alongside periodic monitoring of heart rate, temperature, and respiratory rate as well as observation for signs of urticaria or anaphylaxis allows for early identification of an adverse reaction, such that the flow rate can then be increased significantly if these signs are not seen. This applies to both whole blood and plasma transfusions.

Commercial bovine plasma from BLV- and BVDV-negative donors and with a guaranteed high IgG concentration can be purchased from Lake Immunogenics (Ontario, NY). When highly valuable neonatal calves are treated for sepsis or presented for treatment of other conditions and at high risk for sepsis, plasma can be an important part of the patient's therapy. Although it is expensive to do so, a number of septic and hypoproteinemic adult conditions may also benefit from bovine plasma therapy. Plasma can also be harvested from appropriately selected donor cattle by a very similar technique as described for blood collection, but this requires added equipment to centrifuge and separate the plasma from the whole blood. The more time-consuming closed system previously described may be better suited to maintaining sterility during the collection of whole blood for subsequent plasma harvesting, but by the use of a vacuum system one can still obtain several liters of blood from a donor cow through a 14-gauge, 13-cm catheter in less than 1 hour (see Fig. 2.21).

After centrifugation and separation into sterile blood transfer bags (Teruflex, Terumo Corporation, Somerset, NJ), one can obtain approximately two-thirds of the original whole blood volume as plasma. The authors have found that allowing the blood to stand for 12 to 18 hours under refrigeration before centrifugation appears to increase the yield. In our hospitals, plasma is stored for later use for up to 12 months from the time of collection; thawing should be done slowly at no more than body temperature, never by microwave or scalding, hot water.

Cerebrospinal Fluid Collection

Cerebrospinal fluid may be collected from either the atlanto-occipital (AO) or lumbosacral space (LSS) in cattle, and veterinarians should be familiar with both sites because a patient's status may dictate a preferential site. Recumbent or severely depressed patients may have CSF collected from either site. However, ambulatory patients usually are tapped at the LSS because an AO tap usually requires sedation or anesthesia for safety. Suspected diagnoses also may influence the decision of site selection. When meningitis or encephalitis is suspected, an AO tap may be preferred, but with a suspected spinal abscess or lymphosarcoma, the LSS may be chosen. Although tapping "close to the lesion" is often a clinical preference, we have found little concrete evidence that this approach makes a significant difference in diagnostic yield for CSF. With the exception of rare spinal abscesses or lymphosarcoma masses that have been tapped into at the LSS, abnormalities of the CSF usually will be reflected in the fluid, regardless of collection site; the LSS, for example, is a reliable location for diagnostic CSF sampling for cattle with meningoencephalitis due to listeriosis.

Atlantooccipital collection usually is easier than LSS collection, but AO collections require that the patient be recumbent, depressed, or sedated sufficiently to make the procedure possible without risk of iatrogenic injury. The area from the poll cranially to the axis caudally is clipped and surgically prepared (Fig. 2.22). The prepped area is usually 15 to 20 cm in length and 5 to 10 cm in width. The external occipital protuberance (cranial) and a line drawn transversely across the cranial aspects of the wings of the atlas (caudal) serve as landmarks.

Approximately equidistant from these landmarks, on the dorsal midline, is the site for AO CSF collection. The patient's head is ventroflexed so that the muzzle is pushed toward the brisket. The patient's neck should be straight, not turned to the side. An 8.75-cm, 18-gauge needle with stylet is preferred for adult cattle or bulls, and a 3.75-cm, 20-gauge needle is used for neonatal calves. The needle is advanced ventrally, carefully but directly. The exact direction (slightly cranial or slightly caudal) will vary based on the selected site of the puncture. The most common displacement is to advance too far cranially such that the needle encounters the skull. This does not pose a major problem and allows the veterinarian to "walk" the needle off the skull caudally into the AO space. The distinct decrease of resistance encountered when the needle perforates the dura mater and enters the subarachnoid space must be anticipated carefully and the stylet withdrawn to check for CSF whenever the administrator suspects that the space has been entered. When the patient is in lateral recumbency, fluid will flow for collection without aspiration. Although the AO site is usually 5.0 to 7.5 cm ventral to the skin (in adult cattle) and on the median plane, distance estimates are not helpful because the cranial- or caudal-angle variations may add 2.5 cm versus a direct perpendicular approach. Practice on cadavers is the best way to become experienced with CSF collection techniques.

Lumbosacral space puncture in cattle is not as difficult as in horses because the needle travels much less distance from the skin to the LSS in cattle. The LSS usually is palpable on midline as a depression caudal to the L6 vertebral dorsal spine and cranial to the dorsal spine of S2 (S1 is not usually palpable). The site also is medial to the tuber sacrale and intersects a transverse line drawn from the caudal aspects of the tuber coxae. This area and a surrounding 15- to 20-cm square area is surgically clipped and prepared before puncture. An 8.75-cm, 18-gauge spinal needle with stylet is sufficient for most cattle, but a longer needle may be necessary for cows weighing more than 750 kg and adult bulls (Video Clip 2.02).

A scalpel puncture of the skin over the selected site may greatly decrease skin resistance on the spinal needle in adults, thus making adjustments in needle position easier. The needle is advanced ventrally and usually 10 to 15 degrees cranial or caudal on the median plane. The needle must remain perpendicular to the long axis. A less distinct "pop" accompanies puncture of the dura at the LSS than at the AO site, but a distinct decrease in resistance usually is felt as the subarachnoid space is entered. The patient frequently jumps, kicks, or otherwise reacts to the needle entering the subarachnoid, thereby signaling a successful placement of the needle. This response is transient, and CSF may be aspirated from the needle after the patient relaxes. As opposed to AO puncture, LSS puncture usually requires that the CSF be aspirated rather than collected free-flow because of gravitational differences in the techniques and any actual CSF pressure differences that may exist. A majority of adult cattle can undergo LSS CSF sampling with restraint in a head catch and local anesthesia in the skin and subcutis only. In calves, it is worth considering performing a LSS cerebrospinal tap while recumbent with the calf positioned sternally with the hind limbs extended forward (Fig. 2.23).

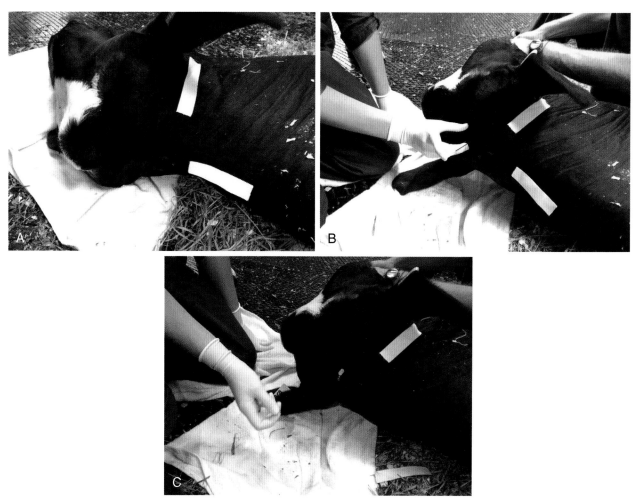

• **Fig. 2.22** Procedure for obtaining cerebrospinal fluid (CSF) from the atlantooccipital site in a mature cow. **A,** Tape identifies anatomic landmarks of wings of atlas and dorsal spinous processes of cervical vertebrae on midline. **B,** Eighteen-gauge, 8.75-cm spinal needle inserted on midline toward the commissures of the lips with the head ventroflexed by an assistant. **C,** Spontaneous flow of CSF.

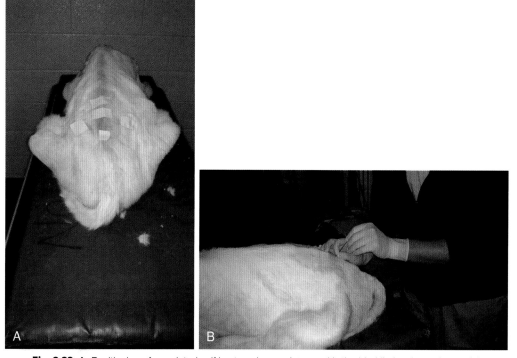

• **Fig. 2.23** **A,** Positioning of a sedated calf in sternal recumbency with the hind limbs drawn forward for a lumbosacral space (LSS) tap. Tape marks are on the dorsal spinous processes of the lumbar vertebrae, S2 and tuber coxae on each side. **B,** Slight cranial angulation of the spinal needle as it is advanced perpendicular to the long axis of the calf.

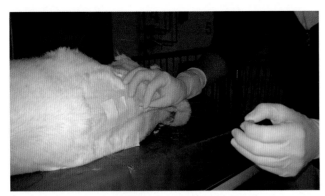

• **Fig. 2.24** Alternative positioning of a sedated calf for a cerebrospinal fluid tap in the lumbosacral space in lateral recumbency.

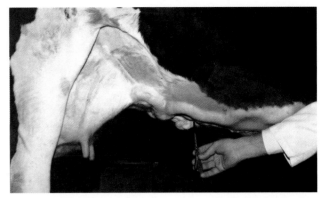

• **Fig. 2.25** A pointer is directed to a potential abdominal paracentesis site on a longitudinal line between the ventral midline and the right mammary vein. Obvious subcutaneous blood vessels should be avoided when selecting a site.

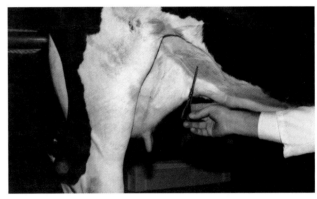

• **Fig. 2.26** A pointer is directed to the alternative site for attempted abdominal paracentesis when sites between the midline and right mammary vein are unsuccessful.

This may require light sedation depending on the neurologic signs being demonstrated. Some colleagues prefer to perform LSS CSF sampling in calves with the patient in lateral recumbency (Fig. 2.24). Generally, in calves, it is often unnecessary to provide local anesthesia to the skin and subcutis, nor to perform a stab incision. Smaller gauge spinal needles (8.75 cm, 20 or 22 gauge) are adequate in calves. Manual compression of both jugular veins by an assistant will increase CSF pressure and in some cases make the collection easier.

Aseptic technique during CSF collection is imperative to protect both the patient from iatrogenic infection and the veterinarian from zoonoses such as rabies. CSF is aspirated slowly into sterile syringes and then placed in ethylenediaminetetraacetic acid (EDTA) tubes (for cytology) and sterile tubes for culture. If the animal is in lateral recumbency gravity collection into appropriate tubes can be done. Although not an absolute requirement, the stylet can be replaced before the needle is withdrawn.

Specific abnormalities of the CSF are discussed in Chapter 13. Our laboratory considers normal CSF values for cattle to be:

Pressure >200 mm H_2O
Protein <40 mg/dL
Nucleated cells <5 per μL

Abdominal Paracentesis

Abdominal paracentesis (AP) is used to collect peritoneal fluid as an ancillary aid toward diagnosing cattle with abdominal disorders. The most common indication for AP in cattle is to rule in or out the existence of peritonitis in a patient. Extraction of abdominal fluid (AF) also may be helpful for other purposes such as to provide exfoliative cytology when visceral lymphosarcoma or other tumors are suspected, confirm intraabdominal blood loss, detect rupture of the urinary bladder when suspected, and confirm ascites.

Because healthy cattle often have little AF, several sites of collection may have to be attempted before a successful AP is performed. The most common site for AP is the intersection of a longitudinal line between the ventral midline and

right mammary vein and a transverse line drawn midway between the umbilicus and xiphoid. If this site is unsuccessful, then a site on the same longitudinal line but closer to the umbilicus or most pendulous portion of the abdomen may be attempted (Fig. 2.25). As a last resort, the lower right abdomen just lateral to the lateral support ligaments of the udder may be an attempted site for AP (Fig. 2.26). If this site is used the needle should be inserted perpendicular to the contour of the abdominal wall and held in place by the veterinarian once fluid begins to flow. It is important that an assistant be ready to catch the initial fluid, which may come out in a single spurt or intermittent drips, as red cell contamination is common if the needle is left in place for 30 or more seconds. The left abdomen should not be used because the rumen fills the entire left abdomen in most cows and may extend somewhat to the right of midline as well. Abdominal ultrasound examination is very helpful in evaluating location, amount, and echogenicity of AF and can be used to determine proper location for the AP.

During clipping and surgical preparation of an AP site, large SC vessels should be noted and avoided during needle puncture of the abdomen. The patient should be restrained by a halter and tail restraint for AP. If more restraint is required nose tongs can be used. In adult cattle, a 16- or

18-gauge, 3.7- to 5.0-cm sterile needle is popped through the skin and then advanced carefully until it pops through the parietal peritoneum. Alternatively, a blunt 14-gauge, 5.0-cm sterile stainless steel teat cannula can be used following a small scalpel puncture of the skin at the selected site. In addition to minute advancements of the needle, the needle hub should be twisted to vary the location of the needle opening. When successful, fluid dripping or flowing from the needle is collected in EDTA tubes and prepared for cytologic examination. Additional fluid can be collected for culture if indicated. In calves, a 2.5-cm, 20-gauge or 18-gauge, 3.75-cm needle is recommended, and great care should be practiced to avoid puncture of a viscus. Normal AF in cattle is light yellow in color and has less than 5000 nucleated cells/μL and total protein below 2.6 g/dL.

The most common error occurring during AP in cattle is entering a viscus. This not only contaminates the needle, but also the intestinal contents may be confused with AF and subsequently sent for analysis. In addition, leakage of ingesta from iatrogenic intestinal punctures may result in subclinical or clinical peritonitis, especially in calves. Normal periparturient cattle occasionally have increased amounts of AF that is a physiologic transudate. This fluid needs to be differentiated from fluid associated with peritonitis and from allantoic fluid.

In general, when peritonitis is suspected, a large volume of AF indicates a grave prognosis. For example, cattle having diffuse peritonitis from abomasal perforation tend to have large volumes of AF—so much so that nucleated cell counts of this fluid may fall within the normal range (≤5000/μL) because of the dilutional effect of this massive inflammatory exudate on the relatively limited neutrophil pool of cattle. Although the protein value of this fluid will be elevated (>3.5 g/dL), consistent with an inflammatory peritonitis, the low cell count creates confusion. Therefore the volume and protein levels of the AF (in addition to a decline in plasma protein levels) are the major parameters used to assess diffuse peritonitis, especially acute diffuse peritonitis. Ultrasound examination can also be very helpful in the evaluation of AF volume, location, and distribution in peritonitis cases. Localized peritonitis caused by traumatic reticuloperitonitis or smaller perforating abomasal ulcers may yield normal "textbook" values for AF. Localized peritonitis tends to cause a suppurative exudate confined by fibrin and therefore should have elevated protein and nucleated cell counts. This fluid also may have a foul odor; be colored dark yellow, reddish, or orange; and have flecks of fibrin present. Frequently, it is difficult to obtain AF from cattle with localized peritonitis because of "walling off" or loculation of the fluid by fibrin. Therefore several sites may have to be tried before fluid or at least the most abnormal fluid is obtained. Similarly, samples obtained from different sites may have greatly varying compositions (Fig. 2.27) because of lessening degrees of peritonitis at greater distances from the site of origin. The use of ultrasonography to identify pockets of AF also may be useful when taking samples of fluid and provides very

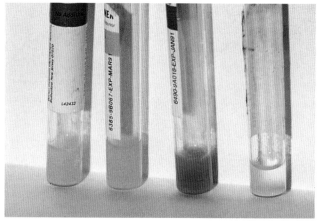

• **Fig. 2.27** Abdominal fluid samples collected from different abdominal sites of a cow having localized peritonitis secondary to a perforating abomasal ulcer. Although all samples had elevated nucleated cell counts and total protein values, the samples closer to the site of peritonitis (tubes on the left) had greater abnormalities.

valuable ancillary information for a patient suspected of having peritonitis.

Due to this variability, AF obtained by AP is an ancillary aid, not an absolute diagnostic tool. Frequently, the values obtained from analyses of AF fall into the gray zone of normal versus abnormal. Various authors argue over the cellular contents of "normal" bovine AF. Cell count references may be found that range from less than 5000/μL to less than 10,000/μL. The reported ratio of neutrophils, mononuclear cells, and eosinophils found in normal bovine AF also varies. Despite these limitations, AP may yield diagnostic information that allows differentiation of surgical versus medical conditions of some patients, especially if peritoneal fluid lactate is higher than blood lactate. Abdominal paracentesis is specifically indicated in cattle whenever peritonitis is included in the differential diagnosis. In addition, patients suspected of having abdominal neoplasia, hemoperitoneum, uroperitoneum, and ascites should have AP performed.

Contraindications for AP include extreme abdominal distention caused by distention of viscera that would necessitate surgical exploration regardless of AF values and extreme abdominal distention associated with a viscus that might be punctured during AP.

Thoracocentesis and Pericardiocentesis

Thoracocentesis seldom is performed in cattle simply because large-volume accumulations in the pleural cavity are not nearly as common as in horses. Bacterial bronchopneumonia commonly causes fibrinous anteroventral bronchopneumonia with some exudative fluid, but the volume seldom is significant enough to warrant thoracocentesis for drainage. In addition, the tendency of cattle to develop fibrinous adhesions between the visceral and parietal pleurae makes pleural fluid difficult to collect when loculated within a labyrinth consisting of small pockets of exudate.

Occasional cases of pleural fluid accumulation have been observed; they occur secondary to lymphosarcoma or other neoplasms, thoracic trauma, lung abscessation, and acute perforation of the diaphragm by ingested hardware. Thoracic abscesses tend to be unilateral and may originate either from a primary thoracic site of infection or from a previous migration of hardware from the reticulum into the thorax. Thoracocentesis is an essential ancillary aid for diagnosis of these conditions.

Thoracocentesis is performed on the hemithorax which is considered to harbor the most fluid, as determined on auscultation, percussion, and ultrasound examination, if available. Usually auscultation and percussion are sufficient for diagnosis of pleural fluid accumulation in field situations because thoracic ultrasonography and radiography may not be available. In performing thoracocentesis in the absence of ultrasound guidance, the fifth intercostal space in the lower third of the thorax between the elbow and the shoulder is clipped and surgically prepared. The cow is restrained by halter and tail restraint. If the patient is not in respiratory distress, then mild sedation or local infiltration of the site with 2% lidocaine may be helpful. If the patient is suffering respiratory distress, then it is best to be direct and minimize sedation or additional needle punctures.

For diagnostic purposes, an 18-gauge, 8.75-cm spinal needle with stylet is an excellent choice for thoracocentesis. In small or average-size cattle, a 14-gauge, 5.0-cm blunt-tip stainless steel teat cannula may be used after scalpel puncture of the skin. For drainage of fluid or evacuation of thick exudates such as those present in a thoracic abscess, a 20- or 28-Fr chest trochar with stylet may be required. Previous scalpel puncture of the skin will be essential to allow thoracocentesis with these large trochars. Thoracocentesis of adult bulls and large, mature dairy cows often requires incision of the subcutis and outer intercostal musculature to pass an appropriately large-diameter chest trochar for drainage (Fig. 2.28).

Thoracic drainage of air may also be a lifesaving procedure for cattle with pneumothorax. The approach and equipment needed for tube placement are exactly the same as for fluid centesis, but the location will be much more dorsal. Indeed, the procedure should be performed as dorsally as possible but still below the transverse processes yet within the pleural space to allow for the greatest degree of lung reinflation possible (Figs. 2.29 and 2.30). Radiography, or more usefully ultrasonography, can be used to identify the dorsal extent of the pneumothorax to facilitate tube placement. Ultrasonography can be equally helpful in the identification of the ventral level of the pneumothorax by virtue of the "sliding lung point"; the junction of the aerated lung and free air within the pleural space. This will be seen as a moving area of pleural reflection ventrally that interfaces with an immobile air interface immediately dorsal in the area of free pleural air as the animal breathes. During evacuation, either by continuous flow or by suction, one can also monitor lung reinflation by observing the sliding lung point move dorsally. Many cattle with pneumothorax have diffuse collapse of an entire lung, but the occasional case of compartmentalized pneumothorax or bullous emphysema may

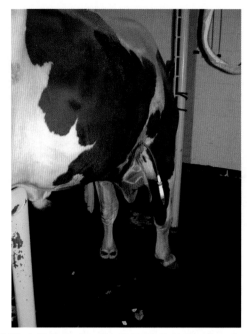

• **Fig. 2.28** A 28-Fr trochar chest tube placed into a thoracic abscess in the right hemithorax of a mature Holstein bull. Note the Heimlich valve to maintain unidirectional flow and avoid pneumothorax.

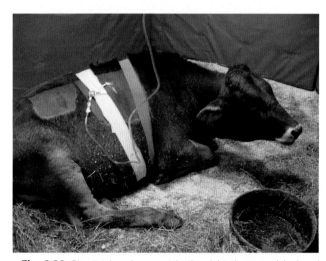

• **Fig. 2.29** Chest tube placement in the right dorsocaudal pleural space of a Brown Swiss heifer with bovine respiratory syncytial virus infection and unilateral pneumothorax. The tubing connects the chest tube to vacuum suction.

be encountered and can be more challenging to diagnose and evacuate without access to diagnostic imaging.

Particular care to avoid cardiac puncture with needles and trochars is essential during thoracocentesis. The initial thrust or force necessary to direct the needle, cannula, or trochar through the chest wall must be immediately dampened as the pleural space is entered. This can be accomplished by holding the instrument with sterile, gloved hands and sterile gauze such that one hand provides the driving force while the opposite hand acts as a "brake" that allows only 4 to 5 cm of the instrument to make initial penetration beyond the skin. Further introduction under less forceful and careful advancement is then possible.

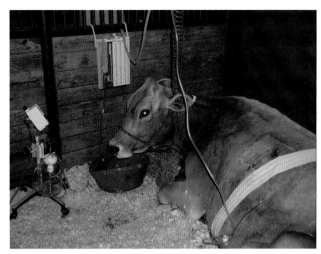

• **Fig. 2.30** Chest tube placement in 6-year-old Brown Swiss cow with left-sided pneumothorax caused by bovine respiratory syncytial virus infection. The tube is connected to a closed continuous-flow evacuation device.

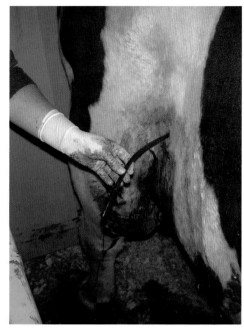

• **Fig. 2.32** Pericardial drainage in a 3-year-old Holstein cow with idiopathic pericardial effusion using a 24-Fr chest trochar.

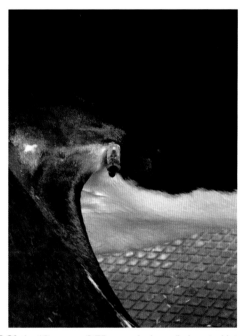

• **Fig. 2.31** An 18-gauge, 8.75-cm spinal needle inserted into the left fifth intercostal space for pericardiocentesis after ultrasonographic identification of a large-volume pericardial effusion in a 4-year-old Holstein cow. The dark hemorrhagic fluid obtained contained numerous lymphoblasts consistent with cardiac lymphosarcoma.

Pericardiocentesis is simply an extension of thoracocentesis and is performed to confirm a diagnosis of pericarditis (Fig. 2.31). Despite what is often tremendous enlargement of the pericardial sac, at least an 8.75-cm needle or trochar should be used to ensure penetration of the pericardium for drainage (Fig. 2.32). Caution must be exercised to avoid cardiac puncture, and the procedure should only be performed after discussion with the owner. Rarely, pericardiocentesis may cause rapid death in a patient with septic pericarditis, not necessarily as a direct result of cardiac puncture but rather because of a rapid alteration in the physiologic gas/fluid pressure gradient within the pericardial sac. Gas produced by bacteria in the pericardium acts to inflate the pericardium away from the heart, thereby lessening possible restrictive pressures. If pericardiocentesis results in a rapid loss of this gas because of needle puncture of the dorsal pericardial sac, then the pericardium and remaining septic fluid may exert a rapid pressure change on the heart in this heretofore "compensated" patient. Therefore, even without cardiac puncture, pericardiocentesis does occasionally cause fatalities. Undoubtedly, pericardiocentesis is best and most safely performed under ultrasound guidance. Many cattle with significant pericardial effusion also have a degree of pleural effusion and the tremendous volumes, partnered with the propensity for cattle to form adhesions and compartmentalize the fluid involved in both cavities, can make it difficult to distinguish between them. For example, cardiac lymphosarcoma, septic reticulopericarditis and idiopathic hemorrhagic pericardial effusion often have significant pleural and pericardial effusions. When pericardiocentesis is performed for purposes of diagnostic cytology from a patient with clinical and ultrasonographic evidence of pericardial effusion, we recommend sampling from the left fifth intercostal space even when there appears to be a "safer" window more caudally or dorsally or on the right. With neoplastic, septic, or hemorrhagic pericardial effusion, the concurrent pleural effusion may have a different cytologic analysis than the primary pericardial disease process. If ultrasonography can be performed simultaneously with the pericardiocentesis, the infusion of 1-2 mL of air into the already advanced needle can help confirm that the needle is indeed in the pericardial space.

After thoracocentesis for diagnostic purposes, needles and cannulas are removed. Thoracic trochars or drains may be anchored in place if continuous or intermittent drainage is anticipated. A Heimlich valve or condom with the closed end cut should be attached to the exposed external end of the drain to prevent pneumothorax when continuous drainage is selected. Most thoracic drain tubes tend to kink as they pass through the intercostal region; this kinking often increases to cause occlusion or necessitate replacement within several days. Continuous drainage of thoracic fluid because of septic processes is also complicated by the speed with which even large-bore chest tubes can become clogged with fibrin and clots.

Abscess Drainage

Abscesses are an extremely common problem in dairy cattle. SC abscesses and IM abscesses are the most common types observed, although mammary gland abscesses also are observed with some frequency.

Subcutaneous abscesses occur over pressure points, limbs, surgical incisions and fascial regions. IM abscesses almost always evolve from dirty injections, but some cases lack a history of any injections and may evolve from skin puncture from a variety of objects in the environment. SC and IM abscesses range from softball to beach ball size.

Abscesses eventually "soften" and drain spontaneously in most cases, but this may require weeks or even months. In addition, the lesions cause patient discomfort or pain; often interfere with locomotion or normal recumbency; and risk secondary problems such as endocarditis, glomerulonephritis, or amyloidosis. Therefore, abscesses should be drained surgically whenever possible because this procedure allows a selection of drainage sites that improve chances of effective and complete drainage and minimize subsequent recurrences and complications.

Although abscesses are much more common than seromas or hematomas, the veterinarian should be careful to rule out these two types of lesions because drainage is contraindicated. After the best site for potential ventral drainage of the suspect abscess is chosen, the skin at this site is clipped and surgically prepped. A 16-gauge, 3.75-cm disposable needle is used to aspirate some material from the lesion. If blood or serum jets from the needle hub, the needle is withdrawn, pressure is applied to the puncture site, and no further therapy is used. More commonly, however, when the needle is introduced, nothing flows from the hub. This dilemma is caused by the thick pus typical of that caused by *Trueperella pyogenes*, which fills most abscesses. Pus can be aspirated by attachment of a syringe or by withdrawal of the needle and observing typically thick yellow-white pus clogging the needle and hub. Although use of a wider bore needle would encourage flow of pus, these needles may be so large as to risk exogenous wicking of bacteria into sterile seromas or hematomas that are tapped. Therefore, the 16-gauge needle seems the best for the initial aspirate in cattle. Ultrasonography can be extremely helpful in distinguishing abscesses from seromas and hematomas and identifying the extent of an abscess as well as the most appropriate site for drainage.

After needle confirmation has been obtained, a scalpel is used to drain the abscess, and a quick and rapid procedure is performed only with simple restraint if judgment dictates or with mild sedation (15–30 mg of xylazine) in most cattle. A liberal incision (≥5.0 cm) is essential for adequate and continued drainage. Large necrotic clumps of tissue and inflammatory debris should be removed manually from the core of the abscess. After initial drainage, the patient's caretaker should be instructed in the following aftercare:

1. Each day the incision should be cleansed, and a gloved hand should be used to open the incision.
2. For large abscess cavities, flushing the cavity with dilute iodophor, hydrogen peroxide, or saline solutions is indicated to encourage removal of necrotic or inflammatory debris for 5 to 7 days.
3. Systemic antibiotics are not necessary in most abscess patients but would be indicated for severe or recurrent cases. Because of the prevalence of *T. pyogenes* and gram-negative anaerobes, β-lactams or oxytetracycline represent good empiric choices.

Liver Biopsy

Although not considered a routine procedure, liver biopsy may be necessary to confirm diffuse liver disease or focal liver lesions identified with the aid of ultrasonography.

Liver biopsy in adult cattle is performed after mild sedation of the patient, if necessary, surgical preparation of a site in the right 11th intercostal space at the level of the mid-paralumbar fossa, local infiltrative anesthesia, scalpel puncture of the skin, and introduction of a Tru-Cut (Tru-Cut Biopsy Needle; Baxter Healthcare Corp., Valencia, CA) biopsy instrument or other liver biopsy needle. The instrument is usually advanced slightly cranial and ventral to the selected site.

The procedure can usually be performed blindly, but without question the use of ultrasonography to identify the exact liver location is extremely helpful to successful biopsy. Liver biopsy can also be performed during a right-sided flank laparotomy.

Mechanical Dehorning

Dehorning of dairy cattle has long been accepted as a routine management necessity in most areas of the United States. Although veterinarians and owners agree that this task should be performed at as early an age as possible, it is inevitable that labor or time constraints develop on some farms with resultant dehorning remaining necessary for cattle 6 to 24 months of age.

Veterinarians must understand and be able to perform proper dehorning technique for various ages of calves and cattle. Laypeople who dehorn livestock almost never adequately attend to details such as local anesthesia, cleanliness or antisepsis, and hemostasis. In addition, complications such as sinusitis and tetanus are much more common when cattle are dehorned by laypeople. A study of dehorning practices in dairy calves in the Canadian province of Ontario identified that when producers dehorn their own animals, local anesthesia is used in fewer than 25% of cases, but the proportion exceeds 90% when veterinarians perform the procedure. There is every reason to believe that these numbers are similar in the U.S. dairy industry. Dehorning techniques will be discussed from their simplest to most complex.

Anesthesia and Restraint for Dehorning

Local anesthesia by cornual nerve blockade is performed before any dehorning technique. This minimizes operative pain to the patient and allows the veterinarian to institute postoperative hemostasis without causing excessive stress or pain to the patient. The cornual nerve is a branch of the zygomatic temporal nerve and runs from the caudal orbit to the horn slightly below the temporal line. The nerve lies deeper near the orbit and more superficial along the caudal portion of the temporal line. Depending on the size of the animal being dehorned, 3 to 10 mL of 2% lidocaine is used to block the cornual nerve with an 18-gauge, 3.75-cm needle. Smaller needles may be acceptable for young calves.

In addition to local anesthesia, some practitioners use sedative analgesics such as xylazine to minimize the need for further restraint. Sedation may be helpful for fractious patients and is definitely indicated for bulls. Dosage depends on the size of the animal, degree of sedation desired, and facilities. Restraint is imperative for effective and proper dehorning. Baby calves simply can be handheld or haltered. Larger calves (older than 4 months) should be tightly secured with a halter and stabilized within a stanchion or held by an assistant whose hip provides a solid object against which the side opposite the dehorning site is positioned. Stanchions or chutes are ideal for calves older than 6 months of age. Such head gates allow the calf to be caught easily and prevent excessive struggling. The calf may be restrained by a halter or nose lead, which allows the calf's head to be pulled to one side and then the other to allow proper positioning for dehorning. A nose lead is preferable to halters in large calves and adults because it provides better restraint and does not interfere with effective hemostasis as a tight halter does, which may either accentuate or mask bleeding because of pressure caudal to the horn region. Adequate anesthesia and restraint for dehorning cannot be overemphasized because without it, the procedure will be prolonged. When the procedure is performed improperly, horn regrowth is possible, patient struggling and apprehension increase, the opportunity for patient injury increases, and handlers and the veterinarian become frustrated. Clients can be particularly intolerant of paying to have the procedure performed on young calves by veterinarians only to have horn scurs or regrowth blemish the appearance of adult cattle, necessitating a second, more challenging procedure, in adulthood.

Electric or Heat Dehorning

This technique is the simplest form of dehorning because it can be done as soon as a horn bud can be palpated in baby calves, requires no hemostasis, and can be performed by one person, and with it, post-dehorning complications are virtually eliminated.

The age for calves is usually 2 to 8 weeks; they are dehorned only if the emerging horn buds are distinctly palpable. One of our colleagues, Dr. Sheila McGuirk at the University of Wisconsin, has been a strong proponent of combining sedation and local anesthesia even for young preweaned calves undergoing heat dehorning. The IM or IV administration of 0.1 mg/kg of xylazine followed by cornual nerve anesthesia approximately 5 to 10 minutes later is her preferred technique. The local anesthetic (3–5 mL of 2% lidocaine) is injected at a point halfway from the lateral canthus of the eye to the base of the horn, immediately underneath the bony ridge of the temporal bone. In larger calves, an additional 1 to 2 mL of 2% lidocaine can be injected immediately caudal to the horn bud for additional anesthesia. Hair should be clipped over, and immediately around, the horn buds to improve thermal contact between the equipment and the skin surface. Electric or battery-heated dehorners that have been preheated before the onset of dehorning then are applied such that they surround the horn bud completely, thereby causing a thermal burn to skin circumferential to the horn and peripheral to the germinal epithelium. The dehorner is rotated slightly under gentle pressure to ensure uniformity of heat distribution. A "copper brown" ring in the burned tissue usually indicates sufficient cautery to prevent horn growth. During the procedure, the calf is held by an assistant or the veterinarian straddles the calf and holds its head to one side while dehorning the contralateral side and then switches hands while the head is pulled to the opposite side. If sedation has been used, it can be helpful to have a reversing agent such as tolazoline (2–4 mg/kg) available in case the animal is still quite sedate several minutes after the procedure has been completed. Although the extra expense and time required to sedate calves may at first seem unnecessary, many individual producers and commercial heifer rearers have come to prefer it over other techniques, citing that the calves appear to recover and resume normal behavior and feeding more quickly. A 4-day meat withhold is currently required if xylazine is used in the United States, and a 1-day withhold is necessary for lidocaine.

There are no significant disadvantages to electric or heat dehorning, but some owners fail to use the technique because of various factors: poor management that allows calves to get too large for effective electric dehorning; aesthetics (i.e., some people cannot stand the odor of burning hair and flesh); or cosmetics—some owners who show cattle believe that gouge dehorning performed at 4 to 12 months of age yields a more cosmetic head for show purposes. Inadequate restraint, poor analgesia, and inexperience regarding the degree of "burn" necessary peripheral to the germinal epithelium to completely prevent growth are common reasons for the procedure to either not go well or be unsuccessful. Electric dehorning with local anesthesia and sedation in preweaned calves is an excellent way of dehorning heifer replacements in the authors' opinion.

Roberts or Tube Dehorners

This instrument, as with electric dehorners, is designed for dehorning young calves that remain in the horn bud stage. After local anesthesia, restraint, or sedation, the tube with a sharpened circumferential edge is applied, twisted while pushed through the skin surrounding the horn bud, and then rotated to flick off the horn bud and surrounding skin. Hemostasis is attained as necessary, and an antiseptic dressing is applied. The method is quick and effective.

Gouge or Barnes Dehorners

After the horn has developed beyond the bud stage and develops an elliptical base, gouge dehorners usually are necessary to ensure complete dehorning and excision of enough skin peripheral to the horn origin to prevent regrowth. Gouge or Barnes dehorners are available in two sizes and can be used in most calves 3 to 10 months of age, depending on breed and size. Wooden or metal tubular handles are available, and an elliptical sharpened metal edge is formed when the handles are held together. Spreading the handles apart causes the sharpened edge to excise skin peripheral to the horn and the horn. The gouge must have a large enough circumference to remove skin circumferential to the horn itself effectively, thus preventing regrowth of the germinal epithelium. The long axis of the elliptical cutting surface is laid over the long axis of the elliptical horn base after the head has been restrained and anesthesia administered. A sharp, quick cut coupled with pushing the cutting edge toward the skull is important to proper dehorning; it will not only cause complete dehorning but also will allow effective hemostasis by exposing bleeding arteries subcutaneously rather than in an interosseous location. Hemostasis is completed by pulling bleeding cornual arteries with artery forceps followed by topical application of an antiseptic spray or solution. Local anesthesia and sedation may be used as previously described. A single appropriate dose of a non-steroidal anti-inflammatory drug may be beneficial in decreasing postoperative pain and improving the immediate post-operative appetite and weight gain.

Keystone Dehorners

Keystone dehorners are necessary for heifers or young bulls with large horn bases and for adult cattle. Large wooden handles operate the guillotine-type blades that remove the horn (Fig. 2.33). Keystone dehorners are heavy, somewhat cumbersome, and dangerous but effective if used properly.

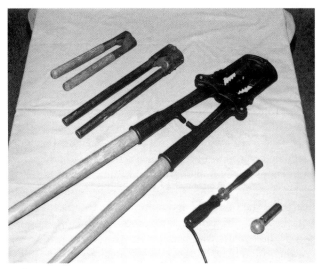

• **Fig. 2.33** A variety of common dehorning instruments. From top to bottom: a small Barnes gouge, large Barnes gouge, Keystone dehorner, electric dehorner, and tube or Roberts dehorner.

To make a "good cut" that effectively removes the horn and a surrounding zone of skin to prevent horn regrowth from the germinal epithelium, the patient has to be well restrained and positioned in a stanchion or head gate. The patient's head is pulled to one side, and the "inside horn" (farther from the veterinarian and closer to the stanchion) is removed. The patient's head then is pulled to the opposite side and the remaining horn removed. Positioning of the Keystone dehorner such that it properly cuts the ventral aspect of a large horn to allow SC exposure of the cornual artery branches requires that the cow's head be tipped toward the veterinarian and the distal portion of the dehorner be pushed closer to the skull. Anesthesia, restraint, hemostasis, and topical antiseptic care are performed as previously described.

In addition to potential complications associated with any open sinus dehorning (acute sinusitis, chronic sinusitis, or tetanus), Keystone dehorning has on rare occasions caused skull fractures in mature adult cattle.

Power Dehorners

Mechanical guillotine-type power-driven dehorners are available commercially. They are used when large numbers of heifers or adults require dehorning or when the veterinarian seeks to reduce the work required in using gouges or Keystone dehorners. The techniques are similar to those described for the Keystone dehorner, and again adequate restraint is essential to proper technique. Extreme care must be exercised in the use of these devices because injuries to assistants or the veterinarian are potential hazards of using any power equipment.

Obstetric Wire

Obstetric wire is used to dehorn bulls and other large cattle that have horn bases too large for Keystone dehorners. Wire frequently is used to dehorn bulls, even yearling bulls, with wide horn bases and horns that protrude perpendicular to the longitudinal plane. Heifers especially have horns that curl upward as they project from the skull, but bulls often have horns that project outward, making it difficult to position dehorners properly to ensure a successful cut. Too often an improper cut with gouges or Keystone dehorners leaves a bull with a shelf of bone on the ventral horn base. This not only allows regrowth of horn ("skurl") but also precludes adequate hemostasis of the cornual artery because the artery is cut transversely and the cut end remains embedded in bone. Wire, on the other hand, can be positioned on skin below the shelf of bone and a proper cut completed as the horn is sawed off, using a sawing motion while holding the wire with obstetric wire handles. As with Keystone dehorners, the inside horn (closer to the stanchion) is removed as the head is tilted toward the veterinarian.

In addition to local anesthesia, it is preferable to sedate bulls and other animals being dehorned with obstetric wire because the procedure requires more time and much more effort for the veterinarian to complete horn removal. Proper removal technique allows hemostasis because the cornual artery is exposed in a SC location. Aftercare is standard.

Dehorning Saws

Box-type saws have been used to dehorn cattle, and the technique is similar to that used with obstetric wire. Saws, like wire, make dehorning more laborious than gouges or Keystone dehorners and are not widely used on dairy cattle.

Cosmetic Dehorning

Cosmetic dehorning is not as popular in dairy cows as in beef cows. Cosmetic dehorning requires careful aseptic technique, is more time consuming, and is more expensive than other techniques. The only advantages of cosmetic dehorning are to allow "shaping" of the head for aesthetic or show value and to attain rapid wound healing resulting from primary closure of the wounds.

The surgical procedure is done after sedation of the patient, local anesthesia, clipping of the entire poll region, surgical prep, and aseptic technique. Skin around the horn and peripheral to the germinal epithelium is incised, undermined, and loosened. Sterile obstetric wire is placed under the skin incision, and the horn is removed at a level below the skin. The skin incision may need to be elongated slightly toward the poll to allow adequate undermining of skin such that skin closure can be accomplished over the area formerly occupied by the horn. Closure with a continuous pattern of heavy suture material is then performed. Preoperative and postoperative antibiotics and tetanus prophylaxis should be considered for patients undergoing cosmetic dehorning.

Hemostasis for Dehorning

Although some veterinarians do not attempt to control bleeding caused by dehorning, fatal blood loss occurs on

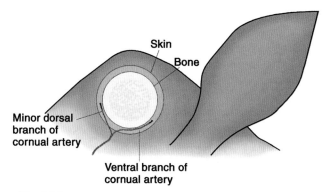

• **Fig. 2.34** Schematic illustration of the cornual artery and typical subcutaneous locations of the ventral and dorsal branches after they are sectioned by a proper dehorning cut. A properly located cut will expose the dorsal and ventral branches within the area shaded pink. These cut ends then are pulled with artery forceps to establish hemostasis.

rare occasions as a complication of dehorning and justifies professional attention to hemostasis. When discussing the technique to be used for dehorning on a farm, some consideration to the transmission of bloodborne infections such as BLV, BVDV, and anaplasmosis should be considered. Bloodless dehorning would obviously be a preferable technique when BLV control is important. Adequate hemostasis only requires that bleeding from the cornual artery be controlled. This can be accomplished only following a proper cut that exposes the cornual artery in a SC location. The cornual artery is a branch of the superficial temporal artery and runs caudally along the temporal line, usually before branching just anterior to the horn into a dorsal and ventral branch. The dorsal branch is smaller and usually is exposed by dehorning on the cranial edge of the cut. The ventral branch is larger and usually is obvious on the ventral aspect of the cut (Fig. 2.34). Improper cuts that fail to remove all of the bone in the ventral aspect of the horn leave the cut ends of one or both of these arteries pulsing blood directly out of the remaining horn. When this occurs, the ends of the arteries cannot be grasped or ligated. Proper cuts expose both branches subcutaneously and allow the arteries to be grasped with artery forceps and "pulled." The ventral branch should be grasped, gently stretched, and pulled caudally until it breaks. If bleeding is still evident in the dorsal branch, this artery should be grasped, gently stretched, and pulled directly dorsal until it breaks. When the ventral branch is stretched sufficiently, it often is unnecessary to pull the dorsal branch because the artery breaks off proximal to the origin of the dorsal branch. Pulling these arteries until they break causes rapid hemostasis because bleeding is thereby confined within tissue or bone and clotting occurs more easily. Proper dehorning technique and adequate anesthesia allow rapid, practical hemostasis.

Castration

Castration seldom is necessary for dairy animals because most male offspring are culled or used as sires. However, owners may request castration of male calves being raised for veal, baby beef, dairy beef, or oxen. Many castration techniques exist; it is beyond the scope of this textbook to delve into all of them and readers are referred to Farm Animal Surgery; Fubini and Ducharme, 2017. We use bloodless techniques with the Burdizzo's emasculatome for bull calves younger than 6 months of age because of the lessened potential for complications and minimal stress on the patient. The Burdizzo's emasculator is applied to two sites on each spermatic cord for 60 seconds per application. The veterinarian should be sure to stretch each testicle when applying the emasculatome so that the penis and urethra are not damaged and to move the spermatic cord being clamped to a lateral location in the scrotum to avoid damaging the blood supply to the entire ventral half of the scrotum.

Other bloodless techniques such as elastrator bands may be used, but these suffer from seasonal concerns such as the presence of maggots in wounds during warm weather and non-seasonal concerns regarding tetanus or improper application.

Many veterinarians prefer surgical castration to ensure complete removal of the testicles. Although bloodless techniques are highly successful when done with proper technique, concern about incomplete castration may influence some owners to prefer surgical castration. Surgical castration can be performed after bilateral scalpel incision on the lateral skin of the scrotum or after excision of the ventral quarter to one third portion of the scrotum. Individual preference dictates open versus closed castration techniques after scrotal incision. Regardless of technique, the use of an emasculator is recommended to minimize hemorrhage. Disadvantages of surgical castration include potential wound complications, maggots, tetanus, blood loss, and a greater stress to the patient. The major advantage is assurance of complete castration.

As with dehorning, recent research suggests that the majority of producers (>80%) who perform castration do so without provision of analgesia. Within the United States the lack of approval for specific analgesic drugs in food animals is another complicating factor, regardless of one's ethical or welfare stance on the subject. In terms of physiologic indicators of pain in young male calves, it appears that there are considerable differences between calves of 8 weeks of age or younger compared with those of 6 months of age or older. It is therefore becoming increasingly difficult to justify performing the castration procedure in calves older than 6 months old without appropriate pain relief.

Nose Ring Placement

Proper placement of a nose ring helps prevent subsequent loss of the ring associated with ripping the ring through the muzzle during restraint. Rings are commonly placed in young bulls as they reach puberty and begin to show dominant or aggressive tendencies. It may be necessary to install a larger nose ring as the bull approaches maturity. Nose rings of several sizes are available commercially. The ring selected for an individual bull should be large enough to allow it to

be grasped easily with fingers or a bull leader and yet not so large as to become easily tangled on objects and torn out.

The nose ring is designed to facilitate restraint, leading, and management of bulls. Without a nose ring, it is impossible to manage individual bulls safely. Group-housed bulls, as observed in some AI studs, do not have nose rings installed because their collective activity and aggressiveness risk trauma that could rip out the ring. Nose rings are inserted as bulls leave the group to be managed individually.

Particularly aggressive or difficult-to-catch bulls may require a short chain leader attached to the nose ring to allow the ring to be grasped more easily.

Nose rings occasionally are installed in heifers that are thought to be sucking teats in group housing situations. These nose rings have a "picket fence" aluminum plate attached that acts as a prod to the heifer being sucked so that such heifers no longer stand and allow the problem heifer to suck them. Nose rings are rarely applied to adult cows but have been used to make particularly aggressive show cows more manageable in the show ring.

Proper installation of a nose ring requires that a nose lead be used to extend the bull's head straight forward. The bull's head should not be turned. With the head fully extended and the nose lead tightly fixed, a no. 22 scalpel blade attached to a scalpel handle is quickly directed through the nasal septum. The back of the scalpel blade should abut the nose leads as the cut through the septum is completed. Dr. R.B. Hillman uses a 1.0- to 1.5-cm trochar rather than a scalpel blade. The trochar stylet acts as a guide for the ring as the trochar is withdrawn and the ring threaded through the nasal septum. Keeping pressure on the nose lead ensures that the ring will be placed as far forward in the nasal septum as possible. This avoids the septum cartilage and potential complications from cartilage injury. Special nose ring pliers that act as combined nose leads, scalpel, and insertion guide are available commercially.

After the septum has been incised, insertion of the nose ring is easily accomplished by projecting the tapered end of the open ring through the incision, closing the ring tightly, and placing the small screw that holds the ring closed tightly in position. Dropping or losing this tiny screw is a common source of frustration and can be avoided by carefully holding the screw between one's teeth until it is needed.

Proper placement of nose rings minimizes the likelihood of nasal and muzzle lacerations caused by the ring being pulled out. Improper placement or excessive tension on a ring can cause this drastic injury and creates an injured bull without any practical means of being restrained or led. Repair of nose ring pullout lesions has been described and is indicated for valuable bulls. Sedation of the patient is coupled with local anesthesia provided by blocking sensory innervation through bilateral blocks at the infraorbital foramina; large mattress sutures of steel or other nonabsorbable material are used in the repair.

Dr. R.B. Hillman has extensive experience in repair of nose ring tears because of his supervision of bull health for the bull stud in Ithaca, New York. He suggests primary closure with large mattress sutures that are preplaced before knotting (so that the entire wound can be seen) followed by simple interrupted sutures to oppose the skin edges. Dr. Hillman prefers heavy sutures. In addition to sedation with xylazine and local infiltration anesthesia, Dr. Hillman restrains the patient by tying it to a tilt table in the standing position so that the head can be restrained securely to the table.

Removal of Dewclaw

Removal of the medial hind dewclaws is sometimes performed on heifer calves on some dairy farms. Managers on these farms believe that this practice minimizes self-induced teat injuries. Although a controversial topic, no question exists that some mature cows or cows with pendulous udders do injure teats with medial dewclaws rather than medial claws of the digit. This can be proved by applying a dye to the medial dewclaw and then observing the cow's udder and teats several hours later to see where contact occurs.

Medial dewclaw removal is performed bilaterally in calves as a prophylactic measure and may be performed unilaterally or bilaterally in adult cows that repeatedly develop self-induced udder or teat injury.

The skin around the medial dewclaw is clipped and surgically prepared. An adult cow should be restrained in a head gate or stanchion and have the limb to be operated raised by a rope as in hoof trimming. Alternatively, a tilt table may be used if available. Calves can be restrained by an assistant or sedated. Local anesthesia via local infiltration, ring block, dorsal metatarsal vein injection after tourniquet application, or specific nerve blocks should be performed. Sedation with xylazine may be helpful—especially in adult cattle—because of the drug's analgesic properties. In baby calves, heavy serrated scissors may be sufficient for removal of the medial dewclaw, and a sterile Barnes or gouge-type dehorner works very well in adult cattle. Care should be taken to avoid injury to deeper structures when amputating the medial dewclaws while being sure to remove a ring of skin peripheral to the dewclaw base so that regrowth cannot occur. After removal, an antiseptic dressing and snug bandage are applied to protect the wound and speed hemostasis. The bandage is removed in 1 week, when it is either replaced or the wound left open and treated topically.

Tail Amputation

At one point in time, it was commonplace to amputate the tail on all cows. The practice had gained popularity through the perception that tail docking improved cow cleanliness, improved udder hygiene, and lessened environmental soiling from tail switching. The practice also is popular with milkers because it prevents tail switching in the face. Tail docking does not correct dirty management practices or lack of bedding. It does not improve upon sound premilking, milking, and postmilking hygiene or technique, and there is no beneficial effect on milk quality. Furthermore, although proponents of tail amputation dispute this, cattle should have a defense against insects that a tail can flick away.

Tails are docked at the level of the ventral vulva or just ventral to the lips of the vulva. This leaves enough tail to protect the perineum and perhaps still allow tail restraint of the animal. An elastrator-type band is used to amputate the tail. The procedure may be performed on calves, heifers, or adult cows. After placement of the band, the tail distal to the band undergoes progressive dry gangrene and falls off in 2 to 8 weeks. The upper limit of this time range is met when bands are placed directly over a coccygeal vertebra rather than closer to an intervertebral location. Wounds that expose bone obviously take longer to heal.

Possible complications include chronic infections, osteomyelitis, ascending neuritis-myelitis, clostridial myositis, and tetanus.

Cattle should not have their tails docked unless the owners are willing to provide excellent insect control measures and practice excellent overall hygiene and cleanliness. Tail docking is not an excuse for dirty management. There have been a number of studies published in recent years examining the effect on fly control and insect avoidance behavior, as well as the animal welfare and pain issues associated with tail docking in cattle. At the current time, tail docking is illegal in several European countries but still permitted in the United States. The available literature suggests that tail docking of calves may cause distress to the animal, and there is no conferred benefit in terms of udder cleanliness or the rate of intra-mammary infections in lactating cows with docked tails compared with those that have not had their tails amputated under conventional free-stall housing practices.

Restraint

Restraint of any species is more art than science. Selection of the proper restraint for a given veterinary procedure requires common sense, judgment, and humane considerations. Experience plays a major role in selection of restraint techniques, and this experience is modified based on factors such as the patient's "personality," the owner's personality, the facilities available, the normal time required for completion of the necessary procedure, and the restraint skills of the assistants or handlers available.

There is an old adage that "the minimum restraint that allows the procedure to be performed quickly and effectively is the correct amount." It would be nice if we never had to restrain cattle, but this is not the case. However, erring on the side of too little restraint risks injury to the veterinarian, handlers, and patient. The potential for professional liability and malpractice suits must be considered with every patient that we, as veterinarians, treat. Too little restraint also may cause the patient to become increasingly apprehensive, wild, and progressively violent because a simple procedure has now become a prolonged adventure. Each time the procedure is restarted in a poorly restrained animal, the animal anticipates the procedure and becomes more violent. In addition, the handler and veterinarian become progressively frustrated, and so lose time and tempers. Too little restraint may result from lack of facilities or lack of knowledge.

Restraint is necessary to protect handlers, assistants, the veterinarian, and the patient itself. Kicking may be a vice or a defense mechanism for cattle. Cattle occasionally kick straight backward but usually "cow kick" by pulling the hind leg forward and then abducting the leg before kicking in a curved lateral and backward stroke. Vicious cows can kick straight back with one or both hind legs, causing severe injuries to handlers. Obviously, if both hind legs kick simultaneously, the cow has to lower her head and put weight on the forelimbs. Such kicks, although uncommon, may deliver a blow as high as a man's face to a person behind the cow and can be devastating. Cows that kick sideways often "crowd" a person that approaches them first; most cows "crowd" people that approach from the side, but not all such cows kick. Being caught between a pipe partition or wall and a cow pushing all her weight against you is not a pleasant experience but is well known to people who handle cattle. Being caught by a mature bull in the same position could be fatal.

Very nervous cattle that bellow and jump about when they anticipate restraint, injections, or handling are dangerous simply because they are frightened. Thus, they may become defensive and, in such a mood, can trap or trample a person.

Most people with even a rudimentary level of animal husbandry realize that cattle kick, but few realize the dangers presented by a cow's head when used in a defensive or aggressive way. A cow's head should never be approached without caution, and a person should stand beyond striking distance of the head unless the head is tightly restrained. Even loosely haltered or held heads can quickly break ribs or cause other damage to handlers. A cow's head only needs about 4 to 6 inches of freedom to generate sufficient force to hurt handlers or cause fractures. Therefore, when restraining a cow's head with a halter or nose lead, the head must be tightly extended with no slack allowed. Similarly, when holding a cow's head for oral examination or to deliver oral medication, the head must be held tightly to the hip and upper body. Angry, demented, or protective (of a newborn calf) cows may attempt to charge, butt, or pin a person to the ground. The cow may charge straight ahead or swing the head back and forth, delivering blows with each change of direction. Not a year goes by when the lay press fails to report fatalities as a result of handlers being mauled or killed by one of their own cattle protecting a newborn calf. Bulls obviously have an even greater potential to maim or kill humans. A dairy bull should never be trusted. Dairy bulls have a long legacy of unpredictability and have seriously injured many experienced dairy handlers who became overconfident or "in a hurry" when working in a bull pen.

Rarely, aggressive or frightened cattle will strike at a human with the forelegs. This usually happens when the cow's head is restrained for an IV injection or some other procedure involving the head or neck. Veterinarians and handlers should take care not to kneel too close to a cow because of this possibility.

Much variation in cattle behavior, handling, and husbandry exists on different farms. Small farms that have conventional housing and a great deal of contact time between the cattle and handlers are less likely to have vicious or wild cattle. However, rough handling, abusive handlers, constant yelling, or beating of cattle can occur in any environment. Free-stall or pastured cattle may be wild and only tractable when previous intense effort by experienced "cow people" has trained them not to fear approach by humans or haltering. The larger the herd, the less likely individual cattle will have been halter trained. Automatic lock-in head gates or stanchions and chutes are necessary to safely handle and treat wild cattle.

An Approach to Dairy Cattle Restraint

Ownership of dairy cattle does not necessarily impart the knowledge, judgment, and techniques needed for proper restraint of these animals. Therefore the veterinarian must balance the need for proper restraint with a consideration of the owner's wishes or suggestions. It is best to allow the owner an opportunity to suggest restraint unless it becomes obvious that the owner's technique will not work. For example, when first visiting a farm, it is courtesy for the veterinarian to say. "Please catch her head up while I prepare this bottle of . . . to give her intravenously." The veterinarian can then observe routine restraint practice on the farm in question. Does the owner prefer a halter or nose lead? Many owners of registered and show cattle always use a halter and consider a nose lead offensive and unnecessary. Therefore a new veterinarian who immediately tries to put a nose lead in cows on this farm might not be called again.

Good dairy people also will warn the veterinarian about dangerous or nervous cows, and this should be an obligation of owners. Veterinarians may need to instruct dairy people in restraint for therapeutics or surgery to ensure safety to humans and beasts.

Cows should be approached slowly and made aware of the approach by verbal communication. Never touch a cow suddenly or move quickly toward her. It is preferable to approach tied cows on the same side that they are milked, given that this may be unknown in free-stall cows. Tied cows often are apprehensive when approached from the off-milking side, and this can be avoided by observing where the vacuum and pipeline stopcocks are located between cows. An assistant or handler should stay at the cow's rear end on the same side as the veterinarian if the veterinarian has to approach the animal's fore end. This prevents "crowding." Gentle cows can be reassured by the handler's scratching the tail head or rubbing the scapula and withers. An assistant should prevent the rear end of the cow from swinging across any posts positioned near the cow when the veterinarian is working near the rear of the cow. Loose cows can be made to stand briefly in a corner or moved into an open area by a person being positioned on each side of the animal. Moving slowly and deliberately without excessive noise is most effective and least likely to upset other cows in the barn. If one cow is roughly handled or mistreated, the entire herd may become apprehensive. Cows in tie stalls or free stalls that move sideways or back and forth should be restrained by a halter so that directional movement is limited.

Restraint of the Head

Rope halters are the most practical and gentle means of restraint. These suffice for most basic restraint and jugular injections, as well as for leading cows. Halters should be attached so that the free end tightens under the jaw and appears on the left side, which is the standard side from which to lead a cow. Positioning two halters on a wild cow to allow two people to lead her from opposite sides is generally worthless, unless the head can be kept in a ventroflexed position lessening forward momentum, because the cow then pulls both people in a straight line. The principle of using one halter allows the leader to pull a wild cow's head to one side, forcing her to circle rather than escape. Nose leads are used when more restraint is necessary because of the cow being wild or when very quick but painful procedures are necessary. Nose leads should not be used to lead a cow because the cow's normal response to nose leads is to pull back against them or to violently charge forward trying to either loosen them or reduce tension exerted by them. Neck straps are helpful to grasp the cow but provide poor restraint for large or wild cows. Bulls often are led by a long rope running from a neck strap or halter through the nose ring or by a snap-on rope attached to the nose ring. Bulls also may be led by a bull leader attached to the nose ring. Whenever bulls are moved, a linear array of partition pipes placed close enough to allow a human to escape, but not the bull, is ideal.

Small- to moderate-sized cows that are calm can be restrained by having one person bend the cow's head around the handler's torso with the aid of a halter or fingers placed in the cow's nose (Fig. 2.35).

Whenever restraining a cow's head, the head should be pulled upward and to the side to gain more leverage. A cow allowed to hold her head too low has more mechanical advantage and thus compromises the restraint and may suddenly swing the head up, striking the person trying to restrain the cow. If additional restraint of the head is needed, grasping the nose with the fingers of a hand (easiest) or applying nose tongs can be helpful for quick venipuncture collections or oral examinations. Blindfolds are advocated as adjuncts to some restraint in Europe, but we have no experience with this technique. Calves may be restrained for injections, venipuncture, and examination by straddling the calf's neck and backing the calf into a corner.

Tail restraint is effective for minor, quick procedures such as IM or SC injections, collecting blood from the middle caudal vein, infusing a quarter, opening an obstructed teat, or draining an abscess. Effective tail

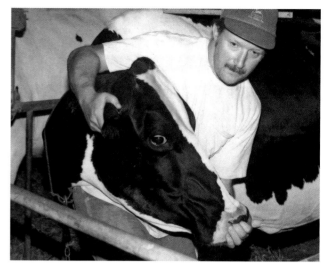

• **Fig. 2.35** Manual restraint for intravenous injections and other minor procedures.

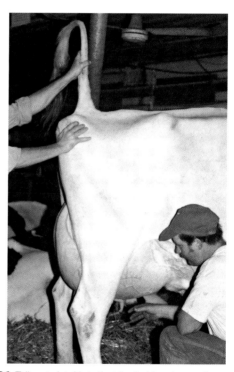

• **Fig. 2.36** Tail restraint. Note that the holder also applies pressure to the cow's hip area on the side where the procedure is being performed. Thus if the cow reacts in a dangerous fashion, she can be pushed away from the person performing the procedure.

restraint is provided with one hand while the opposite hand of the holder applies pressure to the cow's hip area on the same side as the veterinarian works (Fig. 2.36). Tail restraint may be combined with sedative-analgesics or local anesthesia for teat surgery or other more painful procedures. Proper tail restraint discourages kicking and keeps the cow steady. In tie stalls or loose housing, a halter should be applied before tail restraint to prevent excessive side-to-side or back-and-forth movement by the cow. Dry bedding or nonslip surfaces are important adjuncts to

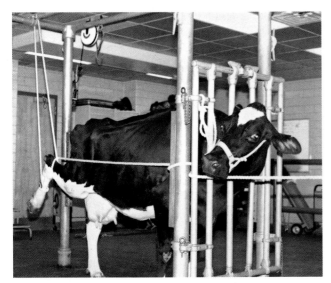

• **Fig. 2.37** Raising a hind limb with the aid of a 30-foot soft nylon or cotton rope equipped with a quick-release honda and an overhead beam or beam hook. The cow is pulled forward in the stanchion, tied with a halter to reduce forward and backward movements, and tied toward the hind limb being lifted if there is a post or support available for her to lean against on the offside. The half-hitch loop in the rope must be maintained in the caudal gastrocnemius region for most efficient mechanical advantage.

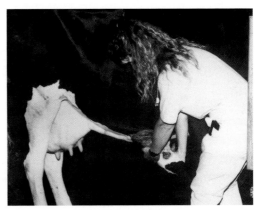

• **Fig. 2.38** Manual lifting of the forelimb for examination of the foot. The patient's head is restrained by a halter and tied toward the opposite side in an effort to reduce weight bearing on the limb being examined. In some instances, a bale of straw or wooden block may be used to rest the limb and reduce back strain for the examiner.

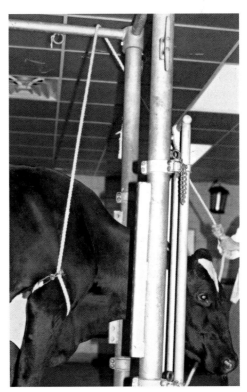

• **Fig. 2.39** Another method to relieve weight bearing or "leaning on the examiner" is to lift the forelimb with the aid of a rope loop taken to the offside over a beam or beam hook and then tied so that the foot is easier to lift and hold. The cow also should be restrained with a halter and tied to the offside.

tail restraint, lest the cow slip backward or sideways while being restrained. Overzealous or sadistic tail restraint by extremely strong individuals can fracture caudal vertebrae, resulting in neurologic deficits to the perineum and tail. In contrast, failure to put some force into raising the tail to a vertical position results in lack of restraint. Therefore judicious pressure and experience are necessary to generate effective restraint by this method.

Antikicking devices seldom are used by veterinarians but are routinely used by milkers for specific cows that repeatedly kick at milking units or milkers. Antikicking hobbles and Achilles tendon (gastrocnemius) clamps are used by some farmers but have largely been replaced by flank clamps that are positioned more safely and easily than hobbles. One other disadvantage of hobbles is that cows that fight these devices tend to "double-barrel" kick by kicking out backward simultaneously with both legs.

Several methods exist to raise a hind limb for hoof trimming. A stanchion or trimming chute provides the ideal restraint for raising hind legs (Fig. 2.37). However, veterinarians should be familiar with other methods because the structure of certain barns may not allow the use of beam hooks or pulleys. Good footing should be available such that the cow can stand on the opposite (non-lifted) hind limb without slipping.

Forelimbs are more difficult to lift and restrain than hind limbs. Regardless of technique, forelimb work contributes to "veterinary back pain" and sweat. A tilt table or portable hydraulic chute with a belly band are obviously preferable for hoof trimming but not always available. Typical techniques for lifting a forelimb are illustrated in Figs. 2.38 and 2.39.

Ropes encircling the flank area or heart girth region that are tightened to effect may restrain some cattle effectively to prevent kicking and excessive movement. Whenever restraining a standing cow for foot care or other therapeutic and surgical procedures, her head should be tied via halter to prevent forward and backward movement. Preferably, the cow's head should be pulled toward the side being worked on.

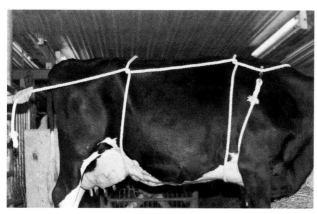

• **Fig. 2.40** Commonly used modification of Hertwig's method to cast a cow. The forward loop is directed between the forelimbs to avoid choking the cow. The forward loop can be secured by either a bowline knot or, as illustrated here, a quick-release honda.

Modifications of encircling flank and heart girth ropes also are used to cast cattle. Several methods have proven valuable, and most practitioners use modifications of Hertwig's method or Szabo's method to cast cattle for ventral abdominal surgery, correction of uterine torsion, or teat surgery (Fig. 2.40). These methods can be used in both sedated and nonsedated cattle.

The cow is the foster mother of the human race. From the day of the ancient Hindoo to this time have the thoughts of men turned to this kindly and beneficent creature as one of the chief sustaining forces of human life.

—**W.D. HOARD, FOUNDER OF HOARD'S DAIRYMAN, COPYRIGHT 1925 BY W.D. HOARD AND SONS, CO.**

Suggested Readings

Ballou, M. A., Sutherland, M. A., Brooks, T. A., et al. (2013). Administration of anesthetic and analgesic prevent the suppression of many leucocyte responses following surgical castration and physical dehorning. *Vet Immunol Immunopath*, *151*, 285–293.

deLahunta, A. (1983). *Veterinary neuroanatomy and clinical neurology* (ed 2). Philadelphia: WB Saunders.

deLahunta, A., & Habel, R. E. (1986). *Applied veterinary anatomy*. Philadelphia: WB Saunders.

Dockweiller, J. C., Coetzee, J. F., Edwards-Callaway, L. N., et al. (2013). Effect of castration method on neurohormonal and electroencephalographic stress indicators in Holstein calves of different ages. *J Dairy Sci*, *96*, 4340–4354.

Edmondson, M. A. (2016). Local, regional, and spinal anesthesia in ruminants. *Vet Clin North Am Food Anim Pract*, *32*(3), 535–552.

Fox, F. H. (1970). *Personal communication*. Ithaca, New York: Cornell University.

Gilbert, R. O., Cable, C., Fubini, S. L., et al. (2017). Surgery of the bovine reproductive system and tract. In S. L. Fubini, & N. G. Ducharme (Eds.), *Farm animal surgery* (pp 439–503). St. Louis: WB Saunders.

Grandin, T., & Shivley, C. (2015). How farm animals react and perceive stressful situations such as handling, restraint, and transport. *Animals (Basel)*, *5*(4), 1233–1251.

Hillman, R. B. (1984). *Personal communication*. Ithaca, New York: Cornell University.

Leahy, J. R., & Barrow, P. (1953). *Restraint of animals* (ed 2). Ithaca, NY: Cornell Campus Store.

Lombard, J. E., Tucker, C. B., van Keyserling, M. A., et al. (2010). Association between cow hygiene, hock injuries and free stall usage on US dairy farms. *J Dairy Sci*, *93*(10), 4668–4675.

Perkins, G. A., Divers, T. J., & Smith, M. C. (2017). Examination of the surgical patient. In S. L. Fubini, & N. G. Ducharme (Eds.), *Farm animal surgery* (pp. 1–22). St. Louis: WB Saunders.

Rosenberger, G., Dirksen, G., Grunder, H., et al. (1979). *Clinical examination of cattle*. Berlin. Verlag Paul Parey, Dirksen G, Grunder H-D, Grunert E, et al, (collaborators) and Mack R (translator): WB Sanders.

Schreiner, D. A., & Ruegg, P. L. (2002). Effect of tail docking on milk quality and cow cleanliness. *J Dairy Sci*, *85*(10), 2503–2511.

Stöber, M. (1988). Surgery for the cattle practitioner: nose ring torn out—nasolabioplastic operation. *Bov Pract*, *23*, 153–155.

PART II

Diseases of Body Systems

3

Cardiovascular Diseases

SIMON F. PEEK AND SEBASTIEN BUCZINSKI

Examination of the Cardiovascular System

The cardiovascular system is assessed by observation of the animal's general state, mucous membrane appearance, and presence of venous distention or pulsation, as well as by examination of arterial pulse quality and rate and auscultation of the heart rate and rhythm.

Inspection of the patient may raise suspicion of cardiac disease if edema is observed in the submandibular space, brisket, ventral abdomen, udder, or lower limbs or if abdominal contours suggest the presence of ascites. Obviously, this requires differentiation from hypoproteinemic states, vasculitis, thrombophlebitis, lymphadenitis, or other less common diseases. Dyspnea, tachypnea, and grossly distended jugular or mammary veins are possible signs of cardiac disease that may be observed during general inspection of the patient. Weakness and exercise intolerance are other signs that require consideration of cardiac disease. In calves, overt congenital abnormalities such as microphthalmos, wry tail, or absence of a tail may also signal the possibility of an accompanying ventricular septal defect (VSD), and ectopia cordis is grossly apparent by inspection of the thoracic inlet or caudal cervical area. However, the majority of congenital heart malformations occur in the absence of other defects. In calves, failure to thrive in comparison with age-matched herdmates, exercise intolerance, and resting tachypnea or dyspnea may suggest a congenital cardiac condition, but confirmation and characterization require auscultation and echocardiography.

During physical examination, the mucous membranes should be evaluated for pallor, injection, or cyanosis. The visual appearance of the oral mucous membranes can vary with normal pigmentation patterns specific to the breed (e.g., Brown Swiss and Channel Islands cattle) and often appear pale to the inexperienced examiner in variably pigmented breeds such as Holsteins. In general, inspection of conjunctival and vulval mucous membrane appearance and refill time is preferable. Cyanosis is rare in dairy cattle with the exception of animals that are dying of severe pulmonary disease. However, cattle having advanced heart failure, right-to-left congenital shunts, and combined cardiopulmonary disease may have cyanotic mucous membranes. Capillary refill time often is prolonged in cattle with advanced cardiac disease.

Close inspection of the jugular and mammary veins for relative distention and the presence of abnormal pulsation is a very important part of every physical examination. Proficiency and practice at palpation of major veins are essential before an examiner can differentiate an abnormal finding from the normal range of variation found in cattle of various ages and stages of lactation. Normally, mammary veins are more sensitive indicators of increased venous pressure than jugular veins and therefore should be palpated routinely during the physical examination. Jugular veins should be observed during the general inspection and again during thoracic auscultation. Jugular veins should not be palpated until the end of the physical examination because many cattle become apprehensive when the neck region is palpated; this apprehension and subsequent excitement could affect baseline parameters or data being collected during the physical examination. This evaluation of the jugular veins, if deemed necessary, should be done at the end of the physical examination during examination of the head.

Mammary veins should be palpated by applying fingertip pressure. First the vein is palpated gently to detect pulsations suggestive of right heart failure; then the vein is compressed against the abdominal wall by gentle fingertip pressure. The amount of pressure necessary to compress the vein against the abdominal wall normally is minimal. When the vein is difficult to compress or, more commonly, seems to roll away from the fingertips, increased venous pressure from right heart failure may be suspected. These evaluations of the mammary veins obviously are subjective techniques but can be helpful adjuncts to other findings when practiced during every physical examination. Although pulsations in the mammary veins are considered abnormal findings suggestive of right heart failure, an occasional healthy older cow with a large udder and rich mammary vein branching may have slight mammary vein pulsation and distention.

Evaluation of the jugular veins for pulsation and distention requires differentiation of the notorious "false"-jugular pulsation commonly observed in thin-necked dairy cattle from true pathologic jugular pulsation and distention. False or normal jugular pulsation is a product of reverse blood flow from atrial contraction at the end of diastole and expansion of the right atrioventricular (AV) valve during systole. Passive jugular filling during systole also may contribute, as does a "kick," or referred carotid artery pulsation. False jugular pulsation arises as a wave that winds its way from the thoracic inlet to the mandible when the cow has her head and neck parallel to the ground. When the head and neck are raised, the false jugular pulse may only ascend a portion of the cervical area or may disappear. A true jugular pulse fills the whole jugular vein rapidly when the head and neck are parallel to the ground or slightly raised. This rapid filling is similar to filling a garden hose with the end held off when water to the hose is turned on full force. In addition, distention of the jugular veins is more obvious with true jugular distention as found in right heart failure (Fig. 3.1). When confusion exists, the jugular vein may be held off near the ramus of the mandible, blood forced distally toward the thoracic inlet by the examiner's hand, and the vein observed (Video Clip 3.1). Emptying the vein in this fashion will eliminate a false jugular pulse, but a true jugular pulse will refill the emptied vein quickly and indicates right heart failure, increased central venous pressure, or right AV valve insufficiency. Some examiners suggest applying light pressure that partially occludes the jugular vein at the thoracic inlet, thereby mildly distending the jugular vein. This is thought to eliminate false (or normal) jugular venous pulsations from a referred carotid arterial impact. In general, the degree of gross distention of the jugular veins in cattle having right heart failure is more impressive than the degree of pulsation (Video Clip 3.2).

Taking the arterial pulse may be helpful in the assessment of cardiac disease. The middle coccygeal artery is the first artery palpated for pulsation during the physical examination. The facial artery is used when treating recumbent (hypocalcemic) cattle, and the median artery is the most convenient to palpate when performing simultaneous cardiac auscultation and pulse monitoring. Pulse rate, rhythm, and quality should be assessed. Pulse quality implies considerations of the size, strength, and duration of the pulse wave and distention of the artery. Most cattle with heart failure have decreased pulse strength, unevenness of the pulse, increased pulse rate, or a pulse rate that is different than the heart rate. Abnormalities in pulse rate or rhythm should alert the examiner to the possibility of cardiac arrhythmias.

Proficiency at auscultation of the heart requires some basic knowledge, willingness to auscultate both sides of the thorax carefully during every physical examination, and patience. Many cattle object to stethoscope placement over the sites on the chest wall necessary for cardiac auscultation and adduct the forelimb tightly against the thorax. This is noticed especially on examining the right side, where cardiac auscultation in cattle requires the stethoscope to be placed very cranial in the axillary area around the third intercostal space (ICS). Dairy bulls and large or fat cows have thick chest walls that reduce the intensity of heart sounds. Heart sounds are easier to hear on the left side of normal cattle. The pulmonic valve region is best heard in the left third ICS at a level between the shoulder and elbow. The aortic valve region near the heart base is best heard in the left fourth ICS at approximately shoulder level. The mitral (left AV) valve region coincides with the cardiac apex and is best heard at the left fifth ICS just above the elbow. The right AV (tricuspid) valve is heard far forward in the right third ICS at a level halfway between elbow and shoulder.

Although clinicians generally discuss two heart sounds in normal cattle, it is possible to hear four heart sounds in some cattle as it is with horses. Although the potential for four heart sounds is somewhat confusing and may be impossible to differentiate in most clinical patients, examiners should be aware of these facts and not overinterpret the significance of auscultating more than two heart sounds. The first heart sound (S1) heralds the beginning of systole, is associated with the final halting of AV valve motion after closing, and is best heard at the apex regions coinciding with AV valves in the cow. A slight splitting of S1 into separate mitral and tricuspid valve components is possible but is rarely audible in normal cattle. S1 tends to be of lower frequency and longer duration than S2.

S2 usually is not as loud as S1 and coincides with aortic and pulmonic valve closure. Current theory suggests that valve closing sounds associated with the generation of S2 result from the sudden halt in valve motion when it closes. Asynchronous closure of the aortic and pulmonic valves results in audible splitting of S2 in many normal cattle, especially during the inspiratory phase of the respiratory cycle.

Although S1 and S2 comprise the major heart sounds for cattle, S3 and S4 have been described. Ventricular vibrations at the end of rapid filling in early diastole are thought

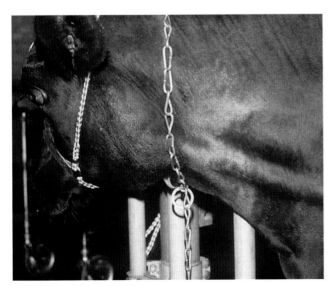

• **Fig. 3.1** Obvious distension of the jugular vein in a cow having heart failure secondary to endocarditis.

to cause S3, a low-frequency sound seldom heard in cattle. S4 sometimes is heard late in diastole and is related to atrial contraction. In cattle with tachycardia, it has been suggested that S4 may in fact closely precede S1 and be mistaken for a split S1. The tripling or quadrupling of heart sounds that resembles a horse's cantering gait is commonly referred to as a gallop rhythm and occurs in the higher range of normal heart rates or when tachycardia exists in some cows. Gallops are diastolic sounds related to atrial contraction (S4 gallop), to ventricular filling (S3), or to both (summation gallop). A prominent and persistent gallop rhythm in a cow with tachycardia may be the first indication of heart disease.

The heart rate of normal adult cattle is 60 to 84 beats/min. Neonatal calves may have normal heart rates as high as 110 to 120 beats/min, but frequently heart rates this high are brought about by the excitement of being handled or in anticipation of being fed. Not everyone agrees on the aforementioned range of normal heart rates for cattle, and several points should be addressed regarding this topic. Oxen and fat, persistently dry cows used only for embryo transfer may have a slower metabolism than lactating dairy cattle. Therefore, somewhat similar to draft horses, these cattle may have heart rates at the low end of the normal range or even less than 60 beats/min. Conversely, healthy but excited, nervous, or aggressive cattle may have heart and pulse rates more than 84 beats/min when approached by any examiner. Therefore, the range of 60 to 84 beats/min really is an average and must be interpreted in light of the patient, its surroundings, and its intended use. Following the work of McGuirk et al. with fasted cattle, a low normal range of 48 beats/min has been proposed. Further studies demonstrated that in normal cattle, a decrease in ruminoreticular fill results in a reflex slowing of the heart rate, predominantly because of an increase in parasympathetic tone. However, fasted healthy cattle seldom are encountered in the world outside of academic settings, and veterinarians are not frequently asked to examine healthy fasted cattle. An exception may be a cow off feed secondary to the classic broken water cup syndrome because she will become anorectic secondary to water deprivation. Sick cattle seldom have a heart rate less than 60 beats/min only because they are anorectic. Sick cattle that do have heart rates less than 60 beats/min usually have a vagal nerve–mediated bradycardia. Therefore, 60 to 84 beats/min is still our preferred normal range for heart rate in adult dairy cattle.

Excited or nervous cattle may have an increased intensity or loudness of the heart sounds in addition to an increased heart rate. Other conditions that increase the intensity of heart sounds may be relative or pathologic. Relative factors include thin body condition, younger animals with thin chest walls, and excitement. Pathologic factors include anemia, the "pounding" heart rate sometimes heard in cattle with endocarditis, and displacement of the heart to a position closer to the thoracic wall by a diaphragmatic hernia or an abscess or tumor in the contralateral hemithorax. "Muffling," or decreased intensity of heart sounds, may occur for relative reasons such as the increased thickness or fat on the chest wall of adult bulls or heavily conditioned

cattle. Muffling also results from pathologic conditions such as pericarditis, pneumomediastinum, diaphragmatic hernia, and displacement of the heart toward the opposite hemithorax by an abscess or tumor in the hemithorax being auscultated. Cattle in shock may have either decreased or increased intensity of heart sounds, depending on the duration and severity of the condition. Whereas "shocky" cows that are weak but still ambulatory tend to have increased intensity of heart sounds, those that are recumbent or moribund have decreased intensity.

Auscultation combined with percussion provides the best subjective means to estimate the position and size of the heart. Heart sounds may radiate over a wider area than normal when transmitted by consolidated lung lobes or pleural fluid or when there is cardiac enlargement.

In calves and thin adult cattle, palpation of the apex beat is possible around the left fourth or fifth ICS at a level halfway between the elbow and shoulder. Palpation of an apex beat on the right side of adult cattle seldom is possible unless profound cardiac disease or displacement of the heart to the right by space-occupying masses has occurred. Deep palpation with the fingertips over the intercostal regions overlying the heart may elicit a painful response in conditions such as endocarditis, pleuritis, traumatic reticulopericarditis, and rib fractures.

As in other species, bovine heart murmurs are classified based on intensity and timing. Intensity may be ranked subjectively on a 1 to 6 basis, with 1 of 6 being a faint, barely detectable murmur; 2 of 6 a soft but easily discernible murmur; 3 of 6 a low to moderate intensity murmur; 4 of 6 moderate in intensity but lacking a thrill; 5 of 6 a loud murmur with a palpable thrill; and 6 of 6 so loud that it can be heard with the stethoscope off the chest and evincing a palpable thrill. Classification relative to timing of the cardiac cycle further defines murmurs as systolic, diastolic, or continuous. Further division is provided by terms such as "early systolic" or "holosystolic." In general, whereas systolic murmurs in cattle reflect AV valve insufficiency or, much less commonly, aortic or pulmonic stenosis, diastolic murmurs reflect aortic or pulmonic valve insufficiency or rarely AV valve abnormalities. Benign systolic murmurs occasionally are heard in excited, tachycardic calves, or cows with anemia, hypoproteinemia, or in those being given rapid intravenous (IV) infusions of fluids. Pathologic systolic murmurs most commonly are found in calves with congenital heart abnormalities such as VSD or tetralogy of Fallot and in adult cows with endocarditis. Continuous murmurs are rare but may be encountered in calves having a patent ductus arteriosus or in cows with pericarditis. The point of maximal intensity for each cardiac murmur may add subjective data as to the valve involved in the cardiac abnormality.

Arrhythmias may be benign, pathologic, or secondary to metabolic disturbances in cattle. Sinus bradycardia and arrhythmia have been confirmed in cattle held off feed, in hypercalcemic adult cattle, and in hypoglycemic or hyperkalemic young calves. Sinus tachycardia may result from excitement, pain, hypocalcemia, and various systemic states such as endotoxemia and shock. Cattle with severe musculoskeletal pain often have normal heart rates while recumbent but have tachycardia when forced to rise and stand. Persistent tachycardia should be considered abnormal and may reflect cardiac disease unless other systemic or painful conditions coexist.

Hyperkalemia may cause a variety of arrhythmias and is most commonly observed in neonatal calves that develop acute metabolic acidosis associated with secretory diarrhea caused by *Escherichia coli* or acute diffuse white muscle disease. Atrial standstill and other arrhythmias have been documented in diarrheic calves having metabolic acidosis and hyperkalemia. Extreme hyperkalemia (>7.0 mEq/L) may lead to cardiac arrest and should be corrected immediately, especially in calves that may require general anesthesia. Because severe hyperkalemia may be associated with pathologic bradycardias, even without confirmatory blood work, the experienced clinician should be alert to the therapeutic need for fluids that will specifically address hyperkalemia in severely dehydrated, diarrheic calves with discordantly low heart rates for their systemic state. Calves with white muscle disease also may have direct damage to the myocardium, which may be manifested by arrhythmias, murmurs, or frank cardiac arrest. Hypokalemia and hypochloremia in cattle with metabolic alkalosis may predispose to the most common arrhythmia of adult cattle—atrial fibrillation.

Hypocalcemia may be present, or contribute to, cattle having abdominal disorders that lead to metabolic alkalosis. Metabolic alkalosis may be a factor that triggers atrial fibrillation in cattle with normal hearts. Atrial fibrillation causes an irregularly irregular rhythm, with a rate that may be normal or increased (88–140 beats/min), depending on the presence of heart disease or the underlying predisposing condition. Atrial fibrillation is associated with irregular intensity of heart sounds. A pulse deficit may be present in any cow with a rapid or irregular cardiac rhythm, especially when the rate exceeds 120 beats/min. Atrial premature complexes (APCs) may also occur in cows with gastrointestinal (GI) disease and electrolyte abnormalities. APCs may precede or immediately follow atrial fibrillation in some cows. Variation in intensity of the first heart sound during auscultation is characteristic of APCs.

Other causes of arrhythmia in adult cattle include cases of lymphosarcoma with significant myocardial infiltration often causing atrial fibrillation, and ventricular or atrial arrhythmias associated with septic or toxic myocarditis. Intravenous administration of calcium solutions is the major drug-related cause of arrhythmias in cattle, but IV administration of antibiotics or potassium-rich fluids occasionally prompts transient arrhythmias.

Sounds auscultated in patients with pericarditis are variable, often confused with murmurs of valvular origin, and tend to change on a daily basis if affected cattle are available for repeated evaluation. Classic pericardial "friction" rubs occur at different stages of each cardiac cycle unlike murmurs, which tend to occur at a distinct, repeatable, phase of each cardiac cycle. Squeaky sounds, often similar to those made in compression of a wet sponge, may also be heard as a result

of pericardial disease. Rubbing sounds caused by contact between fibrin on the visceral and parietal pericardium also may be heard. The heart sounds tend to be muffled, and either free fluid or fluid–gas interfaces may lead to splashing or tinkling sounds or to complete muffling of all sounds. During the acute phase of traumatic reticulopericarditis, the character of the sounds tends to change each day. In those with subacute or chronic disease, muffling of the heart sounds or distinct tinkling or splashing tend to be more consistently present.

Presence of an arrhythmia or murmur alerts the examiner that the heart may be abnormal. However, heart failure may or may not be present. In cattle, right heart failure is more common than left heart failure. The general signs of right heart failure include:

1. Ventral edema—the edema may be diffuse or limited to specific regions such as the submandibular area, brisket, ventral abdomen, udder or sheath, and the lower limbs (Fig. 3.2).
2. Jugular and mammary vein distention with or without pulsations (Fig. 3.3)
3. Exercise intolerance with or without dyspnea
4. Persistent tachycardia
5. Ascites with or without pleural fluid (Fig. 3.4)

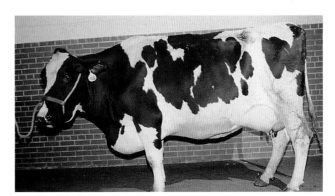

• **Fig. 3.2** Submandibular, brisket, ventral, and udder edema in a cow in right heart failure caused by pericarditis.

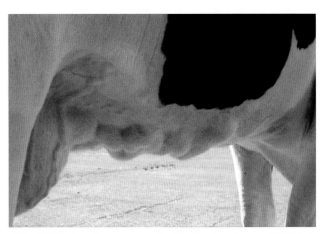

• **Fig. 3.3** Profound mammary vein distention in a 4-year-old Holstein cow with congestive heart failure caused by tricuspid and aortic valve endocarditis. The cow had been markedly hypogalactic for several weeks before this image was taken.

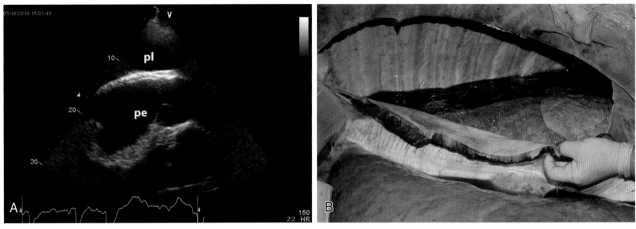

• **Fig. 3.4 A,** Pleural effusion (pl) in addition to pericardial effusion (pe) in a 6-year-old Holstein cow with idiopathic hemorrhagic pericardial effusion and congestive heart failure caused by cardiac tamponade. **B,** Intrathoracic view at postmortem of the same patient demonstrating extravagant pleural fluid.

In addition to the general signs, specific cardiac signs such as a murmur, arrhythmia, or abnormal intensity of heart sounds usually are present and contribute to the diagnosis. Probably the most difficult set of differential diagnoses involves those diseases that result in hypoproteinemia. Hypoproteinemia also causes ventral edema and may cause exercise intolerance and tachycardia. However, hypoproteinemia would not cause jugular and mammary vein distention and pulsation. Therefore, venous distention and pulsation coupled with abnormal heart sounds or rhythm are the key signs when diagnosing heart failure in dairy cattle.

Left heart failure causes dyspnea, pulmonary edema, and exercise intolerance and may lead to cyanosis and collapse or syncope. Specific left heart failure seldom occurs in cattle, but left side failure combined with worsening, antecedent right heart failure may develop as the animal progresses into fulminant congestive heart failure.

Ancillary Procedures

Electrocardiography

The electrocardiogram (ECG) is essential for definitive categorization of arrhythmias in cattle. Vector analysis of ECG tracings to determine cardiac chamber enlargements and other pathology seldom is used in cattle because ventricular myocardial depolarization tends to be rapid and diffuse rather than organized, as in some other species. ECG is also indicated when cattle have variation in heart sound intensity, require monitoring for anesthesia or treatment of cardiac arrhythmias, or show signs of heart failure. Cardiac ultrasonography, however, has largely superseded the ECG as a diagnostic tool in determining chamber enlargement and other cardiac pathology.

The base-apex lead system is most commonly used in cattle. The base-apex lead system results in an ECG with large wave amplitude and is sufficient for evaluating most arrhythmias. The positive electrode is placed on the skin over the left fifth ICS at the level of the elbow, the negative electrode is placed on the skin over the right jugular furrow roughly 30 cm from the thoracic inlet, and the ground

electrode is attached to the neck or withers. The resultant ECG recorded through the base-apex lead system has a positive P wave with a single peak, a QRS complex with an initial positive deflection followed by a large negative deflection, and a variable (positive or negative) T wave (Fig. 3.5).

Echocardiography

Two-dimensional echocardiography and Doppler echocardiography have greatly enhanced our ability to assess cardiac function and visualize anatomic variations and pathologic lesions in cattle. Valvular, myocardial, pericardial, congenital, and acquired lesions can be visualized in real time, measured, and monitored. Qualitative and quantitative assessments of the impact of congenital anomalies and monitoring treatment response of endocarditis, pericarditis, or myocardial lesions are possible with the appropriate equipment and people trained to conduct and interpret a systematic cardiac examination. In short, echocardiography is now an essential component of a full cardiology workup.

Echocardiography for the Evaluation of Heart Disease Detection in Dairy Cattle

Bovine cardiac diseases are most commonly diagnosed when the condition is already advanced and production outcomes have already been affected (decreased milk production, poor reproductive performance, diminished appetite, weight loss or altered growth). The diagnosis of heart disease may be clinically difficult until overt signs of heart failure occur (e.g., peripheral edema, distended jugular veins, or true jugular pulse). However, some cardiac diseases such as endocarditis and VSD may be less commonly associated with clinical signs of heart failure. Routine cardiac auscultation also has its limitations, especially under noisy field conditions or in adults with high body condition score. For these reasons, ancillary tests may be extremely valuable in reaching the definitive diagnosis and to facilitate appropriate case management. Transthoracic echocardiography (TTE) is becoming more available and more readily accessible on farms because of improvements in ultrasound quality, affordability,

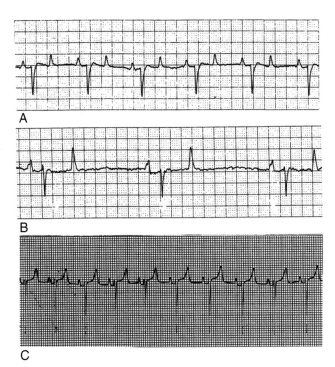

• **Fig. 3.5** **A,** Normal sinus rhythm with a heart rate of 60 beats/min recorded from a 4-year-old Holstein cow. **B,** Sinus bradycardia with heart rate of 36 beats/min recorded from a 6-year-old Brown Swiss cow sick with abomasal ulcers. **C,** Sinus tachycardia with heart rate of 108 beats/min recorded from a 2-year-old Holstein cow with an acute leg injury.

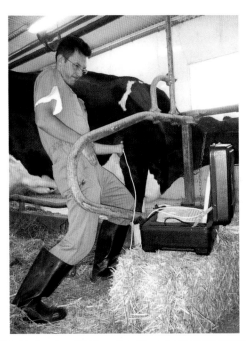

• **Fig. 3.6** Performing right transthoracic echocardiography in a farm setting. The probe is placed cranially between the thorax and right forelimb to access the third to fifth ventral intercostal spaces.

and portability. This imaging technique has the potential to help practitioners reach a definitive diagnosis antemortem, therefore improving case management. Importantly, it can help avoid unnecessary treatments if the prognosis is hopeless as well as differentiate life-threatening conditions (pericarditis secondary to hardware disease) from more benign ones (idiopathic hemorrhagic pericarditis). By contrast with other veterinary species (small animals, horses) in which echocardiographic examination now entails precise calculations of various functional indices or dimensions and can require extensive postgraduate training and expensive equipment and software, bovine echocardiography does not. A great deal of information can be obtained when one knows which views are needed and how to get them. Several of the common cardiac conditions of dairy calves and adult cattle have characteristic ultrasonographic features, and when a veterinarian has become somewhat familiar with the likely image findings for each, a definitive diagnosis can often be reached. Practically speaking, a complete echocardiographic examination can be performed on the farm in about 15 to 20 minutes.

Echocardiographic Technique: Adults and Calves

Transthoracic echocardiography is usually best performed with the individual standing and restrained by a halter. An assistant may also be useful depending on the patient's demeanor to keep the thoracic limb forward during the examination to improve access to the cardiac window on the side in question. The author (SB) generally prefers to put his own leg medial to the forelimb in order to perform a gentle abduction of the cow's limb; this often helps in obtaining better quality images

(Fig. 3.6). TTE is classically performed using "cardiac windows" composed of the ventral third to fifth ICSs on both the right and left sides of the thorax. Ideally, the area is clipped, and ultrasonographic coupling gel is applied. Depending on the context of the examination, a faster technique may be achieved by applying 70% isopropyl alcohol directly to the unclipped skin surface without coupling gel. The author has used this technique increasingly to good effect in recent years. It has the advantage of avoiding unnecessary clipping if there is a high likelihood of sale or culling in the near future and is also more popular with owners of individually valuable cattle during show season! Hair length and body condition (chest wall thickness) can both interfere with the diagnostic quality of images when only alcohol is used. A low-frequency probe (≤3.5 MHz) with good penetration (examination depth >20 cm) is required for adult cows. For calves, a 5 MHz probe is usually adequate because of the smaller size of the thorax. The major limiting factor in performing TTE is the size and shape of the probe compared with the width and accessibility of the relevant intercostal spaces. Many cattle, even those without painful chest walls, resent examination under the elbow and into the axillae, tending to respond by powerful, counterproductive forelimb adduction as the examiner moves the probe forward. Probe rotation, necessary to obtain the standard views, is often challenging, especially in the more cranial ICSs. The phased-array probes (specifically used for echocardiography and therefore more expensive) are optimal; larger sector probes also work quite well but may have limitations for some of the views described in the following section.

Most Important Echocardiographic Views

The views obtained from the right side are generally the most informative, and the examination should always begin on this side. In the author's experience, the long-axis views are the most informative and the easiest to recognize. The four-chamber long-axis view is obtained when applying the transducer parallel to the fourth ICS. This view allows observation of the two ventricles and atria as well as the AV valves (Fig. 3.7). A slight clockwise rotation of the transducer allows observation of the left ventricular outflow tract (LVOT) view. This view is of particular value when aortic problems are suspected and for visualization of the membranous part of the interventricular septum (IVS) (Fig. 3.8) which may be absent or incomplete in cases of VSD.

Continuing the rotation of the probe clockwise or movement of the transducer to the third ICS is necessary to

observe the right ventricular outflow tract (RVOT). This view is required to evaluate the pulmonary valve and pulmonary trunk (Fig. 3.9). If needed, the probe can be applied perpendicular to the ICS to obtain short-axis views of the heart. However, from a practical standpoint, these views are often not very informative. Views from the left side are of special interest when left heart lesions (e.g., mitral valve anomalies) are suspected. The author does not use these views invariably but only when the right-sided views are inconclusive.

Biochemical Assessment of Cardiac Disease

Although rarely analyzed in ambulatory practice, there have been a number of publications in recent years on the use of cardiac biomarkers for the assessment of myocardial injury in the hospital setting. Borrowing from human cardiology in which cardiac troponins have become an essential part of point-of-care assessment in the management of chest pain and the diagnostic and prognostic data set for myocardial ischemia patients, it is appealing to think that there might be similar value to the measurement of cardiac troponin I (cTnI) in cattle with physical examination or ancillary diagnostic findings suggestive of acute cardiac disease. The obvious difference in prevalence of acute myocardial ischemia between cattle and humans means that the number one indication for cTnI measurement in human patients will never be duplicated in cattle. However, bovine cTnI has been examined in association with congenital heart defects in calves, experimental monensin toxicosis, and a variety of primary cardiac conditions such as endocarditis and pericarditis, as well as in dairy cattle with common, noncardiac production diseases. In each of these published studies, commercial human immunoassays were used, and although different manufacturers' kits have been used in different studies, there is a great deal of structural homology between cTnI among mammalian species, suggesting that these

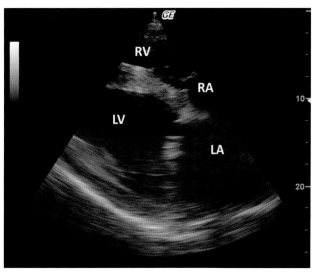

• **Fig. 3.7** Four-chamber long-axis view. This view allows visualization of the two ventricles (LV and RV), the two atria (RA and LA), and the two atrioventricular valves. The thickness of the mitral valve is often difficult to assess from the right because of distortion at such a high depth.

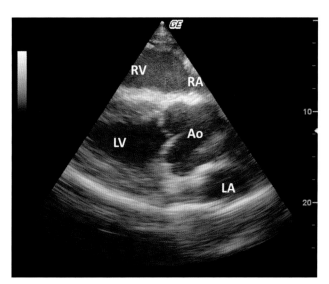

• **Fig. 3.8** Left ventricular outflow tract (LVOT) long-axis view. This view allows visualization of the two ventricles (LV and RV), the two atria (LA and RA), the aortic root (Ao) and the aortic valve. This is the best diagnostic view when one suspects a ventricular septal defect.

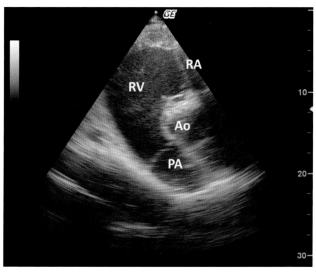

• **Fig. 3.9** Right ventricular outflow tract (RVOT) long-axis view. This view is of particular importance to assess the pulmonic valve, pulmonary artery (PA), right ventricle (RV), right atrium (RA), and aorta (Ao).

assays would very likely accurately detect the bovine protein. Consequently, a normal reference range of 0 to 0.05 ng/mL has been suggested in healthy, lactating dairy cattle when a widely available, handheld point-of-care analyzer was used. Other studies have suggested an upper cutoff point of 0.08 ng/mL when a different, laboratory-based immunoassay was used. Cattle with severe, acute myocardial injury, such as that caused by ionophore toxicosis, show marked increases in cTnI to greater than 1 ng/mL over a 1- to 6-day interval after a single, massive overdose. This quantitative increase is paralleled by echocardiographic, electrocardiographic, and histopathologic evidence of marked myocardial necrosis and cardiac dysfunction. Other studies looking at congenital cardiac defects and acquired cardiac conditions of adulthood (pericarditis and endocarditis) have also demonstrated elevations above normal controls, but there is no useful prognostic information in cattle at this point that can be extrapolated from these data. Other, noncardiac primary intrathoracic diseases, such as pneumonia, and noncardiac intrathoracic abscessation, can also be associated with occasional spikes in measured cTnI. In conclusion, although one can identify acute bovine myocardial injury with the use of cTnI measurement, we are currently uncertain of the kinetics of release and half-life of the released protein and how to prognostically interpret single time point values. The half-life of cTnI is very short in other species eg., one hour in the horse.

Specific Cardiac Diseases in Calves

White Muscle Disease

Myocardial damage from vitamin E and selenium deficiency may occur at any site in the heart and may be focal, multifocal, or diffuse (Fig. 3.10). Signs may develop at any time from birth to 4 years of age but are more common in calves younger than 3 months of age. Specific cardiac signs are variable and include arrhythmias, persistent tachycardia, murmurs, exercise intolerance, cyanosis, dyspnea, congestive heart failure signs, and acute death. Signs may be subtle

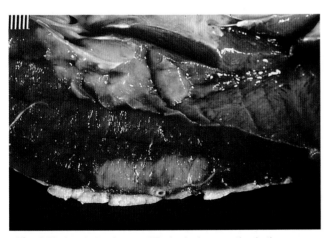

• **Fig. 3.10** A pale focal area of Zenker's degeneration in the myocardium of a calf that died of diffuse white muscle disease.

or dramatic, depending on the magnitude and location of myocardial damage. Sudden death can occur spontaneously, after exercise or even following mere restraint. Other signs of white muscle disease such as stiffness, difficulty in prehension or swallowing, inhalation pneumonia, recumbency, and myoglobinuria may or may not be present. Dyspnea may be directly related to the cardiac lesions or may be caused by Zenker's degeneration in the diaphragm or intercostal muscles. Tachycardia (>120 beats/min) and arrhythmias are the most common specific cardiac signs, but murmurs may be present as well.

Diagnosis can be confirmed by measuring blood selenium values, urine dipstick testing to look for positive "blood" (myoglobin) and protein, and serum biochemistry to evaluate creatine kinase (CK) and aspartate aminotransferase (AST) enzymes. When diagnostic blood samples are obtained after parenteral selenium supplementation, antecedent deficiency can still be confirmed by assaying levels of the enzyme glutathione peroxidase. If the heart is the only muscle involved, serum muscle enzymes may not be greatly elevated; however, the heart seldom is the only "muscle" involved. Because of the necrosis involving the myocardium, acute cases would be expected to have elevated cTnI values.

Treatment should be instituted immediately with vitamin E and selenium injected at the manufacturer's recommended dosage. Although some commercial preparations include label instructions that include IV use, it is suggested that vitamin E and selenium be given intramuscularly (IM) or subcutaneously (SC) to avoid the occasional life-threatening anaphylactic-type reaction seen with these products. The calf should be kept in a small box stall, straw bale enclosure, or hutch so it can move about but not run freely, lest further muscle damage be precipitated. If pulmonary edema is present, furosemide (0.5–1.0 mg/kg) may be given once or twice daily. Concurrent aspiration pneumonia would require intense antibiotic therapy. Vitamin E and selenium injections are repeated at 72-hour intervals for three or four total treatments. Herd selenium status and preventive measures to address the problem should be discussed. Calves that survive for 3 days after diagnosis have a good prognosis.

Hyperkalemia

Cardiac arrhythmias or bradycardia associated with hyperkalemia are primarily observed in neonates having severe, acute diarrhea. Enterotoxigenic *E. coli* causing secretory diarrhea, metabolic acidosis, low plasma bicarbonate values, and hyperkalemia appears to be the most common causative organism. Rotavirus or coronavirus also may be involved in calf diarrhea, but they seldom produce as profound a metabolic acidosis as *E. coli* during the first few days of life.

Less common causes of hyperkalemia include severe diffuse white muscle disease involving heavy musculature of the limbs, ruptured bladders or urachal remnants leading to uroperitoneum, renal failure, urinary obstructions, and nonspecific shock.

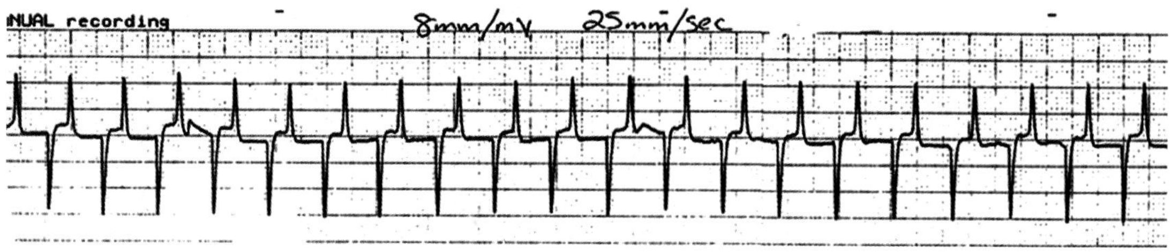

NUAL recording   8mm/mV 25mm/sec

• **Fig. 3.11** Base-apex lead electrocardiographic recording in a calf with a K$^+$ of 8.6 mEq/L. Despite the tachycardia of 130 beats/min, the peaked T waves and flattening of the P waves is very apparent.

Hyperkalemia reduces the resting membrane potential, which initially makes cells more excitable, but gradually (with further elevation in potassium and further reduction in resting membrane potential), the cells become less excitable. Atrial myocytes seem more sensitive to these effects than those within the ventricles. Cardiac conduction is affected, and several characteristic ECG findings evolve in a typical sequence that correlates well with increasing K$^+$ values: ECG changes include peaking of the T wave, shortening and widening of the P wave, prolongation of the PR interval, eventual disappearance of the P wave, widening of the QRS complex, and irregular R-R intervals (Fig. 3.11). Atrial standstill characterized by bradycardia and absence of P waves may occur and has been documented in association with hyperkalemia in diarrheic calves. Further progression may lead to AV block, escape beats, ventricular fibrillation, asystole, and death.

In neonates, hypoglycemia is the major differential diagnosis when bradycardia is present. Septic myocarditis or white muscle disease also may be considered if an arrhythmia is present.

Calves younger than 2 weeks of age that have developed acute diarrhea, are recumbent, dehydrated, and have bradycardia or arrhythmia should be suspected of being hyperkalemic. Obviously only an acid–base and electrolyte analysis and an ECG can confirm this. However, these may not be available in the field. The consequences of underestimating the life-threatening relationship between such elevated K$^+$ levels and pathologic bradycardia in patients are dire.

Calves suspected to be hyperkalemic based on history, physical signs, and arrhythmia or bradycardia, should receive alkalinizing fluids and dextrose. Being neonates, hypoglycemia may contribute to bradycardia when this sign is present. One way to treat metabolic acidosis and hyperkalemia is by IV infusions of 5% dextrose solution containing 150-300 mEq NaHCO$_3$/L. Usually 1 to 3 L is necessary, depending on the magnitude of the metabolic acidosis and bicarbonate deficit. Glucose and bicarbonate help transport K$^+$ back into cells, and the glucose also treats or prevents potential hypoglycemia. After the acute crisis has been resolved, the calf may be safely treated with balanced electrolyte solutions containing potassium. Calves with diarrhea, despite having plasma hyperkalemia, have total body potassium deficits and require potassium supplementation. This may be true even in the acute phase of disease, but when serum K$^+$ is 5.0 to 8.0 mEq/L, this is not the time

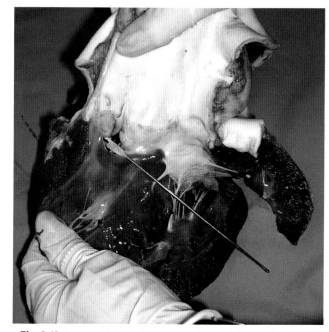

• **Fig. 3.12** Image obtained at necropsy of a calf with ventricular septal defect.

to worry about a "total-body potassium deficit." We have treated hundreds of calves as suggested earlier, and those with a venous blood pH of 7.0 or greater have a good to excellent prognosis unless they have had failure of passive transfer of immunoglobulins and subsequent septicemia. Specific insulin therapy as an adjunct to bicarbonate and glucose to correct hyperkalemia is not necessary in calves.

Congenital Heart Disease

Virtually all forms of congenital cardiac anomaly occur in cattle. Most congenital anomalies appear to be sporadic, but inheritance may play a part in some of the most common malformations. Large retrospective studies indicate that congenital cardiac defects occur in approximately 0.2% of all bovine hearts. The most common congenital anomalies in cattle appear to be VSDs (Fig. 3.12), tetralogy of Fallot, atrial septal defects (ASDs) (Fig. 3.13), and transpositions of the great vessels.

Most congenital cardiac defects cause distinct murmurs. Calves affected with the most common defects such as VSDs, ASDs, tetralogy of Fallot, or aortic or pulmonic stenosis usually have systolic murmurs. Patent ductus arteriosus

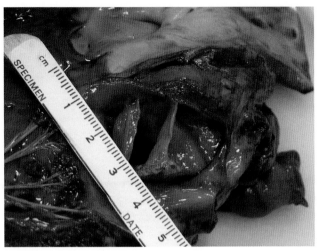

• **Fig. 3.13** Large atrial septic defect in a 3-day-old Holstein calf with multiple congenital heart defects.

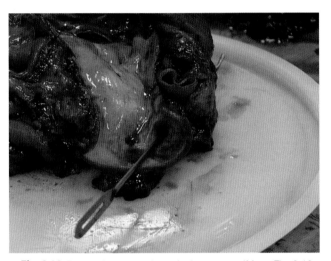

• **Fig. 3.14** Patent ductus arteriosus in the same calf from Fig. 3.13.

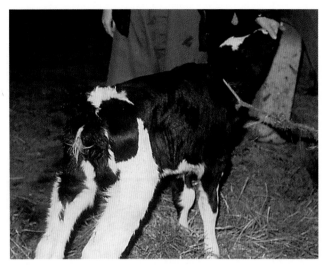

• **Fig. 3.15** Congenital absence of the tail in a 1-day-old Holstein heifer that also had a ventricular septal defect.

(Fig. 3.14), which is rare as a single defect in calves, can cause a systolic or continuous murmur.

Most calves with congenital cardiac defects appear normal at birth but eventually are noticed to have dyspnea, poor growth, or both. Many calves with congenital heart defects are eventually examined by a veterinarian because of persistent or recurrent respiratory signs or generalized ill thrift. The respiratory signs may be real in the form of pulmonary edema associated with heart failure and shunts or be caused by opportunistic bacterial pneumonia secondary to pulmonary edema and compromise of lower airway defense mechanisms. The owners may already have treated the calf one or more times for coughing, dyspnea, and fever, only to have the signs recur. Usually only one calf is affected, thus making enzootic pneumonia an unlikely diagnosis. Regardless of whether pulmonary edema or pneumonia plus pulmonary edema is present, veterinary examination usually detects tachycardia and the cardiac murmur that allows diagnosis. Venous pulsation and distention of the jugular veins may be present, but calves seldom show ventral edema as distinctly as adult cattle with heart failure.

Calves with congenital heart defects that do not develop respiratory signs usually still show stunting compared with herdmates of matched age. The degree of stunting varies directly with the severity of the congenital lesions in regard to blood oxygenation but usually becomes apparent by 6 months of age and is very dramatic in calves that survive to yearlings. Some cattle with small defects survive and thrive as adults, but this is rare.

Ventricular septal defects are the most common defects in dairy calves and are found in all breeds. In Guernseys and Holsteins, VSD may be linked to ocular and tail anomalies. Microphthalmos and tail defects, including absence of the tail, wry tail, or short tail, frequently signal VSD (Fig. 3.15). Sometimes ocular, tail, and cardiac defects all are present in the same calf, but it is more common to find either tail or ocular pathology plus VSD. Depending on the size of the VSD, affected calves have a variable life span. Prognosis for most is hopeless because of eventual respiratory difficulty and stunting. However, calves do, in rare instances, survive to productive adult states. The genetics of these multiple defects (eye, tail, and heart) have not been investigated in Holsteins but have been assumed to be a simple recessive trait in Guernseys.

Echocardiography is of particular value in the characterization of congenital cardiac disease. VSDs are preferentially located on the membranous part of the IVS (i.e., close to the aortic valve). For this reason, when performing echocardiography in neonates, it is important to obtain the LVOT view from the right side to correctly scan this area and observe the defect (Figs. 3.16 and 3.17 and Video Clip 3.3). The size of the defect (<2.5 cm) and velocity of blood flow through the defect (>4 m/s) have been mentioned as positive prognostic factors in horses, but no specific comparable study has been performed in cattle. More complex congenital defects such as tetralogy of Fallot may be more challenging to characterize echocardiographically without the help of an experienced operator. ASDs are less common than VSDs but are similarly identifiable from the right side (Fig. 3.18 and Video Clip 3.4).

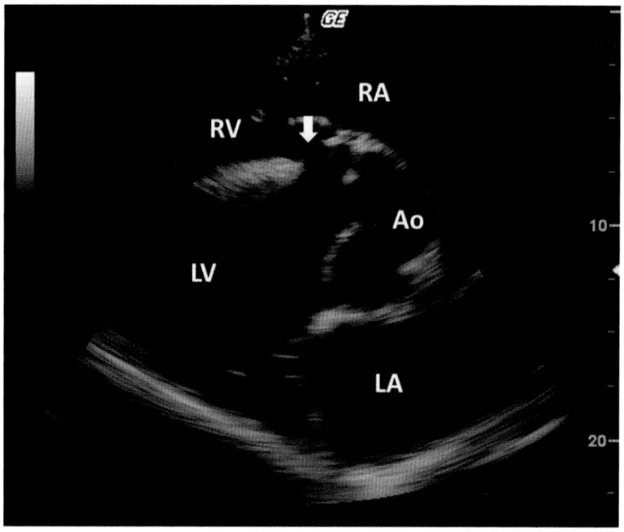

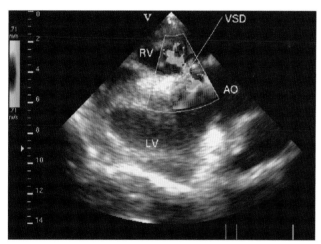

• **Fig. 3.16** Ventricular septal defect in a Holstein heifer, 10 days in milk presented with decreased milk production. The right long-axis left ventricular outflow tract view allows assessment of the membranous part of the interventricular septum. The defect *(arrow)* is observed immediately ventral to the aortic valve. *Ao,* Aorta; *LA,* left atrium; *LV,* left ventricle; *RA,* right atrium; *RV,* right ventricle.

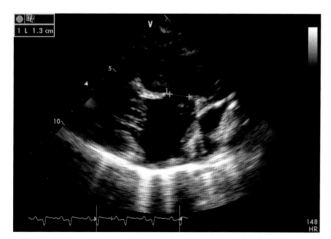

• **Fig. 3.17** Echocardiogram of heifer calf with congenital ventricular septal defect (VSD). *AO,* Aorta; *LV,* left ventricle; *RV,* right ventricle.

• **Fig. 3.18** Right parasternal long-axis echocardiogram of 2-week-old Holstein calf presented for dyspnea and exercise intolerance. Calipers delineate a large atrial septal defect. (Courtesy of Dr. Rebecca Stepien.)

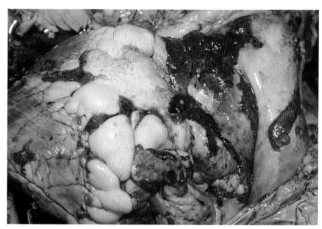

• **Fig. 3.19** Lymphosarcoma in the heart of a cow that died as a result of multicentric lymphosarcoma. Multifocal areas of yellow-red friable tumor infiltrate are present scattered over the epicardium, great vessels, and right atrium.

Tetralogy of Fallot and other multiple congenital defects that allow right-to-left shunting of blood provoke marked exercise intolerance, cyanosis, and dyspnea and may lead to polycythemia secondary to hypoxia. The prognosis for long-term survival is grave in these calves. Ectopia cordis in a calf creates a dramatic sight, with the heart beating under the skin in the neck, but is extremely rare.

Specific Cardiac Diseases in Adult Cattle

Neoplasia

The heart is one of the common target sites of lymphosarcoma in adult dairy cattle. Many cattle with multicentric lymphosarcoma have cardiac infiltration based on gross or histologic pathology, but fewer of these cattle have clinically detectable cardiac disease. When the heart is a major target site, cardiac abnormalities are more obvious. The heart may be the only organ affected with lymphosarcoma. Therefore, detection of cardiac abnormalities coupled with other suspicious lesions (e.g., enlarged peripheral lymph nodes, exophthalmos, melena, and paresis) simply helps to make a lymphosarcoma diagnosis more definite.

Depending on the anatomic location and magnitude of the tumors, cattle with cardiac lymphosarcoma may have arrhythmias, murmurs, jugular venous distention, jugular venous pulsations, or muffling caused by diffuse cardiac or pericardial involvement. Muffling and splashing sounds are possible if a pericardial transudate or exudate is present. The most common site of tumor involvement is the right atrium, but nodular or infiltrative tumors can be found anywhere in the myocardium, pericardium, or epicardium (Figs. 3.19 to 3.21). The color and consistency of the tumors may vary. Mediastinal lymph nodes also are commonly involved. Cattle with signs of heart disease should be thoroughly examined for other lesions consistent with lymphosarcoma. When multiple lesions exist, the diagnosis is easy. However, cattle examined because of vague signs such as hypophagia

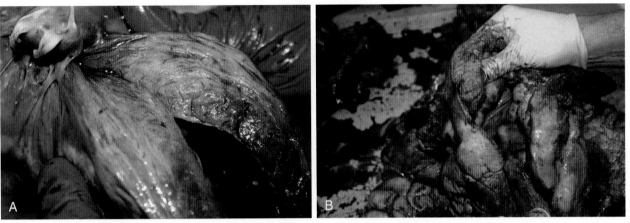

• **Fig. 3.20 A,** Right atrial myocardial infiltration by lymphosarcoma. Note the pale infiltrative neoplasia within atrial wall. **B,** More expansile and proliferative infiltrate within the atrial wall.

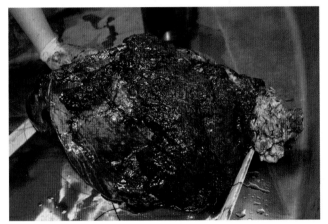

• **Fig. 3.21** Extensive epicardial infiltration by lymphosarcoma in a 7-year-old Holstein cow with a history of idiopathic hemorrhagic pericardial effusion. Note cardiac enlargement caused by congestive heart failure.

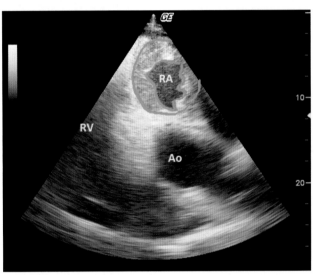

• **Fig. 3.22** Cardiac lymphosarcoma and right atrial thickening (right ventricular outflow tract view). The thickened and irregular atrial wall is surrounded by blue lines. The cow also presented with a homogenous, anechoic pericardial effusion. Pericardiocentesis and cytology confirmed the neoplastic etiology. *Ao,* Aorta; *RA,* right atrium; *RV,* right ventricle.

and decreased milk production that are found to have tachycardia or other cardiac abnormalities can present diagnostic challenges. Although ECGs and thoracic radiographs have seldom helped make a definitive diagnosis, echocardiography may be very helpful to image nodular or large masses of lymphosarcoma. Common echocardiographic findings include varying degrees of pericardial effusion that usually cannot be accurately distinguished from other causes of pericardial effusion by appearance alone (e.g., needs to be confirmed by pericardiocentesis) or the presence of a mass effect in the right atrial wall or atrial wall thickening (Fig. 3.22). In the case of a mass in the right atrial wall, the other important differential diagnosis would be mural endocarditis, although this is very uncommon. Thoracocentesis and pericardiocentesis to obtain fluid for cytologic evaluation are the most helpful ancillary aids when cardiac lymphosarcoma is suspected (Fig. 3.23). A complete blood count (CBC) and assessment of bovine leukemia virus (BLV) antibody status are indicated, but a positive BLV agar gel immunodiffusion (AGID), enzyme-linked immunosorbent assay (ELISA), or polymerase chain reaction (PCR) test does not ensure an absolute diagnosis because most positive cattle never develop

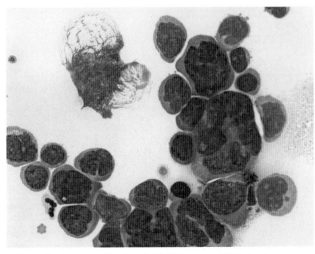

• **Fig. 3.23** Cytology of pericardial fluid from an adult Holstein cow with epicardial lymphosarcoma demonstrating lymphoblasts.

tumors (see the section on lymphosarcoma in Chapter 16). Therefore, simply assuming a cow with a positive BLV test and heart abnormality detected on physical examination has lymphosarcoma may be an incorrect assumption. A double line-positive BLV-AGID may add further weight to the suspected diagnosis, as would the finding of a persistent lymphocytosis (PL) in a CBC. Clinical identification of masses in other locations or cytology from thoracocentesis or pericardiocentesis provides the best means of definitive diagnosis. If both pleural and pericardial effusions can be identified, then pericardiocentesis will often provide a greater chance of identifying exfoliated neoplastic cells in cases of cardiac lymphosarcoma because pleural fluid accumulation may just reflect a transudate associated with poor cardiac function.

Fever usually is absent in cattle with cardiac lymphosarcoma. Occasionally, cattle with large tumor masses in the thorax or abdomen may have fever because of tumor necrosis or nonspecific pyrogens produced by the neoplasms. Secondary bacterial infections of the lungs or other body systems also may lead to fever, which confuses the diagnosis.

The prognosis is hopeless for cattle with cardiac lymphosarcoma, and most cattle with the disease die from cardiac or multisystemic disease within a few weeks to a few months. Successful attempts at chemotherapy have not been reported to our knowledge. One of the contributors (SB) has successfully prolonged life for up to 6 months in a few cattle with cardiac lymphosarcoma by intermittent pericardial drainage. Occasionally, valuable cattle may justify such treatment to allow a pregnancy to be completed or to be superovulated. However, as with many catabolic conditions, owners should be cautioned that maintaining the dam with advanced heart disease for more than a few weeks may produce a gestationally dysmature fetus even if the pregnancy is carried to term or may seriously affect the cow's ability to superovulate or even produce viable oocytes for in vitro fertilization. There is also the risk of vertical transmission of BLV from dam to fetus in utero, which is greater if the dam has clinically apparent tumors. In one late pregnant cow with severe pericardial effusion caused by lymphosarcoma, we were able to maintain the cow for several weeks by surgically opening the pericardial sac into the pleural cavity, which significantly improved venous return to the heart and the overall condition of the cow, permitting delivery of a healthy calf. The cow was also treated with isoflupredone.

Neurofibroma, although uncommon, frequently causes arrhythmia and variable intensity of heart sounds in affected cattle and bulls. Furthermore, the cardiac arrhythmia may coexist with paresis or paralysis caused by neurofibroma masses in the spinal canal. Because lymphosarcoma more commonly causes paresis coupled with cardiac disease, this combination of signs is more suggestive that lymphosarcoma is present. Although perhaps a moot point because both diseases are fatal, further medical workup of patients with neurofibroma fails to provide confirmation of lymphosarcoma. To date, postmortem examination has been the only means of definitive diagnosis for cardiac neurofibroma. Examiners talented in ultrasonography may be able to diagnose these lesions based on the typically gnarled, raised cords of tumor involving the cardiac nerves. One of the authors (SP) has also seen a single case of a neuroendocrine tumor (chemodectoma) in an adult bull, which presented with signs of congestive heart failure associated with a massive, hemorrhagic pericardial effusion and tamponade (Fig. 3.24).

Myocardial Disease

Infections

Septic Myocarditis

Neonatal septicemia caused by gram-negative bacterial organisms, acute infection with *Histophilus somni*, and chronic infections in any age of cattle resulting from *Trueperella pyogenes* are the most common cause of septic myocardial lesions in cattle. Septicemic calves, calves suspected of having

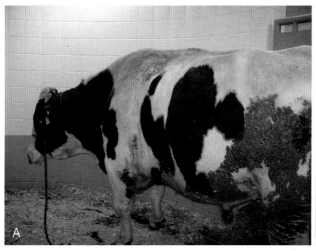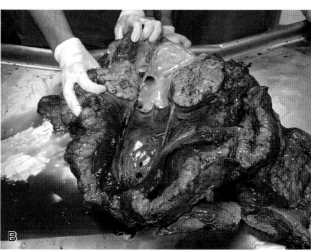

• **Fig. 3.24 A,** Mature Holstein bull presented with signs of cardiac tamponade caused by hemopericardium associated with a large heart base neuroendocrine tumor (chemodectoma). **B,** Gross postmortem image showing the large heart base tumor and extensive local infiltration. (Courtesy of Dr. Howard Steinberg.)

H. somni infection, and calves with chronic infections should be suspected of having septic myocarditis if an arrhythmia or other signs of abnormal cardiac function develop during their illness. White muscle disease, hyperkalemia, and hypoglycemia should also be considered in the differential. Septicemic calves have a guarded prognosis, and septic myocarditis worsens it. Foci of septic myocarditis in adult cattle with chronic, active infection or abscesses associated with mastitis, localized peritonitis, foot lesions, or chronic pneumonia are more commonly identified by pathologists than clinicians. Although tachycardia is likely to be present, this finding often is assumed to result from the primary illness rather than from myocarditis. As with calves, adult cattle with septic myocarditis may have paroxysmal cardiac arrhythmias that alert the clinician to the diagnosis. Definitive diagnosis has been difficult in the living patient, but increased concentrations of troponin I may be used to help diagnose myocardial disease. An ECG showing atrial or ventricular premature depolarizations in a calf or cow with evidence of sepsis or a walled-off infection can be used to lend credence to the diagnosis. Although bovine echocardiography does not have the same diagnostic utility for myocardial disease as it does for endocardial and pericardial conditions, it can still be of some value, particularly in cases of cardiomyopathy or myocardial mass lesions such as lymphosarcoma and myocardial abscesses. In all cases of myocardial injury, whether it is toxic (ionophore, gossypol, other toxic plants), nutritional (white muscle disease) or inflammatory (*H. somni*), disease progression will ultimately be accompanied by cardiac dilation and resultant nonspecific echocardiographic changes if the animal survives the acute injury. Presumably, the right ventricular hypertrophy that accompanies high-altitude pulmonary hypertension in brisket disease of cattle maintained at elevation in the western United States might also be associated with identifiable echocardiographic abnormalities.

Treatment of the primary disease remains the most important part of managing septic myocarditis. If the primary problem and myocardial lesion can be sterilized, the heart may return to normal function. Myocardial fibrosis and scarring may, however, leave the animal with a permanent arrhythmia and increase the likelihood of cardiomyopathy and eventual congestive heart failure.

Septic myocardial disease of adult cattle, as in calves, usually follows septicemia or chronic infections. Septicemic spread of infectious organisms, thrombi, or mediators of inflammation may be involved in the pathophysiology of myocardial injury that occurs in septic cattle. Although relatively uncommon, development of persistent tachycardia with or without an arrhythmia in a patient with infectious disease may suggest myocarditis. Tachycardia is so nonspecific that most veterinarians attribute the tachycardia to the primary disease rather than secondary myocarditis. Only when the myocardial damage causes signs of heart failure does a diagnosis of myocarditis become easier. Acute death is possible. Arrhythmia, if present, must be assessed using ECG alongside blood electrolytes and acid–base status to rule out atrial fibrillation associated with metabolic abnormalities. Adult dairy cattle

are most at risk for myocarditis with acute septic diseases such as severe mastitis, metritis, pneumonia, and infection caused by *H. somni*. Occasional cases also occur secondary to chronic localized infections such as digital abscesses that predispose to bacteremia. Depending on the size and location of the myocardial lesion, clinical signs range from subclinical to overt heart failure. ECG evidence of ventricular arrhythmias would suggest myocardial damage, but supraventricular arrhythmias are possible as well. Unfortunately, definitive antemortem diagnosis is impossible without advanced echocardiographic or invasive cardiac techniques. Treatment must be directed at the primary disease. Minor myocardial lesions away from nodal and conduction tissue may heal or fibrose asymptomatically, whereas large or multifocal lesions may lead to heart failure, persistent tachyarrhythmia, or sudden death. Although rarer than septic myocardial injury it is also possible to see myocarditis secondary to severe anemia in which an ischemic injury caused by insufficient oxygen delivery to cardiac myocytes has occurred. In this instance, it is also easy to attribute the tachycardia to the primary disease, but the observant clinician may pick up on this possibility when a tachyarrhythmia is auscultated or seen on ECG in an animal with peracute to acute hemorrhage.

Toxins

Ionophores such as monensin and lasalocid are capable of damaging myocardial and skeletal muscle when ingested in toxic amounts. Improper mixing of ionophores into rations is the most common error that may lead to toxicity, but accidental exposure to concentrated products also is possible. Obviously, this is a potential concern for calves and heifers being fed milk replacer or feeds containing ionophores. Fortunately, cattle (except for water buffalo) are much more resistant to the toxic effects of ionophores than are horses, but there is a relatively narrow margin of safety, especially in young calves. Abnormal echocardiographic findings have been reported during experimental intoxication with monensin sodium by Varga and coworkers. Decreased cardiac chamber size and altered left ventricular function were evident from 48 to 120 hours after administration when monensin was fed daily at approximately 25 to 50 times therapeutic levels. The authors noted a significant decrease in the left ventricular shortening fraction as well as a decrease in ejection fraction, which, taken together, are indicators of altered systolic function.

Many poisonous plants are theoretically capable of myocardial injury, but in reality, few are likely to be encountered because of increased confinement of heifers and adult cattle. *Eupatorium rugosum* (white snakeroot), *Vicia villosa* (hairy vetch), *Cassia occidentalis* (coffee senna), *Phalaris* spp., and others are capable of toxic myocardial damage. Gossypol also is capable of causing myocardial damage when fed in toxic amounts. This fact is of special concern given the increased incidence of feeding cottonseed to dairy cattle. Copper deficiency, especially when chronic, occasionally has been linked to acute myocardial lesions, resulting in death ("falling disease" in Australia). Although commonly fed as a byproduct to cattle without ill effect, citrus pulp fed as silage caused granulomatous cardiac and lymphoid disease in cattle on one farm. Many other organic and inorganic toxins have the potential for causing myocardial damage but create more obvious pathology in other body systems and thus will not be discussed here.

No specific treatment is available for toxic myocarditis. Common sense dictates identification and removal of the toxin from the environment alongside immediate administration of laxatives, cathartics, or protectants to decrease absorption and accelerate intestinal transit. Vitamin E and selenium administration and specific supportive treatment for cardiac disease should be instituted, but the prognosis for animals already demonstrating signs of congestive heart failure is grave.

Parasitic and Protozoan Infections

Cysticerca bovis may cause myocardial lesions, but these appear rarely in dairy cattle in the northern United States. This is the larval form of *Taenia saginata,* the common human tapeworm. Contamination by human sewage of feedstuffs, pastures, or fields puts cows at risk for this disease.

Although *Toxoplasma gondii* is capable of infecting cattle, clinical disease appears rare because cattle rapidly eliminate the parasite from tissue. Cattle are exposed to, and infected by, *T. gondii* via ingestion of feedstuffs contaminated by cat feces.

Sarcocystis spp. are a relatively common cause of myocardial disease in cattle. Although most infestations are asymptomatic, clinical illness characterized by hemolysis, myopathy, myocarditis, weight loss, rattail, and other signs is possible. *Sarcocystis* spp. require two hosts, and carnivores or humans usually are the hosts that shed sporocysts in fecal material that subsequently contaminates cattle feed (see Chapter 16). Cattle then become the intermediate host as intermediate stages of the parasite invade endothelial cells and later stages encyst in muscle, including the myocardium. Subsequent ingestion by carnivores of beef-containing cysts continues the life cycle.

Histopathologic identification of *Sarcocystis* cysts in myocardium of cattle is very common but seldom deemed clinically significant. Certainly, however, heavy exposure to the organism could provoke significant myocardial damage.

Parasitic or protozoal myocarditis usually requires histopathology or serology for diagnosis. Treatment would be best provided by preventive measures to avoid contamination of cattle feeds by carnivore or human feces.

Inherited Myocardial Disease

A dilated cardiomyopathy has been described in Holstein-Friesians in Canada, Japan, and Switzerland. In Switzerland, the disease affects the Fleckvieh and Red Holstein breeds, too. An autosomal recessive mode of inheritance is suggested, associated with a gene-rich locus on bovine chromosome 18, and it has been traced back to a red factor-carrying Holstein-Friesian bull. This condition manifests itself as heart disease between 19 and 78 months of age. Although most cattle develop clinical signs within 4 years of birth, some have lived for 6 to 7 years.

Most cases are presented because of signs referable to heart failure such as ventral edema, exercise intolerance, inappetance, dyspnea, tachycardia, muffled heart sounds, and jugular and mammary vein distention and pulsation. Although tachycardia is fairly consistent, other auscultation findings such as arrhythmias, murmurs, or varying intensity of the heart sounds may occur in individual cases. Hepatomegaly consistent with chronic passive congestion of the liver secondary to right heart failure is also present in some patients.

Echocardiography and ECG recordings are required for diagnosis. Ultrasonography is the best aid to confirm dilated cardiomyopathy.

Long-term prognosis is hopeless, but affected cattle may be helped in the short term by management with cardioglycosides, and furosemide is indicated if pulmonary edema exists. McGuirk suggests digoxin at 0.86 μg/kg/hr as an IV infusion. This obviously requires diligence, IV catheterization, and hospitalization or else a very attentive owner. Alternatively, 3.4 μg/kg IV every 4 hours may be used but creates greater variation in blood levels and increases the risk of digoxin toxicity. Furosemide is used at 0.5 to 1.0 mg/kg twice daily if pulmonary edema is present. Inappetent cattle may benefit from 50 to 100 g KCl orally each day to maintain potassium levels when being treated with digoxin. Ideally, acid–base and electrolyte status should be assessed daily or every other day by blood sample.

Endocarditis
Etiology

Bacterial endocarditis is the most common valvular or endocardial disease in adult dairy cattle. It also is one of the few treatable heart conditions of cattle. Therefore early suspicion, diagnosis, and appropriate treatment improve the prognosis.

Cattle with chronic infections such as septic musculoskeletal conditions, hardware disease, soft tissue abscesses, lactic acid indigestion, chronic pneumonia, metritis or mastitis, and thrombophlebitis are at risk for bacterial endocarditis. In addition, cattle with long-term IV catheters have increased risk of endocardial infections. Bacteremia appears essential to the pathophysiology of bacterial endocarditis in cattle.

T. pyogenes has been the most common organism isolated from the blood and endocardial lesions of cattle affected with endocarditis, but *Streptococcus* spp., *Staphylococcus* spp., and gram-negative organisms may also cause the disease. A recent report identified *Helcococcus ovis*, a facultative gram-positive anaerobe and member of the family *Peptostreptococcaceae,* in up to one-third of bovine endocarditis lesions in a large study from Europe; many of these cases were mixed infections with other more historically typical species such as *T. pyogenes*. The right AV valve (tricuspid) is the most commonly infected valve with the left AV (mitral valve) being the second most common (Fig. 3.25). Other valves or the endocardium adjacent to valves may also occasionally be the site of infection (Fig. 3.26). Owner complaints regarding affected cattle include recurrent fever, weight loss,

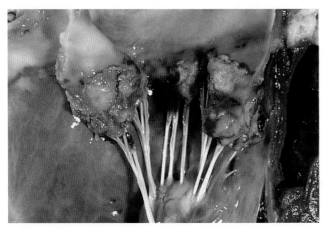

• **Fig. 3.25** Bacterial valvular endocarditis with vegetative lesions in a cow. (Courtesy of Dr. John M. King.)

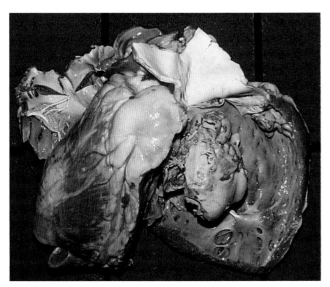

• **Fig. 3.26** Large vegetative endocarditis lesion involving the valves and adjacent endocardium in the ventricle. (Courtesy of Dr. John M. King.)

anorexia, poor production, and sometimes lameness independent of conventional foot or musculoskeletal problems.

Signs

Persistent or intermittent fever, tachycardia, and a systolic heart murmur are the most common signs found in cattle having endocarditis. A "pounding" heart or increased intensity of heart sounds also is common, although the heart sounds may vary in intensity or even be reduced in some patients. Vegetative endocarditis may also occur in the absence of an auscultable murmur, underscoring the diagnostic utility of cardiac ultrasonography in a patient with physical examination findings such as fever and tachycardia with or without arrhythmia that raise suspicion of infectious cardiac disease.

Some cattle with endocarditis appear painful when digital pressure is exerted on the chest wall over the heart region. Fever usually is present, has been present historically, or develops intermittently after initial examination. Some cattle with endocarditis never have fever recorded but do show other signs of illness and a systolic heart murmur or other cardiac signs.

Signs of heart failure may develop along with increased distention and pulsations of the jugular and mammary veins (Fig. 3.27). Tachycardia is a consistent finding, and dyspnea may develop, especially after bacterial showering of the lungs. Arrhythmias are unusual and paroxysmal but may be observed in approximately 10% of patients.

Lameness, often shifting, and stiffness may be observed. Synovitis and joint tenderness sometimes are obvious, but in other patients, exact localization of the lameness is difficult. Bacteremia to joints or epiphyses and immune-mediated synovitis have been suggested as origins of this lameness in patients with endocarditis.

Laboratory Data

Nonregenerative anemia commonly results from chronicity of the primary infection, the endocardial infection, or both. Neutrophilia is common and was found in 24 of 31 cases in one report, and absolute leukocytosis was found in 14 of 31. In this same report, serum globulin values were greater than 5.0 g/dL in 19 of 23 patients with endocarditis that had globulin measured. Elevated globulin was believed to be consistent with the chronicity of infection.

Blood cultures are an important diagnostic test, but echocardiography provides the definitive diagnosis. A patient suspected of having endocarditis should have a series of blood cultures submitted rather than a single time-point sample. Although blood culture results in adult cattle may be negative in as many as 50% of endocarditis patients tested, isolating the causative organism from the bloodstream provides the best opportunity for appropriate and successful treatment with a specific antibiotic. Venous blood cultures should be collected after the jugular vein has been clipped and prepared aseptically. The cow should have been held off systemic antibiotics for 24 to 48 hours before culture, if possible. Although one blood culture attempt is better than none, it is preferable to obtain a series of three to four cultures when economics allow. An appropriate interval between collections of multiple samples has been debated by clinicians for decades. Some clinicians culture only during a fever spike, some at 3- to 30-minute intervals, some at 6- to 8-hour intervals, and some once daily. We prefer to obtain three cultures at 30-minute intervals in febrile patients and at intervals of several hours in nonfebrile patients suspected of having endocarditis.

Diagnosis

Early signs of reduced appetite and production, fever, and tachycardia certainly are not specific for endocarditis. A pounding heart or systolic murmur should suggest the diagnosis and dictate further specific cardiac workup. The diagnosis may be overlooked because of more obvious primary problems such as abscesses, an infected digit or other musculoskeletal infection, suspected hardware disease, or thrombophlebitis because these conditions may also cause fever and nonspecific signs of illness. Therefore heart murmurs, a pounding heart, or

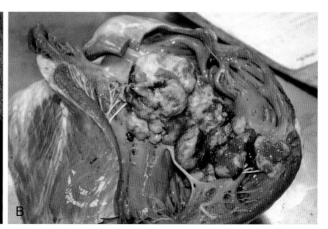

• **Fig. 3.27** Distended jugular vein (**A**) of a mature Holstein cow with extensive endocarditis involving the right atrioventricular valve leaflets and associated endocardium (**B**).

early signs of heart failure in addition to tachycardia merit consideration of the diagnosis of endocarditis. Lameness and stiffness may be difficult to differentiate from primary musculoskeletal disease or the painful stance caused by peritonitis but these can be important clinical signs that aid diagnosis. Because of fever, tachycardia, and sometimes polypnea, cattle having endocarditis often are misdiagnosed with pneumonia or traumatic reticuloperitonitis.

The diagnosis of endocarditis is often suggested by the patient's history and clinical signs. However, a positive blood culture and echocardiography allow definitive diagnosis. Blood cultures, as mentioned previously, may or may not be successful; however, when positive, they allow appropriate selection of antibiotics. Definitive diagnosis based on two-dimensional echocardiography has proved to be one of the most impressive uses of ultrasonography since its more widespread use began about 10 years ago. Veterinarians trained in echocardiography now have a tool to confirm bacterial endocarditis in most patients. The echocardiographic examination should be performed mindful of the fact that endocarditis involves the valvular endocardium in more than 98% of reported cases; mural lesions being extremely rare. As pointed out in a systematic review of published cases by Buczinski et al. (2012), the tricuspid valve is the most commonly affected valve (49.5%) followed by the mitral (29.7%), the pulmonary (13.7%), and aortic (7.5%) valves; information that can be particularly useful in directing the examination when performing echocardiography in cattle with an auscultable murmur. The typical endocarditic lesion will be an irregular valvular thickening with heterogeneous content and a shaggy appearance. Depending on the clinical findings and the resultant, but not invariant, murmur (auscultated in ≈60% of cases), the best views should be selected to image the suspicious valve. Most of time, it is obvious that the valve is abnormal and more than 1 cm thick (Figs. 3.28 to 3.30).

Treatment

Long-term antibiotic therapy is required to cure bacterial endocarditis in cattle. Thus, cattle selected for treatment

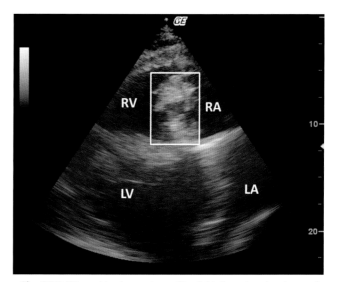

• **Fig. 3.28** Tricuspid valve endocarditis, right, four-chamber long-axis view. The tricuspid valve is irregularly thickened (as outlined by the white box). Secondary right ventricular dilation is suspected based on the relative size of the right and left ventricular (RV and LV) lumina. *RA,* right atrium; *RV,* right ventricle.

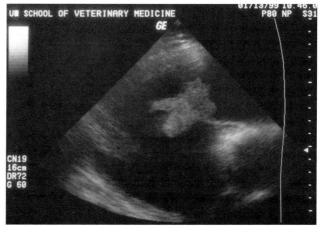

• **Fig. 3.29** Echocardiographic image of endocarditis of the tricuspid valve of a cow.

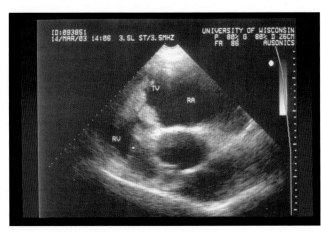

• **Fig. 3.30** Echocardiographic image of vegetative endocarditis of the tricuspid valve (TV) of a mature Holstein cow. *RA,* right atrium; *RV,* right ventricle.

must be deemed valuable enough to justify the cost of antibiotics and discarded milk that will be incurred. A successful blood culture allows selection of an appropriate antibiotic based on sensitivity or mean inhibitory concentration (MIC) values. Because endocarditis in cattle usually is caused by *T. pyogenes* or *Streptococcus* spp., some clinicians assume penicillin will work and do not bother to do blood cultures. This assumption would be a worthwhile gamble if economics dictate that laboratory costs must be minimized.

Therefore, penicillin and ampicillin have historically been the drugs of choice for bacterial endocarditis in cattle caused by *T. pyogenes* and most *Streptococcus* spp. Although ceftiofur has the advantage of limited withdrawal times, depending on formulation, it is more expensive, is not approved for this use and might be overused by some who hope the drug will cure all infections of dairy cattle. Penicillin (22,000–33,000 U/kg twice daily) or ampicillin (10–20 mg/kg twice daily) (both are extralabel dosages) is administered for a minimum of 3 weeks. If gram-negative organisms or penicillin-resistant gram-positive organisms are isolated from blood cultures, an appropriate bactericidal antibiotic should be selected based on MIC or antibiotic sensitivity testing.

Based on work by Dr. Ray Sweeney and others at the University of Pennsylvania, rifampin (rifamycin) has been shown to establish therapeutic blood levels after oral administration to ruminants. Unfortunately, there is significant variability in blood levels between treated cattle, which may limit its treatment potential. Rifampin is a unique antibiotic that gains access to intracellular organisms or walled-off infections by concentrating in macrophages. Rifampin always should be used in conjunction with another antibiotic because bacterial resistance may develop quickly when the drug is used alone. The dosage is 5 mg/kg orally, twice daily for cattle. Although some maintain this dosage is too low, it has seemed effective clinically when used in conjunction with penicillin not only for chronic *T. pyogenes* endocarditis but also for pulmonary abscesses. Therefore, if economics allow, oral rifampin has been reported to improve treatment success in cattle with bacterial endocarditis. Unfortunately, currently within the United States, the Food and Drug

Administration requires that cattle treated with rifampin are not used for either commercial milk or meat production, severely limiting its use. Occasionally, cattle will become significantly anorectic while receiving rifampin (more so than was noted in association with the primary disease), but in many cases, this apparent intolerance to the drug is overcome if administration is discontinued for several days and then reinstituted at the same or lesser dose.

In addition to antibiotic therapy, cattle showing venous distention, ventral edema, or pulmonary edema require judicious dosages of furosemide. Because many patients with endocarditis have reduced or poor appetites, overuse of furosemide may lead to electrolyte depletion (K^+, Ca^{2+}) and dehydration. Therefore when furosemide is used, the drug should be administered on an "as-needed" basis, and 0.5 mg/kg once or twice daily usually is sufficient.

Because cattle with endocarditis often appear painful or stiff and may have either primary musculoskeletal disorders or secondary shifting lameness, aspirin is administered at 240 to 480 grains orally twice daily. Unfortunately, aspirin does not appear to minimize platelet aggregation in cattle and is unlikely to prevent further enlargement of vegetative lesions. Ketoprofen (3 mg/kg IM) has been documented to decrease thromboxane A2 in cattle suggesting it may have some antiplatelet effect. Free access to salt should be denied for cattle showing signs of congestive heart failure.

Antibiotic treatment continues for a minimum of 3 weeks. Positive signs of improvement include increasing appetite and production, as well as absence of fever. The heart murmur persists and may vary as treatment progresses. Resolution of the heart murmur and tachycardia coupled with echocardiographic evidence of resolution of the endocarditis lesions are excellent prognostic signs. Many cows that survive are, however, left with persistent subtle or obvious heart murmurs caused by valvular damage alongside an abnormal echocardiographic appearance to the affected valve. This should not be a concern as long as other signs indicate resolution of infection and heart failure is not present. Cattle with venous distention, ventral edema, or other signs of right heart failure have a worse prognosis than cattle diagnosed before signs of heart failure. However, mild to moderate signs of heart failure should not be interpreted to infer a hopeless prognosis because supportive treatment may alleviate these signs while antibiotic therapy treats the primary condition. Cattle with severe lameness, either as a result or as the cause (i.e., septic joint or tendon) of endocarditis, have a poor prognosis.

The prognosis for patients with endocarditis is guarded at best. Sporadic case reports tend to highlight successfully managed individual cases, but further case series are necessary to suggest accurate recovery rates. Of 31 cattle affected with endocarditis that were admitted to Cornell's hospital between 1977 and 1982, 9 responded to long-term antibiotic (8 penicillin and 1 tetracycline) therapy. Based on these data and the experience of other clinicians, the prognosis is better when the diagnosis is made early in the course of the disease. Repeated echocardiographic examination allows for monitoring and reassessment of the valvular lesions during and

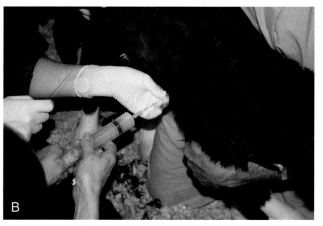

• **Fig. 3.31** Three-week-old Holstein heifer calf with septic pericarditis (**A**). Pericardial sac enlargement was sufficient to allow drainage via the right sixth intercostal space with the calf restrained and the right elbow pulled well forward (**B**).

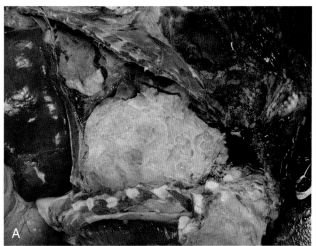
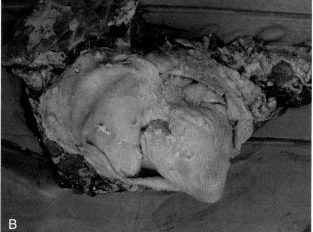

• **Fig. 3.32** Weanling age calf with septic pleuropneumonia (**A**) and septic pericarditis (**B**) associated with *Mannheimia haemolytica* sepsis.

after treatment. With experience and the correct software, ultrasound examination also allows for specific evaluation of cardiac function (e.g., atrial diameter, fractional shortening) that may more accurately assess the degree of cardiac dysfunction and provide valuable prognostic information.

Septic Pericarditis

Etiology

The most common cause of pericarditis in dairy cattle is puncture of the pericardium by a metallic linear foreign body that originated in the reticulum. It is apparent during laparotomy and rumenotomy in cattle that the heart lies very close to the diaphragmatic region of the reticulum. Therefore, traumatic reticuloperitonitis occasionally causes septic pericarditis. Hardware that penetrates the reticulum in a cranial direction may puncture the pericardium or impale the myocardium. It can also infect the mediastinum or puncture a lung lobe. Both the foreign body and the tract of its migration can "wick" bacterial contaminants into the pericardial fluid, resulting in fibrinopurulent pericarditis.

Fibrinous pericarditis can also occur in septicemic calves (Fig. 3.31) or cattle having severe bacterial bronchopneumonia (Fig. 3.32). These forms of pericarditis only occasionally cause clinically detectable fluid accumulation and seldom lead to overt signs of heart failure as are typical in traumatic pericarditis.

Signs

Signs of traumatic pericarditis include venous distention and pulsation, ventral edema, tachycardia, and muffled heart sounds bilaterally (Fig. 3.33). Fever is usually, but not always, present. Tachypnea and dyspnea may be present in patients with septic pericarditis and advanced heart failure. Cattle having traumatic pericarditis are often reluctant to move, appear painful, and have abducted elbows.

Direct pressure or percussion in the ventral chest or xiphoid area elicits a painful response by the cow with traumatic pericarditis. Dyspnea is caused by a combination of lung compression by the enlarged pericardial mass, pulmonary edema, and reduced cardiac output. Auscultation of the heart reveals bilaterally decreased intensity of the heart

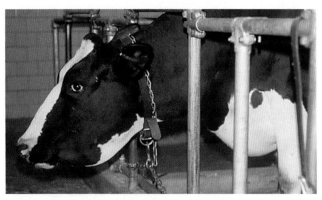

• **Fig. 3.33** Anxious expression and severe ventral edema in a cow with traumatic pericarditis.

sounds. This muffling of heart sounds usually coexists with squeaky, rubbing sounds and splashing or tinkling sounds, but these sounds are not present in all cases. A fluid–gas interface created by gas-forming bacterial organisms in the pericardium creates the most obvious splashing sounds. Lung sounds may not be heard in the ventral third of either hemithorax because of the greatly enlarged pericardial sac displacing the lungs dorsally. In addition to these signs, there are two other very important clinical facts associated with traumatic pericarditis in dairy cattle:

1. Most cows with traumatic pericarditis were observed by the owner to be ill 7 to 14 days earlier and may or may not have been diagnosed with traumatic reticuloperitonitis at that time. Frequently, the signs of illness were vague and nonspecific, and veterinary attention may or may not have been requested. Typically, these cattle improve or appear recovered from this previous illness only to become ill again and have signs of cardiac disease. Certainly not all cattle have this two-phased clinical course, and some have peracute pericarditis or traumatic myocarditis and die within hours or days. When the history supports a two-phased clinical disease, it is assumed the cow transiently "felt better" after the foreign body left the reticulodiaphragmatic area and entered the chest, thereby alleviating the peritoneal pain and inflammation. Subsequently, worsening sepsis in the pericardial sac and eventual heart failure causes the second phase of disease that generally moves the owner to seek veterinary consultation.

2. During the acute and subacute phases of traumatic pericarditis, heart sounds may change on a daily basis. Muffling, tinkling, splashing, rubs, murmurs, and other sounds all may be present on one day, absent the next, and present again later. Pathology is dynamic as the relative amounts of fibrin, purulent fluid, and gas in the pericardium change. Chronic cases, on the other hand, tend to have bilateral muffling of heart sounds and a "far away" tinkling as fluid pus is jostled by heartbeats.

Laboratory Data

If the disease is subacute or chronic, neutrophilia is usually present. Cattle afflicted for longer than 10 to 14 days usually have decreased serum albumin and increased serum globulin; therefore, total protein values are at least high normal and usually elevated. Hyperfibrinogenemia is typically present at all stages of the disease. Other, non-septic causes of pericardial effusion, such as cardiac lymphosarcoma and idiopathic hemorrhagic pericardial effusion, generally have normal fibrinogen and globulin concentrations. Thoracic radiographs, although largely unavailable in the field, often dramatically demonstrate a greatly enlarged pericardium, fluid line, and gas cap above the fluid line. The causative metallic foreign body also may be apparent unless obscured by radiopaque pericardial fluid, fibrin, and the cardiac shadow (Fig. 3.34). Serum liver enzymes may be elevated with pericardial effusions, regardless of the cause, especially when congestive heart failure accompanies the pericardial effusion, often caused by tamponade (Fig. 3.35).

Diagnosis

Although the clinical signs and cardiac auscultation of cattle with traumatic pericarditis usually are sufficient for diagnosis, definitive diagnosis in the field can be accomplished by two-dimensional echocardiography, pericardiocentesis, or both procedures. Thoracic radiographs, if available, also may be definitive. Fluid and fibrin in the pericardial sac are easily visualized with two-dimensional echocardiography (Figs. 3.36 and 3.37). Heavy accumulation of fibrin coats the epicardium and visceral pericardium (Fig. 3.38). This fibrin frequently has the appearance of "scrambled eggs" when seen on postmortem examination (Fig. 3.39). Depending on the severity and stage of the disease secondary ultrasonographic signs of cardiac tamponade can be observed with ventricular collapse during diastole, atrial collapse during ventricular systole or a "swinging heart." Septic pericarditis (either traumatic after hardware disease or secondary to contiguous pulmonary infection), cardiac lymphosarcoma, and idiopathic hemorrhagic pericardial (IHP) effusion are the most common causes of pericardial effusion in cattle. In all cases, a pericardiocentesis under ultrasonographic guidance should be performed to characterize the nature of the pericardial effusion. Other physical examination and clinicopathologic data often heavily suggest the pathogenesis for each of these differentials, but definitive diagnosis is almost always provided by simple cytologic examination of a sample of the effusion.

Pericardiocentesis can be performed with an 18-gauge, 8.75-cm spinal needle or chest trochar of similar length in the left fifth ICS. After clipping and standard preparation of the left thorax, a skin puncture is performed with a scalpel in the fifth ICS just dorsal to the elbow. If continuous drainage is desired, a 20-Fr chest trochar and catheter may be introduced into the pericardium for further drainage. The fluid obtained is purulent and fetid with septic reticulopericarditis. Fibrin clots frequently obstruct flow of the fluid through finer gauge needles or catheters. The purulent fluid greatly exceeds normal values for pericardial fluid (normal; protein <2.5 g/dL, white blood cell count [WBC] ≤ 5000/µL), and neutrophils are the major cellular

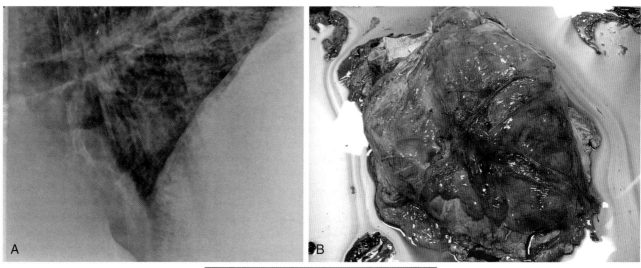

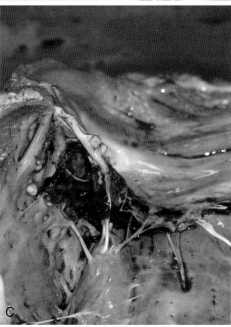

• **Fig. 3.34** Radiographic image (**A**) from an adult dairy cow with reticulopericarditis demonstrating the wire oriented vertically within the enlarged pericardial sac caudal to the heart shadow because of acute penetration. Postmortem appearance of the wire protruding through the outer surface of the pericardium (**B**), and concurrent vegetative endocarditis affecting the same cow (**C**).

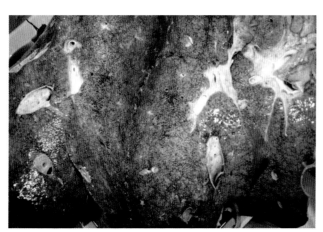

• **Fig. 3.35** "Nutmeg"-like appearance on cut section of a highly congested and enlarged liver from an adult Holstein cow that was euthanized because of congestive heart failure.

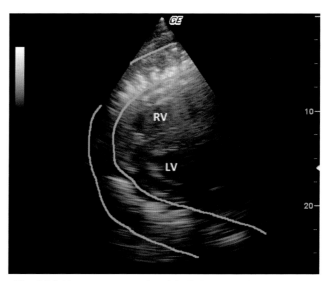

• **Fig. 3.36** Heterogeneous pericardial effusion secondary to traumatic pericarditis. The distended pericardial space is outlined by the *blue lines*. The contents of the pericardial space are heterogeneous compatible with fibrin, pus, and gas, typical of a septic effusion. *LV,* left ventricle; *RV,* right ventricle.

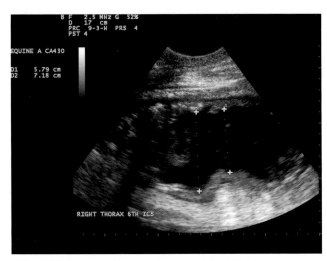

• **Fig. 3.37** Ultrasound image taken from right sixth intercostal space showing an enlarged and thickened pericardial sac containing flocculent and gas-shadowing material associated with septic pericarditis caused by hardware disease in a 6-year-old Jersey cow.

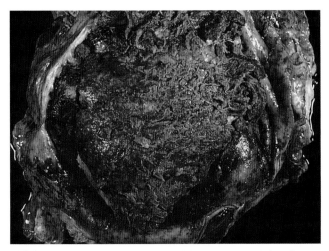

• **Fig. 3.38** Traumatic pericarditis patient's heart and pericardium at necropsy. Purulent fluid has been rinsed away, but the severity of fibrin deposition is apparent because the epicardial surface of the heart is completely covered. The pericardium is also greatly thickened and coated with fibrin. (Courtesy of Dr. John M. King.)

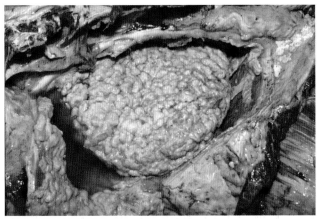

• **Fig. 3.39** "Scrambled egg" appearance of the epicardium and pericardial sac of an adult cow with pericarditis.

component rather than the mononuclear cells normally found in pericardial fluid. Bacteria are easily detected in gram-stained smears of this fluid. With ultrasound guidance, as has become commonplace, it is frequently possible to access the pericardial sac from either the left or the right side (see Fig. 3.31), potentially through several ICSs, so significant is the enlargement and volume of fluid within the pericardium. However, it is advisable that the fifth ICS on the left always be used for diagnostic sampling for cytology. Many cattle with pericardial effusions will also have some degree of pleural effusion, and it can be challenging to differentiate the two spaces ultrasonographically such is the deviation from normal anatomy and the sheer enlargement of the respective spaces. Although septic disease often has comparable cytology in both effusions, this is not always the case for neoplastic disease, nor with idiopathic hemorrhagic pericardial effusion.

The major reason for pericardiocentesis is diagnostic differentiation of traumatic pericarditis from diseases that may create similar signs. Lymphosarcoma with pericardial involvement and fluid accumulation has historically been the major differential diagnosis, but increasing numbers of cases of idiopathic, nonseptic hemorrhagic pericarditis have been documented, in which the clinical signs are similar to those documented with septic pericarditis or neoplastic pericarditis, but the fluid tends to be a sterile hemorrhagic transudate with low to moderate numbers of macrophages, neutrophils, and lymphocytes (see Video Clip 3.5). Cytology of pericardial fluid would clearly differentiate between these diseases. The prognosis for cattle with the idiopathic hemorrhagic condition appears to be better after drainage and antiinflammatory therapy than for pericarditis associated with sepsis or neoplasia (see later section). The presence of flocculent, mixed echogenicity fluid with gas shadowing within the pericardium on ultrasonography is also characteristic for septic pericarditis.

Pericardiocentesis is not without risk. Potential complications include pneumothorax; fatal arrhythmia; cardiac puncture leading to hemorrhage or death; and leakage of pericardial material into the thorax, resulting in pleuritis. Some, but not all, of these complications can be mitigated by performing the procedure using ultrasound guidance. Leakage into the pleural space is possible because most pericarditis patients do not have attachment of the fibrous pericardium to the parietal pleura. Pericardiocentesis performed on one of the author's patients yielded only gas from the needle and was associated with immediate anxiety, dyspnea, and death within 5 minutes. Postmortem examination confirmed that neither hemorrhage nor cardiac injury had occurred. The gas pocket and fluid distending the pericardium had been under positive pressure and may have become somewhat constrictive or altered compensatory mechanisms when suddenly relieved.

Given the poor prognosis usually associated with septic pericarditis, pericardiocentesis is a worthwhile risk to confirm the diagnosis before salvaging a cow suspected to have the disease. The fact that idiopathic hemorrhagic pericarditis carries a much more favorable prognosis further emphasizes the diagnostic relevance of the procedure in a patient with pericardial effusion.

Treatment

Treatment of traumatic pericarditis in dairy cattle usually is nearly hopeless. Medical therapy with systemic antibiotics and drainage of the pericardial sac rarely, if ever, permanently cures affected cattle. Therefore most therapeutic efforts have included surgical approaches. Thoracotomy and pericardiectomy or pericardiotomy have been performed in many fashions in an effort to provide drainage, search for the foreign body, and prevent fluid or later constrictive damage to the heart (see Video Clip 3.6). Sporadic case reports and third-hand stories attest to the occasional success of pericardiectomy and fifth rib resections, but success is not common. Authors recommending rib-splitting thoracotomy and pericardiectomy reported that five of nine clinical patients recovered. Results from Cornell University, as reported by Ducharme and coworkers, are much more pessimistic with only one of seven surviving following thoracic surgery. Pericardiocentesis followed by fluid drainage may result in clinical improvement with prolongation of life to reach a short-term goal such as calving. Despite a poor prognosis, surgery remains the treatment of choice for valuable cattle with septic reticulopericarditis.

To improve a patient's chances of survival, surgery should be performed as early in the course of the disease as possible. Cattle with severe ventral edema and obvious heart failure are not good candidates for surgery. Removal of the causative wire during the thoracotomy may be difficult but obviously is desirable. Usually the wire is mostly or completely in the thorax and would be difficult or impossible to remove through rumenotomy. However, we have observed patients with acute reticuloperitonitis and acute traumatic pericarditis from a single metallic foreign body that was still lodged in the reticulum and was removed through rumenotomy. These patients had clinically detectable pericardial effusions and radiographic evidence of foreign body penetration of the pericardium. Rumenotomy and intensive bactericidal systemic antibiotics are sometimes sufficient treatment of peracute or acute pericarditis in such cases. If pericarditis worsens despite systemic antibiotics and rumenotomy to retrieve the foreign body, thoracotomy may then be considered. Rumenotomy probably is most indicated in acute cases for which it is hoped that some portion of the metallic foreign object remains in the reticulum. Unfortunately, it is difficult to know this without the benefit of radiographs, and an unsuccessful rumenotomy in the field may further compromise the patient.

It is very disturbing that these "valuable cows" unfortunate enough to develop traumatic pericarditis were not administered a magnet prophylactically at some time in their lives by their owner. The routine administration of a magnet to heifers of breeding age and bulls before 2 years of age should be part of routine herd health in dairy cattle.

Idiopathic Hemorrhagic Pericardial Effusion
Etiology

Over the past decade, we have seen a seemingly new form of pericardial disease manifest itself in dairy cattle in the northern United States and Canada. The initial reports of the condition were case reports or small case series of individual adult cattle presented to university teaching hospitals with signs of congestive heart failure associated with substantial volumes of hemorrhagic pericardial fluid. Diagnostic workup of these cases demonstrated that cytologically the effusion was neither neoplastic nor septic but merely hemorrhagic and that extended survival times could be achieved with pericardial drainage and parenteral corticosteroid administration. In many cases, the effusion would resolve with such treatment, and cattle would return to milk production or reproductive use for a variable period from several months to years. In the past decade, it has increased in prevalence to the point that at the time of writing, it is now the most common cardiac condition of cattle presenting to the University of Wisconsin's Large Animal Hospital. Subsequent literature has highlighted that many of these cattle go on to develop an unusual form of cardiac lymphosarcoma principally involving the epicardium in the months to years after initial presentation for cardiac disease. Occasionally, cattle have epicardial lymphosarcoma at the time of initial presentation, but we have seen cattle for whom the delay in progression from initial treatment of the nonneoplastic hemorrhagic pericardial effusion to euthanasia for epicardial lymphosarcoma has been in excess of 3 years. The gross appearance of the epicardial neoplasia is quite strikingly different to that seen with classic cardiac lymphosarcoma involving the myocardium. It seems extremely rare for cattle with cardiac lymphosarcoma to have neoplastic infiltration of both myocardial and epicardial locations, although both may show infiltration of thoracic or mediastinal lymph nodes locally. In cases when cattle have been euthanized or died with the disease, without any gross or histologic evidence of lymphosarcoma, the epicardial surface of the heart has a network of highly vascular fibroelastic connective tissue, which is presumably the source of the hemorrhagic effusion (Fig. 3.40). Fulminant cases of epicardial lymphosarcoma have variably florid and highly extensive amounts of this highly vascular connective tissue within which it appears the neoplasia has developed, raising the possibility that it behaves as a "scaffold" for transformed lymphocytes (Figs. 3.41 and 3.42). Affected cattle are reliably BLV positive.

Because this condition is the most treatable of the primary cardiac conditions of dairy cattle, early recognition and appropriate therapy carry the greatest chance of returning the patient to production for an extended period. We have not seen the condition in animals younger than 2 years of age, although first lactation heifers can certainly be affected. It can be seen in either lactating or dry animals, although many are in mid to late lactation at the time of diagnosis. A large retrospective study of 125 cases demonstrated a median age and days in milk of 47 months and 262 days, respectively. Many affected cattle have been producing expected levels of milk

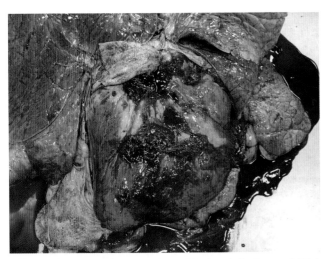

• **Fig. 3.40** Postmortem appearance of the heart of a 2-year-old Holstein heifer euthanized for idiopathic hemorrhagic pericardial effusion. The epicardium is covered with highly vascular, proliferative epicarditis, but there was no neoplastic infiltrate histologically.

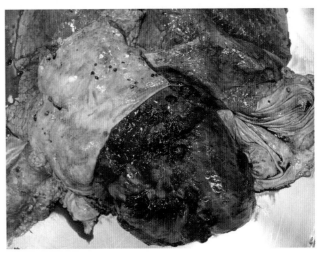

• **Fig. 3.42** Pericardial sac opened to demonstrate epicardial lymphosarcoma in a 3-year-old Holstein cow with a 9-month history of idiopathic hemorrhagic pericardial effusion.

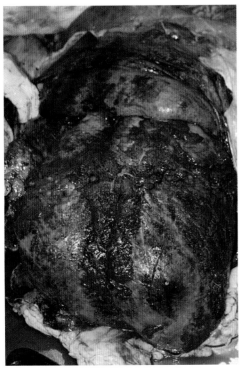

• **Fig. 3.41** Postmortem appearance of the heart of a 7-year-old Brown Swiss cow euthanized approximately 2 years after initial presentation and treatment for idiopathic hemorrhagic pericardial effusion. At the time of death, there were lymphoblasts in the pericardial fluid, and histologically, the epicardial surface was diffusely infiltrated by lymphosarcoma.

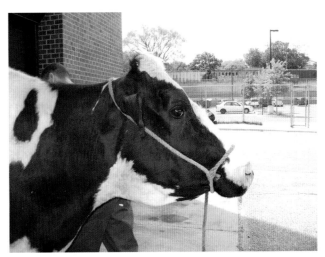

• **Fig. 3.43** Mild submandibular edema in an 8-year-old Holstein cow presented with muffled heart sounds and idiopathic hemorrhagic pericardial effusion.

immediately before diagnosis and are often average- to high-producing animals compared with herdmates. However, the stage of lactation at which animals appear to be commonly affected certainly puts them into a group for whom there may not be such intense health-related oversight unless they are individually valuable or daily milk weights are recorded and checked. In several instances we have investigated this as a herd problem with multiple animals affected over the course of many months.

Signs

The presenting signs typically point toward a cardiac condition with observant producers noticing jugular distention, alongside variably severe submandibular and brisket edema in combination with a seemingly acute reduction in appetite and milk production over 24 to 72 hours (Fig. 3.43). Peripheral vessels such as the superficial mammary veins may also be inappropriately distended and turgid for the stage of lactation. Cattle are typically afebrile or demonstrate only a low-grade fever and have high normal to mildly elevated heart rates. Respiratory rate and effort are usually also mildly increased. Because of the presence and frequently large volume of pericardial effusion, one might expect obvious muffling of heart sounds or a washing-machine type murmur on cardiac auscultation, but it has been our experience that this is not invariable. Certainly, muffling would instantly raise the clinician's suspicion of pericardial disease, but it has been humbling to image the heart of affected cattle ultrasonographically and reveal the extravagant depth of pericardial fluid that had not been anticipated after ordinary stethoscope examination.

Diagnosis

The definitive diagnosis requires exclusion of other causes of cardiac disease and peripheral vein distention, especially septic pericarditis and pericardial effusion associated with more classical cardiac lymphosarcoma. This is most readily achieved by echocardiography and pericardiocentesis. Routine hematology and biochemistry can be useful for exclusionary purposes in that there is an absence of hyperfibrinogenemia, mature neutrophilia, and hyperglobulinemia such as one would expect with septic pericarditis caused by hardware disease. There may well be a significant and persistent lymphocytosis in cattle with this condition who are also BLV positive, which may also be true in cases of right atrial lymphosarcoma. Biochemical abnormalities are infrequent, although many cattle demonstrate elevations in gamma-glutamyl transferase likely associated with passive hepatic congestion of cardiac origin. Pericardial fluid reliably appears bloody, typically has a packed cell volume (PCV) of between 10% and 15%, with a mildly elevated total protein, and a cytologic mixture of nondegenerate neutrophils, macrophages, and small lymphocytes. The latter usually represent the majority of the cells on cytologic examination even if the cow does not have a peripheral lymphocytosis. These small lymphocytes are phenotypically unremarkable in the majority of cases at the time of first diagnosis, but as mentioned earlier, over time this can transition into an obviously lymphoblastic population. Transabdominal ultrasound examination often confirms hepatic congestion, intrahepatic vessel prominence, and commonly a moderate degree of ascites. Thoracic ultrasonography and echocardiography are highly informative and the effusion(s) so marked that either a medium-frequency sector scanner or lower frequency cardiac probe can be used. Echocardiographic findings from either side of the chest include a large volume of predominantly anechoic fluid within the pericardial sac (5–25 cm in depth) (see Video Clip 3.7) often accompanied by a moderate but smaller volume of pleural fluid (see Fig. 3.4). The latter is more likely in individuals with a particularly large volume of pericardial effusion. The epicardial surface of the heart is often coated with more hyperechoic-appearing tissue that projects like fronds of seaweed into the more anechoic fluid within the pericardium, having an ultrasonographic appearance reminiscent of fibrin. The anechoic nature of the pericardial fluid is notably different from that seen with septic pericardial disease, which tends to be more heterogeneous and frequently contains gas shadows (compare Figs. 3.4 and 3.37). Cardiac function is often obviously impaired on echocardiography with poor contractility and low ejection fractions most likely caused by tamponade.

Treatment

Successful treatment of this condition has been achieved both by systemic corticosteroids alone and through a combination of pericardial drainage and systemic corticosteroids. The best results that one author has achieved (SP) in terms of long-term survival have been subsequent to pericardial drainage combined with dexamethasone administration (0.1 mg/kg) over 3 days. In pregnant cattle, isoflupredone acetate at standard, labeled doses can be substituted for the more abortifacient dexamethasone. Understandably, grade cattle may not justify pericardial drainage, and we have experienced good results with steroid use without drainage on the farm, although survival times for commercial cattle treated in this way tend to be measured in terms of months to 1 year. If pericardial drainage is performed, it is wise to concurrently administer an antibiotic such as ceftiofur or ampicillin parenterally.

Cor Pulmonale

Etiology

Conditions of right heart dilatation, hypertrophy, and subsequent failure caused by pulmonary hypertension and increased pulmonary vascular resistance often are referred to collectively as cor pulmonale. This condition is uncommon and sporadic in dairy cattle. Most cases of cor pulmonale occur in cows known to have chronic pneumonia, bronchiectasis, and pulmonary abscesses secondary to bacterial bronchopneumonia, consolidated anteroventral lung lobes from previous pneumonia, or chronic lungworms. Severe chronic interstitial pulmonary disease, although rare, may also result in cor pulmonale in mature cattle with diffuse pulmonary fibrosis. Occasionally, calves with chronic pulmonary disease or those with congenital defects leading to chronic hypoxia and pulmonary hypertension may also develop this problem, but this represents a very small fraction of all calves with even severe or repeated bouts of conventional bronchopneumonia. In calves in which we have observed it, the radiographic and pathologic interpretation of the calf's disease has included both concurrent interstitial disease as well as the more common bronchopneumonia. In cases of cor pulmonale, pulmonary hypertension initially may result from alveolar hypoxia and subsequent precapillary vasoconstriction. Chronic hypoxia and pulmonary hypertension in cattle may provoke hypertrophy of medial smooth musculature within pulmonary arteries and arterioles, causing further work for the right ventricle. We have treated only one adult Holstein cow that had confirmed primary pulmonary hypertension suggesting that it is a very rare condition in the northern and Mid western United States.

The most common example of cor pulmonale is "brisket disease" or "mountain sickness" of beef cattle. This disease can occur in dairy cattle, and in fact Holsteins have been reported to be particularly sensitive. However, on a practical basis, to our knowledge, few dairy cattle in the United States are at risk because of a lack of exposure to high altitudes. Brisket disease may be seen at elevations of 1600 m (5249 ft) above sea level and tends to have an increasing incidence at elevations above 1600 m. Definite genetic resistance or susceptibility is documented, and affected cattle must be returned to low altitudes early in the course of the disease to survive. Concurrent ingestion of certain plants such as *Astragalus* spp. and *Oxytropis* spp. (locoweed) is known to accentuate and accelerate brisket disease in animals at high elevations.

Pulmonary hypertension secondary to pulmonary and bronchial arteritis recently was observed as an endemic problem in a group of dairy calves. Periarteriolar sclerosis and vasculitis were identified pathologically and explained signs of right heart failure observed in the calves. Although unconfirmed, monocrotaline, a pyrrolizidine alkaloid, was suspected as the cause by the authors.

Signs

Dyspnea, tachycardia, ventral edema, and venous distention and pulsation characterize cor pulmonale. Therefore, the signs are similar to those found in other common heart diseases of cattle and require differentiation from cardiomyopathy, endocarditis, lymphosarcoma, pericarditis, and myocarditis.

Murmurs or a gallop rhythm may be auscultated, depending on valvular function, the degree of myocardial hypertrophy, or cardiac chamber dilation. Heart sounds have normal or increased intensity. Greatest attention should be directed toward the lungs to determine chronic abnormalities (e.g., consolidation determined via auscultation, radiography or ultrasonography, or interstitial disease via radiographs) that may explain the right heart failure. Affected cattle appear more ill as the degree of dyspnea progresses.

Diagnosis

A history of chronic pulmonary disease (or exposure to high altitude), ruling out other cardiac diseases, and finding signs consistent with right heart failure provide suggestive evidence of cor pulmonale. Microscopic examination of stained blood smears may reveal the presence of vacuolation in the cytoplasm of the lymphocytes in cattle with clinical signs caused by locoweed poisoning. Two-dimensional echocardiography may add further evidence if right ventricular hypertrophy and dilatation is proved. Echocardiographic visualization of the pulmonary outflow tract may provide suggestive findings of enlargement and dilation with a diameter similar to that of the aorta. Increased pulmonary arterial pressures, confirmed by cardiac catheterization, are diagnostic but limited to research facilities. Tracheal washes, thoracic ultrasonography, and thoracic radiography may contribute to an understanding of the pulmonary problem in suspected cases, especially cattle with chronic pneumonia, *T. pyogenes* pneumonia, abscesses, or diffuse pulmonary fibrosis. Measurement of arterial blood gas concentrations may confirm the presence of underlying hypoxemia.

Treatment

In cattle affected with primary chronic pulmonary disease, treatment of the primary lung disease coupled with furosemide therapy may be beneficial. Cattle known to have had pneumonia in the past and mild but persistent chronic respiratory signs thereafter may benefit from a tracheal wash to establish cytologic and cultural aids to antibiotic treatment of the chronic lung problem. Baermann's technique should be performed if chronic lungworm infestation is suspected. Cattle at high altitude suspected to have brisket disease should receive oxygen and be moved to lower altitudes.

Furosemide is administered at 0.5 to 1.0 mg/kg twice daily as a diuretic. Although digoxin may be considered in these cases, cattle that require digoxin require hospitalization and incur significant expense. Therefore, use of digoxin seldom is practiced. If digoxin is required for a select case, the recommended dosage is 0.86 μg/kg/hr IV.

Arrhythmias

Etiology

Arrhythmias in adult cattle can be caused by a variety of drugs, myocardial insults, myocardial lymphosarcoma, and metabolic abnormalities. In calves, myocarditis, hyperkalemia, hypoglycemia, and white muscle disease have been discussed previously as factors involved in the pathogenesis of arrhythmias.

Myocarditis may be the most difficult of the adult cow causes to diagnose definitively and therefore is suspected when other known causes are eliminated. Toxic myocardial damage from ionophores and plant toxins, as well as septic or inflammatory mediators (myocardial depressant factor, tumor necrosis factor), must be considered when arrhythmias appear in cattle without GI, electrolyte, or other typical predisposing factors. Cattle with lymphosarcoma of the myocardium, most commonly involving the right atrium, often present with tachyarrhythmias with or without other concurrent signs of cardiac disease on physical examination. It is therefore worthwhile considering this differential whenever the clinician is presented with an adult cow (>2 years of age) that has a tachyarrhythmia (frequently atrial fibrillation) for which no other metabolic, GI, or toxic explanation is forthcoming. Clinical signs consistent with lymphosarcoma in other anatomic locations (abomasum, spinal cord, retrobulbar) are only occasionally found but should be thoroughly investigated. The identification of peripheral lymphadenopathy or PL is supportive, but not definitive.

Calcium solutions are well recognized as being capable of causing cardiac arrhythmias or even death when administered IV to cattle. Both hypocalcemia and hypercalcemia have been associated with arrhythmias, and arrhythmias associated with hypercalcemia are thought to be mediated by vagal stimulation. In fact, arrhythmias associated with hypercalcemia may be abolished by atropine. However, atropine seldom is used for this purpose because of its negative effects on the GI tract of cattle. Atrial fibrillation has been associated with hypocalcemia and has been reported after treatment of cattle with neostigmine (mostly for ileus)

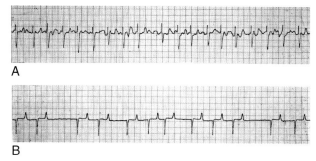

A

B

• **Fig. 3.44** Electrocardiographic recording from two different cows showing characteristic changes of atrial fibrillation. Both **A** and **B** demonstrate an irregular rhythm with normal QRS complexes but no P waves. In **A**, the f (fibrillation) waves are coarse, and the heart rate is more rapid than in **B**, which demonstrates relatively fine f waves along with a normal heart rate. In both tracings the intervals between QRS complexes are irregular, a typical feature of atrial fibrillation.

that may have provoked increased vagal tone. Hypocalcemia and hypokalemia in cattle with primary GI diseases seem to be major risk factors for the development of atrial fibrillation and atrial premature contractions (APCs) in adult dairy cattle.

Oxytetracycline in propylene glycol vehicles may cause decreased cardiac output and stroke volume, as well as decreased heart rates and aortic pressures. Systemic hypotension and cardiac asystole also have been observed when these drugs are given IV to awake, healthy calves. It is common knowledge among bovine practitioners that oxytetracycline, especially when prepared in propylene glycol vehicles, should ideally be administered slowly and diluted with saline or dextrose to avoid hypotension, collapse, or death in both calves and adult cattle.

Atrial fibrillation is the most common arrhythmia occurring in adult dairy cattle (Fig. 3.44). One report suggests that APCs in cattle with GI disease may occur as commonly as atrial fibrillation. APCs often were associated with hypocalcemia and sometimes with hypokalemia in that study. APCs probably reflect vagotonia associated with abdominal distention or GI diseases and are characterized using ECG by abnormal premature P waves (P′) from depolarization at an atrial site different from the sinus node. APCs usually result in a normal QRS-T on the ECG unless they enter the ventricle when it is partially refractory or if the AV node is refractory to excitement. In any event, it appears that APCs may precede or predispose to atrial fibrillation. Sporadic irregularities rather than the irregularly irregular rhythm of atrial fibrillation are auscultated during APCs in cattle.

Although atrial fibrillation may occur with or without underlying heart disease, it usually is a secondary event unrelated to primary heart disease. There may be a normal or fast heart rate, depending on the severity of the underlying condition, but the rhythm is always irregular with variation in the intensity of heart sounds and pulse deficits when the heart rate is rapid. There is an absence of P waves and presence of f (fibrillation) waves demonstrated by ECG recordings (see Fig. 3.44).

Signs

Clinical signs related to APCs and atrial fibrillation are nonspecific unless underlying primary heart disease is present, in which case general signs of heart failure also may be observed. Close observation of the jugular vein may reveal occasional abnormal pulsations in cows with APCs. Signs of heart failure, such as venous distention or ventral edema, usually are not present in cattle with atrial fibrillation, except in advanced cases that have progressed to congestive heart failure. Because most cows with either APCs or atrial fibrillation have a primary GI or other medical disorder, the signs vary in each case. Without question, cattle with abomasal displacement and other diseases characterized by abdominal distention are most frequently affected by atrial fibrillation. Specific signs of APCs or atrial fibrillation are associated with cardiac auscultation. Sporadic arrhythmias and variations in the intensity of S1 typify APCs. Although the heart rate varies, perhaps dependent on the primary disease, it often is within the normal range. Atrial fibrillation, on the other hand, leads to more obvious abnormalities in cardiac auscultation. Marked irregularities in rhythm, tachycardia, and dramatic variations in the intensity of heart sounds are obvious. Pulse deficits may be present in cattle with rapid heart rates, and an absence of the S4 has been reported. Although exercise intolerance is possible with atrial fibrillation, cattle seldom show this sign because they are not "raced."

Cattle confirmed to have atrial fibrillation or some other arrhythmia associated with cardiac lymphosarcoma that also have outward signs of congestive heart failure have a guarded to poor prognosis, and such individuals seldom survive more than a few weeks to a few months.

Diagnosis

Although cardiac auscultation is highly suggestive, an ECG is necessary to make a definitive diagnosis of APCs (Fig. 3.45) or atrial fibrillation in cattle (see Fig. 3.44). The increased availability of cTnI testing, usually through local human hospitals, or by using "stall-side" commercial kits (i-STAT) designed initially for people but with diagnostic utility in cattle, provides a useful adjunctive tool for the workup of cattle with suspected myocardial insult. Elevations in cTnI (see earlier section) do not identify the cause of the myocardial injury, and as yet we do not know the kinetics of release or the half-life of the protein in cattle; however, it has become an active focus of current research and the source of several publications. Key ECG findings in each condition are listed below and shown in the figures:

APCs : Abnormal premature P waves (P′);
   Normal QRS-T unless occurring during refractory
   period of ventricle or AV node; Sporadic

Atrial fibrillation : Absence of P waves;
   F waves may be apparent;
   "Irregularly irregular" rhythm;
   Tachycardia (usually); Pulse deficit

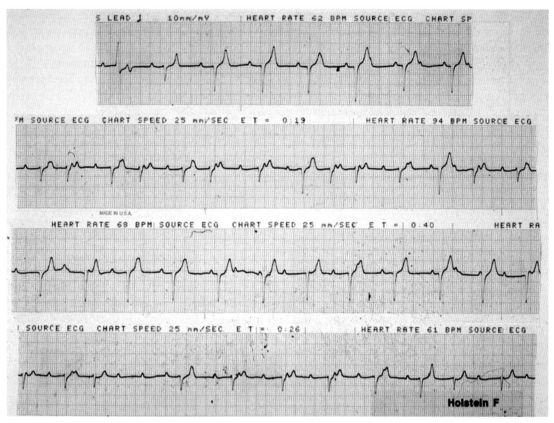

• **Fig. 3.45** Electrocardiographic recording from a cow with atrial premature contractions associated with concurrent gastrointestinal disease.

Treatment

Specific anti-arrhythmic treatment of atrial fibrillation in cattle seldom is necessary because resolution of the patient's primary medical or GI problem generally results in a return to normal sinus rhythm. Medical or surgical treatment of the primary problem coupled with correction of existing acid–base and electrolyte abnormalities is indicated for cattle whose problems include atrial fibrillation.

Routine administration of oral or SC calcium solutions as indicated and oral supplementation with 50 to 100 g of KCl orally, twice daily for 3 to 5 days, are excellent empiric and supportive treatments for cattle with abomasal displacements or other causes of abdominal distention that also have APCs or atrial fibrillation.

Occasionally atrial fibrillation persists several days to several weeks after resolution of the primary problem. Persistent atrial fibrillation raises concerns, lest the long-term condition lead to eventual heart failure. Heart failure has been suspected to result from prolonged (a course of years) atrial fibrillation in horses. Similar suspicions exist in cattle, but we know of no work that confirms this theory pathologically. In addition, cattle with atrial fibrillation that persists more than 1 month after resolution of a GI or medical problem may in fact have myocardial disease causing atrial fibrillation or acquire heart disease because the noncontracting atria will develop progressive dilation that eventually results in tricuspid and mitral valve regurgitation. It also is possible that some cows with persistent atrial fibrillation

had it before the onset of their medical or GI disease. Therefore, discussions of appropriate criteria on which to base treatment are subjective. If medical or surgical therapy for the primary illness fails to resolve the atrial fibrillation, it is difficult to know how much the arrhythmia might contribute to any ongoing inappetence, depression, and decreased milk production. It seems that cattle, similar to horses, can be remarkably tolerant of chronic atrial fibrillation provided there is not concurrent, significant cardiac disease. The fact that chronic atrial fibrillation will ultimately lead to cardiomyopathic changes and deteriorating cardiac function means that there would be circumstances under which an attempt to convert cattle back to sinus rhythm should occur.

If atrial fibrillation persists for 5 days beyond treatment or resolution of the primary problem, it is thought by some that it should be treated with quinidine therapy. This may be premature in cattle that are clinically improved by resolution of their primary problem. It is our opinion that therapeutic intervention in cattle that are improving should be delayed at least 14 days because spontaneous resolution may occur during this time. Failure of cattle to resolve atrial fibrillation spontaneously may result from ongoing medical, GI, acid–base, or electrolyte abnormalities. Treatment with quinidine, or digoxin followed by quinidine, may be expensive and requires careful clinical and ECG monitoring to avoid toxic side effects.

However, if atrial fibrillation persists beyond a reasonable time after resolution of a primary illness or is thought to be partially responsible for vague signs of illness in a patient or is thought to risk eventual heart failure, treatment may be considered. The following treatment protocols have been suggested:

1. Simple atrial fibrillation that has persisted despite resolution of primary disease:

   Quinidine 48.0 mg/kg in 4 L of saline or lactated Ringer's solution administered at a rate of 1 L/hr IV. Balanced fluids may be given concurrently via the opposite jugular vein.

2. Atrial fibrillation that is complicated by extreme tachycardia or that has not responded to previous quinidine therapy:

   Digoxin 0.86 µg/kg per hour or 11.0 µg/kg thrice daily IV for 4 to 5 days. After this time, quinidine is administered as in (1) above.

   Digoxin—loading dose 22.0 µg/kg once followed by 0.86 µg/kg/hr for 2 to 4 days. After this time, quinidine is administered as in (1) above.

In all treatment protocols, side effects of quinidine such as diarrhea, rumen hypermotility, and tachycardia must be anticipated. Signs of quinidine toxicity may also include arrhythmias other than atrial fibrillation, prolonged QRS complexes, or collapse. If signs of toxicity appear in the form of pronounced tachycardia, the rate of infusion should be slowed or stopped. Intravenous sodium bicarbonate also may be administered. Some cattle are reported to show blepharospasm and ataxia just before conversion to normal sinus rhythm.

Cattle having atrial fibrillation that persists despite attempted conversion therapy may have ongoing primary illnesses, myocardial disease, or vagotonia that interferes with conversion to normal rhythm. Prognosis remains guarded for these patients and for untreated atrial fibrillation patients that remain in atrial fibrillation for more than 30 days after apparent successful resolution of their primary GI or medical disease.

Diseases of the Veins

Thrombosis and Phlebitis

Etiology

Traumatic venipuncture and perivascular reactions to irritating drugs from attempted IV therapy are the major causes of venous thrombosis and thrombophlebitis. Dextrose solutions and calcium solutions that contain dextrose are the greatest offenders because of the tissue reaction that develops around hypertonic dextrose solutions. Tetracycline, phenylbutazone (not to be used in dairy cows older than 20 months of age in the US), and IV sodium iodide also are capable of causing severe thrombophlebitis when inadvertent perivascular leaking occurs.

Traumatic or repeated venipuncture may result in simple thrombosis, thrombophlebitis, or septic thrombophlebitis. Poor restraint, improper preparation of the vein for venipuncture, inexperience in venipuncture, and inappropriate selection of needles for IV therapy increase the risk of injury to veins. The common use of disposable 14-gauge needles for jugular venipuncture in cattle has increased the incidence of venous injury because these needles are only 3.75 cm (1.5 in) long—too short to be placed properly for adult cattle. Furthermore, these same needles are extremely sharp and can lacerate the intima of the vein if the cow moves at all. Prolonged use of indwelling IV catheters risks both thrombophlebitis and septic thrombophlebitis, but catheter materials have improved over recent years such that less thrombogenic polyurethane or antimicrobially coated catheters are available for longer term use and use in patients deemed to be at greater risk for thrombosis. Septic thrombophlebitis of any cause creates a major risk for endocarditis in cattle.

Dehydrated cattle and endotoxic cattle are especially prone to thrombosis during attempts at venipuncture. The normally thick bovine skin becomes even more difficult to penetrate when the animal is severely dehydrated. This is especially true in neonatal calves that are severely dehydrated by diarrhea. Repeated attempts at venipuncture in these patients may injure the vein and cause thrombosis. Endotoxic patients and septicemic patients that are predisposed to coagulopathies may develop venous thrombosis very easily. Platelet activation and other coagulation factors may contribute to venous thrombosis in such cattle, even when an experienced clinician performs venipuncture. In some endotoxic or septic patients, gelatinous or "Jell-O–like" clots appear at the site of venipuncture within seconds of entering the intima of the vein. Further attempts at venipuncture often result in extension of the thrombus along the length of the vessel.

Although the jugular is the most commonly damaged vein in dairy cattle, mammary and tail veins may sustain damage occasionally. It is contraindicated to perform venipuncture in the mammary vein except in dire emergencies or when both jugular veins have been thrombosed. Injury to the mammary vein not only damages the vein but also causes persistent udder edema of both the forequarter and hindquarter on that side and will negatively impact future production or udder symmetry in the case of show animals.

Although most thromboses, thrombophlebitis, and septic thrombophlebitis are iatrogenic because of the aforementioned conditions, occasional cases develop spontaneously. Neonatal calves always are at risk for umbilical vein omphalophlebitis and subsequent septicemic spread of bacteria to distant sites. In adult cattle, the mammary vein is the most common vein to sustain spontaneous thrombosis, and this usually occurs during the dry period. Trauma by other cows butting the patient or simple pressure thrombosis caused by preparturient udder and ventral edema or excessive abdominal weight when lying on hard surfaces may contribute to this condition. Spontaneous thrombosis or rupture of the perineal vein and caudal udder hematoma formation may also occur in the region of the rear udder support and escutcheon (see the section on Udder Hematomas in Chapter 8).

Signs

Signs associated with simple thrombosis include palpable soft or firm clots within the vein. The vein may appear grossly distended by the thrombus or be of normal diameter. When the vein is held off below the thrombus, a fluid wave of blood cannot be ballotted within the vessel. Acute thrombi tend to be soft or "Jell-O–like," but chronic or subacute thrombi may be firm to the touch. Edema may be apparent as a result of poor venous return in areas "downstream" from the thrombus. Therefore, facial edema may appear with jugular thrombosis and ipsilateral udder edema with mammary vein thrombosis. Thrombosis may cause the patient mild pain, but it is not as painful as thrombophlebitis. "Needle tracks" or palpable swelling may be apparent in the skin overlying the site of thrombus formation.

Thrombophlebitis causes more obvious swelling in and around the affected vein. A perivascular component to the swelling and pain are more likely than with simple thrombosis (Fig. 3.46). Palpable warmth to the swelling may be present, and SC edema usually appears downstream from the lesion. It may be difficult to differentiate a sterile thrombophlebitis from a septic thrombophlebitis. In general, fever and inappetence are more common with septic thrombophlebitis. Both may be painful and warm, and when the jugular vein is involved, the patient may be reluctant to raise or lower its neck or eat. Ipsilateral Horner's syndrome develops in some cattle with jugular thrombophlebitis. Thrombophlebitis of the mammary vein causes marked ventral abdominal pain over the site and severe ipsilateral udder and ventral edema (Fig. 3.47). Because septic thrombophlebitis predisposes to bacterial endocarditis in cattle, careful auscultation of the heart is indicated in all cases (Fig. 3.48). Tissue necrosis associated with extremely irritating drugs (e.g., 50% dextrose, 20% sodium iodide, and phenylbutazone) placed perivascularly or resulting in thrombophlebitis eventually will cause sloughing, cellulitis, or sterile abscess formation. Bacterial contamination of such lesions ensures abscess formation and eventual drainage.

Severe thrombophlebitis involving the tail vein may result in sloughing of the entire tail (Fig. 3.49).

Diagnosis

Clinical signs usually suffice for diagnosis. Two-dimensional ultrasound may be used to confirm the diagnosis, assess the extent of thrombosis, and detect fluid or pus accumulations that may be drained in cases of septic thrombophlebitis.

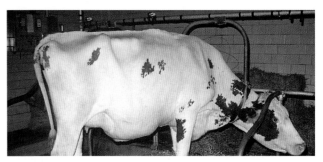

• **Fig. 3.47** Thrombophlebitis of the right mammary vein in a Holstein cow secondary to owner-administered oxytetracycline and dextrose.

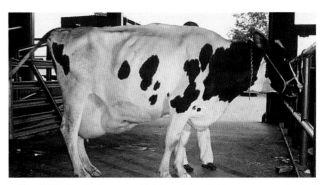

• **Fig. 3.48** Septic thrombophlebitis of the right mammary vein that resulted in cellulitis cranial to the udder and septic endocarditis. Attempted blind stitching of an abomasal displacement caused the original venous damage.

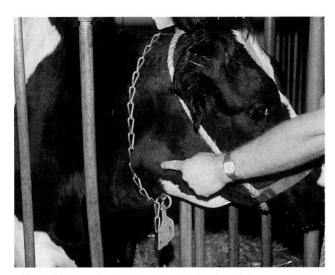

• **Fig. 3.46** Thrombophlebitis of the right jugular vein in a cow that had repeatedly been administered dextrose by the owner.

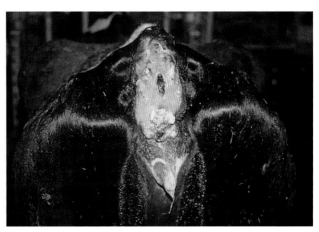

• **Fig. 3.49** Tail slough secondary to perivascular injection of the tail vein.

Treatment

Simple sterile thrombosis requires no treatment other than avoidance of further injury to the vein. In acute cases, cool compresses may be applied to the site overlying the thrombus, but this only minimizes hematoma formation. If simple thrombosis is complicated by perivascular leakage of a treatment that risks thrombophlebitis, SC tissues around the swelling should be injected with normal saline in an effort to dilute the drug deposited in the perivascular region. In addition, warm compresses should be applied to the area several times daily.

Sterile thrombophlebitis is best managed by warm compresses and oral aspirin therapy (240–480 grains orally, twice daily for adult cows). Sterile thrombophlebitis may or may not eventually slough or abscess. Cases caused by irritating drugs are more likely to slough or abscess. Signs of improvement include stabilization or reduction in the degree of swelling, improved appetite and production, and less pain on palpation.

Septic thrombophlebitis requires more aggressive and intensive therapy lest further complications such as endocarditis occur. Warm compresses several times daily, systemic bactericidal antibiotics, and oral aspirin therapy are indicated. Unless culture results from a draining abscess or catheter tip indicate otherwise, procaine penicillin 20,000 to 30,000 U/kg IM or SC twice daily should be chosen because of its activity against *T. pyogenes*. When septic thrombophlebitis associated with IV catheters occurs, the catheter tip should be cultured after its removal from the vein. An effort should be made to avoid further IV therapy in all patients having thromboses or phlebitis because injury to one vessel may predispose to multiple thromboses. When IV therapy is essential for patient management, extensive care and aseptic technique are essential for future placement of IV catheters or injections. Therapy for septic thrombophlebitis usually is long term (several weeks), and relapses are common if therapy is halted prematurely. Occasional cattle with septic thrombophlebitis may have intermittent fever, depression, and inappetence, as well as swelling and pain at the site of venous injury. Such chronic thrombophlebitis is not as common as in horses but may benefit from surgical removal of the affected area of vein. Positive signs for cattle being treated for septic thrombophlebitis include normal temperature; increased appetite and production; reduced pain, swelling, and heat at the site; and decreasing amounts of drainage in cases with sloughing or abscessation.

The prognosis for simple thrombosis is fair. If further injury to the vessel is avoided, some veins recannulate with time. The prognosis for thrombophlebitis is guarded, and most affected veins do not recannulate. In addition, SC edema of the tissue downstream to the vein injury is more common and requires a longer time to resolve. In some cases involving the mammary vein the edema and asymmetry of the udder never completely resolve despite apparent resolution of the thrombophlebitis. This is a particularly frustrating outcome in show cattle.

Prevention

Good restraint, proper technique and equipment, and clinician experience are the best ways to avoid iatrogenic vein injuries. Careful preparation of the selected vein and cutdowns through the skin with small scalpel blades are very important aids when injecting or catheterizing a vein in a known high-risk patient such as a severely dehydrated or endotoxic cow (see Chapter 2). Consideration of catheter type is important, especially in "at-risk" patients and those for whom a long-term indwelling catheter is anticipated. It is the opinion of many veterinarians that the milk vein should be "off limits" for IV injections, particularly in show cattle.

Lacerations

Etiology

Mammary vein lacerations are the most common life-threatening venous laceration in dairy cattle. Sharp objects or barbed wire are the usual cause of injury, and blood loss can be profound unless the animal is attended to quickly.

Signs

Whereas small lacerations or penetrations lead to mild blood loss and hematoma formation, complete lacerations can lead to massive blood loss and exsanguination. Other than the obvious venous bleeding from the site, clinical signs are those associated with blood loss anemia. Weakness, polypnea, tachycardia, anxiety, and pallor of mucous membranes indicate a life-threatening degree of blood loss. Heart rates greater than 120 beats/min and respiratory rates greater than 60 breaths/min usually are associated with severe blood loss. These parameters, coupled with extreme pallor of the mucous membranes and weakness, dictate a need for whole blood transfusion.

Diagnosis

The diagnosis is self-evident. Because blood loss is peracute, the PCV should not be used as a decisive parameter when assessing the need for a whole blood transfusion. Peracute blood loss does not allow time for physiologic reestablishment of plasma volume, and a cow with peracute severe blood loss may die with a normal PCV. Many clinicians rely more on the respiratory rate, heart rate, mucous membrane color, and degree of weakness to judge the severity of the blood loss.

Treatment

Initial treatment includes temporary hemostasis by hemostats, ligatures, clothespins, locking pliers ("mole grips"), or nylon ties followed by a complete physical examination to determine the severity of blood loss. If transfusion of whole blood is indicated (heart rate >120 beats/min, respiratory rate >60 breaths/min, and extreme pallor of membranes), at least 4 L of fresh whole blood should be administered. After transfusion, surgical correction of the laceration with fine sutures or ligation of the vein should be performed.

For mammary vein lacerations if the physical status of the patient tolerates it, the cow should be placed in dorsal recumbency to allow the wound to be explored, extended, and assessed before repair or ligature placement.

Because phlebitis and septic thrombophlebitis are potential complications, systemic bactericidal antibiotics such as penicillin or ceftiofur at standard dosages should be given and continued for 5 to 7 days. A belly wrap applied with self-adherent tape is useful as a pressure wrap after surgery.

Caudal Vena Caval Thrombosis

Caudal vena caval thrombosis secondary to rupture, or outgrowth, of abscesses near the hilus of the liver into the caudal vena cava is the most common clinically impactful consequence of enteric origin liver abscesses in dairy cattle. Thrombi may form at the site of abscess rupture into the caudal vena cava or lodge between the heart and diaphragmatic region of the vessel. Thromboemboli can traverse the right heart to lodge in the pulmonary arterial circulation, potentially leading to acute death, acute respiratory distress, or the more common respiratory sequelae of caudal vena caval thrombosis syndrome with subsequent epistaxis, hemoptysis, anemia, and pneumonia. Endocarditis of the right heart valves is another common sequela. Further discussion of this syndrome is covered in Chapter 4.

Congenital Anomalies

Congenital portosystemic anastomoses have been identified in calves and usually result in poor growth and neurologic signs. They are further discussed in Chapter 13.

Diseases of the Arteries

Rupture

Rupture of major arteries is relatively rare in cattle. Occasional uterine artery tears occur in parturient cattle and are of unknown etiology. Trauma to the artery is suspected and may result from the vessel being trapped in the pelvis as extensive traction is placed on the calf during dystocia. The uterine artery also may experience extreme traction in some severe uterine torsions. Occasional cows having uterine prolapse suffer rupture of the uterine artery and exsanguinate (Fig. 3.50).

Copper deficiency has been suggested but seldom is confirmed as a cause of arterial rupture because it causes degeneration of the tunica elastica within arteries. Deficiency of the enzyme lysyl oxidase, which contains copper, may prevent normal cross-linking of collagen and elastin. Although the aorta seems most at risk for rupture in copper deficiency, Drs. Charles Guard and John M. King have investigated several herds in New York that have had multiple cows die acutely from arterial rupture of the mesenteric arteries or aorta. Histopathology of arteries from affected cattle suggests copper deficiency, but copper levels have not been

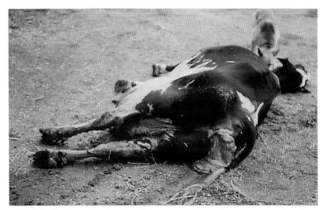

• **Fig. 3.50** Fatal uterine artery rupture and self-induced uterine amputation in a cow that stumbled as a result of hypocalcemia and stepped on her prolapsed uterus.

confirmed to be deficient. Therefore, copper deficiency, although suspected, has not yet been proven. Major arterial rupture usually is fatal.

Aneurysms

An example of aneurysmal pathology in adult dairy cattle is presented by pulmonary artery aneurysms that develop proximal to septic thromboemboli in individuals with caudal vena caval thrombosis syndrome. These aneurysms later contribute to hemorrhage into the airways after dissection by septic thrombi that abscess.

We have observed several adult dairy cattle with persistent or intermittent colic that subsequently were shown to have mesenteric arterial aneurysms. Surgical removal of the aneurysm may be possible in some cases, but these cattle are likely to develop arterial rupture and exsanguination eventually. If several cows are affected simultaneously, a toxin such as moldy clover or sweet vernal hay, which can prolong clotting times, should be suspected. For isolated cases, the reason for the abdominal hemorrhage is generally unproven, although copper deficiency has again been proposed as a causative factor.

Arterial Hypertrophy

Hypertrophy of the tunica media of pulmonary arteries and arterioles and subsequent pulmonary hypertension occurs as a response to prolonged hypoxia in high-altitude disease or brisket edema of cattle. This situation leads to right heart failure and is further discussed under cor pulmonale earlier in this chapter.

Vasculitis

Although of nonspecific etiology, vasculitis may occur in conjunction with many infectious, parasitic, and immune-mediated diseases. In dairy cattle, malignant catarrhal fever is a cause of classic generalized vasculitis. Bovine viral diarrhea virus, bluetongue virus, *Salmonella* spp., *H. somni*, and *Erysipelothrix rhusiopathiae* are other potential causes of vasculitis in cattle.

Disorders of the Erythron

Evaluation of the erythron with CBC, stained blood smears, PCV, hemoglobin, and other parameters is primarily useful to clinicians monitoring anemia in cattle. It should be emphasized that the PCV for healthy lactating dairy cattle is lower than in many other species (see Table 1.2). Anemia usually is suspected based on physical examination findings and may be confirmed, quantified, and differentiated as to type based on evaluation of the erythron and leukon. Although a single CBC often allows classification of anemia into a regenerative or nonregenerative category, serial CBC analyses are required to follow trends in the erythron. Blood loss anemia and hemolytic anemia are "regenerative anemias," and anemias caused by chronic disease are termed "nonregenerative." Regenerative simply implies bone marrow response to anemia through increased erythropoiesis. Regenerative anemias in cattle frequently result in overt microscopic evidence of increased erythropoiesis such as increased anisocytosis, polychromasia, reticulocytosis, and occasionally even nucleated red blood cells (RBCs). In addition, an increase in mean corpuscular volume (MCV) and decreased mean corpuscular hemoglobin concentration (MCHC) are typical in regenerative anemias. Complete nonregenerative anemia would occur from a bone marrow disorder such as bracken fern toxicity. Neutropenia and thrombocytopenia would be seen before anemia in bracken fern–poisoned cattle.

Physiologic hemoconcentration occurs with dehydration in calves and adult cattle. Because anemia may be counterbalanced by hemoconcentration, interpretations of PCV in sick cattle must always be made with consideration of the hydration status. True polycythemia (persistent elevation of PCV despite normal hydration) is rare but may occur as a result of familial, geographic, and pathologic conditions. Peracute severe blood loss as might occur in mammary vein lacerations or some abomasal bleeding ulcers does not immediately lower the PCV because physiologic dilution of hematocrit by renal and intestinal absorption of fluid requires at least 12 to 24 hours. Therefore, the degree of acute, obvious blood loss in a patient can be assessed best clinically by evaluating heart rate, respiratory rate, strength in rising and walking, and mucous membrane pallor.

Definitions

Anisocytosis; variation in size of RBC; normal to some degree in cattle; increases in regenerative anemias.
Polychromasia; variable staining (toward blue) in Wright's type stains; indicates "young" RBC or reticulocytes still containing DNA.
Basophilic stippling; blue granules, again indicative of DNA; also may be observed in chronic lead poisoning.
Nucleated RBC; not unusual in cattle with severe but responsive anemia.
Heinz bodies; precipitated hemoglobin deposits on the edge of RBC; observed in some hemolytic anemias. New methylene blue stain is helpful for detecting Heinz bodies and polychromasia in smears.
Poikilocytosis; uncommon in cattle RBC.
Mean corpuscular volume:

$$MCV = \frac{PCV \times 10}{RBC \text{ count in millions/}\mu L}$$

Increase = Usually regenerative anemia

False increase = Blood not spun sufficiently for accurate PCV

Mean corpuscular hemoglobin:

$$(MCH) = \frac{Hb\ (g/dL) \times 10}{RBC \text{ count in millions/}\mu L}$$

Increase = Increased number of reticulocytes

= Hemolysis

Mean corpuscular hemoglobin concentration:

$$MCHC = \frac{Hb\ (g/dL) \times 10}{PCV}$$

Decrease = Responding anemia with reticulocytosis

= Hemolysis

False decrease = Blood not spun down sufficiently

Polycythemia

Relative polycythemia resulting from hemoconcentration is extremely common. Absolute polycythemia results from an absolute increase in PCV (usually ≥60%) that is repeatable, not associated with hemoconcentration, and does not lower in response to fluid therapy. Absolute polycythemia (absolute erythrocytosis) may be primary or secondary. Primary polycythemia, also known as polycythemia vera, is a rare myeloproliferative condition that usually causes excess production of WBCs and platelets as well as RBCs. Plasma erythropoietin is decreased below normal levels in polycythemia vera. Regardless of cause, progressive polycythemia eventually interferes with tissue oxygenation because of hyperviscosity and reduced cardiac output.

Secondary polycythemia is more common than primary polycythemia in cattle and implies a physiologic response to increased erythropoietin. Generally, increased erythropoietin is a response to chronic tissue hypoxia. Therefore, secondary polycythemia tends to occur in animals kept at high altitudes and in calves having congenital cardiac defects with right-to-left shunts. The chronic hypoxia associated with brisket disease or high-altitude disease of cattle is capable of inducing polycythemia (see section on cor pulmonale). Tetralogy of Fallot and other severe congenital cardiac defects that create or progress to right-to-left shunting of blood also may cause secondary polycythemia.

Congenital polycythemia in Jersey cattle has been described as a recessive defect. These cattle are thought to have increased erythropoietin of unknown origin and the condition has been grouped within the secondary polycythemias.

Clinical signs associated with polycythemia are dyspnea, exercise intolerance, tachycardia, tachypnea, and very injected maroon or muddy-red membranes. Calves affected with polycythemia do not grow properly, regardless of whether the cause is cardiac or inherited. Funduscopic examination allows confirmation of hyperviscosity (Fig. 3.51) in the retinal vessels. Retinal vessels are greatly increased in diameter, and the stars of Winslow (choriocapillaries on end) are very obvious. The hematocrit is consistently elevated over 55% and often greater than 60%.

Treatment is impractical in most patients with polycythemia. This is especially true regarding congenital heart defects and inherited forms of the disease. Particularly valuable cattle with high-altitude hypoxia may benefit from phlebotomy and a return to lower altitudes. The practicality of the matter, however, dictates that although extremely dyspneic cattle are most likely to benefit from phlebotomy, these animals may die if restrained. If phlebotomy is accomplished, the PCV should be decreased below 50%, the animal moved to lower altitude, and symptomatic therapy given. Suspected hereditary polycythemia cases should be investigated genetically, and family members should be culled.

Anemia

Blood Loss Anemia

In addition to sporadic trauma and surgical procedures that result in severe blood loss, a long list of differential diagnoses exists for blood loss anemia in cattle. However, several common causes deserve comment.

Bleeding abomasal ulcers may cause acute or subacute blood loss in adult cattle. Melena is associated with most abomasal ulcers causing significant blood loss (Fig. 3.52). Bleeding abomasal ulcers that result in clinically significant anemia are not common even though abomasal ulceration is commonly found on necropsy of sick cattle. Bleeding ulcers causing clinical signs of anemia are more common in adult cows than in calves, where perforations are most common. Abomasal bleeding also may occur in association with chronic abomasal displacement in cattle. This combination of chronic abomasal displacement with ulceration is most common in dry cows, bulls, and heifers that are not observed as closely as lactating cattle. Thus the abomasal displacement may have existed for days to weeks before diagnosis. The distention and ileus of the displaced abomasum, coupled with large volumes of hydrochloric acid, contributes to mucosal injury and subsequent ulceration with bleeding.

Lymphosarcoma of the abomasum may cause abomasal ulceration, hemorrhage, and blood loss anemia. The clinical signs may be difficult to differentiate from bleeding abomasal ulcers unless other signs of lymphosarcoma are detected during the physical examination.

Acute splenic rupture caused by infiltration of the spleen by lymphosarcoma may cause severe acute or peracute hemoperitoneum with resultant signs of blood loss anemia.

Caudal vena caval thrombosis syndrome may cause blood loss anemia after abscesses resulting from septic thromboemboli lodged in pulmonary arterioles erode into airways or lung parenchyma. Subsequent hemorrhage results in hemoptysis and epistaxis. Melena or fecal occult blood may be detected if the affected cow swallows sufficient quantities of blood. Epistaxis and blood loss also may occur as a result of granulomatous rhinitis, skull trauma and invasive neoplasia of the upper respiratory tract (usually adenocarcinomas of the respiratory epithelium).

Parasites are another cause of blood loss anemia. Lice are the most common ectoparasite to cause anemia in both calves and adult cattle in the northern United States. In other geographic areas, fleas (*Ctenocephalides felis*) and ticks also may cause significant blood loss. Thanks to modern heifer

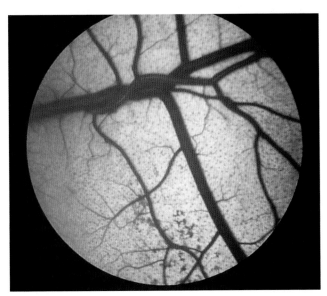

• **Fig. 3.51** Dorsal view of the fundus of a calf that had polycythemia secondary to tetralogy of Fallot. The fundic vessels are greatly accentuated as is typical of hyperviscosity syndrome.

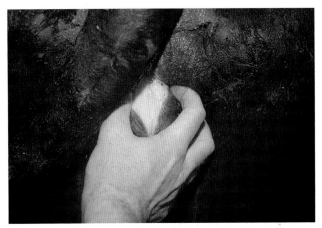

• **Fig. 3.52** Extreme pallor of the vulvar mucous membranes in a cow that had severe blood loss associated with a bleeding abomasal ulcer.

management systems and routine deworming, endoparasites are uncommon but may result in blood loss, especially in pastured heifers. *Eimeria bovis* may cause life-threatening anemia as a result of intestinal blood loss in weanling through yearling age cattle. *Anaplasma marginale* or *Theleria* infection may cause fever, jaundice, and anemia associated with severe extravascular hemolysis. With hemolytic disorders PCV is decreased but there is usually no decrease of plasma protein. By contrast, in severe hemorrhage of more than a few hours duration both PCV and plasma protein concentrations decrease.

Pyelonephritis in cattle may result in anemia by either blood loss (acute and uncommon) or by nonregenerative mechanisms (chronic and common). Cattle having blood loss associated with acute pyelonephritis also may have colic and stranguria as a result of blood clots obstructing the ureters or urethra (see Chapter 11) and usually have fever. Anemia of chronic infection or perhaps that associated with decreased erythropoietin production caused by chronic pyelonephritis may be involved in the anemia observed in such patients. Blood loss anemia, sometimes severe, also occurs in association with thrombocytopenia caused by type 2 bovine viral diarrhea virus (BVDV) infection. Affected animals often have obvious petechial and ecchymotic hemorrhages on their oral, vulval, and conjunctival membranes (see section on thrombocytopenia).

Acquired or congenital defects in hemostasis may cause blood loss and resultant anemia by a variety of mechanisms. When hemostatic dysfunction exists, simple bruising, insect bites, injections, and other minor trauma may cause significant blood loss.

Rupture of the uterine artery during parturition or after uterine prolapse and sporadic rupture of other major arteries are other causes of acute blood loss. Occasionally, vaginal hemorrhage associated with dystocia can be significant enough to cause severe life-threatening anemia. Self-induced trauma or laceration of a prolapsed uterus with subsequent hemorrhage has been observed in dairy cattle. Manual removal of a corpus luteum through rectal palpation to induce heat has fortunately fallen out of favor with bovine practitioners. This procedure occasionally resulted in severe blood loss or exsanguination.

Winter dysentery very occasionally causes severe blood loss from the colon in first-calf heifers. Affected heifers have fresh clots of whole blood and severe dysentery and may require whole blood transfusions.

Nonregenerative Anemia (Anemia of Chronic Disease)

Chronic infections and neoplasms are the most common primary conditions associated with inadequate erythrocyte production or nonregenerative anemia. Chronic pneumonia with abscessation, chronic pyelonephritis, multiple abscesses secondary to musculoskeletal problems, endocarditis, and visceral abscesses may cause nonregenerative anemia. Nonregenerative anemia caused by chronic inflammation is mostly the result of hepcidin release from

the liver causing macrophage sequestration and malabsorption of iron resulting in secondary iron deficiency. Serum iron concentration is moderately decreased as is total iron-binding capacity (TIBC) and transferrin. The PCV in these cases is generally not lower than 18%. Primary iron-deficiency anemia may rarely cause severe weakness in milk-fed calves when PCV decreases below 14%. It is characterized as a microcytic and hypochromic anemia. Serum iron is extremely low, and iron-binding capacity is normal or high in affected calves. Treatment with blood transfusion is usually curative.

Cattle with chronic renal disease may have depressed erythropoietin synthesis resulting from renal impairment to help explain their nonregenerative anemia. Chronic protein-losing nephropathies such as amyloidosis and glomerulonephritis also may have a nonregenerative anemia and hypoproteinemia.

Lymphosarcoma may result in anemia through several mechanisms; nonregenerative anemia simply because of diffuse neoplasia, nonregenerative anemia caused by myelophthisis in sporadic adult cattle or calves with the juvenile form of lymphosarcoma, and blood loss anemia resulting from neoplastic ulceration of the abomasum or splenic rupture.

Bone marrow depression by chronic bracken fern intoxication may result in nonregenerative anemia plus blood loss anemia secondary to thrombocytopenia and subsequent hemorrhage (Fig. 3.53). In regions where enzootic hematuria occurs in cattle pastured in bracken fern, blood loss anemia commonly accompanies the bladder lesions. Chronic bovine viral diarrhea virus infection may rarely cause nonregenerative anemia, although BVDV-associated anemia is more commonly associated with acute disease, thrombocytopenia, and blood loss. This is typically associated with a PCV of less than 15%.

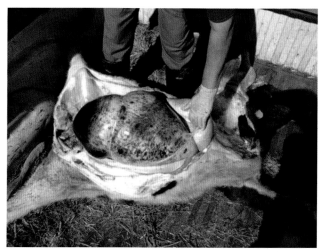

• **Fig. 3.53** Necropsy of a 5-month-old Holstein calf found dead in the pasture. Petechial and ecchymotic hemorrhages were immediately visible upon opening the abdomen. Other calves in the pasture were found to have hemorrhages, and complete blood count evaluation revealed severe neutropenia and thrombocytopenia. Bracken fern was plentiful in the pasture and had been eaten by the calves. (Photo courtesy of Dr. Jennifer Nightingale)

Anemia Through Hemolysis

Hemolytic anemias are associated with either intravascular or extravascular erythrocyte destruction (see Chapter 16 for specific causes discussed in more detail). Although extravascular erythrocyte destruction is more common in most species, cattle have several forms of hemolytic anemia caused by intravascular destruction of erythrocytes. A common cause of intravascular hemolysis in calves is water intoxication. Calves watered intermittently that are then given plentiful supplies of water may overdrink to the point that severe decrease in serum osmolality occurs and RBC lysis follows. The presence of hemoglobinuria alongside the history are diagnostic. Low-grade fever also may be present resulting from RBC destruction, and neurologic signs develop in extreme cases. Similarly, IV administration of hypotonic solutions is an occasional complication observed in adults or calves when electrolytes are not added or are added in insufficient quantities to large fluid containers (for example, 20 L of sterile water will reliably cause this problem in an adult cow) before administration. Fever, trembling, hair standing on end, and hemoglobinuria are the four clinical signs that identify the therapeutic error.

Intravascular destruction of RBC occurs in babesiosis (piroplasmosis, tick fever or red water fever) in cattle; this disease has been eradicated from the United States. Fever, anemia, depression, icterus, hemoglobinuria, and other signs associated with anemia can occur in young cattle with leptospirosis. *Leptospira interrogans* Pomona, *Leptospira interrogans* Icterohaemorrhagiae, and *Leptospira interrogans* Grippotyphosa are the most common disease-producing serovars in young cattle. Bacillary hemoglobinuria caused by *Clostridium novyi* type D *(Clostridium hemolyticum)* is another infectious disease that causes intravascular hemolysis in cattle.

One of the authors (TD) has seen *Theileria buffeli* cause intravascular hemolysis in North American dairy cattle. High fever, tachycardia, diarrhea, jaundiced membranes, dark-colored urine, and lymphadenopathy are other clinical findings. Asymptomatic cows may also be in the herd, and the reason why one cow develops severe disease is unknown. Concurrent lymphosarcoma has been sometimes blamed for the onset of *T. buffeli* disease, but *Theileria* spp. can transform lymphocytes to have the appearance of lymphosarcoma, so the association is unclear. The life cycle of *Theileria* includes two intracellular developmental stages; intralymphocytic schizonts and intraerythrocytic piroplasms. Piroplasms can be identified in the red blood cells in stained blood smears but cannot always be differentiated from other blood parasites such as *Babesia* spp. Several hematologic and biochemical changes associated with bovine theileriosis have been reported such as anemia (regenerative), leukopenia, neutropenia, lymphocytosis, and hypo- or hyperproteinemia. Hyperbilirubinemia, increased liver enzymes, and dark urine are all related to the hemolytic process. Treatment with tetracycline and imidocarb has been unsuccessful.

Heinz body hemolytic anemia results from a variety of oxidizing agents that denature hemoglobin. Complexes of globin, a protein, are then observed microscopically as Heinz body inclusions in RBC. Although rare in dairy cattle, Heinz body anemia has been observed in selenium deficiency and in cattle grazing on rye grass (*Secale cereale*), onions, and *Brassica* spp. Hemoglobinuria generally is also observed in cattle with these diseases.

Postparturient hemoglobinuria may develop when lactating dairy cattle are fed a ration deficient in phosphorus. Intravascular hemolysis and hemoglobinuria associated with hypophosphatemia tend to appear during the first month of lactation. A depletion of adenosine 5′-triphosphate (ATP), secondary to phosphorus deficiency, may be involved in the RBC lysis in this condition. A recent report by Grunberg et al suggests that hypophosphatemia is not the actual cause of the hemolytic disorder.

Extravascular hemolysis occurs as a result of immune-mediated RBC destruction in anaplasmosis in cattle. Hemoglobinuria does *not* occur with this form of hemolysis. Severe anemia, jaundice, fever, weakness, weight loss, and decreased production are the typical findings. Autoimmune hemolytic anemia, as described in other species, is rare or has yet to be documented in cattle other than the RBC destruction that occurs with protozoal RBC parasites. *Mycoplasma wenyonii* may rarely cause severe immune-mediated anemia in cattle. Pitting edema of the hind limbs, teats, and udder along with a mild to modest anemia are the characteristic findings. The organisms are seen on the surface of erythrocytes or free in the serum during a Wright's stained cytologic examination. If milk production is affected by the disease, treatment with tetracyclines is generally successful. Autoimmune RBC destruction has been suspected in some cattle with lymphosarcoma, but definitive documentation has not yet been provided. Neonatal isoerythrolysis does not occur naturally in cattle, but the disorder has been observed as a consequence of vaccination of dams against anaplasmosis and babesiosis with products of cattle origin. Subsequent passive transfer of maternal antibodies against specific blood types to calves from these cattle results in some calves showing isoerythrolysis.

The anemia sometimes present in cattle having the inherited disease erythropoietic porphyria ("pink tooth") (see also Chapter 7) is thought to be hemolytic in origin, although several other factors may be involved.

Determination of when an anemic patient requires whole blood transfusion must be made primarily based on the physical examination and secondarily based on PCV. In peracute blood loss, the PCV may be misleadingly high despite obvious pallor, tachycardia, polypnea, weakness, and other general signs that would indicate the need for a transfusion. When acute or subacute (24–72 hr) blood loss causes anemia, the usual PCV associated with the need for transfusion is in the range of 12% to 14%. With subacute or chronic hemorrhage or hemolysis, and assuming normal hydration, a PCV greater than 14% seldom requires an immediate transfusion. A PCV of less than 14% usually coincides with heart rates greater than 100 beats/min, respiratory rates of greater than 60 breaths/min, obvious mucous membrane pallor, jaundice if a hemolytic process is present, and weakness. Heart rates that are greater than 120 beats/min and pounding, respiratory rates over 60 breaths/min, and obvious pallor all dictate a need for transfusion regardless of the PCV. An increase in blood lactate is a good marker for inadequate tissue oxygenation in cattle with hemolytic anemia and may serve as a transfusion guide.

Chronic blood loss and nonregenerative anemias seldom require transfusions, and the slow, gradual development of anemia seems to allow physiologic compensation for the reduced numbers of RBCs. Cattle with chronic anemias may have PCV values of 9% to 10% without appearing in an anemic crisis.

Diseases of the Leukon

Cattle are unique in regard to their leukogram and its response to various diseases and stresses. Certain conditions, especially peracute inflammatory or endotoxic diseases, cause consistent changes in the leukogram, but other diseases, although infectious in origin, may be associated with normal or variable leukograms that shed little light on the patient's primary problem. Despite having requested leukograms on thousands of bovine patients in academic referral hospitals, we find that the majority of these leukograms, regardless of the cause of illness, have been within normal limits. Despite this fact, the leukogram or, better yet, serial leukograms occasionally may aid greatly in the diagnosis and prognosis for a bovine patient. WBC reference ranges used at the New York State College of Veterinary Medicine for adult cattle are listed in Chapter 1.

Stress and glucocorticoids reliably alter the leukogram to create neutrophilia, lymphopenia, and eosinopenia. The numbers of monocytes appear variable. Concurrent inflammatory diseases may alter this typical "stress leukogram." For example, a cow with acute coliform mastitis that has been treated with dexamethasone may have a normal neutrophil count because of glucocorticoid-induced neutrophilia counterbalancing the expected neutropenia normally found in endotoxemia. This same cow could have a left shift with band (immature) neutrophils present and a lymphopenia in the absence of steroid administration. Cattle and their leukograms are exquisitely sensitive to exogenous corticosteroids. A single injection of 20 mg or more of dexamethasone usually results in a stress leukogram characterized by neutrophilia, lymphopenia, and eosinopenia within 24 hours. Calves occasionally may have neutrophil counts of 20,000/µL or more after administration of dexamethasone. In addition to altering numbers of neutrophils, corticosteroids can also alter the function of neutrophils in a negative fashion. Whereas glucocorticoids are well known for their ability to be immunosuppressive, a single ketosis treatment dose of 0.02 mg/kg dexamethasone is not associated with clinically significant immune function impairment. Neutrophil function may be impaired in cattle with retained fetal membranes and with other common periparturient diseases such as ketosis and fatty liver. Selenium and copper deficiency are also associated with negative alterations in granulocyte function.

A "degenerative left shift" wherein neutropenia coexists with the appearance of band neutrophils is typical of cattle with severe acute inflammation or endotoxemia. This helpful and, for the most part, consistent leukogram result is seen in dairy cattle affected with severe coliform mastitis, acute *Mannheimia hemolytica* pneumonia, severe salmonellosis, severe postpartum gram-negative mastitis, and perforating abomasal ulcers that cause diffuse peritonitis. A simplistic explanation of this phenomenon revolves around the fact that cattle have a limited bone marrow neutrophil pool to draw on in an acute emergency. Although the degenerative left shift remains a negative prognostic indicator and yet a consistent indicator of severe infection or endotoxemia, it is so typical in cattle that it must be tempered by the patient's signs and response to treatment before using it as the sole basis of a prognosis. Cattle that have a degenerative left shift will often have a return to normal neutrophil numbers within 4 to 7 days after successful treatment of their acute infection. This time lapse may simply reflect the time necessary for resolution of a severe infectious insult. If the infection requires more than 1 week for resolution, rebound neutrophilia usually will occur. Chronic infections may cause a neutrophilia, but many cattle with chronic infections such as visceral abscesses, musculoskeletal infections, chronic peritonitis, and other diseases, frequently have normal neutrophil numbers despite having obvious infection. Neutrophilia seems more likely in resolving acute or subacute infections than in chronic infection. Certainly, some cattle with chronic infections have neutrophilia, but the magnitude of the neutrophilia seldom is dramatic. It is rare to see an adult cow with more than 18,000 to 20,000 neutrophils per microliter unless exogenous corticosteroids have been administered to the animal.

Neutropenia also may be found during severe viral infections such as BVDV infection. Acute BVDV infection causes a leukopenia as a result of neutropenia, lymphopenia, or both. Because acute BVDV infection also adversely affects neutrophil function in addition to sometimes reducing absolute numbers, naive cattle acutely infected with BVDV have a reduced ability to respond to concurrent or secondary infections until they form antibodies and resolve the BVDV infection. The immunosuppressive effect of acute BVDV infection and the potential for greater morbidity and mortality to be associated with concurrent infectious diseases such as salmonellosis or pasteurellosis should not be overlooked diagnostically during a herd outbreak of enteric or respiratory disease.

Absolute lymphopenia occurs in conjunction with stress, exogenous corticosteroid administration, some viral diseases such as BVDV, and some acute severe infections or endotoxemias. Frequently, it is difficult to know whether the lymphopenia is associated directly with the disease or simply represents stress associated with a disease. Although eosinopenia should accompany lymphopenia when the cause is stress or corticosteroid administration, eosinophil counts have limited value in this regard. Absolute lymphocytosis that is transient is rare in dairy cattle and when present usually is associated with a neutrophilia in patients recovering from acute infection. Lymphocytosis that is persistent and repeatable usually indicates infection with BLV. PL is a condition that develops in association with BLV infection in certain lines of cattle. The Bendixen method of control of BLV was based on elimination of cattle with PL until a more modern understanding of the disease evolved. This method proved successful because it was eventually determined that PL cows have greater levels of viremia than most BLV positive cows without PL and are the predominant virus spreaders within a herd. Cattle that are BLV positive and have PL may be at greater risk of developing lymphosarcoma than cattle that are BLV positive without PL, but this is controversial. In one study, PL was present in as many as one third of cattle infected with BLV. However, these percentages may vary in individual herds because genetic predispositions appear to affect the trait of PL in response to BLV infection. The lymphocytosis in cattle with PL is generally refractory to stress or corticosteroid treatment. Lymphocyte counts may range from 30,000/μL to 150,000/μL in cases of PL associated with BLV infection (Fig. 3.54). True lymphocytic leukemia does occur in a very small percentage of cattle that develop lymphosarcoma after infection with BLV, and in such cases, lymphoblasts may be observed peripherally.

Eosinophils seldom are of diagnostic significance when interpreting the leukon of cattle. Geographic and management variations may alter the "normal numbers" expected as a result of parasite load and other conditions. Eosinopenia concurrent with lymphopenia is consistent with stress or exogenous corticosteroid administration. Eosinophilia is rare in dairy cattle. Eosinophilia is thought to indicate heavy parasitism, histamine release, or occasionally, immune-mediated or allergic diseases. Unfortunately, eosinophil numbers seldom convey useful clinical data. The same is true of basophils.

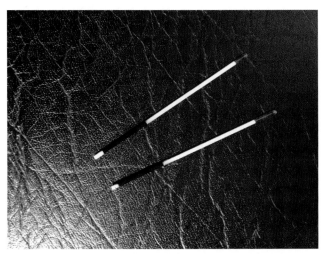

• **Fig. 3.54** Hematocrit tube showing remarkable buffy coat in a bovine leukemia virus–positive, mature Holstein cow with a persistent lymphocytosis of 125,000/μL. (Courtesy of Dr. Sheila McGuirk.)

Monocytosis may be of some value in cattle because it generally is associated with chronic infection. For example, a cow having chronic peritonitis may have a misleadingly normal neutrophil count with no left shift but also may have a monocytosis. Monocytosis, although not specific, should at least raise the clinician's index of suspicion for chronic infection. Although monocytosis is not a consistent finding in the peripheral blood of ruminants infected with *Listeria monocytogenes,* as in humans and rodents so infected, some cattle with listeriosis do have a classical monocytosis. (The name *L. monocytogenes* evolved from the tendency of monogastric animals to have a peripheral monocytosis in response to infection with the organism.)

Bovine Leukocyte Adhesion Deficiency (Bovine Granulocytopathy Syndrome)

Etiology

A fatal syndrome consisting of poor growth, chronic or recurrent infections, and persistent, extreme neutrophilia was first observed in Holstein calves during the latter part of the 20th century. Affected calves had persistent neutrophil counts exceeding 30,000/μL, and some had counts exceeding 100,000/μL. Such calves were initially described subjectively as having a leukemoid blood response that required differentiation from myelogenous leukemia. Despite their neutrophilia, these calves seemed unable to mount a normal defense against common pathogens and minor infections. Although these leukemoid calves sometimes survived for several months, most died before 1 year of age. The true incidence of the disease was impossible to estimate because many "poor-doing" calves eventually die in field situations without ever having a CBC or other diagnostics performed. A genetic immune-deficiency trait was suspected based on clinical observation of the condition in full siblings in a cohort of embryo transfer offspring.

Reports from the United States and Japan on selected calves with the disorder suggested a granulocytopathy, and comparative studies of a canine granulocytopathy in Irish Setters and a leukocyte adhesion deficiency in humans brought about further suspicion of an inherited disorder in these "leukemoid calves." Subsequently this was confirmed and termed bovine leukocyte adhesion deficiency (BLAD) by Kehrli et al. as a genetic disease in Holsteins that represents a severe deficiency of neutrophil Mac-1 (CD11b/CD18). Recessive homozygotes are affected, and heterozygote carriers have intermediate amounts of the Mac-1 β subunit (CD18), but are clinically normal. The molecular basis is a single point mutation (adenine to guanine) at position 383 of the CD18 gene, giving rise to an autosomal recessive mode of inheritance. Despite more than adequate circulating neutrophils, affected calves cannot effectively fight infections because their neutrophils have deficient β2 integrin expression, preventing adherence to vascular endothelium and subsequent migration into tissue sites of inflammation.

Signs

Affected calves have chronic or persistent infections and poor growth (Fig. 3.55). Signs may appear early in life, although some calves live for several months. Relative exposure to a variety of routine pathogens may dictate somewhat the apparent age of onset reported by client histories. Diarrhea and pneumonia are typical signs, but persistent ringworm lesions, persistent keratoconjunctivitis, gingival ulcers, loose teeth, tooth abscesses, poorly healing dehorning wounds, and other lesions also are common. Infections thought to be clinically minor respond poorly or not at all to appropriate therapy. Recurrence of signs and multiple health problems are typical.

Diagnosis

Persistent leukocytosis caused by neutrophilia without a remarkable left shift is a hallmark of the disease. To date most affected calves studied have had greater than 30,000 neutrophils/μL in their peripheral blood. Although myelogenous leukemia is a consideration, neutrophil function tests differentiate these diseases because neutrophils in myelogenous leukemic patients have decreased neutrophil alkaline phosphatase activity. In addition, the truly leukemoid blood picture is characterized as a regenerative left shift, but BLAD calves have primarily a mature neutrophilia. Furthermore, ex vivo tests of adhesion-dependent responses such as chemotaxis and phagocytosis can differentiate between BLAD animals and those with severe, chronic neutrophilia without β2 integrin deficits. Affected calves must be differentiated from calves with chronic abscessation of the thorax or abdomen and calves persistently infected with BVDV that show similar poor growth and apparent reduced resistance to routine pathogens.

Failure to confirm persistent infection with BVDV and ruling out visceral abscessation via radiography, ultrasonography, and serum globulin values support the diagnosis. Definitive diagnosis alongside identification of carriers can be achieved by restriction analysis of PCR-amplified DNA from a suspect individual to allow discrimination between normal, carrier (heterozygote), and affected (homozygote) animals.

Currently, artificial insemination (AI) sires are being tested and identified as either carriers or noncarriers of

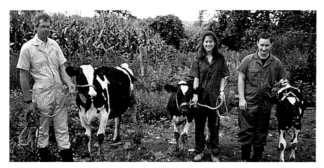

• **Fig. 3.55** A normal heifer and two animals affected with bovine leukocyte adhesion deficiency. All three animals were 8 months of age and had been raised on the same farm. (Courtesy of Dr. Robert O. Gilbert.)

BLAD. The routine genetic screening and identification of carriers by AI companies worldwide will eventually lead to the eradication of the disease. It is rare to non-existent now.

Treatment

Treatment is only palliative, and most affected calves die before 1 year of age. The exact age of onset, progression, and true incidence are unknown because most sick calves never have a CBC performed. Theoretically, it is possible that many BLAD calves die early in life and that only those that survive to develop chronic disease associated with poor growth are suspected to have the disease. Because variable expression of the glycoprotein deficiency is possible in homozygote recessives and in heterozygotes, it also is possible that mild forms of disease and prolonged survival occur. The proportionate decrease in β2 integrin expression demonstrated by heterozygotes does not appear to result in any clinical significance however, and heterozygote carriers have comparable growth and performance compared to non-carrier, normal cattle.

Disorders of Coagulation

Inherited

A factor XI deficiency has been described in Holstein cattle and appears to be a recessive trait. Homozygote recessives bleed excessively or repeatedly after injuries or routine surgical procedures such as castration or dehorning. Hematomas commonly occur at venipuncture sites and may lead to venous thrombosis. Routine coagulation profiles may not show in vitro clotting abnormalities in heterozygote carrier cattle even though such animals have less factor XI than normal.

Acquired

Thrombocytopenia

Etiology

Thrombocytopenia is the most common cause of abnormal coagulation in dairy cattle. Cattle normally have between 100,000 and 800,000 platelets/μL of blood. Platelet survival time is thought to be 7 to 10 days, and megakaryocytes in the bone marrow are the precursors of circulating platelets. Thrombocytopenia may result from decreased platelet production, increased platelet destruction, sequestration, or consumption.

Decreased platelet production generally implies a bone marrow insult. Therefore, hemorrhage caused by thrombocytopenia may be the first clinically detectable sign of true pancytopenia. This is the situation with chronic bracken fern toxicity in cattle. Thrombocytopenia and leukopenia tend to be profound long before affected animals become anemic because of the longer normal life span of erythrocytes compared with granulocytes and platelets. Similarly, thrombocytopenia caused by decreased thrombopoiesis has been reported in association with intoxications resulting from ingestion of trichloroethylene-extracted soybean meal, prolonged furazolidone treatment (in calves), and suspected mycotoxin ingestion in Australian cattle.

Decreased survival of platelets is probably the most common reason for clinical thrombocytopenia. Infectious diseases cause decreased platelet survival via several mechanisms. For example, an immune-mediated thrombocytopenia has been reported in cattle with East Coast fever, and although not specifically immune mediated, the thrombocytopenia that occurs in association with certain strains of type 2 BVDV results from decreased platelet survival after viral infection. Thrombocytopenia in adult cattle and veal calves with natural acute BVDV infection has been observed, and studies confirm a thrombocytopenia beginning 3 to 4 days after experimental infection with some type 2 strains of the virus. Platelet numbers in these cattle then decrease progressively over the next 10 to 14 days (Fig. 3.56). Animals that survive this acute BVDV infection show a return to normal platelet numbers in conjunction with an increase in serum antibody titers against BVDV. It is worth pointing out that this syndrome is a consequence of certain type 2 BVDV strains infecting naive, yet immunocompetent, animals and is not a characteristic manifestation of mucosal disease nor typically seen in persistently infected cattle.

Infectious diseases also may initiate disseminated intravascular coagulation (DIC) with subsequent consumption of platelets. DIC has been suggested as the cause of thrombocytopenia in acute sarcocystosis and can be observed clinically in a variety of septicemic and endotoxic states in cattle. Septic metritis and septic mastitis are the most common endotoxic diseases to cause thrombocytopenia in adult cattle (Fig. 3.57). Thrombocytopenia in these cattle may either be caused directly by DIC or decreased platelet survival for other reasons. In neonatal calves, thrombocytopenia is most commonly observed in association with neonatal calf septicemia due to failure of passive transfer.

Therefore, infectious diseases may result in thrombocytopenia for a variety of reasons. However, these reasons usually affect platelet survival rather than production. Increased destruction, decreased life span resulting from platelet infection, consumption, vasculitis, and unknown factors contribute to thrombocytopenia in association with these infectious diseases. With the exception of BVDV infection and a few other diseases in which thrombocytopenia has been reproduced experimentally, most thrombocytopenia cases are sporadic and associated with a variety of disorders.

Trauma rarely has been associated with thrombocytopenia in cattle and may lower platelet numbers either by consumption or unknown mechanisms. We have confirmed occasional adult cattle with udder hematomas and cattle that are bleeding into a quarter as thrombocytopenic. It is not known whether the thrombocytopenia in these cattle represents cause or effect, but these patients showed no other evidence of systemic disease. One of the editors (TJD) treated a calf with skull and orbital trauma that apparently resulted in profound orbital hemorrhage secondary to thrombocytopenia (Fig. 3.58). The calf completely recovered after a whole blood transfusion and replacement of the proptosed globe.

Immune-mediated thrombocytopenia—or thought to be immune mediated—rarely is observed in ruminants. Perhaps "idiopathic" thrombocytopenia is a better term because clinicopathologic confirmation of true immune-mediated thrombocytopenia seldom is possible in ruminants. Although perhaps more common in goats, idiopathic thrombocytopenia has rarely developed in calves having no evidence of infectious disease, trauma, bone marrow depression, and so forth. Morris states, "The diagnosis of idiopathic thrombocytopenia must be based on small vessel hemorrhagic diathesis and severe thrombocytopenia in a horse with normal coagulation times and no other evidence of DIC." Although this statement refers to horses, it may also pertain to cattle because, in general, specific reagents to detect platelet-associated immunoglobulin G, serum antiplatelet activity, and other confirmatory tests either have not been developed or are unavailable to most veterinarians.

Signs

Petechial hemorrhages on mucous membranes coupled with other signs of hemorrhage that may occur from small vessels anywhere in the body typify thrombocytopenic bleeding. Ecchymotic hemorrhages may accompany the

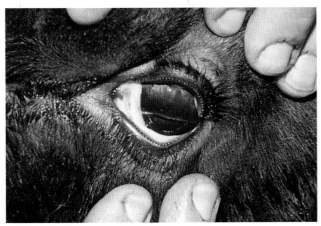

• **Fig. 3.56** Subconjunctival hemorrhage and hyphema in a calf with thrombocytopenia secondary to bovine viral diarrhea virus infection.

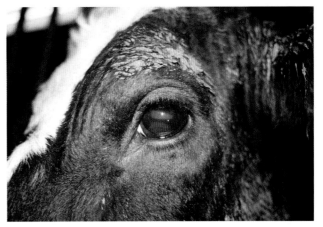

• **Fig. 3.57** Hyphema associated with thrombocytopenia and DIC in an adult cow suffering from acute coliform mastitis.

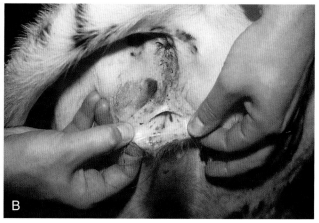

• **Fig. 3.58** **A,** Proptosed globe secondary to orbital hemorrhage in a calf with thrombocytopenia after entrapment and struggling. **B,** Petechial hemorrhages visible on the vulvar mucous membranes of the same calf as in Fig. 3.58, *A.*

petechial hemorrhages on mucous membranes such as the conjunctival, nasal, oral, or vulvar mucosa. Bleeding may occur from the skin at sites of injections or insect bites. Venipuncture causes bleeding, hematoma formation, and possible venous thrombosis. Epistaxis is common in cattle with thrombocytopenia and other signs of bleeding frequently accompany inflammation or injury to specific sites. For example, cattle with thrombocytopenia associated with acute BVDV infection frequently have fresh blood or clots of blood in their feces because of the irritation of diarrhea. Hyphema, scleral hemorrhages, and hematomas may occur secondary to minor trauma, especially in stanchioned cattle. Melena and hematuria also are possible signs.

Clinical bleeding seldom appears until platelet counts drop below 50,000/µL and usually occurs when platelets are less than 20,000/µL. Obviously, stress, trauma, and hydration status may influence the incidence of bleeding at platelet values less than 50,000/µL. Many cattle with confirmed platelet numbers of less than 20,000/µL show no evidence of, or tendency for, bleeding. However, if stressed, traumatized or subjected to multiple injections, venipuncture, bone marrow aspirates, rectal examinations, and so forth, these same cattle will begin to bleed.

Diagnosis

Absolute diagnosis of bleeding resulting from thrombocytopenia depends on:
1. Platelet count (usually <50,000/µL)
2. Ruling out DIC and other coagulopathies

Although it may be difficult in field situations, confirmation of thrombocytopenic purpura necessitates a coagulation panel to confirm normal values for prothrombin time (PT), activated partial thromboplastin time (APTT), thrombin time, fibrinogen, and fibrinogen degradation products (FDPs). Bleeding time and clot retraction are abnormal. In essence, DIC is the major differential diagnosis, and the aforementioned tests differentiate primary thrombocytopenia from thrombocytopenia secondary to DIC.

After the diagnosis of thrombocytopenia is confirmed by laboratory studies, clues to the cause of this disorder should be sought. Septicemia, endotoxemia, and recent trauma may be clinically obvious, whereas ingested toxins or parenteral drugs may require careful historical data and evaluation of the patient's environment. When no predisposing factor or cause can be determined, "idiopathic" or immune-mediated thrombocytopenia is the diagnosis by exclusion. Fortunately, this latter category is very rare in cattle.

Bone marrow aspirates or biopsy are indicated whenever the etiology of thrombocytopenia remains obscure, granulocytopenia coexists with thrombocytopenia, or thrombocytopenia has been chronic or recurrent.

Treatment

Thrombocytopenia resulting in clinical bleeding requires therapy with a fresh whole blood transfusion and treatment of any primary condition. Ideally, blood donors should be free of BLV and persistent BVDV infection. The volume of transfused blood is somewhat dependent on the degree of concurrent blood loss and the size of the patient. The standard empiric quantities are a minimum of 1 L for a calf and 4 L for an adult cow, but greater volumes may be essential for severely anemic patients. Blood transfusions are "first aid" for thrombocytopenia, and the success of transfusion completely depends on whether platelet loss or lack of production will continue.

Specific and supportive therapy for primary causes such as endotoxemia, septicemia, trauma, and localized infections may allow a single whole blood transfusion to suffice for treatment of thrombocytopenia secondary to these disorders. Similarly, calves or cattle with acute BVDV infection that are thrombocytopenic and bleeding usually require only one transfusion. These BVDV patients often have their lowest platelet counts approximately 14 days after infection. Immunologically speaking, therefore, they are near recovery, and humoral antibodies are peaking at this same time. Whole blood transfusion and supportive care can save many of these patients.

The prognosis must be grave for patients having both thrombocytopenia and granulocytopenia because a pancytopenic disorder should be suspected. Chronic bracken fern toxicity, furazolidone toxicity in calves, and other conditions that broadly depress bone marrow are difficult to correct. Supportive therapy, whole blood (collected in plastic) or platelet-rich plasma transfusions, and antibiotics to protect against opportunistic infections are indicated in these patients. Bone marrow aspirates are essential to confirm the diagnosis.

If a primary cause cannot be found and idiopathic thrombocytopenia is diagnosed, the clinical course is more difficult to predict. Idiosyncratic drug reactions should be ruled out by history, and drugs having the potential to cause thrombocytopenia should be discontinued. The patient must be monitored with daily platelet counts and physical examination to determine whether bleeding is continuing or a transfusion is necessary as a lifesaving procedure. Fecal occult blood, Multistix evaluation of urine, and inspection of mucous membranes are important means of monitoring idiopathic thrombocytopenic patients. Further whole blood transfusions are often not indicated unless signs of bleeding appear or the patient is showing signs of severe anemia and hypoxia. Idiopathic thrombocytopenia patients that have persistent or recurrently low platelet counts of less than 25,000/µL and bleeding should have bone marrow aspirates evaluated. If the bone marrow is normal, low-dose corticosteroids may be used in an effort to increase platelet numbers by increasing thrombocytopoiesis and counteracting a variety of immune mechanisms that may contribute to platelet destruction. Dexamethasone is preferable in our experience and may be therapeutic at doses as low as 0.05 mg/kg once daily. Most adult patients can be further reduced to 0.02 mg/kg once daily after 5 days. Most patients requiring corticosteroids for suspected immune-mediated thrombocytopenia can be weaned off medication within 30 days and do not tend to relapse.

Disseminated Intravascular Coagulation

Etiology

Disseminated intravascular coagulation is a complex coagulopathy characterized both by bleeding and excessive intravascular thrombosis. This apparent contradiction leads to a dramatic, and usually fatal, clinical progression. It does not occur spontaneously by itself but as a complication of some other primary illness. Cattle experiencing septicemia, endotoxemia, exotoxemia from clostridial infections, and other severe localized infections are at greatest risk for DIC. Septic mastitis and septic metritis are probably the two most common infections to cause DIC in adult dairy cattle. In calves, neonatal septicemia and severe enteritis are probably the two most frequently encountered causes. Fortunately, DIC is uncommon in cattle.

Clinical signs of bleeding and thrombosis represent overstimulation of coagulation within vessels that eventually depletes coagulation factors to such a degree that bleeding evolves as a major sign. Fibrinolysis is excessive, and localized or regional tissue hypoxia occurs as a result of thrombosis.

Subsequent major organ dysfunction (liver, kidney, brain, gut) may ensue. Because a serious primary disease already exists in patients that develop DIC, patients are further predisposed to organ failure and shock.

Products of inflammation (platelet–activating factors) or infectious agents (endotoxin, clostridium α toxin) that encourage procoagulant activity or damage vascular endothelium may activate DIC. However, the exact mechanism by which DIC occurs is unknown, and it is impossible to predict those patients who will have DIC complicate their already potentially life-threatening primary disease.

Signs

Rapid systemic deterioration in conjunction with vascular thrombosis and hemorrhage should cause suspicion of DIC in patients with serious primary inflammatory or GI disease. Hemorrhages may be manifest as petechiae, ecchymoses, hematomas, or bleeding from body orifices. Melena or frank blood clots in the feces may appear, especially in cattle with enteritis. Microscopic or macroscopic hematuria may be present. Bleeding from injection sites and rapid venous thrombosis after venipuncture are typical signs. Epistaxis, hyphema, hemarthroses and visceral hematomas occasionally occur. Renal failure is common (see Chapter 11).

Major organ failure may be caused by reduced perfusion associated with thromboses. Lesser degrees of ischemia may cause renal (infarcts or tubular nephrosis), GI (bleeding), neurologic (bleeding into central nervous system), hemarthroses, or other signs.

As the patient's condition further deteriorates, venous thrombosis may frustrate therapeutic attempts to improve the systemic state.

Diagnosis

Coagulation profiles and platelet counts are essential tests to confirm clinical suspicions of DIC in a patient to differentiate it from other causes of thrombosis and hemorrhage. In all instances, a patient already seriously ill from a primary disease becomes "sicker" and has signs of thrombosis and bleeding. Because both may be caused by similar predisposing causes, DIC must be differentiated from simple thrombocytopenia. Other causes of bleeding such as hepatic failure, warfarin toxicosis, and inherited coagulopathies can only be ruled out by laboratory tests.

The diagnosis of DIC is not made on the basis of a single laboratory value but on a collection of abnormal laboratory results combined with clinical evidence and history of a primary illness known to be associated with DIC in that particular species. Historically, textbooks have discussed the following as being consistent with the diagnosis of DIC:
1. Decreased platelet counts
2. Prolonged PT, APTT, and thrombin time
3. Elevated FDPs
4. Prolonged bleeding time
5. Decreased antithrombin III

In human medicine a diagnostic algorithm can be used that allocates a numerical score based on the severity of abnormalities in platelet count, FDP (total FDP or D-dimer), PT prolongation, and fibrinogen concentration, alongside the presence of a primary disease known to be associated with DIC. Realistically, it is unusual to have all of these parameters satisfied in a bovine patient suspected of having DIC. For example, the PT and APTT may or may not be outside the normal reference range for the laboratory and if abnormal may be only slightly prolonged. In addition, FDP results in large animals with DIC usually fall in the intermediate (10–40 µg/mL FDP) or suspicious range rather than being obviously elevated. Decreased fibrinogen levels are not typical of DIC in cattle and if identified may actually suggest liver disease. Therefore, clinical cases of bovine DIC may only fulfill two or three of these parameters for diagnosis. Patients fitting many of the textbook parameters usually are in an advanced state and have a grave prognosis. Most bovine DIC patients have thrombocytopenia and intermediate FDP (10–40 µg/mL) results and may have slight prolongation of PT or APTT.

Treatment

Treatment of patients with DIC is perhaps as poorly understood as the disease itself. Without question, intense treatment for the primary condition must continue. Intravenous fluids are essential to counteract hypotension, poor tissue perfusion, and major organ failure. Nonsteroidal antiinflammatory drugs, especially flunixin meglumine (0.5 mg/kg body weight twice daily), may be helpful to patients having underlying gram-negative infections or enteric disorders. Severe thrombocytopenia or continued bleeding dictates replacement of clotting factors even though this may provide further substrate for ongoing coagulation. Therefore, fresh whole plasma or, more likely in the field, fresh whole blood may be indicated.

Other therapies, such as heparin and corticosteroids, have been suggested, but there appears to be no scientific confirmation of their value in treating DIC, and in fact they may have deleterious effects in patients with DIC.

The prognosis for cattle with DIC is guarded to grave. Unfortunately, most patients with confirmed DIC die.

Coumarin Anticoagulants, Dicoumarol Toxicity, and Diffuse Hepatocellular Disease

Etiology

Rodenticides such as warfarin and brodifacoum that are coumarin derivatives, coumarin-containing sweet clover (*Melilotus* spp.) or sweet vernal grass (*Anthoxanthum odoratum*) forages that have become moldy, and diffuse hepatocellular disease may cause hemorrhage resulting from lack of liver origin clotting factors. Coumarin competes with vitamin K1, a precursor of clotting factors II, VII, IX, and X. Excessive fungal growth during improper curing of sweet clover or sweet vernal grass forages causes coumarin to be converted to dicoumarol and results in a decrease in liver production of the aforementioned clotting factors. Diffuse hepatocellular disease also may prevent normal synthesis of these factors, but this is rare and generally seen only in advanced hepatic failure.

Because factor VII has a shorter plasma half-life than factors II, IX, and X, a prolonged PT tends to be the earliest laboratory coagulation abnormality found in patients with coumarin or dicoumarol toxicity. Subsequent prolongation of APTT and activated clotting time occurs as the disease progresses. Obvious external blood loss, hematomas, or occult internal hemorrhages causing profound anemia may appear in affected cattle.

Accidental ingestion of rodenticides containing coumarin derivatives or ingestion of sweet clover forages that are moldy tend to cause sporadic or endemic coagulopathies, respectively.

Toxicity of a given amount of ingested coumarin may be enhanced by hypoproteinemia, drugs that are highly protein bound (thus freeing more coumarin from protein binding), reduced hepatic function, and insufficient vitamin K in the diet.

Clinical signs tend to occur within 1 week of the ingestion of the toxic agent.

Signs

Ecchymotic hemorrhages, hemarthroses, hematomas (especially over pressure points), epistaxis, melena, hematuria, and prolonged bleeding from injection sites or insect bites (Fig. 3.59) all are possible signs. Although not common,

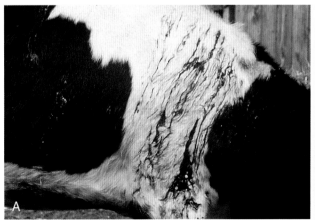 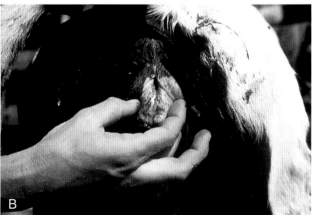

• **Fig. 3.59 A,** Streaks of blood originating from fly bites over the withers area in a calf that had eaten warfarin rodenticide. **B,** Petechial and ecchymotic hemorrhages of the vulvar mucous membranes of the same calf as in Fig. 3.59, *A.*

petechial hemorrhages may be observed in some patients. In addition, moderate to severe anemia may be apparent resulting from internal or external blood loss and is apparent based on mucous membrane pallor, elevated heart rate, and elevated respiratory rate. Hypoproteinemia also is present when blood loss has been severe. Other less common clinical signs simply reflect bleeding into unusual locations as a result of incidental trauma. For example, seizures or neurologic signs may result from skull trauma. Prolonged bleeding may become obvious after minor surgical procedures such as dehorning in otherwise subclinical cattle.

Diagnosis

Clinical signs, history of exposure to sweet clover or sweet vernal forages, or potential exposure to a coumarin-type rodenticide coupled with a prolonged PT and possibly prolonged APTT support the diagnosis when no other clotting abnormalities are identified. Platelet counts also should be normal. The absence of biochemical evidence of hepatic failure rules out liver disease. Analysis of blood, liver, or feedstuffs for dicoumarol may be available at some diagnostic or toxicology laboratories.

Treatment

All affected animals should receive vitamin K1 (1.0 mg/kg SC or IM). Treatment should be repeated twice daily and continue for at least 5 days. Affected animals that are severely anemic should receive 2 to 6 L of fresh whole blood in transfusions from healthy donor cattle (see also Chapter 2).

Vitamin K3 is not a substitute for K1 and in fact may be toxic. Most vitamin K3 products (menadione sodium bisulfite) have been taken off the market because of toxicity to domestic animals and humans.

Affected feed should be discarded and remaining feed inspected before allowing cattle access to it. Rodenticides should be managed carefully to avoid accidental ingestion.

Causes of Fatal Peracute Hemorrhage in Cattle

Sudden death resulting from exsanguination may result in cattle from a variety of causes. When called to examine or necropsy a previously healthy animal that develops peracute anemia or dies from blood loss, the veterinarian should consider several diseases:
1. Obvious external blood:
   - Laceration of a major vessel such as occurs with mammary vein laceration
   - Caudal vena caval thrombosis with obvious bleeding from the mouth and nose
   - Bleeding from the abomasum with obvious melena
2. Occult or internal blood loss:
   - Manual removal of a corpus luteum during rectal palpation
   - Rupture of the spleen secondary to massive enlargement of the organ with lymphosarcoma

- Rupture of a uterine or mesenteric vessel (consider both reproductive causes and copper deficiency). Mesenteric vessel rupture may be an endemic herd problem
- Rupture of vaginal artery during parturition or dystocia; may have some evidence of external hemorrhage from caudal reproductive tract, but blood may "pool" within uterus beyond view
- Peracute abomasal hemorrhage without obvious melena
3. Toxicity and coagulation disorder such as sweet vernal or sweet clover hay that may interfere with vitamin K–dependent coagulation factors.

Thrombosis

Arterial and venous thromboses are generally associated with septic causes, such as vena caval and related pulmonary thrombosis; jugular and vena caval thrombosis associated with septic phlebitis; uterine, mammary, or intestinal thrombosis associated with infectious or inflammatory diseases of those organs; and septic splenic thrombosis. Endocarditis may result in thrombosis of renal or pulmonary arteries. *Claviceps purpurea,* the cause of fescue foot or ergotism, may cause thrombosis of limb, ear, and tail arteries. Severe frost bite of distal extremities, especially in septic calves, may also cause vascular thrombosis of distal extremities (Fig. 3.60). The prognosis for frostbitten extremities can be determined after rewarming the affected sites and assessing the severity of necrosis and thrombosis. Rewarming the frostbitten area as quickly as possible to salvage as much tissue and function as possible is suggested. The use of circulating water at 40°C is recommended. Do not allow the water to get too hot or too cold. Avoid premature termination of the rewarming process. Remember to treat pain associated with rewarming and provide antibiotic and surgical treatments as needed. Mechanical trauma (from over-vigorous massaging or rubbing), rewarming at too high temperatures, and allowing refreezing are

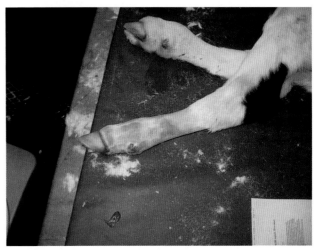

• **Fig. 3.60** Frostbite of the rear limbs in a septic calf. The foot remained cold and discolored after warming the legs and giving intravenous fluids, which suggested arterial thrombosis. The calf was then euthanized, and thrombosis was confirmed.

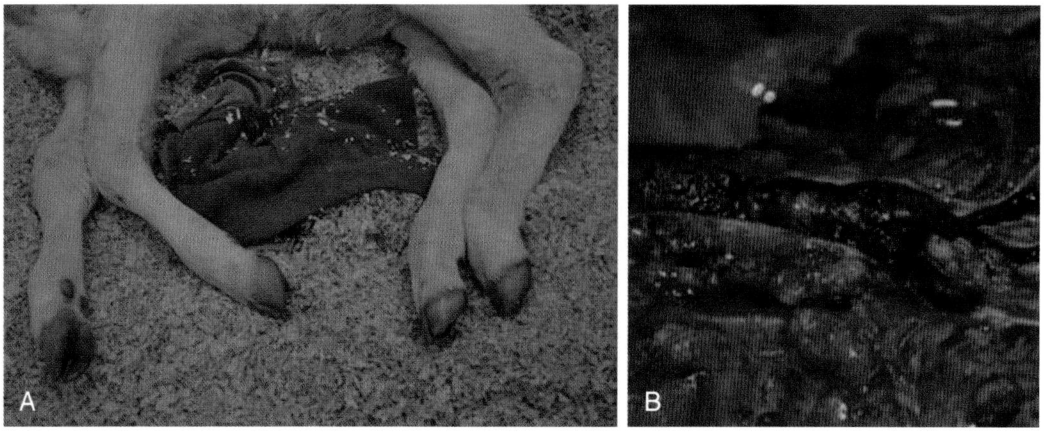

• **Fig. 3.61 A,** A 3-week-old calf with acute onset of progressive posterior paresis that has rapidly advanced to recumbency and the inability to stand. Both distal rear limbs felt cold, there was dark discoloration of the coronary band and hoof, and the calf did not respond to stimuli to the distal extremity. **B,** Necropsy of the calf showing aortoiliac thrombosis.

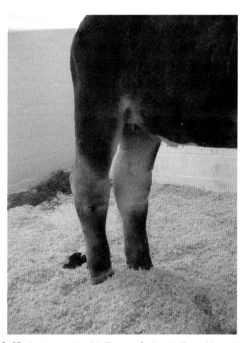

• **Fig. 3.62** A 14-month-old Brown Swiss heifer with a history of chronic leg swelling but without fever or pain on palpation of the limb. The limbs felt cold to the touch, and pitting was noticeable when pressure was applied to the leg. The owners first noticed the edema when the calf was approximately 2 months of age.

Lymphatic Disorders

Congenital lymphedema is described in several breeds of cattle, with the description in Ayrshire cattle being the first in veterinary medicine. In some patients, the signs may not be noted until the calf is several months of age, so *primary lymphedema* would be the preferred term for those cases. The disease is characterized by edema of the hind limbs (Fig. 3.62) and sometimes the forelimbs, tail, and prepuce. Lymphatic system lesions may include hypoplasia and aplasia of lymph vessels and prescapular, iliofemoral, and popliteal lymph nodes. Chronic edema is associated with thickening and fibrosis of tissues, making successful treatment highly unlikely.

Acknowledgment

We would like to thank Dr. Sheila McGuirk, Professor Emerita at the University of Wisconsin, for her contribution in the previous edition of Diseases of Dairy Cattle.

some of the commonest errors in treatment. Anticoagulants such as heparin may be of some value in decreasing further thrombosis but can have side effects; aspirin, however, has minimal effects on coagulation in cattle. Tissue plasminogen activator could be injected proximal to the thrombosis if the thrombosis is acute but it is very expensive.

Aortic and iliac artery thrombosis (Fig. 3.61) may occur in young calves (<6 months of age), resulting in an acute onset of posterior paralysis. The distal limb(s) feel cold below the stifle and may be hyporesponsive to stimuli. Serum CK levels are often 10,000 IU/L to 30,000 IU/L in affected calves. Successful treatment for aortic and iliac artery thrombosis in calves has not been reported.

Suggested Readings

Anderson, D. C., Schmalsteig, F. C., Finegold, M. J., et al. (1985). The severe and moderate phenotypes of heritable Mac-1 LFA-1 deficiency: their quantitative definition and relation to leukocyte dysfunction and clinical features. *J Infect Dis, 152,* 668–689.

Anderson, D. C., & Springer, T. A. (1987). Leukocyte adhesion deficiency: an inherited defect in the Mac-1 LFA-1 and p150, 95 glycoproteins. *Annu Rev Med, 38,* 175–194.

Araujo, F. R., Silva, M. P., Lopes, A. A., et al. (1998). Severe cat flea infestation of dairy calves in Brazil. *Vet Parasitol, 80,* 83–86.

Baird, J. D. (1988). Dilated cardiomyopathy in Holstein cattle: clinical and genetic aspects. In *Proceedings: 6th Annual Veterinary Medicine Forum (American College Veterinary Internal Medicine)* (pp. 175–177).

Bartol, J. M., Thompson, L. J., Minnier, S. M., et al. (2000). Hemorrhagic diathesis, mesenteric hematoma, and colic associated with ingestion of sweet vernal grass in a cow. *J Am Vet Med Assoc, 216,* 1605–1608.

Braun, U. (2009). Traumatic pericarditis in cattle: clinical, radiographic and ultrasonographic findings. *Vet J, 182*(2), 176–186.

Braun, U., Lejeune, B., Rauch, S., et al. (2008). Ultrasonographic findings in 22 cattle with pericarditis traumatica. *Schweiz Archiv Tierheilk, 150*(6), 281–286.

Buck, W. B. (1975). Toxic materials and neurologic disease in cattle. *J Am Vet Med Assoc, 166*, 222–230.

Buczinski, S. (2012). Echocardiographic findings and clinical signs in dairy cows with primary cardiac lymphoma: 7 cases (2007-2010). *J Am Vet Med Assoc, 241*(8), 1083–1087.

Buczinski, S., Fecteau, G., & DiFruscia, R. (2006). Ventricular septal defects in cattle: a retrospective study of 25 cases. *Can Vet J, 47*(3), 246–252.

Buczinski, S., Francoz, D., Fecteau, G., et al. (2010a). Heart disease in cattle with clinical signs of heart failure: 59 cases. *Can Vet J, 51*(10), 1123–1129.

Buczinski, S., Francoz, D., Fecteau, G., et al. (2010b). A study of heart diseases without clinical signs of heart failure in 47 cattle. *Can Vet J, 51*(11), 1239–1246.

Buczinski, S., Tolouei, M., Rezakhani, A., et al. (2013). Echocardiographic measurement of cardiac valvular thickness in healthy cows, cows with bacterial endocarditis, and cows with cardiorespiratory diseases. *J Vet Cardiol, 15*(4), 253–261.

Buczinski, S., Tsuka, T., & Tharwat, M. (2012). The diagnostic criteria used in bovine bacterial endocarditis: a meta-analysis of 460 published cases from 1973 to 2011. *Vet J, 193*(2), 349–357.

Buntain, B. (1980). Disseminated intravascular coagulopathy (DIC) in a cow with left displaced abomasum, metritis and mastitis. *Vet Med Small Anim Clin, 75*, 1023–1026.

Callan, R. J., McGuirk, S. M., & Step, D. L. (1992). Assessment of the cardiovascular and lymphatic systems. *Vet Clin North Am Food Anim Pract, 8*, 257–270.

Carlson, G. P. (2002). Diseases of the hematopoietic and hemolymphatic systems. In B. P. Smith (Ed.), *Large animal internal medicine* (3rd ed.). St. Louis: Mosby.

Carlson, G. P. (2002). Heinz body hemolytic anemia. In B. P. Smith (Ed.), *Large animal internal medicine* (3rd ed.). St. Louis: Mosby.

Carlson, G. P., & Kaneko, J. J. (1976). Influence of prednisolone on intravascular granulocyte kinetics of calves under nonsteady state conditions. *Am J Vet Res, 37*, 149–151.

Constable, P. D., Muir, W. W., 3rd, Bonagura, J. D., et al. (1990). Clinical and electrocardiographic characterization of cattle with atrial premature complexes. *J Am Vet Med Assoc, 197*, 1163–1169.

Constable, P. D., Muir, W. W., 3rd, Freeman, L., et al. (1990). Atrial fibrillation associated with neostigmine administration in three cows. *J Am Vet Med Assoc, 196*, 329–332.

Corapi, W. V., Elliot, R. D., French, T. W., et al. (1990). Thrombocytopenia and hemorrhages in veal calves infected with bovine viral diarrhea virus. *J Am Vet Med Assoc, 196*, 590–596.

Corapi, W. C., French, T. W., & Dubovi, E. J. (1989). Severe thrombocytopenia in young calves experimentally infected with noncytopathic bovine viral diarrhea virus. *J Virol, 63*, 3934–3943.

Crispin, S. M., Douglas, S. W., Hall, L. W., et al. (1975). Letter: warfarin poisoning in domestic animals. *Br Med J, 2*, 500.

D'Angelo, A., Bellino, C., Alborali, G. L., et al. (2006). Aortic thrombosis in three calves with Escherichia coli sepsis. *J Vet Intern Med, 20*, 1261–1263.

Divers, T. J. (2005). Blood component transfusions. *Vet Clin North Am Food Anim Pract, 21*, 615–622.

Ducharme, N. G., Fubini, S. L., Rebhun, W. C., et al. (1992). Thoracotomy in adult cattle: 14 cases (1979-1991). *J Am Vet Med Assoc, 201*, 86–91.

Dyson, D. A., & Reed, J. B. H. (1977). Haemorrhagic syndrome of cattle of suspected mycotoxin origin. *Vet Rec, 100*, 400–402.

Evans, E. T. R. (1957). Bacterial endocarditis of cattle. *Vet Rec, 69*, 1190–1206.

Evans, I. A., & Howell, R. M. (1962). Bovine bracken poisoning. *Nature, 194*, 584–585 [London].

Evans, W. C. (1964). Bracken fern poisoning of farm annuals. *Vet Rec, 76*, 365–369.

Ferrer, J. F. (1979). Bovine leukosis: natural transmission and principles of control. *J Am Vet Med Assoc, 175*, 1281–1284.

Firshman, A. M., Sage, A. M., Valberg, S. J., et al. (2006). Idiopathic hemorrhagic pericardial effusion in cows. *J Vet Intern Med, 20*, 1499–1503.

Fox FH: Personal observation, 1968, Ithaca, NY.

Fox, F. H., & Rebhun, W. C. (1983). Warfarin poisoning with complications in a heifer. *Vet Med Small Anim Clin, 78*, 1611–1613.

Fraser, B. C., Anderson, D. E., White, B. J., et al. (2013). Assessment of a commercially available point of care assay for the measurement of bovine cardiac troponin I concentration. *Am J Vet Res, 74*, 870–873.

Fregin, G. F. (1970). Arial fibrillation in the horse. In *Proceedings: 16th Annual Convention American Association Equine Practitioners* (pp. 383–388).

Frelier, P. F., & Lewis, R. M. (1984). Hematologic and coagulation abnormalities in acute bovine sarcocystosis. *Am J Vet Res, 45*, 40–48.

Gabor, L. J., & Downing, G. M. (2003). Monensin toxicity in preruminant dairy heifers. *Aust Vet J, 81*, 476–478.

Gentry, P. A. (1984). The relationship between factor XI coagulant and factor XI antigenic activity in cattle (factor XI deficiency). *Can J Comp Med, 48*, 58–62.

Gentry, P. A., & Ross, M. L. (1986). Failure of routine coagulation screening tests to detect heterozygous state of bovine factor XI deficiency. *Vet Clin Pathol, 15*, 12–16.

Gentry, P. A., Tremblay, R. R. M., & Ross, M. L. (1989). Failure of aspirin to impair bovine platelet function. *Am J Vet Res, 50*, 919–922.

Giger, U., Boxer, L. A., Simpson, P. J., et al. (1987). Deficiency of leukocyte surface glycoproteins Mo1 LFA-1 and Leu M5 in a dog with recurrent bacterial infections: an animal model. *Blood, 69*, 1622–1630.

Gilbert, R. O., Grohn, Y. T., Guard, C. L., et al. (1993). Impaired post partum neutrophil function in cows which retain fetal membranes. *Res Vet Sci, 5*, 15–19.

Goldman, L., & Ausiello, D. (2004). The chronic leukemias. In J. B. Wyngaarden, & L. H. Smith, Jr. (Eds.), *Cecil textbook of medicine* (22nd ed.). Philadelphia: WB Saunders.

Gross, D. R., Dodd, K. T., Williams, J. D., et al. (1981). Adverse cardiovascular effects of oxytetracycline preparations and vehicles in calves. *Am J Vet Res, 42*, 1371.

Grunberg, W., Mol, J. A., & Teske, E. (2015). Red blood cell phosphate concentration and osmotic resistance during dietary phosphorous depletion in dairy cows. *J Vet Intern Med, 29*, 395–399.

Gunes, V., Atalan, G., Citil, M., et al. (2008). Use of cardiac troponin kits for the qualitative determination of myocardial cell damage due to traumatic reticuloperitonitis in cattle. *Vet Rec, 162*, 514–517.

Hagemoser, W. A., Roth, J. A., Lofstedt, J., et al. (1983). Granulocytopathy in a Holstein heifer. *J Am Vet Med Assoc, 183*, 1093–1094.

Harrison, L. R. (1979). A hemorrhagic disease syndrome of the vealer calf. In *Proceedings: 21st Annual Meeting American Association Veterinary Laboratory Diagnosticians* (pp. 117–125).

Hayashi, T., Yamane, O., & Sakai, M. (1976). Hematological and pathological observations of chronic furazolidone poisoning in calves. *Jpn J Vet Sci, 38*, 225–233.

Howard, J. L. (1999). Monensin, lasalocid, salinomycin, narasin. In J. Howard, & R. A. Smith (Eds.), *Current veterinary therapy—food animal practice* (4th ed.). Philadelphia: WB Saunders.

Hoyt, P. G., Gill, M. S., Angel, K. L., et al. (2000). Corticosteroid-responsive thrombocytopenia in two beef cows. *J Am Vet Med Assoc, 217*, 717–720, 674.

Irmak, K., Sen, I., Col, R., et al. (2006). The evaluation of coagulation profiles in calves with suspected septic shock. *Vet Res Commun, 5*, 497–603.

Jain, N. C. (1986). *Schalm's veterinary hematology* (4th ed.). Philadelphia: Lea & Febiger.

James, L. F., Hartley, W. J., Nielsen, D., et al. (1986). Locoweed oxytropis-sericca poisoning and congestive heart failure in cattle. *J Am Vet Med Assoc, 189*, 1549–1556.

Jeffers, M., & Lenghaus, C. (1986). Granulocytopaenia and thrombocytopaenia in dairy cattle—a suspected mycotoxicosis. *Aust Vet J, 63*, 262–264.

Jensen, R., Pierson, R. E., Braddy, P. M., et al. (1976). Brisket disease in yearling feedlot cattle. *J Am Vet Med Assoc, 169*, 513–520.

Jesty, S. A., Sweeney, R. W., Dolente, B. A., et al. (2005). Idiopathic pericarditis and cardiac tamponade in two cows. *J Am Vet Med Assoc, 226*, 1555–1558, 1502.

Jubb, K. V. F., Kennedy, P. C., & Palmer, N. (1985). *Pathology of domestic animals* (3rd ed.). (vol. 3). New York: Academic Press, Inc.

Kehrli, M. E., Jr., Schmalstieg, F. C., Anderson, D. C., et al. (1990). Molecular definition of bovine granulocytopathy syndrome: identification of deficiency of the Mac-1 (CB11b/CD18) glycoprotein. *Am J Vet Res, 51*, 1826–1836.

Kimeto, B. A. (1976). Ultrastructure of blood platelets in cattle with East Coast fever. *Am J Vet Res, 37*, 443–447.

King JM: Personal communication, 1968, Ithaca, New York.

Krishnamurthy, D., Nigam, J. M., Peshin, P. K., et al. (1979). Thoracopericardiotomy and pericardiectomy in cattle. *J Am Vet Med Assoc, 175*, 714–718.

Kutzer, P., Schultze, C., Englehardt, A., et al. (2008). Helcococcus ovis, an emerging pathogen in bovine valvular endocarditis. *J Clin Microbiol, 46*(10), 3291–3294.

Labonte, J., Roy, J. P., Dubuc, J., et al. (2015). Measurement of cardiac troponin I in healthy lactating dairy cows using a point of care analyzer (iSTAT-1). *J Vet Cardiol, 17*, 129–133.

Lacuata, A. Q., Yamada, H., Nakamura, Y., et al. (1980). Electrocardiographic and echocardiographic findings in four cases of bovine endocarditis. *J Am Vet Med Assoc, 176*, 1355–1365.

Littledike, E. T., Glazier, D., & Cook, H. M. (1976). Electrocardiographic changes after induced hypercalcemia and hypocalcemia in cattle: reversal of the induced arrhythmia with atropine. *Am J Vet Res, 37*, 383–388.

Litwak, K. N., McMahan, A., Lott, K. A., et al. (2005). Monensin toxicosis in the domestic bovine calf: a large animal model of cardiac dysfunction. *Contemp Top Lab Anim Sci, 44*, 45–49.

Mason, T. A. (1979). Suppurative pericarditis, treated by pericardiotomy in a cow. *Vet Rec, 105*, 350–351.

McGuirk, S. M. (1991). Treatment of cardiovascular disease in cattle. *Vet Clin North Am Food Anim Pract, 7*, 729–746.

McGuirk, S. M., & Bednarski, R. M. (1986). Bradycardia associated with fasting in cattle. In *Proceedings: 4th Annual Veterinary Medicine Forum* (2) (pp. 10–29, 10–32).

McGuirk, S. M., Bednarski, R. M., & Clayton, M. K. (1990). Bradycardia in cattle deprived of food. *J Am Vet Med Assoc, 196*, 894–896.

McGuirk, S. M., Muir, W. W., Sams, R. A., et al. (1983). Atrial fibrillation in cows: clinical findings and therapeutic considerations. *J Am Vet Med Assoc, 182*, 1380–1386.

McGuirk, S. M., & Shaftoe, S. (1990). Alterations in cardiovascular and hemolymphatic system. In B. P. Smith (Ed.), *Large animal internal medicine*. St. Louis: CV Mosby.

McGuirk, S. M., Shaftoe, S., & Lunn, D. P. (1990). Diseases of the cardiovascular system. In B. P. Smith (Ed.), *Large animal internal medicine*. St. Louis: CV Mosby.

Mellanby, R. J., Henry, J. P., Cash, R., et al. (2009). Serum cardiac troponin I concentrations in cattle with cardiac and non-cardiac disorders. *J Vet Intern Med, 23*, 926–930.

Morley, P. S., Allen, A. L., & Woolums, A. R. (1996). Aortic and iliac artery thrombosis in calves: nine cases (1974-1993). *J Am Vet Med Assoc, 209*, 130–136.

Morris, D. D. (1988). Recognition and management of disseminated intravascular coagulation in horses. *Vet Clin North Am Equine Pract, 4*, 115–143.

Muller, M., Platz, S., Ehrlein, J., et al. (2005). [Bacterially conditioned thromboembolism in dairy cows—a retrospective study of 31 necropsy cases with special consideration of the causative complex] (German). *Berl Munch Tierarztl Wochenschr, 118*, 121–127.

Nagahata, H., Noda, H., Takahashi, K., et al. (1987). Bovine granulocytopathy syndrome: neutrophil dysfunction in Holstein Friesian calves. *Zentralbl Veterinarmed A, 34*, 445–451.

Nicholls, T. J., Shiel, M. J., Westbury, H. A., et al. (1985). Granulocytopaenia and thrombocytopaenia in cattle. *Aust Vet J, 62*, 67–68.

Ogawa, E. R. I., Kobayashi, K., Yoshiura, N., et al. (1987). Bovine postparturient hemoglobinemia: hypophosphatemia and metabolic disorder in red blood cells. *Am J Vet Res, 48*, 1300–1303.

Otter, A., Twomey, D. F., Crawshaw, T. R., et al. (2003). Anaemia and mortality in calves infested with the long-nosed sucking louse (Linognathus vituli). *Vet Rec, 153*, 176–179.

Owczarek-Lipska, M., Denis, C., Eggen, A., et al. (2009). The bovine dilated cardiomyopathy locus maps to a 1.0 Mb interval on chromosome 18. *Mamm Genome, 20*, 187–192.

Peek, S. F., McGuirk, S. M., Gaska, J., et al. (2012). Idiopathic hemorrhagic pericardial effusion as a precursor to epicardial lymphosarcoma in three cows. *J Vet Intern Med, 26*(4), 1069–1072.

Pipers, F. S., Rings, D. M., Hull, B. L., et al. (1978). Echocardiographic diagnosis of endocarditis in a bull. *J Am Vet Med Assoc, 172*, 1313–1316.

Power, H. T., & Rebhun, W. C. (1983). Bacterial endocarditis in adult dairy cattle. *J Am Vet Med Assoc, 181*, 806–808.

Pringle, J. K., Bright, J. M., Duncan, R. B., Jr., et al. (1991). Pulmonary hypertension in a group of dairy calves. *J Am Vet Med Assoc, 198*, 857–861.

Pritchard, W. R., Rehfeld, C. E., Mizuno, N. S., et al. (1956). Studies on trichlorethylene-extracted feeds. I. Experimental production of acute aplastic anemia in young heifers. *Am J Vet Res, 17*, 425–429.

Radostits, O. M., Gay, C., Blood, D. C., et al. (2007). *Veterinary medicine. A textbook of the diseases of cattle, sheep, pigs, goats and horses* (10th ed.). London: Saunders. [with contributions by Arundel J.H., Gay C.C].

Rebhun, W. C., French, T. W., Perdrizet, J. A., et al. (1989). Thrombocytopenia associated with acute bovine virus diarrhea infection in cattle. *J Vet Intern Med, 3*, 42–46.

Reimer, J. M., Donawick, W. J., Reef, V. B., et al. (1988). Diagnosis and surgical correction of patent ductus venosus in a calf. *J Am Vet Med Assoc, 193*, 1539–1541.

Renshaw, H. W., & Davis, W. C. (1979). Canine granulocytopathy syndrome: an inherited disorder of leukocyte function. *Am J Pathol, 95*, 731.

Rosenberger G. (1979). *Clinical examination of cattle*. Dirksen G, Grunder H-D, Grunert E, et al (collaborators) and Mack R (translator) (Eds.), Berlin: Verlag Paul Parey.

Roth, J. A., & Kaeberle, M. L. (1982). Effect of glucocorticoids on the bovine immune system. *J Am Vet Med Assoc, 180*, 894–901.

Roth, J. A., & Kaeberle, M. L. (1981). Effects of in vivo dexamethasone administration on in vitro bovine polymorphonuclear leukocyte function. *Infect Immun, 33*, 434–441.

Scott, E. A., Byars, T. D., & Lamar, A. M. (1980). Warfarin anticoagulation in the horse. *J Am Vet Med Assoc, 177*, 1146–1151.

Step, D. L., McGuirk, S. M., & Callan, R. J. (1992). Ancillary tests of the cardiovascular and lymphatic systems. *Vet Clin North Am Food Anim Pract, 8*, 271–284.

Stockdale, C. R., Moyes, T. E., & Dyson, R. (2005). Acute postparturient haemoglobinuria in dairy cows and phosphorus status. *Aust Vet J, 83*, 362–366.

Suzuki, K., Uchida, K. E., Niehaus, A., et al. (2012). Cardiac troponin I in calves with congenital heart disease. *J Vet Intern Med, 26*, 1056–1069.

Sweeney, R. W., Divers, T. J., Benson, C., et al. (1988). Pharmacokinetics of rifampin in calves and adult sheep. *J Vet Pharmacol Ther, 11*, 413–416.

Takahashi, K., Miyagawa, K., Abe, S., et al. (1987). Bovine granulocytopathy syndrome of Holstein-Friesian calves and heifers. *Jpn J Vet Sci, 49*, 733–736.

Tennant, B., Asbury, A. C., Laben, R. C., et al. (1967). Familial polycythemia in cattle. *J Am Vet Med Assoc, 150*, 1493–1509.

Tennant, B., Harrold, D., Reina-Guerra, M., et al. (1969). Arterial pH, PO2, and PCO2 of calves with familial bovine polycythemia. *Cornell Vet, 59*, 594–604.

Van Biervliet, J., Krause, M., Woodie, B., et al. (2006). Thoracoscopic pericardiotomy as a palliative treatment in a cow with pericardial lymphoma. *J Vet Cardiol, 8*, 69–75.

Varga, A., Angelos, J. A., Graham, T. W., et al. (2013). Preliminary investigation of cardiac troponin I concentration in cows with common production diseases. *J Vet Intern Med, 27*, 1613–1621.

Varga, A., Schober, K. E., Walker, W. L., et al. (2009). Validation of a commercially available immunoassay for the measurement of bovine cardiac troponin I. *J Vet Intern Med, 23*, 359–365.

Vrins, A., Carlson, G., & Feldman, B. (1983). Warfarin: a review with emphasis on its use in the horse. *Can Vet J, 24*, 211–213.

Weldon, A. D., Moise, N. S., & Rebhun, W. C. (1992). Hyperkalemic atrial standstill in neonatal calf diarrhea. *J Vet Intern Med, 6*, 294–297.

Wessels, J., & Wessels, M. E. (2005). Histophilus somni myocarditis in a beef rearing calf in the United Kingdom. *Vet Rec, 157*, 420–421.

4

Respiratory Diseases

SIMON F. PEEK, THERESA L. OLLIVETT, AND THOMAS J. DIVERS

Diseases of the Upper Airway

These disorders are characterized by inspiratory dyspnea. The increased resistance to airflow caused by upper airway obstructions often creates audible inspiratory noise and results in referred airway sounds through the tracheobronchial apparatus. Sounds that have been "referred" to the lower airway from an upper airway obstruction may be misinterpreted as lower airway in origin in such cases unless the upper airway is examined and the trachea auscultated. If the respiratory sounds can be heard without a stethoscope, they are most likely originating from the upper respiratory tract. The upper airway examination should include detection of airflow from both nostrils, close examination of soft tissues of the head, and oral examination if necessary. Severe upper airway obstruction can cause open-mouth breathing and head extension as the affected cow tries to decrease the resistance to airflow (Fig. 4.1).

Mechanical or Obstructive Diseases
Congenital

Etiology and Signs

Congenital disorders, including pharyngeal cysts of respiratory epithelial origin, nasal cysts, cystic nasal conchae, skull anomalies, laryngeal malformations, and branchial cysts, have been observed in calves and adult cows. Inspiratory dyspnea with audible snoring sounds or stertorous breathing is a sign common to most of these problems. The condition may be present at birth or is most often observed within the first few months of life. The degree of dyspnea associated with these abnormalities tends to be progressive as a result of either enlargement of the lesion (cyst) or worsening upper airway edema and swelling from the mechanical overwork associated with respiratory efforts to move air through an airway narrowed by a malformation. Environmental conditions of high heat and humidity may markedly exacerbate the dyspnea.

Diagnosis

Specific diagnosis requires physical examination, including visual inspection of the nares and oral cavity, endoscopy, and skull radiography (Fig. 4.2). In addition, aspiration for cytology and cultures may be indicated for cystic lesions. Most cystic lesions become secondarily infected.

Treatment

The method of treatment depends on the specific lesions found. Cystic conditions may be the most treatable because surgical removal offers some hope of being curative. Simple drainage or drainage with cautery of cystic lesions is not likely to be successful. Therefore referral of such cases to veterinary surgeons experienced in upper airway surgery is recommended so that complete excision of the secretory epithelium can be completed. Other conditions such as laryngeal malformations and skull anomalies have a poor prognosis.

Regardless of the cause, symptomatic or supportive treatment may be necessary before diagnostic procedures are performed in calves with severe dyspnea, lest the stress of examination or endoscopy induce anoxia. A tracheostomy should be considered to allow safe diagnostic manipulation. Misinterpreting anoxic patient-struggling as wildness requiring additional physical restraint is a frequent, and potentially fatal, error in judgment made by inexperienced clinicians. When a dyspneic animal struggles during examination, usually it is anoxic, frightened, and extremely anxious. All restraint of the head and neck should be relaxed, and the animal should be allowed to "get its breath." Continued restraint during these situations may result in asphyxiation of the animal.

Although the prognosis for congenital lesions varies with the specific diagnosis, generally it is guarded to poor.

Acquired

Etiology and Signs

Acquired mechanical or obstructive lesions of the upper airway may occur in calves or adult cattle. Most of the lesions represent enlargement or inflammation of tissues and structures external to the airway itself. Impingement into the upper airway by soft tissue masses such as pharyngeal abscesses, laryngeal or pharyngeal branchial cysts, retropharyngeal cellulitis, necrotic laryngitis, pyogranulomatous swellings (e.g., wooden tongue), enlarged lymph nodes, neoplasms, foreign bodies, or enlarged maxillary sinuses comprise the majority of lesions. Pharyngeal abscesses and necrotic laryngitis are probably the most common acquired causes of obstruction. Pharyngeal abscesses and retropharyngeal cellulitis may occur after traumatic injury to the mouth when an animal is treated with oral medication requiring the use of a balling

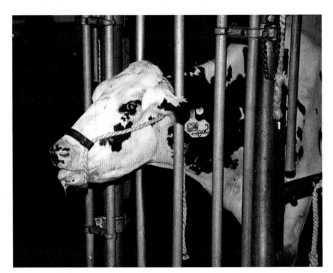

• **Fig. 4.1** Open-mouth breathing and neck extension in adult Holstein with retropharyngeal abscessation, upper airway obstruction and pain associated with iatrogenic trauma.

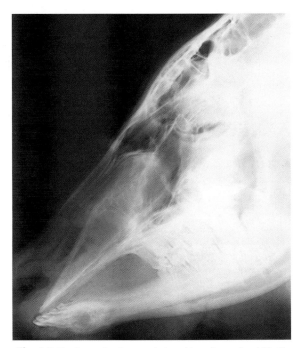

• **Fig. 4.2** Radiograph of a conchal cyst in a 6-month-old heifer.

gun, speculum, or other device in either adults or calves (Fig. 4.3). These lesions may also arise in calves with no history of iatrogenic pharyngeal trauma or oral medication.

Regardless of the cause, progressive inspiratory dyspnea is the primary sign observed in affected cattle. Fever may be present with pharyngeal abscesses, cellulitis, or chronic maxillary sinusitis. Unilateral nasal discharge or reduced airflow from one nostril may be present with maxillary sinusitis or unilateral neoplasms of the nasal pharynx or maxillary sinus. Lymphadenopathy may be present as a primary sign in neoplastic conditions, such as juvenile lymphosarcoma and adult lymphosarcoma (Figs. 4.4 and 4.5), or as a secondary sign in cases of soft tissue infections. Unilateral Horner's syndrome and progressive exophthalmos have been observed in

slow-growing adenocarcinomas of respiratory epithelial origin in the nasopharynx (Fig. 4.6). Cattle with unilateral nasal obstruction often show more obvious respiratory signs during hot weather. One cow with Horner's syndrome would demonstrate open-mouth breathing only on hot days because of the nasal mucosal vasodilation and edema (Fig. 4.7).

A fetid odor may exist on the breath caused by chronic inflammation or tumor necrosis in some cattle. The owner may report a progressive course of stertorous breathing eventually leading to open-mouth breathing. Inflammatory lesions often have a more acute course than neoplasms, but this is a generality rather than a rule. Obvious external swelling may be present in certain conditions such as chronic maxillary sinusitis, pharyngeal or retropharyngeal abscesses, and lymphosarcoma.

Diagnosis

A complete physical examination followed by manual and visual inspection of the oral cavity is the first diagnostic procedure. Relative equality of airflow and the odor of the breath should be evaluated at the nostrils. If chronic maxillary sinusitis is suspected, the upper premolar and molar teeth should be examined closely for abnormalities.

Endoscopy should be performed in an effort to identify a specific lesion or the anatomic region of impingement of tissue into the airway. When performing endoscopy in a calf or cow with severe upper airway dyspnea, most of the mucosal surfaces (e.g., soft palate, larynx, and respiratory pharynx) will be edematous from exertional or labored respiratory efforts. This edema should not be misinterpreted as the causative lesion (see Video Clip 4.1).

Skull radiographs may be necessary if physical examination and endoscopy fail to identify a lesion. Radiographs are helpful for definitive diagnosis of sinusitis or nasal or sinus cysts and for identifying the location of soft tissue masses such as abscesses or tumors. In addition, radiographs help to identify metallic foreign bodies and abscessed tooth roots in cases of chronic maxillary sinusitis.

Diagnostic ultrasonography, if available, may help in the assessment of soft tissue swellings and laryngeal cartilage abnormalities. This technique also has been used to locate retropharyngeal abscesses and nonmetallic foreign bodies so that external drainage may be performed safely.

In the case of obvious or palpable swellings of the head or pharynx, aspirates for cytology and culture are indicated. Similarly, biopsies for histopathology are indicated for solid masses or enlarged lymph nodes where neoplasia is suspected.

Treatment and Prognosis

Treatment is most successful when external compression of the upper airway can be cured through treatment of an inflammatory lesion. Pharyngeal or retropharyngeal abscesses should be drained either by manual pressure during oral examination or externally under ultrasound guidance with liberal incisions that avoid vital structures. Internal drainage is preferred unless the abscess is close to the skin surface. External drainage is technically difficult for deep pharyngeal abscesses located more than a few centimeters below the skin surface. Vagus nerve damage,

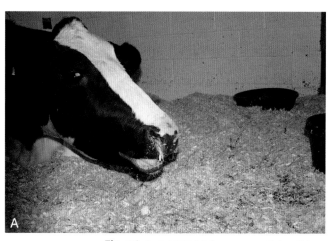
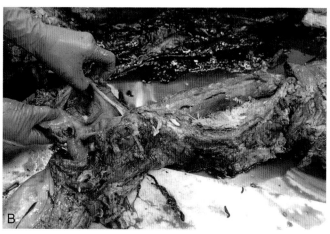

• **Fig. 4.3** **A,** Adult Holstein open-mouth breathing with an extended neck and upper airway stridor associated with pharyngeal laceration. **B,** Post mortem image of the same animal demonstrating laceration in pharynx (held by gloved left hand) and feed material that accumulated outside the cervical esophagus coincident with severe gangrenous cellulitis.

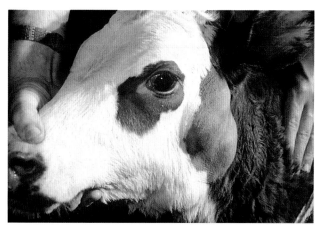

• **Fig. 4.4** Juvenile lymphosarcoma in a 4-month-old Milking Shorthorn calf presented because of inspiratory dyspnea.

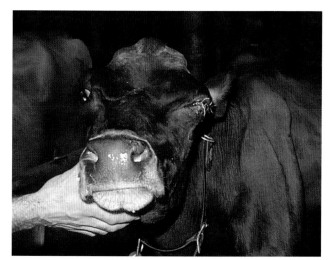

• **Fig. 4.6** Aged Jersey cow with an adenocarcinoma of respiratory epithelial origin. The mass caused reduced airflow through the left nasal passage, left-sided Horner's syndrome, and exophthalmos. The eyelids have been sutured together to protect the eye.

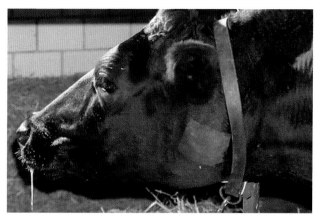

• **Fig. 4.5** Adult Holstein with a lymphosarcoma mass in the pharyngeal area that caused inspiratory dyspnea.

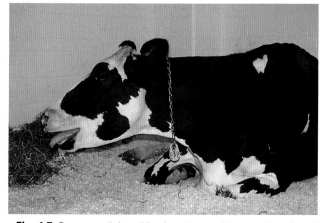

• **Fig. 4.7** Open-mouth breathing in a 5-year-old cow with unilateral Horner's disease (etiology unknown). The cow had no respiratory difficulties during the winter months.

vascular injury, salivary duct laceration, and acute cellulitis are potential complications associated with opening abscesses. The salivary duct was severed in one calf we treated, and saliva flowed from the incision for a couple of days after which the salivary flow stopped and the calf had a complete recovery. If drainage is not liberal, abscesses tend to recur. If recurrence is obvious, culture and sensitivity coupled with drainage through multiple sites are indicated. Daily flushing of the drainage sites is important. Systemic antibiotics should be administered for 1 to 2 weeks after drainage; *Trueperella pyogenes* and *Fusobacterium* spp. are the most common organisms cultured, so β-lactams are the most commonly used antibiotic class.

Chronic maxillary sinusitis should be treated by trephination of the sinus, removal of any teeth that have infected roots, daily flushing of the sinus with dilute disinfectants or sterile saline, and appropriate systemic antibiotics for 1 to 2 weeks.

In general, neoplasms have a hopeless prognosis, and the animal should not be treated. Juvenile lymphosarcoma often causes upper airway dyspnea via enlarged pharyngeal lymph nodes. Occasional adult-form lymphosarcoma cases have one or more very large (10–20 cm diameter) pharyngeal or mediastinal lymph nodes that will cause dyspnea. Lymphosarcoma usually results in death within 1 to 6 months of diagnosis. Adenocarcinomas originating in the respiratory epithelium in older cattle (i.e., more than 8 years of age) may have an insidious but progressive course over months to years. Therefore, unlike cattle with lymphosarcoma, these animals may be allowed to survive for some time to deliver another calf or to undergo superovulation and embryo transfer. Only if the animal stops eating, develops severe respiratory distress, or is suffering from exposure damage from an exophthalmic eye will euthanasia be necessary. Cattle affected with primary squamous cell carcinoma, metastatic squamous cell carcinoma, or osteosarcoma originating in a sinus, bone, or periocular location occasionally may have enough tumor mass or lymph node metastases to develop inspiratory dyspnea. Cattle with squamous cell carcinomas frequently have a fetid breath odor from the primary tumor and should not be made to suffer unduly.

Inflammatory Diseases

Allergic Rhinitis

Also called summer snuffles, allergic rhinitis occurs primarily in yearling or adult cattle turned out on pasture in the spring and summer. This condition also has been described as a familial problem in a group of Holstein-Angus cattle. Affected cows do not act ill but have a bilateral thick nasal discharge (Fig. 4.8, *A*) and nasal pruritus with variable but often progressive degrees of nasal stertor and increased respiratory rate and effort. Affected cattle may rub their noses so frequently that foreign bodies may become trapped in the nasal cavity, and significant self-induced trauma may ensue. Diagnosis is based on clinical signs; endoscopic examination of the nasal and nasopharyngeal cavity (Fig. 4.8, *B* and *C*); and when indicated, cytology of nasal mucus, tracheal aspirates or nasal biopsy, all of which contain large numbers of mononuclear cells and eosinophils (Fig. 4.8, *D*). Treatments generally include removing the affected animals from the pasture, or if

that is not possible, the administration of corticosteroids to nonpregnant heifers. Improvement in clinical signs is generally noted within 5 to 7 days after removal from pasture.

Granulomatous Rhinitis

Diffuse nasal granulomas are uncommon in dairy cattle in the northern United States. *Rhinosporidium* is the most common cause of granulomas that are observed. The granulomas develop on the nasal mucosa through the turbinate region, and as they enlarge, the nasal airway is progressively compromised. Therefore signs include a progressive inspiratory dyspnea, nasal discharge, and nasal pruritus.

Frequently, epistaxis is reported by the owner. Inspection at the nares with the aid of a focal light source allows observation of tan or brown granulomatous masses in the nasal region. Endoscopy further defines the lesion. Biopsy for tissue culture and histopathology is indicated to determine the exact cause of the nasal granulomas.

Treatment consists of sodium iodide solution intravenously (IV; 30 g/450 kg once or twice at 24-hour intervals) followed by 30 g of organic iodide powder orally each day until signs of iodism occur. Although permitted in some countries such as Canada, parenteral sodium iodide is not approved for use in lactating dairy cattle in the United States.

Granulomas Caused by Actinobacillus lignieresii or Actinomyces bovis

Etiology and Signs

Actinobacillus lignieresii granulomas within the nasal cavity usually are unilateral masses within the external nares and appear as red, raised, fleshy masses that bleed easily and look very similar to *Rhinosporidium* granulomas (Fig. 4.9). Signs include a progressively enlarging mass in one nostril, progressive decrease in airflow, and inspiratory dyspnea as the lesion enlarges to occlude the nostril completely. These granulomas may originate at the site of nose-lead lesions of the mucosa near the nasal septum or at other mucosal sites of soft tissue injury from restraint, foreign bodies, or fibrous feed.

Progressive inspiratory dyspnea and nasal discharge are found in patients having granulomas deeper in the nasal cavity, larynx, pharynx, or trachea. *Actinomyces bovis* was responsible for multiple tracheal granulomas in a cow treated at the New York State College of Veterinary Medicine.

Diagnosis

Granulomas can be confused with tumors on gross inspection. Therefore diagnosis requires biopsy for histopathology and tissue culture. Sulfur granules may be observed grossly on cut surface and suggest the diagnosis. Although usually found near the external nares, granulomas caused by *A. lignieresii* or *A. bovis* could occur anywhere in the upper airway or trachea because these opportunists reside in the oral cavity and pharynx. When soft tissue infection occurs after injury to the mucosa, both organisms produce similarly appearing granulomas. Endoscopy and radiographs are necessary to identify deeper granulomas at locations other than the external nares.

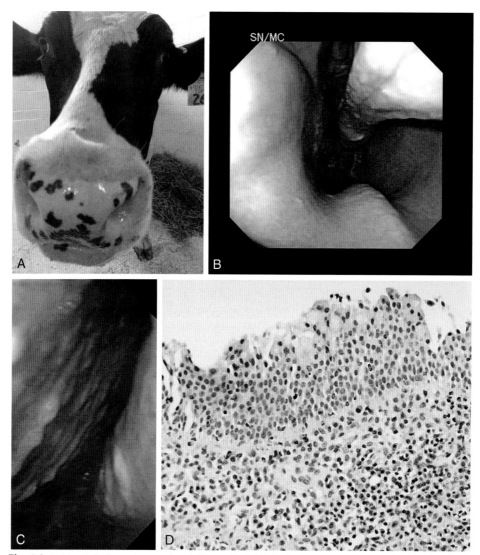

• **Fig. 4.8** **A,** Nasal discharge in a pastured 17-month-old Holstein heifer with a 3-week history of progressive nasal stertor and discharge caused by allergic rhinitis. **B,** Endoscopic examination of the heifer's nasal cavity showing multiple nodular lesions in the nasal mucosa. **C,** Close-up photo of the nodular lesions seen in the nasal mucosa via endoscopy. **D,** Histopathology of a biopsy taken from the nasal mucosa of the same heifer showing a pronounced mononuclear–eosinophilic reaction.

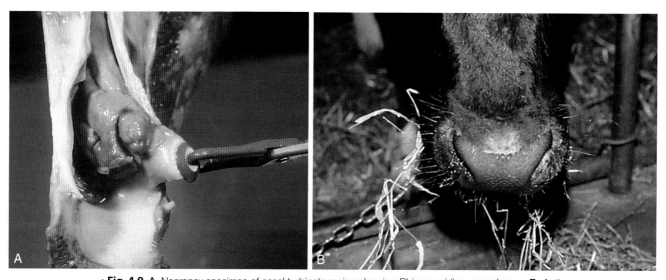

• **Fig. 4.9** **A,** Necropsy specimen of nasal turbinate region showing *Rhinosporidium* granulomas. **B,** *Actinobacillus* nasal granuloma in a Holstein cow.

Treatment

Treatment for granulomas caused by *A. lignieresii* consists of excisional biopsy to debulk the mass to the level of nasal mucosa and sodium iodide therapy until iodism is observed. Usually this requires IV sodium iodide (30 g/450 kg) initially and at 2- to 3-day intervals for several treatments or oral organic iodide (30 g/450 kg) daily after the initial IV dose. Cryosurgery has been used successfully on these granulomas after debulking. In severe or recurrent cases, antibiotic therapy may be necessary in addition to sodium iodide. Penicillin and ampicillin have been used to treat infection caused by *A. lignieresii*. Whenever possible, an antibiotic should be selected based on organism culture and sensitivity results. Usually the prognosis is good.

Granulomas caused by *A. bovis* are much more difficult to treat because this organism is poorly responsive to sodium iodide therapy. Treatment with penicillin (22,000 U/kg intramuscularly [IM] once a day), in conjunction with sodium iodide, may be effective. Surgical debulking of soft tissue granulomas also is indicated. The prognosis for lesions caused by *A. bovis* is guarded because of the limited clinical knowledge regarding treatment of this organism, and the fact that many owners may not treat for a sufficient time.

Frontal and Maxillary Sinusitis

Etiology and Signs

Frontal sinusitis in calves and adult cattle may be acute or chronic. Acute frontal sinusitis is more common and usually follows sharp dehorning techniques. Older calves and mature cattle dehorned by laypeople are most at risk because of nonsterile equipment and techniques. Signs of acute sinusitis include fever (103.0° to 106.0°F [39.4° to 41.1°C]), unilateral or bilateral mucopurulent nasal discharge, depression, and headache type pain characterized by partially closed eyes, an extended head and neck, head pressing or resting the muzzle on support structures (interestingly, cattle with severe skeletal or mild to moderate visceral pain can also often be found pressing their muzzles against an object, which suggests this must be a pain relief point), and sensitivity to palpation on percussion of the sinus. When acute sinusitis follows recent dehorning, purulent drainage or heavy scabs may be observed at the wound in the cornual portion of the sinus. A multitude of bacteria such as *T. pyogenes, Pasteurella multocida, Escherichia coli,* and anaerobes may contribute to acute frontal sinus infection. Tetanus is another possible complication of acute frontal sinusitis if wound debris or scabs occlude the cornual opening to allow an anaerobic environment.

Maxillary sinusitis is rare in cattle, especially compared with horses, but as in the equine species, it can be a spontaneous primary condition or occur secondary to diseased teeth roots. Secondary maxillary sinusitis related to dental disease is only likely to become more unusual in dairy cattle as the average age of dairy animals becomes younger. Occasional secondary cases may also present in association with osteomyelitic conditions of the skull such as lumpy jaw (Dr. Mike Livesey, University of Wisconsin, 2017, personal communication). Extension of frontal sinusitis associated with dehorning into the more rostral maxillary sinus is also possible. The most common presenting signs are chronic, purulent, unilateral nasal discharge; it is very rare to see facial asymmetry, but affected cattle may sometimes show resentment

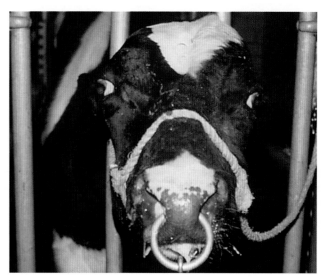

• **Fig. 4.10** Chronic frontal sinusitis in a mature bull. The bull died from septic meningitis caused by the sinusitis.

and sensitivity during percussion of the skull over the maxillary sinus region on the relevant side. As mentioned in the previous section, they may also have mild upper airway noise caused by a reduction in air flow on the affected side.

Chronic frontal sinusitis does not develop until months to years after dehorning and may be completely unassociated with dehorning because it occasionally occurs in animals dehorned by noninvasive techniques, polled animals, or animals with horns. Ascending respiratory tract infections, as in other species, are a cause of chronic frontal sinusitis and usually are caused by *P. multocida*. Chronic frontal sinusitis associated with old dehorning complications such as low-grade infection, bony skull fragments, or sequestra typically is associated with infection by *T. pyogenes* or mixed infections that may include *T. pyogenes, P. multocida,* anaerobes, or miscellaneous gram-negative organisms. Signs of chronic frontal sinusitis include gradual loss of condition and production that may be persistent or intermittent. Unilateral nasal discharge usually is observed, again as a persistent or intermittent complaint. Additional signs include head pressing, an extended head and neck, partially closed eyes, or resting of the muzzle on inanimate objects, all of which signal headache or pain. Intermittent or persistent fever is present. Bony expansions of the sinus may occur, causing asymmetric facial distortion, especially in cattle that do not have significant nasal discharge because of occlusion or obstruction of the opening of the ethmoidal meatus into the nasal cavity. In fact, some cattle have intermittent bony swelling of the sinus that becomes less apparent during times of sinus drainage and subsequent nasal discharge. Palpation or percussion of the frontal bone overlying the affected sinus causes pain, and the patient may be extremely apprehensive when the examiner approaches the head. Bony expansion of the sinus may result in ipsilateral exophthalmos and decreased air movement through the ipsilateral nasal passage (Fig. 4.10). Neurologic complications, including septic meningitis, dural abscesses, and pituitary abscesses, are possible in neglected cases as a result of erosion through the bony sinus. Tetanus is another potential complication. Occasionally, cattle with chronic frontal sinusitis have developed orbital cellulitis, pathologic exophthalmos, or facial abscesses from infectious destruction of the postorbital diverticula of the sinus, allowing soft tissue infection of the orbit (Fig. 4.11).

Diagnosis

In acute cases, diagnosis is based on signs, history, and palpation and percussion of the sinus. Ancillary data include bacterial culture and susceptibility testing to ensure proper antibiotic selection. Radiographic imaging (Fig. 4.12) and computed tomography (CT) provide helpful information regarding the extent of the lesion; severity of any accompanying osteomyelitis; and in the case of CT, greater detail regarding the possible involvement of deeper soft tissues of the head. Diagnostic imaging studies are also of great value in the evaluation of chronic nasal discharge associated with maxillary sinus infection (Fig. 4.13).

The diagnosis of chronic cases may be possible based purely on clinical signs coupled with palpation and percussion of the sinus. As with acute sinusitis, imaging can be very helpful in the evaluation of highly suspect cases prior to surgical intervention. When mature animals are affected, however, it is important to rule out neoplasia and other differentials. Drilling into the frontal sinus with a Steinmann's pin and collection of purulent material for cytology and bacterial cultures will confirm the diagnosis (Fig. 4.14). Sedation and local anesthesia allow this procedure to be performed with minimal patient discomfort.

Treatment

In individuals with acute frontal sinusitis, treatment requires cleansing of cornual wounds, lavage of the sinus with saline, or saline and mild disinfectant solutions, and appropriate systemic antibiotics for 7 to 14 days. Penicillin usually suffices, but selection of a systemic antibiotic is better based on culture and susceptibility testing. Tilting the patient's head to allow the sinus to fill and then twisting the head to empty the sinus facilitate lavage and drainage. Systemic analgesics such as aspirin or flunixin meglumine greatly aid patient comfort. The prognosis is good.

Treatment of chronic frontal sinusitis requires trephination of the sinus at two sites to allow lavage and drainage. One site is at the cornual portion of the sinus, and the second is located over the affected sinus approximately 4.0 cm from midline and on a transverse line connecting the caudal bony orbits (Fig. 4.15). A third site caudodorsal to the rim of orbit and medial to the temporal ridge has been recommended, but we have found this site to be dangerous because it occasionally results in orbital soft tissue infection as compromised softened bone is penetrated. Further caution regarding trephination of the sinus should be practiced in animals younger than 2 years of age because the rostral and medial rostral portions of the sinus may not be developed in younger animals. Attempts to establish rostral-medial drainage in these

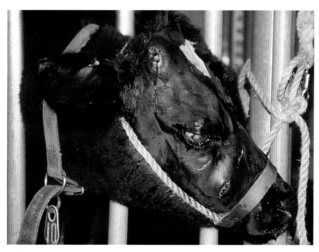

• **Fig. 4.11** Orbital cellulitis, exophthalmos, and facial abscesses secondary to extension of chronic frontal sinusitis into the orbital soft tissue.

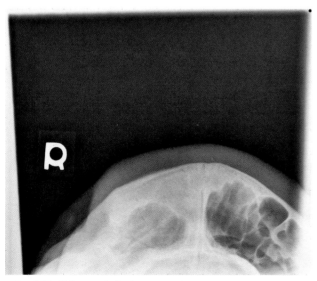

• **Fig. 4.12** Oblique, "skyline" radiograph of frontal region of a yearling Holstein bull that had purulent discharge from dehorning scar (performed at 6 months of age). Note the periosteal reaction and soft tissue opacity in the affected (R) sinus.

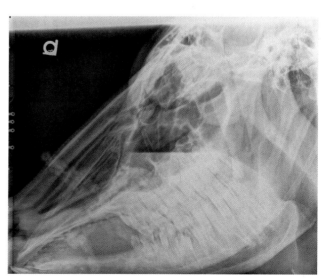

• **Fig. 4.13** Lateral skull radiograph of 5-year-old Jersey bull with chronic unilateral nasal discharge. Note the horizontal fluid line within the maxillary sinus.

animals may risk invasion of the calvarium. Drains may be placed to maintain communication between the two trephine sites and prevent premature closure of the wounds. Trephine holes should be at least 2.0 to 2.5 cm in diameter or they will close prematurely. Liquid pus is a positive prognostic sign, and pyogranulomatous or solid tissue in the sinus is a grave prognostic sign. Antibiotic selection must be based on culture

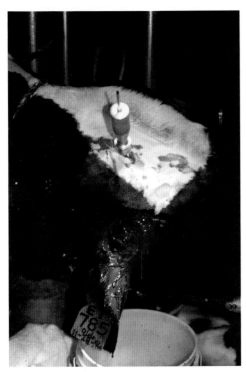

• **Fig. 4.14** Sinus trephination with a Steinmann pin to facilitate sample collection in a bull with chronic sinusitis. Note the caudal trephination flap that has already been made in the dehorning site to facilitate sinus lavage.

and susceptibility testing and should be continued for 2 to 4 weeks. Analgesics such as oral aspirin are used to improve the patient's comfort. Trephination and lavage are also the preferred treatments for primary or secondary maxillary sinusitis, although one will also need to attend to the inciting causes such as diseased tooth roots or maxillary osteomyelitis in secondary cases. It can be anatomically challenging in cattle to adequately access and drain all the somewhat convoluted pockets of the maxillary sinus cavity in affected cattle.

The prognosis is fair to good with appropriate therapy as described earlier unless neurologic signs have been observed. Neurologic signs and orbital cellulitis constitute severe and usually fatal complications of chronic frontal sinusitis. On several occasions, especially in animals younger than 18 months of age, Dr. Rebhun performed enucleation successfully to allow orbital drainage necessitated by severe orbital cellulitis and ocular proptosis in addition to trephination of the affected sinus. Long-term wound care, antibiotics, and nursing are essential if treatment is elected for such complicated cases.

Laryngeal Edema

Laryngeal edema secondary to bracken fern intoxication has been described in calves. Termed the "laryngitic" form, this idiosyncratic response leads to progressive dyspnea without obvious signs of hemorrhage as expected in older animals affected with bracken fern toxicity. Laryngeal edema has also occurred after vaccination of cattle, presumably as part of an adverse immune response. Cattle with persistent upper airway obstruction and dyspnea caused by conditions associated with the soft tissues of the retropharynx or larynx may develop laryngeal edema as a secondary complication. In cases of acute laryngeal edema associated with immune reaction or anaphylaxis, specific therapy with antihistamines, epinephrine (1–5 mL of 1:1000 epinephrine IV or 4–8 mL subcutaneously [SC] or IM) and

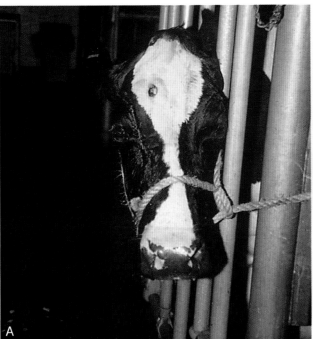
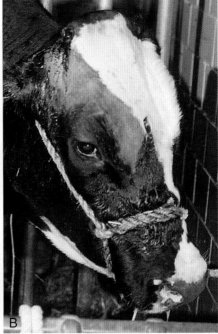

• **Fig. 4.15** A, Trephination sites surgically created to treat chronic frontal sinusitis in a 4-year-old Holstein cow. B, Trephination sites surgically created to treat chronic frontal sinusitis in a 3-year-old Holstein bull.

corticosteroids (mindful of pregnancy status of the animal) (40 mg of dexamethasone or 100–500 mg of methylprednisolone sodium succinate) should be instituted immediately. Almost as quickly as the clinician administers these drugs, a decision as to whether or not a tracheostomy is necessary should be made, but one should not prevaricate for many minutes if the emergency drug treatment does not alleviate the upper airway dyspnea almost immediately. Diuretic therapy is indicated if fulminant pulmonary edema is occurring with anaphylaxis, evidence of which is usually provided when the tracheostomy is placed because individuals with "wet lungs" will remain distressed and tachypneic despite the patent upper airway that has been established. The bovine larynx appears to be rather less dynamically forgiving than the equivalent structure in horses. One of the authors (SP) has treated several cattle with laryngeal edema from anaphylaxis, trauma from intubation, or associated with soft tissue or cartilaginous infections (mainly calves with necrotic laryngitis) that have seemingly recovered from the initial swelling or infectious lesion only to be left chronically with severely diminished arytenoid function. This acquired lack of normal arytenoid abduction has led to repeated bouts of dyspnea and upper airway noise during hot and humid weather, exertion, or even just in response to mild tachypnea. Consequently, this has led to repeated emergency tracheostomy or discussion with the owners regarding the placement of a permanent tracheotomy or a tracheolaryngotomy for long-term resolution. A similar situation sometimes arises with calves that are left with deformed arytenoids after apparent recovery from necrotic laryngitis or laryngeal chondritis.

Necrotic Laryngitis (Calf Diphtheria)

Etiology and Signs

Necrotic laryngitis represents an atypical site of infection by the anaerobe *Fusobacterium necrophorum*, the organism responsible for calf diphtheria. Calf diphtheria is an infection of the soft tissue in the oral cavity after mucosal injury caused by sharp teeth in calves of 1 to 4 months of age. Calves affected with calf diphtheria usually have abscesses in the cheek region and mild salivation and may refuse solid feed (Fig. 4.16). The infection spreads among calves fed from common utensils or feeders or those in such close group contact that they may lick one another. When the larynx becomes infected in the atypical form of this disease, the affected calf

develops a progressive inspiratory dyspnea. Low-grade fever (103.0° to 104.5°F [39.44° to 40.28°C]) may be present along with a painful short cough that is observed when the calf attempts to drink or eat. As the condition worsens over several days, both inspiratory and expiratory dyspnea may be apparent, but the inspiratory component always will be worse. A necrotic odor may be present on the breath.

Audible inspiratory efforts are heard externally. Harsh sounds of airway turbulence are heard when a stethoscope is placed over the larynx; these sounds are also referred down the tracheobronchial tree to confuse auscultation of the lower airway.

Diagnosis

Endoscopy is helpful in confirming the diagnosis. In some calves, the lesions can be seen by using an oral speculum, but endoscopy is much easier and less stressful for the patient. If the calf is in extreme dyspnea or is anoxic or cyanotic, a tracheostomy should be performed before endoscopy (Fig. 4.17). The larynx will be found to be uniformly swollen and may appear to have cartilaginous deformities in chronic cases (Fig. 4.18). The laryngeal opening always is narrowed, and mucosal necrosis will be present in acute cases. Chronic cases may have laryngeal deformity and airway narrowing, but the necrotic, infected cartilage may be covered by normal mucosa (see Video Clips 4.2 and 4.3). If the mucosa appears normal on endoscopic examination performed via the nose and the tracheostomy opening, ultrasound examination of the larynx can be very helpful in detecting the severity of cartilage necrosis (Fig. 4.19). It should be noted that adult cattle may also develop bacterial infections in and around the arytenoid cartilages causing either cartilage necrosis or soft tissue abscess formation (see Video Clips 4.4 and 4.5). Branchial cysts may also occur in cattle and have an appearance similar to layngeal abscess (see Video Clip 4.6).

Treatment

Long-term therapy is required because infection of cartilaginous structures usually exists. Acute cases should be treated with penicillin (22,000 U/kg IM twice daily). A tracheostomy is essential for treatment of calves that have severe dyspnea (Fig. 4.20; see Video Clips 4.7A and B). This provides a patent airway

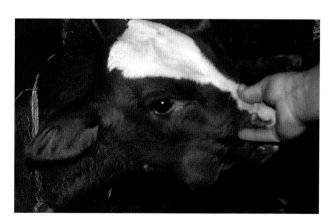

• **Fig. 4.16** Typical cheek abscess observed in calf diphtheria.

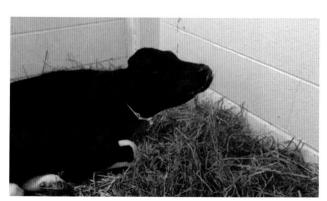

• **Fig. 4.17** A 4-week-old Holstein calf with progressive respiratory noise and cough that presented in respiratory distress. A temporary tracheostomy had to be performed because of the severity of the respiratory obstruction and distress.

and rests the inflamed larynx from further exertional irritation while the infection is controlled. Affected animals can improve from severe respiratory distress and being almost moribund to eupnea in minutes after placement of the tracheostomy. It also allows for easier evaluation of the lower airway; the degree to which bronchopneumonia is worsening the animal's condition is much easier to evaluate by auscultation, if imaging modalities (radiographs or ultrasound) are not available, when one does not have to try to filter out the considerable referred upper airway noise that is typically present before the tracheostomy is placed. The prognosis for acute cases is fair; the goal is to be able

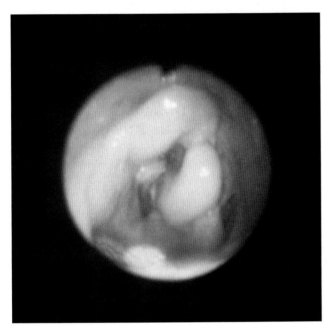

• **Fig. 4.18** Endoscopic view of laryngeal deformity and profoundly narrow laryngeal airway in a 3-month-old Holstein calf that had necrotic laryngitis and chronic laryngeal cartilage infection caused by *Fusobacterium necrophorum*.

to allow the temporary tracheostomy to heal by second intention after it is apparent that normal air flow and eupnea are possible when the temporary tracheostomy is "test" occluded. The temporary tracheostomy, although usually placed under emergency-type conditions, should be located in the proximal third of the neck, close to the larynx. Daily wound care and changing of the tracheostomy tube are critical because the site is usually very "exudative" and prone to purulent discharges that can occlude the airway or become inhaled and travel distally. It is advisable to remove a semicircular part of the adjacent tracheal rings immediately dorsal and ventral to the initial skin incision when placing the tracheostomy tube even if this is performed after a smaller diameter tube has been initially placed for emergency relief. Radiographs can be helpful not only diagnostically but also to give an idea of the diameter of tracheostomy tube that the patient's upper airway can accommodate, although the diameter of the stoma is the usual limiting factor. Radiographs or ultrasonography of the lungs are also helpful to assess the amount of pneumonia (aspiration is common in these cases). Concurrent, severe bronchopneumonia worsens the prognosis markedly and is often suggested by only mild improvement in tachypnea when a tracheostomy is placed.

Chronic cases have a poor prognosis because laryngeal deformity and cartilaginous necrosis have often already occurred or abscesses within the laryngeal cartilage already have developed (Fig. 4.21). Treatment is similar to that described for acute cases but should be extended to 14 to 30 days in patients valuable enough to warrant treatment, or the necrotic cartilage should be surgically removed or debrided. A tracheostomy may be necessary for the reasons listed earlier, and some clinicians recommend concurrent treatment with sodium iodide in the hope of penetrating the deep-seated cartilaginous infection. *T. pyogenes* frequently contributes to, or replaces, *F. necrophorum* as the causative organism in chronic infections because these two organisms are synergistic. For valuable cattle with the chronic form, referral to an expert surgeon familiar with performing a permanent

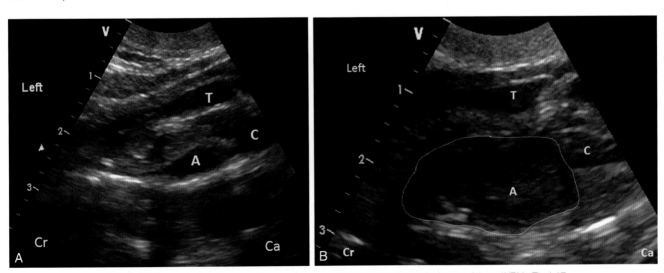

• **Fig. 4.19** Comparative ultrasound images of a normal calf larynx (**A**) with the larynx of the calf (**B**) in Fig 4.17 demonstrating necrosis of the cartilage. An abscess associated with the arytenoid cartilage is identified by the yellow outline. An endoscopic examination performed via the nose and tracheotomy site had not shown any appearance of necrosis, only swelling. A laryngotomy and partial arytenoidectomy were performed, and the calf recovered completely. Ultrasound image key: (T) Thyroid cartilage, (C) Cricoid cartilage, (A) Abscess in arytenoid cartilage, (Cr) cranial, (Ca) caudal (V) ventral. Image courtesy of Dr. M. Cercone.

tracheotomy, the tracheolaryngotomy technique as described by Gasthuys, or a subtotal arytenoidectomy via laryngotomy is recommended. Surgical details are described in the Farm Animal Surgery text, edited by Drs. Fubini and Ducharme.

Anatomic differences in skin redundancy and strap musculature between horses and cattle, even in calves, make surgery more challenging. By removal of the caudal part of the cricoid cartilage and two to three proximal tracheal rings, a permanent tracheolaryngotomy can be established as a long-term solution, and cattle can still thrive after this procedure (Figs. 4.22 and 4.23) but are, of course, susceptible to blockage of, or aspiration into, the stoma. Recently, Nichols and Anderson have described an additional surgical option of partial or subtotal arytenoidectomy via laryngotomy for the long-term management of such calves. Calves can grow

and survive to adulthood. It has been convention to say that these animals cannot calve without assistance because of their inability to forcibly abdominally contract against a closed airway (Valsalva maneuver); that has not been our experience! In dairy calves, the prognosis for animals that undergo such permanent upper airway surgeries must always be guarded, and the treatment goal should preferably be resolution of the condition medically, often with the combined use of a temporary tracheostomy, during the acute stages of the disease.

Tracheal Obstruction

Tracheal obstruction is not common but may occur from either intraluminal obstruction with exudative debris as occurs with infectious bovine rhinotracheitis (IBR) infection or from

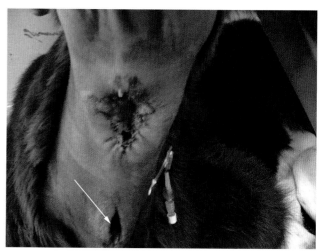

• **Fig. 4.22** Permanent tracheolaryngotomy in 2-month-old calf as a treatment for chronic necrotic laryngitis (ventral view). The image was taken 2 days postoperatively. The more distal stoma *(arrow)* represents site of previous emergency tracheostomy. Note the exudative discharge from the permanent stoma, which will persist for a prolonged period and require wound care.

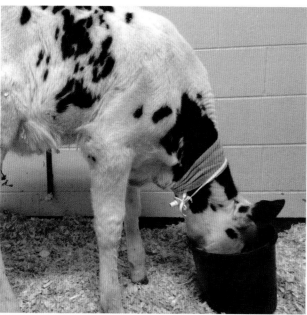

• **Fig. 4.20** Weanling-age Holstein heifer with temporary tracheostomy in place for treatment of severe necrotic laryngitis with chondritis. Immediate relief and desire to eat were associated with tube placement. (Courtesy of Rachel Borchardt.)

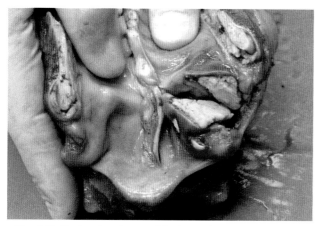

• **Fig. 4.21** Postmortem image of the larynx from a 6-week-old Holstein calf with severe necrotic laryngitis with abscess formation involving the left arytenoid and perilaryngeal tissues. Epiglottis is positioned at the bottom of the image, and fingers are within the proximal trachea.

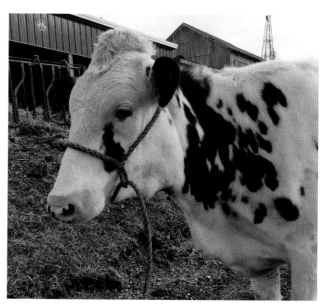

• **Fig. 4.23** Holstein heifer from Fig. 4.20 as a yearling. A permanent tracheolaryngotomy had been created for long-term management 7 months previously. (Courtesy of Rachel Borchardt.)

extraluminal obstruction caused by abscess or lymphosarcoma or as a result of proliferative callus on the first ribs in calves (Figs. 4.24 to 4.26). Congenital tracheal stenosis independent of rib injury has also been reported to occur within the cervical or thoracic portions of the trachea (Fig. 4.27).

The diagnosis is generally easy if endoscopy and radiography can be used to support the clinical examination. Most calves with tracheal obstruction resulting from proliferative rib calluses are several weeks of age when respiratory signs develop and affected calves often have a history of dystocia at birth.

Treatment for intraluminal inflammatory obstruction includes nebulization with acetylcysteine, inhalational antibiotic, and an appropriate bronchodilator (ipratropium inhaler or aminophylline or atropine systemically). Prosthetic repair of tracheal compression caused by proliferative callus formation has been described, but the procedure is technically difficult, and because of the young age of the patient, the prosthesis eventually needs to be removed to permit normal growth of the trachea.

Diseases of the Lower Airway

Bacterial Bronchopneumonia

This remains the most important cause of morbidity and mortality from respiratory disease in dairy calves and adult cattle. Virulent strains of *Mannheimia haemolytica* and *Histophilus somni* are primary pathogens capable of causing acute infections of the lower airway and lung parenchyma. These organisms do not always require the help of environmental and management stressors or other infectious agents to cause life-threatening or fatal pneumonia. Chronic lower airway infections by *P. multocida* and *T. pyogenes* may cause pneumonia in calves either previously infected or co-infected with primary bacterial pathogens (*Mannheimia* and *Histophilus* spp.) or viral or *Mycoplasma* pathogens of the respiratory tract or in animals stressed by shipment, poor management, or ventilation insufficiencies.

Chronic suppurative bronchopneumonia in adult cattle and calves may also be the result of previous aspiration; combinations of *P. multocida*, *T. pyogenes*, *Fusobacterium* spp., and *Mycoplasma* spp. are frequently cultured. Aspiration pneumonia associated with these same pathogens may also be observed in calves with white muscle disease, calves fed via an inappropriately large opening on the nipple of milk feeding bottles, premature calves with inadequately developed protective reflexes of the glottis, and calves with retropharyngeal diseases that interfere with normal upper airway reflexes. Milk-fed calves who are tachypneic or dyspneic because of either upper or lower airway disease, whatever the etiopathogenesis, may also aspirate as a secondary problem as they struggle to swallow properly at very high respiratory rates. Head and neck position during feeding can play a role in increasing or decreasing the likelihood of this occurring, to the extent that hospitalized sick and weak calves that are being fed from a bottle at our institution are routinely encouraged to nurse with the head and neck along a more parallel axis to the ground than is their natural tendency. In general, feeding from a bucket lessens the chances of aspiration.

It is imperative for bovine practitioners to understand the causes, predisposing factors, treatment, control, and prevention of the pathogens associated with bacterial bronchopneumonia, such is the prevalence and impact of the disease. It is by far the most common and significant cause of respiratory disease in dairy calves. When investigating outbreaks of bacterial bronchopneumonia of dairy calves during the first few

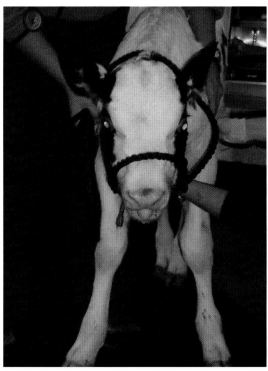

• **Fig. 4.24** A 5-week-old Holstein calf with respiratory distress and a loud honking sound during breathing. This was caused by tracheal compression resulting from a large callus associated with healed rib fractures. The fracture of the ribs had likely occurred during delivery.

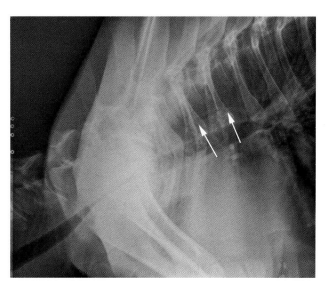

• **Fig. 4.25** Thoracic radiograph of 6-week-old Holstein calf with tracheal compression associated with callus formation over multiple proximal rib fractures *(arrows)* associated with dystocia. The calf had been noted to be persistently tachypneic and exercise intolerant since shortly after birth.

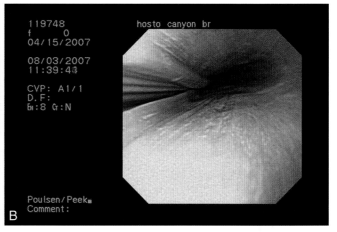

• **Fig. 4.26** Endoscopic images of trachea from calf in Fig. 4.25, proximal to (**A**) and at the level of (**B**) the stenotic segment.

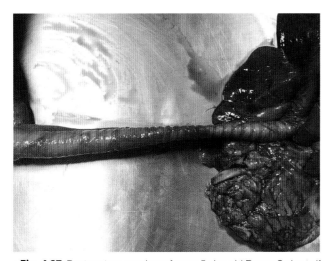

• **Fig. 4.27** Postmortem specimen from a 5-day-old Brown Swiss calf with congenital stenosis affecting the cervical trachea.

weeks of life, it is also critical to incorporate an evaluation of adequacy of passive transfer. There is compelling evidence that adequate transfer of immunoglobulin during the immediate neonatal period is a pivotal determinant of susceptibility to respiratory disease. Greater morbidity and mortality are anticipated with all infectious diseases to include bacterial bronchopneumonia when colostral transfer is suboptimal. When testing total protein by refractometry in calves between 1 day and 7 days of age, the goal is for individuals to be at 5.5 g/dL or higher; on a herd basis, when fewer than 75% of all calves in this age group meet this criterion, then the herd is deemed to have a problem with passive transfer.

In addition, it must be emphasized that the only way to diagnose and control contagious respiratory disease in cattle is to know the exact identity of the pathogens and predisposing causes. This can be accomplished only by careful history, thorough physical examination, collection of appropriate samples, and collaboration with a diagnostic laboratory capable of identifying all known bovine respiratory pathogens. The five major bacterial pathogens of the bovine lower airways currently are *M. haemolytica*, *P. multocida*, *Mycoplasma* spp., *H. somni*, and *T. pyogenes*. They will

be discussed separately. Although other organisms may be involved, they seldom cause herd problems and will not be discussed in detail.

Mannheimia haemolytica

Etiology and Signs

M. haemolytica is a gram-negative rod that may be a normal inhabitant of the upper airway but is not cultured from the upper airway of normal cattle as frequently as *P. multocida*. Several properties of *M. haemolytica* contribute to its pathogenicity. These include a capsule that provides defense against phagocytosis; production of an exotoxin (leukotoxin) lethal to alveolar macrophages, monocytes, and neutrophils; cell wall–derived endotoxin that helps to initiate complement and coagulation cascades; and the ability to reside in the upper airway among other nonpathogenic serotypes and then convert/or overgrow under stressful stimuli to a pathogenic serotype, A1, that is more virulent. The cytotoxicity of the leukotoxin is associated with its ability to bind and interact with β2 integrin leukocyte function–associated antigen 1. Currently, *M. haemolytica* is a leading cause of death as a result of respiratory infection in dairy cattle and calves in most areas of the United States. This organism is a primary pathogen not always needing assistance from other viral or *Mycoplasma* agents to establish lower airway infection, although it is well demonstrated that bovine herpesvirus 1 (BHV1) infection can activate genes that will increase leukotoxin binding, cytotoxicity to bovine mononuclear cells, and the severity of *M. haemolytica* infection. When a virus such as IBR, bovine respiratory syncytial virus (BRSV), or bovine viral diarrhea virus (BVDV) does infect a herd, mortality will be greatly increased if *M. haemolytica* bronchopneumonia is superimposed. In this situation, the bacteria may cause death because the viral infection compromises mechanical and cellular defense mechanisms. Similarly, compromise of the mucociliary clearance apparatus alongside depression of other components of airway defense can be consequences of poor air quality under conditions of poor ventilation, inadequate fresh air changes, and increased partial pressures of inspired noxious gases such as ammonia from soiled bedding. This is true in broad terms for all of the infectious causes of lower airway disease, whether commensal or true pathogen, and serves to emphasize the importance of air quality and ventilation in the prevention and control of pneumonia. The mortality rate may approach 30% to 50% when a virulent *M. haemolytica* infection is superimposed on a preexisting viral infection (e.g., BHV1 or BVDV) in a herd. Cattle that are stressed are at great risk of *M. haemolytica* pneumonia because stress triggers activation of the organism to a more virulent form, permits greater colonization of the virulent strain, and compromises the host defense mechanisms. Corticosteroids, either endogenous or exogenous, impair endotoxin-induced expression of antimicrobial peptides in the upper airway of cattle which would normally be an important part of the host defense response to gram-negative organisms such as *Mannheimia* and *Histophilus* spp. A similar negative effect is noted via endogenous corticosteroid release upon lactotransferrin production, which is another important antimicrobial determinant within the airways. Social group disruption, weaning, and transportation are all established paths to corticosteroid release in calves in particular and are therefore important risks to be aware of when troubleshooting husbandry factors that may be contributing to death losses caused by infection with *M. haemolytica*. Thus, *M. haemolytica* is frequently isolated as the cause of "shipping fever pneumonia" associated with shipment of cattle, transport of cattle to shows, or recent purchase of replacement animals. Classic signs of pneumonia generally develop 1 to 2 weeks after any of these stresses. The morbidity and mortality percentages tend to be much greater for *M. haemolytica* pneumonia outbreaks than if *P. multocida* is found as the cause of "shipping fever".

A great deal of variation in pathogenicity and antibiotic resistance exists amongst isolates of *M. haemolytica*. Therefore, the veterinarian must accept the fact that signs produced by these types may vary from mild to severe. Mild infections or less pathogenic *M. haemolytica* may mimic *P. multocida* with respect to clinical signs and response to therapy, but severe infections may be so drastic as to cause death within hours of the first clinical signs. In rare instances, the death can be so peracute that a toxicity is suspected. A less pathogenic form has been seen causing high fever in recently fresh cows, all of which had a remarkably quick recovery after treatment with ceftiofur.

Signs of acute *M. haemolytica* pneumonia include fever, depression, anorexia, markedly decreased milk production, salivation, nasal discharge, moist painful cough, and rapid respirations (Fig. 4.28). The fever may be as high as 108.0°F (42.22°C) but usually ranges between 104.0° and 107.0°F (40.0° and 41.67°C). Auscultation of the lungs reveals moist or dry rales in the anterior ventral lung fields bilaterally. Bronchial tones indicative of consolidation in the ventral lung fields are observed much more frequently than with acute *P. multocida* infections. Pleuritic friction sounds may be auscultated in some cases because of stretching or compression of fibrinous adhesions between the parietal and visceral pleura. The dorsal lung fields may sound normal on auscultation of animals with mild to moderate *M. haemolytica* pneumonia. In more severe cases, however, the dorsal lung may be forced to overwork because of the ventral lung consolidation. This

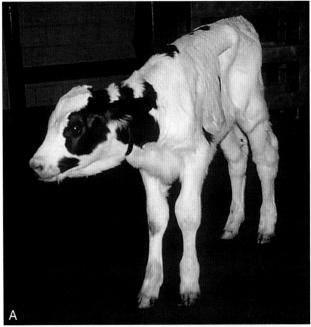

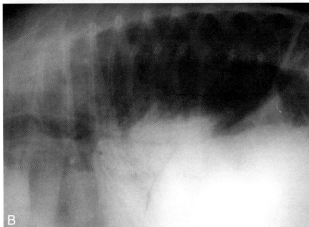

• **Fig. 4.28** **A,** Calf affected with *Mannheimia haemolytica* pneumonia showing an anxious expression, an extended head and neck to minimize upper airway resistance, and ventral edema caused by both albumin loss into the severely infected lungs and gravitational edema. **B,** Thoracic radiographs of the calf. Caudoventral consolidation is highlighted by air bronchograms. Consolidated lesions with air bronchograms give rise to the bronchial tones heard on auscultation.

overwork creates interstitial edema or bullous emphysema on occasion, and these pathologic changes cause the dorsal lung to be abnormally quiet on auscultation. Auscultation of the trachea will reveal coarse rattling or bubbling sounds caused by the inflammatory exudate free in the trachea. Palpation of the intercostal regions over the pneumonic lung causes the animal pain. Occasional cases have an accumulation of transudative or exudative pleural fluid in the ventral thorax unilaterally or bilaterally that causes a total absence of sounds when auscultation is performed.

More severe or neglected cases may show open-mouth breathing (Fig. 4.29), anxious expression, and SC emphysema secondary to tracking of air from bullae rupture in the dorsal lung field and have harsh bronchial tones ventrally with inaudible lung sounds dorsally. Respiratory dyspnea is marked in such cases and affects both inspiratory and expiratory components, with the expiratory component being the most obvious. An audible grunt or groan may accompany each expiratory effort, and the animals are reluctant to move because of hypoxia and painful pleuritis.

A peracute rapidly consolidating form of *M. haemolytica* bronchopneumonia occasionally has been observed in the northern United States and has resulted in high morbidity and mortality within affected herds. The causative *M. haemolytica* has proven extremely resistant to antibiotics. In some instances, it is resistant to all antibiotics approved for use in dairy cows. Signs in acutely affected cattle include high fever (106.0° to 108.0°F [41.11° to 42.22°C]), marked depression, salivation, increased respiratory rate (60–120 breaths/min), complete anorexia and milk cessation, reluctance to move, and an absence of rales when the ventral lungs are auscultated. Profound bronchial tones may be audible bilaterally that indicate consolidation of 25% to 75% of the ventral pulmonary parenchyma (Fig. 4.30), alongside quiet or inaudible sounds in the dorsal lungs where the remaining pulmonary tissue has been subjected to extreme mechanical and physiologic stress to maintain gas exchange. SC emphysema and pulmonary edema are common sequelae in these cattle. Ventral abdominal pain can be elicited in the cranial abdomen as a result of the fibrinous pleuritis present. This pain and absence of rumen activity coupled with the other signs have caused many veterinarians to initially confuse this rapidly consolidating pneumonia with peritonitis caused by hardware or a perforating abomasal ulcer. The major reason for this error is the absence of rales with this form of *M. haemolytica*. Therefore we have had to "retrain" our ears to auscultate carefully for bronchial tones versus normal or harsh bronchovesicular sounds. Careless auscultation of air sounds in the ventral lung field may not discriminate between bronchial tones and vesicular sounds. Acute infection with this form of *M. haemolytica* results in progressive dyspnea and death

in 12 to 48 hours unless the veterinarian is fortunate enough to choose as the first treatment an antibiotic to which the organism is susceptible.

We have also seen this rapidly consolidating form of bacterial bronchopneumonia sporadically in hospitalized cattle, especially calves, in the 1 to 2 days after intubation and ventilation for general anesthesia, when presumably the animal is unfortunate to have a subclinical, preexistent infection that becomes diffusely disseminated during anesthesia (Fig. 4.31). Microbiologic investigation of these cases postmortem have typically yielded pure growths or combinations of *M. haemolytica* or *P. multocida*, but the antimicrobial resistance patterns of the isolates obtained have not typically been very intimidating. The combined stressors of hospitalization, anesthesia, and surgery presumably contribute significantly, but the progression and deterioration have been relentless and the patient's demise inevitable.

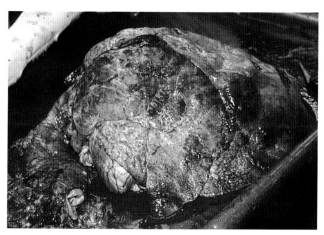

• **Fig. 4.30** Necropsy view of lungs affected by peracute rapidly consolidating *Mannheimia haemolytica* pneumonia. Consolidation exists in over 80% to 90% of the lung parenchyma, and fibrin is obvious on the visceral pleura. The clinical course of the disease was 36 hours.

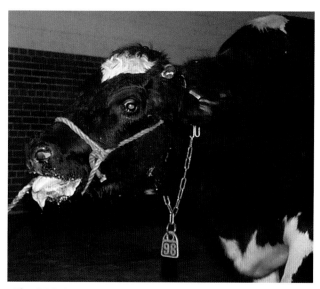

• **Fig. 4.29** Cow affected with severe *Mannheimia haemolytica* pneumonia showing open-mouth breathing, pulmonary edema froth at muzzle, an anxious expression, dehydration, and an extended head and neck to maintain a "straight line" upper airway.

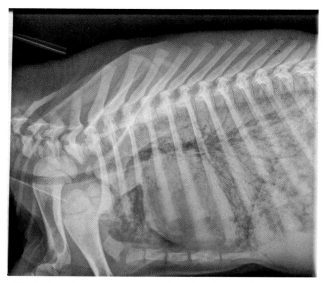

• **Fig. 4.31** Radiograph of a neonatal Holstein calf that underwent general anesthesia and laparotomy at 7 days of age. Radiography was obtained 36 hours after anesthesia and demonstrates marked, diffuse consolidating bronchopneumonia that was ultimately fatal by 48 hours after surgery.

Diagnosis

As with *P. multocida* pneumonia, accurate diagnosis of *M. haemolytica* bronchopneumonia requires culture of the organisms from tracheal wash specimens or bronchoalveolar lavage (BAL) fluid collected from acute, untreated cattle (Figs. 4.32 and 4.33), or postmortem cultures of lung and lymph node specimens. Because mortality is greater for *M. haemolytica* than *P. multocida*, necropsy specimens will often be the source of diagnostic material.

When it is apparent that the disease is epidemic in the herd, the veterinarian should obtain appropriate cultures via

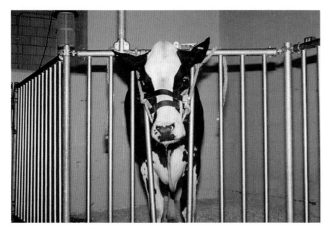

• **Fig. 4.32** A cow being restrained with two halters in preparation for a transtracheal wash. This method of restraint helps keep the head and neck straight during the procedure.

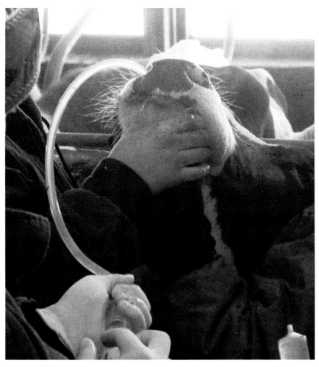

• **Fig. 4.33** Adult cow being restrained for a bronchoalveolar lavage (BAL) procedure. The neck is held in extension during passage of the BAL tube; the presence of the tube in the airway is easily detected by the paroxysmal coughing that is incited as the tube is passed distally from the trachea to the bronchi. (Courtesy of Dr. Sheila McGuirk.)

diagnostic fluid samples or fresh lung tissue at necropsy from several animals so that the delay in accurate diagnosis and receiving information regarding bacterial susceptibility to antibiotics is as short as possible. Tracheal wash; nasopharyngeal swab; BAL fluid; or necropsy specimens also should be cultured, submitted for polymerase chain reaction (PCR), or antigen tested for viral pathogens, *H. somni*, and *Mycoplasma* spp. Serum for viral titers should be collected from several acute cases so that it may be compared with convalescent serum titers in the future if the animals survive. In this way, some viral agents that are difficult to isolate, such as BRSV, may be identified as primary or contributing causes of the respiratory outbreak. Having collected these samples for culture, PCR, antigen testing, and evidence of seroconversion, the veterinarian will now have a basis, albeit retrospective, to identify the pathogens involved and attribute the disease to *M. haemolytica* alone or in combination with other pathogens. This will be of importance for future preventive measures.

Gross pathology specimens show a bilateral fibrinous bronchopneumonia with 25% to 75% or more of the lungs involved. The distribution is anterior/ventral in all cases, and the affected lung is firm, meaty, friable, and discolored. Usually fibrin is present on both the visceral and parietal pleura. Increased amounts of yellow or yellow-red pleural fluid are found frequently. In acute cases with advanced pulmonary parenchymal consolidation or in chronic cases, the dorsal lung may have bullous emphysema or interstitial edema present.

A complete blood count (CBC) from acutely infected cattle usually will show leukopenia characterized by a neutropenia with a left shift as neutrophils move to the site of severe infection. Fibrinogen values are elevated.

Diagnostic imaging has been historically of greatest value for prognosing an individual valuable calf or cow. An estimation of the degree of pulmonary consolidation and any abscess formation may be aided by either radiography (Fig. 4.34) or

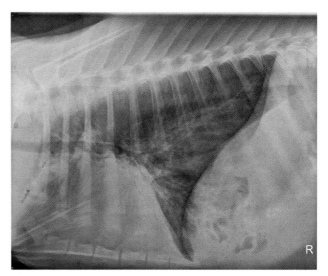

• **Fig. 4.34** Thoracic radiograph of 5-week-old Holstein calf recovering from mild bronchopneumonia associated with *Mannheimia haemolytica* infection. Moderate anteroventral consolidation is present as evidenced by air bronchograms cranial to cardiac silhouette. The calf made a complete recovery.

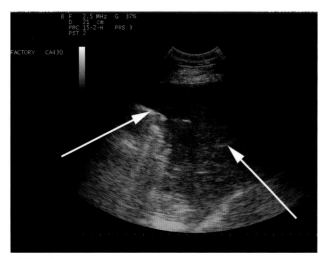

• **Fig. 4.35** Transthoracic ultrasound appearance of severe fibrinous pleuropneumonia associated with *Mannheimia haemolytica* infection. There is a large volume of variably echogenic free pleural fluid *(right arrow)* separating the ventral lung tip *(left arrow)* from the diaphragm and chest wall.

ultrasonography. Although ultrasonographic findings of lobular or lobar pneumonia and anteroventral consolidation can be seen with *M. haemolytica* infection, these are by no means specific to this organism and are seen in association with a number of other etiologic agents, especially other bacteria and *Mycoplasma*. However, if thoracic ultrasonography demonstrates significant pleural fluid and fibrinous pleuropneumonia in cattle with acute, highly febrile disease, then one's index of suspicion should be much higher for *M. haemolytica* (Fig. 4.35). Although less common in dairy than in beef animals, *H. somni* can also give a similar ultrasonographic appearance with fibrinous pleuropneumonia and free pleural fluid, as can severe *P. multocida* pneumonia.

Treatment

Broad-spectrum antibiotics constitute the major therapeutic approach to *M. haemolytica* pneumonia. Again, the veterinarian is forced to use "best guess" judgment when selecting an initial antibiotic in most cases. After collection of appropriate diagnostic samples, antibiotic therapy should commence immediately. Because life-threatening signs usually appear in at least some of the affected cattle, the veterinarian is more likely to select broad-spectrum antibiotics immediately. The currently available antibiotics for dairy cows and calves in the United States are shown in Table 4.1. Even when the causative bacterial organism is known, antibiotic therapy may be unable to cure the patient for a variety of reasons, such as the chosen antibiotic does not reach adequate tissue levels in the lung; the organism is resistant to the antibiotic; the organism is sensitive in vitro but in vitro inhibitory concentrations do not occur in the patient as a result of the dose, frequency of dosage, or other pharmacologic considerations; the drug may not be able to penetrate consolidated lung or work in purulent tissue; and in vitro susceptibility tests may not reflect in vivo success of an antibiotic against a specific organism. Consequently, the Kirby-Bauer disc assay has been criticized as too crude a test compared with mean inhibitory

concentration (MIC) or bactericidal concentration tests that can give a concentration of drug that inhibits or kills an organism. This MIC value then can be compared with known achievable blood and tissue levels of the antibiotic in the patient to determine likelihood of successful treatment. In a recent pharmacokinetic study in six calves, plasma, interstitial fluid (ISF) and pulmonary epithelial lining fluid (PELF) concentrations of ceftiofur (using the ceftiofur crystalline-free acid formulation), enrofloxacin, tulathromycin, and florfenicol were measured in 6-month-old calves to determine the plasma pharmacokinetics of each drug and the likelihood that the drugs would attain levels in bronchial fluid or lung that are above the MIC for common bovine pneumonia pathogens. Based solely on the pharmacokinetic data and previously reported MICs for bovine respiratory pathogens, it was found that drugs such as florfenicol and ceftiofur with high PELF concentrations were expected to be effective in the control of respiratory disease, but those with high ISF concentrations, including enrofloxacin and florfenicol, may be more effective in treatment of active respiratory infections. It was hypothesized that the often reported clinical efficacy of tulathromycin could be related to its antiinflammatory properties. Textbook charts that quote percentages of isolates sensitive to various antibiotics are seldom helpful because both geographic differences in strains and temporal resistance patterns occur. In some instances failure of antimicrobial treatment may also be attributed to the fact that the pulmonary pathology is irreversible or viral, or that *Mycoplasma* spp. or *T. pyogenes* pathogens may coexist to complicate the treatment response. Appropriate withdrawal times for any antibiotic selected for milk and slaughter residues must be known and observed and may shape decisions by the producer as to which antibiotic is chosen so that an immediate slaughter option is maintained.

The industry continues to seek the "silver bullet"—a magic antibiotic that will cure all cases of *Mannheimia* and other bacterial pneumonias. This silver bullet would take away the need for diagnostic work or preventive medicine; excuse management techniques that predispose to pneumonia; and, of course, would only be available through veterinarians. As a profession, we persist in overuse of every new antibiotic that becomes available. We ask these antibiotics to do things that cannot be done while ignoring older time-tested antibiotics and corrective management advice. The silver bullet does not, and will not, exist.

A clinical improvement in response to appropriate antibiotic therapy will appear as better attitude and appetite and a decreasing fever within 24 hours. A decrease of 2°F (1.1°C) or more should be considered clinically indicative of improvement. The body temperature continues to decrease into the normal range over 48 to 72 hours in most cases that have been treated with appropriate antibiotics. Depending on which antibiotic is used, a minimum of 3 days of antibiotic coverage is often required, and more often 5 to 7 days of continuous therapy is necessary and less likely to result in recurrence.

Antiinflammatory medications are used by many veterinarians in conjunction with antibiotic therapy, as discussed in a subsequent section on *P. multocida* pneumonia.

TABLE 4.1   Dosages and Frequencies of Selected Antibiotics for Treatment of Respiratory Disease in Dairy Cattle

Antibiotic	Dose	Frequency	Age
Ceftiofur (as Naxcel)*	1.1–2.2 mg/kg IM or SC	Once daily for 3 days; additional treatments on days 4 and 5 are permitted if response is incomplete	Adult cattle and replacement heifers
Ceftiofur (as Excenel RTU EZ)*	1.1–2.2 mg/kg IM or SC	Once daily for 3 days; additional treatments on days 4 and 5 are permitted if response is incomplete	Adult cattle and replacement heifers
Ceftiofur (as Excenel RTU EZ)*	2.2 mg/kg IM or SC	Every other day for two treatments (48 h apart)	Adult cattle and replacement heifers
Ceftiofur (as Excede)*	6.6 mg/kg in posterior of ear	Once; can be repeated in contralateral ear in 72 h	Adult cattle and replacement heifers
Oxytetracycline HCl alone or in combination with sulfadimethoxine	11 mg/kg IV	Twice daily; use only in well-hydrated cattle	Adult cattle and replacement heifers
Florfenicol (as Nuflor)	20 mg/kg IM (neck only)	Repeated after 48 h	Replacement heifers; not in animals >20 months of age
Florfenicol (as Nuflor or Nuflor Gold)	40 mg/kg SC (neck only)	Single treatment or for control in high-risk cattle	Replacement heifers; not in animals >20 months of age
Florfenicol with flunixin (as Resflor Gold)	40 mg/kg SC (neck only)	Single treatment	Replacement heifers; not in animals >20 months of age
Ampicillin	5–11 mg/kg IM (often used at up to twice this dose in an extralabel manner)	Once daily for up to 7 days	Adult cattle and replacement heifers
Enrofloxacin	7.5–12.5 mg/kg SC	Single treatment	Replacement heifers; not in animals >20 months of age
Enrofloxacin	2.5–5 mg/kg SC	Once daily for 3 days; may repeat on days 4 and 5 if response is incomplete	Replacement heifers; not in animals >20 months of age
Tilmicosin	10–20 mg/kg SC	Single treatment or for control in high-risk cattle	Replacement heifers; not in animals >20 months of age
Tulathromycin	2.5 mg/kg SC in neck	Single treatment	Replacement heifers; not in animals >20 months of age
Gamithromycin	6 mg/kg SC in the neck	Single treatment	Replacement heifers, not in animals >20 months of age and not in dairy veal calves

*All ceftiofur use in the United States must conform strictly to the product license label; no extralabel use is permitted.
IM, Intramuscular; IV, intravenous; SC, subcutaneous.

If corticosteroids are used as part of initial therapy, we believe that 20 mg of dexamethasone or a comparable dose of prednisone for an adult cow is the maximum. This should not be used more than once, and it should not be used at all in pregnant cattle. Currently in our clinics, we do not use any corticosteroids in the treatment of *M. haemolytica* pneumonia. Flunixin meglumine or other nonsteroidal antiinflammatory drugs (NSAIDs) are sound therapeutic agents for use in *M. haemolytica* pneumonia for the first 1 to 3 days of therapy. Excessive doses of NSAIDs or prolonged treatment with these agents should be avoided. Again, aspirin is the safest drug for this purpose (at a dosage of 240–480 grains orally twice daily for an adult cow or 25 grains/100 lb body weight twice daily for calves). Flunixin meglumine at 0.5 to 1.1 mg/kg is the most commonly recommended and only approved NSAID for treating bovine pneumonia and has been documented to improve clinical outcomes when combined with antibiotics compared with antibiotic treatment alone. We do not routinely use the high end of the labeled dose for flunixin (2.2 mg/kg) because of concerns over gastrointestinal (GI) side effects; however, other colleagues feel differently and are prepared to administer it at least once at this dose in the treatment of a critically ill patient.

Antihistamines such as tripelennamine (1 mg/kg twice or thrice daily) are less commonly used these days but are still used by many experienced clinicians as supportive therapy. Atropine may be a useful adjunct in advanced cases showing marked dyspnea, open-mouth breathing, or pulmonary edema. Atropine is used at 2.2 mg/45 kg body weight IM or SC twice daily to decrease bronchial secretions and to act as a mild bronchodilator.

In severe cases, dehydration may be a complication because of toxemia and fever causing depression of appetite and water consumption. In addition, some cattle are so dyspneic that they are unable to take time to drink, lest they become more hypoxic. Any IV fluid therapy that excessively expands the intravascular volume may cause or worsen existing pulmonary edema, consequently the fluid volume administered must be appropriate. Administering fluids through a stomach tube is safer regarding pulmonary edema, but the procedure is very stressful to an already hypoxic and dyspneic animal. Clinical judgment is required for these decisions, and in most cases, it is best to hope that antibiotic therapy will improve the animal within 24 to 48 hours so that the cow or calf may hydrate itself through adequate water consumption. Adequate water and salt, and small amounts of fresh feeds should be used to promote appetite.

Any management or ventilation deficiencies should be remedied immediately, and fresh air is of the utmost importance. It is better that the animals be in the cold fresh air than in a poorly ventilated or drafty but warm enclosure. The worst environmental effects occur when cattle develop *M. haemolytica* pneumonia during hot, humid weather because the additional respiratory effort to encourage heat loss complicates existing hyperpnea. Intranasal oxygen is beneficial for affected cattle being treated in a hospital.

The prognosis always is guarded until signs of clinical improvement are obvious. Cattle improving within 24 to 72 hours have a good prognosis, but those that take more than 72 hours have a greater risk of chronic lung damage or subsequent abscessation.

After endemic *Mannheimia* or *Pasteurella* infection in groups of calves, Drs. King and Rebhun observed occasional calves that developed peracute respiratory distress and dyspnea as a result of proliferative pneumonia 2 to 4 weeks after recovering from confirmed *Mannheimia* or *Pasteurella* pneumonia. At necropsy, resolving anterior ventral pneumonia from the previous *Mannheimia* or *Pasteurella* infection was observed in anterior ventral lung fields, and the remainder of the lung was diffusely firm, heavy, and wet. Histopathology in such cases confirms proliferative pneumonia. Viral cultures, fluorescent antibody (FA) procedures, and serology have been negative for other pathogens, including BRSV, which also may cause a delayed-effect hypersensitivity pneumonia but with different lesions. After observation of a number of these secondary proliferative pneumonia cases in the necropsy room, they were able to clinically recognize and treat several calves with this problem. The calves had a history of being part of a pneumonia outbreak 2 to 4 weeks previously and then apparently recovering. A sudden onset of extreme dyspnea in one recovered calf typifies the clinical situation. Signs include mild fever, open-mouth breathing, and diffusely quiet lungs. The

cause of this disorder is unproven, although increased exposure of the dorsal lung field to inhaled rumen gases after ventral consolidation has been proposed. Treatment consists of atropine (2.2 mg/45 kg twice daily), furosemide (25 mg/45 kg once or twice daily), broad-spectrum antibiotics, and box stall rest in a well-ventilated area. Response to therapy is slow, but survivors gradually improve over 7 to 10 days.

Vaccination of dairy cattle against *M. haemolytica* is performed in many dairy herds, although proof of efficacy is not always agreed upon. A leukotoxin bacterin is most commonly used and will result in serum antibodies against one of the *Mannheimia* leukotoxins. One recent study in calves demonstrated efficacy of a modified live virus (MLV) vaccine combined with the *Mannheimia* leukotoxin antigen in protecting calves challenged with *Bibersteinia trehalosi*, a gram-negative pathogen similar to *Mannheimia* spp. that also has a leukotoxin gene.

Pasteurella multocida

Etiology and Signs

P. multocida is a gram-negative normal inhabitant of the upper airway of cattle and calves. The normal defense mechanisms of the lower airway prevent colonization of the lung by *P. multocida* via physical, cellular, and secretory defenses in the healthy state. *P. multocida* is, however, a likely opportunist any time lower airway defense mechanisms are compromised. Chemical damage to mucociliary clearance, such as is caused by ammonia fumes in poorly ventilated barns, may allow *P. multocida* the opportunity to colonize the lower airway. *P. multocida* also is found in mixed infections of the lung along with *M. haemolytica*, *H. somni*, *T. pyogenes*, *Mycoplasma* spp., and various respiratory viruses of cattle. *Fusobacterium* and other anaerobic organisms may also be concurrently present in chronic suppurative pneumonia of adult cattle. As a general rule, the more chronic the pneumonia in cattle, the more likely *T. pyogenes* is involved.

The strains of *P. multocida* isolated from the lungs of cattle or calves frequently are sensitive to many antibiotics, including penicillin. This is in definite contrast to *M. haemolytica*, in which antibiotic resistance is much more probable. This difference is important regarding treatment and prevention of *P. multocida* pneumonia.

The signs of acute *P. multocida* pneumonia include fever, depression, mild to severe anorexia, a moist cough, increased rate and depth of respiration, and a decrease in milk production commensurate with the degree of anorexia. The fever ranges from 103.5° to 105.5°F (39.72° to 40.83°C) in most cases. Moist and dry rales will be auscultated in the anterior ventral lung field bilaterally and are classical findings in acute cases. Usually the dorsal lung fields are normal. Nasal discharge may be serous or mucopurulent in nature and is more apparent in calves than adult cows. The acute disease may occur in cattle of any age but tends to be more common in weaned calves and other grouped animals. When seen in younger animals, the acute disease usually is indicative of poor ventilation, excessive ammonia fumes, failure of passive transfer of immunoglobulins, or part of a diarrhea–pneumonia complex. All of these predisposing factors are common in dairy calves placed in veal operations or other indoor group housing facilities. *P. multocida* has been found as the cause of neonatal septicemia in calves receiving inadequate colostrum. These septicemic calves may show signs of meningitis, septic uveitis, septic arthritis, septic pericarditis, septic myocarditis and mucopurulent nasal and ocular discharge (Fig. 4.36) in addition to the typical signs of acute *P. multocida* pneumonia.

Acute *P. multocida* pneumonia tends to occur as either an infectious epidemic or endemic disease in groups of housed calves or adult cattle and may affect 10% to 50% of the animals within a group. It is one of the causes of "enzootic pneumonia" in calves, but this is not the preferred term because it gives little information as to the exact cause of the pneumonia. During an acute outbreak, the degree of apparent illness and auscultatable degree of pneumonia will vary greatly among affected cattle or calves. If only one animal in a group is infected, predisposing causes or stress unique to that animal should be sought when establishing a history (e.g., recent purchase, recent calving, possibility of BVDV-persistent infection [Fig. 4.37], transport to a show, sale, or poor ventilatory management).

Chronic pneumonia resulting from *P. multocida* causes signs similar to the acute disease, but bronchial tones indicative of consolidation are frequently limited to the anterior ventral lung fields. The abnormal area may be missed unless the stethoscope is pushed under the shoulder and the calf or cow forced to take a deep breath. In calves this can be accomplished most easily by holding the mouth and nose shut for a short period (Fig. 4.38). Transthoracic ultrasound can also be extremely helpful in the identification of consolidated bronchopneumonic lung lesions (Fig. 4.39; see Video Clip 4.8). Animals affected with chronic pneumonia may have marked exacerbation of dyspnea and an increased respiratory rate (≥60 breaths/min) if housed in poorly ventilated areas or where the environmental temperature exceeds

70.0°F (21.1°C). *T. pyogenes* is a common secondary invader in lungs chronically infected with *P. multocida*.

Diagnosis

P. multocida pneumonia may be suspected after obtaining the appropriate history from the owner and finding typical signs complete with anterior ventral pneumonia and bilateral auscultatable rales. However, confirmation requires culture of *P. multocida* from tracheal wash samples, BAL fluid, or necropsy specimens of acute, untreated affected animals. Neutrophils predominate the white blood cell components of the tracheal wash or BAL fluid, and gram-negative rods may be observed intracellularly in acute cases. The hemogram may show a degenerative left shift typical of acute infection in cattle or may be normal in mild cases. Chronic cases (≥2 weeks) may have neutrophilia, and adult cattle may show hyperglobulinemia in the serum. Many of these more chronic bronchopneumonia cases, especially adult cows with chronic suppurative pneumonia, may have

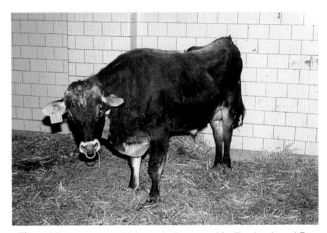

• **Fig. 4.37** This 3-year-old Jersey bull at a stud facility developed *Pasteurella multocida* pneumonia without any environmental stress factors. The bull was later proven to be persistently infected with bovine viral diarrhea virus, which likely resulted in immunosuppression.

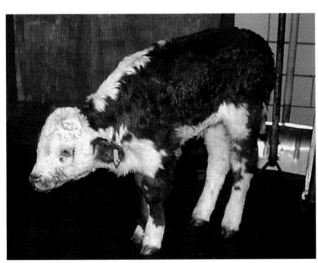

• **Fig. 4.36** Neonatal calf with *Pasteurella multocida* septicemia. In addition to pneumonia, signs included fever, hypopyon, and mucopurulent nasal and ocular discharges.

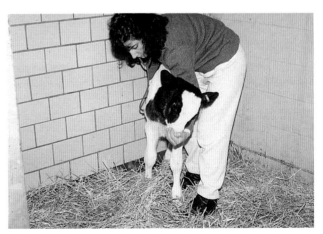

• **Fig. 4.38** An easy method of properly auscultating the lungs in calves. To make the calf breathe deeply, the calf is backed into a corner and one hand is placed over the mouth and nose until the calf struggles, at which time the calf is allowed to breathe. Alternatively, in adult cows, a plastic garbage bag can be used over the cow's nose and mouth to force deep breathing.

mixed infections etiologically with both *T. pyogenes* and *Mycoplasma* spp. commonly co-isolated or demonstrated by PCR.

Gross pathology of fatal acute cases includes bilateral anterior ventral pneumonia with the affected portion of lung being firm and discolored red or blue (Fig. 4.40). Palpation of the firm affected lung is the key to gross pathologic diagnosis. Fibrin may coat the surface of the parietal or visceral pleura but tends to be less than that observed with *M. haemolytica.* Chronic cases show similar firm, pneumonic lung parenchyma but often have bronchiectasis and pulmonary abscesses.

Radiographs seldom are necessary but may be helpful for individual, chronically infected calves or mature cattle to identify abscesses and the degree of consolidation for prognostic purposes. Ultrasound examination helps define the severity of lung involvement and can be used to monitor response to therapy.

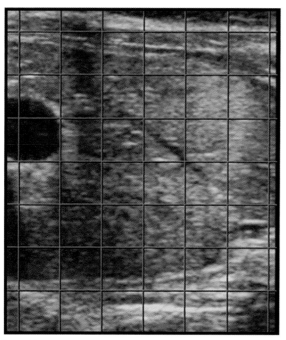

• **Fig. 4.39** Ultrasound image of severe consolidating bronchopneumonia in a calf. Note that tissue has a solid "hepatized" appearance rather than the normal pleural reverberations seen with a healthy aerated lung.

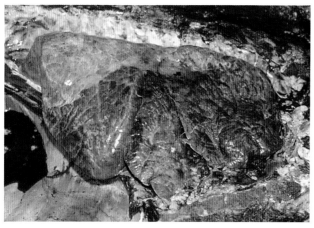

• **Fig. 4.40** Necropsy findings in a calf that was affected with severe cranioventral pneumonia caused by *Pasteurella multocida.*

Treatment

Antimicrobials and changes in husbandry or management constitute the integral components of effective therapy for *P. multocida* pneumonia. Many antibiotics have been used, including penicillin, ampicillin, erythromycin, and tetracycline. Sulfa drugs (trimethoprim–sulfa has been used in calves because it can be individually mixed with milk to bypass the forestomachs) also have been effective when administered either alone or in combination with antibiotics such as penicillin or tetracycline. Ceftiofur, a broadspectrum third generation cephalosporin approved for use in *Pasteurella* pneumonia in cattle, can be effective when the isolate is susceptible, which is frequently the case with *P. multocida,* and often the case with *M. haemolytica,* and *H. somni.* However, the increasing prevalence of *Mycoplasma* spp. co-infection in calves with bovine respiratory disease (BRD), for which the cephalosporin group is ineffective (along with other β-lactams such as penicillin and ampicillin), means that ceftiofur has become less relevant as a first-line antimicrobial choice. Macrolides (tulathromycin, tilimicosin, tildipirosin, gamithromycin), enrofloxacin, and florfenicol have become the most common first-line antibiotics for the treatment of undifferentiated BRD in dairy calves. The practicing veterinarian must often start antibiotic therapy without knowing results of cultures and antibiotic sensitivity tests. Therefore initial treatment is based on previous experience, geographic differences in antibiotic sensitivity, and economic factors. Animals that are febrile, anorectic, and dyspneic require treatment. Other animals that have mild fever and depression but continue to eat and do not act very ill may not require treatment. Individual or small groups of sick animals may be treated empirically if fatalities are not anticipated. However, if an epidemic situation is apparent, it always is best to do transtracheal washes from several animals before any treatment. Having done this, the veterinarian may start empiric therapy cognizant that definitive antibiotic sensitivity results will be forthcoming in about 3 days. It should be mentioned here that although transtracheal washes are recommended as part of a good diagnostic "workup," clinical response to antibiotics does not always correlate with in vitro susceptibility tests. For example, we have attended several calves with severe chronic pneumonia that had been treated with macrolides, β-lactams, and fluoroquinolones with no response but when treated with IV tetracycline and intramuscular penicillin and housed in a well ventilated hospital environment responded remarkably well, often despite in vitro resistance of the pathogen to these drugs (see Video Clips 4.9A and B). The macrolides, fluoroquinolones, and florfenicol all have a spectrum of activity in lung tissue that includes gram-negative organisms such as *P. multocida, M. haemolytica,* and *H. somni* as well as efficacy against *Mycoplasma* spp., and hence they represent sound empiric choices until individual isolate sensitivities are known. Thus, if the animals fail to respond to the initial choice of antibiotic, an alternative, specific antibiotic may be selected based on the sensitivity results as soon as these are available. Strict attention to responsible antimicrobial use, and adherence to federal regulations regarding not only drug withdrawals but also the requirements of the American Medicinal Drug Use Clarification Act (AMDUCA) are critical duties of the veterinarian. Within the United States, veterinarians and producers must be particularly aware of the defined dose, route, and duration restrictions for cephalosporin use in all dairy cattle, alongside the categoric requirement that enrofloxacin only be administered to calves younger than 20 months of age with respiratory disease. The necessity for intravenous administration when using flunixin in lactating cattle is another emphatic requirement in the United States; unfortunately, flunixin has become one of the most common violative tissue residues in cull dairy cows at many slaughter plants because of on-farm perivascular and non-intravenous parenteral administration.

There is, however, a combination injection containing flunixin and florfenicol that is available and labeled for SC administration in nonlactating cattle younger than 20 months of age, but a stand-alone injection of flunixin must always be given IV. Dosages and frequency of administration of the commonly used antimicrobials used to treat pneumonia in cattle are listed in Table 4.1. Regardless of the antibiotic selected, all treated cattle should have temperature and attitudes recorded daily so that 24- and 48-hour evaluations can be assessed. A trend of decreasing temperature into the normal range should proceed at 1° to 2°F per day when an effective antibiotic is used; the attitude, appetite, and degree of dyspnea should improve along with the return to normal body temperature. There has been extensive work done in feedlot cattle examining the efficacies and economics of various antibiotics in pneumonia outbreaks and although this can provide valuable information, dairy practitioners must remember that geographic variations in bacterial serotypes and antibiotic susceptibility exist and that antibiotic resistance is likely to increase in the years to come. Individual treatment generally is easier for dairy animals than for beef animals.

Treatment decisions and the process by which antimicrobial selections are made necessarily differ between adult cattle and calves, especially on larger facilities. Increasingly in calves, on-farm protocols such as the Wisconsin and California clinical scoring systems are used as health screening tools (see later section) that operators can use to identify individuals with an aggregate of physical examination findings that may justify treatment. The specificity of these clinical scoring systems is high, but sensitivity is much lower for individual calf pneumonia detection. These are commonly used for periodic assessments of large groups of calves and have been principally developed with the goal of improving early identification of disease and reflect efforts to diminish the impact of BRD on preweaning heifer morbidity and mortality. Hopefully, individual or groups of adult cattle with either acute or chronic bronchopneumonia caused by

P. multocida would not escape diagnosis because of their clinical signs. Such oversight would be even less likely with *M. haemolytica* because of the greater clinical severity typically seen with this agent. However, timely diagnosis is a ubiquitous and omnipresent challenge in adults as well as calves with milder clinical illness. In adult dairy cattle, the increased observation and daily examination often afforded to recently postparturient cows means that nasal discharge, cough, fever, and tachypnea are all likely to be picked up quite promptly. Indeed, one must be careful not to attribute a diagnosis of pneumonia too frequently merely on the basis of fever and tachypnea, as is quite common. Unfortunately, pneumonia can become a default diagnosis in febrile adult cattle that are breathing faster than normal when the latter is only a physiologic response to true fever of any cause or indeed hyperthermia that may be environmental in origin during hot weather. Identification of mild respiratory disease in dairy cattle beyond the fresh pen can be a challenge. Observation of feeding behavior and monitoring daily milk weight deviations become the tools by which cows beyond early lactation can be identified for further examination, but dry cattle are most easily overlooked on large dairies. We have been involved in several herd investigations of chronic bronchopneumonia in cattle in early lactation when it was highly probable that the onset of respiratory disease in many individuals occurred late in the previous lactation or during the dry period but was missed during the initial stages because of lesser oversight of cattle at these times. It is also worth emphasizing that such chronic bronchopneumonia "outbreaks" in adult cattle are rarely as simple as a single infectious agent that is a new pathogen to the farm; inevitably, the outbreak is multifactorial with components of overstocking, poor ventilation, and nutritional stressors during the transition period often contributing. There has never been, nor will there likely ever be, a replacement for experienced and devoted husbandry that invests time and watchful observation of the individual or groups of cattle for the identification of disease.

Many practitioners use antiinflammatory agents in conjunction with antimicrobial therapy. The goals of antiinflammatory medications are to reduce fever, block specific parts or mediators of the inflammatory cycle, and counteract endotoxins released by the cell wall of causative gram-negative organisms, to result in symptomatic improvement through better appetite and attitude. The two general groups of drugs include corticosteroids and NSAIDs such as aspirin and flunixin meglumine. Corticosteroids have a marked antiinflammatory and antipyretic activity that often leads to a "steroid euphoria" with resultant improved attitude and appetite within 24 hours. Although corticosteroids have these positive effects and also block several parts of the inflammatory cycle, they are dangerous if used repeatedly or in high dosages. Corticosteroids tend to stabilize small vessels and may reduce some of the chemotactic factors and lysosomal enzymes that cause a vicious cycle of increasing inflammation in the lung. However, they also partially or completely inhibit macrophage activation and antimicrobial peptide expression, which are serious detriments to the defense mechanisms of the lower airway. If the veterinarian elects to use corticosteroids, one treatment of low-dose (10–20 mg/450 kg) dexamethasone may be given as part of the initial therapy and should not be used thereafter. This treatment cannot be used in pregnant cows because of the abortifacient qualities of dexamethasone. Corticosteroids have potent antipyretic properties, and this may lead to a false sense of security because the veterinarian may assume that the proper antibiotic has been used based on a decreasing fever 24 hours after treatment when in fact the antibiotic has not been effective, and fever will return 24 to 48 hours later. We do not recommend the use of corticosteroids for bacterial pneumonia.

Nonsteroidal antiinflammatory drugs are safer than corticosteroids in the treatment of bacterial bronchopneumonia in cattle but are not without some disadvantages. Advantages include blockage of some prostaglandin-mediated inflammation within the lung, antiendotoxin effects, and antipyretic activity. Disadvantages include inability to gauge response to specific antibiotics based on body temperature alone as a result of the artificial decrease in fever caused by NSAIDs and the possibility of toxicity manifested by abomasal ulceration or renal damage if treatment is excessive in frequency, dosage, or duration. Aspirin may be the safest of the commonly used NSAIDs in cattle and is given at 240 to 480 grains orally twice daily for an adult animal, but flunixin meglumine at 0.5 to 1.0 mg/kg IV once daily may be the most effective. Aspirin and flunixin meglumine have caused abomasal ulceration when administered for a prolonged time to sick cattle, especially if the animal remains inappetent and has diminished water intake for the duration of treatment. Renal toxicity also is a risk, especially in a dehydrated animal in which the cytoprotective and vascular effects of prostaglandins are essential during reduced renal perfusion. We prefer flunixin when NSAID therapy is selected, but these drugs are adjuncts, not essentials, for the treatment of bronchopneumonia caused by *P. multocida*.

Bronchodilators such as aminophylline have been used in cattle with pneumonia but do not appear to be beneficial clinically except when given by constant infusion (CRI) to calves with respiratory distress. Aminophylline at 5 mg/kg IV over 60 minutes repeated twice daily or 10 mg/kg as a 24-hour CRI can be of considerable benefit in the treatment of severely dyspneic calves with bronchopneumonia. Occasionally, we have used higher doses than this but they can be associated with excitement and agitation, which are obviously undesirable, so it may be helpful to start at this dose and incrementally increase according to tolerance and a demonstrated need by virtue of insufficient clinical response or unimproved blood gases. Aminophylline is well absorbed when given orally to cattle, but we have not had a consistent clinical response when it is given by this route. Atropine given parenterally or ipratropium by inhalation may also be effective bronchodilators. If albuterol could be used in cattle, it might be beneficial because this drug has been shown in other species to act not only as a bronchodilator but also to improve mucociliary clearance. Parasympatholytic

bronchodilators have been shown to be more effective in calves than sympathomimetic drugs.

Antihistamines are used as adjunctive therapy in bovine bronchopneumonia by many practitioners. Drugs such as tripelennamine hydrochloride (1 mg/kg IM or SC twice or thrice daily) are believed to improve the animal's attitude and appetite. These symptomatic observations may be valid, but because histamine has not been shown to be one of the major inflammatory mediators in *Pasteurella* pneumonia, no scientific evidence exists to justify the use of these drugs.

The recognition and correction of management problems or ventilation deficiencies may be as important, if not more so, than any of the previous pharmaceuticals when treating endemic *P. multocida* pneumonia. Because the organism primarily is an opportunist that gains access to the lower airway after insults to the physical, cellular, or secretory defense mechanisms, predisposing causes should be sought and corrected. In calves, poor ventilation, crowding, and poor husbandry relating to excessive ammonia fumes may be sufficient to allow *P. multocida* to descend from its normal habitat of the upper airway and colonize the lungs. Examples include changeable temperature and humidity when calves are grouped during the indoor housing season (especially fall, spring, and during winter thaws), broken fans, failure to clean large pens when calves have been in groups for weeks to months, lungworms, and drafts that the confined calves cannot escape. Fresh air is vital to recovery and should be provided even if it means allowing the animals access to outside air in inclement weather.

In adult cattle, all of these factors apply, but ventilation deficiencies predominate. In modern free-stall facilities, transition cow management practices that add greater stress to an already changeable and stressful period appear to greatly impact the acquisition of acute pneumonia and progression to chronic disease. Frequent pen moves, overstocking, poor ventilation, and concurrent metabolic disease alongside some of the treatments and therapeutic practices used by producers all substantially increase the chances for postpartum respiratory disease to become a herd problem. Bronchopneumonia caused by *P. multocida* alone usually is a management problem. Although it certainly is recognized that previous viral infection or mixed infections (e.g., *Mycoplasma* spp.) can and do predispose to *P. multocida* pneumonia in calves and adult cattle, it must be emphasized that management factors are very important. Secondary *P. multocida* pneumonia, such as that following viral respiratory infection, will be discussed in conjunction with viral diseases. Failure of cattle affected with *P. multocida* pneumonia to respond to appropriate antibiotic therapy based on culture and susceptibility results should alert the veterinarian to the fact that; (1) *P. multocida* is not the only agent involved in the epidemic (i.e., a virus or *Mycoplasma* spp. also may be present or was present, so viral isolation, PCR, paired serology, and so forth are indicated), (2) the predisposing management or ventilation problems have not been corrected, and (3) lungworms should be ruled out.

Vaccination involving *P. multocida* is discussed later in the prevention section within this chapter.

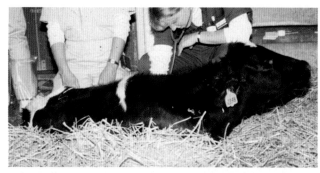

• **Fig. 4.41** A 4-month-old heifer with *Histophilus somni* pneumonia. This heifer was one of several group-housed heifers of similar age with an acute onset fever, cough, and labored breathing. *H. somni* was the only pathogen identified on a tracheal wash sample. All of the heifers had clinical recovery after ceftiofur treatment. Clinical findings would be indistinguishable from those of *Pasteurella multocida* or mild *Mannheimia haemolytica* infection.

Histophilus somni

Etiology and Signs

H. somni has been identified as a pathogen of the lower airway in dairy cattle with increasing frequency. It is occasionally identified as the cause of herd outbreaks of pneumonia in dairy cattle or calves in the northern United States. *H. somni* may be the only pathogen isolated or may be found in conjunction with *Mycoplasma* spp. or *Pasteurella multocida* in diagnostic samples. Although *H. somni* occasionally is isolated from the upper airway of normal cattle as a commensal, this gram-negative organism can occasionally be isolated from the lungs or tracheal wash fluid of clinical pneumonia patients too. A shift in the normal upper airway bacterial flora, stress activation of latent *H. somni* in the upper airway, and factors that negatively impact upper and lower airway defense mechanisms may all contribute to lower airway infection.

The pathogenicity of both *H. somni* and *Mannheimia haemolytica* can be attributed to several shared characteristics: (1) An endotoxin derived from the cell wall lipopolysaccharides; (2) Exotoxins that are lethal or damaging to alveolar macrophages, neutrophils, and vascular endothelium; and (3) Chemotactic factors and possible hemolysins common to *H. somni* and other bacteria that act as inflammatory mediators. Vasculitis is a predominant feature of *H. somni* pathology. *H. somni*–stimulated platelets have been shown to contribute to endothelial cell damage, which may play a role in the pathogenesis of the vasculitis and thrombosis. In addition, *H. somni* has a propensity to cause disease in the heart muscle and sometimes the central nervous system. Involvement of the latter two organ systems appears to be considerably more common in beef cattle than in dairy.

The signs of *H. somni* bronchopneumonia in calves (Fig. 4.41) and adult cattle are indistinguishable from moderate to severe *P. multocida* pneumonia or mild to moderate *M. haemolytica* pneumonia. Affected animals have fever (103.5° to 106.6°F [39.72° to 41.44°C]), an increased respiratory rate (40–80 breaths/min), depression, nasal discharge, occasional hypersalivation, painful cough, and decreased milk production proportional to the degree of anorexia observed.

Dyspnea may be marked in some cases, and these cattle will show anxiety and reluctance to move. Neurologic signs or septicemia caused by *H. somni*, as observed in feedlot animals, is less common in dairy cattle and calves. One reason for this may be that most pneumonia in dairy calves occurs within the first 3 months of life and the neurologic form of *H. somni* only affects cattle older than 4 months of age. If, however, any cattle develop neurologic signs during an outbreak of bronchopneumonia in a herd or group of calves, *H. somni* should be strongly suspected as the cause of the illness.

Auscultation of the lungs typically identifies bilateral anterior ventral pneumonia characterized by moist and dry rales, and bronchial tones indicative of ventral consolidation can be found in up to 50% of cases. Tracheal rales may be auscultated as a result of the heavy mucopurulent exudate found in the trachea. Palpation of the intercostal spaces (ICSs) overlying the pneumonic regions may be painful to the animal.

Diagnosis

Because the signs usually are similar to those of *Pasteurella* and *Mannheimia* pneumonia, the veterinarian should collect appropriate samples (tracheal washes for bacterial culture and antimicrobial sensitivities, or necropsy cultures from lung and lymph nodes) and institute therapy. A failure of response to standard broad-spectrum antibacterial therapy typifies *H. somni* pneumonia. Usually an exact diagnosis as to etiology has to await culture and sensitivity results from diagnostic samples. CBCs are variable and nonspecific, with either a degenerative or regenerative left shift observed and elevated fibrinogen levels. Acute and convalescent serum may be helpful retrospectively if the diagnostic laboratory used for testing has the capability to establish *H. somni* titers.

Postmortem specimens will show firm anteroventral areas of pneumonia bilaterally. Fibrin may be apparent in the visceral and parietal pleura overlying the areas of pneumonia. In some cases, red blotches or hemorrhage are apparent. White microabscesses may be observed also.

Treatment

Although *H. somni* apparently is sensitive in vitro to many antibiotics, including penicillin, clinical results in vivo have been discouraging. Ampicillin and ceftiofur have been commonly used for *H. somni* pneumonia in calves and adult cattle. Ampicillin is used at 11 to 22 mg/kg twice daily by injection for 3 to 7 days in most cases. Just as with *P. multocida*, the increasing likelihood of *Mycoplasma bovis*, or other *Mycoplasma* spp. being involved in undifferentiated BRD and the lack of β-lactam efficacy against this group of organisms may mean that veterinarians preferably select a different first choice antibiotic, such as a macrolide, enrofloxacin, or florfenicol, depending on signalment. Enrofloxacin reportedly has good efficacy against *Histophilus* spp. but currently is not approved for use in lactating dairy cattle in the United States; however, it can be used in calves less than 20 months of age. There are no reports of arthropathy in young calves treated with enrofloxacin. In a recent *H. somni* experimental inoculation metaphylactic study, tildipirosin was superior to tulathromycin.

Response to effective antibiotics will be manifested by a progressive decrease in body temperature to the normal range over 24 to 72 hours. For this reason, the treating veterinarian may find it best not to use NSAIDs or corticosteroids in patients with *H. somni* pneumonia because these drugs decrease the temperature artificially through antipyretic effects and interfere with interpretation of appropriate antibiotic selection.

Just as in *Pasteurella* bronchopneumonia, ventilation or management factors that predispose to altered lower airway defense mechanisms should be corrected immediately. The prognosis is fair to good unless severe pneumonia and marked dyspnea are present.

Trueperella pyogenes: Chronic Suppurative Pneumonia

Etiology and Signs

T. pyogenes is a gram-positive coccobacillus that acts as a ubiquitous opportunist capable of establishing chronic pyogenic infections virtually anywhere in the bovine body. In the lung, it is a secondary invader that usually only establishes infection after suppression of host physical, cellular, or secretory defense mechanisms or as an opportunist that colonizes areas of necrosis such as can occur in the lung after infection with any one of several other infectious agents. Physical factors such as inhalation pneumonia also may allow *T. pyogenes* to infect the lung, and viral, bacterial, or *Mycoplasma* agents may precede infection with *T. pyogenes*. Immunosuppression caused by acute or persistent infection with BVDV has been followed by *T. pyogenes* pneumonia in calves and adult cows. Similarly, calves affected with bovine leukocyte adhesion deficiency (BLAD) frequently have *T. pyogenes* pneumonia. Pulmonary infection is aided by the proteases and hemolysins that the organism produces. These factors contribute to tissue necrosis and inflammatory events that perpetuate the organism's existence. *Fusobacterium* and other pathogenic anaerobic organisms may also be found concurrently with *T. pyogenes*, *P. multocida*, and *Mycoplasma* spp.

Signs are indicative of chronic or recurrent infection, the hallmark of *T. pyogenes* pneumonia. The history usually indicates illness of at least 1 week's duration or recurrent episodes of pneumonia over weeks to months. There may only be one (usually adult cattle) or a few animals (usually calves) affected out of a group or herd. In adult dairy cattle, it seems particularly common for clinical signs to develop after freshening (Fig. 4.42). In some cases, there may be severe SC emphysema over the dorsum, suggesting a rupture of diseased alveoli associated with calving as a cause of pneumomediastinum, SC emphysema, and sometimes pneumothorax. Although chronic suppurative pneumonia should be considered in cattle with dorsal emphysema after calving, similar emphysema may be found sometimes in apparently healthy cattle after calving and, of course, in cattle with interstitial pneumonia. Bullous emphysema and pneumothorax are most commonly associated with BRSV infection of both adults and calves in the United States, but severe, chronic bronchopneumonia with involvement of *T. pyogenes* and extensive ventral consolidation is another common cause of these signs in adults. Affected animals may

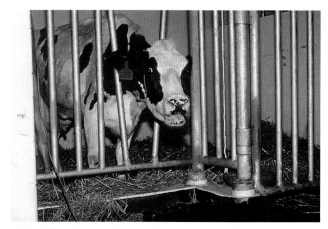

• **Fig. 4.42** A 5-year-old cow with cough and respiratory distress after calving 5 days earlier. The cow had chronic suppurative pneumonia with an acute onset of respiratory signs associated with the stress of calving.

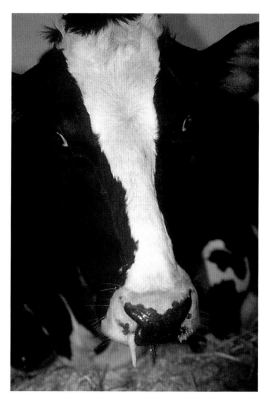

• **Fig. 4.43** This mature Holstein cow presented to the hospital for poor production and weight loss. Although the respiratory rate was within normal limits, the cow coughed after rising; had slight head and neck extension when lying down; and, as seen in this photo, had small and intermittent purulent nasal discharge. *Pasteurella multocida*, *Trueperella pyogenes*, and *Mycoplasma* spp. were cultured from a tracheal wash. The cow improved dramatically after tetracycline therapy.

show low-grade fever (103.0° to 105.0°F [39.44° to 40.56°C]), rapid respiratory rate (40–100 breaths/min), dyspnea characterized by exaggerated inspiratory and especially expiratory efforts (particularly when stressed), head and neck extension when lying down, cough, nasal discharge (Fig. 4.43), rough hair coat, poor body condition (Fig. 4.44), depression, inappetence, or decreased milk production. Some cattle maintain normal respiratory rates but exhibit the other signs. Chronic

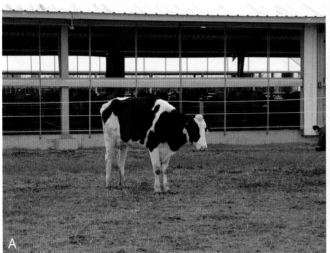
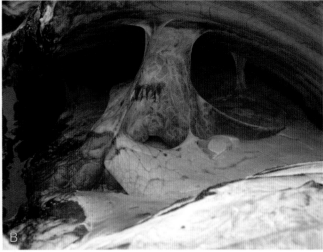

• **Fig. 4.44** **A,** Poor hair coat, hunched back, and ill-thriven appearance of a 3-year old Holstein cow with chronic suppurative pneumonia. **B,** Postmortem image of the thoracic cavity from the same animal showing marked consolidation ventrally (left side of the image) and adhesions to the chest wall.

suppurative pneumonia should always be considered a differential for the "poor doing" cow.

Auscultation of the lungs reveals moist and dry rales in the ventral 25% to 50% of both lungs in calves and one or both lungs in adult cattle, bronchial tones indicative of consolidation in the ventral lung fields, and coarse tracheal rales caused by a thick mucopurulent airway exudate. High environmental temperatures, high humidity, and poor ventilation exacerbate the clinical signs. A fetid smell may be present after a cough if anaerobic bacteria are present. Auscultation during rebreathing, paying close attention to the cranioventral lung fields under the triceps musculature for the presence of bronchial tones indicative of consolidation, is important when investigating possible cases of mild to moderate chronic suppurative bronchopneumonia.

Diagnosis

History and physical signs are very suggestive of *T. pyogenes* pneumonia, but specific diagnosis requires culture of the organism from tracheal wash samples or lung tissue. There may only be one or a few animals affected with signs of chronic pneumonia after a preceding herd endemic of pneumonia caused by other organisms. Chronic or recurrent cases are referred to as "lungers" by some farmers.

Radiography or ultrasonography of the thorax is helpful in establishing a prognosis because lung abscesses, bronchiectasis, and consolidation (sometimes remarkably severe in a single lobe) (Fig. 4.45) are common in the affected lung (see Video Clip 4.8). Because of its diagnostic utility in identifying consolidation and peripheral abscessation, thoracic ultrasonography can be of great value in the diagnosis of these lesions (see Video Clip 4.10). Attention should be directed toward the ventral and cranial ICSs of both hemithoraces.

A CBC may show neutrophilia or be normal. Serum globulin often is in the high range of normal or elevated (>5.0 g/dL), especially in adult cattle. The animal should be screened for persistent infection with BVDV via buffy coat viral isolation

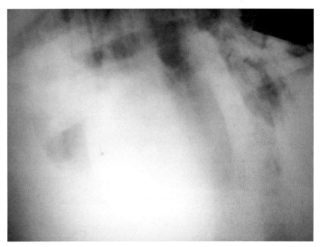

• **Fig. 4.45** Radiograph of a cow with chronic suppurative pneumonia and a dramatic lobar consolidation.

or whole blood PCR particularly if only a single cow or calf in the herd is diseased. Gross necropsy of fatal cases reveals anterior ventral consolidation with areas of purulent bronchiectasis and multiple pulmonary abscesses (Figs. 4.46 and 4.47).

Treatment

Treatment is frustrating, and the prognosis is poor for patients with pneumonia caused by *T. pyogenes.* Other causative organisms such as *P. multocida, M. haemolytica, Mycoplasma* spp., or *Fusobacterium* also may be cultured from the tracheal wash sample. Specific to the involvement of *T. pyogenes,* penicillin is the drug of choice and should be given at 22,000 U/kg twice daily for 7 to 30 days. Although penicillin is effective against *T. pyogenes* in vitro, the in vivo pulmonary infection should be likened to an abscess because of the heavy accumulation of *T. pyogenes* pus in areas of bronchiectasis or encapsulated lung abscesses. If another pathogen, in addition to *T. pyogenes*, is isolated from the tracheal wash sample, appropriate antibiotic therapy should be selected for this organism as well.

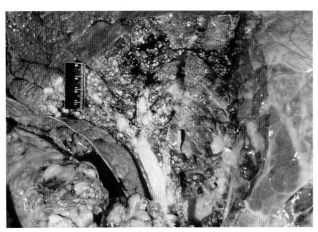

• **Fig. 4.46** Necropsy view of cut section from the cranioventral lung region of a calf showing bronchiectasis and pulmonary abscesses typical of chronic *Trueperella pyogenes* pneumonia.

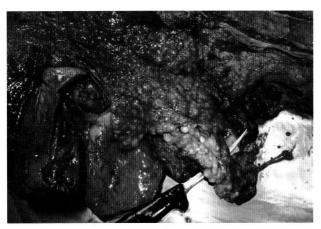

• **Fig. 4.47** Severe, chronic suppurative pneumonia with multiple, nodular *Trueperella pyogenes* abscesses throughout the right ventral lung from a mature Holstein cow with a history of chronic cough, recurrent fever and weight loss.

Ceftiofur, ampicillin, and tetracyclines are other commonly used therapies. Clinical treatment frequently results in short-term improvement followed by relapse, sometimes as distant as 1 year later, when the animal is stressed or subjected to high environmental temperatures, humidity, or poor ventilation. Signs of improvement will be indicated by a consistently normal rectal temperature, improved respiratory function, and improvement in overall body condition and attitude. Many affected animals eventually succumb to the infection or are culled because of poor condition and production.

Mycoplasma Pneumonia

Etiology and Signs

Several species of *Mycoplasma*, including *Mycoplasma dispar*, *M. bovis, Mycoplasma bovirhinis,* and others, have been isolated from the lungs of calves and cattle with pneumonia. In addition, *Ureaplasma* organisms and occasional isolates of *Mycoplasma bovigenitalium* have been found from lower airway infections in cattle. *M. dispar* and *M. bovis* probably are the two major types identified. These organisms may be normal inhabitants of the upper airway in some cattle. Experimentally,

Mycoplasma spp. have caused pneumonia in calves when introduced either into the lower airway or via nasal inoculation. This pneumonia is characterized by peribronchiolar and peribronchial lymphoid hyperplasia and purulent bronchiolitis. Lesions usually are limited to the anterior ventral tips of the lung lobes, and the associated clinical signs are mild. Gross inspection at necropsy reveals ventral areas of lung lobes that are red-blue and firm, appearing almost as atelectatic areas, and that ooze purulent material from the airways on cut sections. *Mycoplasma* pneumonia has been described as a "cuffing pneumonia" because lymphoid hyperplasia appears around the airways and expands with chronicity. *Mycoplasma* organisms have several properties that contribute to their pathogenicity, including inhibition of the mucociliary transport mechanism (at least in humans). In addition, they cause some degree of humoral and cell-mediated immunosuppression in calves and they avoid phagocytosis by attaching to ciliated epithelium above the level of alveolar macrophages.

In our clinics, *Mycoplasma* frequently is isolated from acute and chronic calf pneumonia outbreaks and may be involved in up to 50% of chronic calf pneumonia endemics that we investigate. However, *Mycoplasma* spp. seldom is the only pathogen isolated in these outbreaks, and one or more of *H. somni, P. multocida,* and *M. haemolytica* usually are isolated as well. Because *Mycoplasma* appears ubiquitous on many farms, we wonder whether the *Mycoplasma* infection has been present in the calves' lungs for a long time and contributes to impaired host defense against bacterial and viral pathogens or whether the *Mycoplasma* infection is acute along with the other pathogens. It is also increasingly co-identified with *T. pyogenes* in cases of chronic suppurative bronchopneumonia. In herds with active *Mycoplasma* pneumonia, *Mycoplasma* frequently can be isolated via nasopharyngeal swab from the majority of cows and calves, most of which appear healthy. Therefore the ubiquitous nature of the organism makes it nearly impossible for calves on these farms not to become infected. The subsequent low-grade pneumonia and defense mechanism compromise caused by the *Mycoplasma* infection may precede the onset of clinical pneumonia associated with other bacterial and viral pathogens. How significant *Mycoplasma* spp. is to the entire problem is difficult to determine, but we believe it increases the risk of calfhood pneumonia. In addition to pneumonia, *M. bovis* may also cause otitis media, mastitis, and arthritis once it becomes established in a herd. The spread of *Mycoplasma* spp. can be significantly increased by the feeding of unpasteurized, infected waste milk. Effective control measures for *Mycoplasma* when it is ubiquitous on a premise are challenging and made more so because effective vaccines are not available. In endemic herds, the feeding of unpasteurized waste milk is a known risk factor for transmission of the organism to calves, and this practice should be actively discouraged. Pasteurization removes the risk of *Mycoplasma* spread by this means but only makes economic sense on larger dairies or heifer-rearing operations. When pasteurization is used, periodic quality control assessments by culture are very important to confirm continued equipment efficacy at removing viable *Mycoplasma* spp. from the milk being fed to the calves. Producers should never assume

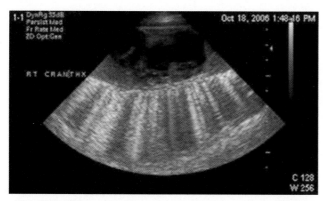

• **Fig. 4.48** Ultrasound findings in the cranial thorax of a 4-month-old Holstein calf with a 2-week history of pneumonic signs and lameness of the left rear leg and marked swelling of the left rear stifle. The calf was euthanized because of a poor prognosis, and *Mycoplasma* spp. were cultured from the pleural fluid (seen above on ultrasonography) and the stifle joint.

that these pieces of equipment remain effective over long periods without checking.

Signs of pure *Mycoplasma* pneumonia may be very mild. In several calf and heifer outbreaks of pure *Mycoplasma* pneumonia, the only signs observed were coughing induced by stress or movement of the animals, a slight increase in the respiratory rate (40–60 breaths/min), and low-grade fever (103.5° to 105.0°F [39.72° to 40.56°C]). Most affected animals continued to eat and experienced only mild depression. Owners reported observing a slight mucopurulent nasal discharge in the animals in the mornings that disappeared after the animals became active, ate, and licked their noses clean. Tracheal washes grew pure cultures of *Mycoplasma*, and no other pathogens were identified by bacterial cultures, viral isolation, PCR, or retrospective paired serology. However, pure *Mycoplasma* is the exception rather than the rule because, in our clinics, *Mycoplasma* usually is isolated in conjunction with other pathogens in the majority of pneumonia outbreaks in which it is involved. Signs of pneumonia in these instances are identical to those described for the other specific bacterial or viral agents isolated. The *Mycoplasma* component does not have any unique clinical features except for its association with otitis media and arthritis in young cattle and perhaps that affected animals sometimes respond poorly to specific antibiotic therapy directed against the bacterial pathogen, especially when the selected antimicrobials have poor efficacy against *Mycoplasma* organisms. When this occurs, a contributory viral or *Mycoplasma* infection should always be suspected. Undoubtedly the association between *Mycoplasma* infection of the lower airways and involvement of this organism with otitis cases in heifer replacement calves preweaning is an increasingly strong one on many farms. It is currently much more common to see comorbid pneumonia and otitis than it is to see the arthritic form in this age of calf. The arthritic form seems to be more common in older, weaned heifers and bulls but can also coexist with the pneumonic form (Fig. 4.48).

Diagnosis

This is totally dependent on demonstration of the organism in diagnostic airway fluid or necropsy samples. The diagnostic emphasis in many laboratories has switched from culture of the organism to identification by PCR. Typically, the primers used are specific to *M. bovis,* but increasingly diagnostic laboratories use additional primer sets for non–*M. bovis* species, too. In pure *Mycoplasma* pneumonia, fatalities are rare, but typical gross lesions of *Mycoplasma* pneumonia appear as red-blue firm areas in the anterior ventral lung. These areas resemble atelectatic areas but are firm, and pus may be expressed from the airways within these firm areas on a cut section. Histopathology demonstrates the "cuffing pneumonia" previously described.

In most instances in which *Mycoplasma* is merely one component of infection, gross necropsy lesions are typical of the other pathogens—usually anterior ventral consolidating bronchopneumonia typical of *Mannheimia, Pasteurella,* or *Histophilus* infection or abscessation caused by *T. pyogenes.* Occasionally, *Mycoplasma* is obtained from lungs showing typical lesions of BRSV, BVDV, or other viral infections.

Treatment

Treatment for *Mycoplasma* pneumonia may be unnecessary in some pure *Mycoplasma* infections because the cattle do not appear extremely ill. In pure infections, oxytetracycline hydrochloride (11 mg/kg once or twice daily) was historically the "go to" antimicrobial, but there is increasing concern over resistance and a lack of clinical response with this antibiotic. Subsequently, other antimicrobial choices such as tulathromycin (2.5 mg/kg SC), florfenicol (20 mg/kg IM in the neck), erythromycin (5.5 mg/kg twice daily), and tilmicosin (10 mg/kg SC) or other macrolides may provide effective therapy in many cases. Enrofloxacin or other fluoroquinolones are reported to be the most effective antibiotic against *Mycoplasma,* but these are not approved for use in lactating dairy cattle in the United States. In vitro antimicrobial testing for *Mycoplasma* spp. is rarely performed or available. As a consequence, antibiotic selection is empiric but should be done mindful of the fact the β-lactams will not work.

When *Mycoplasma* is isolated along with *P. multocida, M. haemolytica, T. pyogenes, Fusobacterium* spp., or *H. somni,* antibacterial therapy should also address the other bacterial pathogens. If the *Pasteurella* or *Histophilus* isolate is sensitive to tetracycline or erythromycin, choosing one of these drugs may provide efficacy against both the bacteria and *Mycoplasma.* Fortunately, if treatment is directed against the bacterial pathogens and ventilation or management factors are corrected, the calves often recover and the *Mycoplasma* infection may not require specific therapy.

At our clinic, we have investigated several chronic heifer and postweaning calf pneumonia problems in which *Mycoplasma* and *P. multocida* or *Mycoplasma* and *H. somni* have coexisted. These problems have been very difficult to solve. In these herds, the *Mycoplasma* infection seems to be ubiquitous and seems to infect calves very early in life. Calf hutches and individual rearing of calves may not be effective in preventing *Mycoplasma* infection in some of these herds, but calf hutches do seem to prevent bacterial infection in the calves pre-weaning. Therefore, as soon as the calves are grouped after weaning, a pneumonia outbreak is caused by both bacterial and *Mycoplasma* components. Every new group seems to be affected, and attempts at prevention appear futile. Isolation of calves to a separate farm after immediate removal from their dams may be the only solution. Other recommendations for prevention of *Mycoplasma* infection in calves include avoiding feeding *M. bovis*–infected milk, using separate feed buckets and bottles for every calf, housing with good ventilation, and preventing calves from direct contact with other cattle.

Bibersteinia trehalosi

In recent years, there has been increased attention given to this organism worldwide, more particularly for its role as a pathogen of small ruminants, especially sheep. Taxonomic reclassification of the organism from its previous allocation as a *Pasteurella* organism within the past decade has been followed by increased reports of the organism being cultured from diagnostic specimens obtained either ante- or postmortem from cases of BRD in dairy calves and adults in the United States. At the current point in time, its role as a primary pathogen is uncertain. Although it can undoubtedly be obtained from the lungs and lower airways of diseased dairy cattle, attempts to reproduce clinical respiratory disease experimentally via direct inoculation have usually been unsuccessful. Whether it can predictably behave as an opportunistic infectious agent of the lower airway, in a manner comparable to *P. multocida*, and clarification of its role in BRD, await further research.

Viral Diseases of the Respiratory Tract

Infectious Bovine Rhinotracheitis

Etiology and Signs

Infectious bovine rhinotracheitis (also known as IBR, BHV1, or "red nose") is an infection of the upper airway and trachea caused by BHV1. Infection may assume many forms in cattle, including respiratory, conjunctival, or infectious pustular vulvovaginitis affecting the caudal reproductive tract; infectious balanoposthitis of the male external genitalia; endemic abortions; and the neonatal septicemic form characterized by encephalitis and focal plaque necrosis of the tongue. Bovine herpesvirus 5 (BoHV5) may also cause outbreaks of encephalitis in young stock. The respiratory form of BHV1 is the most common and may occur alone or coupled with the conjunctival form. DNA variants of BHV1 initially described correlated to specific system disease, but recent genomic mapping has found no basis for these divisions. Abortions may occur in association with any of the forms of the disease, either during the acute disease or in the ensuing weeks after an outbreak. Each infected herd seems to have one predominant clinical form of the disease, but occasional animals may also show signs of other forms during an endemic. Recent work suggests that genetic factors may play a role in the relative resistance of cattle to IBR virus and that this resistance may be mediated by type 1 interferon genotypes.

Similar to many other herpes viruses, BHV-1 virus is capable of recrudescence when previously infected cattle harboring latent virus infection are stressed by infectious diseases, shipment, or corticosteroids. Immunity from natural infection or vaccination is short lived and probably does not

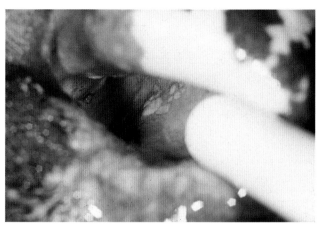

• **Fig. 4.49** Classical infectious bovine rhinotracheitis plaques on the mucosa overlying the nasal septum of a Holstein cow. The view is through the right nares, and a penlight is present in the right lower corner of the image.

exceed 6 to 12 months. Respiratory disease caused purely by IBR is associated with high morbidity but low mortality in susceptible animals. Fatalities seldom result from primary or recurrent IBR infections unless secondary bacterial bronchopneumonia, especially *M. haemolytica*, or concurrent viral infection with BVDV or BRSV occurs. (These viruses are discussed further in this section.) The IBR virus compromises the physical and cellular components of the lower airway defense mechanism by damaging mucociliary transport and the mucus layer and directly infecting alveolar macrophages. Therefore combination infections may result in high mortality rates because of multiple agents compromising lower airway host defense mechanisms and possible immunosuppression, especially with concurrent BVDV infection. As stated previously, BHV1 infection upregulates genes that activate receptors for the leukotoxin of *M. haemolytica* and contribute to the severity of that disease.

Because most dairy cattle and calves currently are vaccinated for IBR, owners and veterinarians sometimes overlook or fail to consider the possibility of IBR infection during acute respiratory outbreaks or herd abortions. However, the confusing array of bovine vaccines available to laypeople, use of outdated or mishandled vaccines, and inadvertent failure to vaccinate individual groups or herds of cattle still predispose to occasional acute outbreaks of IBR.

The clinical signs of the IBR-respiratory form include a high fever of 105.0° to 108.0°F (40.56° to 42.22°C); depression; anorexia; rapid respiration (40–80 breaths/min); heavy serous nasal discharge that becomes a thick mucopurulent discharge during the first 72 hours of infection; a painful cough; a dried necrotic crusting of the muzzle; white plaques visible on the nasal mucosa, mucosa of the nasal septum (Fig. 4.49), and sometimes on the external nares and muzzle (Fig. 4.50); occasional mucosal ulceration of the muzzle and oral mucosa; coarse tracheal rales caused by mucopurulent exudate or diphtheritic membranes in the larynx and trachea; and referred sounds and rales from the upper airway heard over both lung fields (especially in the area of the major bronchi). This fulminant form of clinical IBR has fortunately become quite uncommon in dairy cattle, as vaccine technology and

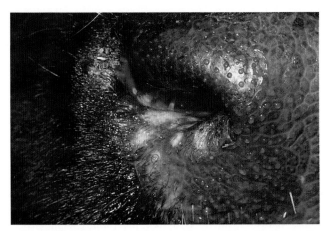

• **Fig. 4.50** Plaques from infectious bovine rhinotracheitis on the mucosa and mucocutaneous junction of the right nares region in a Holstein cow.

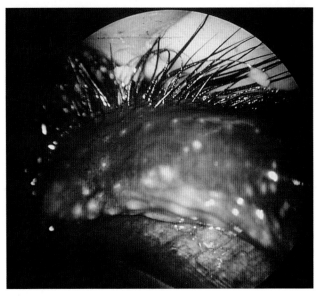

• **Fig. 4.51** Multifocal white plaques on the palpebral conjunctiva of a Holstein cow affected with the conjunctival form of infectious bovine rhinotracheitis.

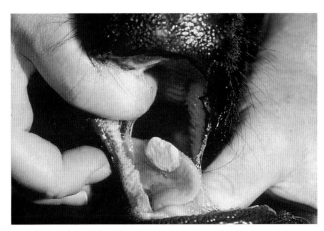

• **Fig. 4.52** White plaque on the tongue of a neonatal calf infected with infectious bovine rhinotracheitis.

widespread and effective vaccination programs have combined to reduce cases of natural disease. Although bronchitis and bronchiolitis occasionally have been observed, most cases do not have pulmonary pathology unless secondary bacterial bronchopneumonia occurs. Bacterial bronchopneumonia usually occurs within 7 to 10 days after acute IBR infection when bacteria complicate the viral illness. Devastating mortality rates may occur in stressed, recently transported or purchased animals that develop IBR infection concurrent with BVDV infection, BRSV infection, or virulent strains of *M. haemolytica* bronchopneumonia. In outbreaks in adult herds, the disease seems to cause the most severe signs in first-calf heifers and may severely affect their future milk production during the remainder of the first lactation.

Affected animals show signs for 7 to 14 days and recover after this time unless secondary infection occurs. Abortions may occur during the acute infection or in the subsequent 4 to 8 weeks. Although fetal death can occur at any stage of gestation, most abortions occur in cows in the second or third trimester of pregnancy. Direct fetal infection or stress and high fever may contribute to the reproductive losses. The conjunctival form sometimes coexists with the respiratory form and is characterized by unilateral or bilateral severely inflamed conjunctivae and serous ocular discharge that becomes mucopurulent within 2 to 4 days. In addition, multifocal white plaques composed of lymphocytes and plasma cells appear grossly on the palpebral conjunctiva (Fig. 4.51). Some cattle also have corneal edema in the peripheral cornea, but ulcerations do not occur (also see Chapter 14). BHV1 has a similar synergistic (increased pathogenicity) role with *Moraxella bovis* in the eye as with *M. haemolytica* in the lung. Calves with the encephalitic form of IBR may demonstrate necrotic plaques on the ventral surface of the tongue or proximal GI tract at necropsy (Fig. 4.52).

Diagnosis

Usually the diagnosis of IBR is based on physical examination when characteristic signs and pathognomonic nasal mucosal plaques are present. Laboratory confirmation is possible by FA techniques during the acute stage (lesions <7 days are best). Scrapings of mucosal lesions and the white plaques in the nasal mucosa should be positive in almost all acute cases. In addition, viral isolation is possible during this time. Undoubtedly, the emphasis for diagnosis in most commercial and state veterinary diagnostic laboratories now rests with PCR, as indeed it does for the majority of viral infections of economic significance in cattle. Amplification of viral DNA using highly specific and sensitive primers for BHV1 can be performed on airway fluid samples, nasopharyngeal swabs, and fresh tissue. This greatly facilitates the accurate and timely diagnosis of BHV1 infection. However, there is one note of caution regarding PCR tests for the diagnosis of BHV1 in that one must obtain an accurate vaccine history when submitting samples or interpreting test results. It is evident (Dr. Keith Poulsen, Wisconsin State Diagnostic Laboratory, personal communication) that recent modified live virus administration can give a false-positive PCR result because of vaccinal virus, on some occasions for up to 14 days after administration. Additional testing using sequencing would be necessary for distinguishing vaccine from field strains. Positive PCR results after IBR vaccination appear to be a more pronounced phenomenon with intranasal products compared with parenterally administered vaccines. We have performed PCR diagnostics on a number of respiratory disease cases when it was only on later questioning that the recent vaccination event was discovered; frequently, vaccination was performed in the face of clinical disease in a sick patient, possibly serving to prolong shedding. Unfortunately, with BHV1, there is also the possibility of latent viral recrudescence from nervous tissue in a sick animal whose primary disease has suppressed its immune system. Individual sick cows with septic mastitis, septic metritis, bacterial pneumonia, and so forth may show typical IBR plaques as a result of recrudescence of latent virus of natural or live vaccine origin during their illness. A diagnosis of primary IBR should not be made in these cattle. Although the plaque represents the only manifestation of BHV1 disease seen in such immunocompromised animals, importantly, they may be a contagious risk for in-contact and naive animals. There are consequently a number of factors to consider when interpreting the significance of a positive PCR result for BHV1, especially in an animal with only limited clinical signs. Paired serum (acute and then convalescent, 14–21 days later) samples provide another means of positive diagnosis.

Necropsy of fatal IBR cases will show diffuse inflammation, necrosis, ulceration, and diphtheritic membranes throughout the nasal passages, larynx, and trachea (Fig. 4.53). Characteristic white plaques will be visible in the inflamed nasal mucosa and sometimes in other areas of the nasopharynx or trachea. Oral mucosal ulceration sometimes occurs. Secondary bacterial bronchopneumonia or superimposed viral infections may mask some IBR lesions.

Bovine Respiratory Syncytial Virus

Etiology and Signs

Bovine respiratory syncytial virus has become one of the most important respiratory pathogens in dairy calves and adult cattle in the past 25 years. The virus certainly may

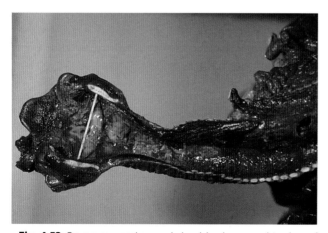

• **Fig. 4.53** Severe mucosal necrosis involving larynx and trachea of a cow that died from infectious bovine rhinotracheitis (IBR). Although fatal cases of pure IBR are rare, the pathology presented highlights the damage to the physical defense mechanisms of the lower airway that predisposes to secondary bacterial pneumonia. (Courtesy of Dr. John M. King.)

have been present for much longer, but new diagnostic procedures, improved technology in virology, and recognition of the virus and its pathophysiology have heightened awareness of this disease. The virus is a pneumovirus within the paramyxovirus family and is distinctly different from the bovine syncytial virus (BSV), which is a spumavirus in the retrovirus family. There is no current evidence that the BSV is a pathogen in cattle. Respiratory disease caused by BRSV was first reported in Europe during the 1970s and has been recognized throughout the United States since the 1980s in endemic form in beef and dairy cattle. Observations from both experimental and natural disease have been reported, and it is now accepted that BRSV was likely the cause of many poorly defined epidemics heretofore diagnosed as "atypical interstitial pneumonia" (AIP) in calves and adult cattle. It also is likely that BRSV infection has preceded, and predisposed cattle to, severe bacterial bronchopneumonia but gone undiagnosed because of overwhelming bacterial lesions.

The virus produces a humoral antibody response, which is helpful both for diagnosis and epidemiologic surveys. Based on surveys completed in several regions of the United States, BRSV infection appears common in cattle because more than 50% of adult cattle surveyed have titers to BRSV. More recent work suggests that up to 70% of calves have now been exposed to BRSV by breeding age. The virus has caused sporadic clinical disease in dairy cattle and calves and probably has gone undiagnosed frequently. Outbreaks of BRSV may be limited to calves, affect only adult cows, or can involve all animals in a herd. Morbidity is high, but mortality as a result of BRSV infection is much lower unless secondary bacterial bronchopneumonia ensues. The virus apparently does not infect alveolar macrophages but may damage physical defense mechanisms of the lower airway, such as mucociliary transport, and may lead to antigen–antibody complexes that subsequently engage complement and result in damage to the lower airway. Although experimental reproduction of the clinical disease has not been consistently successful in challenge studies, recent studies have helped further explain the pathogenesis of the disease. Two- to 6-month-old calves have been successfully infected and have marked production of inflammatory cytokines (tumor necrosis factor, interleukins 6 and 8, and interferon); these are thought to help promote viral clearance but may also have a pathogenic role in causing airway obstruction. Previous work suggests that BRSV alters macrophage function sufficiently to short cycle and depress responsiveness of lymphocytes. In any event, interstitial pneumonia, secondary bacterial pneumonia, airway obstruction, and pneumothorax are very common after BRSV infection. Many unexplained facets of BRSV infection persist despite the proliferation of research on the virus. For example, BRSV infection often arises in herds that appear to have excellent management and have not purchased new cattle, shipped and returned existing cattle, or stressed animals in any apparent way. Where did the infection come from in these herds? Was it latent in a recovered animal, or was it introduced by regular visitors to the farm? Cattle are thought to be the reservoir, but it has not yet been shown how or why the virus activates, replicates, and spreads to cause all clinical epidemics. In closed herds that experience recurrent infections, there appears to be a high degree of sequence variation among BRSV isolates associated with clinical disease, suggesting that BRSV populations may be heterogeneous and relatively diverse, challenging control and prevention even in well-managed herds.

Fortunately, because of increased awareness of BRSV in cattle, bovine practitioners are beginning to suspect the disease based on clinical signs and routinely seek virus identification, histopathologic confirmation of the virus, or serologic confirmation when acute epidemics of respiratory disease occur in cattle.

The signs of acute BRSV range from inapparent to fulminant. In most outbreaks, acute BRSV infection causes high morbidity in the affected group within several days to 1 week. Clinical signs include high fever (104.0° to 108.0°F [40.0° to 42.22°C]); depression, anorexia, decreased milk production, salivation and serous or mucoid nasal

discharge. The degree of dyspnea varies from a merely increased respiratory rate (40–100 breaths/min) to open-mouth breathing. Also, in all but the mildest outbreaks, a percentage of the affected cattle will have SC emphysema palpable under the skin of the dorsum, especially near the withers (Fig. 4.54). Auscultation of the lungs in acute cases may reveal a wide range of sounds. Increased bronchovesicular sounds, bronchial tones, fine crepitation caused by emphysema, and rales (usually as a result of secondary bacterial bronchopneumonia) have been described. Practitioners have found that the lungs may auscultate as diffusely very quiet or almost inaudible in acutely affected cattle in some outbreaks. This has been a very important sign and initially appears in contrast to the outward signs of dyspnea displayed by these cattle. However, the relative deficit of airway sounds fits the existing pathology because pneumothorax or diffuse interstitial pulmonary edema and emphysema compress the small airways and cause the lungs to be quieter than one would expect (Fig. 4.55). This is the same phenomenon that occurs in proliferative pneumonia in which the alveoli and small airways are obliterated or reduced in size. If secondary bacterial pneumonia occurs, bronchial tones or rales are heard in the anterior ventral lung region, and the dorsal and caudal lungs become quieter because of mechanical overwork, increasing the degree of edema and emphysema. Dyspnea is severe in such cases, and affected animals usually show open-mouth breathing and an audible grunt or groan with each expiration (see Video Clip 4.11). This dyspnea is more obvious if affected animals are stressed by handling or being made to move. Despite the high fevers and respiratory distress, affected cattle frequently do not look septic (e.g., severe depression, scleral injection) as with acute overwhelming bacterial pneumonia. There does appear to be some seasonality to outbreaks in the northern United States, with most occurring in the fall or winter.

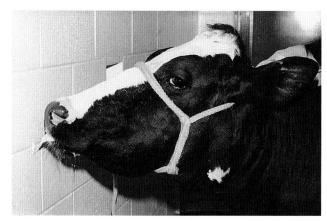

• **Fig. 4.54** A mature cow representative of a herd outbreak with BRSV infection. This cow had respiratory distress and severe subcutaneous emphysema over the chest, back, and face (notice indentation of the halter on the face).

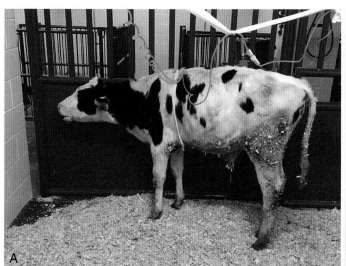

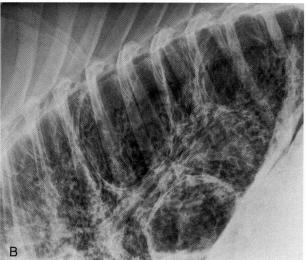

• **Fig. 4.55** A 4-month-old Holstein bull with acute bovine respiratory syncytial virus pneumonia. **A,** Note the open-mouth breathing. **B,** Radiographs of the same bull showing severe diffuse interstitial pneumonia with bullae formation.

A biphasic disease progression may occur in some cattle with BRSV infection. The first stage or phase of the disease is characterized by mild or more serious signs as described earlier. The affected animals apparently improve over the next few days only to develop peracute severe respiratory distress several days to several weeks after their initial improvement. Because these animals initially appeared to have mild disease and responded to treatment, this secondary phase is entirely unexpected. Secondary acute dyspnea is thought to reflect an immune-mediated disease caused by hypersensitivity or a severe T helper 2 response in the lower airway and lung parenchyma and is frequently fatal.

Diagnosis

The signs of BRSV infection in calves or adult cattle may be suggestive of the diagnosis, especially when acute onset, high fever, and SC emphysema are found in several affected animals. These signs are rarely seen in calves younger than 6 weeks, but calves aged 2 to 6 months seem to be most commonly affected. Auscultation of the lungs in acute cases may be helpful if the lungs sound diffusely quiet despite obvious severe dyspnea. The veterinarian must be cautious in diagnosing BRSV based only on the finding of SC emphysema or pneumothorax in some animals. Any severe pneumonia (especially other interstitial pneumonias or severe consolidating bronchopneumonia) can also cause SC emphysema because the only remaining normal lung tissue (dorsal or caudal lung fields) is overworked to the point at which emphysema and interstitial edema are likely. Therefore, SC emphysema may be suggestive of, but not pathognomonic for, BRSV. Thoracic radiographs will commonly reveal findings suggestive of diffuse interstitial pneumonia (Fig. 4.56). As with most of the diseases discussed thus far, laboratory confirmation is the only definitive means to confirm a diagnosis of BRSV. Virus isolation from tracheal wash fluid or necropsy specimens has been used but is often unrewarding because BRSV is quickly cleared, or a rapidly developing secretory antibody neutralizes the virus within the respiratory tract. FA techniques may be used for tracheal wash samples, nasopharyngeal swabs, and necropsy specimens of infected lung. The advent of PCR has made a significant and positive impact on our ability to accurately diagnose BRSV. Both conventional reverse transcription polymerase chain reaction (RT-PCR) assays for the viral genome and real-time RT-PCR for BRSV detection are markedly superior in terms of sensitivity to either immunofluorescence or virus isolation. Diagnostic, multiplex RT-PCR kits that also detect parainfluenza-3 (PI3) and BHV1 are often used but as discussed under the section on BHV1, one has to be careful of false-positive PCR tests when modified live viral vaccines have been recently (<14 days) administered. Serology can be helpful in establishing a diagnosis of BRSV because a marked humoral antibody titer occurs in response to the infection. Baker and Frey emphasize that antibody titers may increase early after acute infection and often peak before 2 weeks postinfection. Therefore, collection of serum on day 1 and day 14 would be important when evaluating seroconversion to BRSV. The same authors state that young calves

may have titers derived from colostrum. These titers, indicative of passive immunity, are only partially protective against BRSV infection but can interfere with vaccinal responses in young calves. Thus, older calves, heifers, or adult animals are better populations to sample.

Gross postmortem findings and necropsy specimens may be very helpful in establishing a diagnosis. This is especially true if death has been acute and secondary bacterial pneumonia has not yet developed to somewhat mask the pulmonary lesions caused by BRSV. Both experimental and natural infection with BRSV produce similar gross lesions consisting of atelectic, consolidated pneumonia with deep red to purple lesions that are "rubbery" on palpation. There is often extensive lobular or lobar consolidation affecting the cranial, middle, and accessory lobes surrounded by lobules of more normal, pink, overinflated lung. The caudodorsal lungs typically fail to collapse and are distended by interlobular, interlobar, and subpleural emphysema and edema (Figs. 4.57 and 4.58). If secondary bacterial bronchopneumonia coexists with BRSV,

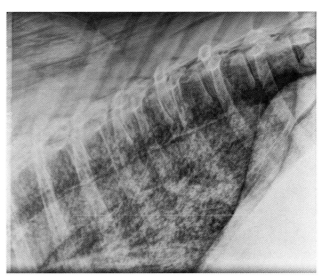

• **Fig. 4.56** Thoracic radiograph of 2-year-old Holstein heifer with diffuse interstitial pneumonia caused by acute bovine respiratory syncytial virus infection.

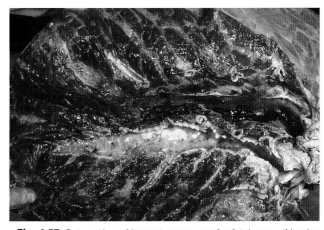

• **Fig. 4.57** Cut section of lung at necropsy of a fatal case of bovine respiratory syncytial virus pneumonia. Interstitial edema and emphysema are apparent. (Courtesy of Dr. John M. King.)

the heavily consolidated anterior ventral lung fields usually are more uniformly dark colored, firm, and fibrin covered (Fig. 4.59). In this instance, typical BRSV lesions of emphysema, edema, and scattered palpably firm areas will still be found in the lung caudal and dorsal to the consolidated areas.

Several times at our clinic, we have obtained *Pasteurella* or *Mannheimia* isolates from tracheal wash specimens that have complicated the course of a BRSV outbreak. Unsurprisingly, cattle in these herd outbreaks failed to respond, or responded unusually slowly, when placed on antibiotics chosen for their specific *Pasteurella* or *Mannheimia* isolate. This poor clinical response can be a signal that another pathogen is contributing to the herd problem.

Treatment

Therapy for acute BRSV infection is symptomatic and supportive. Broad-spectrum antibiotics are indicated to counteract or discourage secondary bacterial bronchopneumonia and should be initiated after collection of diagnostic samples from

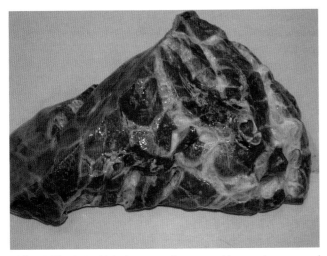

• **Fig. 4.58** Marked lobular separation caused by emphysema and interstitial edema in a cut section of dorsal lung field from a mature bull that had died from acute bovine respiratory syncytial virus infection.

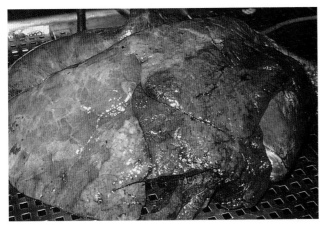

• **Fig. 4.59** Necropsy view of lungs from a fatal case of bovine respiratory syncytial virus combined with secondary *Mannheimia haemolytica*. This combination of pathogens killed 30 of the 55 heifers in the group within 10 days during inclement winter weather.

acutely infected calves or mature cattle. After cultures are completed, specific antimicrobial therapy may be instituted if bacterial pathogens or *Mycoplasma* spp. are isolated.

Nonsteroidal antiinflammatory drugs may be helpful in acute BRSV infections. Aspirin or flunixin may be used at the same dosages mentioned previously. Corticosteroids have been recommended for treatment of BRSV infections in calves. Calves or nonpregnant cattle with respiratory distress but minimal evidence of sepsis may receive some benefit from these drugs in diminishing the pulmonary pathology created by BRSV and, in a few cases, a dramatic improvement in clinical signs can be observed. Corticosteroids can predispose to secondary infections and abortions, and their use should be selective. Antihistamines also have been recommended for treatment of BRSV and may be used (tripelennamine hydrochloride at a dosage of 1 mg/kg IM twice daily).

Any cattle that develop the second phase or stage of BRSV infection, which appears as a hypersensitivity reaction, should receive antiinflammatory medication in addition to broad-spectrum antibiotics. The peracute onset and extreme dyspnea exhibited by these animals is usually fatal; therefore heroic therapeutic measures are indicated. Several drugs may be indicated, and clinical judgment will determine which therapeutic agents will be used. For an adult cow with this form of the disease, drugs that may be considered and their dosages can be found below:

1. Broad-spectrum antibiotics; based upon previous tracheal wash or lung culture results
2. Dexamethasone; 10-20 mg once daily IM or IV (not in pregnant cattle)
3. Antihistamine; tripelennamine hydrochloride 1 mg/kg IM twice daily
4. Atropine; 0.048 mg/kg IM or SC twice daily
5. NSAID; flunixin 1 mg/kg IV every 12 or 24 hours, aspirin 240–480 grains twice daily
6. Furosemide; 250 mg once or twice daily (if severe pulmonary edema is present)

Intranasal oxygen (10–15 L/min) is often used in our hospitals for acute BRSV infection and will frequently decrease the respiratory rate and effort. Nebulization with corticosteroids and antibiotics can be helpful, but a bronchodilator should be administered either before beginning the nebulization or at the same time. Systemic atropine, aminophylline (10 mg/kg as a CRI over a 24-hour period) or inhaled ipratropium can be used for bronchodilation. In animals that develop pneumothorax, evacuation of free air from the pleural space can offer significant improvement. The complete mediastinum of cattle often confines pneumothorax to one hemithorax, but bilateral disease or severe unilateral lung collapse caused by pneumothorax may necessitate evacuation. Details regarding specific treatment of pneumothorax are given later in this chapter.

In summary, the veterinarian must allow for a wide range of severity in BRSV outbreaks. In some mild outbreaks, no animals will require treatment. On the other hand, severe outbreaks complicated by pneumothorax (Fig. 4.60), severe emphysema (Fig. 4.61), or bacterial pathogens may result in 10% to 30% mortality rates despite heroic treatment efforts.

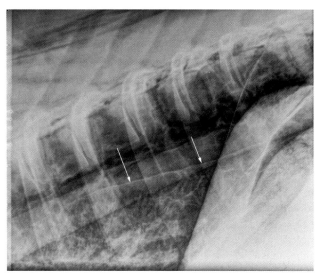

• **Fig. 4.60** Thoracic radiograph of an adult Holstein cow with pneumothorax and lung collapse associated with peracute bovine respiratory syncytial virus infection. *Arrows* indicate the dorsal edge of the collapsed lung. The animal was presented in severe respiratory distress but survived with evacuation of air by chest tube placement and aggressive supportive medical therapy.

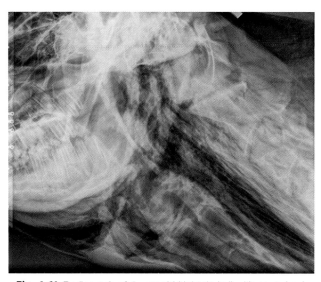

• **Fig. 4.61** Radiograph of 4-year-old Holstein bull with acute bovine respiratory syncytial virus infection, pneumothorax, and massive subcutaneous emphysema. Note the dramatic dissection of air throughout cervical region that had tracked from the thoracic inlet.

Vaccination will be discussed later, but the literature on BRSV vaccination is confusing, with some articles showing protection conferred by inactivated or modified live vaccines, others demonstrating no protection when inactivated vaccines are used, and a few suggesting an adverse immune response on subsequent exposure to the virus in previously vaccinated cattle. Most recently, protection from challenge infection has been demonstrated to be good after the intranasal administration of a MLV vaccine marketed for parenteral administration.

Parainfluenza-3

Etiology and Signs

Experimentally, PI3 virus is capable of infecting the bovine respiratory tract and predisposing infected animals to more severe pneumonia when subsequently exposed to bacterial pathogens such as *M. haemolytica*. After experimental inoculation, the virus infects the upper and lower airways of calves with subsequent damage to ciliated epithelial cells, mucus layer, and mucociliary transport alongside infection of alveolar macrophages. As bronchitis and bronchiolitis ensue, purulent exudate fills some small airways. Despite this pathology, PI3 infection is a mild disease unless complicated by secondary bacterial agents. Based on serologic surveys, most cattle probably have been exposed to PI3 infection as calves. We seldom identify PI3 in bovine respiratory outbreaks in dairy calves or cows in the northern United States. One might argue that this can be explained by virtue of the fact that most dairy animals are vaccinated against this virus, but it seems unlikely that this virus is an important contributor to BRD in the United States.

The signs of PI3 infection include fever (104.0° to 107.0°F [40.00° to 41.67°C]), depression, anorexia, nasal and ocular serous discharge, increased respiratory rate (40–80 breaths/min), tracheal rales, and occasional rales in the lower lung fields. Fatalities are uncommon, and recovery should occur over 7 days.

The signs of PI3 complicated by bacterial pneumonia are simply those of a moderate to severe bacterial bronchopneumonia as previously described under the various bacterial pathogens. Response to specific treatment for the bacterial bronchopneumonia, however, would be less prompt and complete than anticipated for bacterial infection alone.

Diagnosis

The clinical signs of PI3 infection in calves or cattle are not specific enough to allow definitive diagnosis. Therefore, virus isolation or PCR amplification from acutely infected individuals via tracheal wash, nasopharyngeal swabs, or necropsy specimens are necessary to definitively identify the infection. Paired serum samples also are helpful because humoral antibody production is anticipated after infection. Virus isolation attempts may be fruitless if samples are not collected early in the course of the disease, further emphasizing the value of PCR diagnostically.

Fatal cases usually are complicated by secondary bacterial pneumonia, especially *M. haemolytica* or *P. multocida*. Therefore, gross pathology lesions suggest bacterial bronchopneumonia, and a diagnosis of PI3 is easily missed unless the veterinarian requests viral diagnostics or obtains paired serum samples from surviving animals.

Treatment

Treatment must address the frequent secondary bacterial pneumonia. There are no characteristic clinical signs to allow veterinarians to diagnose PI3 specifically.

Bovine Viral Diarrhea Virus

Bovine viral diarrhea virus is one of the major pathogens of dairy cattle and may cause a wide range of lesions or clinical syndromes. This pestivirus from the Flaviviridae family causes fever, mucosal erosions, diarrhea, abortions or reproductive failure, congenital anomalies, persistent infection of fetuses infected between 40 and 120 days of gestation, and many other signs. The disease is discussed fully in Chapter 6. However, BVDV has been incriminated as a "respiratory virus" in cattle, and some strains can certainly be isolated from the lower airway and alveolar macrophages of infected cattle. Some BVDV strains (genotypes 1a and 1b of the non-cytopathogenic biotype) are more commonly found in the lungs of cattle and are frequently associated with respiratory disease outbreaks. All strains of BVDV are immunosuppressive and predispose infected cattle to bacterial or other viral pneumonia. Naive cattle exposed to a type 2 strain may develop severe interstitial pneumonia, thrombocytopenia, bone marrow necrosis, diarrhea, and acute death, sometimes without having mucosal erosions. Additionally, a persistently infected calf or cow may suddenly develop bacterial pneumonia without other predisposing factors, and this scenario should be considered as a possible reason for a single case of bacterial pneumonia in a herd.

During acute BVDV infection, high fevers occur in affected cattle early in the course of the disease. These cattle may show no other signs—no diarrhea, no mucosal lesions—and merely appear depressed and febrile at 106.0° to 108.0°F (41.11° to 42.22°C). Because the high fever necessitates increased physiologic heat loss, some cows have mild increases in their respiratory rate (40–60 breaths/min), but the lungs are normal on auscultation or may have slightly increased bronchovesicular sounds. These cattle are merely in the early stages of acute BVDV infection, and unless a superimposed bacterial infection develops, true clinical pneumonia may not occur. If the animal seroconverts and responds to the BVDV in a normal fashion, no other signs may develop. Some cattle will progress from this early stage of fever with no other overt signs to blatant mucosal lesions and diarrhea 7 to 14 days after the original onset of fever. This situation has been observed in natural outbreaks and with experimental BVDV infection with certain strains of BVDV in naive cattle. Most cattle with BVDV have mild pulmonary lesions or normal lungs grossly and histologically, unless an opportunistic bacterial pneumonia has developed. Naive cattle infected with the type 2 strain, however, may die with severe interstitial pneumonia.

Acute BVDV infection causes profound immunosuppression in affected animals for 7 to 14 days or until they recover. Research documents the negative effects that BVDV infection has on neutrophil, macrophage, and lymphocyte function. Humoral and cell-mediated immune functions are depressed during acute BVDV infection. Furthermore, leukopenia in the peripheral blood is a well-known feature of acute BVDV infection in cattle. Although naive or susceptible cattle fully recover immune function after the development of adequate humoral antibody against BVDV, they are very susceptible to secondary infection during the acute BVDV infection and associated immunosuppression. Alveolar macrophages are frequently infected with BVDV, which would be expected to have a direct negative effect on lung protection against invading bacteria. Therefore, the results can be devastating if a cow or a group of cattle acutely infected with BVDV has the bad fortune to become infected with *P. multocida*, *M. haemolytica*, or *H. somni* at the same time. Bacterial bronchopneumonia may progress rapidly because host defense mechanisms are negligible. In addition, cattle may die so quickly from severe pneumonia that necropsy identifies bacterial pneumonia as the sole cause of death. The existence of BVDV infection will only be confirmed if specific PCR, viral isolation, antigen detection, or immunohistochemistry is performed. Some affected cows develop signs of mucosal disease, or some fatalities demonstrate typical BVDV lesions as well as bacterial pneumonia at necropsy. Other management-related stresses, transportation, pen reorganization, poor ventilation, and so on, may also contribute to the development of bacterial pneumonia during concurrent BVDV infection.

In summary, BVDV by itself rarely causes major respiratory disease except for type 2 infections in naive cattle, which may cause interstitial pneumonia and acute death, sometimes without the typical upper GI tract lesions. Type 1 strains are commonly isolated from the lower airway and pulmonary macrophages in BVDV outbreaks and play a potentially important role in the BRD complex. Acute BVDV infection (any strain) may result in transient immunosuppression that predisposes to severe respiratory infections in cattle concurrently exposed to other respiratory pathogens. This immunosuppressive effect is not limited to the respiratory tract and certainly would also contribute to drastic illness if a cow acutely infected with BVDV experienced septic mastitis, metritis, or salmonellosis.

Bovine Respiratory Coronavirus

The role coronavirus plays in the BRD complex is not clear. There is rather more emphasis placed on it in the literature as it relates to BRD in feedlot cattle than in dairy cattle. Even in feedlot cattle, there is conflicting evidence as to its economic significance as well as its role in clinical disease. Coronavirus is commonly found in outbreaks, either acute or endemic, but can also be commonly found in healthy animals. Experimentally, all of Koch's postulates have been fulfilled with respect to causing respiratory disease in neonatal calves; as such, it may be important, particularly if the farmer describes a "pneumonia–enteritis" complex in 1- to 8-week-old calves. Unfortunately, the frequency with which many diagnostic laboratories can identify bovine coronavirus from diagnostic samples taken from the airways or lungs of both healthy and diseased dairy calves adds further confusion to the issue. Typically, the PCR primers used to identify bovine coronavirus from diagnostic samples do not differentiate between enteric and respiratory strains, so close are they that it requires full sequencing to distinguish them.

Other Viruses

In addition to bovine respiratory coronavirus several other viruses, including adenoviruses (types 3 and 7) and rhinoviruses (bovine rhinitis virus A and B), have been shown experimentally to be potential pathogens of the bovine respiratory tract. Clinically, there are no pathognomonic features of these viruses. Except for coronaviruses, diagnostic laboratories seldom identify these viruses in outbreaks of infectious respiratory disease in cattle or calves.

Control and Prevention of Infectious Respiratory Diseases in Dairy Cattle: General

The control of acute or chronic endemic respiratory disease within groups of calves or adult cattle broadly consists of four components:
1. Definitive diagnosis of the causative agent(s)
2. Specific medical therapy
3. Correction of management, environmental, or ventilation deficiencies that contribute to, or perpetuate, the respiratory disease
4. Preventive medicine, including management techniques and vaccination

Most of these points have been addressed in the discussion of treatment for each of the infectious agents in this section. Field outbreaks of respiratory disease may be limited to individual groups, such as weaned calves, breeding age heifers, milking cows, and dry cows, or may involve all animals on the premises. When only one group is affected, the veterinarian should try to determine what management, environmental, or ventilation conditions might have predisposed this group to the development of clinical disease. It also is necessary to elicit information from the owner regarding vaccination history, previous outbreaks of respiratory disease, recent purchase of animals, recent movement of resident animals to shows, and other facts that may help to explain how the respiratory infection may have become established in a group of animals or the entire herd.

Respiratory viruses, bacteria, and *Mycoplasma* spp. may be involved separately or in combination in these outbreaks. Although severe outbreaks of pure BRSV or Mannheimiosis do continue to occur, the majority of respiratory disease cases in dairy calves and adult cattle that we encounter belong in the category of chronic bacterial bronchopneumonia, often compounded by the presence of *Mycoplasma* spp. In calves, one should also be cognizant of the role that *Salmonella* Dublin can play in respiratory disease outbreaks, especially toward the end of the preweaning period and into group housing! Because many of the bacterial agents discussed in this chapter can be considered ubiquitous in cattle populations one has to consider what stressors or triggers have compromised affected individuals or groups to tip the scales in favor of disease occurrence.

There is no doubting the increasing prominence of *Mycoplasma* infection on many modern dairies, not just as a respiratory pathogen but also as a cause of mastitis and synovitis–arthritis. Many *M. bovis* infections that become chronic and lifelong are acquired in calfhood, and the major manifestations of illness in milk-fed calves are pneumonia and otitis. Feeding of contaminated colostrum or waste milk is thought to be the primary means of transmitting *Mycoplasma* to young calves. Aerosol spread or transmission by direct contact may subsequently occur to calves housed with, or very near, infected cohorts. Use of colostrum

replacer, milk replacer, and pasteurization of waste milk and colostrum are all strategies to reduce exposure of young calves. Heat treating colostrum to less than standard milk pasteurization temperatures is effective in killing important calf pathogens without damaging the immunoglobulins. As colostrum pasteurization becomes more commonplace, it is probable that many dairies will turn to this technique as a means of reducing the pathogen burden that calves are exposed to in the immediate postnatal period. Standard pasteurization procedures are already commonly used to successfully treat waste milk before feeding it to calves. There are no effective vaccines currently available for the prevention of *Mycoplasma* spp. infection in cattle.

Cattle housed in tie stall barns are predisposed to infectious pneumonia when marked environmental temperature and humidity fluctuations occur during the indoor housing season. Late fall and early spring, as well as winter thaws, are the times most likely to vary widely in temperature and humidity. Increased humidity and ammonia accumulation both occur in areas with inadequate ventilation. Ammonia dissolves in the suspended water vapor and is an irritant to the respiratory epithelium. Exhaled bacteria and viruses are included in microscopic droplets of moisture. Prevention of respiratory infections in these settings requires improvement in the ventilation to dilute the pathogens and remove the irritants. If the walls or ceiling accumulate condensation or the odor of ammonia in the barn is noticeable, there is inadequate ventilation. Normally, the inside temperature in these barns in winter should not exceed 50°F (10°C). All modern free-stall barns in cold climates are now curtain sided and these can be adjusted according to weather conditions in the winter to allow adequate fresh air entry for removal of humidity and ammonia. A temperature gradient of only a few degrees between inside and outside is frequently adequate to drive the necessary air exchanges for maintaining air quality inside the barn. A useful resource for facilities design for housing of dairy cattle is provided by the University of Wisconsin through partnerships with private industry; https://thedairylandinitiative.vetmed.wisc.edu

Whenever possible, prevention of infectious respiratory disease in dairy cattle is more desirable than treatment and control measures. Prevention consists both of effective vaccination programs and management designed to reduce the probability of infectious respiratory disease. Currently, highly effective vaccines are available for IBR, PI3, and BVDV. Strong, enduring vaccinal protection against BRSV infection is probably the most sought after advance in the immunoprophylaxis of viral BRD because outbreaks continue to occur in vaccinated herds. More recent MLV products administered intranasally offer the best opportunity for improved prevention and should be incorporated into all herd programs. Vaccines against *H. somni* and *P. multocida*, although available, have equivocal evidence-based literature in terms of disease prevention and economic benefit. The relevance of vaccines for protection against disease caused by opportunistic colonization of lower airways by these commensal pharyngeal organisms will likely always remain contentious. Newer vaccines against *M. haemolytica* that are based on leukotoxins of this bacterium have been proven beneficial in reducing morbidity and mortality rates in cattle. Such commercial products are often combined with antigens of *P. multocida*.

Vaccination strategies for herds should be individually determined and include the assessment of risk for all age groups. Closed herds in isolated settings have a much lower risk of contagious pathogen acquisition than herds that continuously purchase animals or exhibit cattle. However, mortality rates in heifer calves are frequently high enough that many dairies continue to purchase replacement animals merely in order to maintain herd numbers. This need to purchase cattle is only accentuated if the dairy is attempting to expand in size. Regardless, primary immunization requires two doses of vaccine and is best done at an early age. Optimal response to viral vaccines occurs after the waning of colostrally derived antibodies. Thus, current general recommendations are to begin the primary series at about 3 months of age with the second dose administered 2 to 4 weeks later. Recent research indicates the greatest response to immunization against IBR and BVDV occurs if the first two doses are a killed product and the subsequent booster is a modified live vaccine. All major vaccine producers offer combination products with options for killed or modified live virus that provide the four major viral components in a single injection. The *M. haemolytica* leukotoxoids are a distinct product but may be combined with *P. multocida*. Subsequent boosters are administered at frequencies that correspond to the perceived risk and usually at times or ages that offer some convenience to management. The duration of immunity after proper vaccination is mostly not known for each of the components of the routinely used products. Thus, recommendations for low-risk herds may be annual revaccination of the entire herd, but high-risk herds may be given boosters two or three times per year. Alternatively, in many large herds, adults are vaccinated in conjunction with the lactation cycle. For example, a modified live booster is given at 30 days in milk, and killed boosters are given at 120 and 240 days of gestation. When boosters are given at specific points in the lactation cycle, one must be aware of the negative influence that poor reproductive performance or management decisions such as use for embryo transfer or oocyte donation will have on the efficiency of the program. We have seen a number of situations when either on a herd level or for individually valuable cattle, the decision to booster for example at dry-off has meant a 5- to 6-month delay between the booster and the onset of the next lactation, or an early lactation vaccine booster has been separated by over 6 months from the average time of early gestation in the next pregnancy. These circumstances can also contrive to lessen the value of colostrum as a means of adequacy of passive transfer.

Efforts will no doubt continue to develop new immunization products with greater safety, efficacy, and efficiency. Veterinarians are encouraged to remain abreast of these new developments because new knowledge and technologies may make our current practices obsolete.

Control and Prevention of Infectious Respiratory Disease Specific to Dairy Calves

Bovine respiratory disease, particularly in dairy calves, is a multifactorial disease in which a combination of host, agent, and environmental factors contribute to infection of the upper and lower airways by viral and bacterial pathogens. Viruses commonly isolated from calves with respiratory signs and which may cause primary disease include BRSV, BHV1, and PI3. Infection by bovine viral diarrhea virus increases the susceptibility of the calf to disease but is not usually a primary cause of disease. Coronavirus is commonly isolated from the nasopharynx; however, the role of this pathogen in BRD is still under debate. Interestingly, the increasing research use of metagenomics and deep sequencing during the investigation of BRD is serving to rapidly and markedly increase the number of bovine viruses that can be detected in clinical cases. These types of investigations are not yet "routine" for the workup of field cases, but there is undoubtedly a plethora of new viruses (bovine rhinitis A and B, bovine adenovirus, bovine influenza D, and others) in addition to bovine coronavirus that have been previously uncharacterized but that can be found in clinically pneumonic cattle but only rarely in healthy case control animals. The relevance of these agents, as stated with coronavirus, is uncertain from a causal perspective but should be an active area of research in the near future. Viral infection with pathogens often causes destruction of the respiratory epithelium, resulting in impaired mucociliary function and secondary bacterial infection from pathogens normally residing in the nasopharynx. Bacterial respiratory pathogens include *Pasteurella multocida*, *M. haemolytica*, *T. pyogenes*, and less commonly, *H. somni* and possibly *Bibersteinia trehalosi*. *Mycoplasma bovis* is also of increasing relevance in endemic respiratory disease problems in calves. Neutrophilic infiltrates in the bronchial, bronchiolar, and alveolar compartments of the lung are the main pathological changes associated with bacterial bronchitis, bronchiolitis, and bronchopneumonia. Specifics regarding most of these pathogens have been discussed previously.

Clinical cases of BRD typically suffer from some combination of cough, fever, and nasal and ocular discharge. Changes in respiratory pattern and depression can be present in either severe, acute or end-stage, chronic cases. Droopy ears and head tilt occur when calves are comorbid with otitis media or interna. Poor body condition and small stature develop with chronic disease (Fig. 4.62). In general, inappetence is a poor proxy for predicting respiratory disease in calves. Subclinical respiratory disease, or more specifically subclinical pneumonia, is present in dairy calf populations and presents an additional challenge for management.

Respiratory disease affects approximately 12% to 16% of preweaned calves. However, on any given farm, prevalence of BRD can vary markedly from none to nearly all of the calves. This means that BRD is much more of a problem for certain herds. At least 20% to 30% of calves affected by BRD require multiple antimicrobial treatments, and interestingly, compared with veterinarians, producers are twice as

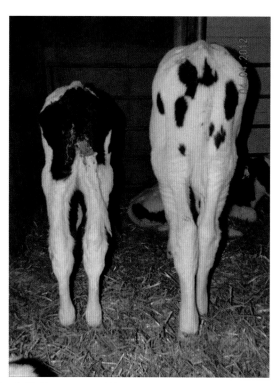

• **Fig. 4.62** Two 5-week-old Holstein calves from a commercial dairy. The calf on the left demonstrates the impact of chronic pneumonia on growth. The calf on the right is a healthy penmate.

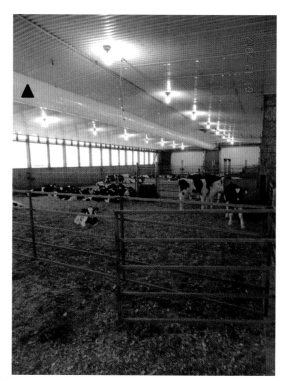

• **Fig. 4.63** Indoor group housing with supplemental air provided through positive-pressure ventilation. The *black triangle* indicates the positive-pressure tube.

likely to retreat. In the United States, 22% of all preweaned calf deaths are the result of BRD, with case fatality rates ranging from 2% to 9%.

Studies have documented reductions in body weight associated with both clinical and subclinical BRD. Calves experiencing BRD are older when they deliver their first calf, are less likely to enter the milking string, and have greater odds of not completing their first lactation. The short-term costs associated with managing BRD are approximately $10 to $16 per calf. Long-term effects increase such estimates by reducing postweaning growth rates, longevity, and future production.

Many risk factors must be managed properly in order to prevent disease. Overcrowding and poor air quality have long been understood to contribute to BRD. Drafts, high ammonia levels, housing with older animals, large herd size, diarrhea, prolonged time to dam separation, and BRSV vaccination have all been reported as risk factors. In enclosed barns, low air bacterial counts within calf pens, solid barriers between calves, and the ability of the calves to nest in deep straw protects preweaned calves from BRD during the winter months in the northern United States. Separating previously sick calves from healthy calves in group housing has also been associated with a lower risk of BRD in the healthy calves. Based on clinical experience, an age difference within a preweaning group pen of less than 7 to 10 days is associated with a lower risk for disease.

When calves are housed in individual hutches outdoors, ventilation is much less of a concern if the calves can freely move in and out of the hutch and bedding is regularly added. However, with the increased prominence of indoor

housing, ventilation must be a priority. Most barns are naturally ventilated and rely on prevailing winds to create air exchanges. In the northern United States, the goal should be approximately four changes per hour in the winter and up to 45 to 60 changes in the summer. Unfortunately, wind is not always present; therefore, these barns require fresh air exchange systems that are supplemented by mechanical ventilation. This is particularly important in the winter when curtains are closed to regulate the barn temperature. Negative pressure, or tunnel ventilation, is not commonly used in calf barns because of problems associated with proper distribution of air within the calf pens, particularly in the winter. Occasionally, "neutral-pressure" ventilation is used by which clean air is pushed in and old air is forced out by mechanical means. The most common method of supplementing fresh air is through positive-pressure ventilation (PPV). In PPV, a fan directs small amounts of clean, fresh air through a distribution tube fitted with strategically sized holes (Fig. 4.63). Old, stagnant air passively leaves the barn through an open ridge, simultaneously removing pathogens and noxious chemicals. Whichever system is used, thorough documentation of the efficacy in achieving the appropriate air exchanges without creating drafts on the calves is essential. Air speed can be quantitatively assessed using anemometers, and air movement can be qualitatively assessed using an insect fogger. These tools help identify drafts as well as areas of dead air. Air sampling units can also be used to culture the pen air at the level of the calf. High-quality pen air should have bacterial counts of less than 30,000 CFU/m^3 on blood agar plates. Pen air exceeding 100,000 CFU/m^3

has been associated with respiratory disease. If an improvement in calf health is not noted after installation, the tubes and associated fans should be reassessed for proper design and installation, and any other possible deficits in management should be investigated, including passive transfer status of the calves, nutritional status, health and biosecurity of new arrivals, vaccination status, commingling, screening methods, treatment protocols, and stocking density. Stocking density has the greatest impact on air quality, and simply increasing ventilation 10-fold does not ameliorate the impact of doubling stocking density. In group pens, preweaned calves should be provided approximately 35 sq ft of bedded space per calf.

In addition to housing and ventilation, the potential association between failure of passive transfer (FPT) and the development of BRD must not be overlooked. This is often an early bottleneck to achieving acceptable levels of BRD in a herd. Although not every calf with FPT will develop BRD, several studies have documented an increased risk in calves with insufficient absorption of maternal immunoglobulins. Passive transfer can quickly be assessed at the herd level by refractometry. Brix refractometry and total protein (TP) refractometry can both be used. Ideally, at least 80% of calves should have evidence of adequacy of passive transfer when tested between 1 and 7 days of age (serum Brix ≥8.4% and serum TP ≥5.5 g/dL).

Maternal antibody levels peak within the calf approximately 24 to 48 hours after ingestion of colostrum and are at significantly lower levels by approximately 3 weeks of age. Often indoor-housed dairy calves are initially treated for BRD around this time. Although maternal transfer of antibody to the newborn calf provides many great benefits, high levels of maternal antibodies are associated with a delayed antigen responsiveness and antibody production by the neonate, as well as selective inhibition of lymphocyte responses. Several studies have shown that administration of a parenteral vaccine in a seropositive calf will not achieve the same immunologic response as that from a seronegative or colostrum-deprived calf.

This potential for maternally derived blockade has been one of the issues causing concern regarding the practice of vaccinating calves during the first few months of life to prevent BRD. However, this should never be used as justification on farm for poor colostral management or timeliness of colostrum delivery nor as a potential "upside" to FPT or partial passive transfer. In general terms, it is also a very weak argument for precocious vaccination protocols in preweaned heifer replacements. That being said, it is worth pointing out that mucosal vaccination via the intranasal rather than by the parenteral route may provide an option to bypass this problem for some infectious agents.

Intranasal vaccination between 3 and 8 days of age with a trivalent viral vaccine against BRSV, BHV1, and PI3 has been shown to be protective against BRSV challenge 9 weeks after vaccination but not at 14 weeks after vaccination, suggesting that the duration of immunity to BRSV is short lived. One of the authors (TO) has also demonstrated that this same viral vaccine can reduce the probability of developing ultrasonographic lung lesions. Recently, an intranasal vaccine against *Pasteurella multocida* and *M. haemolytica* has also become available commercially in the United States, although peer-reviewed literature regarding its efficacy is lacking. In general, vaccination protocols for young calves should be designed keeping in mind the specific infectious pressures for the individual farm, and should never serve as a replacement for good management. Multiple doses of a parenteral, modified live viral vaccine before and/or just after weaning are costly, time consuming, and may negatively impact feed intakes.

There have been recommendations in the face of endemic respiratory disease in calves to hyperimmunize young calves against viral and bacterial diseases by repeated vaccination at 2-week intervals. To date, there is no evidence that this strategy has any merit. Rather, the environmental and management ideas discussed earlier are more likely to provide health and economic returns to the herd. Another widely used strategy for undifferentiated respiratory disease of recently weaned calves is metaphylaxis of the at-risk group. Current practice in many dairies is to wean a group of calves and move them within 1 week or so to group housing. This change, particularly when more than 10 calves in a group are moved at one time, seems to be a trigger for respiratory disease. Control has been achieved in many herds with mass medication at the time of a move with a single injection of a long-acting antibiotic such as oxytetracycline, tilmicosin, tulathromycin, or florfenicol, or by feeding chlortetracycline and sulfamethazine pellets for 5 to 7 days. Herds that practice a more gradual assembly of large groups of calves or that simply have fewer calves seem to be at much lower risk for this problem.

Besides managing the previously mentioned risk factors, there are at least five additional on-farm requirements for effective control of BRD; (1) competent and dedicated personnel, (2) defined screening examinations and diagnostic criteria, (3) consistent and clear treatment and vaccination protocols, (4) a dedicated and permanent place for record keeping in which treatments are always documented, and (5) oversight of records. Increasingly, the majority, if not all, of these are the day-to-day responsibility of farm personnel, not veterinarians. However, there is a pivotal and essential role for veterinarians in the establishment and oversight of each of the first four of the listed items. Periodic reassessment and quality control of each facet of BRD control must involve the veterinarian, and for the veterinarian's input to be most effective and respected, he or she needs to be consistently on farm and up to date. Furthermore, veterinarians have an equally important role to play with respect to responsible use of medications on farm, observance of withdrawal times, and adherence to regulatory specifications regarding legal and illegal drug use.

Personnel responsible for BRD screening should be competent and dedicated. Appropriate training ensures competence and helps the screener understand the purpose of his or her role. As herd size allows, ideally, screeners should not work with adult cattle. This may not be possible in smaller herds, where one person works in multiple management areas. In such situations, precautions, including working with younger animals first, hand washing, use of gloves, and changing coveralls and boots, will help avoid transmission of disease from older cattle to the younger calves. Treatment and vaccination protocols should be based on data gathered from deep nasopharyngeal swabs, tracheal wash, or BAL fluid analysis. Posting these protocols helps ensure consistency, which can only be monitored when records are maintained and oversight is implemented.

Systematic screening can improve early detection rates and initiate treatment decisions, which should reduce the impact of BRD on calf health and welfare and the cost of raising replacement animals. Clearly defining the screening exam and its required frequency ensures regular and consistent examination of all calves at risk of developing respiratory disease. The most widely used system, the Wisconsin Calf Scoring Chart (WCSC), divides the response to respiratory disease into five categories; body temperature, nasal discharge, cough, ocular discharge, and ear position. Each category is assigned 0 to 3 points corresponding to the subjective level of abnormality (0 = normal, 1 = mild, 2 = moderate, and 3 = severely abnormal), and the total number of points is summed to arrive at an overall respiratory score. Calves with two abnormal categories are considered sick, and treatment is recommended. Mortality rates have been shown to immediately decrease, and morbidity rates decrease within 1 to 2 months after implementation of twice-weekly respiratory scoring by producers.

Clinical scoring typically ranks the severity of clinical signs in a subjective manner. More recently, three novel scoring systems have been developed, offering alternatives to the WCSC, using statistical methods instead of subjective judgments to assign weights to describe the severity of the abnormality within each category (e.g., nasal discharge). Each of these systems correctly classified approximately 90% of the animals and required less handling than the WCSC. Although these scoring systems are not intended to act as gold standards for the diagnosis of BRD, they can serve as a useful means of identifying a large proportion of clinically affected calves under some conditions, particularly when one considers that any on-farm scoring technique must be practically useful, repeatable, and consistent in the hands of non-veterinarians. At the very least, such periodic assessments increase observation of calves by attentive individuals who are invested, possibly both personally and financially, in improving calf health. The DART (depression, appetite, respiratory, and temperature) system is another type of screening system that relies on the presence of depression, inappetence, abnormal respiratory pattern, and fever, to indicate when treatment is necessary. Unfortunately, these signs are not consistent in ill calves, and systematic cutpoints have not been well established. However, examination is warranted if a calf does demonstrate these signs. Calves that are standing for excessive periods after feeding when herdmates are resting (or vice versa) should also be evaluated.

The increased utilization of on-farm clinical scoring by non-veterinarians for the timely identification of respiratory disease in calves undoubtedly represents a compromise in terms of precision and accuracy compared with an experienced clinician, particularly if that individual has access to diagnostic imaging. In significant part, clinical scoring is a response to the reality of increased intensification with regard to dairy calf rearing, serving to increase the risk of BRD alongside an increasing awareness and relevancy of the economic impact of respiratory disease in the first 2 months of life. It has coincided with a change in veterinary involvement on many farms from the day-to-day diagnosis and treatment of individual animals to a more population-based approach dictated by the value of individual grade cattle. However, in addition to physical diagnostics, there is substantial benefit to imaging of lung lesions, whether it is via radiography, CT, or ultrasonography.

Unfortunately, radiography and CT are not practical in all but individually valuable calves, so despite their diagnostic utility, it is difficult to envisage any widespread role for these in the near future. However, ultrasonography can be performed using portable, readily available machines without the fear of radiation exposure. Furthermore, ultrasonography provides diagnostic advantages in terms of accuracy over clinical scoring. Recently, the WCSC, thoracic auscultation, and treatment records of 106 calves from 13 Canadian dairy farms were compared with the results of thoracic ultrasonography in a cross-sectional study. Using an ultrasonography cutoff of 1 cm, and lung consolidation as a case definition; the sensitivity and specificity of the WCSC were 55% and 58%, respectively; and the sensitivity of thoracic auscultation compared with ultrasonography ranged from 3% to 17%. This provides strong evidence that both clinical scoring and auscultation underestimate the prevalence of lung lesions in dairy calves compared with thoracic ultrasonography. Importantly, thoracic ultrasonography is no longer the province of referral clinics and university teaching hospitals, and it is increasingly common for it to be used by practitioners on farm for reasons of diminishing equipment cost as well as the fact that medium frequency linear probes that double up for reproductive use are excellent for thoracic ultrasonography.

As long ago as the early 1990s, research began on the diagnostic utility of ultrasonography for BRD. The pathology associated with BRD includes cellular infiltration into the airways, which along with cellular debris, effectively displace air from the lung tissue, resulting in nonaerated or consolidated lung lesions that are easily detectable by ultrasonography. These lesions appear homogeneous and hypoechoic (Figs. 4.39 and 4.64 and Video Clips 4.8 and 4.12). This is in stark contrast to the hyperechoic echogenicity of normal lung, which also displays reverberation artifact (Fig. 4.65 and Video Clip 4.13). Such changes allow for the ultrasonographic detection of lung lesions regardless of the clinical state of the animal. These lung lesions typically have a cranioventral distribution, starting in the cranial aspect of the right cranial lobe or right middle lung lobe and proceeding caudally.

Evidence confirming the accuracy and diagnostic utility of ultrasonography has been forthcoming from several prospective field studies in recent years. An initial small study showed that ultrasonography was a reliable method of confirming clinical bronchopneumonia in 18 Holstein calves up to 5 months of age. In a separate study conducted at the University of Montreal, three observers with varying levels of experience imaged 10 dairy calves (healthy, $n = 4$; treated for BRD, $n = 6$). The inter-observer agreement varied from moderate to almost perfect (kappa = 0.6–1.0) depending on the experience level of the observer. Another study assessing lung

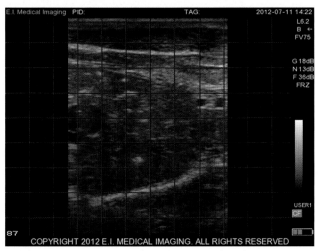

• **Fig. 4.64** Consolidated lung imaged as homogeneous, hypoechoic structure. Note the step in the pleura (top right of image) as the lung deviates around the internal thoracic artery and vein (seen in cross-section in the ventral aspect of the image), which defines this as the cranial aspect of the right cranial lung lobe. This is a lobar pneumonia because the entire lung lobe is consolidated.

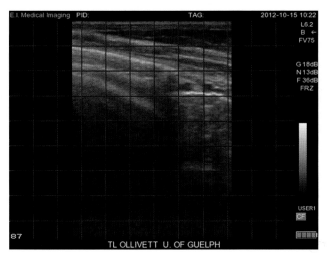

• **Fig. 4.65** Normal gas-filled lung imaged as a hyperechoic line, representing the pleural interface, with reverberation artifact deep to the interface. Interpretations of the lung parenchyma deep to the pleural interface cannot be made when reverberation artifact is present. Note the step in the pleura as the lung deviates around the internal thoracic artery and vein (seen in cross-section in the ventral aspect of the image), which defines this lung lobe as the cranial aspect of the right cranial lung lobe.

lesions post mortem previously identified by ultrasonography after experimental bacterial infection documented excellent agreement between the postmortem examination and ultrasound distribution of lesions. In calves with subclinical lung lesions, the sensitivity and specificity of ultrasonography were an impressive 94% and 100%, respectively. Experimental challenge studies have demonstrated that pathologic changes within the parenchyma of the lung occur as early as 2 hours and peak 6 hours after experimental bacterial challenge and that these changes can already be detected by that time with thoracic ultrasonography.

It is possible to use many different types of ultrasound probes for the identification of lung lesions associated with respiratory disease in dairy calves. In the literature, probe frequency and probe design has ranged from 3.5 MHz sector, 3.5 to 13 MHz linear, 7.5 MHz, and 5 MHz sector. Fortunately, transrectal probes intended for pregnancy diagnosis are slimmer and permit better access to the axillary region and cranial thorax of young dairy calves. These probes, with frequencies varying between 3.5 and 8 MHz, are widely used by bovine practitioners for reproductive purposes, making them preferred for practical, field-based use of ultrasonography in dairy calves, often without the need for added investment in new equipment.

The operator must have a good understanding of bovine lung anatomy and the typical locations of lung lesions in order to perform an accurate ultrasound examination. A systematic approach based on the identification of specific ultrasonographic landmarks will also help prevent detection errors. In general, the recommended ultrasonographic examination extends from the 10th ICS toward the 1st ICS by moving the probe ventrally along the grain of the hair in a dorsal to ventral fashion. The probe should be moved in a slightly caudal direction, staying within one ICS to avoid imaging the rib. Very slight adjustments can move the ultrasound beam onto or off the rib surface or enhance visualization of a lung lesion. The preferred transducing agent is 70% isopropyl alcohol, applied directly to the hair coat with a spray or squirt bottle. The hair does not need to be clipped despite the common recommendations to do so in existing literature.

When scanning the right and left caudal lung lobes from the 10th to the 6th ICS, the diaphragm will mark the ventral border of the lung (Fig. 4.66). The liver can be seen deep to the diaphragm on the right, and the spleen is imaged deep to the diaphragm on the left. The right middle lung lobe is imaged from the right 5th ICS, and the caudal aspect of the left cranial lung lobe can be imaged between the left 4th and 5th ICSs. In both lobes, the ventral image landmark includes a pleural interface that dives deep within the image, as the costochondral junction appears ventrally (Fig. 4.67). The elbow roughly approximates the location of the 5th ICS. The caudal aspect of the right cranial lung lobe is imaged from the right 4th and 3rd ICSs. The heart is the ventral image landmark in both of these locations (Fig. 4.68). The cranial aspect of the right cranial lung lobe is imaged from the right 2nd and 1st ICSs (see Figs. 4.64 and 4.65). These two locations image similarly having an obvious step in the pleural interface as the lung moves around the internal thoracic artery and vein. The pleural step and these two vessels serve as the ventral image landmark on the right side. On the left thorax, the cranial aspect of the left cranial lung is imaged mainly from the 3rd to the 2nd ICSs where the heart is the ventral image landmark. It is noteworthy that the cranial aspect of the right cranial lung lobe can be

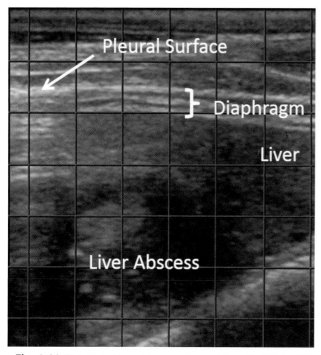

• **Fig. 4.66** The caudal lung lobes are imaged from the 6th to 10th intercostal spaces (ICSs) on either side of the thorax. The diaphragm represents the ventral image landmark within each ICS. On the right, the liver is imaged deep to the diaphragm. On the left, the spleen (not shown) can be imaged deep to the diaphragm.

imaged from the left 2nd ICS as it crosses the thorax in front of the heart (Fig. 4.69). Occasionally, when just the tip is consolidated, it can be imaged only from here.

The cranial aspect of the right cranial lung, the right middle lung lobe, and the caudal aspect of the left cranial lung are most commonly affected by bronchopneumonia. Because bacterial bronchopneumonia rarely affects the caudal lung lobe, the ultrasound examination can be modified to exclude this portion of the lung when the goal is simply to screen calves for this disease. Individual, poor-doing calves should have a complete diagnostic examination performed. Prognosis is worse for individual calves with caudal lung lobe involvement, abscessation, or poor body condition identified during the ultrasound examination. Several studies have reported on the measured depth of the ultrasonographic consolidation over several locations on the thorax. It has been determined that the maximum depth of consolidation is well correlated to the number of locations with consolidation. Categorical scoring systems, however, are easier and more practical for assessing the severity and type of lung lesions versus measuring the amount of consolidation. An easy-to-use, 6-point scoring system is outlined in Table 4.2. Based on comparative histopathology, calves with ultrasound scores of 3 to 5 have lobar bacterial bronchopneumonia. Score 2 lesions are typically viral in nature when the lesions are smaller than 1 cm in diameter. Calves scoring 0 or 1 are typically normal. Lobular lesions (score 2) represent discrete areas of consolidation within otherwise aerated lung (Fig. 4.70 and see Video Clip 4.12). In other words, the normal hyperechoic pleural interface with reverberation artifact can be seen dorsal and ventral to the lung lesion. Lobar lesions indicate that there is full-thickness consolidation of the lung lobe (see Fig. 4.64 and see Video Clip 4.8). In this instance, normal lung cannot be imaged at any point ventral to the start of the lesion. Ultrasound scoring of calves assists the veterinarian

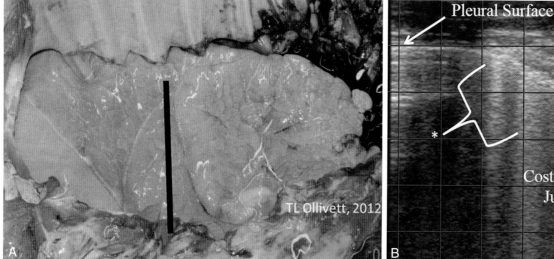
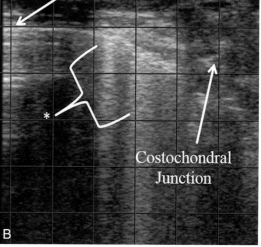

• **Fig. 4.67** The right middle lung lobe (**A**) is imaged from the right 5th intercostal space (ICS), and the caudal aspect of the left cranial lung lobe can be imaged between the left fourth and fifth ICSs. In both lobes, the ventral image landmark includes a pleural interface that dives deep within the image, as the costochondral junction appears ventrally (**B**). The *asterisk* indicates pleural roughening or comet-tail artifacts. The *black bar* indicates the image location.

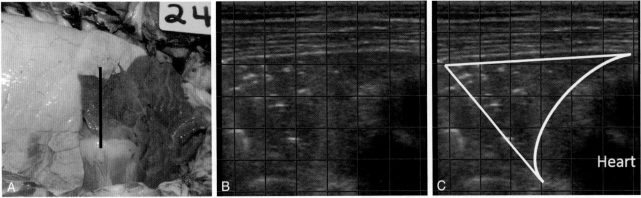

• **Fig. 4.68** Gross specimen (**A**) and ultrasonographic images (**B** and **C**) of the caudal aspect of the right cranial lobe with lobar consolidation in the right fourth intercostal space. Ultrasonographic features of consolidation with homogeneous, non-aerated lung with occasional hyperechoic foci and an absence of normal pleural reverberation artifact can be seen in **B**. Note the liver-like, wedge-shaped appearance of the hypoechoic, consolidated lung dorsal to the heart (*white outline* in C). For images B and C, dorsal is to the left side of the image, ventral is to the right side of image, superficial is at the top of the image, and deep is at the bottom of the image. The *black bar* indicates the image location.

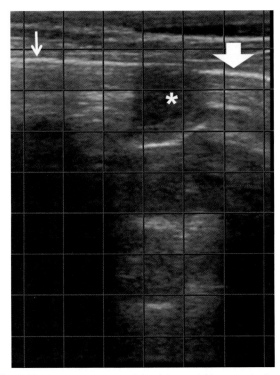

• **Fig. 4.69** The cranial aspect of the right cranial lung can be imaged from the left second intercostal space as it crosses the thorax in front of the heart. Occasionally, when just the tip is consolidated, it can be imaged only from here. The *thin arrow* indicates the left lung, the *thick arrow* indicates the right lung, and the *asterisk* indicates the thymus.

TABLE 4.2	Description of Categorical Scoring System Used for Rapid Detection of Lung Lesions in Dairy Calves	
Ultrasonographic Score	**Description**
0	Very few or no comet-tail artifacts; no hypoechoic consolidation
1	Diffuse comet-tail artifacts; no hypoechoic consolidation
2	Lobular pneumonia with singular or multifocal patchy consolidation
3	Lobar pneumonia with only one lobe entirely consolidated
4	Lobar pneumonia with two lobes entirely consolidated
5	Lobar pneumonia with three or more lobes entirely consolidated

not only with diagnosis and staging severity but also permits assessment of response to therapy and resolution of pneumonia in individual calves. At the farm level, besides determining the prevalence of respiratory tract disease, clinical pneumonia, and subclinical pneumonia, ultrasound scoring can be used to determine if timely diagnosis by cow-side personnel is occurring and whether or not the farm treatment protocols are effective. Thoracic ultrasonography can also improve purchasing and culling decisions.

Parasitic Pneumonia

Dictyocaulus viviparus

Etiology and Signs

Dictyocaulus viviparus is the lungworm of cattle and causes parasitic pneumonia and bronchiolitis in calves and adult cattle. This parasite has a direct life cycle, so infection merely requires management factors that allow a buildup of the parasite in the environment and ingestion of the infective larvae by naive cattle.

Adult lungworms reside in the trachea and bronchi. Eggs produced by female adults hatch either in the trachea or before being passed in the feces. The progression to the infective third stage larvae requires only 5 days, and the larvae are then ingested during consumption of contaminated grass in a

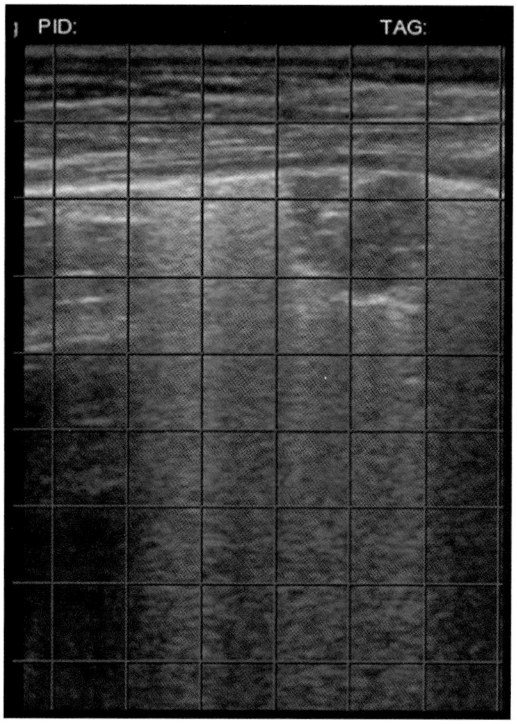

• **Fig. 4.70** Lobular lesions (score 2) are discreet areas of consolidation within otherwise aerated lung. In other words, the normal hyperechoic pleural interface with reverberation artifact can be seen dorsal and ventral to the lung lesion.

pasture or bedding in heavily contaminated box stalls. Ingested larvae traverse the intestinal wall to reside in mesenteric lymph nodes, moult to the fourth stage, and within 1 week migrate to the lungs through lymphatics or blood vessels. The final fifth stage is reached after the larvae arrive in the bronchioles. The prepatent period is approximately 4 weeks because this period is required for the larvae to mature to egg-laying adults.

Signs of primary infection include varying degrees of dyspnea, a characteristic deep and moist cough, and moist rales or crackles heard over the entire lung field. Coughing is more severe and prominent than with most other bovine pneumonias. Diffuse rales rather than rales limited to the anterior ventral lung fields are an important sign that differentiates lungworm from bacterial pneumonias. Severely affected calves or cows will show "heave"-like breathing with visible expiratory and inspiratory effort. In some cases, emphysema is present when heavy airway exudate results in extreme mechanical respiratory efforts. Fever (103.0° to 106.0°F [39.44° to 41.11°C]) may be present in some cases as opportunistic bacteria such as *P. multocida* invade the damaged lower airway and establish a secondary bacterial bronchopneumonia. Fever also may be present simply from exertion involved in breathing during warm weather or in poorly ventilated barns. Usually several animals in a group or the entire herd will show signs, but mortality rates tend to be very low. Affected cattle continue to eat unless severe dyspnea or coughing interferes with their ability to ingest feed. In cases with severe dyspnea, frequent coughing, marked expiratory effort, and open-mouth breathing are noted.

In addition to the signs of primary infection, veterinarians should be aware of the reinfection or acute larval migration

syndrome that occurs in adult cattle previously exposed to the parasite on farms with endemic *D. viviparus*. Although age-related immunity to *D. viviparus* exists in adult cattle in endemic areas, this immunity may be incomplete or may not be able to overcome heavy challenge. Although most ingested larvae are killed or fail to mature in previously infected cattle, heavy exposure apparently allows large numbers of larvae to simultaneously reach the lungs and cause respiratory signs through either an immune-mediated mechanism or from migration of large numbers of larvae into the lung. Signs usually develop 14 to 16 days after exposure to contaminated pastures. Coughing that is frequent and deep, as well as an increased respiratory rate, characterizes the syndrome. Milk production decreases acutely in affected cattle. Rales may not be present. Fecal examinations are usually negative for *Dictyocaulus* with this form because the disease is a result of the L4 migration into the lung.

Diagnosis

In primary infections, the diagnosis is aided by history, physical examination findings, laboratory or postmortem confirmation, and knowledge of the life cycle of the parasite.

The characteristic deep, moist cough and moist rales auscultated throughout the entire lung are the most significant clinical signs, especially if found in a majority of the cattle within a group. As with any parasitic disease, some affected animals ("weak sisters") display more blatant signs than others, but most within the group are affected. History may be very helpful if animals have been placed on pasture recently or confined by group housing (heifers) to pens having a base consisting of several months of manure accumulation.

Baermann's technique performed on fresh manure is indicated for specific diagnosis but is of limited value in prepatent and postpatent infections. Therefore, both Baermann's technique and tracheal washes should be performed on several animals. If larvae are found using Baermann's technique, the diagnosis is confirmed as a patent infection. In prepatent infections, tracheal wash samples may identify parasites, rule out other causes of pneumonia, and allow cytologic confirmation of eosinophilic inflammation typical of parasitic bronchitis and pneumonia. In postpatent infections, tracheal wash cytology also indicates eosinophilic inflammation and may suggest chronic inflammation. Eosinophilic tracheal wash cytology should be highly suggestive of parasitic pneumonia (Fig. 4.71). In temperate areas of the world where the disease is more commonly endemic, milk and serum enzyme-linked immunosorbent assay (ELISA) tests based on a recombinant major sperm antigen of *D. viviparus* are used to identify infection in individuals and groups of lactating cows.

Necropsy findings in fatal cases vary with the stage of infection. In early prepatent infections, microscopic examination of bronchial exudate may be necessary to identify larvae, but in later prepatent infections, the larvae are obvious if the airways are properly opened and inspected. Eosinophilic bronchitis may be confirmed by histopathology. Patent infections are obvious because large numbers of mature parasites up to 8.0 cm in length are found in the airways (Fig. 4.72). Secondary anterior ventral bacterial

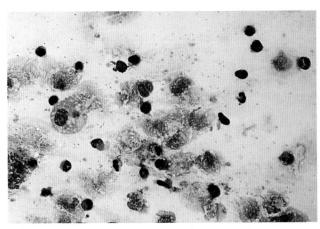

• **Fig. 4.71** Wright-Giemsa stain of tracheal wash from a cow representative of a herd problem of chronic cough and decreased production. Lungworms (*Dictyocaulus viviparus*) were found to be the cause of the disease. The large number of eosinophils on this 40X slide is highly suggestive of lungworm infection.

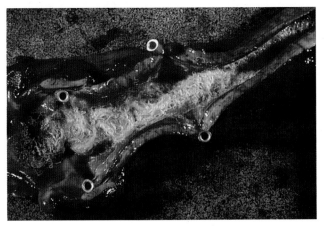

• **Fig. 4.72** Necropsy specimen of trachea from fatal lungworm infection in a calf showing hundreds of *Dictyocaulus viviparus* lungworms. (Courtesy of Dr. John Perdrizet.)

bronchopneumonia may be present, and interstitial emphysema is observed in occasional severe cases. In postpatent infections, chronic bronchitis, bronchiectasis, and secondary bronchiolitis obliterans may be observed.

The reinfection syndrome is characterized by clinical signs of severe coughing in the majority of cattle after their introduction to infected pastures. Tracheal wash samples will reveal eosinophilic inflammation. It is important to note that Baermann's technique will yield negative results. Necropsy lesions in the reinfection syndrome consist of small greenish-gray subpleural nodules, green exudate occluding small airways, and occasional green tinting of the interlobular septa. Histologically, eosinophils predominate, but lymphocytes, plasma cells, macrophages, and giant cells may be observed within the airways.

Treatment

Treatment of primary *D. viviparus* infection consists of an anthelmintic to destroy the parasite and, when necessary, antibiotic therapy to control secondary bacterial infection of the lower airway.

Levamisole phosphate (8 mg/kg body weight, SC or orally), fenbendazole (5 mg/kg orally), albendazole (10 mg/kg orally), and ivermectin (0.2 mg/kg SC) all have been recommended as treatments for primary *D. viviparus* infection in the past. Moxidectin (0.5 mg/kg) and eprinomectin (1 mL/10 kg) as pour-on preparations should also be effective and are currently approved for dairy cattle in the United States. Levamisole has been very effective in our clinics but is no longer approved for use in dairy cattle. Affected cattle should not be allowed back on infected pastures, and confined cattle should be removed from infected manure packs until the pens can be cleaned completely of manure and bedding. Anthelmintic resistance among nematodes in ruminant populations is of increasing concern worldwide, particularly in the more temperate areas where lungworms are more of a consistent problem in pastured dairy cattle. When we have encountered lungworm as a clinical entity in the northern United States, resistance to either the avermectins or benzimidazoles has not appeared to be a significant problem.

Because the most common secondary bacterial invader is *P. multocida*, patients with bacterial bronchopneumonia may be treated with tetracycline, ceftiofur, ampicillin, or penicillin. Secondary bacterial pneumonia may mask the presence of lungworms in calves or heifers. Such animals frequently appear to improve temporarily while on antibiotic therapy but then quickly relapse when antibiotics are withdrawn. Antibiotic therapy in these instances may cause resolution of fever and improved attitude but will not alleviate coughing or severe dyspnea. Only when further diagnostics are pursued in live patients or necropsies are performed in fatal cases will the true diagnosis be obtained and effective treatment instituted.

Although the reinfection syndrome appears to be an immune-mediated disorder, affected cattle appear to respond rapidly to levamisole injections, according to Breeze. Without treatment, continued coughing and production losses persist in the affected animals for weeks.

Control

Control of *D. viviparus* infections requires management decisions regarding contaminated pastures. Because infective larvae have been shown to survive winter conditions, pastures should not be grazed in the early spring. Before being pastured, yearling heifers should be treated with anthelmintics effective against *D. viviparus*, and all animals should be treated routinely with anthelmintics at monthly intervals if the animals are to be placed on contaminated pastures. Targeted strategic anthelminthic treatments are sometimes used in endemic areas in efforts to reduce the development of anthelminthic resistance rather than automatic, repeated deworming based on a calendar date. This approach would also be of benefit from the perspective of diminishing drug resistance among conventional GI nematodes such as *Ostertagia* because on most occasions, deworming treatments during the grazing season try to control multiple nematode populations. Moisture promotes survival and activity of infective larvae. Highlighting this fact, clinical lungworm infections in the northern United States are observed primarily during wet summers. We have seen it as a herd problem in grazing herds, especially when pasture burdens build up during the late summer months from infected heifers and adult cows become reinfected when grazing those same pastures. Similarly, we have observed outbreaks in the lactating herd when they were allowed to graze pasture that had been fertilized with manure from replacement heifers. Whenever possible, extreme care and additional anthelmintic treatment are indicated during wet summers and when animals are pastured in swampy, low-level endemic areas. The use of an irradiated live *D. viviparus* vaccine has been an integral part of lungworm control in other areas of the world for many years but does not form part of the routine vaccination program for dairy cattle in the United States. Increased confinement of cattle in the U.S. dairy industry will likely make this disease less and less common in future years.

Ascaris lumbricoides

Etiology and Signs

Although reported rarely, *Ascaris lumbricoides*, the swine ascarid, has been identified as a natural and experimental cause of pneumonia in cattle. Exposure of susceptible cattle to large numbers of larvae occurs when the cattle are placed in bedded pens, corrals, or poor-quality pastures previously used by pigs.

Clinical signs consisting of elevated temperature, elevated respiratory and heart rates, marked dyspnea, coughing, and an expiratory grunt develop 7 to 14 days after the cattle are exposed to ascarid ova. Auscultation of the lungs may reflect interstitial changes of pulmonary edema and emphysema. Therefore initial increased bronchovesicular sounds may be replaced by decreased sounds as further interstitial pathology and emphysema ensue. The clinical course lasts 10 to 14 days in most cases and occasionally may be fatal.

One experimental study suggested that initial exposure to ascarid larvae resulted in very mild signs, but reexposure resulted in pronounced signs. This may imply an immune-mediated cause or component to the severe interstitial pneumonia.

Diagnosis

Diagnosis of this disease is difficult unless historical information leads to suspicion of exposure to *A. lumbricoides* ova. A tracheal wash sample may demonstrate an eosinophilic inflammatory pattern. Definitive diagnosis requires identification of the parasite or histopathology to reveal the larvae and associated interstitial pneumonia.

Treatment

Treatment is nonspecific and supportive in the hope that the normal life cycle of the parasite will eliminate the larvae. Prevention involves avoidance of environments used by swine.

Caudal Vena Caval Thrombosis and Respiratory Diseases Related to Liver Abscessation

Etiology and Signs

Caudal vena caval thrombosis (CVCT) results in a variety of clinical respiratory syndromes in cattle. The origin is most commonly septic thromboemboli originating from an abscess

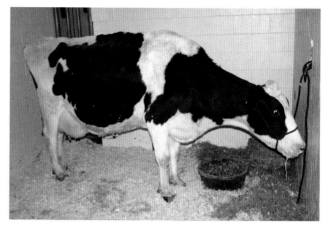

• **Fig. 4.73** A 5-year-old Holstein cow with caudal vena caval thrombosis syndrome associated with a large, nonhepatic, abdominal abscess. The cow presented with open-mouth breathing in respiratory distress.

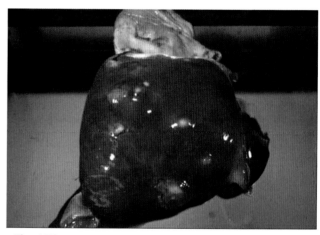

• **Fig. 4.74** Multiple hepatic abscesses that were an incidental finding at postmortem in an adult dairy cow. Abscesses, although multiple, were small and located well away from the hilus. No evidence of embolic showering to other sites was evident at postmortem.

at the hilus of the liver showering the caudal vena cava, right heart, and pulmonary arterial circulation. Potentially, other septic foci that are nonhepatic in origin, such as abdominal abscesses caused by hardware (Fig. 4.73) and deep digital sepsis, can also be the source of the thromboembolic showering. Although most cattle do not show signs of illness when the shower occurs, some cattle experience acute death from massive pulmonary infarction or have an acute onset of profound respiratory distress at the time of a thromboembolic episode. Cattle that have inapparent seeding of the pulmonary arteries or survive an acute respiratory distress episode caused by thromboemboli may eventually develop dyspnea, hemoptysis, and anemia. Epistaxis is the most common clinical sign observed in those cows with hemoptysis.

The classic pathogenesis of CVCT starts in the forestomach or abomasum and involves inflammatory or ulcerative mucosal lesions that allow bacterial seeding of the portal circulation with subsequent formation of liver abscesses. Therefore rumenitis, ruminal acidosis, abomasal ulcers, and similar disorders predispose to the condition. This same pathogenesis is responsible for "sawdust livers" in feedlot beef animals, but in dairy cattle, the abscesses usually are larger and fewer in number. Many dairy cattle have only one abscess. The location is much more important than the number of abscesses, however, because only those at the hilus of the liver or adjacent to the post cava represent significant risk (Fig. 4.74). *F. necrophorum* and *T. pyogenes* are the most common organisms isolated from liver abscesses in dairy cattle. Most cattle with liver abscesses show no clinical signs of illness unless an abscess erodes into the vena cava or multiple large abscesses develop. This disease occurs sporadically in heifers and adult cattle but is rare in calves. This may be the result of calves being fed less intensive diets than heifers or lactating animals.

In CVCT, erosion of a liver abscess into the vena cava with formation of a septic venous thrombosis instigates the clinical disease, and the affected cow may show one of the following syndromes.

Sudden Death Syndrome

Acute rupture of a liver abscess into the caudal vena cava may result in massive release of thromboemboli to the right heart and subsequent pulmonary artery thrombosis, pulmonary infarction, exotoxemia or endotoxemia, and anoxia. Sudden death may result, and this syndrome represents one of the more common causes of acute death in adult dairy cattle. The possibility that this is a potential cause of death with few to no premonitory signs should be kept in mind when performing a field necropsy on an adult cow that has unexpectedly died. Close attention to the perihilar area of the liver and the caudal vena cava should always be part of a thorough gross pathological examination in such cases. This sudden death may represent a hypersensitivity reaction after a previous clinically inapparent thromboembolic episode; however, sudden rupture of a large hilar abscess into the caudal vena cava or embolic movement of an existing large septic thrombus may cause enough direct pulmonary infarction to cause death without the need for a previous sensitizing episode. *F. necrophorum* toxins have also been shown to aggregate cattle platelets, and this may play some role in the development of thrombosis in this condition.

Acute Respiratory Distress Syndrome

This syndrome appears in one animal within a group or herd. The affected cow has peracute onset of respiratory distress, fever, labored breathing, and increased respiratory and heart rates. Pulmonary edema, SC emphysema, and open-mouth breathing also may be observed. Auscultation of the thorax generally reveals reduced airway sounds resulting from pulmonary edema, pulmonary infarction, and bullous emphysema brought on by exertional respiratory efforts. Rales may be auscultated in some instances, but in general, the lungs are quieter than expected given the obviously labored respirations. The key to diagnosis is the fact that only one animal is affected with severe lower airway disease, and to the owner's knowledge, the cow has had no unique stress or previous problems.

Hemoptysis, Epistaxis, Chronic Pneumonia, Anemia Syndrome

This classic syndrome is associated with CVCT in cattle and results from singular or multiple episodes of thromboembolism from the hilar liver abscess and subsequent

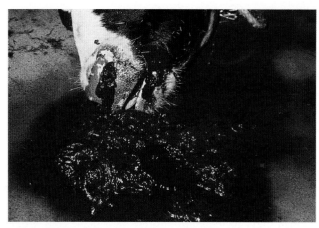

• **Fig. 4.75** Massive pulmonary hemorrhage and acute death in a 3-year-old Holstein cow with hepatic-pulmonary abscesses. The cow was calving when the hemorrhage occurred.

septic thrombosis originating in the caudal vena cava. Septic thromboemboli create pulmonary abscesses at their endpoint in pulmonary arteries, and aneurysms develop proximal to each of these abscesses within the affected pulmonary arteries. Because the pulmonary arterial branches in cattle course close to bronchi, eventual enlargement of the abscesses predisposes to their rupture into airways. Sudden discharge of purulent material into the airway creates septic bronchopneumonia followed immediately by minor or major hemorrhage from the arterial aneurysm now communicating directly into the airway. This hemorrhage may be sufficient to result in hemoptysis and subsequent epistaxis. Affected cattle are unthrifty and frequently have been treated for recurrent bronchopneumonia characterized by fever (103.0° to 106.0°F [39.44° to 41.11°C]), increased respiratory rate, as well as auscultable rales, crackles, or wheezes within localized areas of the lung. Some affected cattle develop endocarditis caused by the septic thrombus in the caudal vena cava persisting as a source of chronic bacteremia through the right heart and pulmonary arteries.

Epistaxis or hemoptysis may be slight and intermittent or may be profound and acute and result in sudden death (Fig. 4.75). Curiously, it seems quite often the case that the appearance of the blood at the nares and mouth in such cases is a vivid, arterial red—a paradoxical finding given that the described pathophysiology involves aneurysmal damage to the pulmonary arterial circulation, which is, of course, the only arterial part of the circulation with a low oxygen tension. Perhaps the close anatomic proximity of the bronchial arteries to the pulmonary circulation or potential extension of pulmonary abscesses into the venous side of the pulmonary capillary network explains the apparent arterial blood loss. Epistaxis associated with coughing and chronic bronchopneumonia in dairy cattle indicates an extremely guarded prognosis because of the irreversible nature of the pathology in CVCT. Other signs such as ascites, generalized visceral edema, and diarrhea are possible if the thrombosis occludes the caudal vena cava and results in portal hypertension. Right heart failure and chronic passive congestion of the liver may also develop in some chronic cases.

Diagnosis of Sudden Death Syndrome

The diagnosis of CVCT requires careful necropsy when sudden death results. In general, affected animals have appeared completely healthy before death. Only one animal is affected in the herd, and the suddenness of death precludes physical examination or ancillary laboratory data. Necropsy will typically reveal a hilar liver abscess with rupture into the caudal vena cava (Figs. 4.76 and 4.77). The lungs may show bullous emphysema, pulmonary edema, pulmonary infarction, and pulmonary arterial thrombosis.

Diagnosis of Acute Respiratory Distress Syndrome

Sudden onset of respiratory distress in a single cow within a herd raises an index of suspicion of acute CVCT. History and physical examination findings should be used to exclude other causes of severe lower airway disease and acute respiratory distress, although this can be challenging. An elevated serum globulin level (>5.0 g/dL) further raises the index of suspicion but cannot confirm the diagnosis. Thoracic radiography, although not widely available in practice, is very helpful to the diagnosis because it usually demonstrates focal or multifocal pulmonary infarction and densities resulting from septic emboli, diffuse pulmonary edema, and bullous emphysema. An enlargement of the thoracic vena cava between the cardiac silhouette and the diaphragm may also be detected radiographically. In field situations, the affected cow is treated symptomatically and gradually may improve over 5 to 10 days. Subsequently, however, these animals usually develop hemoptysis, epistaxis, anemia, and chronic pneumonia typical of the classic signs associated with CVCT. The average lag phase between improvement from the acute syndrome and the onset of epistaxis is 3 to 6 weeks.

Diagnosis of Classical Caudal Vena Caval Thrombosis with Epistaxis, Hemoptysis, Anemia, and Chronic Bronchopneumonia

This form remains the most common clinical syndrome of CVCT. Elevated heart rate, increased respiratory rate, auscultatable rales, persistent or recurrent fever, anemia, and hemoptysis are frequent signs. The owner may have observed epistaxis on several occasions or only once (Figs. 4.78 and 4.79). Some affected cattle bleed out acutely with few premonitory signs. A heart murmur caused by anemia or endocarditis may be present. On rare occasions, generalized edema of the hind parts, ventrum, and udder, as well as ascites may be present in some animals. If edema is generalized, diarrhea caused by GI edema is often also observed. Frequently, serum globulin (>5.0 g/dL) and fibrinogen (>600 mg/dL) are elevated, and a neutrophilic leukocytosis may be present in the hemogram. Thoracic radiography or ultrasonography is helpful in identifying distinct pulmonary abscesses. Transabdominal ultrasonography of the right 8th through 12th ICSs can be useful to identify liver abscesses and allows visualization of the hilus and abdominal caudal vena cava close to the hilus. The causative thrombus may be lodged

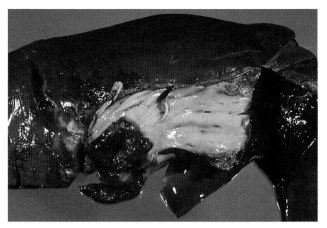

• **Fig. 4.76** Necropsy specimen from a cow that died from rupture of a hilar liver abscess into the postcava. The site of rupture into the postcava is apparent as a rough-edged crater highlighted against the intima of the vein. The purulent remnants of the abscess appear to the left of the crater. (Courtesy of Dr. John M. King.)

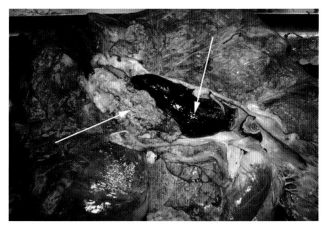

• **Fig. 4.77** Necropsy of a 6-year-old Holstein cow euthanized for severe epistaxis, weight loss, and poor production. Note the large friable abscess *(left arrow)* between the liver and extending through the diaphragm alongside a massive, adherent thrombus *(right arrow)* within the caudal vena cava.

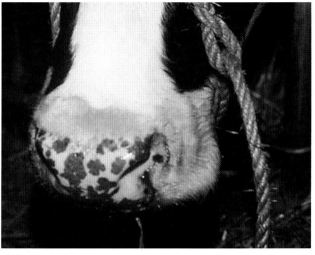

• **Fig. 4.78** Slight epistaxis that was intermittently observed in a cow with caudal vena caval thrombosis.

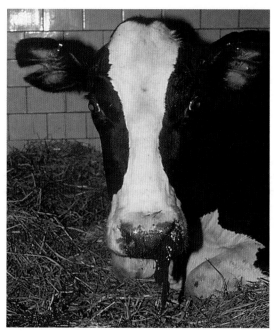

• **Fig. 4.79** Severe epistasis and hemoptysis in a Holstein with caudal vena caval thrombosis (CVCT) that survived for 3 months after initial diagnosis.

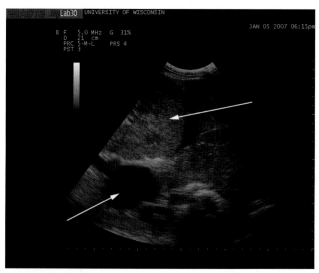

• **Fig. 4.80** Transabdominal ultrasound image of 4-year-old Holstein cow with caudal vena caval thrombosis syndrome. Note the large hepatic abscess *(upper arrow)* and prominent, enlarged caudal vena cava *(lower arrow)* measuring approximately 7 cm in diameter at its widest.

in the caudal vena cava and may also sometimes be visualized ultrasonographically or else its presence inferred by significant intrahepatic vessel enlargement on ultrasonography alongside an increase in the diameter of the perihilar vena cava (normal diameter, 2–5 cm) (Figs. 4.80 and 4.81 and see Video Clip 4.14). Thoracic radiography assists in identifying the severity of pulmonary pathology and may also identify an enlargement of the thoracic vena cava close to the diaphragm in cases of CVCT (Fig. 4.82). Endoscopy will help confirm the origin of hemorrhage in the lower airway and will allow collection of tracheal wash material for cytology and culture if desired.

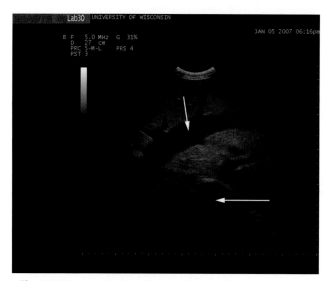

• **Fig. 4.81** Transabdominal ultrasound image of the same cow as in Fig. 4.80 demonstrating prominent, distended intrahepatic vasculature *(upper arrow)* and vena cava *(lower arrow)* caused by a thrombus that was obstructing the caudal vena cava.

Treatment

Therapy for CVCT causing acute respiratory distress is symptomatic and includes:
- Broad-spectrum antibiotics such as oxytetracycline, ceftiofur, or penicillin to control septic thromboemboli. *F. necrophorum* and *T. pyogenes* are the primary organisms found in these abscesses
- Furosemide (250–500 mg IM twice daily per adult animal) if pulmonary edema is present
- Atropine (2.2 mg/45 kg body weight SC twice daily) as a supportive bronchodilator and to dry bronchial secretions
- Aspirin or another NSAID in standard dosages as an antiinflammatory drug. Initially, flunixin meglumine may be used (250–500 mg/450 kg body weight) to counteract possible endotoxemia.

If improvement is observed, the animal should be maintained on long-term antibiotics in the hope that the septic thromboemboli may be sterilized. Rifampin may be added to improve antibiotic penetration, but this represents extralabel drug use and is expensive. Currently, in the United States, the use of rifampin also requires the client to guarantee that neither milk nor meat from that individual will be sold for human consumption, making its use very rare. The prognosis is poor because a large thrombus tends to persist in the caudal vena cava, and constant or intermittent embolic showering is likely to continue. Few cattle have survived long term.

Treatment of CVCT with classic signs of pneumonia, epistaxis, hemoptysis, and anemia seldom is worthwhile because of the extensive pathology that exists. Valuable cattle may be treated with long-term penicillin (22,000 U/kg IM twice daily) and aspirin (240–480 grains/450 kg body weight orally twice daily). Aspirin therapy would be contraindicated in cattle that have already exhibited epistaxis. Penicillin is the antibiotic of choice, given the causative organisms, and aspirin may be safe for long-term use in an effort to discourage

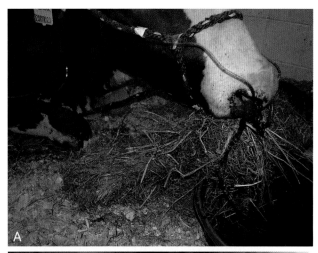

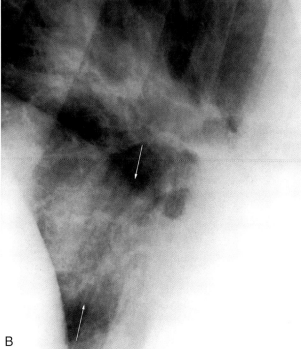

• **Fig. 4.82** Mature Red and White Holstein bull with caudal vena caval thrombosis syndrome presented with marked epistaxis (**A**) and with very enlarged thoracic vena cava on thoracic radiographs (vessel is outlined by *arrows*) (**B**).

further platelet aggregation and thrombosis. When epistaxis has been observed and confirmed to originate from the lower airway, the prognosis is extremely guarded. Attempted therapy may be worthwhile in extremely valuable cattle in the hope that only a few pulmonary arterial abscesses have developed, giving the cow a chance to survive. However, it is rare for a cow with well-defined signs of CVCT to survive. Cattle with CVCT and hemoptysis/epistaxis generally do not survive more than 3 weeks once bleeding is noted.

Control

Prevention or control of CVCT in cattle involves nutritional changes. Highly acidic diets that predispose to clinical or subclinical rumenitis and abomasal ulceration have to be tempered by buffers, prefeeding hay before high-energy

grains such as high moisture corn, or most commonly by feeding total mixed rations. Dairy rations should not be fed to yearling or bred heifers. High production herds are most at risk for rumenitis and abomasal ulceration secondary to intensive feeding of high-energy, acidic diets. Most cattle with liver abscesses are asymptomatic, and those having hilar abscesses that go on to develop CVCT probably suffered initiation of the pathophysiology months to years before the onset of clinical signs. When more than an occasional case of CVCT appears in a herd, immediate evaluation of the herd's nutritional program is in order. One cow in a herd with CVCT is unfortunate but a common clinical problem. More than one cow in the same herd with CVCT, however, signals a potential serious economic loss and requires changes in the feeding program. Evaluation of the herd for subacute rumen acidosis is indicated under these circumstances and is described in Chapter 5.

Inhalation Pneumonia

Etiology and Signs

Inhalation pneumonia occurs when feed materials, milk, or medications enter the trachea; the animal fails to clear the airways of the material; and septic bronchopneumonia ensues. In calves, white muscle disease and iatrogenic inhalation pneumonia are the two most common causes. White muscle disease caused by selenium or vitamin E deficiency may affect the tongue, muscles of mastication, or muscles involved in swallowing and predispose to inhalation of milk or milk replacer as the affected calf tries to drink. White muscle disease may on rare occasion cause similar problems in adult cattle. Iatrogenic inhalation pneumonia in calves follows inadvertent intubation of the trachea with stomach tubes or esophageal feeders or, more commonly, from use of abnormally large holes on the end of nipple bottles that overwhelm the calf's ability to swallow and "flood" the airway. Nipple bottles used to feed calves should only drip milk when the bottle is turned upside down! Prematurity or dysmaturity may also predispose to inhalation pneumonia as a result of incompletely developed laryngeal protective reflexes (Fig. 4.83). Bottle feeding weak calves while recumbent is another common cause of aspiration pneumonia. Inhalation pneumonia may also occur from oral dosing of large volumes of medication (e.g., Pepto-Bismol, mineral oil) with the head held in an elevated position. Inhalation pneumonia also may follow pharyngeal trauma by stomach tubes, esophageal feeders, or balling guns, resulting in dysphagia or neurogenic swallowing deficits. Crude or neophytic use of stomach tubes, feeders, and balling guns by laypeople causes most iatrogenic inhalation pneumonia. Inhalation pneumonia may also occur from aspiration of meconium often associated with a prolonged dystocia (Fig. 4.84).

In adult cattle, milk fever (parturient hypocalcemia) is the most common cause of inhalation pneumonia. A severely hypocalcemic cow not only is recumbent but also may lie in lateral recumbency and thus become bloated. Regurgitation of rumen ingesta may lead to inhalation because the cow's

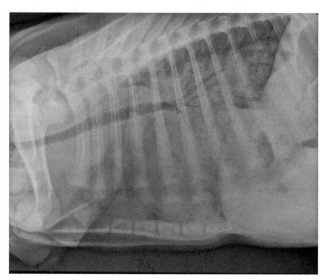

• **Fig. 4.83** Severe aspiration and inhalation pneumonia in a 4-day-old neonatal Brown Swiss calf that had been delivered after protracted dystocia. Thoracic radiographs show severe ventral, consolidating bronchopneumonia consistent with aspiration. The calf had been unable to stand since birth, was tube fed 2 L of colostrum in lateral recumbency, and was then allowed to nurse in recumbency for the next four feedings. It had become progressively more dyspneic but had coughed very little.

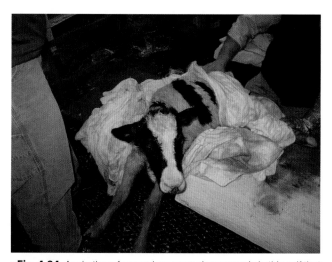

• **Fig. 4.84** Aspiration of meconium caused pneumonia in this calf that was delivered after a prolonged dystocia. Clinical signs of pneumonia began on day 2.

semicomatose state prevents her from clearing the regurgitated ingesta from her pharynx and airway.

Pharyngeal trauma caused by stomach tubes, magnet retrievers, and balling guns may injure vagal nerve branches traversing the pharynx. This neurogenic injury may lead to dysphagia and to defective eructation and regurgitation and may predispose to inhalation pneumonia. Inadvertent intubation of the trachea during attempts at stomach tubing by an unskilled person creates a significant risk of inhalation in adult cattle as in calves. Choke, although rare in dairy cattle today, certainly represents a significant predisposing cause of inhalation pneumonia as well. Cattle that have choked on vegetables or other feedstuffs should be assessed carefully

for early signs of inhalation pneumonia. Occasionally, cattle in dorsal recumbency for surgery, whether under sedation or general anesthesia, may regurgitate and inhale feed material into the trachea and lower airways. Consideration of this potential outcome when deciding on a surgical approach in a high-risk patient makes obvious sense. For general anesthesia, the selection of an endotracheal tube with the correct diameter can help preserve and protect the airway, and holding the cow off feed for at least 24 hours before performing elective surgery in dorsal recumbency may also diminish the risk of aspiration.

Neurologic disease constitutes another potential cause of inhalation pneumonia in cattle. Listeriosis and other diseases that affect the cranial nerves involved in deglutition, mastication, and swallowing food predispose to inhalation pneumonia, although our experience is that aspiration pneumonia associated with listeriosis has rarely caused a clinical problem. Botulism represents an intoxication that may lead to inhalation pneumonia secondary to dysphagia.

Signs of inhalation vary with the relative volume and content of the inhaled material. For example, inadvertent administration of a large volume of fluid into the trachea results in immediate signs of dyspnea, respiratory distress, cyanosis, and repeated coughing. The affected calf or cow will often expel some of the material from the nose or mouth as a frothy liquid before dying within minutes to hours. Smaller volumes of milk (calves with white muscle disease) or feed inhaled into the lower airway cause a septic bronchopneumonia as the microorganisms contained in the causative material proliferate. In this instance, signs are progressive in nature and consist of a fever poorly responsive to antibiotics, dyspnea, rapid respirations, and rales or bronchial tones in both anterior ventral lung fields (unless the animal was in lateral recumbency at the time of inhalation, in which case the major portion of the pathology may occur in only one lung). Rather than groups of animals being affected, as is typical with contagious pneumonia, only an individual animal tends to be affected with inhalation pneumonia. However, when groups of calves are affected with white muscle disease, several calves may be affected with inhalation pneumonia simultaneously. Individual cattle with inhalation of rumen ingesta secondary to milk fever or other problems develop a progressive gangrenous pneumonia with fever, dyspnea, and toxemia. Rapid consolidation of affected lung tissue occurs, and bronchial tones and rales may be auscultated, usually in the cranioventral lung fields.

Radiography, if available, will often demonstrate a classic ventral distribution to the consolidating bronchopneumonia due to inhalation, both cranial and caudal to the cardiac silhouette (Fig. 4.85). In the severest cases, the radiographic lesions may be more diffuse and severe (see Fig. 4.83). Broad-spectrum antibiotic therapy is effective only if the amount of ingesta inhaled was relatively small. In most instances, the course is one of progressive deterioration over several days, ending in death. Sometimes inhalation of saliva or small amounts of water or feed as a result of dysphagia is treatable with broad-spectrum antibiotic therapy. We have

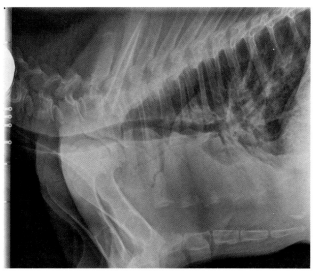

• **Fig. 4.85** Moderate aspiration and inhalation pneumonia in a 9-day-old Holstein calf presented for diarrhea. Radiographs demonstrate consolidating bronchopneumonia cranial and caudal to the cardiac silhouette.

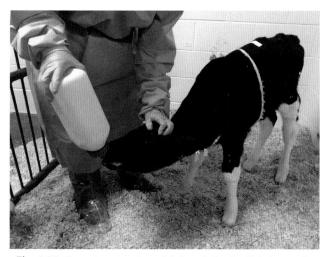

• **Fig. 4.86** Correct posture for a sick, hospitalized calf during nursing. Note the pressure on the calf's poll region to maintain orientation of the head and neck parallel to the ground. Many calves resist this as they recover, wanting to orient the head more perpendicularly, consistent with the orientation of the bottle.

had the best results with cattle that develop some degree of inhalation pneumonia secondary to dysphagia induced by pharyngeal trauma. Because the amount of inhaled material usually is unknown, treatment is indicated unless the animal shows profound dyspnea and cyanosis in which case euthanasia should be elected.

Treatment

Therapy for inhalation pneumonia involves broad-spectrum antibiotics directed against the microbes normally present in the material inhaled. NSAIDs also would be indicated for supportive therapy. Antibiotic therapy should be continued for at least 2 weeks if symptomatic improvement occurs. Persistent fever, depression, dyspnea, and toxemia are negative signs and generally signal a fatal outcome. Cattle with any form of dysphagia should be fed off the ground to lessen the risk of aspiration. In the event of meconium aspiration in a neonate, a single dose of dexamethasone (5 mg/50 kg calf) may be given alongside antimicrobial and other supportive therapy (eg; oxygen if available).

Prevention

Inhalation of certain necrotizing or nonabsorbable chemicals (e.g., mineral oil) is uniformly fatal, and treatment is not indicated. Prevention of inhalation pneumonia can be practiced only when the problem is anticipated and is largely a matter of common sense. Therefore, withdrawing feed from animals with choke, dysphagia, and other known problems may be helpful. Prompt treatment of milk fever or other diseases that may prevent an adult cow from maintaining sternal recumbency is important in preventing aspiration pneumonia. Management practices such as routine or therapeutic drenching of postparturient cattle should only be performed by laypeople who have been properly trained

and provided with appropriate equipment. The feeding of milk to weak, recumbent, premature, or dysmature calves should also be predicated on common sense and an awareness that normal protective airway reflexes may be overcome by impatient feeding practices (e.g., enlarging holes in nipples) or by allowing these calves to nurse with the head and neck hyperextended or dorsiflexed, as appears to be their instinctive habit. Feeding from buckets or a bottle with the head and neck in a neutral position parallel to the ground can lessen the risk of inhalation (Fig. 4.86).

Thermal and Chemical Damage to the Lower Airway

Etiology and Signs

Barn fires and occasionally grass fires in pastures are responsible for thermal and smoke injury to the respiratory tract in cattle. Chemical damage may be mild, as a result of common gases such as ammonia, or severe, as in accidental exposure to anhydrous ammonia.

Thermal damage resulting from excessive heat and smoke inhalation has been well described for comparative species. The pathophysiology involves heat-induced edema and necrosis of the mucosal lining; pulmonary edema and congestion; destruction of the mucociliary apparatus; hyaline membrane formation; and filling of the small airways with proteinaceous fluid, sloughing tissue in the form of diphtheritic membranes, hyaline membranes, and inflammatory cell debris (Fig. 4.87). Pathology tends to be progressive with increasing dyspnea as small airway occlusion develops hours to days after the original thermal and smoke insult. Therefore it is difficult to estimate the severity of the lesions immediately after the fire. Dyspnea characterized by an increased respiratory rate may be the only sign. Cattle with obvious facial burns, muzzle burns, or diphtheritic crusts in the nasal

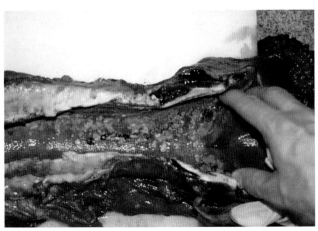

• **Fig. 4.87** Postmortem specimen of trachea from a cow that had died from smoke inhalation during a barn fire. Note the severe tracheal mucosal erosions and diphtheritic damage.

cavity should be suspected of having sustained significant smoke inhalation. Pulmonary edema is an early sign of severe thermal damage and suggests that subsequent pathology with hyaline membrane formation will follow. Other signs in severely affected animals include cough, tachypnea, wheezing, cyanosis, and stridor. In severe cases, respiratory distress will develop 1 to 24 hours after the initial injury, and bacterial bronchopneumonia may develop within 1 to 4 days in cattle that survive the initial thermal injury. Carbon monoxide poisoning is a common cause of death for animals at the time of the fire or shortly thereafter.

Chemical damage resulting from high environmental concentrations of ammonia largely reflects poor management or inadequate ventilation within an enclosure. Excessive buildup of manure and urine without adequate ventilation will allow ammonia fumes to damage the physical defense mechanisms of the lower airway. Secondary bacterial pneumonias are the most common sequelae to this problem. The relevance of ventilation to the prevalence of calf pneumonia in housed calves during the winter months in the northern United States is increasingly evident. The aerial microenvironment and air quality does not have to deteriorate to the level at which the human nose or eyes are irritated for there to be a significant and detrimental impact on the amount and severity of respiratory disease, especially in preweaned calves. During many investigations of calfhood pneumonia over the past decade, the issues of air quality and inadequate passive transfer have proven consistently to be the two most important drivers of respiratory disease in the first 8 weeks of life (see earlier section).

We have also observed a progressive increase in respiratory rate in some hospitalized cattle that have their bedding changed frequently and are kept in deeply bedded stalls for 2 weeks or more. This has occurred in all seasons of the year and does not seem to be simply temperature related. There is no coughing, and tracheal washes have not revealed a cause for the tachypnea. If the cows are put outside, the respiratory rates return to normal in 1 to 3 days.

Anhydrous ammonia is an extremely dangerous chemical that is widely used in agriculture today. It is used as a source of nonprotein nitrogen for forages and fertilization of various crops. The chemical seeks out water when it comes in contact with vegetable matter or tissue. Accidental exposure to anhydrous ammonia can be lethal to animals or humans who come in contact with the material. Because of the intense water affinity of the chemical, anhydrous ammonia seeks moist tissues such as the eye and respiratory tract. As a result of this contact, moist tissue rapidly desiccates followed by necrosis as the chemical dehydrates the tissue. Corneal edema, epithelial necrosis, and corneal stromal burns immediately develop in the eyes. The mucosa of the respiratory tract is burned, and after dehydration, sloughs and diphtheritic membranes fill the airways, leading to hypoxia or suffocation. Pulmonary edema develops rapidly, and death may occur peracutely or be delayed by hours or a few days. Secondary bacterial pneumonias are possible if the animal survives the initial chemical injury.

Insecticides that are fogged into barns for fly control occasionally may induce chemical damage or sensitivity within the lower airway. The exact mechanism of action is not fully understood, but tachypnea, coughing, and mild dyspnea may be observed.

Diagnosis

The diagnosis of thermal or chemical injury is made by the history and physical examination findings. Ancillary information seldom is necessary. Endoscopy and thoracic radiography may provide prognostic information for valuable animals but seldom are used in practice.

Treatment

Major treatment considerations for acute thermal injury of the airway include improved oxygenation and establishment of an adequate airway. If laryngeal edema is so severe as to result in respiratory distress, a tracheostomy may be necessary. A tracheostomy should not be performed unless severe upper respiratory distress is present because the procedure further predisposes to secondary bacterial bronchopneumonia in burn patients. Oxygen administration is indicated if acute dyspnea suggests possible carbon monoxide poisoning.

Judicious dosages of furosemide (25–50 mg/45 kg body weight) may be necessary if pulmonary edema is present. Use of corticosteroids for acute pulmonary distress caused by thermal injury is controversial. Steroids have been proposed as initial therapy to "short cycle" parts of the vicious cycle of inflammation because they decrease mediators of inflammation, stabilize inflamed vasculature, and decrease edema of the upper and lower airway. If steroids are used, they should be given immediately rather than waiting for the subsequent pathology and respiratory distress that will follow thermal injury over the next 24 hours. A single, one-time "shock" dose of 0.1 to 1.0 mg/lb dexamethasone or 200 to 500 mg of prednisolone sodium succinate can be given. Abortifacient properties of dexamethasone need to be considered before it is used in pregnant animals, and a significant risk associated with the use of steroids in the form of possible secondary bronchopneumonia also must be considered. Dr. Rebhun commented that he had treated some barn fire victims with dexamethasone but that the results were hard to interpret.

In one valuable yearling bull, a high dose of corticosteroids was used initially without deleterious consequences, but the bull developed a left displacement of the abomasum within 24 hours of treatment. A cause-and-effect relationship for the exogenous corticosteroids on the displacement never was confirmed but certainly was suspicious. NSAIDs may be used at regular dosages without the additional specific risks presented by corticosteroids. However, NSAIDs probably do not block the ongoing pathophysiology of lower airway disease as effectively as corticosteroids. Prophylactic systemic antibiotics are reported not to influence the subsequent development of bacterial bronchopneumonia. Some literature regarding treatment of thermal and chemical injury to the respiratory tract in humans discourages the use of prophylactic antibiotics for fear of allowing resistant strains of bacteria to emerge in the lower airway. In cattle, especially valuable ones, broad-spectrum antibiotics usually are used on a prophylactic basis, although no controlled data support their use. Tetracyclines may help decrease inflammation via their inhibitory effect on metalloproteinases. Disadvantages of tetracyclines are that they are bacteriostatic, and many commensal organisms may be resistant to the drug. If used, practitioners should be aware of their potential to cause nephrotoxicity, particularly in hemodynamically challenged patients.

If tracheostomies or tracheal washes are performed, extreme care should be taken to minimize iatrogenic introduction of pathogens into the respiratory tract. As in thermal skin injury, *Pseudomonas* spp. and other opportunists are the major bacteria to invade damaged tissue.

Nebulization with antibiotics, bronchodilators, corticosteroids, acetylcysteine, or surfactant has also been used in affected cattle. Acetylcysteine has anticollagenase and antioxidant effects via its glutathione-promoting properties.

In chemical injury resulting from anhydrous ammonia, exposed animals and the entire environment should be sprayed with water to destroy residual fumes. Emergency personnel and fire companies should be summoned immediately so that gas masks and protective clothing are available for people spraying water in the area and repairing the leak. All humans in the area should move upwind and leave the area until the leak and fumes have been controlled. Cattle exposed but still alive should not be stressed and should be allowed immediate access to as much fresh air as possible. No specific treatment is possible. Symptomatic treatment may include furosemide, prophylactic antibiotics, or oxygen

therapy. Animals with chemically injured eyes should have topical antibiotic and atropine ointments applied to the eyes several times daily.

Mycotic Pneumonia

Etiology and Signs

Mycotic or fungal pneumonia usually results from embolic dissemination of fungal organisms from other infected organs such as the rumen, liver, abomasum, or mammary gland. Immunosuppression and immunosuppressive drugs (corticosteroids) predispose to fungal infection, as does intensive antibiotic therapy, which may deplete normal bacterial flora and promote fungal growth. Lactic acid indigestion (toxic rumenitis) remains one of the leading causes of mycotic pneumonia. Pathophysiology evolves from chemical rumenitis through bacterial rumenitis to subsequent mycotic rumenitis, especially if the affected cow has been treated with antibiotics. Embolic infection of the lungs ensues as a result of seeding of the portal circulation and liver from the primary ruminal infection. Similarly, fungal pneumonia has been observed as a sequela to severe septic mastitis in dairy cattle. Intensive antibiotic therapy and overzealous use of corticosteroids predisposed these animals to mycotic infections that became septicemic from the udder and then involved the lungs. Although *Aspergillus* spp. are the most common fungal organisms identified, theoretically any yeast or fungus could be causative.

Signs are nonspecific but consist of persistent fever that is unresponsive to antibiotics (104.0° to 108.0°F [40.0° to 42.2°C]), increased respiratory rate, and variable abnormal lung sounds in one or both lungs. The marked and persistent, often cyclical, fever and the lack of response to antimicrobials are key features of mycotic disease. Rales and increased or decreased bronchovesicular sounds may be heard in individual cases. A primary site of severe infection such as the mammary gland, forestomach, or uterus usually is apparent, or evident from the history, and the respiratory signs may be disregarded or difficult to identify consistently. Multiple organ failure and neurologic signs frequently coexist or develop because of the fungal septicemia. Occasional cases of disseminated fungal disease with fungal pneumonia can be seen in septicemic calves or calves with severe enteritis that have received extensive antibiotic or corticosteroid treatment; similar to adults, affected calves also tend to present with substantial fevers that have been persistent in the face of aggressive antimicrobial therapy.

Diagnosis

The diagnosis is difficult and at best may only be suspected before the death of the individual. Tracheal washings may identify the organisms during cytology or following culture procedures but also may be initially and erroneously disregarded as evidence of environmental upper airway contamination of the tracheal wash sample. However, as

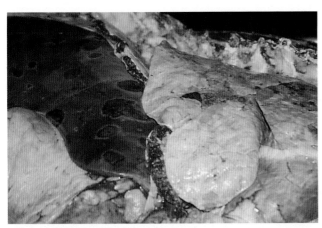

• **Fig. 4.88** Necropsy specimen showing mycotic hepatitis *(left)* and pneumonia *(right)* secondary to lactic acid indigestion. Mycotic lesions appear similar to "targets" with red centers and pale peripheries.

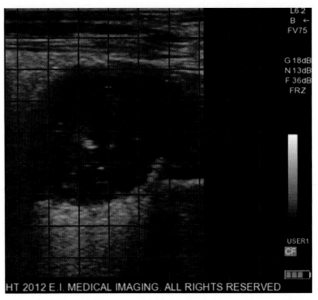

• **Fig. 4.89** Sonogram of caudal lung lobe abscess in 28-day-old Holstein bull calf. Note the mixed echogenicity to abscess content with some hyperechoic gas shadowing present within the luminal center of the lesion.

a generality, it is worth pointing out that cytologic demonstration of fungal elements on tracheal wash fluid is more commonly caused by sample contamination than true mycotic pneumonia.

Gross and histologic pathology confirms the diagnosis. Discolored multifocal areas of pneumonia are present grossly (Fig. 4.88), and hyphae are identified by histopathology.

Treatment

No successful treatment has been described for mycotic pneumonia in cattle, and the primary infection coupled with mycotic pneumonia or mycotic septicemia usually is fatal.

Prevention

Although intensive antibiotic therapy is necessary for certain infections in dairy cattle, practitioners should be aware that chronic localized infections in the udder, uterus, or GI tract that are treated with long-term antibiotics may predispose to yeast or fungal overgrowth and potential embolic spread. Repeated IV therapy by practitioners or laypeople using drugs from contaminated multidose vials also may lead to direct mycotic septicemia, such as occurs occasionally in human abusers of IV drugs.

High or repeated dosages of exogenous corticosteroids are to be condemned in dairy cattle and may represent the most dangerous drugs currently predisposing to fungal infections. There are few, if any, diseases in dairy cattle that require high doses of corticosteroids for effective therapy. Corticosteroid use as initial therapy for severe infectious/inflammatory diseases should not be repeated. The low dosages of corticosteroids (10–20 mg of dexamethasone) used by many veterinarians as daily treatment for ketosis generally are safe if limited to no more than 3 to 5 days but should not be used on several consecutive days in cattle with severe infections such as septic mastitis, septic metritis, pneumonia, or toxic rumenitis.

Space-Occupying Masses in the Thorax, Lung Parenchyma, or Lower Airway

Etiology and Signs

Space-occupying thoracic masses involving the lung parenchyma, visceral or parietal pleura, mediastinum or other structures in the thorax cause subtle or marked progressive dyspnea and may cause signs similar to congestive heart failure. Other clinical signs vary with specific lesions; for example, fever that is only partially or transiently responsive to conventional antibiotic treatment might be present in cattle affected with thoracic abscesses or pleuritis, but fever may not be present at all in thoracic or mediastinal neoplasia.

Inflammatory lesions include thoracic abscesses (Figs. 4.89 and 4.90) and pleuritis (Fig. 4.91, see also Video Clip 4.10). Thoracic abscesses usually are unilateral and when substantial in size may result in detectable absence of lung sounds in the affected ventral hemithorax. Whereas ipsilateral heart sounds may be absent or muffled, contralateral heart sounds are louder than normal and accentuated by the displaced heart's proximity to the contralateral thoracic wall. When small in size, whether single or multiple, thoracic abscesses may be much harder to diagnose; auscultation may not reveal their presence and diagnostic imaging (radiography and ultrasonography) becomes the most helpful diagnostic tool. Fever that is only partially responsive to antibiotics, progressive dyspnea, venous distention and pulsation of the jugular and mammary veins, ventral edema, and a reluctance to move are other signs observed in cattle affected with thoracic abscesses. Etiology of thoracic abscesses sometimes is unknown, but penetration of the thorax by reticular foreign bodies and localized enlarging pulmonary abscesses from previous pneumonia have been confirmed at necropsy in several

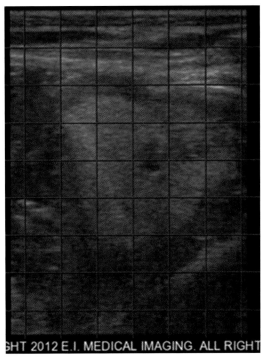

• **Fig. 4.90** Sonogram of the same caudal lung lobe abscess from the bull calf in Fig. 4.89 approximately 2 weeks later, showing more homogeneous appearance to abscess content, suggestive of inspissation.

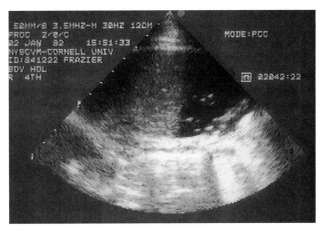

• **Fig. 4.91** Sonogram of the thorax of a cow with septic pleuritis. The white echogenic spots in the black fluid suggest anaerobic infection and gas production.

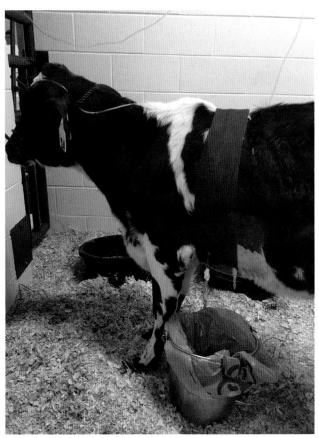

• **Fig. 4.92** A 4-month-old Milking Shorthorn heifer with aseptic pleural fluid being drained from the left hemithorax. Fluid accumulation was associated with pulmonary hypertension and signs of congestive heart failure.

fatal cases. Previous history of pneumonia or hardware disease may suggest the etiology in certain cases, but a specific etiology seldom is determined in surviving cattle. *T. pyogenes* is the organism isolated from most thoracic abscesses, either in isolation or in mixed infections involving gram-negative anaerobes such as *Fusobacterium* spp.

Pleuritis is rare in dairy cattle except when it accompanies severe consolidating bronchopneumonia of bacterial origin such as can occur with *Mannheimia haemolytica* pneumonia. As in other species, fever, progressive dyspnea, absence of lung sounds in the ventral thorax (unilateral or bilateral), and thoracic pain are typical. Although a fibrinous pleuritis with a low volume of free pleural fluid is more common in cattle,

when large amounts of pleural fluid are present, venous distention and apparent pulsations may be present in the jugular and mammary veins. Rare cases of pleuritis resulting from rupture of a parenchymal pulmonary abscess into the pleural space, penetrating thoracic wounds or foreign bodies associated with traumatic reticuloperitonitis, erosion of the diaphragm by an abscess associated with hardware or perforating abomasal ulcer, and rupture of the esophagus secondary to chronic choke or trauma also have been observed.

Pleural effusion may also occur with either nonseptic or septic pericarditis. We have had some patients with pericarditis and pleuritis in whom the cause could not be determined. In one cow with fibrinous pericarditis and pleuritis of mixed cytology on centesis (neutrophils, lymphocytes, plasma cells), a complete cure was achieved after pericardial injection of corticosteroids and systemic antibiotics. Although severe pleural effusion is not common in cattle with right heart failure, we have seen it in a few cases (Fig. 4.92). Pleural effusion of a mild to moderate volume does seem to be quite common in association with idiopathic hemorrhagic pericardial effusion, most likely caused by the cardiac tamponade that accompanies the sometimes massive volume of pericardial fluid. When pleural fluid accompanies pericardial effusion, cytologic evaluation of the two different cavity fluids is not always the same, emphasizing the relevance of pericardiocentesis in the evaluation of primary pericardial disease.

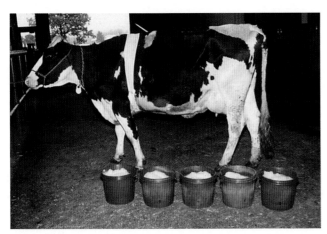

• **Fig. 4.93** A mature Holstein cow with a thoracic seroma or transudate secondary to traumatic injury at the costochondral region of the left thorax. A total of 40 L of transudative fluid had just been removed from the left hemithorax via thoracocentesis. The cow made a complete recovery.

Seromas and hematomas may develop after trauma to the thoracic wall. These masses occasionally extend into the thorax itself. In rare instances, apparent rupture or leakage of the seroma through the parietal pleura occurs. These seromas and hematomas may be associated with rib fractures or traumatic injuries at the costochondral junctions (Fig. 4.93). Dystocia can be a cause of these in neonatal calves. Signs may include progressive dyspnea, increased respiratory rate, venous distention and pulsation, normal temperature, absence of lung sounds ventrally in the affected hemithorax, absence or muffling of heart sounds in the affected hemithorax, and loud pounding heart sounds in the contralateral hemithorax caused by cardiac displacement.

Diaphragmatic hernias may cause dyspnea and absence of cardiopulmonary sounds in the affected thoracic area. Bloat is most commonly observed in cattle having diaphragmatic hernia because the reticulum is usually the herniated organ.

Neoplastic masses may occur in the pulmonary parenchyma, pleura, lymph nodes, or thymus. Cardiac neoplasms are discussed with other cardiac diseases in Chapter 3. Thymic lymphosarcoma may be the most obvious neoplasm within this group. Thymic lymphosarcoma is recognized in cattle between 4 and 24 months of age and causes progressive dyspnea, bloat, or both. It is a sporadic form of lymphosarcoma in cattle, meaning that it is not associated with bovine leukemia virus (BLV) infection. Swelling is often obvious in the distal ventral cervical area and extends through the thoracic inlet. Some thymic lymphosarcoma masses are soft, fluid-like swellings on palpation (Fig. 4.94), but others are firmer. Compression of the trachea, esophagus, and jugular veins results in dyspnea, interference with eructation, and jugular distention that varies with the size of the mass. Compression of the trachea, causing respiratory distress, may also occur in adult cattle with enzootic BLV–associated lymphosarcoma. Adult lymphosarcoma may be associated with tumor formation in the thorax as a result of lymph node, pleural, cardiac, and occasionally pulmonary

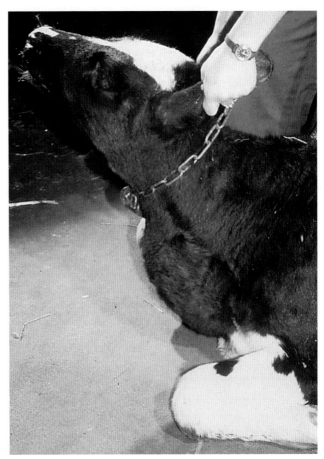

• **Fig. 4.94** Thymic lymphosarcoma in a 6-month-old calf presented because of worsening dyspnea and intermittent bloat.

involvement. Signs vary depending on the tumor numbers, size, and other organs affected. Occasionally, patients with lymphosarcoma have fever caused by tumor necrosis, and this may be a misleading sign because otherwise they should be afebrile. Severe pleural effusion with many neoplastic lymphocytes may occur. The pleural effusion caused by lymphosarcoma is often grossly discolored, having a bloody appearance. Thymomas are rare in cattle.

Primary pulmonary tumors of epithelial origin described as papillary adenomas have been observed in young cattle at slaughter. These were reported as benign, multicentric tumors because metastases were not observed. Signs were not reported because these were incidental findings during slaughter inspection. Several case reports have documented malignant neoplasms such as bronchiolar adenocarcinoma in older cows showing signs of progressive dyspnea. Dr. Rebhun documented one older cow and one bull with massive pulmonary adenocarcinomas that resulted in progressive dyspnea, weight loss, and reduced lung sounds. Mesotheliomas within the thorax originate from the pleura and tend to be multiple. They may enlarge collectively to create signs of progressive dyspnea, decreased lung sounds caused by massive pleural effusion, and weight loss, eventually leading to death. Of the small number of patients with mesothelioma that we have seen, they have all had dual body cavity effusions to some degree with both thoracic (pleural) and abdominal fluid accumulation.

Tuberculosis, although rare in dairy cattle because of regulatory control efforts, should be remembered as a potential cause of progressive dyspnea, coughing, weight loss, and signs of pneumonia. Enlarged thoracic lymph nodes associated with the infection may result in esophageal compression and bloat or obvious respiratory distress from tracheal compression. However, the condition is not commonly associated with significant pleural effusion.

Diagnosis

Diagnosis of space-occupying lesions in the thorax requires careful auscultation to detect differences in lung and heart sounds in each hemithorax. Abscesses, seromas, bronchial cysts, or masses occupying one hemithorax elevate the ipsilateral lung and push the heart toward the opposite hemithorax. Therefore in the affected hemithorax, lung sounds are absent ventrally, and heart sounds are muffled or absent. Auscultation of the opposite hemithorax reveals uniformly increased bronchovesicular sounds and a loud "pounding" heart beat caused by the proximity of the heart to the thoracic wall on this side. Thoracic percussion also may be helpful in detecting the area of involvement. Because cattle affected with these problems often have increased central venous pressure as a result of impaired venous return, they may be confused with heart failure patients. An incomplete physical examination may lead to an erroneous diagnosis such as endocarditis or pericarditis if the examiner only auscultates one hemithorax.

When an abnormality has been identified on physical examination, further diagnostics are indicated. Thoracic radiography and ultrasonography are appropriate if a complete diagnostic workup is to be performed. Blood work may be helpful in the case of thoracic abscesses in that the serum globulin level usually is elevated ($\geq$5.0 g/dL), and neutrophilia may be present. Undoubtedly, ultrasonography has tremendous benefits diagnostically for the evaluation of pleural, cardiac, and mediastinal space-occupying lesions. Because of the extravagant fluid volumes that can be associated with neoplastic lesions in particular, it may be necessary to use low- to medium-frequency probes (2.5–5 MHz) that provide high-quality images at 20 to 25 cm depth to identify deeper space-occupying lesions. Drainage both facilitates cytologic diagnosis and permits better near-field visualization of any masses.

The most direct diagnostic aid remains thoracocentesis with a suitable needle. Although a 5.0-cm needle will enter the pleural space of cattle, it is seldom long enough to invade the capsule of an encapsulated abscess or seroma. Therefore an 8.75-cm, 18-gauge needle is preferred for initial thoracocentesis through the lower fifth or sixth ICS on the affected hemithorax. If fluid or pus is obtained, the material is submitted for cytology and culture. Biopsy of a mass lesion under ultrasound guidance may be indicated.

If thymic lymphosarcoma is suspected, aspirates for cytology or biopsies (True-Cut biopsy needle; Baxter Healthcare Corp., Valencia, CA) are indicated to allow definitive diagnosis. A hematoma of the ventral neck may appear clinically similar to thymic lymphosarcoma, but ultrasound examination and biopsy should allow differentiation of the two. As previously mentioned, some patients with thymic lymphosarcoma have a misleading fluctuant mass in the distal cervical region that appears fluid filled. Aspirate attempts yield no fluid, however, but biopsy will confirm the diagnosis. Biopsy of mediastinal masses that are confined to the thorax are challenging to perform safely, with the risk of iatrogenic cardiac, pulmonary, or great vessel injury being quite high. If accompanied by free pleural fluid, it is always prudent to obtain a sample of this first in hopes of identifying exfoliated neoplastic cells before rushing to a riskier biopsy procedure. Juvenile cattle affected with thymic lymphosarcoma usually are negative for BLV when tested by agar gel immunodiffusion (AGID), ELISA, or PCR.

Pleuritis or pleural effusion may be unilateral or bilateral. Careful auscultation and percussion should lead to suspicion of free pleural fluid because lung sounds usually are absent in the ventral aspect of the affected hemithorax. Dyspnea may be marked in cattle with large accumulations of pleural fluid. Pleural fluid does not displace the heart, as occurs in association with unilateral thoracic masses or abscesses. Therefore heart sounds are audible bilaterally and may appear to radiate caudodorsally by sound conduction through the pleural fluid. Pleural fluid must be differentiated from anterior ventral pulmonary consolidation. Whereas bronchial tones usually are heard in consolidated regions of lungs, absence of sounds is more typical of pleural fluid. Thoracocentesis is indicated to confirm pleural fluid accumulation; any sampled fluid should be analyzed using cytology and culture to differentiate infectious from neoplastic or other causes. Ultrasonography and thoracic radiography, if available, help in the management of a valuable cow affected with this problem. Ultrasonography is an extremely valuable tool for evaluating pleural disease in cattle. As more portable equipment becomes available, an ultrasound machine may be used with increasing frequency as part of the evaluation for sick cows. Ultrasonography can quickly determine whether the patient has pleural effusion, abscessation, consolidation, or pleural surface masses. It can also be used as an aid for collection of samples via needle or biopsy. If available, thoracic radiography is helpful to confirm or deny diaphragmatic hernia.

Thoracic tumors involving the lung parenchyma, pleura, or thoracic lymph nodes are difficult to diagnose unless thoracic radiographs and ultrasonography are available. Signs vary, and dyspnea and progressive weight loss occur despite symptomatic treatment. Thoracic lymphosarcoma may be suspected based on physical signs involving other sites or lymph nodes becoming obviously enlarged. A PCR test for BLV will be positive as will the AGID and ELISA tests in most cows with clinical lymphosarcoma. This does not confirm a diagnosis but does add to the index of suspicion if lymphosarcoma is suspected. Bloat and tracheal compression may occur if mediastinal masses or lymphadenopathy become severe. Thoracocentesis may offer the best means of diagnosis for unusual

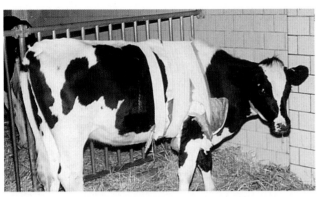

• **Fig. 4.95** Yearling heifer with an encapsulated *Trueperella pyogenes* abscess in the right hemithorax. A chest trochar has been placed to facilitate drainage.

tumors such as adenocarcinomas because exfoliative cytology may help identify the tumor and allow proper prognosis. Thoracoscopy can be performed safely in cattle and allows direct observation of the mediastinal lymph nodes, thoracic portion of the esophagus, and dorsal branch of the vagus nerve, and it could aid in the identification and biopsy of intrathoracic masses.

Treatment

Therapy of unilateral thoracic abscesses and seromas involves drainage of the lesions through the thoracic wall. Because *T. pyogenes* is the usual causative organism of thoracic abscesses, a thick capsule often is present. After the location of the abscess is confirmed by thoracocentesis, a large-bore (20–28 Fr) chest trochar is placed into the abscess cavity (Fig. 4.95). The chest trochar is sutured in place, and the affected cow is started on penicillin (22,000 U/kg twice daily, SC or IM). When ultrasonography is available, it may be used to confirm pleural adhesions between parietal pleura and the abscess, allowing subsequent surgical thoracotomy coupled with rib resection to afford even more efficient drainage and exploration of the cause of the abscess. Complete drainage is the key to successful treatment. Lavage of saline or antibiotic and saline solutions through the indwelling trochar also has been used in some cases. Irritating solutions such as iodine products are contraindicated, however.

Cattle with seromas that are drained in this manner subsequently have a good prognosis. Abscesses require long-term antibiotic therapy and complete evacuation and drainage. Therefore, the affected cow must be of substantial value to justify the medical expenses and associated loss of milk sales for several weeks. Cattle affected with thoracic abscesses may lose significant body condition during early treatment, but absence of fever, decreased venous distention, increased appetite, weight gain, and a return to normal thoracic sounds on auscultation are all signs of improvement.

Treatment for pleuritis and pleural fluid requires drainage of the fluid and appropriate antibiotic therapy to control associated pneumonia. If pleural fluid is caused by effusion from neoplastic conditions, treatment is rarely indicated.

Hardware perforations of the diaphragm may result in frank pleuritis associated with pleural fluid accumulation, thoracic abscessation, or diaphragmatic hernia. When *T. pyogenes* predominates, a thick-walled thoracic abscess develops, resulting in chronic illness. If a mixed infection develops and a fluid pleuritis that is not encapsulated results, the affected cow typically has an acute presentation with large amounts of septic fluid free in the pleural space.

Surprisingly few cattle with bacterial bronchopneumonia develop clinically significant pleural fluid accumulation. Nonetheless, pneumonia remains the most common cause of pleural fluid accumulation. The diagnosis of pleural fluid accumulation unilaterally or bilaterally in a cow affected with severe pneumonia dictates drainage of this fluid. Pleural effusion associated with bronchopneumonia will result in fever unresponsive to antibiotics and marked dyspnea. Drainage is provided by daily thoracocentesis or continuous drainage until negligible quantities of pleural fluid are obtained. Appropriate systemic antibiotics should be selected based on culture and susceptibility results and maintained for at least 1 week beyond the last thoracocentesis. Thoracotomy and drainage may be required in some cases, especially those associated with hardware and a foreign body residing within the abscess.

Pneumothorax

Etiology and Signs

Dyspnea accompanied by increased respiratory rate and effort coupled with absence of bronchovesicular sounds in the dorsal lung fields unilaterally or bilaterally characterizes pneumothorax or bullous pulmonary emphysema. Dyspnea may range from mild to severe. Some adult cattle appear very painful with pneumothorax. When severe dyspnea is present, open-mouth breathing and expiratory groan suggest a bilateral problem. Subcutaneous emphysema may be observed in some affected cattle.

Pneumoretroperitoneum may be appreciated on rectal exam in some cattle with pneumothorax or pneumomediastinum.

Auscultation of the affected hemithorax reveals increased bronchovesicular sounds in the ventral lung fields and absence of lung sounds dorsally. Body temperature is normal unless exertion, high environmental temperatures, or pulmonary inflammation associated with a primary infectious cause (e.g., BRSV) leads to pyrexia. Severe exertion during parturition, exertion during restraint for treatment or surgery, penetrating thoracic wounds, or pharyngeal or laryngeal injury causing a pneumomediastinum that ruptures into the chest may also cause pneumothorax (Fig. 4.96). Primary pulmonary pathology associated with chronic bronchopneumonia and emphysematous bullae formation is the most common cause of pneumothorax in adult dairy cattle in the northern United States. Fever may be present if primary pulmonary inflammation (BRSV, severe bacterial bronchopneumonia, acute bovine pulmonary emphysema [ABPE], among others) contributed to emphysema and resultant pneumothorax. BRSV is the

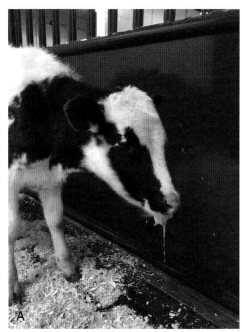
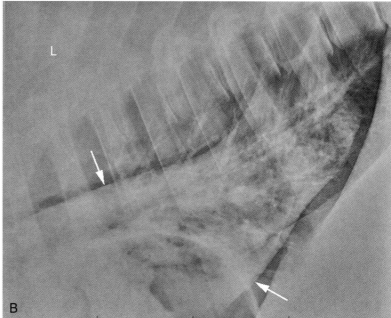

• **Fig. 4.96 A,** A 6-month-old Milking Shorthorn with respiratory distress and severe aspiration pneumonia associated with pharyngeal trauma. **B,** Note pneumothorax with lung collapse and severe pneumonia on a thoracic radiograph. The collapsed lung is highlighted by *arrows*.

most common infectious agent associated with pneumothorax in cattle (see Fig. 4.60). In these inflammatory diseases, auscultation of the ventral lung fields helps to define etiology. Ultrasonography may be helpful in diagnosing the pneumothorax (there is no normal sliding of the dorsal air line) and determining the extent of more cranioventral lung pathology.

Diagnosis

Auscultation and percussion suggest the diagnosis. Pneumothorax must be differentiated from bullous emphysema and pulmonary edema because these two conditions should not be addressed therapeutically by chest drainage. Radiography or ultrasonography will confirm the diagnosis but may not be available. If history, auscultation, and percussion suggest a diagnosis of pneumothorax, thoracic puncture and vacuum evacuation of free air should be attempted through the dorsal 9th or 10th ICS. The presence of free air confirms the diagnosis, and airway sounds should return to the dorsal thorax after evacuation of the free air. Tracheal wash samples for cytology, culture, and BRSV diagnostics may be necessary to assess lower airway infection or inflammation. Care should be taken to avoid causing severe coughing while collecting samples as this could exacerbate the condition.

Treatment

Therapy requires evacuation of air from the affected hemithorax and treatment of any primary problem such as pneumonia, puncture wounds, and so forth. Cattle with pneumothorax resulting from chronic bacterial pneumonia have a guarded prognosis. Following evacuation, rapid improvement in the dyspnea should be anticipated when

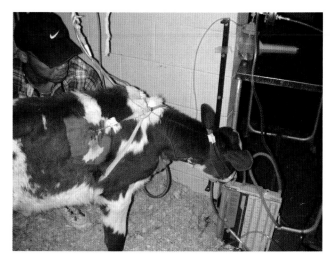

• **Fig. 4.97** A 5-week-old Holstein calf undergoing continuous flow evacuation of right-sided pneumothorax associated with acute bovine respiratory syncytial virus infection. The calf made a full recovery.

pneumothorax is the major problem. The clinician must remember that, except in exogenous puncture of the thorax or ruptured pneumomediastinum, pneumothorax originates from damaged pulmonary tissue that has "leaked" air. Simple evacuation of the free air in the thorax will improve the affected animal temporarily but does not guarantee the problem will not recur. Owners need to be instructed to watch the patient carefully for recurrence of dyspnea if the damaged lung continues to leak. Most cattle, however, respond to one or two evacuations of the thorax. A technique for continuous drainage has been described by Peek and coworkers in cattle that requires hospitalization and confinement (Figs. 4.97 and 4.98).

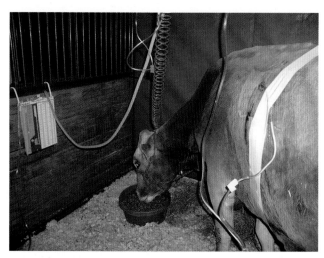

• **Fig. 4.98** A 4-year-old Brown Swiss cow being treated for pneumothorax associated with bullous emphysema and unilateral pneumothorax associated with chronic bronchopneumonia by continuous flow evacuation.

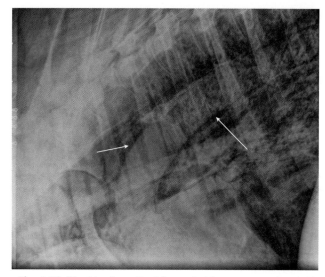

• **Fig. 4.99** "Double silhouetting" *(arrows)* of the aorta associated with pneumomediastinum in an adult cow with bovine respiratory syncytial virus infection and severe interstitial pneumonia.

Pneumomediastinum

Etiology and Signs

Pneumomediastinum most often accompanies severe pulmonary parenchymal diseases that result in emphysema and bullae formation. Subsequent leakage of air into the mediastinum occurs. Several of the causes of pneumothorax mentioned previously are also potential causes of pneumomediastinum. Pneumomediastinum is most common in postpartum cows. In some cases, there is old pulmonary pathology predisposing to the pneumomediastinum, but other cases may simply result from the exertion of calving. Signs may be mild or impossible to separate from those caused by the primary pulmonary pathology. Mild dyspnea, SC emphysema, and bilateral muffled heart sounds are present in most instances. The muffled heart sounds are the only consistent findings and are caused by air insulation of the cardiac sounds. The SC emphysema is mostly on the dorsum of the cow as the air migrates along the aorta and through the lumbar fascial planes. It can also be felt rectally along the aorta.

On rare occasions, respiratory distress may occur within a few minutes after a lidocaine epidural when air may have been heard entering the epidural space for a few seconds before the lidocaine injection. Affected cattle appear apprehensive and restless, have pronounced abdominal effort in breathing, and cough. Although anaphylaxis is often considered, there are no other signs of anaphylaxis, and the cattle slowly recover without treatment in 20 to 30 minutes. This is most likely a result of epidural air acutely entering the mediastinum, causing pneumomediastinum (see Video Clip 4.15).

Diagnosis

Subcutaneous emphysema in a postpartum cow is highly suggestive of pneumomediastinum. The presence of bilateral heart sound muffling requires differentiation of this condition from pericarditis. This differentiation is aided by obvious pulmonary pathology coupled with an absence of signs of heart failure in most cases. If physical examination findings cannot definitively differentiate these problems, ultrasonography and radiography are indicated. Pericardiocentesis is not indicated as an initial procedure because it may subject the patient to unnecessary risks. Thoracic radiographs demonstrate a very clear cardiac and aortic shadow because surrounding air highlights these tissues. "Double silhouetting" of the great vessels on chest radiographs is characteristic of pneumomediastinum (Fig. 4.99). On occasions this radiographic finding may even be incidental in a postpartum cow with no other signs of dyspnea.

Treatment

Specific treatment for pneumomediastinum is not required unless the cow has labored breathing and a probable pneumothorax. Therefore therapy should be directed against any primary pulmonary pathology in addition to oxygen, bronchodilator, and antitussive therapy.

Noninfectious Causes of Acute Respiratory Distress in Cattle

Acute respiratory distress in cattle may occur with a variety of noninfectious pathologic changes. Some causes have well-documented pathophysiology, but others are more poorly defined and controversial. Terminology varies tremendously among pathologists and clinicians, resulting in much confusion regarding these disorders. Most acute diseases discussed here require gross or microscopic pathology to enable positive diagnosis. The clinician cannot differentiate most of these diseases based on physical examination alone. Textbook descriptions have confused the issue by using different synonyms and eponyms to characterize the problem.

Fortunately, as a collected group of respiratory problems, these diseases are uncommon and much less important than infectious causes of respiratory disease in dairy cattle. Therefore they will be described individually as best as possible in this section. Readers should realize that the nomenclature of these diseases has changed in the past and is likely to change in the future. Specific therapy is addressed when indicated. Respiratory distress may also be caused by methemoglobinemia (nitrate toxicity), cyanide toxicity (wilted wild cherry leaf ingestion), or acute and severe hemolytic anemia.

Acute Bovine Pulmonary Edema and Emphysema (Atypical Interstitial Pneumonia, Fog Fever, and Pneumotoxicosis)

Etiology and Signs

This acute disease of cattle classically develops within 2 weeks of the time cattle are moved to lush pasture. The exact composition of the pasture does not seem important because grasses, alfalfa, turnips, kale, and rape all have been incriminated. Consumption of *Perilla* (purple) mint *(Perilla frutescens)* or moldy sweet potatoes may cause identical syndromes. Although not as well documented, we have seen similar clinical and pathological outbreaks associated with grass silages and ryegrass pastures. Affected cattle develop acute, severe respiratory distress characterized by reluctance to move, open-mouth breathing, pulmonary edema, tachypnea, and hyperpnea. Temperatures are normal to only slightly elevated unless environmental temperatures are very high.

The etiopathogenesis of classic "fog fever" is well characterized. Rapid consumption of lush, postharvest pasture leads to ingestion of large amounts of L-tryptophan to which the rumen microbiota is not acclimated. Subsequent transformation of ingested L-tryptophan to indole acetic acid is followed by decarboxylation to 3-methylindole, which is the toxic metabolite of tryptophan. After absorption of 3-methylindole from the rumen into the systemic circulation the cytochrome P450 system metabolizes the chemical, producing pneumotoxicity in Clara cells and type 1 pneumocytes. Experimental studies have confirmed that 3-methylindole is the toxic metabolite of tryptophan involved in classic ABPE. Calves seldom are affected, but adult animals older than 2 years of age in good body condition appear most at risk.

The etiopathogeneses of AIP associated with *Perilla* mint and moldy sweet potato consumption are quite similar. *Perilla* mint is at its most toxic when the plant is flowering and in the seed-producing stage; cattle tend to only consume it when other more palatable pasture components are grazed out; subsequently, the condition is usually seen in the late summer on poor-quality pasture. The toxic principle is *Perilla* ketone rather than 3-methylindole. Cattle can develop identical signs when fed sweet potatoes blighted with the mold *Fusarium solani,* which produces the propneumotoxin 4-ipomeanol. Activation of 4-ipomeanol by pulmonary cytochrome P450 enzyme activity is thought to produce the toxic principle.

Fortunately, ABPE is rare in dairy cattle in the United States because pasture management is more stringent, and pasturing is practiced less commonly in confinement herds than in the beef industry. Dairy practitioners should be aware of ABPE but may never see a herd outbreak of the disease. We have on rare occasion diagnosed this or a similar disease in confined cattle fed silage where the pneumotoxicant was unknown.

Signs

Profound dyspnea, expiratory grunt, reluctance to move, auscultatable evidence of interstitial pneumonia (rhonchi and rales) in the ventral lung field, and quiet lungs dorsally secondary to emphysema and edema characterize the condition. Subcutaneous emphysema may be observed. The morbidity rate may approach 50%, and mortality rates range from 25% to 50%.

Diagnosis and Treatment

Diagnosis is by history, clinical signs, and pathologic study of the lungs from fatal cases. Treatment is seldom helpful, but a variety of drugs have been used in an effort to save badly affected animals. Simple movement or mild restraint may be fatal to these anoxic animals. Therefore treatment is controversial and empiric. Furosemide (0.5–1.0 mg/kg) may lessen pulmonary edema. Atropine (0.048 mg/kg or 1/30 grain/100 lb body weight twice daily), antihistamines, NSAIDs, vitamins A and E, and cortisone all have been used with varying anecdotal results. Animals that are rested, removed from the pasture, and not severely affected usually recover in 1 to 2 weeks. Some cattle may fall into the category of "chronic lungers," with chronic respiratory illness associated with proliferation of type 2 pneumocytes and pulmonary fibrosis.

Prevention

Prevention is the best treatment and may be accomplished by feeding susceptible cattle an ionophore such as monensin (200 mg/head/day) starting several days before they are introduced to lush pasture and for 7 to 10 days after being placed on that pasture. These drugs inhibit the metabolism of tryptophan to 3-methylindole.

Proliferative Pneumonia

Etiology and Signs

Proliferative pneumonia is another cause of acute respiratory distress observed in dairy cattle. This condition occasionally has been observed to cause high morbidity within a herd but usually affects only one or a few cattle within a group. Acute onset of dyspnea characterized by hyperpnea, tachypnea, an occasional cough, open-mouth breathing, and pulmonary edema are observed (Fig. 4.100).

The term *proliferative pneumonia* derives from the characteristic gross pathology consisting of heavy, firm, wet lungs that are diffusely affected. Histologic study of these

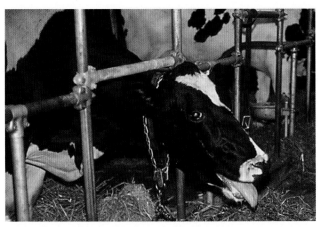

• **Fig. 4.100** A Holstein cow with acute severe dyspnea and open-mouth breathing because of proliferative pneumonia.

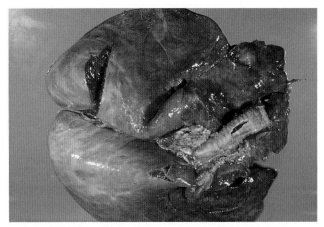

• **Fig. 4.101** Necropsy specimen of the lungs from a calf with acute proliferative pneumonia superimposed on resolving cranioventral bronchopneumonia. (Courtesy of Dr. John M. King.)

lungs reveals obliteration of alveolar spaces by proliferating type 2 pneumocytes and interstitial edema. As such, there are some very comparable clinical and pathological features that are shared by both classic pneumotoxin-associated AIP and proliferative pneumonia. The principal difference is the grazing history in the former and the fact that the pneumotoxins described in the last section tend to affect larger groups of cattle rather than an individual animal or small group.

The gross pathology and histopathology are characteristic. Unfortunately, affected cattle show ante-mortem signs common to many other diseases also characterized by acute respiratory distress. Clinical signs include a low-grade fever (103.0° to 104.0°F [39.44° to 40.00°C]), which may range higher (105.0° to 106.0°F [40.56° to 41.11°C]) as a result of exertion and environmental factors. Auscultation of the lungs reveals diffuse reduction of airway sounds over the entire thorax. Proliferation of type 2 pneumocytes within the alveoli and interstitial edema contribute to the reduced lower airway sounds. Therefore, although the affected cow has severe lower airway dyspnea, the lungs are very quiet on auscultation.

Other diseases, such as ABPE, diffuse pulmonary edema, acute dyspnea associated with embolic showering from a CVCT, nitrogen dioxide inhalation, and other causes of acute respiratory distress, could lead to similar signs.

Not only is the disease difficult to diagnose accurately, but also the exact cause or causes remain unknown. Nitrogen gases have been incriminated, and the disease has similarities to silo filler's disease caused by nitrogen dioxide (NO_2). However, calves and adult cattle that develop proliferative pneumonia frequently have not been exposed to silo gas or other environmental nitrogen gases. Cytochrome P450 enzymatic activity within lung tissue has been demonstrated to be pivotal in the pathogenesis of interstitial pneumonia caused by 3-methylindole, 4-ipomeanol, and *Perilla* mint pneumotoxicosis. It is possible that activation of inhaled or absorbed propneumotoxins by a similar metabolic process plays a role in proliferative pneumonia.

Alternatively, patients with proliferative pneumonia may be unfortunate enough to have a combined pneumotoxin and infectious insult. The question remains: Are all of these individual toxicities completely separate entities in cattle? It seems that the disease known as proliferative pneumonia may be a composite of these toxicities or may be caused by a yet-to-be-determined toxin common within the environment of dairy cattle.

Another form of pathologically confirmed proliferative pneumonia has been observed in dairy calves after previous infection with, and apparent recovery from, *Pasteurella* or *Mannheimia* pneumonia. The disease occurs in a single animal among a group of calves 2 to 4 weeks after apparent recovery from *Pasteurella* or *Mannheimia* pneumonia. This single animal develops an acute severe respiratory distress syndrome with tachypnea, hyperpnea, an elevated heart rate, open-mouth breathing, fever (103.0° to 106.0°F [39.44° to 41.11°C]), and pulmonary edema. An expiratory grunt may also be present. The animal is reluctant to move and may become cyanotic if stressed. The degree of respiratory effort makes it impossible to determine whether the pyrexia is caused by inflammation or exertion. The lungs are very quiet on auscultation and have reduced sounds throughout all fields. If the previous pneumonia resulted in consolidation of anterior ventral lung lobes, bronchial tones may be heard ventrally and reduced sounds elsewhere. Usually both lungs are involved, but occasionally one lung has much more serious lesions. Unless treated quickly and intensively, the calf dies within 24 hours. Gross necropsy reveals diffusely heavy, wet, firm lungs with evidence of resolved or resolving anterior ventral pneumonia (Fig. 4.101). Bacterial products resulting in a delayed hypersensitivity reaction are thought to be the cause of this problem. The 2- to 4-week interval between earlier signs of typical *Pasteurella* or *Mannheimia* pneumonia and subsequent acute proliferative pneumonia, as well as the pathologic lesions, differentiate this syndrome from the "relapse" respiratory distress sometimes observed in

BRSV infections. In addition, paired serum samples do not support BRSV as the cause.

Diagnosis and Treatment

Treatment of proliferative pneumonia is controversial because only lung biopsy or necropsy can definitively confirm the clinical entity at hand. Lung biopsy via a Tru-Cut biopsy needle is a useful diagnostic step to aid diagnosis and treatment in valuable animals. Thoracic radiographs, if available, will demonstrate a diffuse pulmonary edema and mixed alveolar–interstitial pattern. Treatment with atropine has reportedly been beneficial to affected herdmates when endemic proliferative pneumonia has been confirmed by necropsy study (see below). When proliferative pneumonia is confirmed or strongly suspected, the following therapy is suggested:

- Remove affected cattle from any source of toxic plants, nitrogen gases, or fumes; for example, if the only affected cows are confined near a silo chute or manure pit, move them. Affected cattle should be moved only when their ventilation and environment need to be improved. Otherwise, any movement constitutes a severe stress.
- Administer furosemide (0.5–1.0 mg/kg or 25 to 50 mg/100 lb body weight by injection once or twice daily) for the first 2 days of therapy if hydration status allows.
- Administer atropine (0.048 mg/kg or 1/30 grain [2.2 mg] per 100 lb body weight twice daily).
- Administer dexamethasone (10 to 20 mg once daily) for 3 days unless the affected cow is pregnant.
- Administer broad-spectrum antibiotics for 5 to 7 days to protect against secondary bacterial pneumonia.

Respiratory Distress in Newborn Calves

Etiology, Pathophysiology, and Signs

This is a relatively common occurrence and may result from aspiration of meconium, congenital heart disease, white muscle disease, fetal lung pathology, or more commonly from dysmaturity or immaturity of the lung with associated surfactant deficiency. It is especially common in premature, cloned, or in vitro fertilized calves (Fig. 4.102). Calves born in advance of 270 days' gestation are at risk, and the earlier the delivery, the higher the risk. It is true that some calves born as early as 6 weeks premature may have relatively normal pulmonary function, but this is unusual. Regardless of the causative factors, abnormal lung compliance present in these cases causes poor air exchange, hypoxia, pulmonary hypertension, and may eventually lead to right heart failure. Occasionally, rib fractures causing traumatic lung injury or hemothorax may also be a cause of respiratory distress in neonates. Because of protracted labor, these same newborn calves are also at great risk for hypoxemic injury to the central nervous system, GI tract, and other organs; rarely do they acquire or potentially absorb sufficient colostrum and consequently are at further and substantial risk for sepsis. Congenital heart defects may also cause respiratory distress in either newborn or slightly older calves.

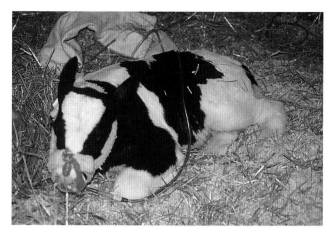

• **Fig. 4.102** A newborn cloned calf with hypoxemia being treated with intranasal oxygen.

Diagnosis

Calves should develop a fairly normal respiratory pattern within the first hour after delivery, whereas newborn calves with respiratory distress syndrome will have labored breathing that does not improve with time. There may be other signs of prematurity (e.g., small size, abnormally fine hair coat) in premature calves. Cloned calves may also have abnormally large umbilical vessels and other abnormalities including ascites. Lung sounds are diffusely harsh and generally do not have rales. The heart rate will be high, but loud murmurs are usually absent unless the respiratory distress is caused by a congenital heart defect. All newborn calves with respiratory distress should have their heart auscultated properly to rule out congenital heart defects. An arterial sample can be collected from the brachial or auricular arteries (Fig. 4.103) to confirm the severity of the hypoxemia. It should be noted that newborn healthy calves may have PaO_2 values of 55 to 60 mm Hg during the first 30 to 60 minutes of life. In many cases with respiratory distress, the PCO_2 will be elevated, and this can be confirmed by a venous sample (>45 mm Hg). If the CO_2 is elevated in a rapidly breathing calf, the PaO_2 will be extremely low. Pulse oximetry is useful in calves after the first hour of life to confirm the hypoxemia and for monitoring therapy. A chest radiograph will reveal diffuse underinflation of the lung and parenchymal collapse. Some premature calves will have moderate to severe respiratory acidosis, hypercapnia, and hypoxemia but because of inappropriate or underdeveloped central responses appear eupneic or only slightly tachypneic. Periodic assessment of preferably arterial blood gases, or at the very least venous blood pH and CO_2 tension, in the first day or two of life in premature calves is therefore recommended. Premature calves with respiratory difficulties can have a rapid downward spiral leading to hypoxic death.

Treatment

Treatment must be early and vigorous if there is hope for survival in neonatal calves with respiratory distress. Premature calves born by cesarean section and not taking a big

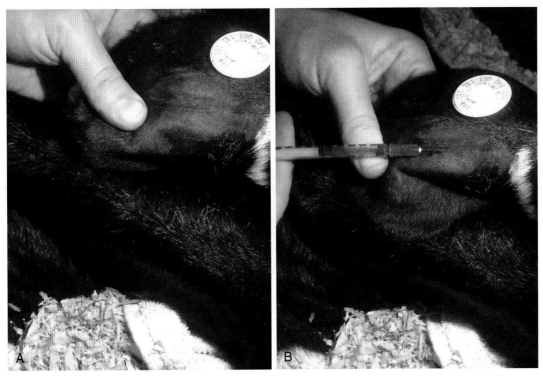

• **Fig. 4.103** Technique for arterial blood gas sampling from auricular artery. The artery is occluded distally along the dorsal edge of the ear to cause the artery to stand out (**A**), and then a heparinized tuberculin syringe with a 25-gauge needle is carefully introduced into the vessel (**B**) and gentle suction applied. (Courtesy of Dr. Chelsea Holschbach.)

breath immediately after delivery are at a high risk of having excessive fluid in the airways, and a loud fluid sound may be notable during labored breathing. Lifting those calves by the hind legs for 10 seconds, suctioning each nostril for 5 seconds, or irritating the nostril with a piece of straw may be helpful in removing excessive fluid from the airways. Prolonged suction or suspension by the hind legs should definitely be avoided because they would make the calf more hypoxic. Vitamin E and selenium should be given IM. Intranasal humidified oxygen must be administered at 5 to 8 L/min as soon as possible in an attempt to improve tissue oxygenation and decrease reflex pulmonary artery constriction (Fig. 4.104). If the calf is premature and the accompanying respiratory distress is severe, nasal cannulas in both nostrils and high-flow humidified oxygen may be needed. This is considered to have a number of physiological advantages compared with standard oxygen therapies, including reduced anatomical dead space, higher FiO$_2$, and positive end-expiratory pressure, which may keep the terminal airways and alveoli open, improving lung compliance. It is best to not let the calves lie in lateral recumbency as this has a negative effect on ventilation and oxygenation.

Newborn calves with respiratory distress are almost always given prophylactic antibiotics and a plasma transfusion if plasma immunoglobulin G is low. One dose of corticosteroid (10 mg of dexamethasone) is often given and empirically does seem to help, especially after meconium

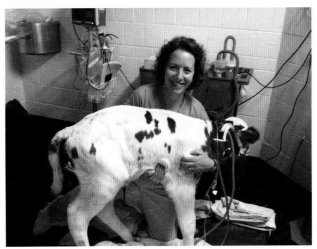

• **Fig. 4.104** A 2-day-old calf with respiratory distress caused by meconium aspiration. The calf is receiving intranasal oxygen through a small tube (*red*) sutured into one nostril. The calf also has an enteral feeding tube for feeding and intravenous fluid line for fluids and medication and a nebulizer in the background for nebulization of surfactant, corticosteroid, bronchodilator, and antibiotics. The calf made a complete recovery with the intensive care treatments.

aspiration. Although it is proven that corticosteroids given to cattle in the last 2 weeks of gestation improve lung function at birth in cesarean section–delivered calves, there is limited proof that postnatally administered steroids will similarly accelerate lung maturation. It may be that

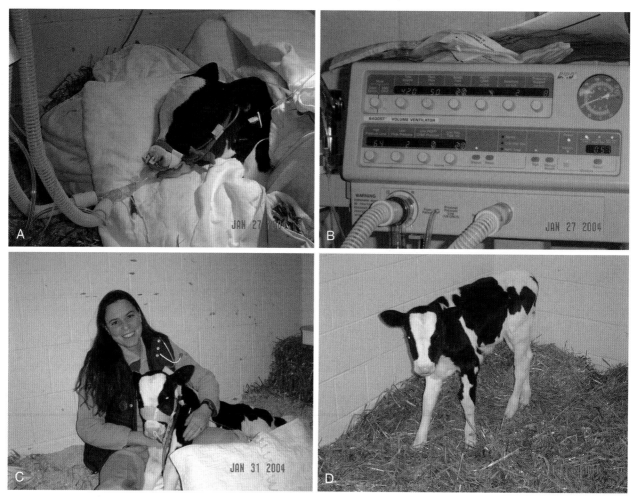

• **Fig. 4.105 A,** A newborn cloned calf with respiratory distress being ventilated with a mechanical ventilator. **B,** Mechanical ventilator settings for this calf. **C,** The calf was weaned off the ventilator 4 days later and is seen here still receiving intranasal oxygen. **D,** Same calf as in A and C ready for discharge.

postnatally administered steroids, if they help at all, inhibit oxidative lung damage in hypoxic calves. If surfactant is available, it should be given to the calf via intratracheal instillation or less commonly by direct tracheal injection, or it can be nebulized. Commercially prepared surfactant is preferred, but we have collected surfactant from healthy donor cows by BAL using 100 mL of sterile saline and then using the top (foamy) part of the collection for intratracheal administration or nebulization. The calf should be turned over in dorsal recumbency for 10 seconds immediately after surfactant is placed in the trachea to facilitate its distribution into all or most areas of the lungs. The surfactant seems to be more effective when given early in the disease process. If a response is noted it may need to be repeated several times as the life of the exogenous surfactant is short. We have also nebulized affected calves with acetylcysteine while they were being administered an aminophylline drip (5 mg/ kg over 2 hours). The aminophylline not only serves as a bronchodilator but also has antiinflammatory properties and helps maintain diaphragm strength. In regions where beta agonist inhalation bronchodilator treatment is legal this might also improve both surfactant production and

mucociliary clearance; however, the treatment is illegal in cattle in the United States.

Fluids (crystalloids and colloids such as plasma) may be given IV as a continuous drip if needed but the calf should not be overhydrated. The calf should be gradually warmed if it is hypothermic. We have also administered thyrotropin-releasing factor or thyroxine (2-5 µg/kg orally once daily) or both, in hopes of increasing surfactant production. Although thyroid hormones are known to be important in prenatal lung development, most studies have been unable to demonstrate a benefit of thyroxine treatment on lung maturation when administered after birth. If pulmonary gas exchange cannot be sufficiently improved with these methods and the owners request further treatment, the calf can be placed on a mechanical ventilator, but this is expensive (Fig. 4.105). It is sometimes more difficult to keep calves quiet on a ventilator compared with foals. Cloned calves with ascites and enlarged umbilical vessels have low survival rates even when placed on the ventilator. A short-term alternative to machine-driven mechanical ventilation is to continuously or intermittently use an Ambu bag to inflate the lung. Another alternative on

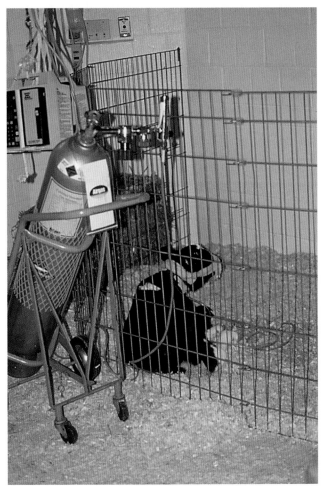

• **Fig. 4.106** A 2-day-old calf with pulmonary hypertension receiving oxygen and nitric oxide.

the farm is to use a commercially sold calf resuscitator/aspirator. Persistent pulmonary hypertension causes progression of right heart failure and sometimes reversion to fetal circulation patterns. The chronic hypoxia results in a mixed acidosis and often multiple organ failure. Nitric oxide (ratio of NO to oxygen, 1:9) can be administered through the oxygen line in hopes of decreasing the pulmonary hypertension (Fig. 4.106).

Prevention of Respiratory Failure in Calves Induced Prematurely

Occasionally, labor in a cow in late pregnancy will need to be induced, most often because of some medical disease of the dam. The likelihood of respiratory distress caused by premature delivery may be decreased by the administration of glucocorticoids and prostaglandin F2α to the dam. If the calf is at less than 260 days' gestation, this treatment might not improve lung function. If the premature delivery must occur before 260 days of gestation, then a 7-day induction protocol should be used if the dam can be kept humanely alive for that period. Induction begins with administration of 5 mg of dexamethasone intramuscularly every 12 hours for 4 days. On day 5, the dose of dexamethasone is doubled

to 10 mg every 12 hours. In some cows, parturition occurs on day 6; in the remainder, 40 mg of dexamethasone and an abortigenic dose of prostaglandin F2α is given once on day 6. The cow must not be suffering during this time!

Other Less Common Causes of Respiratory Distress

Silo Filler's Disease (Nitrogen Dioxide Poisoning)
Etiology and Signs
Fumes of NO_2, a heavy yellow gas produced by anaerobic fermentation of fresh silage, may cause the same lower airway damage in exposed cattle as in humans. Because the gas is heavier than air, it lies on top of recently ensiled material, especially corn silage, and seeks out lower locations such as silo chutes. The major risk to farmers occurs when workers enter a silo chute or silo without first starting the blower in the silo loader to "wash out" NO_2. Cattle confined next to the silo chute are most at risk and may receive chronic low-exposure toxicity or severe acute toxicity. Gaseous NO_2 seeks water that then converts it to nitric acid, which is highly tissue damaging. In the respiratory tract, nitric acid causes acute chemical injury similar to anhydrous ammonia and subsequent obliterative bronchiolitis and interstitial fibrosis.

Affected cattle that have been chronically exposed to NO_2 have a chronic dry cough and increased respiratory rate greater than 40 breaths/min but few other symptoms. Cattle with severe acute exposure have a moist cough, more severe dyspnea (increased rate and effort), and pulmonary edema.

Diagnosis
Careful observation and history may be the key to diagnosis because the signs are nonspecific. Lung biopsy or necropsy is the only absolute means of diagnosis.

Treatment
Corticosteroids may be used judiciously in affected cattle. Cattle are very sensitive to dexamethasone, and 10 to 20 mg/day for a few days would be appropriate therapy. Risk of secondary infection and abortifacient properties of dexamethasone need to be considered. Atropine and furosemide may also be indicated at previously described doses.

Farmer's Lung: Hypersensitivity Pneumonitis (Extrinsic Allergic Alveolitis)
Etiology and Signs
Hypersensitivity pneumonitis may occur in cattle and result in respiratory distress or chronic respiratory disease. In humans, many specific inhalant antigens may cause similar symptoms, but frequently *Micropolyspora faeni* and related organisms are incriminated. Wet hay that ferments excessively remains the biggest cause of this condition in farmers and cattle. The resultant dusty, moldy hay releases tremendous numbers of spores when bales are opened into the faces of humans and animals. Large round bales also have been observed to cause the problem occasionally. A delayed hypersensitivity reaction is suspected.

Signs of acute experimental exposure include a sudden decrease in appetite and milk production, coughing, cranioventral pulmonary rales bilaterally, and transient fever. In natural cases, chronic cough without obvious illness remains the most common sign when this disease has been recognized in the northern United States. Usually more than 50% of the herd is affected, and herd production decreases 10% to 25% because affected cattle cough enough to interfere with normal consumption of feed. Auscultation of the lungs may reveal a few wheezes or may be normal. Signs lessen but do not stop entirely when animals are fed outdoors or go to pasture. Confinement and feeding the causative hay indoors accentuate the signs. Death is rare, but occasionally severe chronic cases have developed right heart failure. With the feeding of total mixed rations and the reduction in lifespan of dairy cattle in the United States, this disease has become less common. However, sporadic cases continue to be seen, not so much as a herd issue but as an individual, older multiparous cow problem on traditional stanchion and tie stall farms. We occasionally see a similar clinical syndrome in a hospitalized cow that is bedded heavily and has frequent bedding changes.

Diagnosis

The diagnosis can be aided by history, observation, lack of profound illness in affected cattle, and exclusion of other causes of lower airway disease. Tracheal wash samples suggest lymphocytic inflammation with macrophages, lymphocytes, and some plasma cells. The serum of affected cattle may be analyzed for precipitins to *M. faeni* and to other antigens known to be associated with the condition in humans. When results are positive, this is suggestive but not definitive evidence because many normal cattle have positive antibodies.

Lung biopsy also may be a very helpful diagnostic aid if the value of the affected cow precludes necropsy. Necropsy inspection of the affected lungs reveals gray spots indicative of lymphocyte accumulations around small airways in the interstitium. Histopathology shows infiltration of lymphocytes and plasma cells in the interalveolar septa. Provocative testing using the hay in question provides subjective, causative evidence. Lungworms definitely should be ruled out by Baermann's technique, tracheal wash cytology, and necropsy if necessary.

Treatment and Control

When a large percentage of the herd is affected, corticosteroids do not represent a wise treatment. Corticosteroids benefit acutely affected individual cattle or severe recurrent cases but should not be used on a wide scale. Changes in management constitute both treatment and prevention. Feeding hay outside may give some relief, especially if the bales are opened several minutes or more before the cows are allowed access to the hay. Wetting the hay may be helpful. If economics permit, getting rid of the hay is the best policy and may solve the problem. Farmers who consistently make poor-quality hay should be encouraged to consider haylage or at least include

hay additives during harvesting that inhibit mold growth. Humans working with causative hay should consider the use of surgical masks or protective face masks to prevent symptoms of farmer's lung in themselves.

Bronchiolitis Obliterans

Etiology and Signs

This poorly described condition is observed occasionally in individual animals. A dry cough is the predominant sign in affected cattle, and Dr. Fox (personal communication to Dr. Rebhun) used to highlight the magnitude of the cough by quoting farmers who call only because a cow "coughs so hard she causes the milking machine to fall off." Auscultation of the lungs may reveal wheezes or abnormally quiet lung sounds. Although hyperpnea and tachypnea are present in addition to the dry cough, the affected cow does not otherwise appear ill.

The cause is unknown but probably involves chronic exposure to toxic gases, 3-methylindole, allergens, or other proposed causes of acute respiratory distress in cattle from which the individual has survived but with serious lung pathology. The chronic damage that ensues may result in bronchiolitis obliterans, a pathologic diagnosis.

Diagnosis

Lung biopsy or histopathology after necropsy is required for definitive diagnosis.

Treatment

Dexamethasone often gives some relief to affected animals when administered judiciously at 10 to 20 mg/day. Appropriate contraindications should be considered.

Fibrosing Alveolitis

Etiology and Signs

This is a chronic debilitating respiratory disease of mature cattle. Affected cattle do not act ill but have an obvious increased respiratory rate and effort, as well as obvious coughing. Moist or dry rales may be auscultated over the entire lung field. Morbidity is low, but subsequent mortality is high because the disease is chronic and progressive.

The cause is unknown and may simply be the result of chronic exposure to some of the pneumotoxic materials previously discussed in this section. Chronic exposure to 3-methylindole, NO_2 or other gases, antigens known to cause hypersensitivity pneumonia, survival from smoke inhalation, or unknown factors may result in diffuse fibrosis of the alveoli.

Diagnosis

Gross inspection of the lungs at necropsy reveals diffuse pale, heavy, firm lungs. The lobules are white and fleshy. Obliteration of alveolar air space by type 2 pneumocytes, macrophages, and other cells histopathologically explains the antemortem dyspnea. Lung biopsy is indicated if necropsy is not an option.

Treatment

No treatment is likely to be successful, but antiinflammatory drugs may be tried.

Anaphylaxis and Milk Allergy

Etiology and Signs

Respiratory distress often accompanies anaphylaxis induced by exogenous antigens such as vaccines, antibiotics, local anesthetics and feedstuffs, or endogenous antigens such as α-casein in milk.

In susceptible animals, signs usually develop within minutes after injection of biologics or antibiotics and consist of urticaria, edema of mucocutaneous junctions, and respiratory distress. Signs may be mild, with urticaria predominating, or severe, with collapse quickly following initial signs. Laryngeal edema may occur and be progressive over many hours. Certain biologics have been incriminated more than others in this regard. Antibiotic-induced anaphylaxis has been observed as a result of penicillin, tetracycline, sulfas, and other antibiotics. Penicillin may cause respiratory distress from a true anaphylaxis (usually hives accompany the respiratory distress) or as part of the procaine reaction. A procaine reaction causes hyperexcitement and snorting, but edema is not present because this is not an immunologic reaction. A procaine reaction is rare in cattle in comparison to horses and when it does occur is generally less severe than in horses. Biologics that cause an anaphylactic reaction in more than an occasional cow should be avoided unless suitable alternatives are not available. Many apparent anaphylactic crises may in fact be the result of endotoxins in certain biologics and cattle of certain genetic lines being more susceptible to such vaccine reactions.

Affected cattle appear apprehensive and restless, and their hair stands on end. The heart rate elevates, hives may develop, and frequent attempts to urinate and defecate may alternate with restless treading on the limbs. Dyspnea may be inapparent or obvious, with pulmonary edema, hyperpnea, and respiratory stertor. Cyanosis; cold, clammy skin; and hypotensive collapse ensue in severe cases.

Milk allergy occurs most commonly in Channel Island breeds but may occur in any breed. The onset of signs may follow drying a cow off or a reduction in milking frequency to "bag" a cow for a show. Any delay in the normal milking interval may trigger this reaction in cattle sensitized to their own α-casein. The signs may be mild or severe as previously described. Hives, edema of mucocutaneous junctions, and respiratory signs develop to varying degrees (also see Chapter 7).

A unique syndrome of collapse has been observed by many practitioners in cattle injected with concentrated vitamin E and selenium products. The reaction is observed within minutes of the IM injection, and collapse and dyspnea are the only signs. It is not known whether this represents true anaphylaxis, accidental intravascular administration (most likely), or specific toxicity. Most cases recover, but fatal outcomes may occur in 10% to 20% of the cases.

Diagnosis

History and physical signs suffice for diagnosis.

Treatment

Treatment is commensurate with the severity of disease and consists of drugs such as epinephrine, antihistamines, corticosteroids, and furosemide. Recommended dosages for adult cattle include:

- Epinephrine (1/1000 concentration), 2 to 10 mL IM or SC; 2 to 4 mL can be given IV in severe cases
- Tripelennamine HCl, 1 mg/kg IM or SC
- Furosemide, 0.5 to 1.0 mg/kg IM (if pulmonary edema is present)
- Dexamethasone, 20 to 40 mg IV or IM if the cow is not pregnant
- Flunixin meglumine, 1.1 mg/kg IV

For milk allergy, immediate milking out is indicated along with other symptomatic therapy (see earlier) if the cow shows a serious allergic reaction.

In most anaphylaxis cases, one treatment suffices, but in cattle with severe pulmonary edema or urticaria, several treatments at 8- to 12-hour intervals may be necessary for complete resolution.

Suggested Readings

Abutarbush, S. M., Pollock, C. M., Wildman, B. K., et al. (2012). Evaluation of the diagnostic and prognostic utility of ultrasonography at first diagnosis of presumptive bovine respiratory disease. *Can J Vet Res, 76,* 23–28.

Ackermann, M. R., Brogden, K. A., Florance, A. F., et al. (1999). Induction of CD18-mediated passage of neutrophils by *Pasteurella haemolytica* in pulmonary bronchi and bronchioles. *Infect Immun, 67,* 659–663.

Ahn, B. C., Walz, P. H., Kennedy, G. A., et al. (2005). Biotype, genotype, and clinical presentation associated with bovine viral diarrhea virus (BVDV) isolates from cattle. *Intern J Appl Res Vet Med, 3,* 319–325.

Allan, E. M., Gibbs, A. H., Wiseman, A., et al. (1985). Sequential lesions of experimental bovine pneumonic pasteurellosis. *Vet Rec, 117,* 438–442.

Antonis, A. F., Schrijver, R. S., Daus, F., et al. (2003). Vaccine-induced immunopathology during bovine respiratory syncytial virus infection: exploring the parameters of pathogenesis. *J Virol, 77,* 12067–12073.

Aslan, V., Maden, M., Erganis, O., et al. (2002). Clinical efficacy of florfenicol in the treatment of calf respiratory tract infections. *Vet Q, 24,* 35–39.

Autio, T., Pohjanvirta, T., Holopainen, R., et al. (2007). Etiology of respiratory disease in non-vaccinated, non-medicated calves in rearing herds. *Vet Microbiol, 119,* 256–265.

Bach, A. (2011). Associations between several aspects of heifer development and dairy cow survivability to second lactation. *J Dairy Sci, 94,* 1052–1057.

Bach, A., Tejero, C., & Ahedo, J. (2011). Effects of group composition on the incidence of respiratory afflictions in group-housed calves after weaning. *J Dairy Sci, 94,* 2001–2006.

Baker, J. C., & Frey, M. L. (1985). Bovine respiratory syncytial virus. *Vet Clin North Am Food Anim Pract, 1*(2), 259–275.

Bednarek, D., Kondracki, M., Friton, G. M., et al. (2005). Effect of steroidal and non-steroidal anti-inflammatory drugs on inflammatory markers in calves with experimentally-induced bronchopneumonia. *Berl Munch Tierarztl Wochenschr, 118,* 305–308.

Bednarek, D., Zdzisinska, B., Kondracki, M., et al. (2003). Effect of steroidal and non-steroidal anti-inflammatory drugs in combination with long-acting oxytetracycline on non-specific immunity of calves suffering from enzootic bronchopneumonia. *Vet Microbiol, 96,* 53–67.

Bleul, U. (2009). Respiratory distress syndrome in calves. *Vet Clin North Am Food Anim Pract, 25,* 179–193.

Bowersock, T. L., Sobecki, B. E., Terrill, S. J., et al. (2014). Efficacy of multivalent modified-live virus vaccine containing a *Mannheimia haemolytica* toxoid in calves challenge exposed with *Bibersteinia trehalosi. Am J Vet Res, 75,* 770–776.

Braun, U., Pusterla, N., & Fluckiger, M. (1997). Ultrasonographic findings in cattle with pleuropneumonia. *Vet Rec, 141,* 12–17.

Braun, U., Sicher, D., & Pusterla, N. (1996). Ultrasonography of the lungs, pleura, and mediastinum in healthy cows. *Am J Vet Res, 57,* 432–438.

Braun, U., Hauser, B., Meyer, S., et al. (2007). Cattle with thymic lymphoma and haematoma of the ventral neck: a comparison of findings. *Vet J, 174,* 344–350.

Breeze, R. (1985). Parasitic bronchitis and pneumonia. *Vet Clin North Am Food Anim Pract, 1,* 277–287.

Bryson, D. G., McNulty, M. S., McCracken, R. M., et al. (1983). Ultrastructural features of experimental parainfluenza type 3 virus pneumonia in calves. *J Comp Pathol, 93,* 397–414.

Buczinski, S., Forté, G., & Bélanger, A. (2013). Short communication: Ultrasonographic assessment of the thorax as a fast technique to assess pulmonary lesions in dairy calves with bovine respiratory disease. *J Dairy Sci, 96,* 1–6.

Buczinski, S., Forte, G., Francoz, D., et al. (2014). Comparison of thoracic auscultation, clinical score, and ultrasonography as indicators of bovine respiratory disease in preweaned dairy calves. *J Vet Intern Med, 28*(1), 234–241.

Carbonell, P. L. (1979). Bovine nasal granuloma—gross and microscopic lesions. *Vet Pathol, 16,* 60–73.

Confer, A. W., Fulton, R. W., Step, D. L., et al. (2005). Viral antigen distribution in the respiratory tract of cattle persistently infected with bovine viral diarrhea virus subtype 2a. *Vet Pathol, 42,* 192–199.

Confer, A. W., Snider, T. A., Taylor, J. D., et al. (2016). Clinical disease and lung lesions in calves experimentally inoculated with Histophilus somni five days after metaphylactic administration of tildipirosin or tulathromycin. *Am J Vet Res, 77,* 358–366.

Cornish, T. E., van Olphen, A. L., Cavender, J. L., et al. (2005). Comparison of ear notch immunohistochemistry, ear notch antigen-capture ELISA, and buffy coat virus isolation for detection of calves persistently infected with bovine viral diarrhea virus. *J Vet Diagn Invest, 17,* 110–117.

Dagleish, M. P., Finlayson, J., Bayne, C., et al. (2010). Characterization and time course of pulmonary lesions in calves after intratracheal infection with *Pasteurella multocida* A:3. *J Comp Pathol, 142,* 157–169.

DeDonder, K. D., & Apley, M. D. (2015). A literature review of antimicrobial resistance in pathogens associated with bovine respiratory disease. *Anim Health Res Rev, 16,* 125–134.

Deelen, S. M., Ollivett, T. L., Haines, D. M., et al. (2014). Evaluation of a Brix refractometer to estimate serum immunoglobulin G concentration in neonatal dairy calves. *J Dairy Sci, 97,* 3838–3844.

Donovan, G. A., Dohoo, D. A., Montgomery, D. M., et al. (1998). Associations between passive immunity and morbidity and mortality in dairy heifers in Florida, USA. *Prev Vet Med, 34,* 31–46.

Ducharme, N. D., Desrochers, A., Mulon, P. Y., et al. Surgery of the bovine respiratory and cardiovascular systems. In S. L. Fubini and N. D. Ducharme (Eds), Farm Animal Surgery (2nd ed.) St Louis, Elsevier.

Ducharme, N. G., Fubini, S. L., Rebhun, W. C., et al. (1992). Thoracotomy in adult cattle: 14 cases (1979–1991). *J Am Vet Med Assoc, 200,* 86–90.

Ellis, J. A., Gow, S. P., Mahan, S., et al. (2013). Duration of immunity to experimental infection with bovine respiratory syncytial virus following intranasal vaccination of young passively immune calves. *J Am Vet Med Assoc, 243,* 1602–1608.

Ellis, J., Gow, S., West, K., et al. (2007). Response of calves to challenge exposure with virulent bovine respiratory syncytial virus following intranasal administration of vaccines formulated for parenteral administration. *J Am Vet Med Assoc, 230,* 233–243.

Ellis, J. A., West, K. H., Cortese, V. S., et al. (1998). Lesions and distribution of viral antigen following an experimental infection of young seronegative calves with virulent bovine viral diarrhea virus-type II. *Can J Vet Res, 62,* 161–169.

Ellis, J. A., West, K. H., Waldner, C., et al. (2005). Efficacy of a saponin-adjuvanted inactivated respiratory syncytial virus vaccine in calves. *Can Vet J, 46,* 155–162.

Endsley, J. J., Roth, J. A., Ridpath, J., et al. (2003). Maternal antibody blocks humoral but not T cell responses to BVDV. *Biologicals, 31,* 123–125.

Ewers, C., Lubke-Becker, A., & Wieler, L. H. (2004). *Mannheimia haemolytica* and the pathogenesis of enzootic bronchopneumonia [article in German]. *Berl Munch Tierarztl Wochenschr, 117,* 97–115.

Faber, S., Faber, N., McCauley, T., et al. (2005). Case study: Effects of colostrum ingestion on lactational performance. *Prof Anim Sci, 21,* 420–425.

Fairbanks, K. K., Rinehart, C. L., Ohnesorge, W. C., et al. (2004). Evaluation of fetal protection against experimental infection with type 1 and type 2 bovine viral diarrhea virus after vaccination of the dam with a bivalent modified-live virus vaccine. *J Am Vet Med Assoc, 225,* 1898–1904.

Fingland, R. B., Rings, D. M., & Vestweber, J. G. (1990). The etiology and surgical management of tracheal collapse in calves. *Vet Surg, 19,* 371–379.

Flock, M. (2004). Diagnostic ultrasonography in cattle with thoracic disease. *Vet J, 167,* 272–280.

Foster, D. M., Martin, L. G., & Papich, M. G. (2016). Comparison of active drug concentrations in the pulmonary epithelial lining fluid and interstitial fluid of calves injected with enrofloxacin, florfenicol, ceftiofur, or tulathromycin. *PLoS One, 11,* e0159219.

Francoz, D., Fortin, M., Fecteau, G., et al. (2005). Determination of *Mycoplasma bovis* susceptibilities against six antimicrobial agents using the E test method. *Vet Microbiol, 105,* 57–64.

Francoz, D., Buczinski, S., Bélanger, A. M., et al. (2015). Respiratory pathogens in Québec dairy calves and their relationship with clinical status, lung consolidation, and average daily gain. *J Vet Intern Med, 29,* 381–387.

Fulton, R. W., Briggs, R. E., Ridpath, J. F., et al. (2005). Transmission of bovine viral diarrhea virus 1b to susceptible and vaccinated calves by exposure to persistently infected calves. *Can J Vet Res, 69,* 161–169.

Fulton, R. W., Ridpath, J. F., Confer, A. W., et al. (2003). Bovine viral diarrhoea virus antigenic diversity: impact on disease and vaccination programmes. *Biologicals, 31,* 89–95.

Fulton, R. W., Ridpath, J. F., Saliki, J. T., et al. (2002). Bovine viral diarrhea virus (BVDV) 1b: predominant BVDV subtype in calves with respiratory disease. *Can J Vet Res, 66,* 181–190.

Fulton, R. W., Step, D. L., Ridpath, J. F., et al. (2003). Response of calves persistently infected with noncytopathic bovine viral diarrhea virus (BVDV) subtype 1b after vaccination with heterologous BVDV strains in modified live virus vaccines and *Mannheimia haemolytica* bacterin-toxoid. *Vaccine, 21,* 2980–2985.

Gasthuys, F., Verschooten, F., Parmentier, D., et al. (1992). Laryngotomy as a treatment for chronic laryngeal obstruction in cattle; a review of 130 cases. *Vet Rec, 130*(11), 220–223.

Gevaert, D. (2006). The importance of *Mycoplasma bovis* in bovine respiratory disease. *Tijdschr Diergeneeskd, 131,* 124–126.

Genicot, B., Close, R., Lindsey, J. K., et al. (1995). Pulmonary function changes induced by three regimens of bronchodilating agents in calves with acute respiratory distress syndrome. *Vet Rec, 137,* 183–186.

Gershwin, L. J., Van Eenennaam, A. L., Anderson, M. L., et al. (2015). Single pathogen challenge with agents of the bovine respiratory disease complex. *PLoS One, 10,* e0142479.

Gorden, P. J., & Plummer, P. (2010). Control, management, and prevention of bovine respiratory disease in dairy calves and cows. *Vet Clin North Am Food Anim Pract, 26,* 243–259.

Grell, S. N., Ribert, U., Tjornehoj, K., et al. (2005). Age-dependent differences in cytokine and antibody responses after experimental RSV infection in a bovine model. *Vaccine, 23,* 3412–3423.

Guard, C. L., Rebhun, W. C., & Perdrizet, J. A. (1984). Cranial tumors in aged cattle causing Horner's syndrome and exophthalmos. *Cornell Vet, 74,* 361–365.

Gulliksen, S. M., Jor, E., Lie, K. I., et al. (2009). Respiratory infections in Norwegian dairy calves. *J Dairy Sci, 92,* 5139–5146.

Haines, D. M., Moline, K. M., Sargent, R. A., et al. (2004). Immunohistochemical study of *Hemophilus somnus, Mycoplasma bovis, Mannheimia hemolytica,* and bovine viral diarrhea virus in death losses due to myocarditis in feedlot cattle. *Can Vet J, 45,* 231–234.

Hanthorn, C. J., Dewell, R. D., Cooper, V. L., et al. (2014). Randomized clinical trial to evaluate the pathogenicity of *Bibersteinia trehalosi* in respiratory disease among calves. *Vet Res, 10,* 89–96.

Hasokusuz, M., Lathrop, S. L., Gadfield, K. L., et al. (1999). Isolation of bovine respiratory coronaviruses from feedlot cattle and comparison of their biological and antigenic properties with bovine enteric coronaviruses. *Am J Vet Res, 60,* 1227–1233.

Heins, B., Nydam, D., Woolums, A., et al. (2014). Comparative efficacy of enrofloxacin and tulathromycin for treatment of preweaning respiratory disease in dairy heifers. *J Dairy Sci, 97,* 372–382.

Hill, J. R., Roussel, A. J., Cibelli, J. B., et al. (1999). Clinical and pathologic features of cloned transgenic calves and fetuses (13 case studies). *Theriogenology, 51,* 1451–1465.

Jolly, S., Detilleux, J., & Desmecht, D. (2004). Extensive mast cell degranulation in bovine respiratory syncytial virus-associated paroxystic respiratory distress syndrome. *Vet Immunol Immunopathol, 97,* 125–136.

Jung, C., & Bostedt, H. (2004). Thoracic ultrasonography technique in newborn calves and description of normal and pathological findings. *Vet Radiol Ultrasound, 45,* 331–335.

Kadota, K., Ito, K., & Kamikawa, S. (1986). Ultrastructure and origin of adenocarcinomas detected in the lungs of three cows. *J Comp Pathol, 96,* 407–414.

Karapinar, T., & Dabak, M. (2008). Treatment of premature calves with clinically diagnosed respiratory distress syndrome. *J Vet Intern Med, 22,* 462–466.

Kelling, C. L. (2004). Evolution of bovine viral diarrhea virus vaccines. *Vet Clin North Am Food Anim Pract, 20,* 115–129.

Khodakaram-Tafti, A., & Lopez, A. (2004). Immunohistopathological findings in the lungs of calves naturally infected with *Mycoplasma bovis. J Vet Med A Physiol Pathol Clin Med, 51,* 10–14.

Krahwinkel, D. J., Jr., Schmeitzel, L. P., Fadok, V. A., et al. (1988). Familial allergic rhinitis in cattle. *J Am Vet Med Assoc, 192,* 1593–1596.

Lago, A., McGuirk, S. M., Bennett, T. B., et al. (2006). Calf respiratory disease and pen microenvironments in naturally ventilated calf barns in winter. *J Dairy Sci, 89,* 4014–4025.

Lathrop, S. L., Wittum, T. E., Brock, K. V., et al. (2000). Association between infection of the respiratory tract attributable to bovine coronavirus and health and growth performance of cattle in feedlots. *Am J Vet Res, 61,* 1062–1066.

Lathrop, S. L., Wittum, T. E., Loerch, S. C., et al. (2000). Antibody titers against bovine coronavirus and shedding of the virus via the respiratory tract in feedlot cattle. *Am J Vet Res, 61,* 1057–1061.

Lee, W. D., Flynn, A. N., LeBlanc, J. M., et al. (2004). Tilmicosin-induced bovine neutrophil apoptosis is cell-specific and down-regulates spontaneous LTB4 synthesis without increasing Fas expression. *Vet Res, 35,* 213–224.

Leite, F., Atapattu, D., Kuckleburg, C., et al. (2005). Incubation of bovine PMNs with conditioned medium from BHV-1 infected peripheral blood mononuclear cells increases their susceptibility to *Mannheimia haemolytica* leukotoxin. *Vet Immunol Immunopathol, 103,* 187–193.

Leite, F., Kuckleburg, C., Atapattu, D., et al. (2004). BHV-1 infection and inflammatory cytokines amplify the interaction of Mannheimia haemolytica leukotoxin with bovine peripheral blood mononuclear cells in vitro. *Vet Immunol Immunopathol, 99,* 193–202.

Lockwood, P. W., Johnson, J. C., & Katz, T. L. (2003). Clinical efficacy of flunixin, carprofen and ketoprofen as adjuncts to the antibacterial treatment of bovine respiratory disease. *Vet Rec, 152,* 392–394.

Loneragan, G. H., Gould, D. H., Mason, G. L., et al. (2001). Involvement of microbial respiratory pathogens in acute interstitial pneumonia in feedlot cattle. *Am J Vet Res, 62,* 1519–1524.

Love, W. J., Lehenbauer, T. W., Kass, P. H., et al. (2014). Development of a novel clinical scoring system for on-farm diagnosis of bovine respiratory disease in pre-weaned dairy calves. *Peerj.* http://dx.doi.org/10.7717/peerj.238.

Love, W. J., Lehenbauer, T. W., Van Eenennaam, A. L., et al. (2016). Sensitivity and specificity of on-farm scoring systems and nasal culture to detect bovine respiratory disease complex in preweaned dairy calves. *J Vet Diagn Invest, 28,* 119–128.

Lubbers, B. V., Apley, M. D., Coetzee, J. F., et al. (2007). Use of computed tomography to evaluate pathologic changes in the lungs of calves with experimentally induced respiratory tract disease. *Am J Vet Res, 68,* 1259–1264.

Lundborg, G., Svensson, E., & Oltenacu, P. (2005). Herd-level risk factors for infectious diseases in Swedish dairy calves aged 0–90 days. *Prev Vet Med, 68,* 123–143.

Masseau, I., Fecteau, G., Breton, L., et al. (2008). Radiographic detection of thoracic lesions in adult cows: a retrospective study of 42 cases (1995-2002). *Can Vet J, 49,* 261–267.

Mawhinney, I. C., & Burrows, M. R. (2005). Protection against bovine respiratory syncytial virus challenge following a single dose of vaccine in young calves with maternal antibody. *Vet Rec, 156,* 139–143.

McGuirk, S. M. (2008). Disease management of dairy calves and heifers. *Vet Clin North Am Food Anim Pract*, 24, 139–153.

Michaux, H., Nichols, S., Babkine, M., et al. (2014). Description of thoracoscopy and associated short-term cardiovascular and pulmonary effects in healthy cattle. *Am J Vet Res*, 75, 468–476.

Mevius, D. J., & Hartman, E. G. (2000). In vitro activity of 12 antibiotics used in veterinary medicine against *Mannheimia haemolytica* and *Pasteurella multocida* isolated from calves in the Netherlands [in Dutch]. *Tijdschr Diergeneeskd*, 125, 147–152.

Migaki, G., Helmboldt, C. F., & Robinson, F. R. (1974). Primary pulmonary tumors of epithelial origin in cattle. *Am J Vet Res*, 35, 1397–1400.

Mitra, N., Cernicchiaro, N., Torres, S., et al. (May 5, 2016). Metagenomic characterization of the virome associated with bovine respiratory disease diagnosis in feedlot cattle identified novel viruses and suggest an etiologic role for influenza D. *J Gen Virol*. http://dx.doi.org/10.1099/jgv.0.000492.

Moeller, R. B., Adaska, J., Reynolds, J., et al. (2013). Systemic bovine herpesvirus 1 infections in neonatal dairy calves. *J Vet Diagn Invest*, 25, 136–141.

Morrow, D. A. (1968). Pneumonia in cattle due to migrating Ascaris. *J Am Vet Med Assoc*, 153, 184–189.

Ng, T. F., Kondov, N. O., Deng, X., et al. (2015). A metagenomics and case-control study to identify viruses associated with bovine respiratory disease. *J Virol*, 89, 5340–5349.

Nicholas, R. A. (2004). *Recent developments in the diagnosis and control of Mycoplasma infections in cattle*. Quebec City, Canada: Proceedings of the 23rd World Buiatrics Congress.

Nichols, S., & Anderson, D. E. (2009). Subtotal or partial unilateral arytenoidectomy for treatment of arytenoid chondritis in five calves. *J Am Vet Med Assoc*, 235, 420–425.

Nordlund, K. V. (2008). Practical considerations for ventilating calf barns in winter. *Vet Clin North Am Food Anim Pract*, 24, 41–54.

Nowakowski, M. A., Inskeep, P. B., Risk, J. E., et al. (2004). Pharmacokinetics and lung tissue concentrations of tulathromycin, a new triamilide antibiotic, in cattle. *Vet Ther*, 5, 60–74.

Okada, Y., Ochiai, K., Osaki, K., et al. (1998). Bronchiolar-alveolar carcinoma in a cow. *J Comp Pathol*, 118, 69–74.

Ollivett, T. L., Hewson, J., Schubotz, R., et al. (2013). Ultrasonographic progression of lung consolidation after experimental infection with *Mannheimia haemolytica* in Holstein bull calves. *Proceedings Am Assoc Bov Pract*, 147, Milwaukee, WI.

Ollivett, T. L., Kelton, D. F., Duffield, T. F., et al. (2014). A randomized controlled clinical trial to evaluate the effect of an intranasal respiratory vaccine on calf health, ultrasonographic lung consolidation, and growth in Holstein dairy calves. *Proceedings Am Assoc Bovine Pract*, 147, Albuquerque, NM.

Ollivett, T. L., Caswell, J. L., Nydam, D. V., et al. (2015). Thoracic ultrasonography and bronchoalveolar lavage fluid analysis in Holstein calves with subclinical lung lesions. *J Vet Intern Med*, 29, 1728–1734.

Ollivett, T. L., & Buczinski, S. (2016). On-farm use of ultrasonography for bovine respiratory disease. *Vet Clin North Am Food Anim Pract*, 32, 19–35.

Patel, J. R. (2004). Evaluation of a quadrivalent inactivated vaccine for the protection of cattle against diseases due to common viral infections. *J S Afr Vet Assoc*, 75, 137–146.

Patel, J. R., & Didlick, S. A. (2004). Evaluation of efficacy of an inactivated vaccine against bovine respiratory syncytial virus in calves with maternal antibodies. *Am J Vet Res*, 65, 417–421.

Peek, S. F., Slack, J. A., & McGuirk, S. M. (2003). Management of pneumothorax in cattle by continuous-flow evacuation. *J Vet Intern Med*, 17, 119–122.

Peters, A. R., Thevasagayam, S. J., Wiseman, A., et al. (2004). Duration of immunity of a quadrivalent vaccine against respiratory diseases caused by BHV-1, PI3V, BVDV, and BRSV in experimentally infected calves. *Prev Vet Med*, 66, 63–77.

Platt, R., Burdett, W., & Roth, J. A. (2006). Induction of antigen-specific T-cell subset activation to bovine respiratory disease viruses by a modified-live virus vaccine. *Am J Vet Res*, 67(7), 1179–1184.

Portis, E., Lindeman, C., Johansen, L., et al. (2012). A ten-year (2000-2009) study of antimicrobial susceptibility of bacteria that cause bovine respiratory disease complex - *Mannheimia haemolytica*, *Pasteurella multocida*, and *Histophilus somni* - in the United States and Canada. *J Vet Diagn Invest*, 24, 932–944.

Powers, J. G., Van Metre, D. C., Collins, J. K., et al. (2005). Evaluation of ovine herpesvirus type 2 infections, as detected by competitive inhibition ELISA and polymerase chain reaction assay, in dairy cattle without clinical signs of malignant catarrhal fever. *J Am Vet Med Assoc*, 227, 606–611.

Rabeling, B., Rehage, J., Döpfer, D., et al. (1998). Ultrasonographic findings in calves with respiratory disease. *Vet Rec*, 143, 468–471.

Radi, Z. A., Brogden, K. A., Dixon, R. A., et al. (2002). A selectin inhibitor decreases neutrophil infiltration during acute *Mannheimia haemolytica* pneumonia. *Vet Pathol*, 39, 697–705.

Rebhun, W. C., King, J. M., & Hillman, R. B. (1988). Atypical actinobacillosis granulomas in cattle. *Cornell Vet*, 78, 125–130.

Rebhun, W. C., Rendano, V. T., Dill, S. G., et al. (1980). Caudal vena caval thrombosis in four cattle with acute dyspnea. *J Am Vet Med Assoc*, 176, 1366–1369.

Rebhun, W. C., Smith, J. S., Post, J. E., et al. (1978). An outbreak of the conjunctival form of infectious bovine rhinotracheitis. *Cornell Vet*, 68, 297–307.

Reef, V. B., Boy, M. G., Reid, C. F., et al. (1991). Comparison between diagnostic ultrasonography and radiography in the evaluation of horses and cattle with thoracic disease: 56 cases (1984-1985). *J Am Vet Med Assoc*, 198, 2112–2118.

Reinhold, P., Rabeling, B., Günther, H., et al. (2002). Comparative evaluation of ultrasonography and lung function testing with the clinical signs and pathology of calves inoculated experimentally with *Pasteurella multocida*. *Vet Rec*, 150, 109–114.

Rings, D. M. (1995). Tracheal collapse. *Vet Clin North Am Food Anim Pract*, 11, 171–175.

Ross, M. W., Richardson, D. W., Hackett, R. P., et al. (1986). Nasal obstruction caused by cystic nasal conchae in cattle. *J Am Vet Med Assoc*, 188, 857–860.

Roussel, A. J., Hill, J. R., & Hooper, R. N. (2004). *Clone calves: medical challenges*. Quebec City, Canada: Proceedings of the 23rd World Buiatrics Congress.

Sacco, R. E., McGill, J. L., Pillatzki, A. E., et al. (2014). Respiratory syncytial virus infection in cattle. *Vet Pathol*, 5, 427–436.

Senthilkumaran, C., Hewson, J., Ollivett, T. L., et al. (2015). Localization of annexins A1 and A2 in the respiratory tract of healthy calves and those experimentally infected with *Mannheimia haemolytica*. *Vet Res*, 46, 6–13.

Shahriar, F. M., Clark, E. G., Janzen, E., et al. (2002). Coinfection with bovine viral diarrhea virus and *Mycoplasma bovis* in feedlot cattle with chronic pneumonia. *Can Vet J*, 43, 863–868.

Shin, S. J., Kang, S. G., Nabin, R., et al. (2005). Evaluation of the antimicrobial activity of florfenicol against bacteria isolated from bovine and porcine respiratory disease. *Vet Microbiol*, 106, 73–77.

Slack, J. A., Thomas, C. B., & Peek, S. F. (2004). Pneumothorax in dairy cattle: 30 cases (1990-2003). *J Am Vet Med Assoc*, 225, 732–735.

Stanton, A., Kelton, D., LeBlanc, S., et al. (2010). The effect of treatment with long-acting antibiotic at postweaning movement on respiratory disease and on growth in commercial dairy calves. *J Dairy Sci, 93*, 574–581.

Stipkovits, L., Ripley, P., Varga, J., et al. (2000). Clinical study of the disease of calves associated with *Mycoplasma bovis* infection. *Acta Vet Hung, 48*, 387–395.

Stoffregen, B., Bolin, S. R., Ridpath, J. F., et al. (2000). Morphologic lesions in type 2 BVDV infections experimentally induced by strain BVDV2-1373 recovered from a field case. *Vet Microbiol, 77*, 157–162.

Storz, J., Purdy, C. W., Lin, X., et al. (2000). Isolation of respiratory bovine coronavirus, other cytocidal viruses, and *Pasteurella* spp. from cattle involved in two natural outbreaks of shipping fever. *J Am Vet Med Assoc, 216*, 1599–1604.

Sustronck, B., Deprez, P., Muylle, E., et al. (1995). Evaluation of the nebulisation of sodium ceftiofur in the treatment of experimental *Pasteurella haemolytica* bronchopneumonia in calves. *Res Vet Sci, 59*, 267–271.

Taylor, G., Bruce, C., Barbet, A. F., et al. (2005). DNA vaccination against respiratory syncytial virus in young calves. *Vaccine, 23*, 1242–1250.

Thomas, A., Nicolas, C., Dizier, I., et al. (2003). Antibiotic susceptibilities of recent isolates of *Mycoplasma bovis* in Belgium. *Vet Rec, 153*, 428–431.

USDA. 2010. Dairy 2007, *Heifer calf health and management practices on U.S. dairy operations, 2007*. USDA: APHIS:VS, CEAH Fort Collins, CO #550 0110 2010.

USDA. 2012. *Dairy Heifer Raiser*, 2011. USDA–APHIS–VS, CEAH, National Animal Health Monitoring System (NAHMS), Fort Collins, CO. #613.1012.

Van Donkersgoed, J., Ribble, C. S., Boyer, L. G., et al. (1993). Epidemiological study of enzootic pneumonia in dairy calves in Saskatchewan. *Can J Vet Res, 57*, 247–254.

Vangeel, I., Antonis, A. F., Fluess, M., et al. (2007). Efficacy of a modified live intranasal bovine respiratory syncytial virus vaccine in 3-week-old calves experimentally challenged with BRSV. *Vet J, 174*(3), 627–635.

Vestweber, J. G. (1997). Respiratory problems of newborn calves. *Vet Clin North Am Food Anim Pract, 13*, 411–424.

Virtala, A., Gröhn, Y., Mechor, G. D., et al. (1999). The effect of maternally derived immunoglobulin G on the risk of respiratory disease in heifers during the first 3 months of life. *Prev Vet Med, 39*, 25–37.

Warnick, L. D., Erb, H. N., & White, M. (1995). Lack of association between calf morbidity and subsequent first lactation milk production in 25 New York Holstein herds. *J Dairy Sci, 78*, 2819–2830.

Waltner-Toews, D., Martin, S. W., Meek, A. H., et al. (1986). Dairy calf management, morbidity and mortality in Ontario Holstein herds. I. The data. *Prev Vet Med, 4*, 103–124.

Welsh, R. D., Dye, L. B., Payton, M. E., et al. (2004). Isolation and antimicrobial susceptibilities of bacterial pathogens from bovine pneumonia: 1994-2002. *J Vet Diagn Invest, 16*, 426–431.

Windeyer, M. C., Leslie, K. E., Godden, S. M., et al. (2012). The effects of viral vaccination of dairy heifer calves on the incidence of respiratory disease, mortality, and growth. *J Dairy Sci, 95*, 6731–6739.

Windeyer, M. C., Leslie, K. E., Godden, S. M., et al. (2014). Factors associated with morbidity, mortality, and growth of dairy heifer calves up to 3 months of age. *Prev Vet Med, 113*, 231–240.

Woolums, A. R., Anderson, M. L., Gunther, R. A., et al. (1999). Evaluation of severe disease induced by aerosol inoculation of calves with bovine respiratory syncytial virus. *Am J Vet Res, 60*, 473–480.

Woolums, A. R., Brown, C. C., Brown, J. C., Jr., et al. (2004). Effects of a single intranasal dose of modified-live bovine respiratory syncytial virus vaccine on resistance to subsequent viral challenge in calves. *Am J Vet Res, 65*, 363–372.

Woolums, A. R., Gunther, R. A., McArthur-Vaughan, K., et al. (2004). Cytotoxic T lymphocyte activity and cytokine expression in calves vaccinated with formalin-inactivated bovine respiratory syncytial virus prior to challenge. *Comp Immunol Microbiol Infect Dis, 27*, 57–74.

Zaremba, W., Grunert, E., & Aurich, J. E. (1997). Prophylaxis of respiratory distress syndrome in premature calves by administration of dexamethasone or a prostaglandin F2 alpha analogue to their dams before parturition. *Am J Vet Res, 58*, 404–407.

Zecchinon, L., Fett, T., & Desmecht, D. (2005). How *Mannheimia haemolytica* defeats host defense through a kiss of death mechanism. *Vet Res, 36*, 133–156.

5

Noninfectious Diseases of the Gastrointestinal Tract

SUSAN L. FUBINI, AMY E. YEAGER, AND THOMAS J. DIVERS

Diseases of the Forestomach, Mouth and Esophagus

Simple Acute Indigestion Occurring in the Rumen (or Small Intestine)

Etiology

The term *indigestion* is used to describe a wide spectrum of clinical syndromes in cattle, ranging from excessive fermentation of ingesta and gas production in the bowel to intestinal inflammation and more severe disease forms such as lactic acidosis. As would be expected, the rumen is most often affected by indigestion, although small intestine and cecal indigestion also occur in adult dairy cattle and are discussed concurrently. Changes in intestinal microbiota, intestinal motility, and luminal pH, often resulting from ingestion of feeds that cause abnormal fermentation, are mostly responsible for intestinal indigestion. Ruminal and small intestinal disturbances can occur together or independently. Cecal or hindgut indigestion are also common co-morbidities and may be part of the cecal tympany syndrome; this is discussed later in the chapter. An individual cow (common with small intestinal indigestion) or a few animals (common with ruminal indigestion) can be affected at any one time. The affected cow may be at any stage of lactation, although indigestion seems to be more common in cows in the first weeks after parturition. The causative feed material is usually a component of a total mixed ration. The diagnosis of ruminal or small intestinal indigestion is made by using a combination of history, clinical signs, abdominal ultrasonography (for small intestinal indigestion), rumen fluid analysis, and ruling out other diseases through a complete physical examination. Although the diagnosis of simple indigestion often seems like an "excuse diagnosis" in a cow that is off feed and down in milk, the entity does exist, and the veterinarian should not hesitate to make this diagnosis if other diseases have been eliminated through careful examination. An important differential diagnosis especially for ruminal indigestion is primary ketosis, and this should be ruled out by testing for urinary ketones. The two disorders also may coexist in some recently fresh cattle.

Clinical Signs

Simple ruminal indigestion results in signs of anorexia, decreased milk production, cold extremities, and rumen dysfunction, hence the overlap in terms of presenting signs with primary ketosis during early lactation. Colic is common if there is small intestinal indigestion (Fig. 5.1). Although rumen stasis or hypoactivity is typical, some cattle have increased rumen contraction rates but decreased strength of contractions. The cow's temperature, pulse rate, and respiratory rate are often normal with ruminal indigestion, but tachycardia and tachypnea may develop in cows with small intestinal indigestion associated with colic. Abdominal distension may be present because of mild rumen distension, or gas and fluid distension may be present in the right lower quadrant, representing small intestinal distension. In small intestinal indigestion, enough fluid and gas can accumulate in the small bowel to sometimes cause palpable small bowel distension on rectal examination

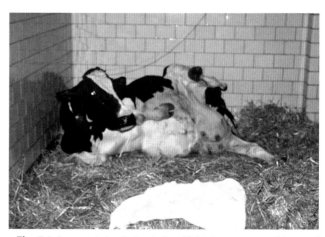

• **Fig. 5.1** Severe abdominal pain in a Holstein cow caused by small intestinal indigestion and bowel distension. The cow developed diarrhea a couple of hours later and was normal the next day.

and put severe tension on the mesentery, resulting in signs of colic such as kicking at the belly, bellowing, violent behavior, getting up and down repeatedly, and treading with the hind feet. In fact, this form of indigestion may be the most common cause of intestinal colic in adult dairy cows! Colic resulting from small intestinal indigestion can sometimes be difficult to differentiate from a mechanical small bowel obstruction. Both may cause colic, succussible fluid in the right ventral quadrant, small intestinal distension on ultrasonography, and palpable small intestines on rectal examination. Extremely distended and tight loops of small intestine, fibrin or crepitus on rectal examination, blood in the stool, absence of manure, and deterioration in cardiovascular status all suggest a physical obstruction rather than simple indigestion. On abdominal ultrasound examination, fluid-filled and dilated loops of small intestine are typical of both indigestion and obstruction, with nonmotile loops of bowel being most suggestive of a physical obstruction or strangulation (Fig. 5.2). With small intestinal indigestion, the fluid responsible for small bowel distension results from stasis associated with indigestion and hypocalcemia. This often progresses to diarrhea within a few hours as the cow responds to therapy or self-initiates more normal gastrointestinal (GI) activity.

Ancillary Data

Laboratory data are seldom helpful in establishing an absolute diagnosis of simple indigestion. Hypocalcemia is the only biochemical abnormality anticipated with mild ruminal indigestion. Hypocalcemia and hypochloremia are common with small intestinal indigestion. With ruminal indigestion, a sample of rumen fluid collected by rumenocentesis or rumen tube can be analyzed. Rumen fluid analysis in cows with indigestion will likely show reduced activity and concentration of large and small protozoa and a prolonged new methylene blue (NMB) reduction time. A NMB reduction test, used to assess the number of functional anaerobic bacteria within the rumen, is performed by adding 0.5 mL of a 0.03% solution of methylene blue stain to 10 mL of fresh rumen fluid in a test tube. The contents are then mixed and the tube is allowed to stand

upright. A robust microbial population will reduce methylene blue to a colorless form (blue disappears) in 2 to 6 minutes. The activity of rumen flora can also be crudely measured by putting a mixture of the fluid in a 10-mL clot vacutainer tube, quickly replacing the stopper on the tube, and evacuating air from the tube with a small needle and syringe. With normal rumen flora and fermentation, a layered mixing effect (bubbles at the top and fluid mixed with fermenting feed below) should occur within 10 minutes. The pH of the rumen sample should also be measured, but if it is collected via an ororumen tube, saliva contamination may confound the results (see further discussion under subacute rumen acidosis).

Treatment

Treatment for simple indigestion follows the two major principles suggested by Udall:
1. Reestablish normal GI motility, pH, and flora by ruminal transfaunation and feeding long-stem fiber.
2. Evacuate the GI tract with the intent of eliminating any potentially toxic causative feed material (e.g., mold, mycotoxins).

These two goals are accomplished by transfaunation when possible, in addition to administration of oral laxative–ruminotoric mixtures and parenteral calcium solutions. Transfaunation fluid can be collected from a healthy cow using the Rosenburg ororuminal collection tube and should be administered to the sick cow in hopes of "repopulating" microbes from the healthy rumen. The phyla Bacteroidetes and Firmicutes comprise the great majority of bacteria in the healthy rumen.

Many laxative–antacid–ruminotoric mixtures are available, and each practitioner may have a favorite. If the rumen has some activity, boluses of these mixtures may be acceptable, but the powdered form of these products should be mixed with warm water and administered through a stomach tube to ensure its distribution if rumen activity is severely depressed. In cases with ruminal tympany, a stomach tube should be passed routinely to relieve gas distension before administering treatment. Excessive treatment with alkalinizing magnesium containing products should be avoided because they can result in hypermagnesemia and metabolic alkalosis, which will further decrease ionized calcium and cause muscular weakness. Parenteral calcium solutions are administered for all cases of simple indigestion because inappetence and GI stasis coupled with continued calcium loss will lead to hypocalcemia. Hypocalcemia results in the clinical sign of cool peripheral parts and exacerbates GI stasis. Hypocalcemia in recently calved cows may, via intestinal stasis, be a risk factor for indigestion rather than a result of the indigestion. For simple indigestion cases, 500 mL of 23% calcium borogluconate intravenously (IV) or divided into four subcutaneous (SC) locations is administered. Magnesium products (sulfate, oxide, or hydroxide) are commonly used as cathartics or alkalinizing products; in dehydrated cattle with low urine production, they may cause hypermagnesemia and clinical weakness when used excessively or repeatedly. Cows that demonstrate severe colic associated with small intestinal indigestion may require a single

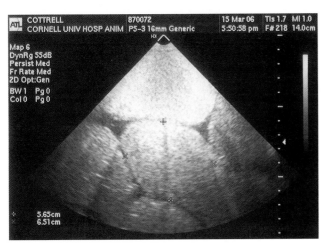

• **Fig. 5.2** Ultrasound image of the abdomen of a cow demonstrating small intestinal distension.

treatment with flunixin meglumine. After treatment, a cow with small intestinal indigestion should regain appetite and pass large amounts of loose manure within 12 to 24 hours. The patient's feces tend to remain watery or looser than normal for 2 to 3 days. Laxative therapy should be continued on a reducing dose basis for 2 to 3 days to ensure complete evacuation of causative feed material from the GI tract.

Subacute to Chronic Rumen Acidosis

Subacute ruminal acidosis (SARA), also called subclinical ruminal acidosis, occurs more commonly (to a possible prevalence of up to 20%) in lactating cows than the acute clinical syndromes of indigestion or ruminal acidosis and derives from modern feeding practices. In brief, feeding excessive amounts of nonstructural carbohydrates (sugars and starches) and rapidly fermentable forages, along with insufficient dietary coarse fiber, allows a degree of rumen acidosis (excess lactic acid and volatile fatty acids) for a transient period after ingestion. During this period of acidosis, small areas of rumen mucosa can be damaged by the same chemical mechanism that causes more widespread lesions in lactic acid indigestion. These small areas of rumenitis may act as entry points for opportunistic bacteria that subsequently ascend the portal circulation and cause liver abscesses. These may be single or multiple and, when located near the hilus of the liver, predispose the cow to caudal vena caval thrombosis syndrome. Dairy cattle seldom develop the "sawdust liver" or miliary liver abscesses of feeder beef animals despite the the shared pathophysiology of rumenitis.

Subclinical ruminal acidosis also may be present on a continual rather than a transient basis in some feeding programs. Immediate clinical signs of the disorder may not be obvious, but computer monitoring will indicate decreased milk production, decreased milk fat percentage, decreased feed consumption, and decreased time chewing cud. In addition to liver abscesses and caudal vena caval thrombosis syndrome that might occur after ruminal acidosis, these herds often have a high incidence of abomasal disease, indigestion, decreased or fluctuating dry matter intakes, decreased time chewing cud (which should be nearly 50% in resting cows), diarrhea, decreased milk production, milk fat depression, lower rumen fill, and low urea nitrogen.

Laminitis may result from release of various mediators, including endotoxins, from rumen microbes destroyed by the pH decreases associated with subclinical rumen acidosis. Mediator absorption is enhanced by chemical damage to the rumen mucosa. When this syndrome is suspected, the veterinarian should collect rumen samples from several cows in the herd to analyze pH and rumen microflora. The abnormal pH indicating SARA will be 5.3 to 5.7 when rumen fluid samples are collected by rumenocentesis from the ventral sac, or 5.5 to 5.9 using an oral probe that can collect 200 mL of fluid from the rumen. A pH less than 6.0 would be suspicious, although a normal pH does not rule out the disease, because the rumen fluid pH will increase to normal following a period of anorexia, and in all cows that are eating, rumen fluid pH varies during the day! Salivary contamination may occur during oral-ruminal collection if a proper ruminal sampling probe is not used or if only a small volume of rumen fluid is obtained. Insufficient fluid volume in a sample is often contaminated with saliva, causing a higher pH than what truly exists in the rumen. Rumenocentesis requires puncture of the rumen through the left flank and provides an accurate assessment of ruminal fluid pH, but there is some, albeit low, risk from the procedure. When testing ruminal pH, practitioners should aim for the nadir in luminal pH; for component-fed herds, this is about 2 to 4 hours postfeeding, but in total mixed ration (TMR)–fed herds, this point is reached about 6 to 8 hours postfeeding. In general, pH meters, appropriately maintained and calibrated before use, should be used whenever possible. Commonly used pH paper is not accurate because the green color of rumen fluid influences the interpretation. Dr. Ken Nordlund at the University of Wisconsin has suggested that that a pH of less than 5.5 in 5 or more cows within a sample size of 12 should be used as an arbitrary cutoff point to define a herd problem with subacute rumen acidosis.

As so well stated by Dr. Ian Lean, correction or prevention of ruminal acidosis requires careful adaptation to diets, well-processed and well-integrated TMR diets, adequate physically effective neutral detergent fiber (peNDF), and limiting and optimizing preformed lactic acid (from silages or high moisture grains and earlage), sugar and starch, and protein. Natural or supplemental buffering of the diet (often magnesium oxide and sodium bicarbonate) is often part of the prevention program, and a nutritional analysis should be performed to aid the dairy farmer, veterinarian, and any nutritional consultants in restructuring the diet to avoid relative acidosis. Sometimes this can be easily accomplished by feeding a small amount of long-stem roughage before the concentrate or TMR, which induces a natural buffering by saliva production before the concentrate or TMR enters the rumen. In other situations (e.g., where component feeding is still being practiced), a switch to a TMR may be indicated. However, the feeding of a TMR does not preclude the opportunity for subacute rumen acidosis! Nor indeed does grazing; in fact, some of the most severely SARA-affected herds that we have experienced have been grazing dairies. Grazing herds appear to be particularly vulnerable to SARA at times of the year when grass is lush and comparatively lower in fiber or in husbandry systems in which concentrate is fed in large amounts at milking time when cattle return from pasture under the erroneous assumption that there is sufficient fiber and buffering emanating from the pasture. Each herd needs to be assessed and corrected on an individual basis, and generalities are not acceptable because feedstuffs, production levels, and management practices vary widely. Ideally, diets should be a balance of rapidly, intermediately, and slowly fermented feedstuffs such that enough fermentable feeds are ingested to meet the cow's energy and protein needs while avoiding the production of excess acid too quickly in the rumen, which could depress pH and fiber fermentation and lead to digestive upset.

Chronic ruminal indigestion of milk-fed calves is well described but is discussed in a subsequent section on bloat.

Moderate to Severe Acute Ruminal Indigestion or Acidosis

Etiology

More severe forms of ruminal indigestion associated with high sugar and starch feeds closely approximate acute ruminal acidosis (lactic acidosis, toxic indigestion). Dramatic increases in ruminal lactic acid occur when excess sugars are fermented by *Streptococcus bovis*. Prior to the increase in ruminal lactic acidosis, high ruminal concentrations of volatile fatty acids (VFAs), especially propionate and valerate, increase in association with excess starch ingestion. A range of clinical signs is possible, depending on the quantity and type of feed material ingested by the cow. Feeding excessive amounts of nonstructural carbohydrates, highly fermentable forages and insufficient dietary coarse fiber are the most common predisposing factors. A history of overingestion of grain or grain silage may exist. Although uncommon in modern dairy management feeding, bolus concentrate has historically been a common prelude to ruminal acidosis in dairy cattle (especially first-calf heifers).

Clinical Signs

Signs of moderate to severe ruminal indigestion, usually resulting from ruminal acidosis, include a dramatic decrease in appetite and milk production, decreased milk fat percentage, complete GI stasis, cool peripheral parts, normal or subnormal rectal temperature, low volume diarrhea in some cases, and normal or elevated heart and respiratory rates. Some affected cows are hypocalcemic enough to be recumbent and unable to rise. It should be emphasized that these cows have more severe signs than simple indigestion cases, including a splashy rumen in some cases, depression, dehydration, and tachycardia. Clinical signs of laminitic lameness or weight loss caused by liver abscesses may occur 2 to 6 weeks later.

Ancillary Data

Hypocalcemia is a consistent finding, and acid–base and electrolyte values vary depending on the degree of lactic acidosis. Azotemia may be present. Ruminal pH may vary from 5.0 to normal depending on the severity of disease, timing of the rumen sample compared with when the high sugar or starch feed was fed, and prior, alkalinizing treatments.

Treatment

Treatment is similar to that described for simple indigestion, but slow IV or SC administration of calcium solutions may be needed for recumbent cattle. Because rumen stasis is more severe and acid rumenitis is present, powdered ruminotoric–laxative–antacid products dissolved in water and 1 lb of activated charcoal administered through a stomach tube are recommended. If rumen fluid is readily regurgitated via the tube, rumen lavage is indicated. If signs of severe indigestion occur within hours of known over ingestion of rapidly fermentable feed material, a rumenotomy may be elected if, in the veterinarian's judgment, the potential for life-threatening lactic acidosis exists. This is a very difficult decision to make because medical therapy often will suffice, and no clear-cut rules exist as to how much of any feed material constitutes a potentially lethal dose. Intravenous fluid therapy with alkalinizing polyionic crystalloids is often beneficial when available. When a continuous infusion of IV fluids is not feasible for practical or economic reasons, small-volume hypertonic fluid administration may be used. However, care should be taken after small-volume hypertonic fluid administration regarding ad libitum access to water. The strong thirst response driven by seven times normal saline infusion can cause some cattle with this condition to drink excessively, leading to further fluid distension of the rumen, thereby exacerbating atony. This can also be problematic in cattle that have undergone rumentomy or large-volume siphoning via a Kingman tube.

Response to therapy should be gradual over 24 to 48 hours, and treatment may need to be repeated at 24-hour intervals. As GI motility returns, loose manure usually is observed. Milk production may be slow to return to previous levels because of the precipitous decrease that occurs with this form of indigestion.

Fulminant Acute Rumen Acidosis

Etiology

Acute rumen acidosis (also called lactic acidosis, toxic indigestion, grain overload, rumen overload, and acute carbohydrate engorgement of ruminants) represents the most severe form of indigestion and is associated with overingestion of rapidly fermentable concentrate feed or the sudden change to a diet containing higher levels of finely ground, rapidly fermentable feeds such as corn or wheat. Clinical examples of this may occur in feedlots when feeder steers are introduced to total concentrate diets rather than being gradually transitioned from high-roughage to high-concentrate feeds. Fortunately, this is less often a herd problem in dairy cattle, but it has occurred when owners have run out of one type of feed and quickly changed to another. Historically, this has happened when owners have switched cattle from pelleted grains containing some fiber to finely ground corn or wheat grains, thus inducing ruminal acidosis. Sudden introduction of highly fermentable small grain silage into the herd can also result in lactic acidosis (both D and L forms). Although rare in modern husbandry systems, sudden, unfettered, accidental access to stores of highly palatable cereal grains may still occur, and the end result provides testimony as to the lack of discernment as well as gluttony of cattle toward these types of feed (Fig. 5.3). Ruminal acidosis may also occur when cattle are fed grain-based silage that has fermented for less than 2 weeks. Another problem that can lead to ruminal lactic acidosis in modern dairy management systems is improper mixing of TMRs. In these cases, equipment failure or human error can lead to stratification of feedstuffs used in the TMR, and cows at one end of the feed line receive mostly roughage, but those at the other end

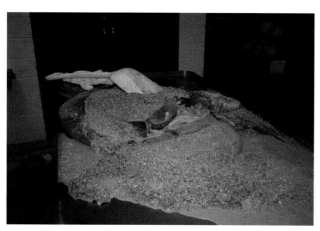

• **Fig. 5.3** Postmortem image with opened rumen demonstrating recent excessive grain (corn) ingestion. The individual was one of a group of heifers that gained unlimited overnight access to grain; all four were found dead the next day. In such severe cases ruminal contents and feces may have a similar appearance.

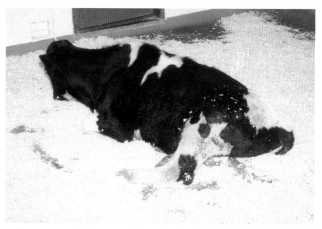

• **Fig. 5.4** A Holstein steer with severe ruminal acidosis after eating recently ensiled oat silage. This steer, one of three affected, was unable to stand, severely dehydrated, obtunded, acidotic, and blind. This individual recovered after being treated with hypertonic saline and thiamine intravenously, draining rumen fluid via oral-rumen tube, and 1 lb of activated charcoal intraruminally.

receive mostly high-sugar, high-starch concentrate. Cattle that overeat grain by accidentally gaining access to grain stores also may develop lactic acidosis. Both the volume and type of concentrate are important, but even a few pounds of a finely ground concentrate such as barley may constitute a dangerous quantity if the cow's rumen flora is unfamiliar with the material. Because management factors often are involved, multiple animals in the herd tend to show signs. A basic understanding of the pathophysiology of ruminal and lactic acidosis is essential for one to understand the signs that occur and be able to institute rational therapy. Within 6 hours of ingestion, the easily fermentable and high-sugar, high-starch concentrate is broken down to volatile fatty acids and both D- and L-lactic acid. Most of this occurs in the rumen, although substantial production of D-lactic acid may also occur in the lower GI tract. The L isomer can be used rapidly, but the D isomer persists and results in D-lactic acidosis. *Streptococcus bovis* is one of several organisms responsible for the excessive lactic acid production. As more and more lactic and volatile acids are produced, the pH of the rumen contents decreases further into the acid range. If sufficient rapidly fermentable starch substrate is available, the rumen pH may decrease to 4.5 to 5.0, destroying most microbes other than *S. bovis*. With very high lactate and histamine content, rumen stasis occurs. *S. bovis* continues to survive at this low pH and perpetuates the problem by producing more lactic acid.

Rapid accumulation of acids osmotically draws water into the rumen, dehydrating the cow and increasing systemic production of L-lactate from enhanced anaerobic metabolism. In addition, the chemical or acid rumenitis damages the rumen mucosa, allowing plasma transudation into the rumen and endotoxin and bacteria escape into the portal circulation.

Clinical Signs

Affected cattle are completely off feed, exhibit drastically decreased milk production, are dehydrated, and have elevated heart (90–120 beats/min) and respiratory rates (50–80

breaths/min). They typically have a splashy, totally static and enlarged rumen; cool skin surface; subnormal temperature; and diarrhea or loose manure, often with whole grain in it. Tachycardia, tachypnea, anorexia, and depression are present in virtually all cases. Affected animals are weak and ataxic and can be recumbent (Fig. 5.4). Because of dehydration, titration of bicarbonate, hypotension, and high levels of D- and L-lactic acid in the rumen and the blood, severely affected cattle have metabolic acidosis and peripheral acidemia. Rumen ammonia and histamine are consistently high in cattle with marked ruminal acidosis and may account for some of the neurologic signs and hypotension, respectively. Abnormally high levels of D-lactate or decreased rumen thiamine production may also cause neurologic signs. Abdominal pain, tachycardia, tachypnea, staggering, recumbency, a marked decline in milk yield, coma and death may occur.

Ancillary Data and Diagnosis

Diagnosis of severe ruminal lactic acidosis is made by combining clinical signs with a detailed history of feeding in the herd. In acute cases, obtaining a rumen fluid sample through a stomach tube or percutaneous left flank puncture or at necropsy examination in acute fatalities will reveal a rumen pH of 4.5 to 5.0. It must be emphasized that cattle with severe ruminal acidosis that survive for 24 hours or more often have rumen pH values that increase to 5.5 to 7.0 because of the buffering effects of swallowed saliva and plasma dilution of the rumen contents. Other laboratory aids include acid–base and electrolyte values that tend to reflect a metabolic acidosis, a neutropenia with left shift in the hemogram, and marked azotemia. This is true even for eventually fatal cases in cows that survive 24 hours or more after ingestion of toxic quantities of grain. The systemic acidosis and acidemia are the result of increases in both D- and L-lactic acid. In some cases, the diarrhea or loose manure that is passed contains whole particles of the causative concentrate and may represent a clinical diagnostic clue.

Treatment

Treatment is difficult, and the veterinarian must decide whether medical therapy will suffice or a rumenotomy will be required. In addition, if signs have been present for 24 hours or more, the amount of rumen mucosal damage has already been determined and may not be affected by any treatment. When more than one cow is affected, the therapeutic difficulties multiply because the professional time commitment and expense of treatment are potentially enormous.

Treatment must correct the rumen acidosis and attempt to discourage further lactic acid production. In an animal with a rumen pH of 5.0 or less, a heart rate greater than 100 beats/min, dehydration greater than 8%, and rumen distension and recumbency indicating a severe grain overload, a rumenotomy should be performed if feasible and the rumen contents evacuated. The rumen is then washed with water and emptied several times to remove as much lactic acid as possible. The cow is treated with laxatives, fresh hay in the rumen, rumen transfaunates if available, parenteral calcium, and IV fluid therapy. IV fluids should initially be hypertonic saline followed by balanced electrolyte solutions such as lactated Ringer's solution, and supplemental sodium bicarbonate is added if acidemia is severe (pH <7.15). Flunixin meglumine should be given to combat excessive prostanoid production and shock. B vitamins should be administered for several reasons, one of which is that some cattle with ruminal acidosis develop polioencephalomalacia. The prognosis for severely affected cattle is poor. Those that survive the initial shock and systemic acidosis may not regain a normal appetite because of ulcerative lesions in the rumen or microbiome disruption and may have more distant complications such as liver abscesses and laminitis.

Other treatments may be attempted for animals showing less severe signs and higher rumen pH values or when the number of animals affected precludes rumenotomies. One method involves passing a large-diameter stomach tube or Kingman tube and lavaging the rumen with warm water several times with the aid of a bilge pump. Several flushes with 10 to 20 gallons of water are necessary, and return flow of fluid must be effective for this treatment to be successful. After lavage, antacid solutions such as 2 to 4 quarts of milk of magnesia, activated charcoal, and ruminotorics are administered, as well as supportive calcium solutions and IV fluids as indicated. Affected cattle should not be allowed to engorge on water because their atonic rumen will only distend again. When rumen activity returns, long-stem hay and free choice water may be made available. Another option that has been used successfully is to simply drain as much rumen fluid (Fig. 5.5) as possible by oral siphon and administer 1 to 2 lb of activated charcoal into the rumen. This appears to be effective in binding rumen toxins (e.g., endotoxin). Additionally, affected cattle should receive SC administered calcium solutions and IV administered isotonic fluids. Cows with moderate to severe rumenitis are generally treated with penicillin (10,000–20,000 U/kg

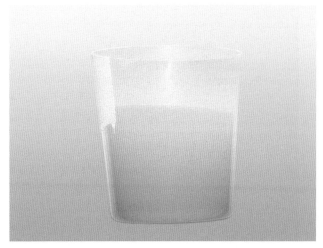

• **Fig. 5.5** Sample of rumen fluid, with a pH of 4.5, obtained from the steer in Fig. 5.4.

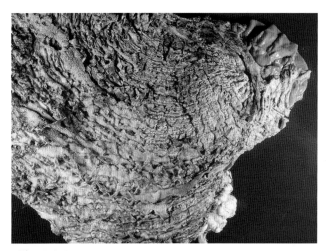

• **Fig. 5.6** Chemical and bacterial destruction of the entire omasal mucosa as a result of lactic acidosis.

administered intramuscularly [IM] or SC once daily for 3-5 days) in an effort to prevent bacteremia and liver abscess formation. Broad-spectrum antibiotics should not be used because they may predispose to fungal overgrowth.

Other treatments are empirical. They include antihistamines, penicillin solutions administered via a stomach tube in an effort to reduce the numbers of *S. bovis* organisms in the rumen, and roughage-only diets until the animals recover. The use of subcutaneously administered antihistamines had long been recommended by Dr. Francis Fox, and a 2014 article by Golder et al confirms that intraruminal histamine may be markedly elevated in cows with severe clinical ruminal acidosis.

Cattle affected with severe ruminal lactic acidosis that survive the acute phase and have their rumen pH return to normal still are at risk for sequelae to the chemical rumenitis that has occurred. During the next several days, bacterial opportunists such as *Fusobacterium necrophorum* may invade the areas of chemical damage, attach to the rumen wall, and cause a bacterial rumenitis (Fig. 5.6). If the animal

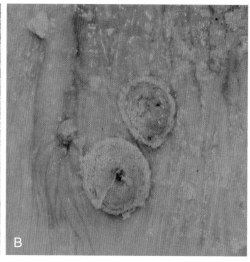

• **Fig. 5.7 A,** Mycotic rumenitis 7 days after acute lactic acidosis in a cow. The *dark areas* represent necrotic rumen mucosa that has sloughed in several focal areas to expose punched-out ulcerative lesions with red peripheries typical of mycotic rumenitis. **B,** Ruminal wall of a cow that demonstrated recurrent fevers 7 to 10 days after acute rumen acidosis. The image demonstrates mycotic plaques on the ruminal mucosal surface. (**A** courtesy of John M. King, DVM.)

lives 4 to 7 days or has been treated heavily with broad spectrum antibiotics or steroids, a mycotic rumenitis may occur in these previously damaged areas (Fig. 5.7). Bacterial and mycotic opportunists invade the damaged rumen mucosa; ascend the portal circulation; and cause embolic infection of the liver, lungs, and other organs, resulting in fever and, in some cases, death (Figs. 5.8 and 5.9). Fever resulting from mycotic infection generally is unresponsive to antibiotic therapy. Embolic infections of the brain may cause bizarre neurologic signs 7 to 14 days after the original clinical signs of lactic acidosis.

Ruminal Bloat

Ruminal bloat can be defined as obvious ruminal enlargement resulting in left-sided abdominal distension in both dorsal and ventral quadrants (Fig. 5.10). When severe, bloat may cause generalized bilateral distension resulting from ventral sac enlargement into the right lower quadrant and crowding of the remaining abdominal viscera into the right dorsal quadrant. Causes of bloat may be divided into acute and chronic disorders. The term *ruminal bloat* is used instead of bloat alone because in young calves a common cause of acute severe bloat is abomasal bloat (abomasitis).

Acute Ruminal Bloat

Etiology

Acute ruminal distension may be caused by either free gas or frothy ingesta. Acute free-gas bloats may occur in association with hypocalcemia and resulting ileus, esophageal obstructions or injuries, pharyngeal injuries that damage the vagus nerve roots controlling eructation, indigestion with tympany, tetanus, and acute localized peritonitis with resultant ileus.

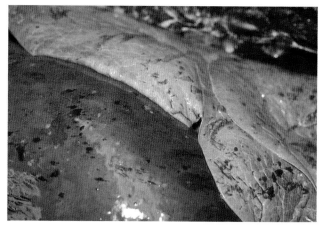

• **Fig. 5.8** Embolic hepatitis and pneumonia secondary to lactic acidosis in a cow. The acute lactic acidosis occurred 7 days before these postmortem findings. The focal lesions in the liver and red areas in the lung represent bacterial and mycotic embolic lesions.

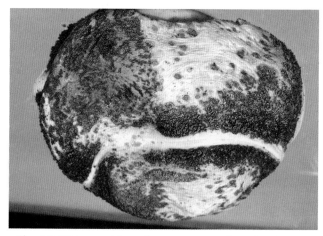

• **Fig. 5.9** Widespread loss of rumen mucosa 2 weeks after acute grain overload. (Courtesy of John M. King, DVM.)

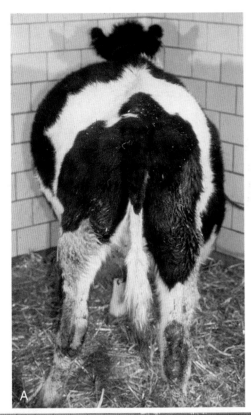

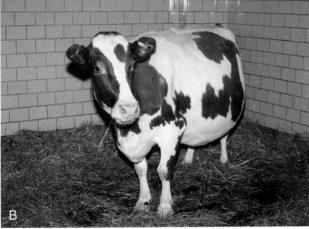

• **Fig. 5.10 A,** Ruminal tympany or bloat in a heifer. The left-sided distension is uniform and extends to the dorsal midline. **B,** Severe ruminal distension with ingesta in a cow with vagal indigestion caused by a perireticular abscess. A lack of respiratory distress, despite the marked distension, is typical of ruminal distension caused by gas or nonfrothy ingesta.

Acute frothy bloat in dairy cattle almost always is associated with indigestion of unknown causes or sudden availability and over ingestion of highly digestible, high protein green forages such as succulent alfalfa or clovers.

Acute bloat can be classified into at least three categories determined by the physical properties causing the bloat:
1. Frothy bloat
   a. Frothy bloat resulting from stable froth of dietary origin that usually is higher in chloroplast membrane fragments and soluble protein. This type of bloat occurs with exposure to succulent legumes and clovers. Certain

genetic strains of cattle may be more prone to frothy bloat than others. Show cows fed calf manna, a highly soluble protein feed, may also develop frothy bloat. Frothy bloat also occurs in some young calves with peritonitis or undetermined causes. This form of bloat is not relieved by a stomach tube.
2. Free-gas bloat
   a. Free-gas bloat occurring secondary to overingestion of grain, which promotes excessive volatile fatty acid production, lower pH, and then lactic acid buildup. This pathophysiology culminates in rumen stasis and free-gas bloat.
   b. Free-gas bloat resulting from mechanical, inflammatory, neurologic, or metabolic conditions that interfere with eructation or affect outflow (e.g., esophageal choke, esophageal motility disorders in calves, vagal indigestion, hypocalcemia, listeriosis, or tetanus).
   c. Free-gas and sometimes fluid bloat occurring in calves after ruminal drinking of milk. This may occur within 30 minutes of milk feeding (usually by bucket), and the rumen fluid may have a putrid smell. Although the bloat is predominantly free gas, simultaneous ballottement and auscultation will produce a fluid "tinkling" in the left ventral quadrant associated with the inappropriately clotted milk. This is part of the clinical syndrome of chronic indigestion in milk-fed calves. In addition to ruminal bloat, affected calves may be depressed, have a poor appetite, be thin with rough haircoat, be weak, and have claylike feces.
3. Fluid and free-gas bloat
   a. Fluid and some gas bloat is seen acutely in calves with clostridial abomasitis-rumenitis and in cows with severe ruminal acidosis. A combination of fluid and gas may also be seen with abomasal outflow disorders, functional or obstructive, and reflux of abomasal contents into the rumen. Passage of an ororuminal tube in these cases has little or no effect on abdominal distension.

We occasionally examine adult cows with subacute (1-3 days) ruminal distension that do not "fit" into the free gas or frothy bloat criteria. Many of these cows have matted ruminal ingesta with a small gas cap to the rumen. In some cases a vagal cause or rarely a diaphragmatic hernia is discovered, while in other cases no etiologic or predisposing cause is found even following a left-sided laparotomy and rumenotomy. Emptying the rumen and feeding the cow small but gradually increasing amounts of grass hay along with oral magnesium sulfate or coffee administration and transfaunation may result in recovery in some cases, but others will unfortunately have recurrence of the problem.

Clinical Signs

Clinical signs of acute ruminal bloat include a combination of acute-onset, typically left-sided distension extending dorsally to the midline with a full paralumbar fossa, and rectal findings of ruminal distension extending into the right abdomen dorsally and ventrally. Dyspnea caused by increased abdominal pressure exerted on the diaphragm and thorax may be moderate to severe with acute frothy bloat.

Free-gas bloat causes a large gas ping on the left upper abdomen extending to the dorsal midline (Fig. 5.11), but respiratory distress is uncommon with free-gas bloat. In some

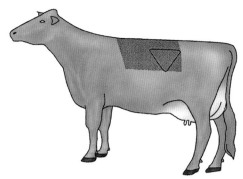

• **Fig. 5.11** Region of ping with rumen tympany or left sided pneumo-peritoneum.

cattle with free-gas bloat, an obvious ping may not be present. If a stomach tube can be passed easily and relieves the bloat, free-gas bloat is confirmed. Other physical signs and signalment data may allow a specific diagnosis of the cause of the bloat. For example, hypocalcemia may be considered if the cow is periparturient and shows signs of normal or subnormal temperature, cool peripheral parts, slow pupillary responses to direct light, recumbency, or weakness. Indigestion with tympany may cause few signs other than free-gas bloat, and signs other than free-gas bloat or signs referable to hypocalcemia require that other diseases must be ruled out. Animals with esophageal obstruction (choke), esophageal injury, or pharyngeal injury with perforation usually present with excessive salivation, an anxious expression, extended head and neck, bloat, and fever. Passage of a stomach tube would be impeded by a choke and be resisted by a cow with pharyngeal or esophageal injury. If left-side abdominal distension and ping are noted over the paralumbar fossa, a high and unusually large left displacement of the abomasum (LDA) should be considered. If the ping over the paralumbar fossa is abomasal, the shape of the organ can often be seen externally, unlike with rumen distension. Very large and high left-sided abomasal displacements (DAs) can often be palpated rectally, and the ping often stops cranially at the 11th rib, unlike with severe ruminal distension, which may ping dorsally from the tuber coxae to the diaphragm. Pneumoperitoneum causing abdominal distension would be expected to ping dorsally on both sides (Fig. 5.11). Frothy bloat is diagnosed based on the typical left-sided distension, less obvious pinging when simultaneous percussion and auscultation are performed, and failure to relieve the distension by passage of a stomach tube. The bloat may progress rapidly if it is frothy, eventually distending both sides of the abdomen to its maximum limit (Fig. 5.12) and causing respiratory distress, hypoxemia, poor venous return of blood to the heart, hypotension, and death.

Treatment

Treatment requires relief of the ruminal distension and correction of the primary cause. In instances of free-gas bloat caused by hypocalcemia, parenteral calcium therapy and passage of a stomach tube are required. Indigestion with tympany requires relief of the gas accumulation with a stomach tube and treatment with a parenteral calcium solution, as

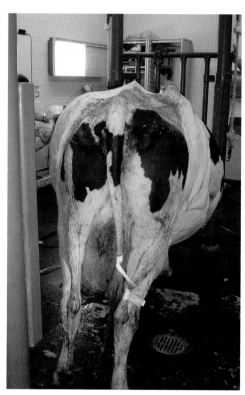

• **Fig. 5.12** Severe abdominal distension, respiratory distress and hypovolemic shock caused by frothy bloat.

well as laxatives, antacids, and ruminotoric mixtures as necessary. In esophageal obstruction or choke, the obstruction must be relieved by gentle manual or mechanical manipulation. Localized peritonitis with secondary ruminal tympany must be treated with antibiotics, stall rest, and a magnet, rumenotomy (for hardware), or dietary changes (perforating abomasal ulcers).

If pharyngeal trauma is suspected, broad-spectrum antibiotics, gentle passage of a stomach tube, and analgesics may be indicated (see the section on Pharyngeal Trauma).

In cases of acute frothy bloat, passage of a stomach tube seldom produces dramatic relief of the rumen distension but does aid in diagnosis and allows treatment with surfactant agents such as Therabloat (poloxalene drench concentrate; Zoetis Inc., Kalamazoo, MI) or vegetable oil to break down the froth. In some frothy bloats, a Kingman stomach tube may permit decompression, but this is not the rule. In severe cases with thoracic compression, passage of a tube may rarely cause sudden death. Oral ruminotoric–laxative–antacid powders in warm water and parenteral calcium solutions also should be administered to encourage rumen emptying. Emergency rumenotomy (see Video Clip 5.1 and Fig. 5.13) is the treatment of choice for progressive and severe frothy bloat. In a hospital environment, hypertonic saline administration, intranasal oxygen, and analgesics (flunixin meglumine) are helpful in stabilizing the cow during standing surgery.

Percutaneous rumen trocharization as a treatment for acute bloat of any cause is contraindicated in the dairy cow except in extreme cases when emergency decompression is necessary. Trocharization in the dairy cow ensures

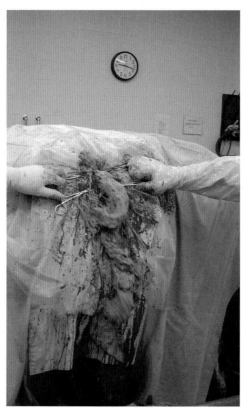

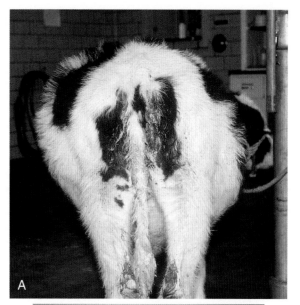

• **Fig. 5.13** Frothy ingesta "exploding" from the rumenotomy site in the cow in Fig. 5.12 (also see Video Clip 5.1).

peritonitis, which may be fatal or may confuse the primary diagnosis by causing fever and signs referable to peritonitis, including bloat, over the following days.

Prevention of acute bloat is possible only for those causes associated with husbandry errors that permit ingestion of causative feedstuffs, including sudden access to lush alfalfa pastures. Fortunately, most dairy farmers are aware of these dangers, and it seldom is necessary to educate owners concerning such hazards and appropriate preventive measures such as gradual introduction to succulent pasture, prefeeding with long-stem hay, pasture surfactant sprays, poloxalene salt blocks, or simple avoidance.

Chronic Ruminal Bloat

Etiology

In calves, most cases of chronic bloat have a dietary or developmental etiology. Low-fiber diets are the usual cause in 2- to 4-month-old calves fed only milk or milk replacers (Fig. 5.14). Otherwise, these affected calves are healthy except for the free-gas bloat that develops shortly after eating. Calves that have been overtreated with oral antibiotics for systemic infections or diarrhea also may develop bloat associated with abnormal rumen flora. Calves affected with diarrhea and treated with methscopolamine or other parasympatholytic drugs may develop a paralytic ileus and subsequent bloat that persists for 24 to 72 hours after the administration of the drug. Although overdosage may have occurred, some

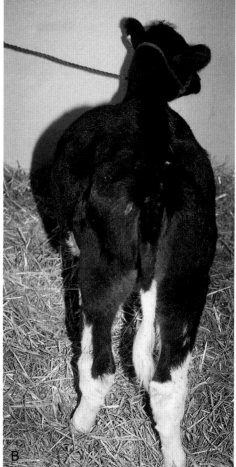

• **Fig. 5.14** **A,** Chronic free-gas bloat in a calf on a low-fiber diet. **B,** Developmental free-gas bloat in an otherwise healthy calf.

calves develop bloat even after using the manufacturer's recommended dosages of methscopolamine.

Calves that have suffered severe bronchopneumonia occasionally develop free-gas bloat from damage to the thoracic portion of the vagus nerve or enlarged thoracic lymph nodes that cause failure of eructation. LDA in calves may cause chronic or intermittent free-gas bloat, thereby confounding a diagnosis of LDA. LDAs in calves often ping more ventral and caudal than in adult cattle with LDA. Intermittent or chronic bloat associated with unthriftiness, inappetence, claylike feces, and abdominal distension occasionally occurs in 3- to 8-week-old dairy calves fed milk (mostly by bucket rather than bottle) (Fig. 5.15, *A*). These calves are called "ruminal drinkers" because they have failure of the reticular groove reflex, causing milk to flow directly into the rumen rather than the abomasum. Ruminal parakeratosis and hyperkeratosis result in addition to metabolic and endocrine abnormalities. The calves may have excessive intestinal production of both D- and L-lactic acid and become severely acidotic, with neurologic signs (see Chapter 13) from the D-lactic acid. The bloat may occur acutely within 1 hour after feeding but may also become chronic, and in some cases, there may be enough milk putrefaction to cause the calf to become quite ill. Passage of a stomach tube may cause reflux of a gray fetid fluid (Fig. 5.15, *B*). Similar putrefaction of milk and free gas accumulation can occur in calves older than 2 months of age that are continuing to receive milk despite already consuming greater than 2 lbs of grain per day. As a consequence of grain feeding to this level or greater, there may already be a postweaning type of ruminal microbiota and an ineffective reticular groove. Calves that have been sick around the time of weaning or older calves for which the owners have decided to reinstate milk feeding because of health issues are at particular risk. This practice may also lead to D-lactic acidosis.

Older calves that have been weaned off milk or milk replacers also may develop chronic free-gas bloat of dietary origin if fed a low-fiber diet. Although this can occur on silage and grain diets, it is much more common in calves fed all-pelleted rations. Up to 10% or more of calves fed all-pelleted rations with no hay supplementation will develop chronic bloat that worsens shortly after they ingest pellets and then drink large quantities of water. There is also a syndrome of free-gas bloat in otherwise healthy calves with no discernible cause; it appears to be a dysfunction of ruminal-reticular movement preventing normal eructation of rumen gas. These calves have a good prognosis if a fistula is placed into the rumen. When the fistula closes, several weeks later, the calves no longer have bloat problems. Many other causes of chronic bloat also exist in postweaning calves but are more difficult to diagnose and treat. These include inherent tendencies of bloat as seen in dwarf animals and inherent defects in forestomach innervation or smooth muscle function.

Other lesions, such as abdominal abscess, umbilical or urachal adhesions, intestinal obstruction, LDA, focal peritonitis, and rarely abomasal impaction (Fig. 5.16), may lead to chronic bloat as well.

Esophageal lesions also must be considered in the differential diagnosis of chronic bloat in the calf. These include pharyngeal and esophageal trauma induced by balling guns, stomach tubes, or esophageal feeders. These lesions may damage the intricate vagus nerve branches responsible for eructation, swallowing, and forestomach motility. Esophageal motility disorders, although rare, should be considered as a cause of bloat in calves with a dilated esophagus (Fig. 5.17). The esophagus can be palpated due to its distension at the thoracic inlet, or it can be seen persistently dilated on ultrasound examination. A barium study (mix barium in feed or preferably give as a bolus after placing a tube with a cuff in the proximal esophagus) is used to confirm an atonic esophagus. Calves with esophageal motility disturbances may also have some regurgitation.

Thymic lymphosarcoma and enlarged mediastinal or pharyngeal lymph nodes resulting from the juvenile form of lymphosarcoma are the most common neoplastic causes of chronic bloat in calves. Diaphragmatic hernias are rare in dairy cattle but can result in acute or chronic rumen distension and bloat (Fig. 5.18). Generally, the reticulum is entrapped in the thoracic cavity through the diaphragmatic rent. Signs include decreased cardiac and lung sounds and dullness during percussion in the ventral thorax (unilateral or bilateral), abdominal distension, bloat, vomiting, and dyspnea. Diaphragmatic hernias may be congenital or

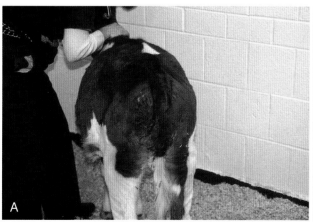
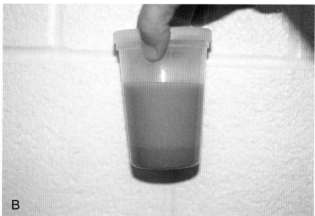

• **Fig. 5.15 A,** Acute ruminal bloat that occurred 1 hour after drinking milk replacer in a bucket. There had been several episodes of bloat in this calf, and its general condition and hair coat are adversely affected. **B,** Rumen ingesta collected from the calf.

acquired as a result of trauma, parturition, or progressive weakening of the diaphragm adjacent to a hardware perforation and reticuloperitonitis.

Chronic ruminal bloat in adult cattle most often involves lesions of the vagus nerve. These lesions may occur anywhere from the brainstem to the pharynx to the abomasum. Causes similar to those described in calves may be involved, as can adult diseases such as listeriosis, hardware, reticular abscesses, liver abscesses, volvulus of

the abomasum, abomasal impaction, advanced pregnancy, and lymphosarcoma. These are discussed further in the section on vagal indigestion.

Forestomach neoplasms primarily include fibropapillomas of the distal esophagus or cardia and lymphosarcoma masses in the forestomach or abomasum. With fibropapillomas, a failure of eructation occurs because the tumor acts like a plug or one-way valve in the distal esophagus, thereby interfering with effective eructation. In cases of lymphosarcoma and abomasal atony following correction of abomasal volvulus (AV), outflow disturbances can result, with reflux of abomasal contents into the rumen, primary failure of eructation, or failure of motility, all potentially contributing to the chronic rumen distension. Rumen chloride content is elevated (>30 mEq/L) with abomasal reflux, and affected cows typically demonstrate moderate to severe hypochloremic, metabolic alkalosis on routine blood work.

Granulomatous lesions caused by *Actinobacillus lignieresii* and *Actinomyces bovis* may cause distal esophageal or reticular lesions that result in chronic bloat or indigestion. However, this is quite unusual.

Cattle with tetanus may have chronic (i.e., of several days' duration) bloat. In this instance, inability of the laryngeal, pharyngeal, and esophageal striated musculature to coordinate the intricate neuromuscular act of eructation because of tetany results in free-gas bloat. Bloat may also be observed in cows with listeriosis, botulism, or other neurologic diseases.

Diagnosis and Treatments

In all cases of bloat, the veterinarian must confirm that the abdominal distension is caused by ruminal distension rather than pneumoperitoneum or LDA. In calves, simultaneous percussion and auscultation, ballottement, and abdominal palpation should differentiate abomasal, small intestinal, and cecal distension from that involving only the rumen. Observation, physical examination, and, if available, ultrasonography are extremely important in the calf because rectal examination is not possible. In adult cattle, rectal

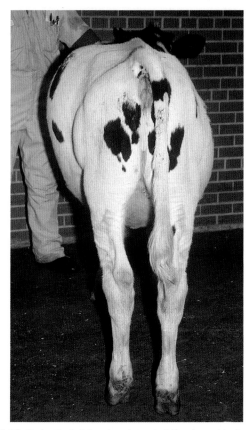

• **Fig. 5.16** Abdominal distension characteristic of vagal indigestion in a calf with abomasal impaction.

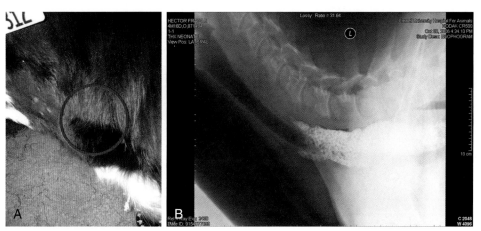

• **Fig. 5.17 A,** A 4-month-old Holstein calf with a 2-month history of chronic bloat and ill thrift caused by megaesophagus (esophageal motility dysfunction). The swelling at the thoracic inlet (marked with the red circle) was caused by distension of the esophagus with feed. **B,** Barium contrast esophagram of the calf.

palpation coupled with other physical findings should easily confirm rumen distension.

The diagnosis of chronic bloat is confirmed by a combination of history and physical examination findings. Other causes of chronic abdominal distension, such as ascites, displacement of the abomasum, cecal distension, and hydrops, should be ruled out. In addition to abdominal auscultation and ballottement, and rectal examination in cows, a stomach tube should be passed to determine whether the bloat is associated with free gas or ingesta. Specific causes of chronic rumen bloat should be sought through physical examination, ancillary data, and surgical exploration of the abdomen if the value of the affected animal warrants this procedure.

Specific treatment depends on the specific cause of the chronic bloat. Because a portion of these cases involve lesions affecting the vagus nerve branches, treatment is discussed later in this chapter under "Vagal Indigestion." Calves with unexplained chronic or intermittent free-gas bloat are best treated by making a temporary rumen fistula (Fig. 5.19). Calves with chronic or intermittent bloat and ill thrift because of ruminal drinking of milk can be weaned or fed via a bottle rather than a bucket. If they become acutely ill in association with feeding milk and bloat, an oral-rumen tube should be passed to drain as much fluid as possible from the rumen, and the calf should be treated with systemic antibiotics and fluids.

Chronic free-gas bloat in tetanus patients may be relieved by gentle passage of a stomach tube or preferably with a surgically created rumen fistula that provides continuous escape of gas and a portal through which to provide feed

and water to the patient. The creation of a therapeutic fistula is an important aid to the successful treatment of tetanus cases because affected animals are typically unable to eructate or swallow, and repeated passage of a stomach tube significantly increases their anxiety and stress level.

Patients with free-gas bloat and ileus secondary to the administration of atropine or methscopolamine require passage of a stomach tube as frequently as necessary. These patients usually improve spontaneously 48 to 72 hours after the last administration of the offending drug.

Cows with chronic ruminal bloat caused by abomasal outflow abnormalities causing reflux of abomasal content into the rumen generally have a poor prognosis.

D-Lactic Acidosis

Etiology

D-lactic acid is produced in the gut by the metabolism of specific substrates, usually simple carbohydrate, by intestinal bacteria. Unlike its isomer L-lactate, which can be produced either by mammalian cells during anaerobic metabolism or by intestinal bacteria, D-lactate is poorly metabolized and potentially neurotoxic. The D-lactic acid syndrome is caused by abnormally high production of D-lactate in either the rumen, small intestine or in the hindgut. Although L-lactate production may be occurring concurrently in many cases, it is the D-lactate that causes pronounced depression. The clinical signs and proposed pathogenesis of these central nervous system (CNS) abnormalities are described in Chapter 13.

Although calves that are "ruminal milk drinkers" have already been discussed within the preceding section on ruminal bloat, they deserve further mention here because the excessive production of D-lactate in the rumen is most commonly associated with milk fermentation. Two forms of ruminal D-lactic acidosis in calves have been described; an acute and a chronic form. The acute form can develop via one of two mechansims; either the reticular groove is bypassed following the force-feeding of milk, allowing large amounts of milk to enter the rumen, or else a primary or

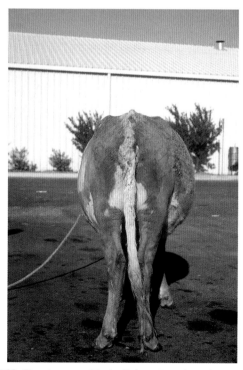

• **Fig. 5.18** Chronic rumen bloat with ingesta and gas in a cow with a diaphragmatic hernia. The reticulum was believed to have been forced through a congenital defect in the diaphragm at calving.

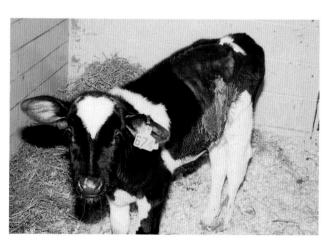

• **Fig. 5.19** Surgically placed rumen fistula in a calf that had chronic free-gas bloat. The ingesta spilling down the side of the abdomen causes no problem.

painful disease condition such as pneumonia or pleuritis, pneumothorax, cough, otitis, or phlebitis of the jugular vein appears to prevent closure of the reticular groove, resulting in milk inappropriately diverting into the rumen. Force feeding milk to calves that already have a functional rumen should be avoided! In the more chronic form of ruminal D-lactate acidosis, the failure of the reticular groove reflex occurs in otherwise healthy calves. This is typically a management problem and is caused by suboptimal feeding practices such as irregular feeding times, poor-quality milk replacer, cold temperature of the milk, reintroducing milk feeding postweaning, or feeding large amounts of milk to older calves with a fully functional rumen, especially those fed from an open bucket. "Spillage" of milk into the rumen again leads to abnormal fermentation and lactic acid production.

Abnormally high production of D-lactate in the hindgut can be a sequela to maldigestion and malabsorption of carbohydrates in the small intestine. The hindgut D-lactic acid syndrome mostly occurs in calves at least 2 weeks of age with small intestinal malabsorption associated with diarrhea and dehydration, although the condition can occur in the absence of diarrhea too. Certainly, many younger calves with diarrhea would be expected to have malabsorption, but these calves may not yet have the sufficiently developed hindgut necessary for large-scale production of D-lactate. Hind-gut lactic acidosis can also occur in adult cattle.

Signs of D-lactic acidosis vary with age of the animal and predisposing cause. Calves that are ruminal drinkers may have ruminal bloat in addition to moderate to severe depression directly associated with the high blood concentration of D-lactic acid. Calves with predominantly hindgut D-lactic acid production may have diarrhea as the predisposing event, so this is commonly part of the patient's recent medical history. Adult cows with hindgut D-lactic acidosis may have decreased appetite; a ping over the spiral colon or cecal area; and foamy, loose manure. Ruminal acidosis also causes variable degrees of D-lactic acidosis, as previously discussed. The most consistent clinical finding with D-lactic acidosis is CNS depression, and the most consistent laboratory findings are metabolic acidosis (low bicarbonate) and increased anion gap.

Treatment

Treatment of D-lactic acidosis should involve bicarbonate-rich fluids given IV or orally to counter the acidosis and alleviate any dehydration. Ruminal drinkers should be weaned or fed smaller amounts of body-temperature milk or properly mixed milk replacer in a bottle. Total daily volume can be maintained by feeding more frequently. For calves with D-lactic acidosis caused by malabsorption or enteritis, fluid therapy and feeding smaller amounts of milk more frequently as suggested above are recommended. Additionally, lactase tablets, cultured yogurt, or probiotics can be added to the milk to improve digestion and absorption and to reestablish normal flora. Adult cows with hindgut acidosis should have the ration evaluated to determine a cause for the excessive starch fermentation in the lower bowel.

Rumen Microbiome and Rumen Transfaunation

The most discussed topic in comparative gastroenterology during the past 5 years has been the intestinal microbiome and how it relates to disease conditions. Metagenomics and the availability of high-throughput sequencing have allowed a great expansion of knowledge in this area, including information on the rumen microbiome. Core microbes, in addition to many diverse noncore flora that likely vary depending on diet and environment, are needed to perform key degradative and fermentative roles in the gut in all species. A more advanced knowledge of the rumen microbiome might provide information for feed and management changes that improve digestibility, decrease methane and ammonia emissions, improve efficiency of nitrogen usage by the rumen, and decrease both ruminal and nutritionally related metabolic disorders. Readers are encouraged to read the reference article by Firkins and Yu (2015) for more in-depth discussion of the rumen microbiome. Information on the core and noncore microbiome of other parts of the intestinal tract in cows and calves is becoming available, but practical applications of this information have not yet been developed.

Bovine veterinarians are well ahead of the curve in providing treatments to normalize the healthy intestinal microbiome, because rumen transfaunation for sick cows has been routinely practiced for several decades. Although veterinarians have generally perceived a clinical benefit of the treatment, there is little scientific documentation to prove such. A PubMed literature search reveals only two articles on rumen transfaunation treatment of sick cows, both by Dr. Lisle George, a classmate of Dr. Rebhun. Dr. George's first article demonstrated the benefits in cows after surgical correction of LDA, showing a lesser degree of ketonuria, greater feed intake, and higher milk yield in transfaunated cows when compared with nontransfaunated cows. In his second publication, he described the clinical value of rumen fluid transfaunation as an effective, practical, and easy method to treat simple indigestion of ruminants. Recommendations for collecting rumen fluid, storage, and volumes transferred were also discussed in that article.

The volume of rumen fluid transferred ranges from 1 L for calves to generally 8 L or more for adult cattle. Collection of large volumes of rumen fluid is most easily accomplished using a rumen-fistulated animal (Fig. 5.20). The empirical but acknowledged value of rumen transfaunation has led a number of large commercial dairies to acquire or establish fistulated cows as an aid to the treatment of sick cattle. The surgery to create a permanent rumen fistula is not straight-forward and requires some experience. It may be advisable for the procedure to be performed only by experienced food animal surgeons, perhaps within a teaching hospital, or a nutritional research institution or department, where it is easier to gain both the technical expertise necessary for the surgery and experience with the required aftercare to ensure a successful outcome. Cornell University has maintained clinically healthy (bovine leukemia virus [BLV]-negative

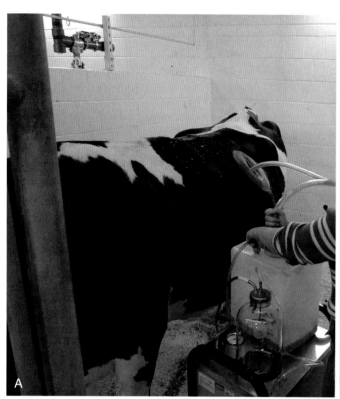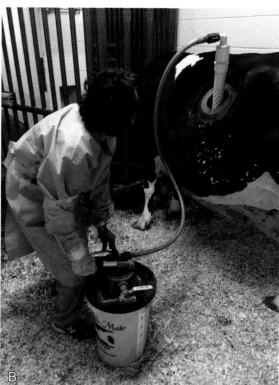

• **Fig. 5.20 A,** Collection of rumen juice from a "fistulated" cow. The probe is placed into the ventral rumen and a vacuum-assisted method of fluid collection is used. **B,** Alternative commercially available system for collecting rumen transfaunate by suction from a fistulated donor.

and bovine viral diarrhea virus [BVDV]-negative) rumen donors in its hospital for more than 40 years; these rumen donor cows also serve as blood donors when needed. Donors are fed only average to good-quality hay such that a normal rumen pH (>6.5) is maintained and they do not become overweight. Each cow has lived to be 9 to 12 years of age, with obesity being the biggest medical problem, since the cows have not been bred nor are they ever in milk.

The collection of rumen fluid is best performed by creating a siphon through a large stomach tube or by vacuum pump. The tube should be placed on the ventral floor of the rumen, where the most fluidy ingesta collects. If there is a large amount of hay in the fluid, it should be strained with a wire screen, to avoid obstructing the pump or tube during transfer to the recipient. Many ruminal fluid collection devices, including the Magrath Cattle Pump System, are commercially available. Alfalfa meal, propylene glycol (4–8 oz), and potassium chloride (1–2 oz) can be added to the transfaunate fluid. If needed, other electrolytes and minerals can also be added. Rumen fluid should be transferred as soon as possible postcollection, but if the fluid cannot be administered within an hour of collection, it is probably best to freeze it. Refrigeration temperature can result in the slow death of anaerobic organisms unless the fluid is maintained in an anaerobic chamber, in which case rumen gases must be continuously removed to prevent explosions! Drs. Whitlock and Kallfelz can attest to this after such an "explosion" in their office. A layer of mineral oil on the surface of

the transfaunate may serve to preserve anaerobic organisms under refrigeration for several hours.

Traumatic Reticuloperitonitis (Hardware Disease)

Etiology

Traumatic reticuloperitonitis following ingestion of metallic foreign bodies is one of the oldest diseases recognized in cattle but still occurs with alarming frequency under modern management. Unlike sheep and goats, cattle do not use their lips to discriminate between very fibrous feed and metallic objects in feedstuffs. Cattle also are given a great deal of chopped feed that may contain wire remnants, machinery parts, and other metallic debris.

Metallic foreign bodies, such as wire and nails, are the most common agents of hardware disease. In most cases, the wires range in length from 5.0 to 15.0 cm and tend to be slightly bent or have a crook at one end. Nails of all sizes also have been recovered from cattle with hardware disease as have, on occasion, hypodermic or blood collection needles. Many clinically normal cows will have metallic objects, sand, cinders, stones, fence staples, and some gravel in their reticulum. After ingestion, these objects drop into the rumen and within 24 to 48 hours are propelled into the reticulum, where they remain because of gravity or entanglement with the reticular mucosa. Nonperforating objects found frequently include nuts, bolts, washers, and short wire fragments (<2.5

cm). Most healthy cows have iron filings attached to their reticular magnet, if they have one, and these generally appear to do no harm, although there is a report of large accumulations of wire bristle attached to magnets causing peritonitis. These objects may be found routinely on radiographic surveys or in slaughterhouse specimens. Therefore, exposure to metallic foreign bodies should be anticipated in dairy cattle. Although perforation may occur randomly at any time in a cow harboring a sharp metallic foreign body, physical factors may contribute to perforation and subsequent clinical signs. The prime example of such a physical factor contributing to perforation is advanced gestation and a heavily gravid uterus. During the last trimester, the combined weight and size of the gravid uterus allows the organ to act like a pendulum as a cow gets up and down; this can apply physical pressure to the rumen and reticulum, contributing to perforation by an existing sharp metallic object. Clinical incidence of hardware disease in cattle in the last trimester of pregnancy is high enough to warrant inclusion of this entity as a differential diagnosis for any acute illness in heavily pregnant or dry cows. Conditions causing tenesmus or straining, such as parturition, also cause increased abdominal pressure, potentially contributing to perforation.

Hardware disease usually occurs in heifers or cows older than 1 year of age. It is not known whether discrimination during prehension or lack of exposure to certain high-risk feedstuffs protects the animal during the first year of life.

In light of the likely exposure of most dairy cattle to metallic foreign bodies in feedstuffs, perhaps the greatest single factor in the causative development of hardware disease is failure to have administered a prophylactic magnet to the animal at 12 to 18 months of age. This should be considered a mandatory component of preventive herd health.

Clinical Signs

When a metallic foreign body perforates the reticular wall, clinical signs develop. These signs are extremely variable and influenced by the anatomic region of perforation within the reticulum, depth of perforation, associated abdominal or thoracic viscera injury by the perforating object, physical features of the causative object, and the affected cow's stage of gestation or lactation. On occasion, significant, repeated ruminal wall perforation by a linear sharp object may lead to clinical signs of peritonitis before the foreign body finds its way to the reticulum. This is uncommon but can be an explanation for clinical and ultrasonographic evidence of left-sided peritonitis and pain in the absence of radiographically demonstrable metallic foreign objects within the reticulum.

Classic hardware disease causing acute localized reticuloperitonitis results in a sudden, dramatic, and often complete anorexia and cessation of milk production. Milk production may decrease to near zero within 12 hours and prompt the owner to seek veterinary attention for the cow. Affected cattle may have fever (103.0° to 105.0°F [39.44° to 40.56°C]), normal to mildly elevated heart and respiratory rates, abducted elbows, an anxious expression, an arched stance (Fig. 5.21), hypomotile rumen with or without mild tympany, little or

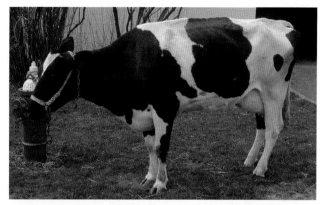

• **Fig. 5.21** Classical appearance of a cow affected with traumatic reticuloperitonitis. The cow has an anxious expression and an arched stance and appears gaunt.

no observed cud chewing, scant dry or loose feces, and signs of abdominal pain localized to the cranial ventral abdomen near the xiphoid. Cattle may be reluctant to ventroflex when their withers are briskly pinched, and a grunt may occur; this is the old "withers pinch test," which is well described in the literature and should be part of the routine physical examination, although sensitivity for detecting hardware is likely low. When the cow is examined within 24 hours of onset, classic cases as described are relatively easy to diagnose. Many clinical cases show more variable signs (e.g., some cows stand up more than normal, but others lie down more than normal) and present more difficult diagnostic challenges. In some cases, vague signs of partial anorexia, decreased milk production, and changing fecal consistency may be observed by the owner and may have been present for some time before veterinary attention is sought. Physical examination may reveal little beyond cranial abdominal pain and ruminal hypomotility or mild tympany suggestive of localized peritonitis. In some mild cases, careful auscultation and observation may reveal treading with the hind feet secondary to the pain associated with localized peritonitis during ruminoreticular contraction. Affected cattle with less obvious signs may "grunt" or grind their teeth while being "poked" by a metallic foreign body embedded in the reticular mucosa or submucosa or one that has penetrated full thickness and continues to cause pain intermittently. Occasionally, cattle affected with hardware disease will "vomit" or regurgitate more material than they can retain as a cud. This represents a neurogenic or pressure-related triggering of the regurgitation reflex from reticular irritation. In these less obvious cases, careful physical examination and attention to detail when assessing abdominal pain are important keys to the diagnosis.

An important point concerning patients with hardware disease is that the body temperature may be normal. This statement is in direct conflict with many textbook descriptions of the disease and seems difficult to explain in light of the obvious peritonitis that exists in these patients. In a review of the case records from more than 200 cattle confirmed by surgery or necropsy to be affected with hardware disease, the body temperature was normal in more than one-half of these

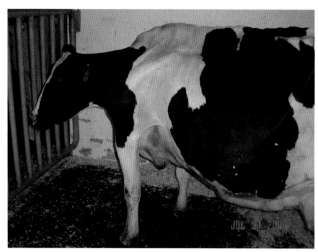

• **Fig. 5.22** A 5-year-old cow with traumatic reticulopericarditis standing with the elbows abducted.

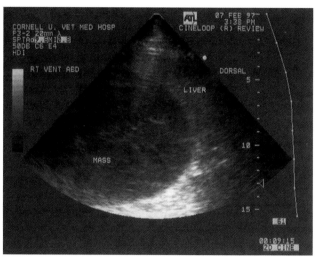

• **Fig. 5.23** Sonogram of a large abscess in the anterior abdomen of a cow with hardware disease.

patients. This may relate to the subacute or chronic nature of the disease in these referral patients, or they may have had an initial fever spike after the acute perforation that was not recorded. The fact remains that the veterinarian may not be called to attend a hardware disease case during the acute phase, and hardware disease should not be ruled out by finding a normal rectal temperature.

Cattle affected with chronic localized peritonitis have signs of weight loss, poor hair coat, intermittent anorexia, decreased milk production, changes in manure consistency, and rumen dysfunction with or without mild tympany. Such cows may have an arched stance and detectable abdominal pain as well.

Cattle affected with traumatic reticuloperitonitis that results in a diffuse peritonitis have much more severe signs than those affected with localized peritonitis. Cattle developing diffuse peritonitis resulting from hardware disease have fever, elevated heart rate (90–140 beats/min), elevated respiratory rate (40–80 breaths/min), total rumen and GI stasis, a total cessation of milk flow and appetite, generalized skin coolness, reduced mucous membrane capillary refill time, and scant loose manure. Affected cattle often have an audible grunt or groan associated with expiration and may stand with elbows abducted (Fig. 5.22). The grunt or groan is most apparent when the animal arises, lies down, or is made to move about. Abdominal pain can be difficult to detect in these patients because the diffuse severe and persistent pain overwhelms any localized attempt to elicit pain by deep abdominal pressure. The animal will be reluctant to rise or move about and in most instances will progress to a shocklike state within 12 to 48 hours. As the animal's condition deteriorates, the body temperature also may plummet from the early fever to normal or subnormal. Risk of diffuse peritonitis is enhanced when a cow develops traumatic reticuloperitonitis in advanced gestation because the weight and movement of the gravid uterus tend to disseminate the peritonitis and make natural attempts at walling off the peritonitis difficult. Diffuse peritonitis caused by abomasal

perforation is the principle differential diagnosis for cows with this presentation and signalment.

Ancillary Data and Procedures

Laboratory tests may be helpful in diagnosing confusing cases. Peritoneal fluid containing elevated total solids and white blood cell numbers supports a diagnosis of peritonitis. A complete blood count (CBC) may or may not be helpful because many patients with hardware disease have normal CBCs, although almost all have elevated plasma fibrinogen levels and rapid glutaraldehyde clotting. Some patients with hardware disease with acute localized peritonitis and most patients with acute diffuse peritonitis will show a degenerative left shift in the leukogram. In chronic hardware disease (lasting >10 days), serum globulin is often elevated (>5.7 g/dL), and the leukogram may be normal or confirm mature neutrophilia. Cows with peracute, diffuse septic peritonitis caused by hardware disease may have hypoproteinemia as a result of fluid and protein loss into the peritoneal cavity, but this does not occur as commonly as with abomasal perforation. Because of forestomach and abomasal hypomotility or stasis, patients with hardware disease often have a hypochloremic, hypokalemic, metabolic alkalosis that varies in severity in direct proportion to the degree of stasis. Cattle affected with subacute or chronic hardware disease that has caused complete rumen stasis may have a metabolic alkalosis with serum chloride values in the 70 to 90 mEq/L range. It is debatable whether the profound alkalosis results solely from the disease present or is accentuated by the commonplace oral administration of ruminotoric-laxative medications before blood collection. Regardless of pathophysiology for alkalosis of this magnitude, the prognosis is not hopeless.

The most helpful ancillary tests are abdominal ultrasonography and reticular radiography (see Video Clip 5.2). Abdominal ultrasonography may often reveal an abnormal pocket of fluid and fibrin in the anterior abdomen (Fig. 5.23). Scanning the left and right sides of the chest wall, lateral to the sternum, caudal to the diaphragm, and up to and

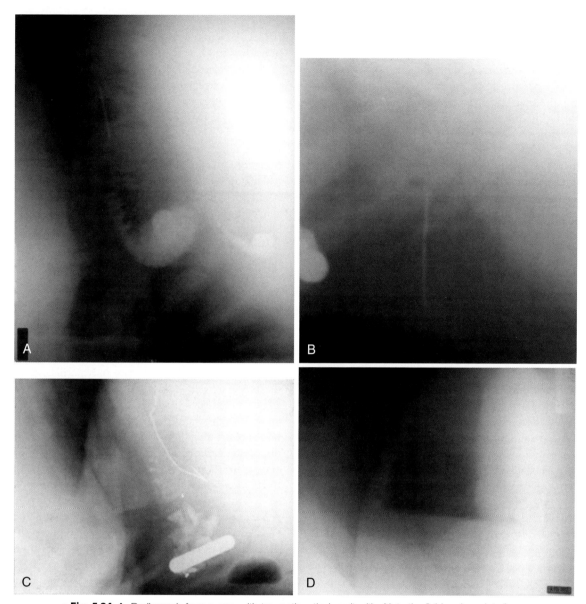

• **Fig. 5.24** **A,** Radiograph from a cow with traumatic reticuloperitonitis. Note the fluid and gas interfaces around a metallic foreign body suggestive of reticular abscess formation. **B,** Radiograph of a cow with a ventrally located draining fistula associated with traumatic reticuloperitonitis. The foreign body was a piece of baling wire. **C,** Abdominal radiograph of a cow with hardware disease showing an abscess (gas) ventral to the reticulum floor. **D,** Radiograph of the anterior abdomen showing a fluid line within a large perireticular abscess.

slightly dorsal to the level of the elbow, will often locate these lesions. Radiography is the best test for confirming metallic penetration of the reticulum (or rarely rumen), the current location of the metal object, and the presence and size of perireticular abscesses (Fig. 5.24). Unfortunately, this is the least available test for the practicing veterinarian because extremely powerful radiographic equipment is necessary to penetrate the reticular region in adult cattle. Radiography of the reticulum has been a useful ancillary procedure in teaching hospitals and referral centers to aid in detecting reticular foreign bodies and abscesses of the reticulum or liver. The procedure is very helpful in confusing cases of abdominal disease or in confirmation of suspected hardware disease. Powerful radiographic units capable of 300 mA and

125 kVp using a 400 ISO speed film-screen combination are necessary for such studies. Experience with such radiographic studies and the subsequent surgical findings allow clinicians to diagnose, determine the need or approach for surgery, and prognosticate more specifically than would be possible without this ancillary aid. A portable unit has reportedly been used to take radiographs of the reticulum in cattle restrained in dorsal recumbency. However, it is difficult to keep cows in that position, and the forced positioning of the cow could worsen the peritonitis.

Diagnosis

The diagnosis of traumatic reticuloperitonitis is based primarily on physical examination and is aided by laboratory tests in less obvious cases. In cattle with obvious signs of peritonitis, perforating abomasal ulcers are the chief differential consideration. Perforating abomasal ulcers tend to cause pain in the midventral abdomen on the right side of midline, are usually associated with fever, and are most common from 2 weeks before freshening up to 100 days postpartum. Acute pyelonephritis, uterine perforation, or necrotic lesions of the cervix or vagina may have a similar presentation to that of hardware disease. With pyelonephritis, the urine may be discolored, rectal examination reveals an enlarged and painful ureter and the patient demonstrates profound stranguria.

Cows with necrotic cervicitis or vaginitis are often febrile and depressed, stand either hunched up or stretched out, and have rumen atony, but unlike hardware cases, they strain and frequently aspirate air into the rectum. If an active magnet is already present in a cow showing signs of peritonitis, abomasal ulceration is more likely than hardware disease. A compass can be used during physical examination to detect an active magnet in the reticulum. The compass is moved slowly into position behind the elbow on the left thoracic wall. A 60- to 90-degree deflection indicates the presence of a strong magnet in the reticulum. In cows with normal rectal temperatures, hardware disease must be differentiated from indigestion and ketosis. This can be based on the absence of abdominal pain in patients with ketosis; not only will cows with hardware have evidence of abdominal pain in addition to ruminal hypomotility but they also demonstrate negative to trace urinary ketones. A cow affected with a musculoskeletal disease such as polyarthritis, laminitis, back pain, or trauma could be misdiagnosed with hardware disease because of an arched stance, weight loss, anorexia, and decreased production. Physical examination should easily differentiate among these diagnoses, however. Peritoneal fluid collection and analysis can be performed to help support a diagnosis of peritonitis, but this diagnostic procedure is rarely necessary or specifically helpful in the diagnosis of hardware.

Treatment

Conservative medical treatment can be successful in many acute cases of traumatic reticuloperitonitis. This treatment consists of a magnet administered orally, systemic antibiotics to control existing peritonitis, and stall rest to aid in the formation of adhesions; other symptomatic therapy such as oral fluids, ruminotorics, calcium solutions, and oral electrolytes also may be helpful. If dehydration is present and metabolic alkalosis is suspected or confirmed, fluid therapy and supplementation with potassium chloride orally (2 to 4 ounces, twice daily) or 40 mEq/L in intravenously administered fluids are indicated. In alkalotic patients, alkalinizing ruminotorics should be avoided. Conservative therapy results should be evaluated within 48 to 72 hours. If the affected cow is beginning to eat and ruminate and production begins to increase, recovery can be anticipated. If the cow is not improving or if appetite and rumen activity wax and wane, rumenotomy may be indicated. After oral administration of a magnet, the magnet first drops into the rumen. The magnet moves to the

desired location in the reticulum only through effectual ruminoreticular contractions. Therefore, if the rumen remains static, it is unlikely the magnet will move into the reticulum to grasp and hold the foreign body. It is revealing to note the number of cattle referred to teaching hospitals that possess a magnet or magnets within the rumen rather than the reticulum when the magnet has been administered as a therapeutic rather than prophylactic aid. If the affected cow already has a magnet at the time signs develop, exploratory laparotomy and rumenotomy may be indicated initially, rather than conservative therapy. This situation may occur when the foreign body is extremely long (>15 cm) and extends off the magnet to a dangerous degree or is not attached to a magnet, as in the case of an aluminum needle. Rumenotomy and object removal should be performed immediately in valuable cows to limit further movement of the object and worsening peritonitis or progression to pericarditis. When laparotomy and rumenotomy are elected, it is best not to explore the serosal surface of the rumen and reticulum if adhesions are obvious, because exploration may encourage dissemination of the peritonitis. During rumenotomy, a careful palpation of the entire mucosal surface of the reticulum is indicated to find the offending foreign body, which may remain only partially embedded in the reticular wall. Left-sided laparotomy and rumenotomy allow for confirmation of the diagnosis, removal of the foreign body or bodies, and drainage of reticular abscesses into the lumen of the reticulum (Fig. 5.25). Even with radiographic or ultrasonographic guidance, it can be challenging to identify and remove some foreign bodies that are embedded within mature, chronic, fibrous adhesions, and reaching a comfort level with abscess drainage by sharp scalpel incision into the reticular wall at the site of the adhesions takes some practice and experience. If there is a large reticular abscess, it could be drained via a ventral percutaneous approach, although cellulitis, reticular fistula, and dissemination of the peritonitis may occur. Particularly valuable animals with traumatic pericarditis or pleural abscess formation may benefit from partial resection of one or more ribs, allowing removal of the foreign body and aggressive abscess drainage (Fig. 5.26). Partial resection of two ribs was performed by Dr. Ducharme in the cow in Fig. 5.26, and the cow made an excellent recovery.

Antibiotic therapy should be continued for a minimum of 3 to 7 days to control existing localized peritonitis and to discourage formation of secondary reticular abscesses at the perforation site. Penicillin, ceftiofur, ampicillin, and tetracycline all have been used successfully for this purpose.

In subacute or chronic cases in which chronic anorexia, dehydration, and severe alkalosis co-exist, IV fluid therapy, antibiotics, and rumenotomy are indicated at the time of diagnosis. Conservative therapy is unlikely to be successful in these patients, and further supportive care with rumen transfaunates, calcium solutions, and long-term antibiotic treatment is often necessary.

Sequelae

Cattle with hardware disease may have myriad complications secondary to perforation and peritonitis. Septic pericarditis

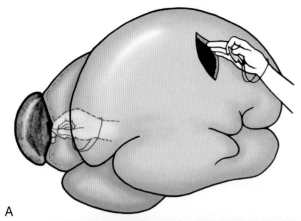

A

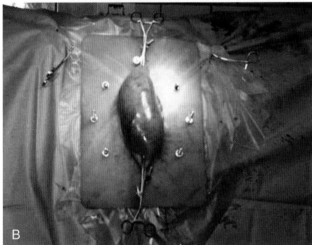

B

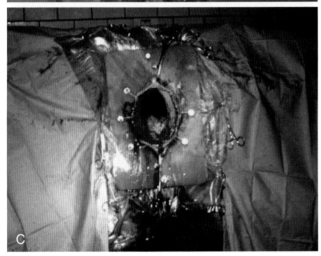

C

• **Fig. 5.25** **A,** A drawing depicting rumenotomy and lancing a perireticular abscess into the reticulum. **B,** Left paralumbar fossa laparotomy with rumen wall attached to a "rumen board." **C,** Same cow as in **B** with the rumen open.

is perhaps the best-known complication and occurs when the metallic foreign body advances in a cranial direction, perforating the diaphragm and pericardium (Fig. 5.27). On rare occasion, pericarditis from a migrating reticular foreign body can occur with no evidence of peritonitis, as was the case in the heifer pictured in Fig. 5.26. Reticular abscesses are fairly common sequelae and often occur on the cranial or

right wall of the reticulum, where they directly, or indirectly, cause dysfunction of the ventral vagus nerve branches and result in signs of vagal indigestion. Signs of vagal indigestion range from mild ruminoreticular disturbances to omasal transport difficulties or abomasal dysfunction or impaction. Septic pleuritis, pneumonia, thoracic abscesses, diaphragmatic hernias, and traumatic endocarditis are less frequent complications of a perforation of the diaphragm. Occasionally, a metallic foreign body, usually a wire associated with a ventral perforation, migrates through the sternum or cranial ventral abdomen, resulting in a reticular fistula or draining tract (Figs. 5.28 and 5.29). Any perforation of the right wall of the reticulum may directly or indirectly, through associated inflammation and adhesions, injure, inflame, or irritate the ventral vagus nerve branches and result in signs of vagal indigestion. Therefore, when hardware disease is suspected as the cause of vagal indigestion, a meticulous search of the right wall of the reticular mucosa is indicated during rumenotomy. Penetration of the liver or spleen can cause abscesses in these organs too.

Prevention

All breeding age heifers or heifers 1 year of age, as well as young bulls, should receive strong prophylactic magnets. Not to recommend this for valuable cattle represents negligence, and the loss of a single valuable dairy cow because of traumatic reticuloperitonitis is inexcusable. Many cows die each year because the owner "forgot" to administer a magnet; in a single month in late 2013, three very valuable cows ($10,000 to $30,000 each), all from different farms, were presented for life-threatening hardware disease at our clinic and none had a magnet, emphasizing that the disease is still extremely common. Although occasional cows pass magnets through the GI tract and some magnets do lose strength, the magnet remains the major means of preventing this disease. The effectiveness of magnets is apparent at slaughterhouses, where an impressive array of metallic foreign bodies are found trapped tightly to magnets. When purchasing magnets, the owner or the veterinarian should assess the strength of the magnet by testing it against metallic objects. Inferior magnets should not be purchased.

Large electromagnetic plates to trap metal can be incorporated into automatic feeding lines or silo unloaders and are available commercially; they are very helpful on large farms with automated feeding assemblies. Use of these plates should be encouraged because they tend to trap many pounds of dangerous sharp metallic objects each year.

Diseases Affecting the Vagus Innervation of the Forestomach and Abomasum: Vagal Indigestion

The vagus nerve may be damaged anywhere along its anatomic course to the forestomach and abomasum. Lesions capable of injuring, inflaming, or destroying the vagus nerve and its branches are discussed by anatomic sequence starting with the brainstem and progressing distally along the course

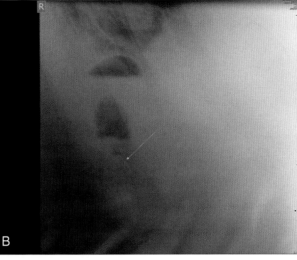

• **Fig. 5.26 A,** A 1.5-year-old Holstein heifer after partial resection of the right fifth and sixth ribs for treatment of both a right sided pleural abscess and traumatic pericarditis. The pericardium is being lavaged with a povidone-iodine (Betadine) solution. **B,** Radiograph of the heifer obtained before surgery showing a mildly radiodense foreign body in the right thorax with gas/fluid interfaces (abscesses) dorsal to the foreign body. There was no ultrasonographic evidence of peritonitis in this cow.

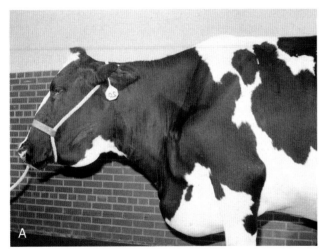

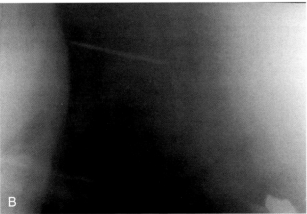

• **Fig. 5.27 A,** A cow with ventral edema, brisket edema, and intermandibular edema caused by pericarditis secondary to traumatic reticuloperitonitis. **B,** Radiograph of the anterior abdomen and ventral thorax of a 96-point cow with acute traumatic reticulitis. The wire has moved into the right thorax and was successfully removed via a standing thoracotomy.

of the nerve. All of these diseases lead to forestomach or abomasal dysfunction to some degree and have been historically included under the term "Vagal Indigestion." Depending on the anatomic area involved and degree of damage to the vagus nerve or its branches, these diseases may cause a wide spectrum of forestomach or abomasal signs. In all cases, ruminal distension is present intermittently or constantly. This distension may be the result of functional or physical outflow obstruction from the forestomach or failure of eructation causing free-gas distension. Physical or functional obstruction of the abomasum or pylorus may prevent outflow with more distal lesions.

The conditions discussed in this section are those that result in the syndrome called vagal indigestion. This syndrome must be thought of as a complex or set of signs secondary to a primary lesion at some point along the course of the vagus nerve.

Clinical Signs

General signs suggesting vagus nerve damage include decreased appetite for several days or more, decreased milk production, abdominal distension that may be constant or intermittent but tends to be progressive, pasty manure that often varies in quantity in direct proportion to appetite and inversely with the degree of abdominal distension, and loss of body condition. Most commonly cattle have rumen hypomotility. Many affected animals develop bradycardia (heart rate, 60 beats/min or less); however, not all cases develop this sign, and its absence should not rule out vagal indigestion. Bradycardia in cattle with vagal indigestion appears to be caused by retrograde irritation of the vagus nerve, with consequent parasympathetic slowing of the heart rate. Bradycardia has also been associated with simple anorexia and a lack of normal rumen fill. Rumen and reticular contractions may be hypermotile, hypotonic, or atonic, and vagal indigestion has been categorized by some authors based on this sign. Although in some cases rumen contractions occur more frequently than normal (3–6 contractions/min), they may be ineffectual. This hypermotility may be initiated because of the distended rumen yet fail to propel ruminoreticular ingesta into the omasum and abomasum, resulting in frothy ruminoreticular ingesta from constant churning activity.

The abdominal distension that develops gives a classical external appearance, with distension in the upper left, lower left, and lower right quadrants as the cow is viewed from the rear (Fig. 5.30). In most cases, this distension results from progressive ruminal enlargement with the ventral sac enlarging toward the right. Therefore, this typical distension results in an L-shaped rumen, as viewed from the rear or palpated per rectum. In severe cases, the rumen ventral sac not only fills the entire right lower quadrant of the abdomen but also may expand into the right upper quadrant such that the rumen assumes a V shape. Extreme distension of the rumen into a V shape occasionally traps gas in the most dorsal region of the expanded ventral sac, and this gas may result in an area of tympanitic resonance in the right upper quadrant. In very rare instances of abomasal impaction, pyloric stenosis, or duodenal stricture, the abomasum may be large enough to account for right lower quadrant distension (Fig. 5.31).

Depending on the primary lesions, signs of vagus nerve dysfunction may appear acutely or have a delayed onset. In most cases, onset of signs and typical abdominal distension occur several days to weeks after the affected cow initially developed signs of illness. Some primary lesions are relatively easy to diagnose, but for others diagnosis requires extensive ancillary data or exploratory surgery. In all cases, primary lesions resulting in the syndrome of vagal indigestion should be sought, because prognosis directly depends on the primary cause. In addition to these general signs of vagal indigestion, specific primary causes are discussed next, and individual signs referable to each are included when pertinent. Table 5.1 summarizes the clinical results of long-term follow-up evaluation for 112 cases of vagal indigestion and illustrates relative occurrence of the various primary disorders.

Vagus nerve nucleus lesions are rare, but occasionally, cattle affected with listeriosis will show vomiting, bloat, and rumen inactivity as early signs, and this may reflect vagus nerve irritation. It also is possible that vomiting or normal regurgitation occurs but cannot be controlled when oral-pharyngeal neuromuscular function is impeded by specific cranial nerve deficits (V, VII, IX, X) at the brainstem level.

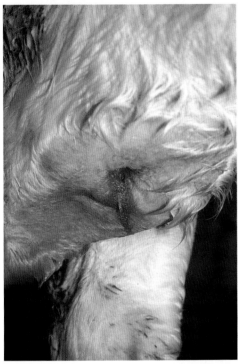

• **Fig. 5.28** Reticular fistula through the sternum of a cow. Ingesta from the reticulum leaked from this fistula secondary to migration of a metallic foreign body.

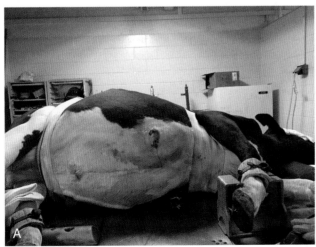
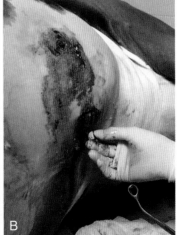

• **Fig. 5.29** **A,** Draining tract to the right of midline in the cranial abdomen of a mature Holstein dairy cow caused by a piece of baling wire. **B,** Percutaneous removal of wire in lateral recumbency. The cow made a complete recovery. Images courtesy of Dr. Sheila McGuirk.

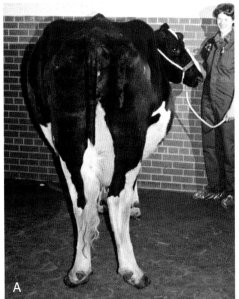
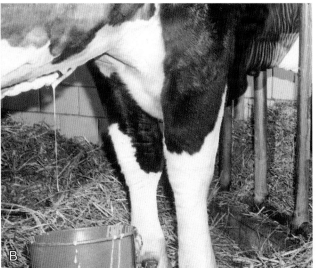
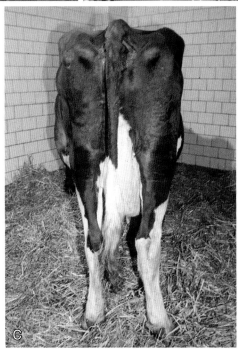

• **Fig. 5.30** **A,** Presurgical vagal indigestion. This cow was found to have a large liver abscess at the time of rumenotomy. **B,** A chest trochar was used to drain the liver abscess after a second surgery performed in the right paramedian area to properly place the trochar. **C,** Postoperative appearance of the cow.

Pharyngeal trauma often results in vagus nerve dysfunction accompanied by typical signs of fever, dysphagia, salivation, an extended head and neck, and soft tissue swelling in the pharyngeal area. This trauma usually results from injudicious or unskilled use of balling guns, dose syringes, stomach tubes, specula, esophageal feeders, or magnet or foreign body retrieval apparatus when treating a cow. Vagus nerve dysfunction may be apparent as ruminal hypomotility, dysphagia, failure of eructation, and subsequent ruminal distension. Bradycardia is present in some cases. The complex neuromuscular act of eructation frequently is altered because vagus nerve branches controlling the pharynx,

larynx, and cranial esophagus are subject to inflammatory or direct traumatic damage in these patients. Retropharyngeal abscesses and pharyngeal foreign bodies may cause signs similar to those caused by pharyngeal trauma but are less common.

Esophageal lacerations from traumatic passage of stomach tubes, esophageal feeders, or magnet or foreign body retrieval apparatus may also lead to severe cellulitis and associated vagus nerve dysfunction. Chemical or septic phlegmon with similar signs of vagus nerve dysfunction may follow perivascular injections of material intended for IV administration in the jugular vein. Fever, salivation, and

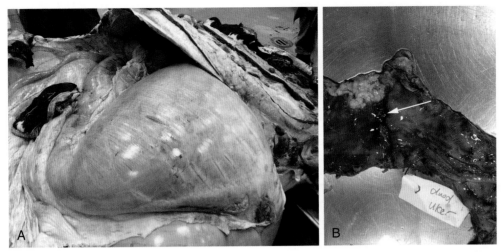

• **Fig. 5.31 A,** Postmortem appearance of grossly distended abomasum from a mature Holstein cow with outward signs of right ventral abdominal distension and the overall "papple" appearance of vagal indigestion. **B,** Postmortem appearance of the mid-duodenum from the cow in **A** showing circumferential linear ulceration pattern (white arrow) that had caused near-complete luminal duodenal obstruction.

TABLE 5.1	Clinical Results of Long-term Evaluation for 112 Cattle Affected with Vagal Indigestion			
	Good	**Moderate**	**Poor**	**Total**
Pharyngeal trauma			1	1
Pneumonia			1	1
Fibropapilloma	1			1
Actinomyces granuloma		1		1
Lymphosarcoma			2	2
Toxic rumenitis			3	3
Traumatic reticuloperitonitis	13	3	16	32
Reticular abscess	10	1	4	15
Abomasal ulcer (perforating)	3	3		6
Right displacement abomasum	4			4
Right torsion abomasum	3	3	20	26
RDA and perforating ulcer			1	1
Left displacement abomasum			1	1
Omasal impaction			1	1
Abomasal impaction			2	2
Abdominal abscess			1	1
Diffuse peritonitis	1		7	8
Advanced pregnancy			1	1
Idiopathic	1		1	2
	33	8	71	112

"Good" indicates remained in herd and returned to, or exceeded, previous production levels. "Moderate" indicates remained in herd but was culled within one lactation cycle. "Poor" indicates died or was culled within 1 month of treatment.
RDA, Right displacement of the abomasum.

severe inflammatory swelling in the cervical region and signs of Horner's syndrome may accompany any signs of vagus nerve damage in these patients. Chronic choke may lead to esophageal necrosis and similar signs, along with profuse salivation and reflux of ingested food or water.

Occasionally in calves and adult cattle, severe bronchopneumonia results in apparent inflammatory damage to the vagus nerve traversing the mediastinum. It is not known whether this syndrome involves direct inflammation of the nerve or indirect pressure from enlarged lymph nodes. In any event, the affected calf, or less commonly cow, develops signs of abdominal distension, ruminal tympany, and inappetence despite apparent response of the pneumonia to broad-spectrum antibiotic therapy. Usually signs of ruminal tympany develop several days after the onset of the pneumonia. Passage of a stomach tube in these patients relieves and resolves a free-gas bloat, but the bloat recurs as a chronic problem and results in weight loss because the animal eats only during those times when the bloat is relieved. Failure of eructation seems to be the major cause of this recurrent free-gas bloat. Occasional cases of frothy-type bloat may occur in association with chronic bronchopneumonia in adult cattle, when pneumonic pathology involves thoracic branches of the vagus nerve.

Neoplasms such as thymic, juvenile, or adult lymphosarcoma, neurofibromatosis, and pulmonary carcinomas sometimes may result in signs of vagus indigestion resulting from extraluminal compression of the esophagus or pressure on the vagus nerve and subsequent failure of eructation with chronic free-gas bloat. Lesions at the cardia include fibropapillomas, other neoplastic processes, and granulomas caused by *Trueperella pyogenes* or *A. lignieresii*. Generally, lesions in this area mechanically occlude the distal esophagus during attempts at eructation or regurgitation and cause signs of vagal indigestion.

Most lesions involving the reticulum are located on the right or medial wall of the reticulum. These lesions damage the ventral vagus nerve branches with inflammation, pressure, or direct trauma. Traumatic reticuloperitonitis, reticular abscesses, liver abscesses, severe toxic rumenitis, and neoplasms such as lymphosarcoma are included in this group. Some authors include adhesions of the cranial and medial reticulum in this category and imply that mechanical dysfunction results from these adhesions. Most authors, however, believe that neurogenic damage to the ventral vagus branches must also occur even if adhesions are present. In this category, the prognosis seems to vary depending on the cause (Table 5.1). Traumatic reticuloperitonitis carries a variable prognosis based on the degree of peritonitis and involvement of the ventral vagus branches (13 of 32 cases had good outcomes), but reticular abscesses carry a more favorable prognosis (10 of 15 cases had good outcomes) presumably because they tend to cause vagus nerve dysfunction by pressure on the nerve. This pressure dysfunction is alleviated by surgical drainage. Rapid resolution of the clinical signs of vagal indigestion may similarly be seen following draining of a liver abscess that was pressing on the vagus nerve (see Fig. 5.30).

Lesions of the forestomach distal to the reticulum or involving the abomasum include a diverse group of problems such as lymphosarcoma and other neoplasms, diffuse peritonitis, peritonitis caused by perforating abomasal ulcers, abdominal abscesses, vagus nerve damage, vascular thrombosis secondary to right-sided AV, omasal impaction or displacement, and chronic or severe abomasal impaction. In general, the prognosis is poor for cattle with signs of vagal indigestion secondary to these lesions (see Table 5.1) because of the extent of the pathology, the possibility of multiple sites being affected, and the likelihood of persistent functional and mechanical outflow disturbances. In referral practice, a disproportionate number of cattle with right-sided AV are treated. Many of these cattle have been affected for 24 hours or longer before referral, and thus are at high risk for subsequent signs of vascular thrombosis and vagus nerve dysfunction. Usually these cattle appear to improve for 24 to 72 hours after surgical correction of their AV but then begin to show signs of an outflow disturbance. They subsequently develop bradycardia, ruminal distension, scant manure, poor appetite, and abdominal distension typical of an L-shaped rumen. Their prognosis is extremely poor.

In most cases distension following right-sided AV also involves the forestomach compartments even though the abomasum was the primary problem. Recent work helps explain this syndrome. Because volvulus involves the abomasum, omasum, and reticulum, either neurogenic damage by stretching the ventral vagus branches or thrombosis of major vessels supplying the lesser curvature of the abomasum, omasum, and reticulum may result from prolonged volvulus. Most cattle that develop signs of vagal indigestion after right-sided abomasal displacement and volvulus never recover despite attempts at therapy. Rumenotomy is seldom suggested for cows with vagal indigestion secondary to right-sided AV because the primary pathology is thought to be mostly irreversible. Vagus nerve damage secondary to right-sided volvulus has an extremely poor prognosis, with only 3 of 26 patients having a good outcome (see Table 5.1). Right-sided DAs and volvulus should be corrected on an emergency basis to minimize chances of vagus nerve damage or subsequent outflow disturbance. Valuable cattle that begin to develop symptoms of vagal indigestion after correction of right-sided volvulus of the abomasum by omentopexy may be considered for abomasopexy after rumenotomy to ensure proper abomasal alignment that may improve outflow. The prognosis, however, remains guarded to poor.

The diagnosis of vagal indigestion is based on subacute to chronic history, typical abdominal distension, rectal findings of an L- or V-shaped rumen, and bradycardia (when present). The diagnosis is incomplete, however, until a primary cause of vagus nerve dysfunction is determined. The primary lesion is obvious in some instances, such as pharyngeal trauma, esophageal laceration, and vagus nerve dysfunction secondary to reticular abscess or recent surgical correction of right-sided volvulus of the abomasum. In other instances, especially those with less common abdominal lesions or when associated with advanced pregnancy,

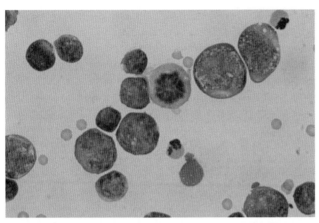

• **Fig. 5.32** Cytologic appearance of peritoneal fluid from a bovine leukemia virus–positive 5-year-old Holstein cow with abomasal lymphosarcoma. Note the large lymphoblasts with prominent nucleoli and mitotic figures. The sample was obtained from the right paramedian location immediately under the greater curvature.

the primary diagnosis may be difficult to determine unless exploratory laparotomy and rumenotomy are performed. Abomasal and sometimes ruminal impactions unrelated to any apparent vagus nerve injury occur sporadically. Abomasal impactions are a cause of decreased appetite and production in dairy cattle, and most have complete recovery after medical or surgical treatments and are likely unrelated to vagus dysfunction. Cows with abomasal impactions associated with vagus nerve dysfunction are much less amenable to treatment.

Clinical Pathology

In all cases, a thorough physical examination (including a rectal examination) should be performed. If physical examination fails to reveal the primary lesion, ancillary tests may be helpful. CBC may indicate chronic or acute inflammation or suggest lymphosarcoma based on persistent lymphocytosis. Serum total protein, albumin, and globulin should be assessed. Elevated serum globulin may suggest reticular or liver abscess. Abdominal paracentesis is difficult to perform in cattle with vagal indigestion because the tremendous rumen distension leaves virtually no space for separation of the visceral and parietal peritoneum. Nevertheless, with ultrasonography as an aid, abdominal fluid analysis may indicate peritonitis or lymphosarcoma. The right cranial paramedian location can be a rewarding location from which to obtain diagnostic fluid containing exfoliated neoplastic cells in cases of abomasal lymphosarcoma; possibly up to 50% of abomasal lymphosarcoma cases will have neoplastic cells in the peritoneal fluid (Fig. 5.32). Acid–base and electrolyte status is helpful in determining relative degrees of alkalosis. The clinician should not conclude, however, that severe alkalosis always indicates primary abomasal or pyloric disease because some cattle with subacute to chronic traumatic reticuloperitonitis have severe alkalosis. Somewhat surprisingly, most patients with vagal indigestion have either normal acid–base and electrolyte values or mild hypochloremic, hypokalemic alkalosis despite their

apparent outflow disturbance. A marked hypochloremic (chloride <75 mEq/L) metabolic alkalosis would be most supportive of a pyloric or proximal small bowel obstruction or renal failure. Gamma glutamyl transferase is elevated in approximately 50% of cows with liver abscess but overall has poor sensitivity and specificity for this disease.

Ancillary Tests

Abdominal ultrasonography is very helpful in evaluating cattle affected with vagal indigestion. Ultrasonography can help determine the nature of abdominal fluid, detect the presence of fibrin, or locate an intraabdominal abscess. Ultrasonography can also be useful to image the abomasal wall to determine the size of the viscus and search for any evidence of neoplasia. Because of the poor sensitivity and specificity of biochemical markers of liver disease in cattle with liver abscess(es), transabdominal ultrasonography is the most useful ancillary test in making a diagnosis of liver abscessation. If facilities are available, radiographs of the reticulum are very helpful in detecting foreign body perforation of the reticulum, and radiographs of the pharynx or thorax can aid in the diagnosis of pharyngeal or thoracic lesions. If bovine lymphosarcoma is suspected, serum should be submitted for a BLV agar-gel immunodiffusion test, enzyme-linked immunosorbent assay, or whole blood for a polymerase chain reaction test, and a peritoneal centesis should be performed followed by cytologic examination for neoplastic lymphocytes as previously described.

Treatment

Some primary etiologic disorders carry (neoplasms, vagal indigestion secondary to right-sided volvulus of the abomasum, and diffuse peritonitis) a sufficiently negative prognosis that exploratory surgery may not be necessary or indicated. Similarly, medical causes of vagal indigestion such as pharyngeal trauma, severe pneumonia, and other definable lesions that result in failure of eructation may only require symptomatic therapy for the primary problem. In cases of pharyngeal trauma or cellulitis, for example, broad-spectrum antibiotics, antiinflammatories, and analgesics would be indicated. If failure of eructation persists in these instances, however, use of a rumen fistula may alleviate chronic bloating and provide a means of administering feed and water during the prolonged recovery. If the value of the affected cow warrants treatment and the suspected primary problem is abdominal in location, surgical intervention is necessary. Left-sided exploratory laparotomy and rumenotomy offer the best means of making a definitive diagnosis of the primary cause for the vagus nerve dysfunction. In addition to the diagnostic and prognostic advantages of a rumenotomy, a therapeutic benefit is realized because the massively distended rumen may be emptied. This temporarily reduces the weight of the organ and relieves pressure receptor dysfunction caused by massive distension of the rumen.

After rumenotomy, rumen and reticular pressure receptors may be better able to instigate effective forestomach contractions if indeed the vagus nerve damage has not been extensive or permanent. After surgery, transfaunation and slow reintroduction of feed should be performed. In a few cows, the passage of a Kingman tube before surgery may permit dramatic emptying of the rumen fluid, making the rumenotomy and exploratory examination easier for both the cow and the surgeon.

Adequate hydration and correction of acid–base or electrolyte deficits should be achieved by IV fluid therapy before surgery. If peritonitis is suspected, broad-spectrum antibiotics should be used as well. Usually oral medications or fluids are contraindicated because of existing functional outflow disturbance, although the administration of 1 lb of coffee by orogastric tube to adult cattle has occasionally had some dramatic effects on the passage of ingesta from the forestomach compartments and abomasum. Parenteral calcium solutions are indicated for patients that are hypocalcemic secondary to reduced intestinal uptake coupled with continued calcium loss resulting from milk production.

As complete an exploration of the abdomen as possible should be attempted during left flank celiotomy. If extensive adhesions are found in the abdomen or around the reticulum, these adhesions should not be manipulated or broken down because this would be painful and may act to disseminate the existing peritonitis. After exploration of the abdominal viscera, rumenotomy should be performed and the ruminal contents evacuated. Careful search of the forestomach compartments should be conducted with particular care devoted to the reticulum, cardia, and reticulo-omasal orifice. The reticular mucosa should be lifted to detect adhesions between the visceral and parietal peritoneum. The abomasum and omasum should be palpated through the wall of the rumen. Abomasal impactions or extensive adhesions caused by perforating abomasal ulcers may be palpated at this time. Anatomic dislocation of the abomasum or pylorus associated with extensive adhesions also may be detected. In average-sized cattle, the surgeon may pass a hand into the omasal orifice to palpate the interior of the omasum and, occasionally by directing a hand ventrally, the interior of the abomasum. A methodical search of the reticular mucosa should be completed to rule out traumatic reticuloperitonitis and to detect any foreign bodies or tumors in the reticulum. Fibropapillomas should be removed. Palpation of the caudal esophagus will detect the occasional tumor or granuloma that may occur in this region. Reticular abscesses and liver abscesses resulting in vagus nerve dysfunction tend to be located along the right or medial wall of the reticulum, although the anterior-posterior orientation varies in each case. Usually reticular abscesses will be attached firmly to the reticular wall by adhesions, although liver abscesses generally are not. Large reticular or liver abscesses give the impression, based on palpation, that two omasums are present in affected cows. Usually the abscess is located anterior to the omasum. If a reticular abscess is confirmed by firm adhesion of the mass to the reticulum and by an aspirate, the surgeon should proceed with drainage of the abscess into the reticulum by lancing the abscess as shown in Fig. 5.25, A. When a liver

abscess is confirmed (see Fig. 5.30, B and C), a second procedure through a ventral abdominal approach to establish drainage is indicated if the owner elects further attempts at therapy. After exploratory survey of the forestomach compartments is completed, transfaunate from a healthy cow's rumen should be administered and the rumen and body wall closed. If vagus nerve dysfunction characterized only by free-gas bloat exists, a rumen fistula may be placed surgically during closure of the abdomen; this will allow escape of rumen gas until healing of the primary condition occurs. After the exploratory examination, if vagal indigestion signs are believed to be caused by advanced pregnancy, the cow may need to be aborted at an appropriate time.

Postoperative care is dictated largely by the exploratory rumenotomy findings. The primary cause of the vagus nerve dysfunction should be treated specifically. If active peritonitis or an abscess is present, broad-spectrum antibiotic therapy would be indicated. Fluid and electrolyte balance should continue to be assessed and treated. Daily rumen transfaunates, if available, should be administered. A laxative diet with adequate fiber (e.g., grass or grass and alfalfa hay) should be fed along with any other feedstuffs that may stimulate the cow's appetite. Parenteral calcium solutions are indicated if hypocalcemia is present. Recovery is slow but progressive; even in cattle that respond to therapy, complete recovery usually requires weeks. Positive signs include an improved appetite and milk production, lack of recurrent bloat, increased manure production, lack of rumen distension on rectal examination, and weight gain. Negative prognostic signs include a continued poor appetite, scant fecal production, recurrent bloat, and rumen and abdominal distension. Cattle that have had large amounts of ingesta removed from the forestomachs during surgery should not be allowed free access to feed, and particularly water, in the immediate postoperative period. Most cattle with substantial peritonitis will not want to eat or drink very much at this time anyway, and in many cases, they look significantly worse for the first 24 to 48 hours after surgery. However, the occasional individual will gorge or drink excessively in the postoperative period and rapidly redistend the rumen if allowed ad libitum access.

Left Flank Abdominal Exploratory Laparotomy and Rumenotomy

This common surgical procedure (see Fig. 5.25) provides direct access to the rumen of cattle, and indications for medical and research purposes have been reviewed by Fubini and Ducharme. In some instances, the rumen is so enlarged that it precludes any meaningful intraabdominal palpation. After routine preparation and left flank incision, the abdomen may be explored to some extent before rumenotomy. The surgeon should bear in mind that adhesions—especially those associated with the reticulum or abomasum—represent a potentially septic focus. Manipulation of such adhesions may lead to dissemination of infection and subsequent diffuse peritonitis. Depending on the size of the cow being explored, some of the abdominal viscera may be palpated by extending an arm over or caudal to the rumen. Usually, however, the right cranial abdomen is out of reach from this approach.

On performing a rumenotomy in cases of vagal indigestion or hardware disease, the interior of the rumen should be cleared of as much ingesta as possible. This allows the surgeon to palpate the abdominal viscera through the wall of the rumen similar to the technique used in rectal palpation. The reticulum should be searched meticulously for foreign bodies. The wall of the reticulum should be grasped and inverted to detect adhesions. The distal esophagus should be entered to detect neoplastic or granulomatous masses. The reticulo-omasal orifice should be entered with several fingers or the whole hand to palpate the interior of the omasum. In smaller cows, the surgeon may be able to advance through the omasum into the abomasum at this time. The omasum and abomasum should be palpated through the wall of the rumen. Abdominal abscesses associated with the reticulum, liver, or umbilical remnants likewise may be identified by palpation through the rumen wall.

If a reticular abscess is identified and is definitely adhered to the wall of the reticulum, aspiration to confirm abscess content followed by incisional drainage of the abscess into the reticulum should be performed. Intraoperative ultrasonography with the probe held up against the mucosa of the reticulum by the surgeon can be particularly helpful in identifying or confirming the presence and extent of perireticular abscesses and suspicious palpation findings. If an abscess is identified but is found not to be adherent to the forestomach, it should be located carefully and approached by a second abdominal surgery for definitive drainage or marsupialization, assuming the cow's value dictates a second procedure.

In cattle suspected of having hardware disease, identification of the reticular adhesions helps confirm the diagnosis and directs the surgeon's search for the causative foreign body. Methodical palpation of every "honeycomb" mucosal division in the reticulum should be performed. On many occasions in the teaching hospital, several surgeons have palpated for a foreign body and been unable to identify the object until aided by a more experienced surgeon. In these instances, the foreign body has been found lying flush to the reticular wall, having perforated several mucosal ridges, or has penetrated the wall to such a depth that only the very end of the wire or nail is palpable. Certainly, many foreign bodies have been found to have fully penetrated and exited the reticulum to lie outside the organ. In these instances, efforts to retrieve tiny metallic objects are futile unless a ventral exploratory procedure is deemed possible. On rare occasions, it has been possible to retrieve foreign bodies from a ventral approach when previous rumenotomy or ultrasonography has identified the object and its surrounding fibrous tissue. Several of these attempts have resulted in frustration, however, because of diffuse adhesions making removal of the foreign body impossible or because of the unintended creation of diffuse peritonitis after radical procedures. Probably only foreign bodies definitely palpated or

visualized with radiography or ultrasonography ventral or caudal to the reticulum warrant a second abdominal exploratory procedure from a ventral approach, or a thoracotomy if the foreign body has migrated from the abdomen into the thorax. In a teaching hospital setting, it is recommended that the first person who finds a foreign body remove it rather than leaving it for a student or trainee to palpate. Too often, the foreign body "disappears".

Cows showing signs of vagal indigestion that are found to have primary reticuloperitonitis almost invariably have had perforation of the right or medial wall of the reticulum. The perforation, localized peritonitis, and associated inflammation in this location cause direct or indirect damage to the ventral vagus nerve branches on the medial wall of the reticulum. Therefore, the methodical search for the foreign body should be concentrated on the right wall of the reticulum.

On very rare occasions, placenta, plastic material, or other nonmetallic foreign objects are found trapped in the reticulo-omasal orifice. Rumenotomies have had to be performed to retrieve balling guns, parts of balling guns, Fricke specula, stomach tubes, parts of esophageal feeders in calves, and other pieces of equipment swallowed by cattle during the administration of oral medications by laypeople and veterinarians alike. Before closure of the rumen, a good-quality magnet should be placed in the reticulum. In some instances, it may be indicated to transfaunate the cow by administering rumen juice from a healthy cow into the rumen of the patient before closure.

An uncommon complication of a laparotomy and rumenotomy is infection at the laparotomy site. If the site is noticed to be swollen and painful, antibiotic therapy should be continued and if necessary 1 or 2 ventral sutures should be removed to permit drainage and flushing of the wound with a disinfectant.

Listeriosis and Forestomach Dysfunction

Occasionally, cattle affected with meningoencephalitis caused by *Listeria monocytogenes* show rumen stasis and vomition as early signs (see Chapter 13 for complete discussion of listeriosis). These signs may result from direct inflammation of the vagus nucleus in the brainstem that stimulates excess regurgitation, or they may be the result of an inability to retain regurgitated rumen ingesta because of inflammation involving cranial nerves such as V, IX, X, and XII. Cattle with listeriosis that have complete dysphagia will develop very firm rumen contents that may cause abdominal pain when deep abdominal pressure is exerted by the examiner. This pain has been confused with pain caused by peritonitis when the affected cow's cranial nerve deficits were not recognized, leading to misdiagnosis of peritonitis.

Regurgitation

Regurgitation, or the discharge of food from the mouth and occasionally from the nose, may occur immediately after eating or as cud is being chewed and swallowed. Normal rumination is a form of regurgitation, but the regurgitated bolus is not expelled from the mouth. Cattle that regurgitate may suddenly stop eating or chewing their cud, extend the neck momentarily, and after a brief episode of retching, eject partially chewed food mixed with saliva or cud. Regurgitation must be differentiated from vomiting, which is often characterized by a short period of restlessness followed by a considerable amount of forestomach ingesta exiting the mouth or nose with force. Regurgitation is most commonly a result of an esophageal disorder, such as motility disorders in calves, injury to the esophagus, or extraluminal compression, often affecting the intrathoracic part. Pharyngeal trauma and pharyngeal masses may also cause regurgitation. Regurgitation may occur in calves with otitis interna or media caused by inflammation extending beyond the tympanic bulla with involvement of the vagus or glossopharyngeal nerve in that area. With sufficient regurgitation, the cow or calf may develop acidosis and hypophosphatemia caused by a loss of saliva. Regurgitation should also be differentiated from quidding, which is simply dropping food from the mouth while chewing. This is mostly associated with fractured teeth, fractured mandible, tooth abscess, foreign body in the mouth, and so on. Nasal regurgitation of milk in calves should always suggest a congenital defect of the hard or soft palate; spontaneous oral regurgitation of milk shortly after feeding in a calf from birth may also suggest a persistent right aortic arch or other congenital lesion involving the esophagus.

Disorders of the Mouth

The most common mouth disorders in dairy cattle are viral mucosal diseases, lumpy jaw, oropharyngeal trauma and wooden tongue, each of which is discussed in more detail in Chapter 6. Dental disease per se appears to be much less common in dairy cattle than in horses. Tooth root abscesses in ruminants, although uncommon, are thought to be caused by injury to the gingiva predisposing to infection of the premolar and molar teeth during eruption at 1.5 and 3 years of age respectively. *Trueperella pyogenes* is the most common organism isolated. Affected cattle may be asymptomatic until a soft swelling is noted over the ventral aspect of the mandible or over the rostral maxilla. The softness of the swelling and bacterial culture results should easily rule out lumpy jaw. Surgical drainage of the abscess, removal of any loose or damaged teeth, and penicillin treatment are generally curative. A fractured tooth, fractured jaw, or a foreign body caught in the mouth may also cause signs such as excessive salivation, quidding, and difficulty chewing. Fractured teeth and foreign body injury to the mouth can be diagnosed with a visual and manual exam using a speculum to hold the mouth open. Fracture of the jaw is not rare in cattle and is best diagnosed by radiographic imaging. Repair of mandibular fractures is described in detail in the chapter on surgery of the digestive system in the *Farm Animal Surgery* text edited by Drs. Fubini and Ducharme. Tumors of the mouth are rare in dairy cattle but include hamartomas in newborn calves, viral papillomas in young cattle, and rarely squamous cell

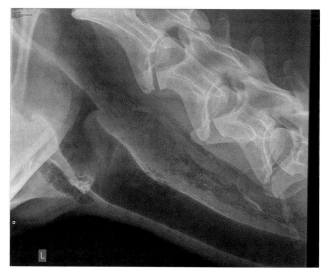

• **Fig. 5.33** Radiograph of the cranial cevical region in a 5-year-old Holstein cow with mild bloat, decreased appetite, and absence of cud regurgitation caused by an esophageal perforation. The cause of the perforation was not known, but the esophageal ulceration seen on endoscopy resolved and the cow recovered within 1 week after antimicrobial therapy. Moderate, dissecting gas shadowing can be seen ventral to cervical vertebral bodies.

carcinomas in very old cows. Dr. Wayne Wratten, a former student of Dr. Rebhun's, once manually removed a large papilloma from the pharynx of a yearling heifer that he examined for upper airway obstruction. Neoplasia of the jaw and teeth are uncommon in cattle, but both fibrosarcoma of the jaw and odontogenic myxomas may cause firm swelling of either the mandible or the maxilla. Both have a poor prognosis.

Esophageal Disorders

Esophageal disorders of dairy cattle include trauma from stomach tubes, esophageal feeders, or balling guns; ulcerative mucosal lesions from BVDV, malignant catarrhal fever, or infectious bovine rhinotracheitis; parasitic infections; ingested chemical or foreign body injury; intra- or extraluminal obstruction; and motility disturbances such as congenital achalasia or from injury or extraluminal compression causing physical or neurogenic dysfunction. Intraluminal obstruction of the esophagus is rare in cattle but may occur from eating apples, corncobs, or potatoes or other root crops. In calves, obstruction may occur when esophageal feeding tubes are broken off in the esophagus.

The most common clinical signs of esophageal disorders are salivation, regurgitation, and ruminal bloat. Esophageal endoscopy can be particularly valuable in confirming many of the above mentioned disorders. With esophageal rupture, crepitus from subcutaneous gas can often be palpated in the neck at the level of, and rostral to, the site of perforation. With smaller perforations, the amount of palpable gas may be minimal, but radiographs may demonstrate marked gas along the esophagus (Fig. 5.33).

The treatment and prognosis of esophageal perforations and rupture depend on the cause and extent of the injury. Small perforations may heal with antibiotics. Larger

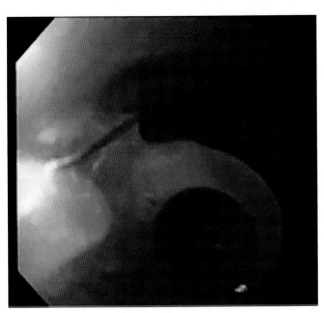

• **Fig. 5.34** Endoscopic view of the esophagus of a 1-day-old calf and a broken esophageal feeder tube. The accident occurred during the administration of colostrum to the calf. A snare was used to gather the tube and pull it from the esophagus (see Video Clip 2.1).

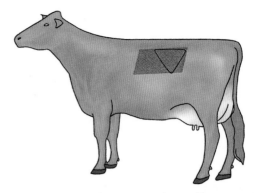

• **Fig. 5.35** Area of tympanic resonance observed in rumen collapse.

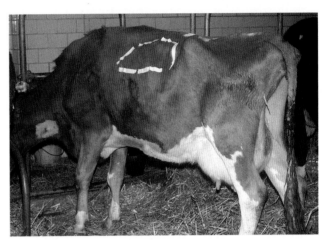

• **Fig. 5.36** Area of tympanic resonance in a cow with rumen collapse secondary to septic metritis.

perforations that leak feed material are generally considered to carry a grave prognosis, and if treatment is attempted, it would require surgical drainage of feed material and cellulitis in the neck in addition to an esophagostomy with placement of an esophageal feeding tube below the rupture site or a rumen fistula for feeding. For calves with esophageal feeders broken and caught in the esophagus, the tube can usually be felt by external palpation along the jugular furrow and may be removed endoscopically using a wire snare passed through the scope (see Video Clip 2.1 and Fig. 5.34). The calf can either be tranquilized with a light dose of xylazine and the scope with snare passed through the mouth to remove the tube, or the scope with snare can be passed through the nose in an unsedated calf and the tube snared and pulled into the pharynx, where a forceps inserted into the mouth can grasp the tube for removal. In some calves, the broken feeder tube may not lodge in the esophagus but pass into the rumen. If endoscopic equipment is not available, rumenotomy will permit removal of those tubes lodged in the rumen or the distal esophagus.

Rumen Void Syndrome

Rumen void is a poorly understood syndrome that has also been called "rumen collapse." It is observed sporadically in cattle with severe inflammatory diseases such as septic metritis, septic mastitis, or severe pneumonia causing complete anorexia of several days' duration. Chronically anorectic patients with other conditions such as peritonitis may also occasionally present with rumen void. Physical examination usually identifies the primary inflammatory disease and a large area of tympanic resonance in the left upper quadrant of the abdomen. Simultaneous percussion and auscultation

reveal a "ping" localized to the dorsal one-half to one-third of the left abdomen. This ping extends dorsally beyond the transverse processes of the lumbar vertebrae and includes the area of the paralumbar fossa and an area cranial to the paralumbar fossa covering up to four to five rib spaces (Figs. 5.35 and 5.36). The abdomen is not distended on the left side, but this ping creates great confusion because the other differential diagnoses of LDA, ruminal tympany, and pneumoperitoneum must be considered. Importantly, no fluid can be detected by ballottement in patients with rumen void, and the absence of this finding lessens the likelihood of a LDA. Rectal examination is necessary to confirm the problem and will reveal a collapsed dorsal sac of the rumen with no palpable rumen in the dorsal left quadrant and the left kidney pulled ventrally into the midabdomen (rather than slightly to the right of the dorsal midline as is normal). The dorsal sac of the rumen is not gas distended, ruling out ruminal tympany, and the rectum is not tightly compressed around the examiner's arm, ruling out pneumoperitoneum. Before the syndrome was recognized, standing laparotomies were performed on several cattle with pings caused by rumen collapse. These laparotomies merely revealed a collapsed dorsal sac and the left kidney pulled ventrally and medially into the midabdomen. Although it is not understood why a ping occurs in these cattle, the characteristic clinical signs now allow diagnosis and avoid subjecting an already very ill cow to surgery.

After a diagnosis of rumen collapse has been made and other causes of left-sided abdominal pings have been ruled out, treatment should be directed toward the primary disease. Systemic antibiotics are indicated for septic metritis, septic mastitis, or pneumonia. Furthermore, local antibiotic therapy, along with evacuation of septic secretions, is indicated for mastitis and metritis patients. If endotoxemia is suspected, it should be treated with nonsteroidal antiinflammatory drugs (NSAIDs). Supportive therapy for hypocalcemia or ketosis should be used if indicated. Dehydration and acid–base and electrolyte abnormalities should be corrected, and rumen stasis may be treated by ruminotorics, oral fluid and electrolyte therapy, or rumen transfaunates.

If therapy for the primary inflammatory disease is successful, the affected cow will begin to eat. The ventral extent of the ping will be located more dorsally each successive day during recovery as the rumen begins to fill and return to its normal position in the left upper quadrant. The prognosis is excellent if the primary disease is managed successfully because rumen collapse is merely a physiologic sign of prolonged anorexia rather than a pathologic GI disorder.

Vomition

Vomition is observed sporadically in dairy cattle and may result from dietary or physical conditions. The most common cause of vomition is hyperacidity of the diet, which usually affects only one cow in the herd. Why only one animal is affected is unknown. Such cows remain healthy, continue to eat, and do not show signs of distress despite vomiting once or more daily. It is important to determine when the vomiting has occurred in relation to the time the animal ingested a given feed. Buffering by feeding roughage before the offending grain or silage or adding alkalinizing buffer to the feedstuff usually stops the problem. In rare instances, withdrawal of the causative feedstuff is necessary.

Vomiting also may be rarely observed in cows with traumatic reticuloperitonitis due to repetitive irritation of the reticulum. There is a greater likelihood of this when the foreign body is located in the cranial reticulum near the cardia or is free in the ventral abdomen. One cow with intermittent vomiting was found to have a wire that had apparently migrated from the reticulum to a subcutaneous location in the xiphoid area. The wire was removed through a skin incision, and the vomiting stopped. Whether, or how, this irritation triggers receptors involved in regurgitation is unknown. In addition to vomiting, these cattle usually are ill with signs consistent with traumatic reticuloperitonitis. Treatment is as described in the section on traumatic reticuloperitonitis. Similar irritation that triggers the regurgitation reflex may be observed with distal esophageal or reticular warts and in diaphragmatic hernia. Rumen or reticular ulcers can also cause vomition; the vomited ingesta were hemorrhagic in one case we have seen.

Similarly, some cattle affected with vagal indigestion will vomit. These cows usually have advanced signs of abdominal and rumen distension. Regurgitation may be associated with

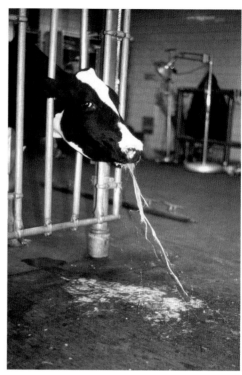

• **Fig. 5.37** Vomiting and depression were the most noticeable clinical signs in this adult cow with listeriosis.

the release of a large amount of liquid rumen ingesta that cannot be retained in the oral cavity and therefore appears as vomition. It is also possible that attempts at regurgitation in the presence of greatly increased intraruminal pressure may predispose to vomiting.

As previously mentioned, dairy cattle affected with listeriosis may vomit in the early stages of the disease (Fig. 5.37). This is thought to represent either irritation of the vagus nerve caused by inflammation of the vagus nucleus or inability to retain regurgitated ingesta as a result of cranial nerve deficits involving V, IX, X, and XII.

Vomiting has been observed in calves with white muscle disease, pharyngeal injury or mass, and esophageal motility disturbances. An unusual cause of vomiting in calves is dysphagia resulting from pharyngeal muscular dysfunction in which they may not be able to control regurgitated material. This may also be seen in calves with otitis media or interna. Inhalation pneumonia is a common sequela in calves so affected. Poisonous plants or toxins may cause vomiting in dairy cattle exposed to *Eupatorium rugosum*, *Hymenoxys* spp., *Andromeda* spp., *Oleander* spp., *Conium* spp., and other toxic plants. Legume forages contaminated with *Rhizoctonia* mold may cause excessive salivation in cattle, although this is much less common in cattle than in horses. Because of modern management systems, however, dairy cattle are infrequently exposed to plants causing vomition or salivation. Vomiting has also been reported in cattle with arsenic poisoning and other mechanical or chemical irritation to the reticulorumen mucosa, including ruminal acidosis.

Dairy cattle with severe parturient hypocalcemia may vomit as a result of increased intraruminal pressure and loss

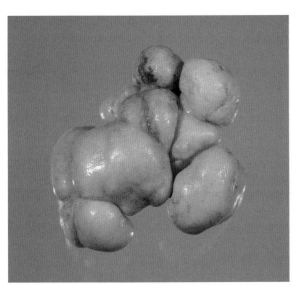

• **Fig. 5.38** Fibropapilloma removed from the reticulum adjacent to the cardia. This mass acted as a valve to interfere with eructation and create signs of vagal indigestion in a cow.

of smooth muscle tone. Due to their comatose state these animals are at greater risk for inhalation pneumonia compared with cattle that vomit because of other causes.

Passage of stomach tubes, especially large-diameter stomach tubes (4.0–5.0 cm in diameter), may stimulate vomiting in some dairy cattle. This may be caused by pharyngeal or reticular irritation or be associated with the cow's primary disease (e.g., hardware disease) that has prompted the clinician to pass a stomach tube in the first place. If this repeatedly occurs and the cow needs to be tubed for feeding, a smaller tube passed through the nasal cavity will usually permit feeding without regurgitation.

Forestomach Neoplasia

Fibropapillomas are relatively common in the distal esophagus, reticulum, or rumen of young dairy cattle (Fig. 5.38) but are seldom large enough or positioned so as to cause clinical problems. Large fibropapillomas located in the distal esophagus or cardia region may act as an impediment to eructation, thereby causing intermittent or chronic bloat. Bovine papillomaviruses (BPV-5, -1, and -2) usually are the cause of alimentary tract warts in cattle. These viruses cause fibropapillomata in the oral cavity, esophagus, and forestomach compartments. In some parts of the world, ingestion of carcinogens such as bracken fern may encourage malignant transformation of fibropapillomas to carcinomas or squamous cell carcinomas. Cattle affected with forestomach fibropapillomas are healthy otherwise and have normal appetites when not bloated. Rumenotomy offers the best means of diagnosis and surgical removal in such cases and has been performed successfully for fibropapillomas and fibromas. Seldom is the diagnosis suspected before rumenotomy, although endoscopy may be used to examine the distal esophagus in suspected cases. The papillomas are typically easy to remove, and one with

a thin stalk in the pharynx was removed by simply pinching the stalk.

The other major neoplasm of the forestomach compartments is lymphosarcoma. Although more commonly found in the abomasum, lymphosarcoma may form singular or multiple lesions in the wall of the forestomach compartments and associated lymph nodes. In these instances, forestomach dysfunction characterized by bloat or signs of vagal indigestion may appear. The diagnosis may be suspected if other target organs, peripheral lymph nodes, or visceral masses palpated per rectum are identified, and a definitive diagnosis reached by cytologic examination. Neoplastic cells are found in the peritoneal fluid of approximately 50% of cattle with abomasal lymphosarcoma, but it is unknown what the diagnostic utility of abdominocentesis is for forestomach masses. In most cases, however, the lesions can be identified on ultrasound examination (see Video Clip 5.3) or at the time of abdominal exploratory laparotomy. Treatment is rarely attempted. We have successfully used either isoflupredone or prednisone (alcohol base, 1 mg/kg IM daily) to improve clinical signs in late pregnant cattle such that the cow might survive long enough to deliver a term calf. Although this has been successful in a few cases, the owners should be informed that the calf will likely be infected with BLV, and depending on the stage of gestation and body condition of the dam at diagnosis, the calf may also have significant in utero growth retardation and be gestationally dysmature, even at term.

Rumen Fistulas as a Therapeutic Tool

Creation of rumen fistulas has been used as a surgical means of treatment for chronic or recurrent free-gas bloat in dairy cattle and calves. For this procedure to be most effective, definitive diagnosis of the primary cause of free-gas bloat should be made. Therefore, rumenotomy often precedes the rumen fistula procedure in cows. The cow or calf most likely to benefit from creation of a rumen fistula is one that is healthy and appetent whenever free-gas bloat is not present (failure of eructation). Thus, if passage of a stomach tube easily relieves free-gas bloat in the patient and returns the animal to a normal appearance and attitude, a rumen fistula may be considered a reasonable alternative to repeated passage of a stomach tube in cattle with chronic or recurrent free-gas bloat. It is not an effective procedure for chronic frothy bloat conditions, which are often caused by peritonitis, reflux of abomasal contents, or abomasal groove disorders.

Failure of eructation because of previous reticuloperitonitis, pharyngeal trauma, or other causes of apparent vagal indigestion may benefit from this procedure if rumenotomy excludes other causes and definitely identifies the rumen distension as primarily a free-gas type. Similarly, calves that have had severe bronchopneumonia and that subsequently develop chronic free-gas bloat, possibly from vagus nerve irritation or inflammation in the thorax, may benefit from this procedure if their pneumonia responds to antibiotic therapy. Rarely, no lesions are found by exploratory procedures and rumenotomy in chronically bloated patients, and rumen fistulas are fashioned in the hopes of "buying time" for the animal and avoiding frequent passage of a stomach tube to relieve the free-gas distension. Rumen fistulas have a high success rate in 2- to 6-month-old calves with idiopathic free-gas bloat.

Cattle with certain medical disorders also may benefit from the creation of a rumen fistula. The most common indications for this are pharyngeal trauma or lacerations and tetanus. In cases of pharyngeal trauma or lacerations, the animal usually has dysphagia, fever, and pharyngeal pain. The cow also may have forestomach dysfunction caused by injury to vagus nerve branches in the pharyngeal region. Therefore, ruminal dysfunction or failure of eructation sometimes occurs. If the clinical recovery time is expected to be prolonged or if chronic free-gas bloat develops in such a patient, the rumen fistula will allow feeding, watering, and an escape route for rumen gas during recuperation. This also avoids frequent passage of a stomach tube in a cow that already has a very painful pharynx. In patients with tetanus, free-gas bloat and inability to eat are common signs. Passage of a stomach tube to hydrate, feed, and debloat cows affected with tetanus is a painful and frightening experience for the animal. Therefore, creation of a rumen fistula after sedation and local anesthesia early in the course of the disease allows a nonstressful means to feed and water the patient and to prevent bloat. A complete surgical description is available in a recent surgery text (*Farm Animal Surgery*, edited by Drs. Fubini and Ducharme).

Diseases of the Abomasum

Abomasal Displacement

Abomasal displacements are the most commonly detected abdominal disorder and represent the most common reason for abdominal surgery in dairy cattle.

Etiology

Displacement may occur to the left (LDA) or to the right (RDA) side, but in the United States, most displacements are to the left. Peak occurrence for displaced abomasum (DA) is during the first 6 weeks of lactation, but they may occur sporadically at any stage of lactation or gestation. Bulls and calves of any age may also be affected with DA. DA in calves before weaning usually occurs as RDA, but after weaning, calves may experience displacement to either side. RDA has been observed in calves as young as 3 days of age.

Abomasal displacements in calves, bulls, heifers before calving, and dry cows may be chronic because of lack of suspicion of DA in these groups, as well as management factors that contribute to less careful observation when compared with milking cows. Although DAs occur most commonly in pluriparous cows, the condition is also common in first-calf heifers, and lactating cattle of any age may be affected. The

exact pathophysiology of DA is unknown. However, several factors may contribute to the development of DA:
1. Excessive production of volatile fatty acids caused by modern diets consisting of highly acidic feed materials such as corn silage, haylage, and fermentable grains such as high-moisture corn.
2. GI stasis caused by metabolic or infectious diseases such as hypocalcemia, hypokalemia (may be a predisposing factor but more commonly is a result of DA), ketosis, retained placenta, metritis, mastitis, and indigestion. These factors are extremely important in the early postparturient period when GI stasis with or without endotoxemia may be accompanied by abomasal stasis and gas production. These associated diseases also decrease the size of the rumen because of decreased appetite and may allow DA (especially LDA) to occur.
3. Twinning and dystocia appear to increase the risk for many periparturient disorders, including DA.
4. The deeper body capacity that has been selected for in modern dairy cows may allow more room in the abdomen for movement of the abomasum. Some lines of cattle and families of dairy cattle appear to have a higher incidence of DA than others. This has been especially apparent since embryo transfer was popularized.

A combination of these factors may be involved in any one case, but when a high incidence of DA occurs in a herd, investigation of the feeding regimen and management is in order. Several elements of dairy cow management including nutrition and housing are important in controlling incidence of ketosis and DA. Intensive detection of subclinical ketosis followed by treatment with propylene glycol has been shown to decrease the risk of DA and ketosis. Providing ruminal buffers, prefeeding hay before fermentable feeds, and use of TMR may all help decrease frequency in herds with a previously high incidence of DA. Similarly, herds with a high incidence of postparturient metritis may benefit from a cleaner calving environment, evaluation of selenium status, and dry cow nutritional analysis. Management procedures that create undue stress or diet changes during the periparturient period have been shown to contribute to DA. Lastly, through a full evaluation of breeding and calving programs, the incidence of twinning and dystocias should be minimized.

Clinical Signs

Dairy cattle that develop simple LDA or RDA generally lose their appetite for high-energy feeds and show a decrease of 30% to 50% in milk production. Therefore, the initial chief complaint from the owner is "off feed and down on milk." With the more widespread use of ruminating monitors, it may be noted that a decline in time ruminating might occur 1 to 3 days before the onset of a ping, allowing a more aggressive diagnostic approach (increased number of and more extensive examinations potentially including ultrasonography) searching for the DA. Inspection of the cow with a "simple" DA may merely reveal an animal with a dull appearance and mild dehydration. Temperature, pulse and

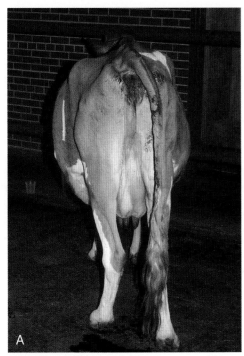

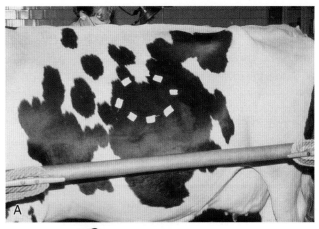

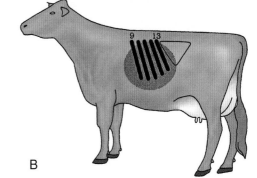

• **Fig. 5.40** **A** and **B**, Typical area of tympanic resonance indicative of a left displacement of the abomasum.

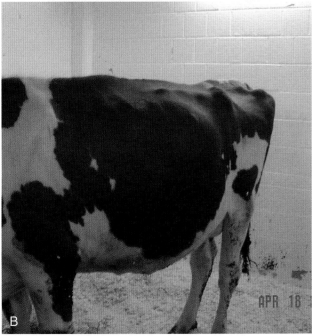

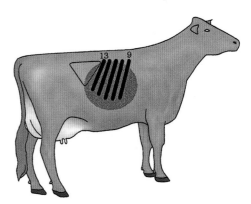

• **Fig. 5.41** Typical area of tympanic resonance indicative of a right displacement of the abomasum.

• **Fig. 5.39** **A**, "Sprung" rib cage caused by left displacement of the abomasum (LDA) in a Guernsey cow. **B**, An even more dramatic "sprung" rib cage caused by an LDA. The abomasum of this cow could be palpated rectally.

respiratory rates are normal. Rumen contractions are present and moderate in strength but may not be externally visible. A "sprung" rib cage (Fig. 5.39) may be present on the side of the displacement as the cow is inspected from the rear. This may be easier to appreciate with LDA because the rumen is no longer palpable in the left paralumbar fossa as the DA pushes the rumen to the right and balloons under the left rib cage. Simultaneous auscultation and percussion will reveal an area of high-pitched tympanic resonance (ping) under the rib cage on the left or right side, corresponding to the location of the DA. Usually this ping lies on a line from the tuber coxae to the elbow but may be of varying size. The ping should extend cranially at least to the ninth rib and often to the eighth rib (Figs. 5.40 and 5.41). (This requirement is especially important for RDA because proximal colon distension, displaced omasum, and cecal gaseous distension may be confused with RDA.) Differentiation of right-sided pings is discussed further in upcoming sections. Ballottement coupled with auscultation will confirm the presence of a large fluid-filled viscus under the rib cage, because a fluid wave creates a splashing sound with this technique (most dramatic with RDAs). Some LDAs have minimal succussible fluid. A large DA may be visible as a quarter-moon or half-moon distended viscus appearing caudal to the 13th rib in the paralumbar fossa when viewed from the side (Figs. 5.39, *B* and 5.42). In most cases, rectal palpation of simple DAs will not be possible; however, volvulus of the abomasum is often palpable per rectum. In extremely large LDAs or RDAs, it may be possible to just palpate the greater curvature of the abomasum, but this is not typical.

Although most DAs conform to the aforementioned anatomic ping location, variants do occur and deserve mention. The typical location of LDA in calves is caudal to the rib cage and extends dorsally into the paralumbar fossa (Fig. 5.43). The chief complaint for calves with LDA is chronic or intermittent bloat. The ping and fluid present in the LDA in a calf are easily missed if the examiner confines "pinging" and ballottement to the area of the left rib cage. Rarely, LDAs in adult cattle are also identified in this location (Fig. 5.44, *A*). Additionally, LDA and rumen pings may coexist, causing more rostral location of the LDA and adding some confusion to the diagnosis (Fig. 5.44, *B*). Rumen pings should not extend as ventral as the ping of an LDA and will not have the fluid succussion nor high-pitched resonance of a typical LDA. Presence or absence of auscultable

or palpable rumen contractions can be helpful in differentiating between a confusing rumen or LDA ping; if rumen contractions are present, strong, and palpable, then the ping is less likely to be a rumen ping. If the ping is relatively large and the rumen is against the body wall (based on rectal and external palpation), these findings would be more supportive of a ruminal ping rather than an LDA.

Other uncommon locations for LDA include; (1) caudal to the left elbow in the area of the ruminoreticular junction, which might indicate the omentum is torn; (2) dorsal to the rumen in cattle with an empty rumen or rumen collapse; or (3) in the lower (ventral) left side of the abdomen (in adult cattle, any ping heard low on the left side of the abdomen should be considered to be a LDA). Because of this variety in location, examiners should keep an open mind regarding clinical variations and ping over the entire left abdomen during the physical examination before ruling out LDA. It should be remembered that some LDAs do not ping consistently (the old "truck ride and no ping" phenomenon), and a ping may not be found at all in LDAs with concurrent rupture of an ulcer (often chronic displacements) or when the abomasum is trapped in a very unusual position such as between the rumen and the uterus in cows with twins or cranial and dorsal to the reticulum; this last position has been confirmed only once by Dr. N.G. Ducharme and Dr. T. Divers after a

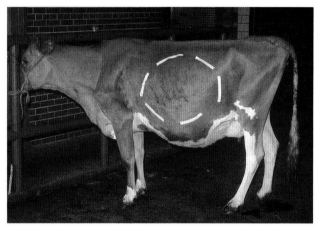

• **Fig. 5.42** Large left displacement of the abomasum extending into the paralumbar fossa caudal to the 13th rib.

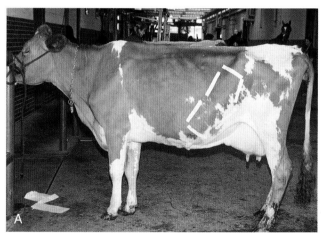

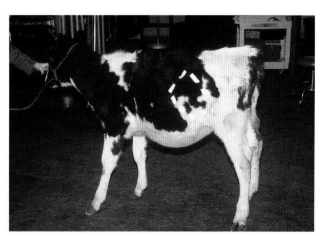

• **Fig. 5.43** Typical location of a ping in a calf with a left abomasal displacement.

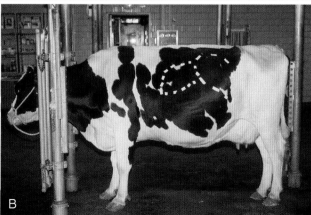

• **Fig. 5.44** **A,** Guernsey cow with left displacement of the abomasum in caudal location. **B,** Coexisting left displaced abomasum and ruminal gas in a cow.

radiographic finding of a gas-distended viscus in this area of a cow with intermittent anorexia. No tell-tale ping was present on either side of the abdomen in this animal.

Signs of fever and pneumoperitoneum in a cow with LDA should alert the clinician to the possibility of abomasal perforation in addition to the displacement. Such cattle are found to have the abomasum adherent to the parietal peritoneum adjacent to the ulceration. A guarded prognosis must be offered, and surgical repair is best attempted from the ventral right paramedian approach.

Urinary ketones frequently are positive in cattle with DA. This ketosis may be the primary cause of a depressed appetite and rumen motility predisposing to DA or secondary in a patient with DA that refuses high-energy feeds while continuing to produce milk. The strength of the urine ketone reaction may have some weak diagnostic utility in distinguishing between primary and secondary ketosis in cows with DAs, with strong reactions more likely an indication of primary ketosis.

Concurrent diseases such as metritis, mastitis, pneumonia, pyelonephritis, hypocalcemia, and musculoskeletal problems should be identified by completion of a thorough physical examination and treated appropriately. Although the diagnosis of a DA is rather straightforward, ultrasound examination to identify the location of the abomasum can be used to confirm or rule out a DA. With LDA, the abomasum is seen between the left abdominal wall and the rumen. It contains a rather homogeneous fluid with ingesta ventrally and a variably sized gas cap dorsally. The abomasal folds can often be seen in the fluid and ingesta image. In cattle with RDA the liver is displaced medially from the right abdominal wall by the abomasum, and the abomasum has an ultrasonographic appearance similar to that described for an LDA.

After a DA has been diagnosed, the value of the cow should be determined in light of past and present productivity, associated diseases, and genetic potential. If the cow's value dictates therapy, medical and surgical treatment should be planned to correct the DA. There are very few situations in which at least some treatment of an LDA will not automatically occur after diagnosis; the low likelihood of a poor outcome and the relatively low cost and simplicity of treatment typically prevail in decision making. However, with large RDAs and particularly with AV, there is a greater relevance to pragmatic discussion about outcome with the client, especially in a grade cow. Presurgical evaluation of such patients is appropriate with regard to prognosis; this is discussed in a later section.

Clinical Pathology

Cattle affected with DA without other concurrent diseases have a characteristic hypochloremic, hypokalemic metabolic alkalosis. With simple DA, metabolic alkalosis is mild to moderate and seldom requires intensive electrolyte correction. In chronic DA or in cattle with DA and associated diseases contributing to more drastic anorexia, acid–base and electrolyte disorders may require more vigorous therapeutic efforts. Table 5.2 shows normal values and approximate ranges of acid–base and electrolyte abnormalities in DA patients. Abdominal paracentesis is indicated if concurrent ulceration and displacement are suspected.

When laboratory tests are available and indicated, acid–base and electrolyte values constitute the most meaningful data for affected cattle that appear to be excessively dehydrated or weak or have chronic histories. Cattle that are severely ketotic and therefore ketoacidotic may occasionally have a blood pH in the acid range, a high anion gap, and a lower bicarbonate value than expected in cattle with simple DA. Assessment of urinary ketones always is indicated for cattle with DA and may help explain unexpected variations from the anticipated metabolic alkalosis found in most cattle with simple DA.

TABLE 5.2	Approximate Acid–Base and Electrolyte Status of Cattle with Displaced Abomasum (DA) and Abomasal Volvulus (AV)				
	pH	Cl⁻ mEq/L	K⁺ mEq/L	HCO₃⁻ mEq/L	Base Excess
Normal venous blood	7.35–7.50	97–111	3.7–4.9	20–30	-2.5–+2.5
Typical left DA	7.45–7.55	85–95	3.5–4.5	25–35	0–10
Typical right DA	7.45–7.60	85–95	3.0–4.0	30–40	5–15
Large right DA	7.45–7.60	80–90	3.0–3.5	35–45	5–20
Typical AV	7.45–7.60	75–90	2.5–3.5	35–50	10–25
Advanced AV	7.45–7.65	60–80	2.0–3.5	35–55	10–35
Very advanced AV with abomasal necrosis*	7.30–7.45	85–95	3.0–4.5	15–25	-10–0
Typical LDA with severe ketosis†	7.15–7.30	85–95	3.5–4.5	15–30	-10–0

*These cattle have very large AV and clinically severe dehydration, high heart rate, and weakness, and may appear to be in shock. Therefore, the acid–base and electrolyte status seems inconsistent. In fact, tissue necrosis and shock have superimposed metabolic acidosis on the preexisting metabolic alkalosis of typical or advanced AV.
†These cows do not appear to have serious abomasal problems and are not greatly dehydrated or weak. The acid–base status seems to contradict the anticipated metabolic alkalosis typical of a left displacement of the abomasum (LDA) but can be explained by the severe ketoacidosis that affected the venous pH, anion gap, and so forth. The cows may be so ketoacidotic that nervous ketosis should be anticipated.

Paradoxic aciduria has been described as a consequence to prolonged or severe metabolic alkalosis associated with DA. This probably relates to hypochloremia, causing decreased passive sodium reabsorption in the proximal tubule along with dehydration, resulting in increased sodium and water reabsorption in the distal nephron, and most importantly, potassium depletion to such a degree that hydrogen ions must be excreted in the urine (to offset the increased sodium resorption) instead of potassium. Although interesting as a physiologic event, it does not change fluid and electrolyte therapy in our hospital because we always assume cows with DA have whole-body potassium deficits except in rare cases of oliguric renal failure.

Medical Treatment

In simple DA, economic factors, concurrent diseases, or veterinary and management time constraints may temporarily or permanently rule against surgical correction and dictate medical therapy. Although not as successful as surgery, medical therapy may be attempted in simple LDAs. We recommend surgery for the correction of RDA but in circumstances where economics or owner and veterinary uncertainty exist then the following medical treatment would worth trying for a possible RDA too. Medical therapy usually includes oral laxatives, ruminotorics, antacids, or cholinergic medications designed to stimulate GI motility and encourage evacuation of the GI tract. Calcium solutions should be administered SC or IV (slowly) if the patient is judged to be hypocalcemic. Potassium chloride (2–4 oz twice daily) may be administered orally in gelatin capsules, added to drinking water, or added to water administered by stomach tube. Some practitioners recommend the use of 0.5 to 1 lb of coffee mixed with warm water and administered via stomach tube. Although rarely performed anymore, "rolling" can be performed in addition to the medical treatment for simple LDA (but never for RDA or AV).

The cow may be cast onto either side and then rolled into dorsal recumbency with the help of two or three people. We advocate rolling the cow preferentially onto the right side first from sternal and then rolling her in a clockwise fashion (as viewed from behind) into dorsal. The cow is rocked gently from side to side while in dorsal recumbency and maintained in this position for 2 to 5 minutes. During this time, the LDA should float or "balloon" to the ventral midline, returning to a normal position. The longer the cow remains on her back, the more gas and sequestered fluid will escape the distended organ. The cow is then rolled down on the left side so that the rumen is always in contact with the left parietal peritoneum; this prevents immediate recurrence of the LDA. The cow is then forced to stand immediately. This procedure should *never* be performed on cattle with simple RDA because this may predispose to AV. We would also caution against this approach in the rare case of a heavily pregnant cow with LDA.

After medical therapy alone or medical therapy, including rolling, the cow should be encouraged to eat as much hay as possible to fill the rumen with roughage. This may act as a physical deterrent to recurrence of LDA, as well as to encourage ruminal and GI motility in the case of either

LDA or RDA. Highly acidic feed components should be added to the diet only gradually until full intake resumes. If concurrent diseases exist (e.g., metritis, mastitis, or ketosis), they must be treated at the same time, or the likely success of medical treatment for the DA is severely compromised.

In one study performed in our practice, 30 of 100 cattle with simple LDA remained corrected for an entire lactation after one or two medical treatments that involved rolling and symptomatic medications. Although this study is not highly significant or highly successful, it illustrates the fact that medical therapy may hold some value when surgery is not deemed possible, practical or economic.

The clinician must remember that after a diagnosis is made and correction of DA has occurred, the GI tract has mechanically and functionally returned to normal. Therefore, oral fluids and electrolytes usually suffice for correction of acid–base, electrolyte, and hydration abnormalities in cattle with simple DA. Potassium chloride may be administered in drinking water, through a stomach tube, or in gelatin capsules to help correct existing or suspected electrolyte abnormalities. It is common practice to administer 2 to 4 oz of potassium chloride orally, twice daily, to cattle formerly affected by DA, after correction. Cattle that are weak should be suspected of having hypokalemia (<3.0 mEq/L) and may require more intensive IV fluid therapy and potassium supplementation, although increased urine production from rapidly administered IV fluids may enhance potassium losses. When supplementing potassium chloride, 1.0 g yields approximately 14 mEq.

To illustrate, assume a cow has severe metritis, LDA, inappetence, and weakness to such a degree that manual assistance by tail lifting is required to help her to rise. Hypokalemia should be suspected to be part of the reason for her weakness. Subsequent plasma electrolyte analysis determines $Cl^- = 85$ mEq/L and $K^+ = 2.5$ mEq/L. The cow weighs 600 kg (1320 lb). Consider that plasma potassium ideally should be increased to 4.5 mEq/L. Therefore, the cow needs a minimum of 2.0 mEq of potassium per liter of extracellular fluid (ECF) to be corrected. This cow would need 360 mEq (25 g) of potassium chloride to return extracellular levels to 4.5 mEq/L (using 30% of body weight as the conversion factor for total body ECF). With IV administration, the potassium chloride should be delivered at a concentration of 40 mEq/L in crystalloids. However, 98% of the body K^+ is intracellular, and plasma concentrations may poorly reflect total-body needs. It has been estimated that for every 1 mEq/L decrease in plasma K^+ from normal, there is a 10% decline in total body K^+. For a 500-kg cow, this would equate to 2500 mEq, or nearly 175 g (6 oz) of K^+. Therefore, a more practical, safer and more efficient way to replace K^+ is via oral supplementation. Potassium chloride may be given in gelatin capsules added to drinking water or administered via balling gun or rumen gavage. Using the oral route, 2 to 4 oz (1 oz = 420 mEq) of potassium chloride is administered, once or twice daily, after repair of the LDA and treatment of metritis until the cow regains strength and appetite.

Occasionally, cows with hypokalemia fail to respond to potassium supplementation or saline-based fluids and develop progressively worsening hypokalemia despite intensive attempts to provide potassium. These cattle become weaker and often recumbent and may show neurologic signs when serum potassium is less than 2.0 mEq/L. Affected cattle that do not respond to potassium supplementation and have low serum potassium values despite resolution of hypochloremia and alkalosis are frequently cows that have been treated aggressively for ketosis with glucose and corticosteroids, particularly extralabel doses of isoflupredone. Cattle that have potassium values less than 2.5 mEq/L should be considered critical patients, and intensive potassium supplementation should be provided orally (sometimes up to 1 lb), 80 mEq/L slowly IV, or both. A specific predisposing factor to the development of severe hypokalemia and recumbency has been the repeated use of the drug isoflupredone acetate; however, not all cases appear to be associated with the administration of this combined mineralocorticoid–glucocorticoid drug. Some cases are associated with repeated treatments of dexamethasone. A more detailed discussion on severe hypokalemia can be found in Chapter 15.

Surgical Correction

This discussion addresses available surgical options for simple DA. Individual training and experience of the veterinarian will dictate which surgical procedure will be chosen. Other factors, including concurrent disease, stage of gestation, and economic value of the animal, may further alter the decision as to the surgical procedure pursued. Advantages and disadvantages of each procedure will be discussed.

Right paramedian abomasopexy allows the best access to the abomasum and allows it to be inspected completely and relocated to the correct anatomic position. In a cow with fever, pneumoperitoneum, and LDA, this procedure will allow access to the greater curvature and the ability to oversew an ulcer, if present. If performed properly, abomasopexy should result in a permanent adhesion of abomasum to parietal peritoneum. Nonabsorbable sutures are recommended for the abomasopexy procedure to ensure permanent adhesion formation.

Disadvantages of abomasopexy include the additional labor necessary to roll and restrain the affected cow in dorsal recumbency, the risk of incisional hernia or fistula formation, incisional infection resulting from contamination of the incision site, regurgitation during recumbency, and concern about ventral parturient edema and superficial abdominal vessels associated with the mammary circulation in cattle with large udders. The procedure is also contraindicated in cattle concurrently affected with acute or chronic bronchopneumonia or certain musculoskeletal injuries, and in late gestation cows. In one study, cows that had DAs corrected with the paramedian approach did not lie down as much and had higher heart rates than cows with DAs corrected by the standing right flank approach, suggesting that paramedian surgery causes more postoperative pain. Despite the list of disadvantages, this procedure has been used successfully in thousands of cattle and is the procedure of choice for valuable cattle because

it minimizes the risk of future DA and ensures correct anatomic relocation of the organ. Attention to presurgical preparation and surgical detail minimizes the chance of incisional problems after abomasopexy.

Right flank omentopexy is a standing procedure that is favored by many clinicians for surgical correction of simple LDA or RDA. It can be performed with minimal assistance, allows manual reposition of the abomasum, and has few incisional risks. As in any procedure done with the animal standing, minimal risk of regurgitation exists so that there is no fear of operating on a DA cow with concurrent problems such as pneumonia or musculoskeletal disorders that may be worsened during dorsal recumbency. Among the disadvantages are that the entire abomasum frequently is not available for inspection, the repositioning is relative rather than absolute, the integrity of the omentopexy may be affected by tears in the omentum of excessively fat cows, and future RDA is possible despite an intact omentopexy. Preexistent adhesions to the ventrolateral body wall, subsequent to ulceration, and significant sand ingestion weighing down the body of the abomasum can be occasional hurdles to the successful completion of an omentopexy. In the rare instance of LDA in a heavily pregnant cow, left or right flank approaches may be considered, or alternatively, it may even be worth considering performing a bilateral approach with two surgeons to more simply and quickly pass the deflated abomasum ventrally under the rumen and gravid uterus before performing a right-sided omentopexy or pyloropexy.

In right flank pyloropexy, the surgeon incorporates a small portion of the seromuscular part of the pylorus of the abomasum into the closure of the right flank incision, creating a direct fixation of the viscus. This has the advantage of not relying totally on the fatty omentum for stabilization. However, it is important not to go too close to the pylorus because this is the narrowest part of the abomasum. Furthermore, this is only recommended if there is not excessive tension on the pylorus. As with any abdominal surgery, a potential complication from a right sided omentopexy or pyloropexy is infection at the surgical site. Such infections can generally be successfully managed by drainage, flushing the infected area with disinfectants and systemic antibiotic treatment. On rare occasion infection spreads between the body wall and peritoneum but the incision site itself appears normal. This condition is described in more detail at the end of this chapter.

Left flank abomasopexy is used by some surgeons to correct LDA. It has the advantages of a standing procedure as listed earlier and incorporates an abomasopexy through a continuous suture placed in the greater curvature of the LDA. The suture is placed such that each end of the nonabsorbable suture is left long and can be attached to a large needle. These two needles then are directed through the right paramedian ventral abdominal wall in the desired location. The abomasum is repositioned by the surgeon, and the long suture ends are tied by an assistant to the outside of the body wall. Disadvantages include the possibility of exogenous infection following the sutures into the peritoneal cavity, malposition

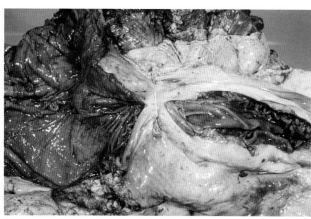

• **Fig. 5.45** Blind stitch complication. The suture has completely obstructed the abomasum at the pylorus, resulting in the cow's death.

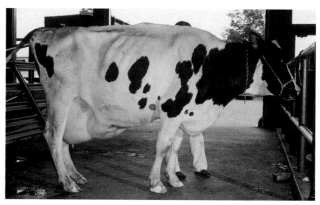

• **Fig. 5.46** Phlebitis of the right mammary vein after blind-stitch abomasopexy. This cow died because of endocarditis secondary to this phlebitis.

of the organ or sutures based on limited accessibility of the abomasum via the left flank in some cattle with LDA, and failure of the abomasopexy if the abomasum is not tightly apposed to the parietal peritoneum or if the sutures break. Care must be taken to avoid iatrogenic damage to branches of the superficial mammary vein when needles are passed through the paramedian part of the body wall to the outside when performing this procedure alone. A word of caution with this approach; in particularly large multiparous dairy cows it can be almost impossible to reach the right paramedian position from a left flank incision. A mirror-image procedure through the right flank has been recommended by some practitioners for correction of RDA in cattle.

Blind tack abomasopexy and toggle-pin abomasopexy have been applied by practitioners when economics dictate an inexpensive and quick alternative to more definitive surgical procedures in cattle affected with LDA. The cow is cast and rolled into dorsal recumbency as described before, and the gas-distended abomasum located by simultaneous auscultation and percussion in the right paramedian area. In the blind tack procedure, after minimal preparation of the surgical site, a large half-circle upholstery needle attached to nonabsorbable suture is driven through the abdominal wall into the abomasal lumen and back out the abdominal wall. The suture is then tied. One or more sutures are placed in this fashion.

The toggle-pin procedure is similar in that two separate toggle pins attached to sutures are placed through a sharp cannula driven into the abomasal lumen. The ends of the sutures then are tied together. Proponents of this technique cite the advantage of being able to obtain abomasal contents through the cannula to confirm the low pH fluid as abomasal rather than ruminal in origin. This is rarely done; however, as it is possible to smell the characteristic odor of abomasal gas through the cannula for confirmation. Advantages are speed and low cost. Disadvantages are innumerable but include missing the abomasum, obstructing the abomasal body or pyloric region with an encircling suture (Fig. 5.45), suturing the abomasum in a malposition, allowing leakage from the abomasal lumen into the peritoneal cavity, puncturing the wrong organ, phlebitis from injury to the mammary vein (Fig. 5.46), and risking peritonitis via

endogenous (abomasal contents) or exogenous (skin, hair, environment) contamination of the peritoneal cavity.

Severe complications have been documented subsequent to blind tack and toggle-pin procedures. We continue to see cattle referred because of complications such as toggle pins placed in the cecum, proximal colon, and rumen. Many of these complications have fatal outcomes even after referral and exploratory laparotomy in an often-futile attempt to correct the problem. Therefore, these procedures cannot be recommended for valuable dairy cows.

In defense of these procedures, in the hands of an experienced practitioner, they can be a very cost-effective and labor-saving option in grade cattle. Complications of the toggle-pin procedure can be lessened by prompt identification of a problem in the immediate days after the abomasopexy, promptly removing the suture or toggle if a problem is noticed in the day or two after the procedure, and making sure that the toggle sutures are not left in place too long (>10–14 days). Cows with simple LDA will show a marked increase in appetite and production in the 48 to 72 hours after the procedure; however, cattle with iatrogenic malpositioning of the abomasum, penetration of another viscus, or significant peritonitis usually appear worse over this time period. At the very least, releasing the sutures and, at best, exploring the cow at this time may be indicated, but economics frequently dictate that conservative medical treatment is the chosen approach. Cattle that require an exploratory for toggle complications generally have a guarded to poor outcome.

A few veterinary teaching hospitals use laparoscopic repair of LDAs, but this technique is not common practice. It is described in the *Farm Animal Surgery* text by Fubini and Ducharme.

Regardless of the procedure used, a short course of treatment with NSAIDs and antibiotics may hasten the recovery of the cow.

Abomasal Volvulus After Right Displacement of the Abomasum

Abomasal volvulus or right-sided volvulus of the abomasum is a serious, life-threatening condition in dairy cattle and is characterized by moderate to severe dehydration, hypochloremic, hypokalemic alkalosis, and mechanical obstruction of abomasal outflow.

Etiology

Although it develops after RDA, the incidence of AV after RDA is not known. Certainly, it does not follow in all cases of RDA, because many cattle can be affected with RDA for days or even weeks without the complication of AV. Although the gas and fluid distension present in neglected RDA probably predispose to volvulus of the organ, it remains that many cattle with AV have acute (24- to 48-hour) histories of illness and most likely have not had long-standing RDA before AV.

Abomasal volvulus may occur in cattle of any age or either sex. Most adult dairy cows with AV develop the disorder during the 6 weeks after calving, similar to the peak occurrence of DA. Young calves (preweaning) that are affected with RDA frequently develop AV with marked bilateral abdominal distension and unfortunately sometimes are erroneously diagnosed with ruminal bloat. The exact mechanism and direction of AV have been debated, but anatomic dissection studies confirm rotation around the lesser curvature that involves the abomasum, omasum, and reticulum. The resultant malposition places the omasum medial to the abomasum and the reticulum caudal to the omasum and medial to the abomasum.

Clinical Signs

Cattle affected with AV usually appear much more depressed, dehydrated, and anxious than cattle with simple DA. Appetite and milk production decrease acutely and dramatically after development of AV. Physical examination reveals normal temperature, a heart rate that varies from bradycardia (<60 beats/min) to as high as 110 beats/min, normal or reduced (caused by severe alkalosis) respiratory rate, cool peripheral parts, an anxious expression (Fig. 5.47), and dehydration (Fig. 5.48). Frequently, the distended abomasum appears as right-sided abdominal distension or a "sprung rib cage" as viewed from the rear of the cow (Fig. 5.49). The AV may be so large as to extend caudally behind the 13th rib, causing an obvious quarter-moon or half-moon distension that is visible and palpable in the right paralumbar fossa. Simultaneous auscultation and percussion will produce a large area of tympanic resonance under the right rib cage. The area of "ping" usually extends cranially to the 9th or 8th rib and caudally to the 13th rib or into the paralumbar fossa as discussed previously (Figs. 5.50 to 5.52) and may be larger than the ping associated with a simple RDA (Fig. 5.53). Combined ballottement and auscultation will confirm a large fluid wave within the AV on the right side. Rarely, the ping includes the entire paralumbar fossa or an extreme cranial location (Fig. 5.54), and this may indicate omental tearing with loosening of the abomasum from its attachments. Cecal dilatation, distension of the spiral colon, or pneumorectum or pneumoperitoneum may occur simultaneously with RDA, causing some confusion in the interpretation of the "pings" (Fig. 5.55).

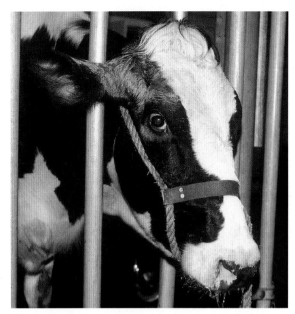

• **Fig. 5.47** Anxious expression in a cow with abomasal volvulus.

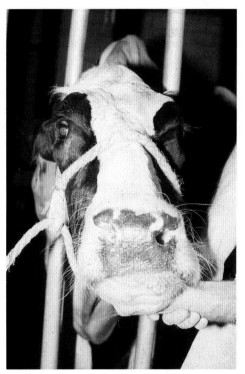

• **Fig. 5.48** Severe dehydration (sunken eyes) in a Holstein cow with abomasal volvulus.

In some cattle, it is difficult to differentiate RDA from early AV based on the physical examination! So often have we diagnosed right DA pre-operatively only to find a volvulus during surgery and vice versa. In general, cattle with AV are moderately to severely dehydrated, often with sunken eyes; have cool extremities; and appear more anxious than cattle with simple RDA. In addition, the examiner is more likely to palpate the distended abomasum per rectum in AV than in RDA. If the abomasum can be palpated per rectum in AV, the distended greater curvature can be felt lying against the right flank area at arm's length. The greater omentum is palpable

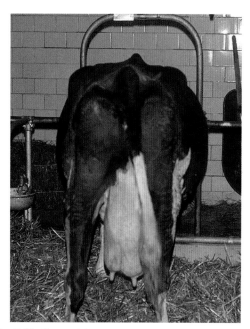

• **Fig. 5.49** "Sprung" rib cage in a cow with abomasal volvulus.

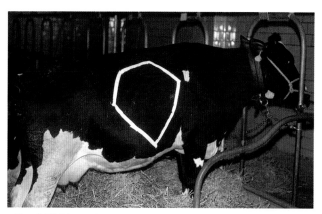

• **Fig. 5.50** Tympanic area resulting from abomasal volvulus in a Holstein cow.

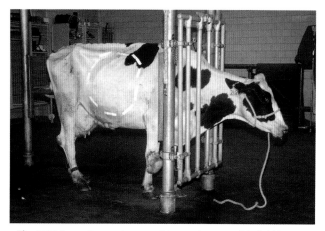

• **Fig. 5.51** Large tympanic area of gas and succussible fluid in a cow with an abomasal volvulus.

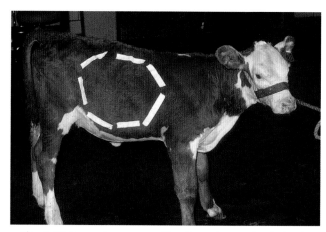

• **Fig. 5.52** Tympanic area resulting from abomasal volvulus in a 4-week-old Hereford calf.

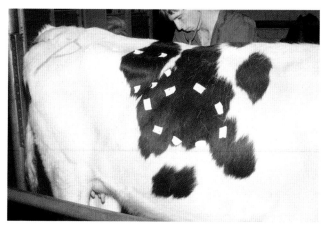

• **Fig. 5.53** Typical areas of ping in a cow with both a right abomasal displacement and pneumorectum (more caudal and dorsal tape).

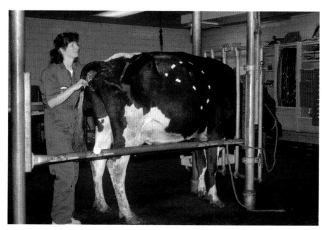

• **Fig. 5.54** Marked cranial location of ping from a right displaced abomasum and omental tear.

covering the organ in most instances, and this seems to help differentiate it from a distended cecum or proximal colon.

Furthermore, it is difficult on rectal examination to get one's hand and arm between the abomasum and lateral body wall with an RDA or AV. With cecal distension, the examiner can usually palpate both the medial and lateral surface of the distended viscus, and it is more easily reached due to its more caudal location.

Slow, extremely shallow respirations occasionally are observed in cattle affected with AV. This physical sign often signals severe metabolic alkalosis with respiratory

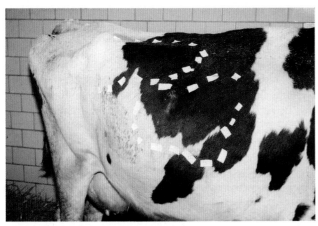

• **Fig. 5.55** Holstein cow with abomasal volvulus and cecal dilatation. Only by rectal examination could the more caudal-dorsal ping be determined to be cecal dilatation instead of pneumorectum, pneumoperitoneum, or gas in the descending colon.

compensation as the animal attempts to retain carbon dioxide through decreased respiratory effort. Bloat also is observed in some cattle affected with AV and is probably secondary to either the true mechanical outflow disturbance created by the abnormal positioning of the abomasum and pylorus or ileus caused by hypocalcemia.

Clinical Pathology

Cattle affected with AV typically have hemoconcentration and moderate to severe hypochloremic, hypokalemic, metabolic alkalosis. Serum chloride concentrations range from 80 to 90 mEq/L in early cases to 65 to 80 mEq/L in neglected or severe cases. Plasma chloride values and base excess show a roughly direct correlation with the clinical prognosis in most cases. In extremely advanced AV, however, devitalization of the affected organs, shock, and lactic acidosis produce metabolic acidosis that overwhelms the previous metabolic alkalosis, masking the laboratory severity of the metabolic disorder! Therefore, a cow with a large AV, severe dehydration, cool peripheral parts, AV palpable per rectum, and weakness but having measured acid–base and electrolyte values in the normal or metabolic acidosis range likely has a grave prognosis. Marked elevation in plasma L-lactate could indicate poor systemic or abomasal perfusion. It has been reported that AV cows with L-lactate levels greater than 6 mmol/L have a poor prognosis and treatment may not be warranted. This decision should not be based solely on a single point of care test because the value of the cow must be considered along with experience that some cows with L-lactate levels greater than 6 mmol/L have a good outcome. Measurement of L-lactate can be performed stall-side within 2 to 3 minutes. If metabolic acidosis is present but hypochloremia and hypokalemia also are present, the possibility of severe ketoacidosis should also be investigated and the prognosis adjusted accordingly. Respiratory acidosis is often present because of respiratory compensation (hypoventilation) for metabolic alkalosis or severe abdominal distension, which may compromise the depth of respiration. Examples of anticipated or approximate acid–base and electrolyte values are provided in Table 5.2.

Although many publications have detailed statistical correlations of prognosis for cattle with AV based on acid–base and electrolyte, anion gap or lactate values, clinicians must not fail to look at the patient and integrate the clinical examination findings when offering a prognosis. A cow should never be denied surgical repair based only on laboratory values if her physical parameters are fair to good. In general, whereas the prognosis varies directly with chloride levels and hydration status, it varies inversely with preoperative heart rate, duration of AV, plasma lactate, and anion gap. If the cow has metabolic acidosis and is recumbent, the prognosis is extremely grave.

Although ketosis and hypocalcemia may be present and require treatment in those with AV, they usually are overshadowed by acid–base and electrolyte abnormalities. Serum sorbitol dehydrogenase (SDH) or glutamate dehydrogenase (GLDH) elevations in cows with LDA could suggest hepatic lipidosis, but with AV, such elevations may be the result of systemic hypotension or an inflammatory response. CBC and peritoneal fluid analysis are rarely helpful in cattle affected with AV unless the condition is advanced to a point at which tissue necrosis, transudation, or exudation create a left shift in the hemogram and elevated white blood cell numbers and protein in the peritoneal fluid.

Treatment

The most important treatment for AV is early recognition and correction. AV, as opposed to simple LDA or possibly RDA, is a progressive disorder, and the eventual outcome is dictated largely by the duration and nature of volvulus. Early suspicion by the owner with subsequent early diagnosis and surgical correction by a veterinarian provides a favorable prognosis in most instances. Cattle affected with AV for longer than 24 hours probably have a less than 50% survival rate after surgical correction, and cattle affected longer than 48 hours generally have an extremely poor prognosis. These guidelines must be coupled with the physical examination findings because it is possible that a cow could have had an RDA for 24 to 36 hours and have developed AV in the 12 hours before diagnosis, thus making the prognosis less severe.

Treatment consists of surgical correction of the volvulus and medical correction of dehydration and electrolyte and acid–base disturbances. Surgical treatment consists of either right flank omentopexy or right paramedian abomasopexy, depending on the preference and judgment of the surgeon. Other surgical approaches are contraindicated because they offer no direct means of access to the affected abomasum, omasum, and reticulum. The surgeon will encounter the omasum lying medial to the abomasum and the reticulum caudal to its normal location because of volvulus involving the lesser curvature of the abomasum, omasum, and reticulum. The right flank approach is less stressful, less likely to cause regurgitation, allows direct access to the volvulus for abomasotomy to drain gas and fluid if necessary, allows easier anatomic realignment of omasum and abomasum, and can be done with less help. The major advantage of right paramedian abomasopexy is exact relocation of the abomasum once correction of the volvulus is completed. This helps ensure that the greatly distended abomasum and pylorus will remain well positioned postoperatively as opposed to the right flank omentopexy, after which a greatly distended abomasum may tend to remain slightly displaced to the right. Abomasopexy is arguably more difficult for an inexperienced surgeon in AV cases because of the anatomic challenges and because it may allow regurgitation in patients with severe ruminal and abomasal distension. In either approach, manipulation of the omasum can be helpful when correcting the volvulus. The omasum is lifted or pushed dorsally and laterally in an attempt to reposition both the omasum and abomasum.

Replacement of the abomasum is facilitated by removal of the gaseous distension via suction. In those with severe AV and more than 10 L of fluid present, abomasotomy (pursestring a stomach tube into the viscus) to relieve fluid distension may be necessary and is more easily accomplished through a right flank surgical approach. Rehydration and correction of acid–base or electrolyte deficits may be performed postoperatively in early cases, but it may be necessary to address some of these needs preoperatively in severe cases, lest hypokalemia and hypotension progress to diffuse muscular weakness. In early cases or cattle with AV that have mild dehydration, oral fluids (20–40 L of water) and potassium chloride supplementation (30–120 g orally, twice daily) suffice for medical needs postoperatively, because the GI tract has been realigned and should have normal absorptive capacity. With moderate to severe dehydration and metabolic alkalosis, 1 to 2 L of IV hypertonic saline or 20 to 60 L of IV physiologic saline with 40 mEq/L of potassium chloride may be necessary to correct existing deficits. From a practical standpoint, oral administration can be used after the AV is surgically corrected, except in extremely severe cases in which ileus of the forestomach compartments persists postoperatively. Oral fluids are probably contraindicated preoperatively because they may worsen abdominal distension before surgery. Associated hypocalcemia or ketosis and any concurrent diseases should be treated as indicated. In our hospital, it is routine practice to administer 500 mg of flunixin meglumine, 1 to 2 L of hypertonic saline IV, and 500 mL of calcium SC before surgically correcting an AV and to monitor ionized calcium after surgery. Transfaunation after surgery may also be helpful. Peri- and post-operative broad spectrum antibiotics are indicated. The duration of their use will be dictated by any encountered problems during surgery such as abdominal contamination, whether or not an abomasotomy was necessary, the appearance of the abomasum at surgery and any anticipated incisional problems. A pragmatic delay regarding antimicrobial selection and use may be elected until the prognosis for the patient is established at surgery.

Prognosis and Sequelae

As in any surgery, incisional complications are a potential problem after celiotomy in cattle. These are recognized by swelling and drainage at the site. Routine surgery to correct a DA with a flank or ventral paramedian approach rarely is followed by complications, though it is possible especially if there were multiple surgeons, the procedure was lengthy, or there was contamination. In cows with AV that requires drainage of fluid followed by pexy, there is more potential for incisional problems if the wall of the viscus was devitalized. Postoperative ultrasonographic evaluation of the body wall and incisional area is very helpful in determining if intervention is needed. Some degree of edema and dependent fluid accumulation is to be expected; however, if it becomes excessive or the surgical incision becomes hot and painful, ventral drainage may be indicated.

Most surgeons leave a few interrupted sutures at the ventral aspect of the incision, which can be easily removed to establish drainage if necessary. This is particularly true for large flank incisions with lots of dead space, such as those after cesarean section. Failure to drain an incisional infection can result in a large retroperitoneal abscess.

Two major complications of AV—direct damage to vagus nerve branches and vascular thrombosis along the axis of the volvulus in the lesser curvature—are responsible for most poor results or deaths after surgical correction and medical therapy. Most cattle that survive surgery for AV and receive fluid therapy appear dramatically improved in appetite and attitude following this treatment for 24 to 72 hours. Clinical experience, however, indicates that a good prognosis cannot be offered until at least 96 hours postoperatively. Vagus nerve damage or vascular thrombosis (Fig. 5.56), if present, usually results in failure of abomasal outflow by this time. If AV is diagnosed and properly treated within 1 to 4 hours after onset of clinical signs, these complications are much less common than in patients in which the AV is not surgically corrected for 24 hours or more. Either complication results in progressive abdominal distension, dehydration, bradycardia, decreased appetite, decreased fecal production, ineffectual rumen contractions, and weight loss that mimics the signs of vagal indigestion (Fig. 5.57). The aforementioned signs respond poorly to symptomatic therapy, but the cattle may survive for weeks before death occurs (see the section on vagal indigestion).

Occasionally, cattle with severe AV and subsequent abomasal devitalization die of abomasal perforation and diffuse peritonitis within 72 hours postoperatively, but this complication is rare in contrast with the two previously described complications that cause a slower deterioration.

Without question, early recognition of illness by an experienced owner, coupled with early diagnosis and surgical intervention by an experienced veterinarian, improves the prognosis for cattle affected with AV. Cows with AV that are recumbent and cannot rise, even after correction of hypocalcemia, are often acidotic and have an extremely poor prognosis.

Abomasal Ulcers
Etiology

Abomasal ulcers in dairy cattle and calves constitute common clinical problems. Intensive management and highly acidic, high-energy, finely ground diets consisting of concentrates and silage probably contribute to the pathogenesis of abomasal ulcers in adult cows. Abomasal ulcers occur frequently in herds fed high-moisture corn and corn silage

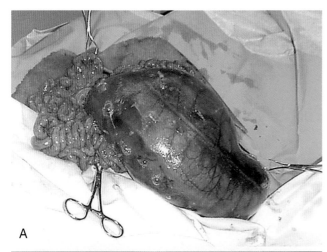

A

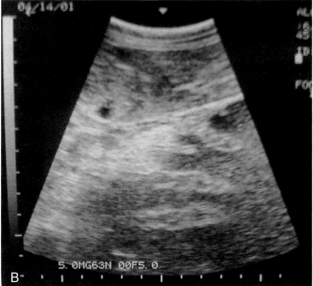

B

• **Fig. 5.56** **A,** Purple discoloration of an abomasum with severe vascular compromise secondary to abomasal volvulus. **B,** Ultrasound image of the right abdomen of the cow showing the distended abomasum and abomasal folds.

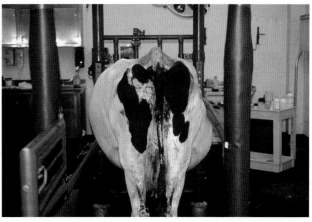

• **Fig. 5.57** Vagal signs in a cow after correction of an abomasal volvulus. This is generally a poor prognosis, but luckily this cow survived.

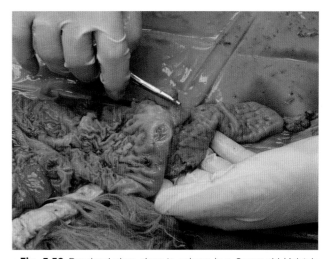

• **Fig. 5.58** Duodenal ulcer close to pylorus in a 3-year-old Holstein dairy cow. Antemortem the cow had been extremely colicky, but no other explanation for the signs of abdominal pain were noted at necropsy.

as a major portion of the diet. Stress, although poorly defined, also contributes to the pathogenesis in recently fresh cows. Additionally, higher-producing cattle seem predisposed to abomasal ulcers, and it is possible that the greater proportion of cardiac output going to the udder may cause a relative underperfusion of the abdominal viscera, which could predispose to abomasal ulceration. Most clinically detectable abomasal ulcers in dairy cattle occur within the first 4 to 6 weeks of lactation, which is a time of negative energy balance despite high-concentrate diets, and of hypocalcemia with potential for delayed intestinal motility. The second most common time in adult dairy cattle seems to be just before freshening and may be related to increased plasma cortisol and decreased abomasal perfusion caused by shunting of a higher percentage of cardiac output to the uterus and fetus.

Young, rapidly growing calves are also frequently affected by abomasal ulceration and perforation. In many cases, predisposing factors may be difficult to determine, although feeding of large volumes of milk in only two daily feedings may be involved in the pathogenesis, because more frequent feeding of milk will maintain a higher "under the curve" pH. In some calves with abomasal perforations, shavings or trichobezoars may be found in the forestomachs and abomasum but are not necessarily causative. Calves and adult cows treated with NSAIDs may also develop abomasal ulcers; we have commonly seen this in young calves receiving flunixin and in bulls being treated with NSAIDs for prolonged periods for musculoskeletal disorders. Lymphosarcoma may also cause bleeding abomasal ulcers in adult cattle. Ulceration is most common in the fundic region in adult cattle and in the pyloric antrum in milk-fed calves. On rare occasions, adult cattle and calves with abomasal ulceration may also develop proximal duodenal ulcers. The predisposing factors presumably overlap. The editors' experience is that isolated duodenal ulceration in the absence of concurrent abomasal disease, most commonly ulcerative abomasal disease, is extremely rare (Fig. 5.58). The clinical signs are indistinguishable in most cases, but it may be that the degree of colic or abdominal pain demonstrated by the patient can be

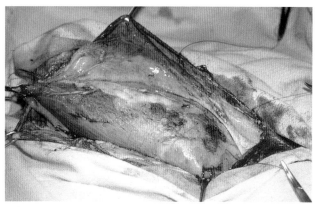

• **Fig. 5.59** Fibrinous localized peritonitis on the abomasal serosa from a small perforating ulcer discovered during abomasopexy.

greater in cases of isolated duodenal ulceration, especially in adults. On occasions, particularly in calves, the ulcerated duodenal mucosa will perforate, giving rise to localized, usually mild, peritonitis. Whether the perforated duodenum heals with extraluminal adhesion formation or merely with internal mucosal repair, some cases become "obstructed" because of stricture formation or entrapment of the duodenum in adhesions; these cattle and calves present similarly to a vagal indigestion case with progressive abdominal distension and concomitant severe hypochloremic, metabolic alkalosis (see Fig. 5.31). The affected section of the duodenum may be several inches from the pylorus, making a paramedian approach in adults very challenging for diagnosis and any attempt at surgical correction.

Clinical Signs

Clinical signs are mostly determined by whether the ulcers cause perforation or severe bleeding. Ulcers rarely cause both, except with chronic DAs. Whereas young calves most commonly have perforating ulcers, there appears to be a relatively equal incidence of perforating and bleeding cases in lactating cattle.

Perforating abomasal ulcers may be seen in calves, bulls, older heifers, and milking cows at any stage of lactation or gestation. They are most common in cows during the first 6 weeks of lactation. Because the clinical syndrome can vary tremendously depending on the size, site and number of perforations, this discussion is divided into perforations that cause localized peritonitis and those that cause diffuse peritonitis. Perforating ulcers that cause localized peritonitis in cattle produce a syndrome similar to traumatic reticuloperitonitis. An acute leakage of abomasal contents occurs but is walled off by the omentum and development of fibrinous adhesions (Fig. 5.59); and the abomasum becomes adherent to the parietal peritoneum, or to the omentum (or both). The septic reaction from the perforation may also be trapped and localized between the abomasum and diaphragm, sometimes causing infection of the pleural cavity by extension many months later. Cows with localized peritonitis caused by a perforated abomasal ulcer are anorectic to a variable degree, usually febrile with a fever of 103.0° to 105.0°F (39.44° to 40.56°C), exhibit rumen hypomotility

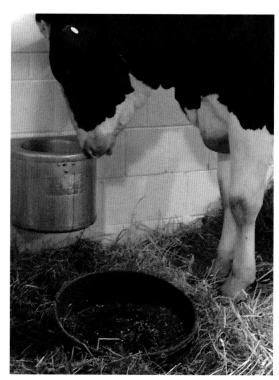

• **Fig. 5.60** A 2-year-old heifer with peritonitis found nose pressing. This is a nonspecific sign of severe pain in cattle.

or stasis, and have painful abdomens. Anatomic localization of pain is achieved more easily in acute cases. The cow will be reluctant to move, and deep palpation of the ventral abdomen usually will localize a painful area of the midventral to the right of the midline. Occasionally, some affected cattle will grind their teeth and press their nose against an inanimate object (Fig. 5.60). In subacute or chronic cases, pain may be difficult to localize, thereby making the differentiation of this syndrome from traumatic reticulitis difficult. In calves, the same signs are present, but ruminal tympany is more common secondary to ileus because of the localized peritonitis. Calves with perforating abomasal ulcers seem to be more likely to develop diffuse peritonitis than adult cows. Ultrasound examination may be helpful in determining the extent of the peritonitis. If the cow is known to have a magnet in her reticulum (either by history, radiographs, or by confirmation with a compass), abomasal ulceration is much more likely than hardware; conversely, if the cow is in the mid- or late lactation stage, abomasal ulceration is less likely than hardware. Symptoms vary widely depending on the size of the perforation and the resulting amount of localized peritonitis present.

Cattle and calves affected with ulcers that cause diffuse peritonitis are much different on initial presentation from those with localized peritonitis. Massive leakage of abomasal contents (Figs. 5.61 to 5.63) prevents localization of the infection. Signs include acute complete anorexia, complete stasis of the forestomach and distal GI tract, fever (typically 104.0° to 106.5°F [40.0° to 41.39 C]) that may be present for only a few hours, cold skin and peripheral parts, dehydration, a reluctance to move, an audible grunt or groan with each expiration if the animal is forced to move or rise,

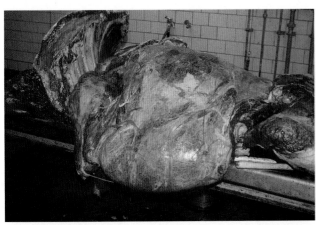

• **Fig. 5.61** Diffuse peritonitis with large sheets of fibrin coating all the viscera after abomasal perforation.

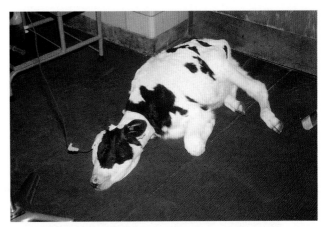

• **Fig. 5.64** A 3-week-old calf with an acute onset of septic shock caused by a perforated ulcer.

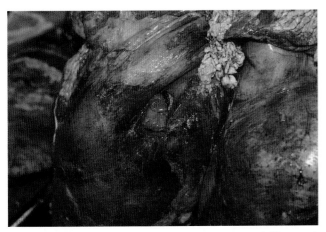

• **Fig. 5.62** Large perforating abomasal ulcer that caused diffuse peritonitis and death in a cow. Abomasal mucosa protrudes through the full-thickness ulcer.

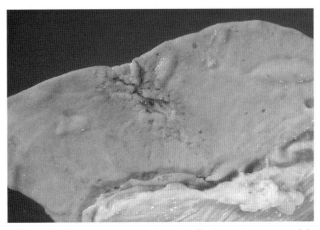

• **Fig. 5.65** Abomasal mucosal ulceration. Such a lesion may result in mild hemorrhage from the abomasum. (Courtesy of John M. King, DVM.)

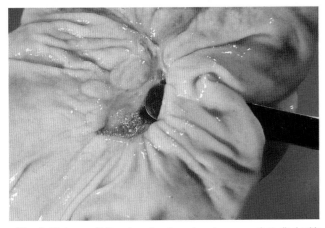

• **Fig. 5.63** Large (3.0-cm) perforating ulcer in a cow that died with diffuse peritonitis. (Courtesy of John M. King, DVM.)

evidence of generalized abdominal pain, pulse rate elevated to 100 to 140 beats/min, severe depression, and progression to recumbency. Basically, the animal is in a state of septic shock similar to that seen with severe coliform mastitis. Calves with perforated abomasal ulcers are often either found dead or, if alive, are recumbent (Fig. 5.64) and have abdominal distension and respiratory distress. The entire course of the disease can be peracute, with death occurring within 6 hours, or can be extended to 36 to 72 hours or longer if medical support is provided. The prognosis is grave, and if the body temperature begins to decrease or is subnormal when the animal is first attended, the animal usually dies within 12 to 36 hours.

Bleeding abomasal ulcers are uncommon in calves compared with perforating ulcers. In adult cows, bleeding ulcers or perforating ulcers can be seen at any stage of lactation but are most common during the first 6 weeks of lactation. Bleeding abomasal ulcers can be categorized by the extent of abomasal hemorrhage and the severity of subsequent anemia.

Abomasal ulcers with slight bleeding (Fig. 5.65) are the most difficult to diagnose because signs are not profound. Whereas asymptomatic cattle that have mild bleeding may pass small, tarry, partially digested blood clots intermittently in the manure, symptomatic cattle show mild chronic abdominal pain, periodic grinding of the teeth, capricious appetite, and the intermittent presence of occult blood in the manure. Such symptomatic cattle appear interested in feed but stop eating after a few mouthfuls, as if interrupted by abdominal discomfort. The diagnosis is difficult and is

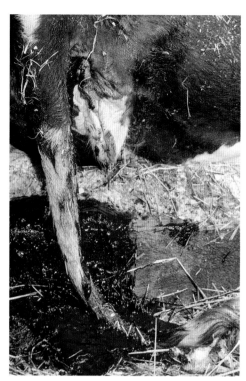

• **Fig. 5.66** Black tarry feces (melena) caused by a bleeding abomasal ulcer.

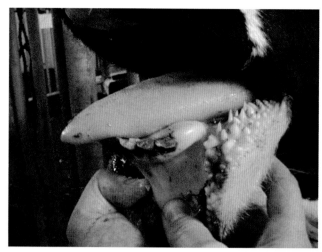

• **Fig. 5.67** White mucous membranes of the mouth in a Holstein cow with bleeding abomasal ulcers and a packed cell volume of 14%.

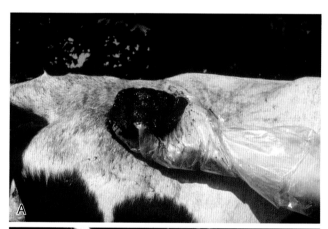

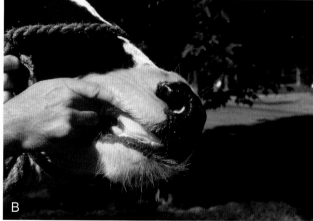

• **Fig. 5.68** Melena (**A**) and pale membranes (**B**) of a cow with bleeding abomasal ulcers and a packed cell volume of 11%.

made by elimination of other diseases, coupled with a normal abdominal paracentesis and positive fecal occult blood. A fecal occult blood test should be performed on a sample obtained before a rectal examination to avoid false-positive results.

Cattle with bleeding abomasal ulcers causing major hemorrhage have normal temperatures but show obvious melena (Fig. 5.66) and partial to complete anorexia. When complete anorexia and severe depression are apparent, the cow usually shows all the cardinal signs of massive blood loss. These signs include pale to chalk-white mucous membranes (Fig. 5.67), a weak pulse elevated to 100 to 140 beats/min, rapid and shallow respirations, weakness, and cool extremities. A typical sweetish odor of digested blood can be detected around the melena-stained perineum or tail. The diagnosis usually only requires physical examination if melena is obvious (Fig. 5.68). Manure may be normal in consistency or, more commonly, loose. A packed cell volume (PCV), total serum protein, and evaluation of hydration status can be used for ancillary and confirmatory purposes.

Although most abomasal ulcers are predominantly either bleeding or perforating, occasionally an animal demonstrates signs consistent with both perforation and bleeding. Long-standing displacement of the abomasum predisposes to both perforation and bleeding. Therefore, this syndrome tends to occur in animals not observed closely or not thought to be likely candidates for DA (heifers, bulls, and dry cows). These animals are often kept in group housing and are not observed as carefully; partial anorexia in a single animal sometimes could go unnoticed for days or weeks.

Chronic distension of the displaced abomasum contributes to physical stretching or tearing of the abomasal mucosa and diminished perfusion. Furthermore, constant exposure of the compromised mucosa to large amounts of retained hydrochloric acid propagates ulceration. Hemorrhage results from multiple mucosal erosions and ulcerations that can deepen to cause major submucosal hemorrhage or frank perforation. Clinical signs include anorexia, partial

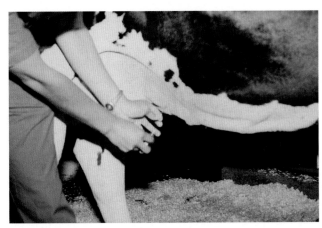

• **Fig. 5.69** A common location for performing a peritoneal centesis in a cow.

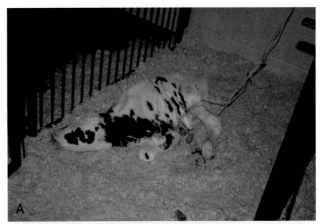

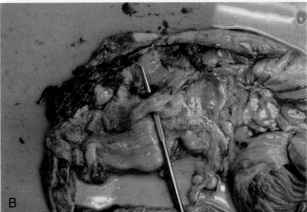

• **Fig. 5.70** Moribund 2-week-old Holstein calf (**A**). The calf had been improving on supportive therapy for diarrhea before rapidly deteriorating coincident with development of an abdominal effusion and signs of shock. Postmortem image (**B**) from the calf in **A** showing full-thickness abomasal perforation that communicated with the peritoneal cavity, causing diffuse septic peritonitis.

to complete ileus, melena, fever, elevated pulse rate, and evidence of abdominal pain. Displacement of the abomasum may be present, and abdominal pain will be most intense when pressure is exerted in the region of the displacement. Signs of pneumoperitoneum and fever also may be present if perforation has occurred.

Laboratory Data

The best ancillary aids to diagnosis of perforating ulcers causing localized peritonitis is ultrasound examination and abdominal paracentesis, which typically demonstrate increased peritoneal effusion with fibrin alongside elevated numbers of white blood cells (>5000–6000/μL) and protein (>3.0 g/dL). Although it would be helpful to see bacteria either free or intracellularly within either neutrophils or macrophages, this is an unusual finding because the adult bovine has such an inherent ability to "wall off" localized peritonitis with fibrin. The peritoneal tap can most easily be performed on the right side just in front of the udder to the side of the mammary vein (Fig. 5.69); an 18-gauge, 1.5-inch needle should be directed perpendicularly into and through the abdominal wall until fluid is obtained. A fetid smell to the fluid and low plasma protein suggest more diffuse peritonitis and a poor prognosis. Ultrasound examination can be of value in detecting pockets of fluid and fibrin here and at other locations prior to abdominocentesis. CBCs and serum biochemistry seldom are helpful in making a diagnosis, although an inflammatory and degenerative leukogram in combination with an abnormally low chloride may be seen in some cases.

Similarly, in cattle affected with perforating ulcers that cause diffuse peritonitis, abdominal paracentesis confirms the diagnosis. A large amount of inflammatory exudate is obtained easily. The total solids and total protein always are elevated (>3.0 g/dL protein), but the white blood cell count may be surprisingly low (<10,000/μL) within the peritoneal fluid of some acute cases. This low count, despite obvious massive peritonitis, is simply dilutional because the affected cow usually has gallons of exudate in the abdomen. A neutropenia with left shift frequently is present in the leukogram, and serum albumin and total protein values are low

because of loss of protein into the peritoneal cavity. A similar dilutional effect on protein and cell levels in abdominal fluid is observed in calves with diffuse peritonitis caused by abomasal perforation.

For cattle suspected of having bleeding abomasal ulcers, PCV and total protein are the major laboratory aids. Performing a fecal occult blood test is rarely needed because of the obvious melena. Rarely, the bleeding may be so acute that PCV and plasma protein do not accurately predict the severity of the blood loss; mucous membrane color, heart rate, and degree of weakness, in addition to measuring blood lactate, will provide a more accurate assessment.

Diagnosis

The diagnosis of perforating abomasal ulceration is based on physical signs, ruling out other causes of peritonitis, and the abdominal paracentesis. Obviously, without exploratory surgery or necropsy (Fig. 5.70), the diagnosis of abomasal ulceration is not truly confirmed. The correlation, however, between clinical signs observed in past nonsurvivors or in survivors that had surgery allows a high index of clinical suspicion for abomasal perforation. Diagnosis of bleeding abomasal ulcers is based on clinical signs of pale mucous membranes, a high pounding heart rate, melena, and low PCV and protein. In calves, primary perforating abomasal ulcers can be distinguished from abomasitis–ulcer syndrome by the abomasal fluid and gas distension within the abomasum with the abomasitis syndrome. Transabdominal ultrasonography can be helpful in adult cattle (Video Clip 5.4) but is particularly useful in calves with diffuse peritonitis, in which a large volume of anechoic abdominal effusion with fibrin can be visualized. Ultrasound examination can also help direct the abdominocentesis to areas of fluid accumulation in cases with low-grade peritonitis and adhesions.

Treatment

The management of perforating abomasal ulcers causing localized peritonitis requires both dietary changes and medical therapy. The cow should be held off silage, high-moisture corn, and finely ground concentrates for 5 to 14 days or until clinical evidence of maintained improvement occurs. A more fibrous diet including high-quality hay should be substituted. If ketosis becomes a complicating factor as high-energy feeds are withdrawn, a coarse calf grain or whole oats can be fed judiciously. Medical therapy includes stall or box stall rest and broad-spectrum antibiotics for 7 to 14 days (or until a normal temperature has been present for at least 48 hours) to control the peritonitis present.

In valuable cattle or calves, IV histamine type 2 blockers can be administered (e.g., 1.5 mg/kg of ranitidine every 8 hours) or a proton pump blocker (1.5 mg/kg of pantoprazole IV or SC every 24 hours). Calves that are still nursing may be given small amounts of milk frequently mixed with antacids or alternated with alkalinizing oral electrolyte solutions. H2 receptor antagonists or proton pump blockers can be given orally in milk-fed calves to increase abomasal pH. If other complications such as hypocalcemia or ketosis are found during the course of the disease, adult cows should be treated symptomatically. Corticosteroids and NSAIDs are contraindicated because they may contribute to further ulceration; we have observed this to be the case, especially with the use of aspirin, phenylbutazone (bulls only), or flunixin meglumine in cattle.

Most patients require 5 to 14 days for recovery; dietary management should continue until the cow is fully recovered and totally appetent. For calves, or on farms with a herd problem of perforating ulcers in calves, more frequent feeding is recommended in addition to measures designed to prevent infectious intestinal disorders.

Management of abomasal ulceration with diffuse peritonitis is difficult and often unsuccessful because of the massive septic peritonitis present. Most commonly, therapy includes high levels of broad-spectrum antibiotics, continuous IV fluids specifically addressing the animal's current acid–base and electrolyte status, and other supportive drugs as necessary. Because of the shocklike state of these animals, most affected calves and cattle are acidotic rather than alkalotic; and the clinician may favor a balanced crystalloid fluid such as lactated Ringer's solution for IV administration instead of saline. Peritoneal lavage should be considered. Few cattle

or calves survive this problem, and massive abdominal adhesions are expected sequelae. Also, if lactating, these cows usually dry off for the remainder of the lactation.

Not all cows with diffuse peritonitis after ulcer perforation die on the day of the perforation. Some cows survive for a few days, but if progressive abdominal distension, complete anorexia, and a progressive decrease in plasma protein are noted, they seldom survive beyond a week despite the most intensive therapy.

It is the consensus of most experienced clinicians that perforating abomasal ulcers are best handled medically rather than surgically unless concurrent DA is present or a calf has both abomasitis syndrome and focal ulceration. Many reasons exist for this opinion. One is that fibrinous adhesions form quickly in the cow's abdomen; therefore, even through a right paramedian abdominal incision, it may be difficult to expose or explore the abomasum sufficiently to surgically oversew or resect the affected area. Another reason is that the ulcerations can be multiple, and resection of all affected abomasal wall may be impossible. In diffuse peritonitis, the shocklike state of the cow generally results in death during surgery. The only cases that are considered for surgery are those with peracute histories (seldom seen in a referral hospital) or cows that do not appear to be responding to medical therapy but have not developed findings suggestive of diffuse septic peritonitis such as abdominal distension or a precipitous decrease in plasma protein.

Such surgical candidates have often stabilized over the first 24 to 72 hours of medical treatment only to develop fever, rumen stasis, acute abdominal pain, and symptoms of further abomasal leakage as if fibrinous adhesions have not adequately walled off the perforation. Calves with peracute signs of diffuse peritonitis caused by large perforating ulcers may also undergo surgery in an effort to find and oversew the causative ulcer.

In calves with abomasitis, emptying the abomasum and oversewing ulcerations combined with medical treatments can be successful. Medical therapy for shock, coupled with such surgery, has resulted in a few survivors. Some calves with abomasal ulceration or duodenal ulceration present with a more chronic history because of peritoneal adhesions involving the abomasum and/or duodenum or a resultant duodenal stricture. Often the abomasum is distended because of a failure of ingesta transit through the pylorus or proximal duodenum subsequent to anatomic occlusion or malpositioning of the pylorus and proximal small intestine (Fig. 5.71). It is rarely possible to safely break down such adhesions intraoperatively to reestablish aboral flow, so these calves become candidates for heroic bypass surgery with resection and anastomosis. This is a challenging surgery and one associated with a high risk for recurrent ulcer disease and repetition of the clinical signs. Interestingly, this seems to be in contrast with adult cattle with obstructing pyloric and duodenal adhesions secondary to presumed duodenal ulceration. Breaking down the adhesions in some of these adult patients can provide almost instant and prolonged recovery.

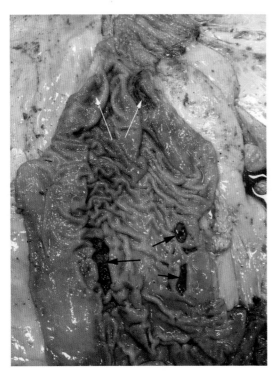

• **Fig. 5.71** Postmortem image of the abomasum and pylorus of a 3-week-old Brown Swiss calf with both abomasal *(black arrows)* and pyloric ulceration *(white arrows)*. The abomasum was markedly distended before being opened because of mucosal adhesions between the damaged tissue at the level of the pylorus.

Usually, abomasal ulcers with only slight bleeding can be managed easily by changing the diet as previously described and, although they are of unproven efficacy, by administering oral antacid protectants or astringents. Concurrent inflammatory or metabolic diseases, if present, also should be treated. It is very important to keep the cow ruminating, so the provision of a high-quality, age-appropriate feed that emphasizes forages is pivotal. By keeping the patient eating such a diet, a higher pH of rumen fluid will flow into the abomasum and naturally buffer the lower pH there.

Abomasal ulcers with major hemorrhage are life-threatening and must be treated by both medical and dietary means. Dietary management and oral antacid protectants (in calves) should be used as described under treatment of perforating ulcers. The major medical therapeutic decision is whether a whole-blood transfusion is necessary. If the mucous membranes are chalk white, the pulse rate is greater than 100 beats/min in adults or 120 beats/min in calves, and the respiratory rate is elevated, a blood transfusion usually will be necessary to allow time for the individual to compensate and respond to its blood loss anemia as the ulcer heals. As in any massive blood loss situation, whole-blood transfusion is the only treatment that will stabilize the patient, although isotonic crystalloids are indicated in addition to the whole blood to maintain perfusion pressure. Whole blood is used to improve both oxygen-carrying capacity and perfusion pressure, and crystalloids help improve perfusion. In cattle with bleeding abomasal ulcers, hypertonic IV fluids should be used only in those patients with life-threatening

hypotension, because the fluid expansion may disrupt clot formation as a result of rapid increases in blood pressure. In Dr. Rebhun's experience, a cow with normal hydration and subacute blood loss (24–72 hours) has a transfusion "trigger point" at a PCV of 14%. With peracute hemorrhage, which rarely occurs in cattle with bleeding ulcers, PCV and plasma protein concentrations are not good indicators of blood loss in the first 12 to 18 hours of hemorrhage. Therefore, clinicians must always base the need for transfusion on clinical signs of pallor, increased heart rate, and increased respiratory rate along with PCV. Cows with PCV less than 14% usually have high respiratory rates, a pulse rate more than 100 beats/min, and extremely pale mucous membranes and need a transfusion. Hydration status can greatly affect these parameters, and a dehydrated cow with a PCV of 16% to 17%, for example, still may require a transfusion. These guidelines apply to cattle that have experienced fairly rapid blood loss over 24 to 72 hours, not cattle that have chronic anemia with physiologic compensation, which may be able to survive with a PCV of 8% to 9%. In chronic cases blood lactate measurement can be a helpful parameter in decision making regarding transfusion; if the blood loss has stopped (demonstrated by a stable PCV) and the blood lactate is <2 mmol/L, then a transfusion may not be necessary.

Routine transfusion in our clinics totals 4 to 6 L of whole blood from a healthy cow to the affected animal. Larger volumes may be given provided the donor can tolerate, or is treated for, the volume depletion. Because the multiple blood types present in cattle make a transfusion reaction unlikely, cross-matching is not done. An appropriate blood donor would be BLV and BVDV-negative animal. Usually one transfusion is sufficient to stabilize the cow until dietary and medical treatment aid healing of the abomasal ulceration. Also, cattle generally have a bone marrow that is very responsive to blood loss; the patient tends to self-correct and stabilize quickly after a transfusion has eased the critical situation. Although such cases are uncommon, some cattle require two or more transfusions over the first few days of treatment; one cow we treated even required seven transfusions during 8 days of continued blood loss from her abomasum! If multiple transfusions over a period of several days are needed, a cross-match is then recommended. Although transfusions require professional time, they are lifesaving in most cases (even in the cow transfused seven times) and thus are worthwhile, especially for a valuable dairy cow. Also, they need not be overly time-consuming if the practitioner has the basic equipment necessary and is well practiced in collecting and administering blood.

Aminocaproic acid (40 mg/kg every 6 hours for one day) can be administered intravenously over 20 minutes to cattle with ongoing hemorrhage in hopes of decreasing fibrinolysis and stabilizing the clot. Although we have used this treatment in cattle with bleeding abomasal ulcers, there are certainly no controlled studies in cows to prove efficacy.

Abomasal bleeding can occur secondary to DAs, especially chronic displacements. If melena, anemia, and DA are

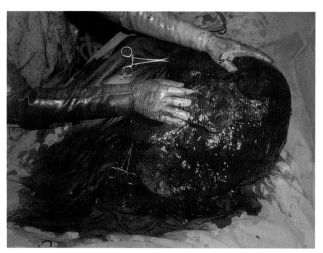

• **Fig. 5.72** Massive adhesions on the surface of an abomasum with a perforating ulcer secondary to chronic left displacement. The surgeon has successfully separated the adherent abomasum from the parietal peritoneum and delivered the organ through a ventral midline incision. The organ would now be examined for any leakage of ingesta, over-sewed as appropriate, and an abomasopexy performed.

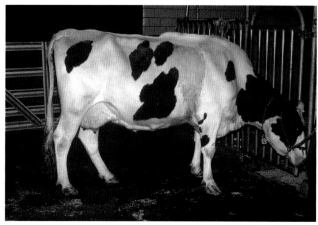

• **Fig. 5.73** A 6-year-old Holstein cow with septic pleuritis caused by a perforated abomasal ulcer during late pregnancy with adhesions to the diaphragm and eventual necrosis of the diaphragm after calving.

all present, the cow should be stabilized, and the severity of its anemia should be assessed. If the PCV is greater than 14% and a transfusion is deemed unnecessary, the DA should be corrected surgically as soon as possible. If the PCV is less than 14% and the cow shows other physical signs of severe anemia (high heart rate, weakness, elevated blood lactate), a blood transfusion should be performed before, or at the time of, surgical correction of the DA. Surgical correction of the DA relieves abomasal distension and acid pooling in the abomasum, and hemorrhage usually stops within 24 to 48 hours postoperatively. Thus, the DA appears to contribute most significantly to hemorrhage in these cases and warrants prompt surgical correction.

In cases of ulcers that are bleeding and that have also per-forated, physical examination should confirm the presence or absence of concurrent DA. If left or right displacement is present, the abdomen should be explored surgically from the right paramedian approach. If the abomasum is adhered in an abnormal position by adhesions resulting from per-forating ulcers, it will be necessary to decide whether the adhesions can be broken down manually without rupture of the abomasum. Then an attempt to dislodge the abomasum from adhesions to the parietal peritoneum is made, and if this is successful, abomasopexy and ulcer resection (or over-sew) can be completed (Fig. 5.72). Surgical replacement of the organ to its normal location generally will result in marked improvement in the abomasal ulcer symptomatol-ogy within 24 to 48 hours.

Dietary changes and broad-spectrum antibiotics should be used for 7 to 14 days after surgery in these difficult cases. Histamine H2 receptor blockers or proton pump inhibi-tors are not commonly used in the therapy of abomasal ulceration in adult cattle, primarily because of prohibitive costs. Research in mature sheep suggests that ranitidine may elevate abomasal pH significantly. Unfortunately, the

dosage of ranitidine required was so high as to be imprac-tical and unaffordable. In calves, ranitidine could be used IV (1.5 mg/kg every 8 hours) or orally (10 mg/kg every 8 hours) mixed in milk. Oral omeprazole (4 mg/kg every 24 hours) could also be used in milk-fed calves. Frequent feed-ing of milk via bottle will itself help increase abomasal pH and might be equally or more valuable than treatment with a H2 blocker or proton pump inhibitor. The pH can be fur-ther increased by adding commercially available antacids to the milk. Sucralfate may also have an additional protective effect and should be mixed in milk feedings four times daily. We have treated several valuable adult cows and calves with pantoprazole (1 mg/kg of pantoprazole IV every 24 hours or 1.5-2 mg/kg SC every 24 hours), but efficacy in ruminants has not been documented.

Prognosis and Discussion

The prognosis for cattle and calves with perforating aboma-sal ulcers that cause localized peritonitis is good with dietary and medical management. It is important to con-tinue broad-spectrum antibiotics until the peritonitis is well under control. When fully recovered for 7 to 14 days, there does not appear to be a tendency for recurrent ulceration, and the animal may return to the herd as a productive indi-vidual. The most difficult patients are dry cows with large gravid uteri. These cows seem to have difficulty forming effective adhesions around the perforation. In addition, the gravid uterus may force the abomasum more cranially in the abdomen to lie against the diaphragm. Therefore, if a perfo-rating ulcer occurs in a dry cow, the abomasum may remain in this position, which would be considered anatomically abnormal in a lactating cow. Such cows may show variable appetites when placed on intensive rations after calving. In addition, we have observed two such dry cows with perfo-rating ulcers with localized peritonitis and adhesions to the diaphragm that subsequently developed septic pleuritis due to septic erosion through the diaphragm (Fig. 5.73). For these reasons, cows in an advanced state of pregnancy may have a more chronic course, may be more prone to multiple

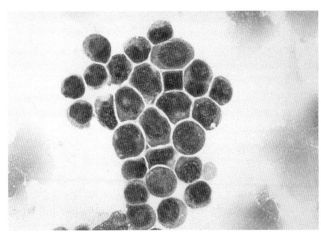

• **Fig. 5.74** Neoplastic lymphocytes in the peritoneal fluid from a 2-year-old Holstein bull with a non–bovine leukemia virus associated lymphosarcoma of the abomasum.

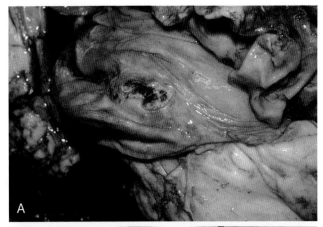

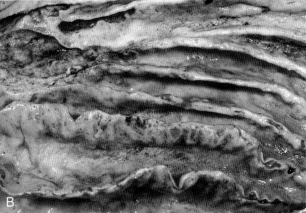

• **Fig. 5.75** A and B, Necropsy views of the mucosal surface of an abomasum infiltrated with lymphosarcoma. A deep ulcer that had caused melena in this cow is apparent.

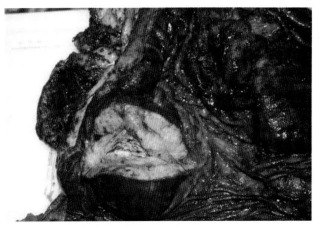

• **Fig. 5.76** Gross postmortem image of abomasal lymphosarcoma from a 5-year-old bovine leukemia virus–positive Holstein cow. Both diffuse wall infiltration and larger nodular masses (seen on cut section) were present within the abomasum. Exfoliated neoplastic cells were present in abdominal fluid (see Fig. 5.32).

episodes of ulceration and may subsequently develop diffuse peritonitis, omental abscesses, or other complications. Consequently, they should only be given a poor to fair prognosis.

The prognosis for cattle with perforating abomasal ulcers that cause diffuse peritonitis is grave. Most of these cases in cattle and calves result in death. Some animals can be normal at night and dead "suddenly" by the next morning. Others live long enough to be diagnosed but die within 24 to 48 hours despite supportive therapy. Infrequent survivors may be left with massive abdominal adhesions despite several weeks of broad-spectrum antibiotics before stabilizing. The current lactation, if the cow is milking, is ruined. Thus, only extremely valuable dairy cattle warrant intensive and protracted treatment.

The prognosis for cattle with bleeding abomasal ulcers is good if the condition is diagnosed before severe anemia develops. Dietary and medical therapy as discussed earlier usually will result in a cure within 7 to 14 days. Even in animals that require blood transfusions, the prognosis is good if the clinician and the owner are willing to spend the time and money necessary for effective treatment. Adult cattle with bleeding ulcers secondary to NSAID treatments seem to have a good prognosis following simple discontinuation of the ulcerogenic drug and instigation of medical and dietary management.

Occasionally, lymphosarcoma can cause severe hemorrhage with subsequent melena as the tumor infiltrates the abomasum. Although other lesions of lymphosarcoma usually are obvious on physical examination of affected cattle, rare cases have no other lesions detectable at the time that anemia and melena are present. These animals do not respond to blood transfusions and die within a few weeks despite treatment. Neoplastic cells (Figs. 5.32 and 5.74) may be observed on peritoneal fluid in approximately 50% of cattle with abomasal lymphosarcoma in which bleeding or evidence of pyloric obstruction are the predominant clinical findings. At necropsy, typical lesions of lymphosarcoma are found (Figs. 5.75 and 5.76). On very rare occasions, abomasal perforation may occur. A thorough physical examination to rule out lesions of lymphosarcoma in other anatomic predilection sites is always indicated for cattle

that have melena. Serologic or PCR testing for BLV status may be indicated, but results must be interpreted carefully (see the section on BLV in Chapter 16) because of the tests' low predictive value for neoplasia. Only on very rare occasions will abomasal lymphosarcoma be found in a non–BLV-infected patient (Fig. 5.74). Right paramedian

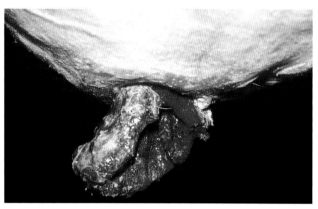

• **Fig. 5.77** Abomasal fistula secondary to an abomasopexy.

abdominocentesis may reveal lymphoblasts and is a valuable procedure to perform in cattle with signs consistent with GI bleeding caused by abomasal ulceration that are outside of the usual signalment range for early lactational ulcers.

Bleeding abomasal ulcers causing melena in calves are rare and sporadic, but perforating abomasal ulcers are quite common. The reason for this discrepancy between calves and adult cows is not known. Calves experiencing sepsis and concurrent enteritis or receiving parenteral nutrition appear to be at greatest risk for spontaneous abomasal ulcers that perforate.

The prognosis for cattle affected with ulcers that both bleed and perforate is poor. Because these cases tend to be chronic, or neglected, or involve concurrent DA, the lesions can be severe. If displacement of the abomasum is present and can be corrected surgically, the prognosis for the ulcers improves. However, if the perforating ulcers have locked the abomasum in a displaced position or caused a great deal of peritonitis, the prognosis must be guarded to poor. Each of these cases must be assessed individually for treatment and prognosis.

Abomasal Fistulas

Abomasal fistulas infrequently develop following surgical abomasopexies or blind abomasopexy procedures such as the blind stitch and toggle-pin techniques. Intimate adhesion of the abomasal visceral peritoneum to the parietal peritoneum, coupled with intraluminal suture placement (unintentional during abomasopexy or intentional during blind procedures), can cause abomasal contents to seek an outlet through the body wall following the path of the incisional line (abomasopexy) or through-and-through sutures (blind stitch, toggle pin). In either event, the abomasopexy sutures have penetrated the abomasal lumen to allow egress of ingesta. Eventually, the incisional line weakens or breaks down in surgical abomasopexy patients, allowing abomasal contents and mucosa to protrude to the exterior. In through-and-through techniques, the same phenomenon may occur as abomasal ingesta follows the nonabsorbable sutures through the body wall and abomasal mucosa migrates along the suture to the outside. In some cases, the mucosa eventually prolapses to the exterior and presents as a hemorrhagic, edematous mucosal surface (Fig. 5.77). Blood loss may be severe at this time.

The diagnosis is made by observation and knowledge of a history of abomasopexy. If blood loss appears severe, laboratory data may be necessary for assessment of PCV and plasma protein in anticipation of whole-blood transfusion. If the fistula has been chronic, acid–base and electrolyte status should be assessed, because chronic chloride loss may have occurred, leading to advanced metabolic alkalosis. The prognosis depends somewhat on the size of the area that must be resected to correct the fistula but should be guarded in all cases.

Treatment consists first of medical therapy with systemic antibiotics, whole blood (if necessary) or balanced-electrolyte solutions, as dictated by physical examination and laboratory data. Second, the abomasal fistula requires surgical resection using an en bloc abdominal wall resection that includes the abomasal adhesion to the parietal peritoneum. Hemostasis and closure after en bloc abdominal wall resection present time-consuming problems for the surgeon. Fistulas through abomasopexy incisions are often complicated by incisional hernias that also require resection, thereby creating a larger abdominal wall defect. Successful primary closure of the site after en bloc resection has been reported. In severe cases with huge body wall defects and infection, closure can be accomplished by through-and-through tension mattress sutures using heavy surgical steel and quill sutures. Postoperatively, the wound is bandaged and the cow maintained on systemic antibiotics until the incisional area heals completely "from the inside out" over a 2- to 4-week period. General anesthesia is highly desirable for these procedures.

Abomasitis, Abomasal Tympany, and Abomasal Ulceration Syndrome in Calves

Etiology

This is a clinical syndrome with characteristic clinical signs and pathological findings in nursing calves of which the exact etiology(s) remains unproven. *Clostridium perfringens* type A, *Sarcina* spp., and *Salmonella* Typhimurium DT104 have all been incriminated. Although outbreaks of the syndrome have been described in nursing beef calves and lambs, in dairy calves, it is mostly sporadic but may become endemic on a farm.

Clinical Signs

Affected calves are milk-fed calves, often 2 to 6 weeks of age, and develop acute abdominal bloat, anorexia, rapidly progressive depression leading to recumbency, and frequently shock. Affected calves may have diarrhea or colicky signs, although these are inconsistent findings. On clinical examination, the calves show noticeable distension (Fig. 5.78) on both sides of the abdomen and have variably sized pings with easily succussible fluid throughout the ventral abdomen. The fluid- and gas-distended abomasum may be seen throughout the right and left ventral abdomen on ultrasound examination, and a smaller gas-filled rumen may be visualized externally or imaged via ultrasound examination pushed to the top of the left

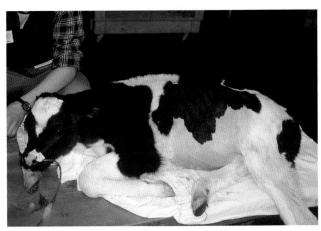

• **Fig. 5.78** Abdominal enlargement due to abomasal distension and shock in a 6-week-old calf with acute abomasitis, tympany, and abomasal ulceration. After surgical drainage of the abomasum, suturing of two abomasal ulcers, and intensive medical therapy, the calf recovered.

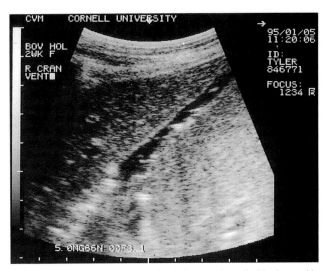

• **Fig. 5.79** Ultrasound image of the abdomen of a calf with abomasitis showing marked edema *(black)* of the abomasal wall. The liver is seen between the body wall and the abomasum.

paralumbar fossa. Affected calves have tachycardia, cold extremities, and other signs of shock or poor perfusion. The progression of clinical signs can be rapid. It is our impression that the disease is more common in bucket-fed calves than in bottle-fed calves. We have seen a similar, if not identical, syndrome in 1- to 3-day-old calves in whom we hypothesize that mixing high-starch colostral supplements into milk or milk replacer may be an important predisposing management factor.

Laboratory Findings

Severely affected calves frequently have a metabolic (high lactate, high anion gap) acidosis. Other abnormalities include low serum chloride, azotemia, elevated PCV, and immature and toxic-appearing neutrophils. With severe abdominal distension or depression, respiratory acidosis due to hypoventilation may accompany the metabolic acidosis and cause marked systemic acidemia with a pH of 7.0 or less. True renal azotemia with acute renal failure can also be seen in severe cases, likely associated with sepsis, exotoxemia, and hypotensive shock.

Diagnosis

The diagnosis is based on the age of the calf; the characteristic clinical findings; and laboratory evidence of acidosis, dehydration, and sepsis. The differential diagnosis includes displaced abomasum; acute peritonitis caused by a conventional perforating abomasal ulcer; and ruminal bloat, either idiopathic or resulting from ruminal milk accumulation. Calves with ruminal bloat are generally not as sick as calves with abomasitis and do not have the amount of succussible fluid characteristically found with the abomasitis syndrome. Evidence of ruminal drinking and abomasitis may be concurrent in some calves, but this is not characteristic. Ultrasound examination often demonstrates an edematous and thickened wall of the abomasum (Fig. 5.79), alongside marked enlargement of the viscus. Significant abdominal effusion is rarely noted in calves with nonperforated

abomasitis, but its presence should raise suspicion of full-thickness perforation and suggest a grave prognosis.

Treatment

Calves with progressive signs associated with abomasitis should be treated intensively with colloids, crystalloids, and systemic antibiotics. Unfortunately, many are already moribund even at the time of first examination. Colloids (plasma or hetastarch) may have particular benefit in severely affected calves because there is evidence of systemic inflammatory shock, leaky capillaries, and a predisposition to intestinal wall and pulmonary edema. Systemic antibiotics are indicated because there is high potential for translocation of *Clostridium* spp. or other intestinal bacteria from the gut to other organs. An oral-gastric or rumen tube should be passed because in some cases, a large amount of fetid fluid is refluxed, which improves the clinical condition of the calf. It is unclear whether this reflux is a consequence of the primary abomasal condition or if rumen putrefaction plays a role in the disease in some calves. In many cases, there is minimal to no reflux. Regardless, penicillin is often administered orally in an attempt to decrease intestinal clostridial overgrowth. There is a technique of percutaneous abomasal puncture described for lambs that have severe abomasal tympany, but this is untested by us in calves. In relatively early cases of the disease, rolling of the calf on its back and puncturing the abomasum may allow enough deflation that motility is regained, and the calf recovers. We have performed this procedure prior to anesthetic induction as part of our attempts at presurgical stabilization of some calves and would recommend that serious consideration be given to laparotomy after such percutaneous abomasal decompression to address the inevitable leakage that can occur. *C. perfringens* C and D antitoxin is frequently given SC or orally, but its efficacy is unproved. Etiologically, the association with *C. perfringens* type A gives credence intuitively to the use of antitoxin; unfortunately, there are no commercially available sources of type A antitoxin in North America, and the degree to which anti-C and D antitoxin will cross-protect is unknown but highly dubious.

If the calves do not respond promptly to fluid therapy and passage of the oral-rumen tube or abdominal distension and signs of shock do not rapidly improve, a laparotomy (right paracostal or right ventral paramedian approach) to empty the abomasum and oversew any apparent abomasal ulceration sites can be performed. If there are no abomasal perforations and hypotension can be reversed, the calves may have a fair to good prognosis. Affected calves may die quickly from acute peritonitis or severe hypotension, or some may linger after surgery and die several days later from peritonitis and adhesions.

Preventive recommendations are unknown, although it seems as if "greedy" nursers are most often affected, which suggests that either ruminal drinking or abomasal stasis may allow overgrowth of the causative organism. Because the problem can be endemic on some farms, a concentrated effort at routine disinfection of equipment, proper handling of the milk or milk replacer to avoid bacterial contamination, feeding milk or well mixed milk replacer at body temperature, use of bottle rather than bucket for feeding, isolation of affected calves, and disinfection of their stalls all seem pertinent. Several farms that have had multiple cases of abomasitis in calves have prevented further cases by administering oral penicillin mixed in the milk or, in situations when the age at onset is predictable, as is often the case, by use of parenteral penicillin metaphylactically. Dividing the milk into an increased number of feedings may also be helpful. Vaccination of adult cattle or calves with *C. perfringens* type C and D products should not be expected to provide significant protection against any of the incriminated organisms, but recently a *C. perfringens* type A toxoid has become available and could be tried. Anecdotal field observations have suggested that the condition may be more common in calves fed according to accelerated milk replacer programs, particularly when ad libitum access to water is denied. The problem of abomasitis and tympany has assumed such severe and repeatable significance on some farms in the northern United States that it may represent their most significant cause of calf morbidity and mortality.

Prophylactic husbandry measures as described, even alongside metaphylactic use of β-lactam antibiotics, have often been the most effective means of control. On rare occasion, we have seen a similar, sporadic abomasitis condition in adult cows that appears similar to braxy (*Clostridium septicum*).

Abomasal Impaction
Etiology

Primary abomasal impaction in adults may be caused by extremely fibrous feed or pica with subsequent heavy ingestion of sand, nut shells, or rocks, or it may be idiopathic. Primary abomasal impaction resulting from extremely fibrous feeds and lack of water as seen in wintered beef cattle is rare in dairy cattle. Secondary causes, which are more common, include pyloric outflow disturbances secondary to ventral vagus nerve injuries, vascular or neurogenic damage secondary to AV, abdominal adhesions, pyloric masses or adhesions, and lymphosarcoma. Traumatic reticuloperitonitis and peritonitis associated with perforating abomasal ulcers are the most common predisposing causes of abomasal impaction at our clinic. These conditions may create either neurogenic or mechanical abomasal outflow disturbances. Other hospitals have diagnosed this condition more commonly in early lactation cows, often without a known etiopathogenesis but mostly involving the pyloric antrum. The presumed higher incidence in early lactation cattle might suggest that abomasal hypomotility caused by subclinical hypocalcemia, hypokalemia, or high intraluminal concentrations of volatile fatty acids is a predisposing factor. Dairy cows on sand bedding or a gravel dry lot may develop abomasal impaction from those sources and abnormal diets, or occasionally, recurrent herd issues with ketosis may predispose the cattle to eat excessive sand or gravel.

In calves, idiopathic abomasal impaction may be observed in any breed but is most common in Guernseys. Calves with peritonitis occurring for any reason may also develop abomasal impaction secondary to abdominal adhesions. Neurogenic damage to the vagus nerve in calves with AV or chronic DA also provides a risk for subsequent abomasal impaction.

Clinical Signs

Signs are not specific and are similar to those observed in all patients with vagal indigestion. Progressive abdominal distension may occur over days to weeks, and the patient has an intermittent appetite, reduced manure production with frequently loose or watery feces, weight loss, and decreased milk production. Diarrhea is common because primarily small volume, highly acidic, fluid ingesta escapes the abomasum, bypassing the impaction. Abdominal distension, if present, is similar to that of vagal indigestion, with high left, low left, and low right distension. In other cases, the signs are not pronounced, and decreased appetite is the only clinical finding. Rumen contractions may be absent to normal or even increased in frequency. In calves, the firm, enlarged abomasum sometimes can be palpated externally or visualized with ultrasound, but the former is less commonly possible in adult cattle. Rectal examination of adult cattle usually finds enlargement of the rumen dorsal and ventral sacs. Rarely, the enlarged abomasum may be palpated in the right lower quadrant, but usually the enlarged or lifted up ventral sac of the rumen occupies this position.

Cattle with abomasal impaction sometimes grind their teeth and may show evidence of pain in response to deep pressure in the midabdomen. Temperature, pulse rate, and respiratory rate usually are normal unless bradycardia secondary to vagus nerve irritation is present.

Ancillary Data

Varying degrees of metabolic alkalosis are possible depending on the degree of hydrochloric acid retention or reflux into the forestomach. Surprisingly, most dairy cows with abomasal impactions have only moderate or no metabolic alkalosis, perhaps resulting from the insidious chronic progression of the disease, location of the impaction, and less than complete obstruction to fluid outflow.

Diagnosis

The diagnosis of abomasal impaction is made during right-side exploratory laparotomy or left-side laparotomy and rumenotomy. For cattle showing signs of vagus nerve injury, the diagnosis usually is made by palpation of the abomasum through the also distended rumen during rumenotomy. A majority of cattle with abomasal impaction have impactions of the pyloric antrum alone, but more severe cases have impaction of the abomasal body and pyloric antrum.

Treatment

Passage of a stomach tube through the reticulo-omasal orifice into the abomasum during rumenotomy allows mineral oil or dioctyl sodium succinate (60–80 mL of a 25% solution) to be delivered to the impaction. However, a one-time medical treatment such as this is rarely expected to work if there is vagus nerve injury. Laxatives, ruminotorics, and laxative feeds seldom are successful in affected cattle, although coffee (1 lb given in the rumen) has helped some patients. Definitive treatment for vagal indigestion or abomasal impactions may require abomasotomy performed on a recumbent patient, usually through a low right paracostal or ventral right paramedian approach. The prognosis is guarded for all nerve injury–associated abomasal impactions, but some patients may be helped if specific causative lesions such as localized adhesions or malposition of the organ can be corrected. Abomasal impactions secondary to peritonitis of any type carry a poor prognosis. Idiopathic abomasal impactions may carry a good prognosis with massage via right flank laparotomy and ororuminal administration of mineral oil, coffee (1 lb), or magnesium products for 2 to 5 days. Normal serum calcium and potassium should be maintained! Cows with antrum impactions alone have a better prognosis than those with abomasal body impactions. Motility "enhancers" such as bethanechol (0.07 mg/kg SC), lidocaine constant-rate infusion (CRI) (1.3 mg/kg slow bolus followed by 0.05 mg/kg/min) or erythromycin (8–10 mg/kg IM once to twice daily) can be attempted. Erythromycin is most effective, but in the United States, the use of an antimicrobial for this purpose is illegal. Electrolyte-containing fluids should be administered IV to correct any dehydration, electrolyte and acid-base abnormalities. If the cow is stable, this treatment and oral laxatives can be continued for 2-3 days in hopes that surgery can be avoided.

Abomasal Neoplasia

The most important tumor involving the abomasum is lymphosarcoma. The abomasum is one of the favorite "target" regions for lymphosarcoma in cattle. The tumor may invade the wall of the abomasum diffusely or in multifocal fashion (Figs. 5.75, 5.76, and 5.80). The pyloric region may be

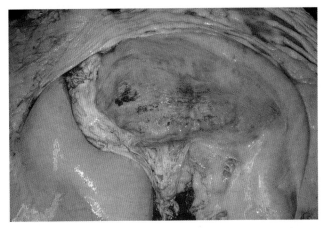

• **Fig. 5.80** Necropsy view of an abomasum infiltrated with lymphosarcoma. The corrugations and raised areas are neoplastic lesions.

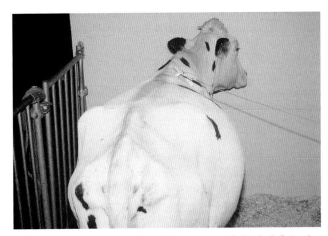

• **Fig. 5.81** Slowly progressive and now severe abdominal distension caused by pyloric obstruction from pyloric lymphosarcoma, resulting in abomasal and forestomach compartment distension.

obstructed, resulting in an outflow disturbance from the abomasum and forestomach compartments. On rare occasion, biliary outflow may be obstructed, causing icterus and marked elevation in gamma glutamyl transferase. Serum chloride is almost always low (sometimes <70 mEq/L), and rumen chloride is quite high (>60 mEq/L) if the lymphosarcoma is obstructing the pylorus. Affected cows may show progressive abdominal distension (Fig. 5.81) and eventually become so weak they cannot rise. We have treated a small number of pregnant cows with lymphosarcoma with isoflupredone acetate (Predef 2X) at 20 to 30 mg IM daily (for no more than 3 consecutive treatments for fear of inducing hypokalemia) or prednisolone (1 mg/kg daily) and on rare occasion obtained enough improvement that the cow remained alive until the calf was born. Owners were made aware of the fact the calf was at high risk of being infected with BLV and may also be genetically predisposed to developing the neoplasia. In valuable and terminally ill cows, ovary or oocyte harvesting (except for cows in late pregnancy) is commonly requested. In some cases, melena is the only sign observed as the neoplasia progresses to cause abomasal ulceration and hemorrhage. The diagnosis can usually be made by knowledge of the age of the cow (usually 4 years or older), clinical signs, evidence of tumorous disease elsewhere in the cow, BLV status, ultrasound examination of the abomasum (may reveal diffuse involvement), and cytologic examination of peritoneal fluid and blood. Although most adult dairy cattle with abomasal lymphosarcoma in the United States are BLV- positive, some cases may occur in virus-negative cattle. A low percentage of cows with lymphosarcoma have blast cells in the peripheral blood, but approximately 50% of cows with abomasal lymphosarcoma have tumor cells in the peritoneal fluid. Definitive diagnosis in some cases may require a right-side laparotomy and biopsy. Adenocarcinomas of the abomasum also have been described but are very rare.

Displacement of the Omasum

In the past few years, we have seen a few cows with displacement of the omasum into the upper right abdomen, either just behind or just in front of the last rib. These cases were first brought to our attention by Dr. Chuck Guard and were confirmed on exploratory laparotomy and at necropsy in at least 6 cases. Cows often have a several-day history of decreased appetite and production and mild abdominal distension just cranial to the right paralumbar fossa (Fig. 5.82). A small ping can be heard in some of the cases over the area of the displacement, often high on the 13th rib, somewhat mimicking RDA. Ultrasound examination can help distinguish between the two conditions, as can measurement of serum chloride. The omasum was palpated rectally on a couple of the cows. An appropriate surgical repair method has not been determined at this time, but one excellent cow survived for more than 2 years after documentation of the disorder by laparotomy.

Obstructive Diseases of the Small Intestine

Mechanical obstructive diseases of the small intestine are not as common as forestomach and abomasal disorders, but they occur regularly enough to warrant concern in the differential diagnosis of abdominal distension in the cow and calf, especially if colic is also present. The various obstructions are discussed as a group, with additions when appropriate concerning specific obstructive disorders.

Etiology

The cause of small intestinal obstructions such as volvulus, torsion, and intussusception is seldom apparent, although predisposing factors may be identified retrospectively during exploratory laparotomy or necropsy in affected cattle. For example, it is relatively common to find a potential nidus of aberrant intestinal motility such as an *Oesophagostomum* spp. nodule or small polyp at the site of an intussusception in an adult cow. Intussusceptions are more common in calves than in cows and may occur in association with infectious diarrhea. Complete torsions at the mesenteric root have been observed after the casting and restraint of cattle for surgical procedures as well as following treatment of uterine torsion

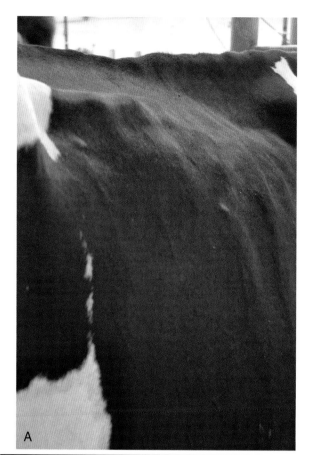

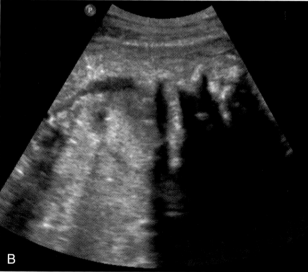

• **Fig. 5.82** **A,** A 4-year-old Holstein cow with distension of the right dorsal abdomen near the 13th rib caused by omasal displacement. **B,** Ultrasound image of the same cow showing distended viscus proven to be omasum on exploratory surgery. The omasal leaves are often elongated with chronic distension.

by the "flank in the plank" technique. Similarly, fibrous bands from adhesions or umbilical remnants traversing the abdomen may predispose to intestinal entrapment and subsequent obstruction, especially in calves. Growing calves, especially those irritated by lice, may become obstructed by trichobezoars. In some herds, intraluminal obstructions are more common because of hemorrhagic bowel syndrome

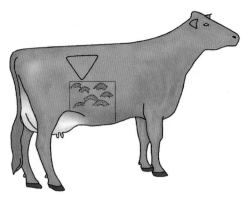

• **Fig. 5.83** Typical area for small intestinal fluid distension.

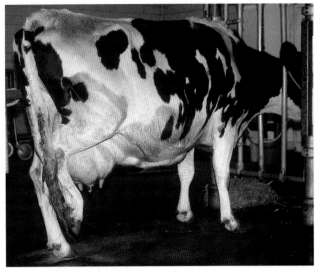

• **Fig. 5.84** Colic characterized by kicking at the abdomen in a cow affected with intussusception. The wet hair on the right lower flank has been caused by the cow's right hind foot contacting the abdomen at this site.

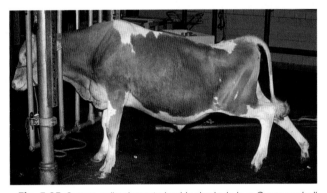

• **Fig. 5.85** Severe colic characterized by lordosis in a Guernsey bull affected with small intestinal volvulus.

(HBS). Although uncommon, fecal impactions of the small intestine (most commonly ileum) do occur in cattle. Duodenal obstruction caused by duodenal sigmoid flexure volvulus has been reported in adult dairy cattle, most commonly in cattle that had a prior omentopexy or pyloropexy. We have also seen a similar syndrome of proximal duodenal obstruction caused by adhesions or post-ulcerative stricture.

Clinical Signs

The general signs of small intestinal obstruction in cows are distinct and include:
1. Acute onset of anorexia and GI stasis
2. Abdominal distension, especially of the right ventral quadrant with obstructions (mechanical or functional) other than those of the proximal duodenum
3. Colic
4. Absence of manure production
5. Fluid-distended bowel can be identified by ballottement and auscultation in the right ventral quadrant of the abdomen (Fig. 5.83) with obstructions (mechanical or functional) other than those involving the proximal duodenum
6. Rectal or ultrasound findings of distended loops of small bowel
7. Progressive deterioration in the general physical status as regards hydration, attitude, and heart rate for strangulating causes

These signs allow the diagnosis of small intestinal obstruction to be made with assurance in most cases. Rapid determination of mechanical obstruction is then important so that surgical treatment or slaughter may be discussed. Obviously, variations exist in the signs depending on the duration of obstruction, the age of the patient, and the type of obstruction present. Dehydration begins early in small intestinal obstruction and progresses rapidly. Metabolic alkalosis may be mild in distal small intestinal obstruction or severe in duodenal obstruction (i.e., serum chloride concentration often <70 mEq/L). The heart rate tends to increase progressively because of pain and deteriorating hydration status but may be misleadingly normal in some small intestinal obstructions for which the cow has received analgesics or in cases of long-standing (>24 hours) intussusception when the patient is no longer showing signs of colic. Hypocalcemia may occur secondary to absence of appetite, GI stasis, and continued, albeit modest, milk production.

Severe colic is observed in patients with torsion of the root of the mesentery, volvulus of various types, torsion of the distal flange of the small intestine, internal herniation of the small intestine through the visceral layer of the greater omentum in adults or epiploic foramen in calves, and extraluminal obstruction by fibrous adhesions or bands in all ages of cattle or remnants of umbilical vessels in calves. Cecal volvulus, which generally also causes small intestinal distension, is another common cause of severe colic in cattle. Severe colic in cows is characterized by kicking at the abdomen (Fig. 5.84), bellowing, lordosis (Fig. 5.85), and reluctance to stand for even a few seconds (Fig. 5.86) and by the animal throwing itself down. Less severe colic may be noticed in intussusception with kicking at the abdomen, treading with the hind feet, swishing the tail, and a preference for recumbency. We need to remember that the most common cause of colic in the adult dairy cow is small intestinal indigestion and that colic is not always caused by an

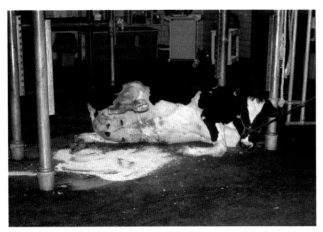

• **Fig. 5.86** Marked abdominal pain in a cow with mesenteric volvulus.

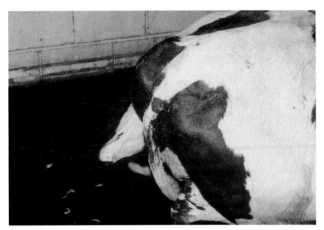

• **Fig. 5.87** "Raspberry-colored" manure typical of that passed from devitalized small intestine.

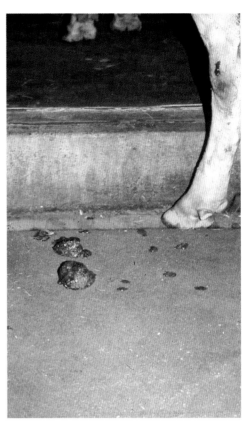

• **Fig. 5.88** Scant manure with flecks of blood passed from a cow with intussusception.

intestinal problem, such as with uterine torsion. Except for *C. perfringens* enteritis, calves rarely demonstrate marked colic with infectious bacterial, parasitic, or viral diarrheas, although calves with marked abomasal tympany/abomasitis can be very colicky too. Cattle affected with intussusception may show colic during the first 12 to 24 hours of obstruction but thereafter have minimal signs of colic with anorexia, absence of manure, dehydration, and abdominal distension as the only outward signs of obstruction. This makes rectal or ultrasound examination imperative for diagnosis, because cattle with intussusception may survive several days or up to 1 week with complete obstruction. Intraluminal obstructions from other causes; HBS, ileal impaction, and trichobezoars, similarly may only cause colic signs early in the course of the disease.

Confusion may result if a cow affected with small intestinal obstruction passes any manure. Certainly, manure distal to the obstruction may be passed early in the course of intestinal obstruction of any type, but in general, cattle with small intestinal obstructions pass no manure and will not eat. Occasionally, red or raspberry-colored bloody mucus or blood clots descend the intestinal tract from the site of an intussusception (Figs. 5.87 and 5.88) and appear at the

rectum or are found on rectal palpation. This is an especially helpful sign in the calf with suspected obstruction because thorough rectal examination is impossible. Not all cases of intussusception show this blood-stained mucus, nor is the finding always limited to intussusception, a notable differential being HBS. Abdominal distension worsens progressively in small intestinal obstructions and consists of two major components:

1. The small intestine proximal to the obstruction fills with fluid and gas, resulting in distension of the right lower abdominal quadrant, and is detectable by simultaneous ballottement and auscultation, except in cases with very proximal obstruction.
2. The forestomach and abomasum distend secondary to the intestinal obstruction because of failure of normal outflow and reflux of small intestinal contents. This results in left-sided abdominal distension of a degree that is proportional to the duration of obstruction. The more proximal the small bowel distension, the more likely and promptly this secondary change will occur.

Rectal examination findings of distended loops of small bowel provide the key to diagnosis in cattle affected with small intestinal obstruction. In addition, tight mesenteric bands, volvulus at the mesenteric root, or the intussusception (Fig. 5.89) itself, may be palpated in some patients. Unfortunately, rectal examination is not possible in calves and may be very difficult to use diagnostically in large cows in advanced gestation because the gravid uterus occupies so great an area. In

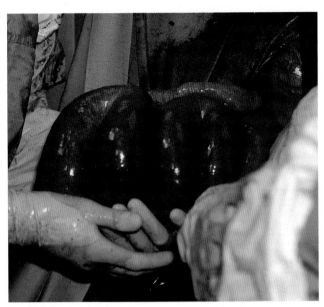

• **Fig. 5.89** Intussusception in a cow. The coiled appearance of the affected bowel is typical.

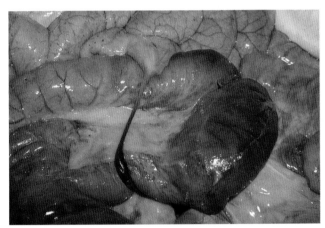

• **Fig. 5.90** A segment of small intestine trapped by a band of undetermined origin in a 3-week-old "colicky" calf.

these cases, the cow or calf may need to undergo exploratory laparotomy to confirm the diagnosis. In young calves, entrapment of a segment of the bowel by an umbilical structure or another band is not unusual (Fig. 5.90). On rare occasion, an infectious enteritis such as one caused by *C. perfringens* will be associated with focal small intestinal inflammation and hemorrhage, resulting in bowel obstruction. Passage of blood-stained diarrhea may precede the obstruction (Fig. 5.91). Ultrasonography is an important and highly informative tool for evaluating cattle (adults and calves) with suspected small intestinal obstruction. Distended small intestines are usually readily visible in the right flank. The intestinal wall may be thickened or thin walled, and with strangulating lesions there is little to no motility within the distended loops. If sedimentation is noted in the small intestine during ultrasound exam, this would suggest a surgical problem. With intraluminal obstruction such as a blood clot caused by the HBS, motility may be increased or normal early in the obstructive disorder, but eventually hypomotility will ensue.

Hemorrhagic bowel syndrome has been one of the most common causes of small intestinal obstruction in our hospital in recent years. Most of the other causes of small intestinal obstruction are sporadic and occur in individual cows; however, HBS can occur as a cluster of cases and occasionally become an endemic challenge on some farms. The cause of the syndrome is not known, but it is most common in third lactation cows, and the median time between parturition and onset is 3 to 4 months. Some farms have a relatively high incidence of the disease, but other farms have no cases. Farms that feed the highest-energy diets seem to be at greatest risk for having cows with HBS. The disease appears to be disproportionately common in the Brown Swiss breed, but it has been seen in all of the conventional North American dairy breeds and even in bulls. We have worked with several pedigree Brown Swiss farms where the annual prevalence rate is as high as 10% in adult cattle. A more in-depth discussion of this condition can be found in Chapter 6.

Differential Diagnosis

The differential diagnosis for signs of small intestinal obstruction includes diseases that may result in colic:

1. Simple indigestion with gas and fluid distension of the small intestine is the major differential for small bowel obstruction. Occasionally, cattle with indigestion have fluid and gas distension of the small intestine and subsequent tension on the mesentery preceding passage of this fluid ingesta as diarrhea. These cattle may show extreme colic and be easily misdiagnosed with intestinal obstruction. They tend to have GI stasis, abdominal distension, increased heart rate, slight dehydration, hypocalcemia, hypochloremia, and either absent or scant manure production, at least initially. Usually they do not have tightly distended loops of bowel per rectum. On ultrasound examination, the small intestine is dilated, but some motility is often present, especially after hypocalcemia is corrected. These cows may begin to pass liquid manure on their own with resultant remission of signs or do so after symptomatic therapy with laxatives, ruminotorics, flunixin, and calcium solutions. It is extremely important to recognize that a cow passing substantial quantities of manure does not have a small bowel obstruction. Most cows with small bowel obstruction will not eat, although a small number will eat a few bites. Although many cows with colic do not require surgery because of the high incidence of small intestinal indigestion, colic caused by enteritis in calves is not common, and a higher percentage of calves showing obvious colic signs have structural obstruction and require surgery.

2. Acute pyelonephritis and other painful urinary tract problems such as renal calculi or ureteral calculi could cause signs of colic and thus may be confused with small intestinal obstruction. However, no abdominal distension is evident externally, no distended small bowel is palpated per rectum, and the cow usually is passing manure. Examination of the urinary system and urinalysis lead to proper diagnosis (see Chapter 11).

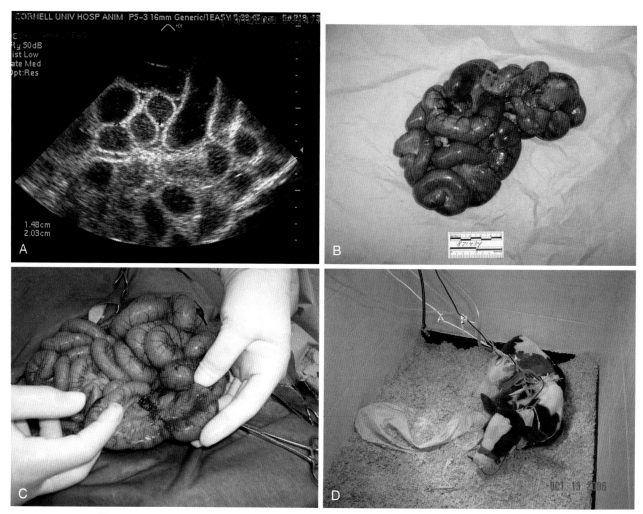

• **Fig. 5.91** A 5-day-old Red and White Holstein calf with a 1-day history of hemorrhagic diarrhea followed by decreased passage of manure, abdominal distension, and colic. **A,** Abdominal ultrasound examination of the calf showing markedly distended loops of small intestine. **B,** A section of jejunum that was removed because of severe adhesions obstructing the lumen of the jejunum. **C,** Anastomoses after resection. **D,** Postoperative treatment of the calf including a blood transfusion. The calf made a complete recovery with no complications.

3. Cecal distension or volvulus may lead to signs of mild to even severe colic. This colic can be as violent as that observed in small intestinal obstruction, although it is more common for the cow to be treading the hind feet and kicking at the abdomen only occasionally. Abdominal distension involves the upper and lower right quadrants, and rectal examination is diagnostic for cecal distension or volvulus. Small intestinal distension proximal to a cecal volvulus may contribute to the observed colic.

4. Occasionally, patients with a very large RDA or right-sided AV demonstrate moderate colic. A very large right-sided ping (extending from the paralumbar fossa cranially to beyond the 9th rib) is found, and there is no rectal or ultrasonographic evidence of small intestinal or cecal distension.

5. Uterine torsion during the middle or final trimester of pregnancy causes mild colic with treading of the hind limbs. Rectal and vaginal examination will confirm this diagnosis.

6. Hematomas of the mesentery may also manifest as acute colic, as can the very rare case of acute hemabdomen from other causes. In many of these cases, the life-threatening blood loss will provide a clinical and clinicopathologic picture of acute hemorrhagic shock (severe pallor, tachycardia, tachypnea, anemia) on top of the signs of pain. Rectal examination of cattle with mesenteric hematomas is nondiagnostic, and the ultrasound examination is frequently nonspecific, showing mild to moderate ileus but no significant small bowel distension. If intraabdominal hemorrhage is confined to the mesentery, then it can be impossible to see via transabdominal ultrasonography, but in cases of true hemabdomen a thorough ultrasound examination can be diagnostic (Fig. 5.92).

7. Organophosphate toxicity can cause colic secondary to hypermotility of the bowel.

Treatment

The only treatment for small bowel mechanical obstruction is right-sided exploratory laparotomy, identification of the anatomic malposition, and correction thereof. Because

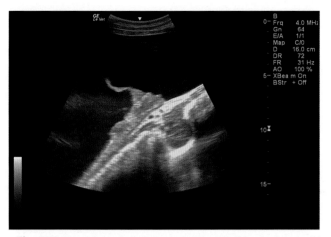

• **Fig. 5.92** Transabdominal ultrasound of the left side of a 5-year-old Holstein cow that presented with acute colic, anemia (packed cell volume, 13%), and mild abdominal distension. A large volume of swirling, anechoic fluid (hemorrhage) was identified between the rumen and left body wall. Transfusion and symptomatic care led to complete recovery.

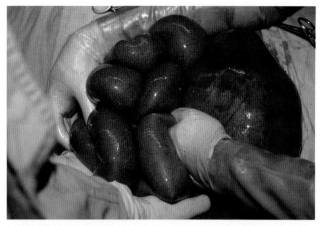

• **Fig. 5.93** Distended loops of a small intestine proximal to an intussusception in a cow.

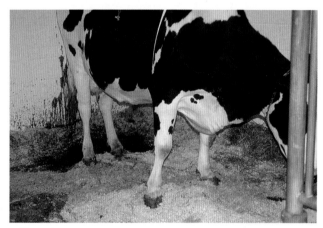

• **Fig. 5.94** "Bloody" manure passed from a "colicky" cow believed to have hemorrhagic bowel syndrome. The cow passed blood in the manure for less than 12 hours and then recovered after fluid therapy and flunixin.

the prognosis varies tremendously depending on the exact obstruction identified, economics may dictate slaughter as an option for affected cattle deemed of marginal value, advanced cases, or those rapidly approaching a shocklike state. If the value of the animal dictates surgical exploration, a decision regarding on-farm surgery versus referral must be reached. Small bowel surgery in cattle is difficult under the best of circumstances and often requires trained assistants or multiple surgeons when complications occur or bowel resection is required.

Before surgery or during preparation, IV fluids and analgesics such as flunixin meglumine (1.1 mg/kg) should be administered to help stabilize the patient. Calves should be positioned in left lateral recumbency. If laboratory facilities exist, acid–base and electrolyte status, PCV, and plasma proteins should be assessed preoperatively to assist fluid therapy recommendations. In complicated cases in which resection of bowel is anticipated, most surgeons prefer left lateral recumbency and general anesthesia for adult patients.

The small bowel should be examined or "run" from the duodenum to the ileum or vice versa to identify the exact anatomic lesion. Difficulties revolve around the large amount of dilated small bowel that often needs to be exteriorized, manipulated, and replaced or resected (Fig. 5.93). Excessive manipulation will lead to further intestinal injury and ileus. Some conditions such as abdominal fibrous bands, slight torsions of the mesentery, and volvulus of the distal flange require only anatomic repositioning or resection of the causative band.

Although several cows with HBS have survived with medical therapy (Fig. 5.94) or flank laparotomy (Fig. 5.95) and drainage of the clot without resection, the prognosis, even with surgery, is guarded. Dr. Peek has reported one of the highest survival rates (58%) and found manual massage of the clot provided a more favorable outcome than did enterotomy. Likewise, ileal impactions are best treated by laparotomy and massage of the ingesta into the cecum.

Other problems such as complete torsion of the mesentery (Fig. 5.96), mesenteric tears with entrapped bowel, volvulus of the intestine, and intussusception are more difficult and may require resection and anastomosis. Postoperatively, continued IV fluids, broad-spectrum antibiotics, calcium and potassium solutions, and judicious use of analgesics may be required. If resection and anastomosis have been necessary, broad-spectrum antibiotics should be used for 3 to 7 days. After resection and anastomosis and before final closure, some surgeons use peritoneal lavage of warm, balanced electrolyte solutions and bactericidal antibiotics.

The patient should begin to pass loose feces within 4 to 24 hours postoperatively. Intensive aftercare may be required, including colloid and crystalloid therapy and even partial parenteral nutrition in some cases, especially in calves. The major complications include further deterioration in blood flow and oxygenation of part of the small intestine, peritonitis, anastomosis breakdown, and adhesions that result in obstruction or abscess formation. A patient that maintains a normal temperature, has returning appetite, and continues to pass manure during the first 5 to 7 days postoperatively has a favorable prognosis.

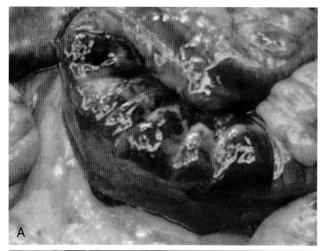

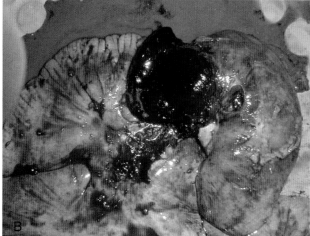

• **Fig. 5.95 A,** Small intestine at the time of surgery in a "colicky" cow with hemorrhagic bowel syndrome. **B,** Blood clot in the lumen of the intestine of the cow in **A.**

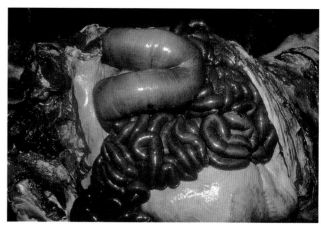

• **Fig. 5.96** Complete 360-degree torsion of the mesentery in a cow.

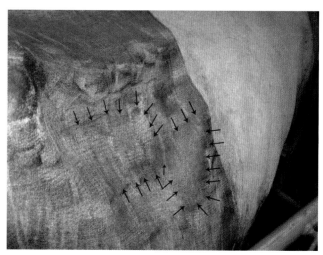

• **Fig. 5.97** Visibly distended viscus (spiral colon) in a 4-year-old Jersey cow with abdominal fat necrosis causing bowel obstruction. *Arrows* outline two segments of distended bowel that can be seen in the paralumbar fossa.

Miscellaneous Causes of Small Intestinal Obstruction

Fat Necrosis

Fat necrosis may be observed in any breed of cattle and is characterized by hard masses in the mesentery and omentum that gradually cause partial or complete extraluminal intestinal obstruction. Most commonly, rectal constriction occurs, establishing a risk for iatrogenic rectal injury during palpation. Affected cattle usually are overconditioned middle-aged to old animals. Before complete obstruction, affected cattle frequently have diarrhea, because the intestinal lumen is constricted from external pressure. Partial anorexia, loose manure followed by little or no manure, and occasional abdominal distension or mild colic (Fig. 5.97) characterize this vague illness. Hard masses associated with the omentum and mesentery and around the small intestine, rectum, or colon can sometimes be palpated per rectum to confirm a diagnosis of fat necrosis (Figs. 5.98 and 5.99).

The differential diagnosis includes lymphosarcoma, intestinal adenocarcinoma, and abdominal abscesses. It is worth

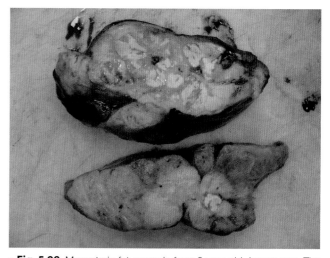

• **Fig. 5.98** Mesenteric fat necrosis from 8-year-old Jersey cow. The cow was presented with colic and abdominal distension alongside the absence of fecal production for 24 hours. Multiple, very firm masses were palpable per rectum; at postmortem examination, numerous areas of mesenteric and omental fat necrosis were identified.

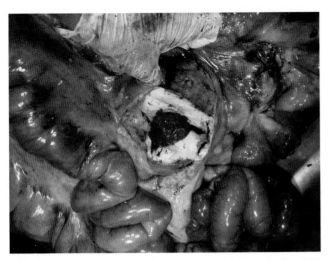

• **Fig. 5.99** Area of fat necrosis from same patient as in Fig. 5.98 encircling and extraluminally obstructing the distal colon.

emphasizing that lesions of fat necrosis feel exceptionally hard, even compared with neoplasia, on rectal palpation. In valuable cattle, ultrasound-guided biopsy or exploratory laparotomy and biopsy to confirm the disease may be warranted. The prognosis for cattle affected with fat necrosis usually is hopeless, but in rare cases localized masses have been identified that were amenable to resection and anastomosis of affected bowel. This disease is more common in fat, pastured beef cattle than in dairy cattle.

Neoplasia

Partial to complete intestinal obstruction has been observed in cattle affected with intestinal adenocarcinoma, lymphosarcoma, and, rarely, other tumors. Signs, as in fat necrosis, are vague. If obstruction becomes complete, abdominal distension and colic may be observed. Metabolic alkalosis can be marked in proximal small intestinal obstructions secondary to neoplasia. Physical examination may allow an index of suspicion for lymphosarcoma, but intestinal adenocarcinoma seldom is diagnosed short of exploratory laparotomy. If palpable per rectum, adenocarcinomas tend to be hard, but lymphosarcoma is merely firm and may have associated visceral lymphadenopathy. The prognosis is hopeless for lymphosarcoma and poor for adenocarcinoma unless all of the involved intestine can be resected.

Small Intestinal Lesions Associated with Reproductive Tract Pathology

Adhesions of the small intestine secondary to puncture of the dorsal cranial vagina by infusion pipettes most commonly occur when laypeople attempt to infuse the uterus of a recently postparturient or multiparous cow that has a uterus too heavy to retract. The ensuing chemical or bacterial peritonitis can involve the omental sling or small intestine through adhesions. Partial or full intestinal obstruction can result if extensive adhesions develop. Treatment consists

of systemic broad-spectrum antibiotics and time. The prognosis varies with the degree of adhesion present. The affected cow should have complete reproductive rest and only be palpated once monthly to assess and evaluate her condition.

Traumatic rupture of the small intestine during calving was described by Dr. John King, now deceased professor emeritus of pathology at the New York State College of Veterinary Medicine. Most of these cattle die within 24 hours after calving. Lesions consist of rupture of the small intestine with subsequent massive fibrinous peritonitis. Apparently, during labor and straining, a loop of bowel is trapped in the pelvic region by fetal pressure, and further pressure during fetal extraction leads to rupture.

At our hospital, we observed a multiparous cow that became anorectic and mildly colicky immediately after calving. The cow would tread with her hind feet, occasionally kicked at her abdomen, and preferred to lie down. She temporarily regained an appetite and continued to pass manure for 1 week in response to symptomatic therapy but then relapsed with reduced manure production, inappetence, colic, and fever. Small bowel distension was found on rectal palpation. Surgical exploration confirmed a localized perforation of the small intestine that the mesentery had walled off as an abscess. Resection of the affected bowel resulted in full recovery. It was theorized that during calving, this cow had experienced severe bruising and compromise of a loop of small bowel but the injury had not been sufficient for complete laceration.

Prolapse of the intestine through uterine rupture can follow dystocia or prolapse of the uterus. In general, the prognosis is hopeless, and the affected animal should be slaughtered. Heroic efforts may be indicated for valuable cattle, but the complicated surgery required, coupled with obvious peritonitis, makes survival unlikely.

Diseases of the Cecum and Proximal Colon

Cecal Dilatation and Volvulus
Etiology

Although much less common than abomasal disorders, cecal disorders constitute a common cause of GI dysfunction in dairy cattle.

Many of the same theories proposed to explain DA could be used to explain cecal dilatation or subsequent volvulus. Volatile fatty acid production occurs in the cecum just as in the abomasum.

Modern diets consisting of high concentrate and silage levels provide a large amount of substrate for volatile fatty acid production throughout the cow's GI tract, and hindgut fermentation and acidosis disorders have likely been underdiagnosed in the past in dairy cattle. Additional factors such as hypocalcemia, endotoxemia secondary to metritis or mastitis, and indigestion that result in GI ileus further predispose to cecal dilatation. In simple cecal dilatation, the cecum distends with gas and fluid to a variable degree and the apex begins to rise in the abdomen from its normal location toward or into the pelvic inlet. Further distension of the organ leads to rotation of the cecum, which tends to occur in a clockwise direction, as viewed from the right side, or a ventral or dorsal retroflexion. Although cecal dilatation–volvulus–retroflexion may occur at any stage of lactation or gestation, the majority of cases occur early in lactation at the same time as the peak of metabolic disorders and DAs. Cecal dilatation and volvulus also may occur in calves and bulls, especially those fed highly fermentable concentrate such as high moisture corn. Many experienced practitioners note that there are a surprising number of normal, healthy dairy cattle in which a mild to moderate degree of cecal dilatation can be palpated during routine reproductive examination, suggesting that the condition can be subclinical in some individuals.

Clinical Signs

Inappetence, reduced manure production, and mild to moderate abdominal distension are the usual complaints and initial observations in cattle affected with cecal dilatation. Milk production decreases commensurate with the appetite reduction. Affected cattle have a normal body temperature, respiratory rate, and a normal to slightly elevated heart rate. As cecal dilatation progresses, mild to moderate colic manifested by treading in the hind limbs or kicking at the abdomen may be observed. Rumen contractions weaken and become less frequent, and intestinal motility is decreased. A right-sided ping will be detected by simultaneous percussion and auscultation. This ping will develop in the right paralumbar fossa and may extend one to three rib spaces cranial to the fossa (Figs. 5.100 and 5.101). In advanced cases, the ping may extend into the mid- or ventral right caudal abdomen. Fluid may be detected by ballottement in a distended viscus within the right upper quadrant. Right-sided abdominal distension is often apparent when the cow is viewed from the rear or from the right side. In early cases, this distension causes the right paralumbar fossa to appear "full." In advanced cases, both the upper and lower right abdominal quadrants appear distended, and an outline of a portion of the body of the cecum and sometimes the ascending colon may be seen in the right paralumbar fossa. In cattle affected for more than 24 hours, or in severe cases, dehydration may be mild to moderate, and cool peripheral parts, suggesting hypocalcemia, may be apparent. Rectal examination provides the key to diagnosis because the dilated cecum is easily palpable in the right caudal abdomen in most cases, and frequently with cecal dilatation, the apex of the cecum is directed into the pelvic inlet such that the veterinarian palpates the organ or the ascending colon as soon as the wrist enters the rectum. If rotation of the body of the cecum has already occurred, more than one loop of cecum and spiral colon may be palpable rectally in the right and central caudal abdomen. A serum chloride concentration can also be

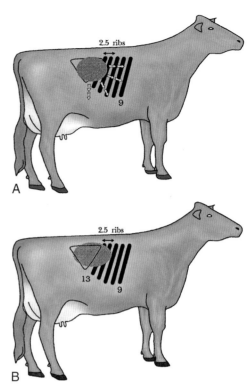

• **Fig. 5.100** **A,** Area of tympanic resonance and "ping" resulting from mild cecal dilatation. The size of the ping *(arrows)* may increase if cecal dilatation worsens or cecal volvulus is present. **B,** Ping associated with distension of the proximal or coiled colon.

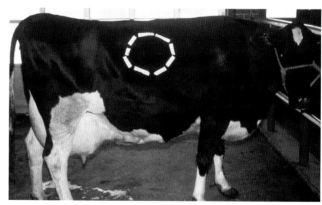

• **Fig. 5.101** Area of tympanic resonance in a cow with cecal dilatation. This ping includes the last three ribs and the cranial portion of the right paralumbar fossa. Rectal examination would be essential to differentiate cecal dilatation from benign colonic distension and right displacement of the abomasum or abomasal volvulus.

useful. Cattle with right-sided abomasal disorders typically are hypochloremic, but cattle with cecal disease do not usually have dramatic changes in serum chloride.

In those with cecal volvulus, the signs are more remarkable and obvious. Milk production, appetite, and manure production decrease dramatically. Affected cattle are moderately to severely dehydrated; have obvious right abdominal distension, ruminal distension, and stasis; have an elevated heart rate (80–100 beats/min); and have a large ping in the right caudal abdomen expanding from the paralumbar fossa cranially at least three rib spaces and often ventral to the

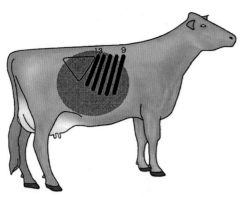

• **Fig. 5.102** Area of tympanic resonance or "ping" typical of very large cecal volvulus or abomasal volvulus.

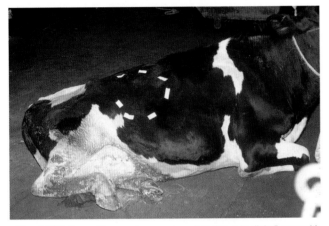

• **Fig. 5.103** Area of tympanic resonance (ping) in a "colicky" cow with cecal volvulus. Succussible fluid was easily detected in the right flank.

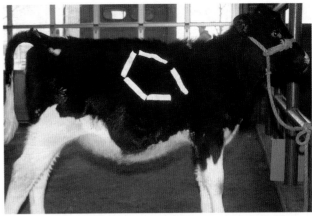

• **Fig. 5.104** Area of tympanic resonance in a calf with cecal dilatation. Because the calf was too small for rectal examination, it would have been difficult to differentiate cecal dilatation from right displacement of the abomasum because the area of ping extended from the cranial paralumbar fossa forward to rib nine.

paralumbar fossa. Additionally, fluid is easily detected by ballottement combined with auscultation. In some cases, the ping is so expansive that differentiation from AV is necessary (Fig. 5.102). Rectal examination reveals dilatation of the cecum with rotation or volvulus alongside dilatation of the proximal colon and may reveal a distended ileum because the cecal volvulus kinks the ileocecal region. Rectal examination also rules out the major differential diagnosis, AV. Ultrasound examination can help differentiate cases when it is not clear whether the problem is cecal volvulus or AV, or in those rare cases when the cecum cannot be identified upon rectal palpation (most likely ventral retroflexion). Small intestinal distension is present with cecal volvulus. Additionally, cows with cecal volvulus can be very colicky, which is less commonly the case in those with AV (Fig. 5.103).

In calves, right-sided abdominal distension, anorexia, greatly decreased manure production, dehydration, and an elevated heart rate (80–120 beats/min) characterize cecal dilatation and volvulus. A large ping may be detected over the right caudal (and sometimes simultaneously over the left) abdomen, including the right paralumbar fossa and several rib spaces cranial to the fossa (Fig. 5.104). Fluid may be heard to splash in a large viscus on ballottement of the right abdomen. Mild colic with treading, lying down, and kicking at the abdomen are common. Rectal examination

is not possible because of the size of the patient, and the condition may be difficult to differentiate from AV in animals of this age. Ultrasound examination is helpful in distinguishing between the two disorders. As in adult cattle, however, the uniform distension of the paralumbar fossa and the outline of a distended tubular viscus in the flank area suggest cecal distension. In contrast, AV usually causes a half-moon viscus distension projecting into the paralumbar fossa caudal to the right 13th rib. Of particular importance in calves is the fact that cecal dilatation or volvulus may progress to necrosis and peritonitis within a relatively short time (24–72 hours) because of the more fragile nature of the calf's intestinal tract. In such cases, fever and abdominal pain are detected in addition to the other clinical signs.

Laboratory Data

Laboratory data seldom are diagnostic in cecal distension or volvulus. Mild to moderate metabolic alkalosis is the rule because a physical obstruction of the GI tract has occurred. This obstruction may be partial in cecal distension, with mild alkalosis in some cases, or complete in cecal volvulus, with more dramatic metabolic alkalosis. Rumen chloride will be increased in some cases, possibly caused by the enlarging cecum compressing the duodenum. Metabolic acidosis only occurs in advanced cases of volvulus with bowel necrosis. Abdominal fluid is normal except in advanced cases, in which protein levels exceed normal limits because of vascular compromise and edema in the mesentery and cecum. In addition, rare calves that have cecal perforation or leakage will have abdominal fluid values consistent with peritonitis.

Differential Diagnosis

The major considerations in the differential diagnosis are RDA and right AV. In general, abomasal problems cause a more cranial ping and abdominal distension under the right rib cage rather than the caudal abdomen and paralumbar fossa. Adhesions and dilation of the spiral colon and a rare case of omasal dilatation may be confused with a cecal volvulus. Small intestinal obstruction should be considered in cattle passing no feces and showing signs of colic, but right-side abdominal distension is mild in adult cows with small intestinal obstruction (distension may be more pronounced in calves). Rectal examination should allow differentiation of these problems.

Treatment

For cecal patients with dilatation, the clinician must decide whether medical treatment will suffice or if a surgical exploratory procedure is necessary. The best candidates for medical therapy meet the following conditions:

1. Normal or slightly elevated heart rate and good general demeanor
2. Some manure production and appetite (usually for roughage)
3. Mild to nonexistent dehydration
4. Normal abdominal shape or only mild to moderate abdominal distension, with the cecal apex palpable in the pelvic inlet per rectum
5. Probable hypocalcemia, which may be easily treated

For these patients, medical treatment consists of daily laxative ruminotorics; transfaunation; rehydration if needed; calcium and potassium solutions as needed; and treatment of any concurrent problems such as ketosis, metritis, or mastitis. Daily laxatives seem more effective (clinical impression) when administered mixed with warm water using a stomach tube rather than merely as oral boluses. Increases in appetite, manure production, and milk production are positive signs after treatment. Highly fermentable feeds should either not be offered or be offered only in limited quantities. Treatment must continue for 3 to 7 days and should not be stopped after initial signs of improvement, lest relapse occurs. The cecal distension is monitored by rectal palpation or ultrasonography, and the organ seldom returns to normal size and position in less than 4 days. If the animal continues to improve, continued medical therapy usually resolves the problem. To avoid masking signs of abdominal pain, analgesics are not used.

The following clinical signs are present in patients with cecal dilatation, retroflexion or volvulus that require surgical intervention:

1. Cecal torsion or retroflexion of the cecum based on rectal palpation
2. Consistently elevated heart rate
3. Little or no manure production and appetite
4. Detectable dehydration
5. Moderate to marked abdominal distension with the cecum and proximal colon very distended when palpated per rectum; in some cases, only the distended colon can be palpated
6. Colic
7. Recurrent cecal dilatation that has been proved consistently refractory to medical therapy

Intravenous fluid therapy and IV flunixin meglumine (0.5–1.0 mg/kg) are administered preoperatively. Perioperative antibiotics are appropriate. Surgical treatment consists of right flank laparotomy followed by typhlotomy. A long

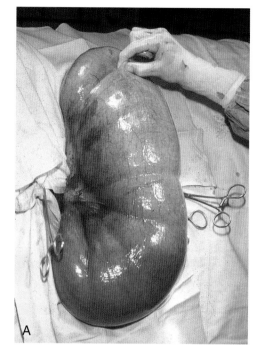
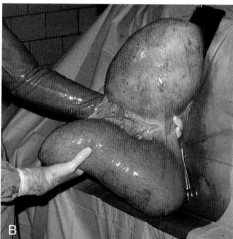

• **Fig. 5.105** **A,** Cecal dilatation as seen when the organ is exteriorized through a right flank laparotomy incision. **B,** The cecum (ventral) and proximal colon being exteriorized in a cow with cecal dilatation.

flank incision is indicated because the cecal diameter may approach 18 to 30 cm in severe cases, and delivery of this greatly distended organ into the incision is difficult if the incision is too small. On entry into the abdomen, the cecum is gas decompressed in situ by a needle attached to tubing and a suction apparatus. This alleviates some of the distension. After the cecum is externalized (Fig. 5.105), a typhlotomy at the apex should be performed (Fig. 5.106), the cecum emptied, the proximal colon and ileum "milked" of ingesta (Fig. 5.107), and a double-layer closure used for the typhlotomy.

In advanced cases with cecal necrosis or in patients with recurrent cecal dilatation or volvulus, a partial typhlectomy may be necessary. Complete typhlectomy in cattle is a difficult procedure because of the intimate apposition of the ileum to the cecal base, which is continuous with the

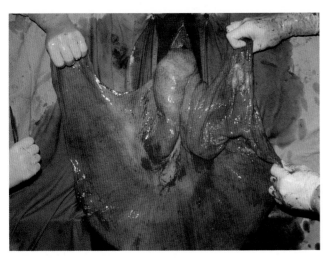

• **Fig. 5.106** A large flaccid cecum after typhlotomy for cecal volvulus in a cow. The apex of the cecum appears at the left, and the proximal colon appears in the right upper area.

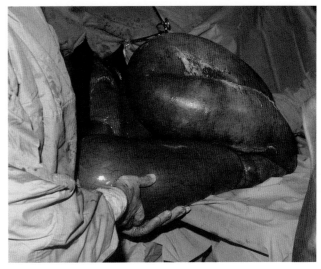

• **Fig. 5.108** Infarcted cecum and fibrin on the visceral peritoneum of the cecum in a cow affected with severe cecal volvulus. These lesions necessitated typhlectomy.

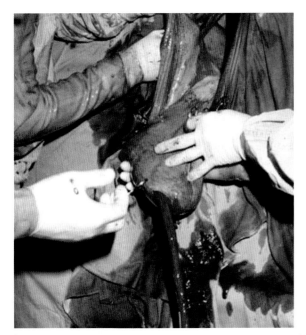

• **Fig. 5.107** Typhlotomy and cecal content drainage in a cow with cecal volvulus.

proximal colon. Therefore, in most instances, a partial typhlectomy removing the apex of the cecum and leaving the ileocecal region intact is performed to minimize the "balloon effect" and lessen the chances of future recurrences. In advanced cecal or cecocolic necrosis (Fig. 5.108), complete typhlectomy and ileocolic anastomosis is the only alternative. This is an extremely difficult procedure for all but the most experienced surgeon. However, typhlotomy, rather than the more complicated typhlectomy, usually is indicated for first-time surgical patients because recurrence rates for cecal dilatation with volvulus are only reported to be approximately 10%.

Postoperatively, supportive therapy with laxative ruminotoric mixtures can be given on a daily basis for several days,

and rectal palpation should be performed at 24- to 48-hour intervals to assess the degree of cecal distension. Loose manure for 48 hours is typical and desirable postoperatively. Antibiotic therapy is indicated for 3 to 7 days for typhlotomy patients, and broad-spectrum antibiotic therapy for 5 to 14 days is indicated for typhlectomy patients. Highly fermentable feeds should be reintroduced gradually. The prognosis is favorable for patients with cecal distension and volvulus. Complications include recurrence in approximately 10% of the patients and the possibility of peritonitis or adhesions in those that underwent complicated surgical procedures.

Hindgut Acidosis

Microbial fermentation of carbohydrates in the hindgut of dairy cattle is responsible for 5% to 10% of total-tract carbohydrate digestion. Gressley (2011) has suggested that when dietary factors cause abnormal, excessive flow of fermentable carbohydrates from the small intestine into the hindgut, hindgut acidosis can occur. The cecum does not have the protective factors of the rumen (saliva or a large protozoal population) to buffer excessive acid production associated with highly fermentable carbohydrate loads, and although hindgut acidosis occurs most commonly in association with subacute ruminal acidosis, it may also occur independently. Hindgut acidosis is characterized by increased rates of production of short-chain fatty acids, including lactic acid, decreased digesta pH, and damage to the gut epithelium as sometimes evidenced by the appearance of mucin casts in feces (Fig. 5.109). This hindgut acidosis may predispose to cecal dysfunction and allow translocation of endotoxins and amines from the cecum, causing systemic inflammatory responses and increasing the risk of laminitis. Clinical signs of hindgut acidosis are similar to those seen in subacute rumen acidosis, including reductions in feed intake, milk fat depression, and watery, foamy, and mucus-mixed

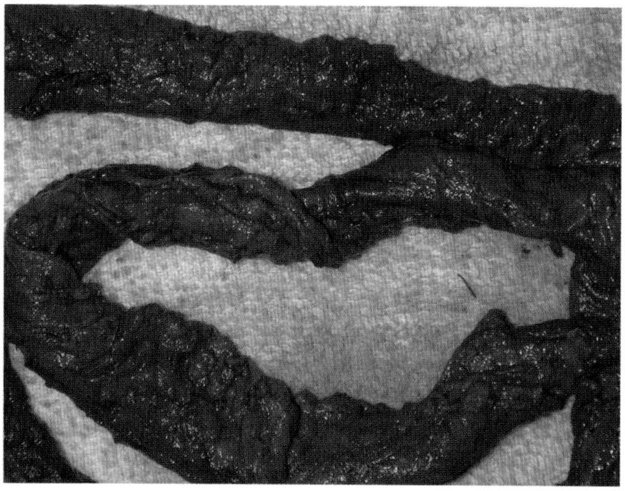

• **Fig. 5.109** Extensive intestinal mucin cast from adult Holstein with severe hindgut acidosis; the cow also passed a lot of undigested grain along with this remarkable cast.

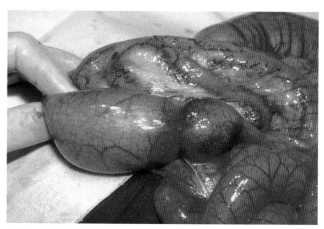

• **Fig. 5.110** Intussusception of the descending colon in a 2-week-old Holstein calf. The calf had diarrhea for 3 days and then an acute onset of colic and sudden absence of feces. On ultrasound examination, the cecum was distended with fluid. Surgery with intestinal resection and anastomosis was successful.

feces, indicating excessive fermentation in the hindgut. Large amounts of undigested grain may be observed in the manure. Prevention of hindgut acidosis includes feeding diets with higher particle size, such as diets high in forage and lower in grain, in hopes of decreasing excessive flow of fermentable substrates to the hindgut.

Colonic Obstructions

Colonic obstructions are sporadic in dairy cattle. In general, they are caused by regional inflammation resulting in adhesions or by masses. Intraperitoneal injections through the right paralumbar fossa are one cause of nonseptic or septic peritonitis that can result in partial or complete colonic obstruction. Concentrated dextrose solutions injected in this fashion are capable of inducing significant chemical peritonitis, resulting in adhesions and intestinal obstruction. Any intraperitoneal injection that penetrates the duodenum or proximal colon can allow leakage of ingesta with localized septic peritonitis and similar signs of obstruction. Fever is usually present in patients with septic peritonitis. Similar inflammation or abscessation occasionally results from previous surgical procedures performed through the right flank, perimetritis, rupture of the uterus, or rectal perforation and peritonitis.

Spiral colon intussusception can also occur in calves (but not adults) and should be considered in those with diarrhea that suddenly pass no manure and exhibit progressive abdominal distension (Fig. 5.110). Calves with small colon obstruction will have fluid distension of the cecum that can be easily visualized by ultrasound examination. Space-occupying masses such as fat necrosis or neoplasia also may result in colonic obstruction in mature animals (see Fig. 5.99).

Clinical Signs

Cattle affected with colonic obstructions have vague signs of anorexia, low-volume production of loose manure, and decreased milk production. If the obstruction is complete,

abdominal distension may be present. A ping is present in the right paralumbar fossa consistent with colonic or cecal distension. In cattle that have had intraperitoneal injections, the history may be helpful, and "needle tracks" with dried blood matting the hair below the injection site may be observed in the right paralumbar fossa. Rectal examination determines whether distended proximal colon, cecum, or fibrinous or fibrous adhesions are present. Fever often is present in those cattle with localized septic peritonitis. Rectal examination and ultrasonography also are beneficial in the diagnosis of fat necrosis because hard masses may be palpated or imaged in the right upper abdominal quadrant. In calves with spiral colon intussusception, a large homogeneous fluid-filled cecum can be visualized on ultrasound examination.

Treatment

In cattle with injection reaction obstructions, immediate therapy is symptomatic and consists of antibiotics, anti-inflammatories and analgesics. If this regimen is not successful after several days of treatment, a right paralumbar fossa exploratory celiotomy is indicated. Adhesions of the visceral colonic peritoneum and parietal peritoneum should be anticipated and a decision reached as to the practicality or feasibility of surgical bypass of the lesion. A similar determination is required for cattle affected with fat necrosis. An advantage of "simple" colonic obstruction compared with that associated with fat necrosis is that there are generally no other lesions of an obstructive nature affecting the GI tract; unfortunately, there may well be multiple areas of fat necrosis such that a thorough exploratory or consideration of potential progression of currently unobstructive lesions in the future must be made. Fat necrosis tends to be progressive over time.

Prognosis

Unless medical therapy alleviates the signs of obstruction, the prognosis is poor. Colonic bypass surgery is technically difficult, and only extremely valuable animals are candidates.

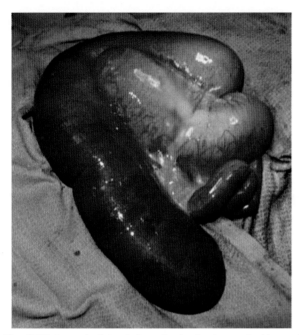

• **Fig. 5.111** Severely distended proximal colon in a calf with atresia coli.

The prognosis for cattle affected with fat necrosis that causes rectal or colonic obstruction is extremely poor.

Atresia Coli

Atresia coli is the most frequent congenital intestinal malformation of dairy calves, affecting mainly the ascending colon at the level of the spiral loop. This sporadic congenital defect results in complete obstruction of the GI tract, and signs usually appear by 1 to 3 days of age. Unfortunately, many cases are not brought to the veterinarian's attention until day 4 or 5, or later. The etiology is unknown, but damage from early pregnancy palpation of the embryo has long been suggested as a possibility. However, a strong counterargument to this is provided by reliable information on several cases in affected calves that were never palpated as early embryos. Comparative literature suggests compromised vasculature during early embryogenesis as a likely cause.

Clinical Signs

Abdominal distension (Fig. 5.111) and absence of manure production signal this diagnosis. The anal sphincter and rectum appear normal, which distinguishes the condition from atresia ani. The owner may report some early passage of mucus after birth followed by no manure after that time. Affected calves appear normal at birth and are usually willing to drink colostrum. Within 24 to 72 hours, however, they go off feed, with rapid development of abdominal distension and depression, and begin to dehydrate. Rarely, a calf will remain apparently healthy for 5 to 7 days. Calves with atresia coli usually have a normal temperature, elevated heart rate, and detectable fluid on ballottement of the right lower quadrant. Colic may be observed. The differential diagnoses for atresia coli in calves also includes atresia recti (discussed later) and a rare case of atresia jejuni.

Laboratory Data

Blood work to evaluate PCV and plasma proteins is indicated, as are acid–base and electrolyte analyses. Some assessment of passive transfer of immunoglobulins also should be made before treatment, because many calves with atresia coli have inadequate immunoglobulin levels despite proper and timely administration of colostrum. This observation suggests compromised absorption directly or indirectly associated with the atresia. If fever is present, an abdominal paracentesis may be indicated.

Treatment

The only treatment is to bypass the defect surgically by anastomosing the proximal spiral colon to the descending colon distal to the atresia. Excessive attempts to determine colonic patency by means of passage of tubes or probes into the rectum are contraindicated. Before surgery, the calf may need to be stabilized with fluid and electrolyte supplementation, glucose, plasma or whole blood (if failure of passive transfer has occurred), and antibiotic therapy. The surgical procedure has been described in a number of surgical texts (see Fubini and Ducharme, *Farm Animal Surgery*, 2nd edition). Technical difficulties include possible anatomic confusion and the anastomosis of a relatively large-diameter section of proximal colon to the small-diameter descending colon. The major surgical complication is peritonitis, but medical complications such as neonatal enteritis, pneumonia, or septicemia also are possible. Electrolyte imbalances such as hyponatremia may also occur in association with the reintroduction of milk; this seems to be random and the cause is not known. Lidocaine is sometimes used as a CRI for ileus, but newborn calves have delayed hepatic metabolism of lidocaine, and toxic levels can result, causing seizures. We have observed this on two occasions when the "standard" equine dose for treating ileus was used. Both calves recovered within hours following treatment with diazepam to control seizures and discontinuing the lidocaine CRI.

The survival rate is probably no better than 50% even in the hands of an experienced surgeon. Therefore, only extremely valuable calves should be treated. If owners elect treatment, referral to surgeons experienced in this repair is highly recommended. Calves with a good prognosis have great appetite and pass manure soon after surgery. Calves that have ileus and abdominal distension and pass limited manure may "linger" but have a guarded to poor prognosis. There do not seem to be any motility drugs that are of benefit in these calves. Growth rates may be compromised, at least initially, in some animals that do survive the surgery.

Benign Distension of the Proximal Colon
Etiology

Benign distension of the proximal colon results in gas and fluid accumulation in the proximal colon with a subsequent ping detected in the right paralumbar fossa region. The extent of this ping varies (Fig. 5.112) but includes the right paralumbar fossa and in some cases reaches two to three rib spaces cranial to the paralumbar fossa. The location of this ping leads to confusion

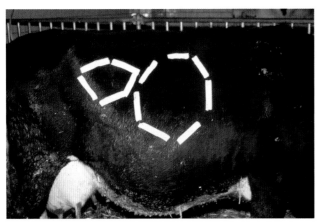

• **Fig. 5.112** Two distinct areas of tympanic resonance in a cow affected with right displacement of the abomasum but also having benign colonic distension (caudal area). Ileus or passage of some gas and fluid from the displaced abomasum into the lower gastrointestinal tract during transportation may have resulted in the benign colonic distension in this case.

in differential diagnosis, and many cattle with benign colonic distension are diagnosed erroneously as having RDA or cecal dilatation. In fact, benign distension of the proximal colon simply reflects GI stasis, which may occur in septic or endotoxic conditions or due to hindgut acidosis or as a result of a primary GI obstruction. Because the region of this ping can overlap that of a cecal dilatation, a rectal examination should be performed to rule out cecal dilatation. In cattle with benign proximal colonic distension, rectal palpation reveals mild to undetectable colonic distension. If palpable at all, the loops of colon are fluctuant and soft rather than pathologically distended. In addition, there is no external right-sided abdominal distension.

This syndrome usually occurs as a secondary consequence of GI stasis and is not a primary diagnosis. After rectal examination confirms this finding, the animal must be reassessed and a different primary diagnosis sought. Despite the caudal location of the ping associated with benign distension of the proximal colon, this ping is commonly misdiagnosed as an RDA. It must be emphasized that the RDA ping extends cranial to at least the ninth or even eighth ribs, unlike a benign proximal colon ping, which never extends more than three rib spaces cranial to the right paralumbar fossa.

Occasionally, pings associated with the proximal and descending duodenum occur when small intestinal obstruction, ileus or recent DA has been present. This distension causes a ping along the course of the duodenum as illustrated in Fig. 5.113. This ping is most obvious in cattle that have been rolled or recently transported to correct a preexisting LDA.

Diseases of the Descending Colon and Rectum

Extraluminal Compression of the Rectum
Etiology
Extraluminal compression of the rectum occasionally may accompany pelvic inflammatory or mass lesions. Signs are

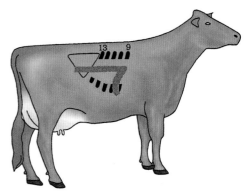

• **Fig. 5.113** Ping resulting from distension of the proximal and descending duodenum.

disparate because of variable underlying causes, but straining to defecate and narrow liquid streams of feces are observed in most cases, regardless of other specific signs. The most common diseases that cause extraluminal rectal compression are listed in Table 5.3 alongside diagnostic aids, treatments, and prognoses. Pelvic adhesions caused by rectal or vaginal injury during natural service are unusual in dairy cattle because of the preferential use of artificial insemination. However, occasional breeding accidents or injury may occur in heifers when dairy farms use bulls at pasture or in free stalls. Unless egregious and visibly witnessed, they do not come to veterinary attention until subsequent reproductive examination and palpation, by which time the adhesions are often mature and reproductively catastrophic. Postinjury hematomas and abscesses are also possible under such circumstances.

Diagnosis
Rectal examination confirms the diagnosis in most cases. It may be difficult to differentiate lymphosarcoma from fat necrosis unless other signs of lymphosarcoma are found during the physical examination. Reproductive ultrasonography can be useful to better characterize any pelvic or caudal abdominal masses that have been palpated during a conventional rectal examination and to evaluate the ultrasonographic appearance and echogenicity of any contents. A history of recent calving, presence of fever, and rectal and vaginal examinations confirm perimetritis. Pelvic abscesses may result from dystocia, uterine perforation during infusion with a pipette, or *T. pyogenes* abscesses that have ascended the lymphatics from deep musculoskeletal abscesses in the hind limb.

Vaginal examination should be performed to ascertain whether adhesions exist between the pelvic masses and the vagina. If adhesions are present, diagnostic aspiration, biopsies, and subsequent surgical drainage of abscesses may be performed through the vaginal wall. If adhesions between the mass lesions and vagina are absent, caudal flank abdominal exploratory surgery is necessary to confirm the diagnosis and attempt drainage of the abscess.

Postparturient pelvic hematomas are extremely common in primiparous cattle and possible in multiparous cattle. Dystocia is the usual cause. Hematomas can be singular or

TABLE 5.3 Causes of Extraluminal Compression of the Rectum

Disease	Diagnostic fetaures/findings	Treatment	Prognosis
Fat necrosis	Diffuse hard masses surrounding rectum on rectal examination	None	Hopeless
Lymphosarcoma	Firm masses in pelvis, often associated with the reproductive tract or pelvic lymph node enlargement	None	Hopeless
Perimetritis	Firm uniform pelvic soft tissue swelling; most prominent ventral to the rectum associated with reproductive tract but also surrounding the rectum and restricting movement Fever Occurs within a few days after parturition (usually with a history of dystocia)	Intensive systemic antibiotics and analgesics	Poor
Abscesses	Rectal findings of large fluctuant or firm masses attached to reproductive tract or associated pelvic lymph nodes	Drainage Antibiotics Iodides	Fair to good with drainage; poor for multiple abscesses
Hematomas	Firm, often multiple masses within the pelvis Dystocia in history Very common in heifers	Rest	Good; most resolve in 30–60 days

multiple and may be found at any location in the pelvic region, although most occur in the ventral or lateral pelvic areas. Treatment is not necessary. Rarely, a massive hematoma may develop secondary to dystocia and cause severe anemia and rectal compression.

Laboratory Aids

In confusing cases, ancillary aids such as cytology from aspirates or biopsies may be indicated. Serum globulin levels usually are elevated in cattle affected with pelvic abscesses. Although laboratory aids seldom are necessary in patients with perimetritis, in severe cases, the acute overwhelming infection usually results in a degenerative left shift in the hemogram, elevated fibrinogen, and a decrease in serum albumin secondary to protein loss into the massive cellulitis.

Treatment

Pelvic abscesses causing extraluminal rectal compression have a fair to good prognosis depending on location. In singular large abscesses, drainage may be attempted per vagina, assuming solid adhesions to the vagina exist, or via laparotomy. Appropriate systemic antibiotics should be administered after drainage. Penicillin at 22,000 U/kg once or twice daily is suitable when *T. pyogenes* is isolated from the abscesses. Organic iodide powder may be fed at 1 oz/day for 2 to 3 weeks for its nonspecific antimicrobial activity in thick-walled abscesses. If drainage is not possible without contamination of the peritoneal cavity, the prognosis is poor, but long-term penicillin therapy (3–6 weeks) and oral iodide powder for a similar length of time may be tried. The addition of rifampin to the antibiotic regimen may also be considered to improve abscess penetration, although this represents extralabel drug use. Currently, in the United States the use of rifampin requires the client to guarantee that neither milk nor meat from that animal will ever enter the human food

chain and so its use is discouraged. Furthermore, the absorption of the drug is variable, and the drug is quite expensive.

Treatment of perimetritis is not highly successful but includes broad-spectrum intensive antibiotic therapy to control the mixed bacterial flora likely found in such cases. Analgesics such as flunixin meglumine also are indicated.

The prognosis for lymphosarcoma and fat necrosis is hopeless. Pelvic hematomas require no treatment other than rest and once-monthly rectal palpation to assess resolution. Most resolve within 30 to 60 days after freshening. Rarely, massive hematomas that cause anemia may require whole-blood transfusions and carry a poor prognosis.

Rectal Lacerations

Etiology

Rectal lacerations result from ignorant roughness by neophyte examiners, frustrated or angry attempts at palpation on poorly restrained animals, and sadism. Occasional rectal lacerations have been blamed on inadvertent penile damage to the rectum during attempts at natural breeding. Inexperienced examiners cause most rectal lacerations. Although rectal lacerations are much less common in cattle than in horses, they occur frequently enough to emphasize the need for gentle, well-lubricated rectal palpation. Plastic sleeves are to blame for some of the rectal lacerations that occur in dairy cattle. Neophyte examiners should be trained with rubber gloves and sleeves; it is easier to palpate carefully and gently with a rubber glove than with a plastic sleeve. Even experienced examiners using plastic sleeves often inadvertently cause rectal mucosal irritation and bleeding that might have been avoided with the use of more lubricant, more patience, and a glove worn over the rectal sleeve.

Rectal lacerations in cows generally are not graded, as are equine rectal tears, but a simple classification system would include mucosal injuries, submucosal and muscular layer injuries, and full-thickness injuries. Fortunately, the latter are extremely rare.

Clinical Signs

If rectal laceration occurs during rectal examination, signs are immediately apparent in the form of fresh blood on the sleeve as it is withdrawn from the rectum and subsequent tenesmus. If the veterinarian has not been present for the causative rectal examination, subsequent signs will depend on the depth of the rectal injury and the time elapsed since injury. In injuries of less than full thickness, tenesmus, inappetence, and blood-stained fecal material may be present. Attempts at repeated rectal examination in cattle with preexisting rectal tears will be greatly resisted with tenesmus and often bellowing. Partly because of the association with persistent tenesmus but also because of the obvious requirement for prior rectal palpation, veterinarians should be prepared for considerable pneumorectum to complicate the initial assessment of significant rectal injury. Patience, epidural anesthesia, and only the most careful attempts to manually resolve this pneumorectum are advised.

In full-thickness injuries, the cow will become febrile, with GI ileus, tachycardia, and an arched stance. Septic peritonitis has occurred, and if the rectal tear communicates fully with the peritoneal cavity, the cow will usually die within 24 hours. In heifers that are examined and sent back to pasture, where they are not closely observed, apparent sudden death may occur, and the exact cause will escape detection unless a necropsy is performed. If a full-thickness rectal tear remains retroperitoneal, the cow will still typically be febrile, have tenesmus, stand with an arched stance, and have GI ileus. Again, rectal palpation will be greatly resisted. These animals will survive longer (2–7 days) than cattle with full-thickness lacerations directly entering the peritoneal cavity, but death is still the usual outcome.

Diagnosis

Unless present for the causative injury, the veterinarian may not be confident of a diagnosis until a rectal examination is done. As soon as the rectal injury is palpated or suspected by the rapid appearance of blood on the examiner's sleeve and severe tenesmus, the rectal examination should be terminated. For obvious reasons most tears occur in the floor of the rectum. The veterinarian should administer epidural anesthesia immediately and perform a gentle rectal examination using either a rubber sleeve or a bare arm with plenty of lubrication. The extent of the injury then can be palpated gently and a diagnosis and prognosis reached. If no history of previous rectal examination exists and there is no possibility of a natural service breeding accident, the veterinarian must keep in mind the possibility of sadism and decide judiciously if and when to discuss this with the owner and authorities. Ultrasonography can be very valuable in assessing the presence and extent of peritoneal effusion and ileus involving more proximal intestine.

Treatment

If only mucosal injury has occurred, rest from rectal examinations for a minimum of 1 week along with laxative feeds (silage or green chop) are indicated. Epidural anesthesia may be required for 24 to 48 hours in some cases with extreme tenesmus. Epidural catheters can be easily placed in cattle and offer an easy route for repeated administration of lidocaine. The prognosis is favorable.

If the injury extends to submucosal or muscular layers, rest from rectal examinations for a minimum of 1 month and provision of a laxative diet are imperative. Broad-spectrum antibiotics might be considered for these cases because of the risk of bacterial translocation. Again, epidural anesthesia may be required for 1 to 4 days to minimize tenesmus in individual cattle that strain excessively such that they refuse feed and water because of the vicious cycle of straining–more pain–straining.

After 1 month of rest, an experienced examiner should perform a rectal examination and assess rectal integrity. The prognosis is often favorable, but only an experienced veterinarian should palpate such cows in the future. If full-thickness rectal lacerations communicate with the peritoneal cavity, the cow should be slaughtered, because fecal material will have entered the abdomen, and the prognosis is hopeless. If full-thickness rectal lacerations communicate with the retroperitoneal space in the pelvic region, the prognosis is usually poor. However, some cattle with small full-thickness rectal lacerations in this area have healed after systemic broad-spectrum antibiotics, a very laxative diet, and rest from rectal examinations. The laxative diet and species difference in fecal consistency preclude the necessity for flushing or manual evacuation of the injured area free of impacted fecal material as might be necessary in a horse with a similar injury.

Rectovaginal Constriction in Jersey Cattle

Rectovaginal constriction is a simple, autosomal recessive defect that results in constriction at the anorectal region and vulva–vestibule region. Fibrous tissue at these areas prevents rectal examinations and leads to dystocia. Jersey cattle with this defect also appear especially prone to severe parturient udder edema.

Atresia Ani

Atresia ani is seldom encountered in dairy cattle. Affected calves show signs shortly after birth because they are unable to pass manure. Abdominal distension, depression, colic, tenesmus, and weakness will be observed if the condition is undiagnosed until 24 hours or more after birth. The rectal lumen usually bulges subcutaneously in the normal region of the anus when the abdomen is compressed. Although simple cutaneous puncture often allows fecal passage, these incisions often become fibrosed leading to anal stricture, tenesmus, and abdominal distension. A rectal pull-through procedure has been advocated for best long-term results. Although heritability has not been documented, the ethics of performing this procedure in an animal with breeding potential are questionable. We have also seen this condition in dairy breeds co-present with congenital defects of the external genitalia.

Rectovaginal Fistula

Rectovaginal fistula is a congenital condition that may occur either solely or more commonly with atresia ani in calves. It can, of course, occur, as can more distal, communicating perineal defects, as an acquired condition subsequent to dystocia. Surgical repair of post dystocia rectovaginal fistula is described in the 2nd edition of *Farm Animal Surgery* edited by Drs. Fubini and Ducharme.

Constipation

Constipation is uncommon in cattle and, when observed, generally points to neurologic deficits or painful conditions that interfere with defecation. Neurologic conditions often are associated with trauma to the sacral area or severe spinal cord damage that results in atony and hypoalgesia of the anus. Possible causes of nontraumatic caudal spinal cord injury include lymphosarcoma, neurofibroma, and ascending cauda equina myelitis associated with tail head cellulitis secondary to perivascular leakage of irritant drugs intended for coccygeal administration. Poor aseptic technique during repeated epidural administration is another possible cause of ascending myelitis.

Fractures of the base of the tail involving the sacrococcygeal junctional area may cause severe enough pain or neurologic defects to result in the cow showing signs of constipation. The most common cause of tail fractures in cattle is being ridden by other cows or bulls during standing estrus. Sadistic tail restraint that fractures the tail may also cause severe pain, constipation, tail head swelling, and flaccidity of the tail.

Treatment for tail fractures is symptomatic in most cases and includes analgesics, antiinflammatories, and laxative diets. Aspirin (240–480 grains orally twice daily), flunixin meglumine (1 mg/kg IV), or meloxicam (0.5 mg/kg orally once daily) may be used for analgesia for 3 to 5 days. Systemic dexamethasone (10–30 mg IM once daily) or epidural administration of 5 mg of dexamethasone may be helpful in acute cases (if the animal is not pregnant) to help reduce inflammation in the spinal nerves. Permanent tail paralysis may persist and result in a soiled perineum and tail, as well as possible vulvovaginal fecal contamination, which interferes with fertility. Surgical repair may be possible for show animals or very valuable breeding animals in which a fractured tail would be cosmetically unacceptable or potentially interfere with breeding.

Pneumorectum

Pneumorectum may be caused by conformational defects in the perineum, rectovaginal lacerations after dystocia, dyspnea, tenesmus for any reason, or rectal examination allowing air to enter the rectum. Pneumorectum usually does not require treatment because it does not cause illness unless it persists and becomes severe, in which case one or more epidurals may

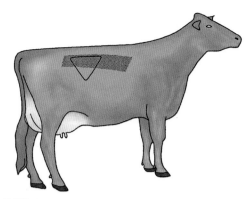

• **Fig. 5.114** Area of typical tympanic resonance associated with a pneumorectum "ping".

be needed as treatment. Cows can get into a vicious cycle of "sucking" air and straining until they become anorectic; Dr. Whitlock called this malignant tenesmus. When a rectal examination is essential for diagnostic purposes (e.g., pregnancy) in a cow affected with pneumorectum, the examiner must know how to gently evacuate the air from the rectum. This may be accomplished by a gentle sweeping of the rectum until a contraction band can be grasped and pulled caudally to express the air from the rectum. The procedure may need to be repeated several times to complete evacuation and is quite successful except in instances of severe rectal irritation and tenesmus.

Persistent air sucking and tenesmus may occur in some cows after rectal palpation, although no rectal laceration has occurred; this appears to be particularly common in cows with retained placenta or vaginal injury after calving but can occur in almost any cow after rectal palpation.

Repeated lidocaine epidurals, lidocaine infused into the rectum, and appropriate treatment of vaginal or cervical irritation are often required to break the cycle.

Pneumorectum can also result in a right-sided abdominal ping that may be confused with other causes of right-sided abdominal distension (Fig. 5.114). Because the rectum traverses the right upper abdominal quadrant, the ping occurs from the tuber coxae through the right paralumbar fossa and extends a variable distance cranially. The ping may extend to the dorsal midline. Although this finding creates a broad differential diagnosis (cecal distension, benign colonic distension, pneumoperitoneum) based on external percussion and auscultation, rectal examination should quickly identify pneumorectum and rule out other causes of tympanic resonance.

Miscellaneous Abdominal Disorders

Pneumoperitoneum

Etiology

Pneumoperitoneum is defined as the presence of air or free gas in the peritoneal cavity. Although the most common cause of this condition is laparotomy, particularly flank surgery, other causes such as perforation or rupture of distended abdominal organs may result in pneumoperitoneum. Clinically appreciable pneumoperitoneum appears to be more commonly associated with abomasal perforation rather than traumatic

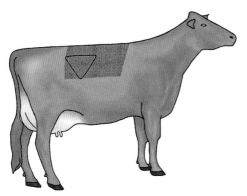

• **Fig. 5.115** Area of tympanic resonance associated with a right-sided pneumoperitoneum "ping".

TABLE 5.4	How to Differentiate Pneumoperitoneum from Other Pings	
Side	**Key Aid**	
Left		
Ruminal tympany	Rectal examination or stomach tube	
Rumen collapse	Rectal examination No abdominal distension in rumen collapse	
Right		
Cecal dilatation	Rectal examination—not bilateral	
Benign colonic distension	Rectal examination—not bilateral—no abdominal distension in benign colonic distension	
Pneumorectum	Rectal examination	
Right abomasal displacement (RDA)	Fluid present in RDA (ballottement) and RDA located midabdomen and cranial rather than dorsal third, as in pneumoperitoneum	

perforation of the reticulum. Pneumothorax or pneumomediastinum also occasionally progresses to involve the abdomen, thereby creating air either in the retroperitoneal space as detected by rectal exam or true pneumoperitoneum.

Clinical Signs

Pneumoperitoneum causes mild to marked bilateral abdominal distension and a ping bilaterally in the upper third of the abdomen extending to the dorsal midline (Fig. 5.115). Although more easily heard on the right side because of the rumen mass filling the left abdomen, this ping generally is detectable to some degree on both sides. Fluid is not present when ballottement of the abdomen is performed over the area of the ping. When rectal examination is performed, the examiner will find the rectum uniformly compressed against the hand and arm by the pressure of air free in the peritoneal cavity. It is difficult or impossible to grasp structures through the wall of the rectum such that the examiner must just "touch" various organs with the fingertips. The rumen is difficult to palpate or auscultate through the left paralumbar fossa because free air lies between the parietal peritoneum and visceral peritoneum of the rumen.

Although these signs are present in all cases of pneumoperitoneum, other concurrent signs will be specific for distinct causes of pneumoperitoneum. For example, fever and abdominal pain also will exist in cattle with pneumoperitoneum secondary to a displaced abomasum that has developed a perforating ulcer. Cattle with pneumoperitoneum of originally thoracic origin would be dyspneic in addition to showing the aforementioned signs. Uterine perforation during dystocia and penetrating abdominal wounds are other causes of pneumoperitoneum that would have additional distinct signs or historical features.

Diagnosis

The diagnosis is made by physical examination and rectal findings. This disorder must be differentiated from other causes of abdominal distension by careful auscultation or percussion and rectal evaluation (Table 5.4). When the ping is present bilaterally, there seldom should be confusion. If a cow has had laparotomy surgery recently, the cause should be obvious. A cow with LDA or RDA that suddenly develops signs of pneumoperitoneum and fever should be suspected of having a perforating abomasal ulcer.

Treatment

In mild cases of pneumoperitoneum after exploratory surgery, no treatment is necessary. In moderate to severe cases, affected cattle have such severe distension that discomfort and lack of appetite may result. Therefore, the free air in the abdomen should be evacuated by suction through needle puncture in the right paralumbar fossa. Introduction of a 1.5- or 2-inch needle perpendicular to the abdominal wall will usually suffice. The needle can be attached to a portable suction machine to speed evacuation of the air.

If pneumoperitoneum and fever are present in cattle with a recent history or physical signs of LDA or RDA, surgery through the ventral right paramedian approach should be performed in an effort to secure the abomasum and oversew the perforating ulcer (Fig. 5.116). Some cattle will remain displaced to the left or right after the perforation has occurred, allowing adhesions of the displaced abomasum to the parietal peritoneum. In these cattle, the typical ping and fluid content of a displaced abomasum will be present along with the signs of pneumoperitoneum and fever. The pneumoperitoneum may mask or confuse the diagnosis of DA in such instances until the air is evacuated through aspiration or at surgery (Fig. 5.117). Localized abdominal pain also may be present in the area of the displacement when perforation coexists. Right paramedian laparotomy to best gain access to the abomasum is recommended, but the prognosis is guarded because the abomasum may be affixed to the body wall by fibrinous adhesions and is prone to rupture or leak contents through the perforating ulcer when surgical manipulations detach the organ from the body wall. Systemic and peritoneal lavage antibiotics are indicated as supportive therapy.

Prevention

Prevention of severe pneumoperitoneum is only possible for animals at risk secondary to exploratory laparotomy and is

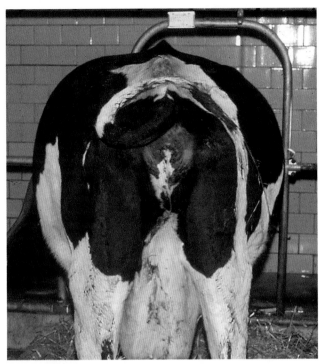

• **Fig. 5.116** Pneumoperitoneum in a cow that historically had simple left displacement of the abomasum before shipment to our hospital. The cow had fever present at admission as well. Immediate surgical exploration from the right paramedian approach confirmed a small perforating abomasal ulcer, which was oversewn and an abomasopexy performed.

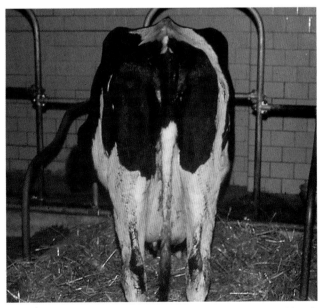

• **Fig. 5.117** Postoperative view of the cow shown in Fig. 5.116; this animal made a full recovery after surgery and supportive antibiotic therapy.

accomplished by an attendant pushing on the opposite side of the cow's abdomen to evacuate the air before final closure of the peritoneal sutures by the surgeon. Rapid identification and correction of simple DA can help prevent a chronically displaced abomasum from developing a concurrent ulcer with subsequent pneumoperitoneum and localized peritonitis.

Uncommon Causes of Peritonitis

Well-known causes of peritonitis in dairy cows include traumatic reticuloperitonitis, perforating abomasal ulcers, improperly performed blind tack and toggle-pin procedures, and uterine rupture following dystocia. Less frequent causes of peritonitis exist, but because of both their rare occurrence and high mortality rate, discussion of these will be limited.

Small Intestinal Rupture

Small intestinal rupture results in rapid clinical deterioration and often appears as sudden death. It may be observed in neonatal calves that apparently have been stepped on by their dam or other adult cows. It also occurs in adult cattle during parturition when a loop of small intestine is entrapped and subsequently squeezed between the maternal pelvis and the fetus within the birth canal.

Uterine Perforation by Pipette Injury

Pipette injuries of the uterus result in peritonitis or abscessation involving the uterus and are caused by neophytic or overaggressive attempts at uterine infusion, especially when attempting to infuse a cow suffering from septic metritis less than 2 weeks post partum when the cervix and uterus cannot possibly be elevated into the pelvis for routine infusion. This lesion is typically non–life threatening, but it can limit the animal's future reproductive use and value.

Vaginal Perforation

Perforation of the vagina has been observed after natural mating, pipette injuries, dystocia, or sadism. The prognosis varies with the degree of contamination introduced by the offending object.

Abdominal Abscesses

Although reticular and liver abscesses are well recognized and have been discussed as potential causes of vagal indigestion, other abdominal locations may harbor abscesses. These include the umbilical remnants or region and the omental bursa. Perforating abomasal ulcers are the most common cause of omental bursitis, bursal abscesses, or walled-off omental abscesses. Perforations of the visceral surface of the abomasum may allow ingesta to enter the omental bursa, the potential space between the superficial and deep sheaths of the greater omentum. Abscesses also may develop subsequent to rumen trocharization or after rumenotomy. Signs are not specific but include progressive inappetence, decreased milk production, abdominal distension, and usually fever that is incompletely responsive to antibiotic therapy. Ruminal abscesses can also be seen secondary to toxic rumenitis or rumenocentesis, but these tend to be confined to the wall of the organ. Occasional full-thickness ruminal perforations with associated peritonitis will occur because of penetrating foreign bodies, but this is not as common as traumatic reticuloperitonitis. More commonly, walled-off large abscesses may

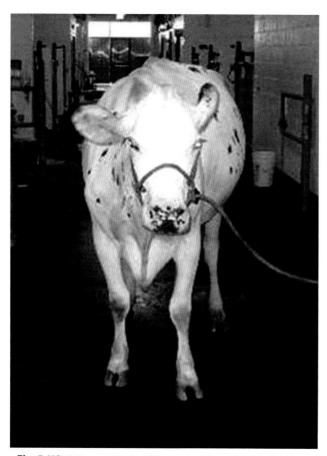

• **Fig. 5.118** A 3-year-old cow with severe abdominal distension caused by a perforated abomasal ulcer and prolonged omental bursitis.

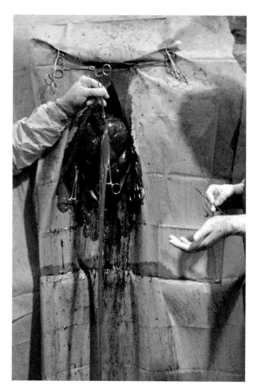

• **Fig. 5.119** Drainage of omental bursitis in a cow that had a perforated abomasal ulcer.

form between the rumen wall and body wall after rumenotomy, left-sided cesarean section, rumen trocharization, or left flank repair of LDA. These abscesses can become very large, but there may be minimal abdominal enlargement and the skin incision may have healed perfectly. A similar but more extensive condition may be found on the right side of the abdomen between the body wall and omentum after right flank repair of a DA or right-sided cesarean section. Cows often appear ill sooner with abscesses on the right because the infection spreads along the body wall and omentum more quickly than on the left, and the small intestine often adheres to the inflamed or infected omentum. Laboratory data may be helpful in the diagnosis because serum globulin often is elevated, serum albumin is decreased, and the abdominal fluid usually reflects inflammation with elevated total solids (>3.5 g/dL) and an elevated white blood cell count. Ultrasonography is extremely helpful in localizing the lesion such that surgical drainage may be attempted. Infection that spreads between the peritoneal membrane and body wall following laparotomy may have multiple pockets and be difficult to drain. The fluid generally possesses a fetid smell and has a mixed population of bacteria. Appropriate antibiotic therapy is based on results of culture and sensitivity testing of fluid from the abscess. The prognosis is poor.

Omental bursa abscesses (Fig. 5.118) may be so large as to create a detectable fluid wave on ballottement of the right

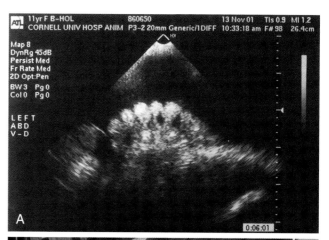

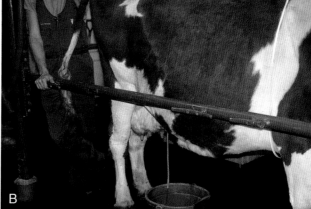

• **Fig. 5.120** A, Ultrasound image revealing massive peritoneal effusion in an 8-year-old Red Holstein cow with mesothelioma. B, Drainage of the neoplastic peritoneal fluid seen in A.

abdomen and a dull right-sided midabdominal ping resulting from gas accumulation dorsal to the large volume of purulent fluid (Fig. 5.119; see Video Clip 5.5).

Neoplasia of the abdomen other than lymphosarcoma is rare. Tumors such as mesothelioma (Fig. 5.120) are occasionally seen and may cause massive peritoneal effusion.

Idiopathic Eosinophilic Enteritis

Idiopathic eosinophilic enteritis is a rare but well-documented cause of chronic diarrhea and weight loss in adult cattle. The clinical signs and age are nearly identical to those seen with Johne's disease. Plasma albumin, although consistently low in clinical cases of Johne's disease, often remains within the normal range in cattle with eosinophilic enteritis. In addition to Johne's disease, the differential diagnosis includes intestinal lymphosarcoma, lymphocytic or plasmacytic inflammation, chronic intestinal irritants such as sand or gravel, liver flukes, peritonitis, and intestinal amyloidosis. Confirmation of the diagnosis is by biopsy of the small intestine and finding eosinophilic inflammation and edema within the intestinal wall. Blood eosinophil count is normal. One-month treatment with systemically administered corticosteroids has been attempted in a very few cases, and a favorable response was observed.

Suggested Readings

Abutarbush, S. M., & Naylor, J. M. (2006). Obstruction of the small intestine by a trichobezoar in cattle: 15 cases (1992-2002). *J Am Vet Med Assoc, 229*, 1627–1630.

Adaska, J. M., Aly, S. S., Moeller, R. B., et al. (2014). Jejunal hematoma in cattle: a retrospective case analysis. *J Vet Diagn Invest, 26*, 96–103.

Ahmed, A. F., Constable, P. D., & Misk, N. A. (2001). Effect of orally administered cimetidine and ranitidine on abomasal luminal pH in clinically normal milk-fed calves. *Am J Vet Res, 62*, 1531–1538.

Ahmed, A. F., Constable, P. D., & Misk, N. A. (2002). Effect of feeding frequency and route of administration on abomasal luminal pH in dairy calves fed milk replacer. *J Dairy Sci, 85*, 1502–1508.

Ahmed, A. F., Constable, P. D., & Misk, N. A. (2005). Effect of orally administered omeprazole on abomasal luminal pH in dairy calves fed milk replacer. *J Vet Med A Physiol Pathol Clin Med, 52*, 238–243.

Azizi, S., Mohammadi, R., & Mohammadpour, I. (2010). Surgical repair and management of congenital intestinal atresia in 68 calves. *Vet Surg, 39*, 115–120.

Braun, U., Nuss, K., Knubben-Schweizer, G., et al. (2011). The use of ultrasonography for diagnosing the cause of colic in cows. A review. *Tierarztl Prax Ausg G Grosstiere Nutziere, 39*, 289–298.

Bertone, A. L. (1990). Neoplasms of the bovine gastrointestinal tract. *Vet Clin North Am Food Anim Pract, 6*, 515–524.

Boulay, G., Francoz, D., Doré, E., et al. (2014). Preoperative cowside lactatemia measurement predicts negative outcome in Holstein dairy cattle with right abomasal disorders. *J Dairy Sci, 97*, 212–221.

Braun, U. (2009). Traumatic pericarditis in cattle: clinical, radiographic and ultrasonographic findings. *Vet J, 182*, 176–186.

Braun, U., Beckmann, C., Gerspach, C., et al. (2012). Clinical findings and treatment in cattle with caecal dilatation. *BMC Vet Res, 8*, 75.

Braun, U., Forster, E., Steininger, K., et al. (2010). Ultrasonographic findings in 63 cows with haemorrhagic bowel syndrome. *Vet Rec, 166*, 79–81.

Braun, U., Milicevic, A., Forster, E., et al. (2009). An unusual cause of traumatic reticulitis/reticuloperitonitis in a herd of Swiss dairy cows nearby an airport. *Schweiz Arch Tierheilkd, 151*, 127–131.

Braun, U., Pusterla, N., & Anliker, H. (1998). Ultrasonographic findings in three cows with peritonitis in the left flank region. *Vet Rec, 142*, 338–340.

Braun, U., Schmid, T., Muggli, E., et al. (2010). Clinical findings and treatment in 63 cows with haemorrhagic bowel syndrome. *Schweiz Arch Tierheilkd, 152*, 512–522.

Braun, U., Schnetzler, C., Dettwiler, M., et al. (2011). Ultrasonographic findings in a cow with abomasal lymphosarcoma: case report. *BMC Vet Res, 7*, 20.

Brenner, J., & Orgad, U. (2003). Epidemiological investigations of an outbreak of intestinal atresia in two Israeli dairy herds. *J Vet Med Sci, 65*, 141–143.

Breukink, H. J. (1986). Clinical consequences of ruminal drinking in veal calves. In *Proceedings: 14th World Congress on Diseases of Cattle* (pp. 1157–1162).

Breukink, H. J. (1991). Abomasal displacement, etiology, pathogenesis, treatment and prevention. *Bovine Pract, 26*, 148–153.

Bristol, D. G., & Fubini, S. L. (1990). Surgery of the neonatal bovine digestive tract. *Vet Clin North Am Food Anim Pract, 6*, 473–493.

Carlson, S. A., Stoffregen, W. C., & Bolin, S. R. (2002). Abomasitis associated with multiple antibiotic resistant *Salmonella enterica* serotype Typhimurium phage type DT104. *Vet Microbiol, 85*, 233–240.

Cebra, M. L., Cebra, C. K., Garry, F. B., et al. (1998). Idiopathic eosinophilic enteritis in four cattle. *J Am Vet Med Assoc, 212*, 258–261.

Chapman, W. L., & Smith, J. A. (1982). Abomasal adenocarcinoma in a cow. *J Am Vet Med Assoc, 181*, 493–494.

Constable, P. D., Nouri, M., Sen, I., et al. (2012). Evidence-based use of prokinetic drugs for abomasal disorders in cattle. *Vet Clin North Am Food Anim Pract, 28*, 51–70.

Constable, P. D., St. Jean, G., Ring, D. M., et al. (1991). Preoperative prognostic indicators in cattle with abomasal volvulus. *J Am Vet Med Assoc, 198*, 2077–2085.

Constable, P., Grünberg, W., Staufenbiel, R., et al. (2013). Clinicopathologic variables associated with hypokalemia in lactating dairy cows with abomasal displacement or volvulus. *J Am Vet Med Assoc, 242*, 826–835.

Constable, P. D., Ahmed, A. F., & Misk, N. A. (2005). Effect of suckling cow's milk or milk replacer on abomasal luminal pH in dairy calves. *J Vet Intern Med, 19*, 97–102.

Constable, P. D., Hiew, M. W., Tinkler, S., et al. (2014). Efficacy of oral potassium chloride administration in treating lactating dairy cows with experimentally induced hypokalemia, hypochloremia, and alkalemia. *J Dairy Sci, 97*, 1413–1426.

Constable, P. D., St. Jean, G., Hull, B. L., et al. (1997). Intussusception in cattle: 336 cases (1964-1993). *J Am Vet Med Assoc, 210*, 531–536.

Constable, P. D., Miller, G. Y., Hoffsis, G. F., et al. (1992). Risk factors for abomasal volvulus and left abomasal displacement in cattle. *Am J Vet Res, 53*, 1184–1192.

Cramers, T., Mikkelsen, K. B., Andersen, P., et al. (2005). New types of foreign bodies and the effect of magnets in traumatic reticulitis in cows. *Vet Rec, 157*, 287–289.

Davidson, H. P., Rebhun, W. C., & Habel, R. E. (1981). Pharyngeal trauma in cattle. *Cornell Vet, 71*, 15–25.

Dirksen, G. (1979). Digestive system. In G. Rosenberger (Ed.), *Clinical examination of cattle*. Berlin: Verlag Paul Parey.

Dirksen, G., Doll, K., Einhellig, J., et al. (1997). Abomasal ulcers in calves: clinical investigations and experiences [article in German]. *Tierarztl Prax, 25*, 318–328.

Dirksen, G., & Stöber, M. (1962). Contribution to the functional disorders of the bovine stomach caused by the lesions of the nervus vagus-Hoflund's syndrome summary. *DTW Dtsch Tierarztl Wochenschr, 69*, 213–217.

Divers, T. J., & Smith, B. P. (1979). Diaphragmatic hernia in a cow. *J Am Vet Med Assoc, 175*, 1099–1100.

Doll, K., Klee, W., & Dirksen, G. (1998). Cecal intussusception in calves [article in German]. *Tierarztl Prax Ausg G Grosstiere Nutztiere, 26*, 247–253.

Ducharme, N. G. (1983). Surgical considerations in the treatment of traumatic reticuloperitonitis. *Compend Contin Educ Pract Vet, 5*, S213–S224.

Ducharme, N. G. (1990). Surgery of the bovine forestomach compartments. *Vet Clin North Am Food Anim Pract, 6*, 371–397.

Ducharme, N. G., Arighti, M., Horney, F. D., et al. (1988). Colonic atresia in cattle: a prospective of 43 cases. *Can Vet J, 29*, 818–824.

Ducharme, N.G., Desrochers, A., Fubini, S.L., et al. (2017). Surgery of the bovine digestive system. In S.L. Fubini & N.G. Ducharme (Eds.), Farm Animal Surgery (2nd ed.). St. Louis:Elsevier..

Ducharme, N. G., Smith, D. F., & Koch, D. B. (1982). Small intestinal obstruction caused by a persistent round ligament of the liver in a cow. *J Am Vet Med Assoc, 180*, 1234–1236.

Dunlop, R. H., & Hammond, P. B. (1965). D-Lactic acidosis of ruminants. *Ann N Y Acad Sci, 119*, 1109–1132.

Edgson, F. A. (1952). Bovine lipomatosis. *Vet Rec, 64*, 449.

Figueiredo, M. D., Nydam, D. V., Perkins, G. A., et al. (2006). Prognostic value of plasma L-lactate concentration measured cow-side with a portable clinical analyzer in Holstein dairy cattle with abomasal disorders. *J Vet Intern Med, 20*, 1463–1470.

Firkins, J. L., & Yu, Z. (2015). Ruminant nutrition symposium: how to use data on the rumen microbiome to improve our understanding of ruminant nutrition. *J Anim Sci, 93*, 1450–1470.

Fox, F. H. (1980). The esophagus, stomach, intestines, and peritoneum. In H. E. Amstutz (Ed.), *Bovine medicine and surgery* (2nd ed.). Santa Barbara, CA: American Veterinary Publications.

Fubini, S. L., Ducharme, N. G., Erb, H. N., et al. (1989). Failure of omasal transport attributable to perireticular abscess formation in cattle: 29 cases (1980–1986). *J Am Vet Med Assoc, 194*, 811–814.

Fubini, S. L., Ducharme, N. G., Murphy, J. P., et al. (1985). Vagus indigestion syndrome resulting from liver abscess in dairy cows. *J Am Vet Med Assoc, 186*, 1297–1300.

Fubini, S. L., Erb, H. N., Rebhun, W. C., et al. (1986). Cecal dilatation and volvulus in dairy cows: 84 cases (1977–1983). *J Am Vet Med Assoc, 189*, 96–99.

Fubini, S. L., Gröhn, Y. T., & Smith, D. F. (1991). Right displacement of the abomasum and abomasal volvulus in dairy cows: 458 cases (1980–1987). *J Am Vet Med Assoc, 198*, 461–464.

Fubini, S. L., & Smith, D. F. (1982). Failure of omasal transport due to traumatic reticuloperitonitis and intraabdominal abscess. *Compend Contin Educ Pract Vet, 4*, S492–S494.

Fubini, S. L., Smith, D. F., Tithof, P. K., et al. (1986). Volvulus of the distal jejunoileum in four cows. *Vet Surg, 15*, 410–413.

Fubini, S. L., Yeager, A. E., Mohammed, H. O., et al. (1990). Accuracy of radiography of the reticulum for predicting surgical findings in adult dairy cattle with traumatic reticuloperitonitis: 123 cases (1981–1987). *J Am Vet Med Assoc, 197*, 1060–1064.

Garry, F. B., Hull, B. L., Rings, D. M., et al. (1988). Prognostic value of anion gap calculation in cattle with abomasal volvulus: 58 cases (1980–1985). *J Am Vet Med Assoc, 192*, 1107–1112.

Golden, H. M., Denman, S. E., McSweeney, C., et al. (2014). Ruminal bacterial community shifts in grain, sugar and histidine challenged dairy heifers. *J Dairy Sci, 97*(8), 5131–5150.

Gressley, T. F., Hall, M. B., & Armentano, L. E. (2011). Ruminant nutrition symposium: productivity, digestion, and health responses to hindgut acidosis in ruminants. *J Anim Sci, 89*, 1120–1130.

Grymer, J., & Ames, N. K. (1981). Bovine abdominal pings: clinical examination and differential diagnosis. *Compend Contin Educ Pract Vet, 32*, S311–S318.

Grymer, J., & Johnson, R. (1982). Two cases of bovine omental bursitis. *J Am Vet Med Assoc, 181*, 714–715.

Habel, R. E. (1956). A study of the innervation of the ruminant stomach. *Cornell Vet, 46*, 555–633.

Habel, R. E., & Smith, D. F. (1981). Volvulus of the bovine abomasum and omasum. *J Am Vet Med Assoc, 179*, 447–455.

Hagan, H. A. (1921). Fat necrosis in cattle. *J Am Vet Med Assoc, 59*, 682.

Herrli-Gygi, M., Hammon, H. M., Zbinden, Y., et al. (2006). Ruminal drinkers: endocrine and metabolic status and effects of suckling from a nipple instead of drinking from a bucket. *J Vet Med A Physiol Pathol Clin Med, 53*, 215–224.

Hund, A., Dzieciol, M., Schmitz-Esser, S., et al. (2015). Characterization of mucosa-associated bacterial communities in abomasal ulcers by pyrosequencing. *Vet Microbiol, 177*, 132–141.

Jafarzadeh, S. R., Nowrouzian, I., Khaki, Z., et al. (2004). The sensitivities and specificities of total plasma protein and plasma fibrinogen for the diagnosis of traumatic reticuloperitonitis in cattle. *Prev Vet Med, 65*, 1–7.

Jarrett, W. F. H., Campo, M. S., Blaxter, M. L., et al. (1984). Alimentary fibropapilloma in cattle. A spontaneous tumor, nonpermissive for papillomavirus replication. *J Natl Cancer Inst, 73*, 499–504.

Kleen, J. L., Hooijer, G. A., Rehage, J., et al. (2004). Rumenocentesis (rumen puncture): a viable instrument in herd health diagnosis. *Dtsch Tierarztl Wochenschr, 111*, 458–462.

Kmicikewycz, A. D., Harvatine, K. J., & Heinrichs, A. J. (2015). Effects of corn silage particle size, supplemental hay, and forage-to-concentrate ratio on rumen pH, feed preference, and milk fat profile of dairy cattle. *J Dairy Sci, 98*, 4850–4868.

Koch, D. B., Robertson, J. T., & Donawick, W. J. (1978). Small intestinal obstruction due to persistent vitelloumbilical band in a cow. *J Am Vet Med Assoc, 173*, 197–199.

Kumar, A., & Saini, N. S. (2011). Reliability of ultrasonography at the fifth intercostal space in the diagnosis of reticular diaphragmatic hernia. *Vet Rec, 169*, 391–393.

Kumar, P., Nagarajan, N., Saikumar, G., et al. (2015). Detection of bovine papillomaviruses in wart-like lesions of upper gastrointestinal tract of cattle and buffaloes. *Transbound Emerg Dis, 62*, 264–271.

Kunz-Kirchhofer, C., Schelling, E., Probst, S., et al. (2010). Myoelectric activity of the ileum, cecum, proximal loop of the ascending colon, and spiral colon in cows with naturally occurring cecal dilatation-dislocation. *Am J Vet Res, 71*, 304–313.

Lean, I. J., Golder, H. M., & Hall, M. B. (2014). Feeding, evaluating, and controlling rumen function. *Vet Clin North Am Food Anim Pract, 30*, 539–575.

Leipold, H. W., Watt, B., Vestweber, J. G. E., et al. (1981). Clinical observations in rectovaginal constriction in Jersey cattle. *Bovine Pract, 16*, 76–79.

Lombardero, M., & Yllera Mdel, M. (2014). An unusual colon atresia in a calf: at the junction of the distal loop and transverse colon. A brief overview. *Organogenesis, 10,* 312–316.

Lorenz, I., & Gentile, A. (2014). D-lactic acidosis in neonatal ruminants. *Vet Clin North Am Food Anim Pract, 30,* 317–331.

McArt, J. A., Nydam, D. V., & Oetzel, G. R. (2012). Epidemiology of subclinical ketosis in early lactation dairy cattle. *J Dairy Sci, 95,* 5056–5066.

McArt, J. A., Nydam, D. V., & Oetzel, G. R. (2012). A field trial on the effect of propylene glycol on displaced abomasum, removal from herd, and reproduction in fresh cows diagnosed with subclinical ketosis. *J Dairy Sci, 95,* 2505–2512.

McDuffee, L. A., Ducharme, N. G., & Ward, J. L. (1993). Repair of sacral fracture in two dairy cattle. *J Am Vet Med Assoc, 202,* 1126–1128.

McFadden, A. M., Christensen, H., Fairley, R. A., et al. (2011). Outbreaks of pleuritis and peritonitis in calves associated with *Pasteurella multocida* capsular type B strain. *N Z Vet J, 59,* 40–45.

McGuirk, S. M., & Butler, D. G. (1980). Metabolic alkalosis with paradoxic aciduria in cattle. *J Am Vet Med Assoc, 177,* 551–554.

Melendez, P., Krueger, T., Benzaquen, M., et al. (2007). An outbreak of sand impaction in postpartum dairy cows. *Can Vet J, 48,* 1067–1070.

Mohammedsadegh, M. (1994). Effect of isoflupredone acetate on pregnancy in cattle. *Vet Rec, 134,* 453.

Newby, N. C., Pearl, D. L., LeBlanc, S. J., et al. (2013). The effect of administering ketoprofen on the physiology and behavior of dairy cows following surgery to correct a left displaced abomasum. *J Dairy Sci, 96,* 1511–1520.

Newton-Clarke, M., & Rebhun, W. C. (1993). Diaphragmatic herniation causing respiratory signs in a heifer. *Cornell Vet, 83,* 205–209.

Nuss, K., Lejeune, B., Lischer, C., et al. (2006). Ileal impaction in 22 cows. *Vet J, 171,* 456–461.

Owaki, S., Kawabuchi, S., Ikemitsu, K., et al. (2015). Pathological findings of hemorrhagic bowel syndrome (HBS) in six dairy cattle cases. *J Vet Med Sci, 77,* 879–881.

Palmer, J. E., & Whitlock, R. H. (1984). Perforated abomasal ulcers in adult dairy cows. *J Am Vet Med Assoc, 184,* 171–173.

Pardon, B., Vertenten, G., Cornillie, P., et al. (2012). Left abomasal displacement between the uterus and rumen during bovine twin pregnancy. *J Vet Sci, 13,* 437–440.

Pardon, B., Vertenten, G., Durie, I., et al. (2009). Four cases of omental herniation in cattle. *Vet Rec, 165,* 718–721.

Parker, J. L., & Fubini, S. L. (1987). Abomasal fistulas in 8 dairy cows. *Cornell Vet, 77,* 303–309.

Pearson, H. (1977). Intestinal obstruction in cattle. *Vet Rec, 101,* 162–166.

Peek, S. F., Santschi, E. M., Livesey, M. A., et al. (2009). Surgical findings and outcome for dairy cattle with jejunal hemorrhage syndrome: 31 cases (2000-2007). *J Vet Med Assoc, 234,* 1308–1312.

Penner, G. B., Oba, M., Gäbel, G., et al. (2010). A single mild episode of subacute ruminal acidosis does not affect ruminal barrier function in the short term. *J Dairy Sci, 93,* 4838–4845.

Pitta, D. W., Pinchak, W. E., Dowd, S., et al. (2014). Longitudinal shifts in bacteria diversity and fermentation pattern in the rumen of steers grazing wheat pasture. *Anaerobe, 30,* 11–17.

Rager, K. D., George, L. W., House, J. K., et al. (2004). Evaluation of rumen transfaunation after surgical correction of left-sided displacement of the abomasum in cows. *J Am Vet Med Assoc, 225,* 915–920.

Rebhun, W. C. (1980). Vagus indigestion in cattle. *J Am Vet Med Assoc, 176,* 506–510.

Rebhun, W. C. (1982). The medical treatment of abomasal ulcers in dairy cattle. *Compend Contin Educ Pract Vet, 4,* S91–S98.

Rebhun, W. C. (1987). Rumen collapse in cattle. *Cornell Vet, 77,* 244–250.

Rebhun, W. C. (1991). Differentiating the causes of left abdominal tympanitic resonance in dairy cattle. *Vet Med, 86,* 1126–1134.

Rebhun, W. C. (1991). Right abdominal tympanitic resonance in dairy cattle: identifying the causes. *Vet Med, 86,* 1135–1142.

Richardson, D. W. (1984). Parovarian-omental bands as a cause of small intestinal obstruction in cows. *J Am Vet Med Assoc, 185,* 517–519.

Roussel, A. J., Brumbaugh, G. W., Waldron, R. C., et al. (1992). Abomasal and duodenal motility of cattle after administration of prokinetic drugs. In *Proceedings: 11th Annual American College Veterinary Internal Medicine Forum* (p. 960) [Abstract].

Ruf-Ritz, J., Braun, U., Hilbe, M., et al. (2013). Internal herniation of the small and large intestines in 18 cattle. *Vet J, 197,* 374–377.

Rutgers, L. J. E., & Van der Velden, M. A. (1983). Complications following use of the closed suturing technique for correction of left abomasal displacement in cows. *Vet Rec, 113,* 255–257.

Sattler, N., Fecteau, G., Helie, P., et al. (2000). Etiology, forms, and prognosis of gastrointestinal dysfunction resembling vagal indigestion occurring after surgical correction of right abomasal displacement. *Can Vet J, 41,* 777–785.

Smith, D. F. (1978). Right-side torsion of the abomasum in dairy cows: classification of severity and evaluation of outcome. *J Am Vet Med Assoc, 173,* 108–111.

Smith, D. F. (1982). Surgical repair of atresia coli in a calf. *Compend Contin Educ Pract Vet, 4,* S441–S445.

Smith, D. F., & Donawick, W. J. (1979). Obstruction of the ascending colon in cattle. I. Clinical presentation and surgical management. *Vet Surg, 8,* 93–97.

Smith, D. F., Erb, H. N., Kalaher, K. M., et al. (1982). The identification of structures and conditions responsible for right side tympanitic resonance (ping) in adult cattle. *Cornell Vet, 72,* 180–199.

Smith, G. W., Ahmed, A. F., & Constable, P. D. (2012). Effect of orally administered electrolyte solution formulation on abomasal luminal pH and emptying rate in dairy calves. *J Am Vet Med Assoc, 241,* 1075–1082.

Steen, A. (2001). Field study of dairy cows with reduced appetite in early lactation: clinical examinations, blood and rumen fluid analyses. *Acta Vet Scand, 42,* 219–228.

Stengärde, L., Holtenius, K., Tråven, M., et al. (2010). Blood profiles in dairy cows with displaced abomasum. *J Dairy Sci, 93* 4891–4699.

Stengärde, L., Hultgren, J., Tråven, M., et al. (2012). Risk factors for displaced abomasum or ketosis in Swedish dairy herds. *Prev Vet Med, 103,* 280–286.

Stock, M. L., Fecteau, M. E., & Garber, J. R. (2012). What is your diagnosis? *J Am Vet Med Assoc, 241*(10), 1279–1281.

Stocker, H., Lutz, H., Kaufmann, C., et al. (1999). Acid-base disorders in milk-fed calves with chronic indigestion. *Vet Rec, 145,* 340–346.

Stocker, H., Lutz, H., & Rusch, P. (1999). Clinical, haematological and biochemical findings in milk-fed calves with chronic indigestion. *Vet Rec, 145,* 307–311.

Stöber, M., & Dirksen, G. (1977). The differential diagnosis of abdominal findings (adspection, rectal examination and exploratory laparotomy) in cattle. *Bovine Pract, 12,* 35–38 [This paper was originally published in German in *Berl Munch Tierzaztl Wochenschr* 89:129–133, 1976].

Tithof, P. K., & Rebhun, W. C. (1986). Complications of blind-stitch abomasopexy—20 cases (1980–1985). *J Am Vet Med Assoc, 189,* 1489–1492.

Trent, A. M. (1990). Surgery of the bovine abomasum. *Vet Clin North Am Food Anim Pract, 6,* 399–448.

Troutt, H. F., Fessler, J. F., Page, E. H., et al. (1967). Diaphragmatic defects in cattle. *J Am Vet Med Assoc, 151,* 1421–1429.

Tulleners, E. P. (1984). Avulsion of the jejunum, with vaginal evisceration in a cow. *J Am Vet Med Assoc, 184,* 195–196.

Tulleners, E. P., & Hamilton, G. F. (1980). Surgical resection of perforated abomasal ulcers in calves. *Can Vet J, 21,* 262–264.

Udall, D. H. (1954). *The practice of veterinary medicine.* Ithaca, NY: published by the author.

Vergara, C. F., Döpfer, D., Cook, N. B., et al. (2014). Risk factors for postpartum problems in dairy cows: explanatory and predictive modeling. *J Dairy Sci, 97,* 4127–4140.

Vogel, S. R., Nichols, S., Buczinski, S., et al. (2012). Duodenal obstruction caused by duodenal sigmoid flexure volvulus in dairy cattle: 29 cases (2006-2010). *J Am Vet Med Assoc, 241,* 621–625.

Whitlock, R. H. (1976). Cecal volvulus in dairy cattle. In *Proceedings: International Congress on Diseases of Cattle, 1,* 60–63.

Wittek, T., Constable, P. D., & Morin, D. E. (2005). Abomasal impaction in Holstein-Friesian cows: 80 cases (1980-2003). *J Am Vet Med Assoc, 227,* 287–291.

Wittek, T., Furll, M., & Constable, P. D. (2004). Prevalence of endotoxemia in healthy postparturient dairy cows and cows with abomasal volvulus or left displaced abomasum. *J Vet Intern Med, 18,* 574–580.

Wittek, T., Grosche, A., Locher, L. F., et al. (2010). Diagnostic accuracy of D-dimer and other peritoneal fluid analysis measurements in dairy cows with peritonitis. *J Vet Intern Med, 24,* 1211–1217.

6

Infectious Diseases of the Gastrointestinal Tract

SIMON F. PEEK, SHEILA M. McGUIRK, RAYMOND W. SWEENEY, AND KEVIN J. CUMMINGS

Calves

Escherichia coli

Escherichia coli is a normal inhabitant of the gastrointestinal (GI) tract of warm-blooded animals and ubiquitous in the farm environment. Disease caused by *E. coli* in calves may present as enteric or septicemic illness and is an important cause of neonatal mortality in dairy calves. Failure of passive transfer and management practices that allow exposure of neonatal calves to large numbers of *E. coli* are of central importance in the pathogenesis of disease. Because of substantial genotypic and phenotypic variation, it is possible to subgroup *E. coli* into a large number of different serotypes. The commensal *E. coli* are important members of the normal gut microbiota, and only a small fraction of the total *E. coli* population in nature are classified as pathovars or pathotypes. Modern analytical methods have permitted more detailed identification of virulence associated factors and elucidation of specific virulence mechanisms in the classification of pathogenic serotypes of these gram-negative organisms. Broadly speaking, *E. coli* are classified based on several serologic and antigenic parameters, including cell wall or somatic (O) antigens, capsular (K) antigens, pilar or fimbrial (F) antigens, and flagellar (H) antigens. Heretofore, pilus antigens were sometimes classified as K antigens, but recent reference to pilus antigens as F antigens reduces confusion in this area. Among the diarrheagenic pathotypes of *E. coli* the most significant in neonatal calves are the enterotoxigenic *E. coli* (ETEC), which is the most commonly confirmed noncommensal pathotype of *E. coli* in cattle. Enteropathogenic (EPEC), enterohemorrhagic (EHEC), and Shiga toxin–producing *E. coli* (STEC) are pathotypes that are also isolated from diarrheic calves, but their role in neonatal calf diarrhea remains more controversial because they can also be found in healthy individuals. Increasing concern about zoonotic illness and antimicrobial resistance among these pathotypes of *E. coli* is impossible to ignore if one works in the cattle industry, dairy cattle in particular being identified as important reservoirs for zoonotic ETEC, EHEC, and STEC disease.

Septicemia (Septicemic Colibacillosis, Colisepticemia)

Etiology

Colisepticemia in neonatal calves can be considered a disease of poor management. Failure of passive transfer is the primary risk factor for this disease. Colostral transfer of immunoglobulins may be compromised by short dry periods, preparturient leaking of colostrum, assumption that a calf has nursed colostrum just because it is left with the dam for 24 hours, primiparous heifers that have poorquality colostrum, and many other factors. Provision of an inadequate immunoglobulin mass can be a problem with both commercial colostrum substitutes or replacers as well as dam or farm sourced colostrum. In addition, poor maternity area and poor calf pen hygiene promote exposure of calves to the multitude of strains of *E. coli* capable of causing septicemia, the majority of which are commensal. Filthy conditions; calving areas that are dirty, wet, overcrowded, or overused; and failure to dip navels are additional factors that predispose to this problem. Sanitation and hygiene with respect to collecting, storing, and administering colostrum are important factors in the provision of adequate passive transfer and the prevention of colibacillosis.

Invasive *E. coli* of many subgroups are capable of opportunistic, septicemic infection of neonatal calves. Various reviews suggest an involvement of a multitude of possible *E. coli* types. Variations may be explained by geographic or environmental differences.

Calves with less than 500 mg IgG/dL are very prone to septicemic *E. coli,* and those with 500 to 1000 mg IgG/dL are defined as having partial failure of passive transfer (FPT) and are also at increased risk. Adequate transfer of passive immunoglobulin that ensures at least 1000 IgG mg/dL serum (10 mg/mL serum) or preferably 1600 mg/dL serum is likely to prevent the disease.

Septicemia caused by *E. coli* most commonly occurs from 1 to 14 days of age. The onset of disease tends to occur earlier in this time frame when calves are exposed to high numbers of *E. coli* soon after birth (i.e., in the maternity pen). Poor or nonexistent transfer of passive immunoglobulins to the calf also hastens the onset of disease. Invasive *E. coli* may gain entrance through the navel, intestine, or nasal and oropharyngeal mucous membranes. After invasion and septicemia occur, clinical signs develop rapidly and usually are apparent within 24 hours. Calves with partial FPT or those exposed to less virulent *E. coli* strains may develop more chronic signs of disease over several days.

Septicemic calves shed the causative *E. coli* in urine, oral secretions, nasal secretions, and later in the feces, provided they survive long enough to develop diarrhea. Thus, transmission may occur among communally housed calves, crowded calves, or uncleaned maternity stalls because of the heavily infected secretions of sick and septicemic calves. Because septicemic calves can shed large numbers of the organism before clinical signs are evident, contamination of communal pens and common-use feeding devices (e.g., esophageal feeding tubes) and direct contact with the infected calf or its feces or urine may promote spread of infection. Infected calves allowed to remain in the maternity area will amplify the level of environmental contamination, thereby placing other neonates born in that area at risk. Similar amplification may occur in calf housing areas and reinforces the biosecurity need for spatial and temporal separation between occupants, as well as the appropriate and routine disinfection of calf housing.

Clinical Signs

Peracute signs of depression, weakness, tachycardia, and dehydration predominate when highly virulent strains of *E. coli* cause septicemia. Affected calves usually are less than 7 days of age and may be less than 24 hours old. Although often present early on, fever is usually absent by the time obvious clinical signs of fulminant disease occur, when endotoxemia and the resultant poor peripheral perfusion often render the animal normothermic or hypothermic. Exceptions to this rule are calves with peracute disease that collapse when exposed to direct sunlight on hot days; such calves can be markedly hyperthermic. Signs of dehydration are mild to moderate in most cases. The suckle reflex is greatly reduced or absent, and the vasculature of the sclerae is markedly injected. Petechial hemorrhages may be visible on mucous membranes and extremities, particularly the pinnae of the ears (Fig. 6.1). The limbs, mouth, and ears are cool to the touch. Affected calves show progressive weakness and lethargy, often becoming comatose before death. Diarrhea is often seen but may not be apparent in peracute cases.

Evidence of localization of infection in certain tissues may become apparent in cases that survive the acute disease. Hypopyon may be present, as may uveitis, which is evidenced by miotic pupils with increased opacity to the aqueous fluid ("aqueous flare"). Hyperesthesia, paddling, and opisthotonus (Fig. 6.2) are signs suggestive of septic

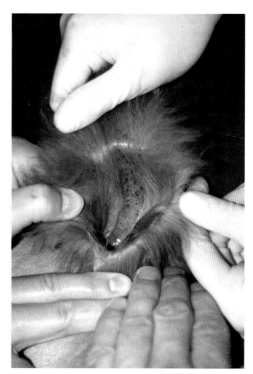

• **Fig. 6.1** Ear of 5-day-old Jersey calf demonstrating petechial hemorrhage associated with *Escherichia coli* septicemia.

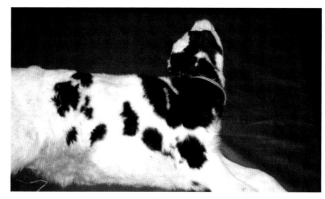

• **Fig. 6.2** Seven-day-old Holstein calf with opisthotonus associated with *Escherichia coli* meningitis and septicemia as a result of failure of passive transfer.

meningitis. Diarrhea may be present in some calves with colisepticemia. Lameness may result from bacterial seeding of joints or growth plates. Signs of omphalophlebitis may be present. Weakness, poor body condition, and recumbency secondary to weakness or joint or bone pain may be present in chronic cases. These localized and less fulminant infections may occur in slightly older calves (>7 days of age). Fever is often present in calves with joint ill or meningitis.

Clinical signs of acute septicemia may be difficult to differentiate from those of acute ETEC infection because dehydration, weakness, and collapse may be common to both. Age at onset can be valuable in the differentiation of ETEC infections because calves are most often within the first 72 to 96 hours of life with this condition and frequently less than 48 hours old. Furthermore, septicemic calves tend to be less dehydrated and have less watery diarrhea than calves with ETEC diarrhea; also, diarrhea tends to develop in the terminal stages of septicemia. Historical data may indicate other neonatal calves have recently shown similar signs or died at less than 2 weeks of age. Other differential diagnoses for acute colisepticemia include hypoxia or trauma during birth, simple hypothermia or hypoglycemia, septicemia caused by *Salmonella* spp., and congenital defects of the central nervous or cardiovascular systems. Polyarthritis caused by *Mycoplasma* spp. is an important differential diagnosis for septic arthritis secondary to colisepticemia but tends to be seen in considerably older calves. Salt poisoning, hypoglycemia, congenital neurologic disorders, traumatic injuries, and intoxications (e.g., lead) should be considered as differential diagnoses for meningitis secondary to colisepticemia. We have also seen several herds in recent years with young calves presenting with neurologic signs indistinguishable from meningitis for which the ultimate diagnosis was ionophore toxicity caused by overdosing before feeding milk replacer. Failure of passive transfer and meningitis were not involved.

Ancillary Data

Calves with peracute *E. coli* septicemia often have elevated packed cell volumes resulting from dehydration and endotoxic shock. The total white blood cell (WBC) count is variable but is frequently low or within normal ranges. Generally, a left shift is observed, and toxic changes (e.g., azurophilic cytoplasm, nuclear hypersegmentation, and Dohle bodies) are often apparent on cytologic examination of blood neutrophils. Plasma fibrinogen concentration is variable. Hypoglycemia is a common finding, and metabolic acidosis, although common, usually is less severe than in calves recumbent as a result of ETEC. In fact, an acid–base and electrolyte determination that does not demonstrate a severe metabolic acidosis in a recumbent, diarrheic, dehydrated calf less than 14 days of age usually portends septicemia. Blood cultures provide the greatest specific diagnostic aid, but results may not be forthcoming in time to help the patient.

Acutely, subacutely, and chronically septicemic calves may have detectable clinical signs of localization of infection that allow a more definitive diagnostic test (e.g., cerebrospinal fluid [CSF] tap for patients showing signs of meningitis or arthrocentesis to confirm septic arthritis) (Fig. 6.3). In chronic cases (calves 2 weeks of age or older), the serum immunoglobulin concentration (and serum total globulin concentration) may be normal or increased as a result of de novo synthesis of antibodies in response to the well-established bacterial infection.

Diagnosis

Whenever clinical signs suggest the diagnosis, the calf's serum immunoglobulin levels should be analyzed. Although adequate levels of IgG do not rule out the disease, calves with IgG of 1600 mg/dL or more based on a single radial immunodiffusion test are highly unlikely to develop septicemic *E. coli* infection. Specific laboratory evaluation of immunoglobulin

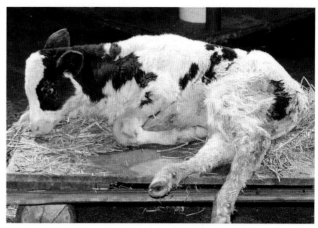

• **Fig. 6.3** A 1-week-old calf affected with subacute *Escherichia coli* septicemia. The calf has fever, diarrhea, dehydration, and a septic carpal joint. The calf had inadequate immunoglobulin levels.

levels is preferable to field techniques when confirmation of FPT is essential but may not provide timely results for practitioners. Therefore, even though dehydration may falsely elevate blood protein levels, these field techniques may be useful. Adequate immunoglobulin levels are suggested by serum total protein of 5.5 g/dL or more in calves less than 7 days of age. The use of a Brix refractometer is a simple, inexpensive on-farm tool for the monitoring of neonatal dairy calf immunity levels. A plasma value of 10% or more can be used to classify calves with successful transfer of passive immunity. Other reports have found that using a Brix percentage of 8.5% or less had optimal sensitivity (100%) for detecting failure of adequate immunoglobulin transfer. Previous literature has suggested that serum γ-glutamyl transferase (GGT) activity greater than 200 IU/L in 1 day old calves could be used as a cut-off point for adequacy of passive transfer. However, values for serum GGT can vary widely in healthy and sick calves and measurement of serum GGT should not be used as a gold standard in measuring colostral absorption. The development of visible turbidity in the 18% solution of sodium sulfite turbidity test is a reliable test for adequate passive transfer. A commercial turbidimetric assay (Midlands Bio-Products, Boone, IA) is available for on-farm determination of IgG concentration in serum samples from neonatal calves.

Blood cultures provide definitive diagnosis of bacteremia but usually provide this information too late to be of practical value. When multiple calves are affected, however, blood cultures can help to differentiate *E. coli* septicemia from septicemia caused by other pathogens (e.g., *Salmonella* spp.); this differentiation is relevant for determining the source of infection and initiation of preventive measures. Furthermore, antimicrobial sensitivity testing of blood culture isolates may aid in directing therapy, especially if a common etiologic cause is identified. Clinicians and producers should be aware of the differences between pathotypic strains of *E. coli* (e.g., ETEC) capable of producing severe disease in calves with adequate passive transfer and the everyday, commensal, and environmental *E. coli* often associated with sepsis caused by FPT. This is an important distinction, lest clients concentrate preventive efforts and management on specific vaccination programs rather than colostrum and neonatal calf management.

Treatment

Treatment of peracute *E. coli* septicemia usually is unsuccessful because of overwhelming bacteremia and endotoxemia in the patient. Signs progress so quickly that most septicemic calves are recumbent and comatose by the time of initial examination. Shock, lactic acidosis, hypoglycemia, and multiple organ failure are common in peracute cases.

If treatment is attempted, correction of endotoxic shock and acid–base and electrolyte abnormalities, effective antimicrobial therapy, and nutritional support are the primary goals. Intravenous (IV) balanced electrolyte solutions should contain dextrose (2.5%–10%), and sodium bicarbonate (20–50 mEq/L) if the plasma bicarbonate concentration is (<10 mEq/L), to address hypoglycemia and metabolic acidosis respectively. Adjustments of the concentration of dextrose and sodium bicarbonate in polyionic fluids can be guided by subsequent serum chemistry results. Maintaining normoglycemia in some peracute and acute septicemic calves can be extremely challenging due to consumption of administered glucose by bacteria. Antimicrobials used to treat neonatal septicemia should be bactericidal and possess a good gram-negative spectrum, such as ceftiofur, trimethoprim-sulfa, or ampicillin. Parenteral administration is necessary to achieve effective blood concentrations. Aminoglycosides such as gentamicin or amikacin can be used alone or in conjunction with the synergistically acting beta-lactam antibiotics (e.g., ceftiofur, penicillin, or ampicillin). Unfortunately, it is not uncommon to find *E. coli* cultured from blood or tissue of calves with septicemia resistant to ceftiofur, ampicillin and gentamicin. The use of potentially nephrotoxic aminoglycosides in a dehydrated patient with prerenal azotemia must be weighed against the potential bactericidal activity of the drugs. Given the present concerns regarding aminoglycoside use in food animals in the United States, use should be limited to situations in which other antibiotics have proven ineffective or in patients for which in vitro susceptibility testing has revealed an absence of approved, labeled alternatives. Furthermore, a minimum 18-month slaughter withdrawal must be enforced for calves that receive aminoglycosides. Use of fluoroquinolones (e.g., enrofloxacin, danofloxacin) and florfenicol in dairy calves is currently not permitted for anything other than respiratory disease under federal law in the United States.

If the previous therapy stabilizes the patient, a transfusion of 1 to 2 L of whole blood from (preferably) a bovine leukemia virus (BLV) and most importantly, bovine viral diarrhea virus (BVDV) negative cow should be performed because FPT is either assumed or confirmed. This translates to a dosage of 20-40 mL of whole blood per kilogram for the calf. Bovine plasma may also be used at the same dosage rate as whole blood and is currently commercially available in the US (Lake Immunogenics, Ontario, NY). Nutritional support ideally entails frequent feedings of small volumes of whole milk or good-quality milk replacer. Partial or total parenteral nutrition (TPN) may be considered for valuable calves, particularly those with concurrent and significant enteritis. Deep, dry bedding; good ventilation; and good nursing care are essential adjuncts to medical treatment.

Specific sites of localized infection also may require specific therapy. As an example, patients manifesting seizures because of meningitis may require diazepam (initial 5 mg dose for a neonatal calf, increasing by 5 mg increments, to effect) to control seizures. Calves with septic joints often require joint lavage. In many cases, especially chronic ones, arthrotomy is necessary to remove fibrin clots and more inspissated material from infected joints.

Chronic cases usually are cachectic; have polyarthritis, bronchopneumonia, and diarrhea; and have an extremely poor prognosis. Although recumbent, weak, dehydrated, and emaciated, these patients tend to have relatively normal acid–base and electrolyte values, so fluid therapy is often of limited value.

Prevention: Colostrum and Management

Sporadic cases of *E. coli* septicemia are unfortunate events, but endemic neonatal calf losses resulting from this disease demand a thorough evaluation of management regarding dry cows, periparturient cows, and newborn calves. There are two basic questions that require answers: (1) Are newborn calves being fed sufficient volumes of high-quality colostrum soon enough after birth? And (2) is the environment likely to harbor large numbers of *E. coli* during the periparturient and neonatal period? In other words, two facets of the dairy operation must be carefully critiqued: colostrum management and the hygiene of the maternity area and neonatal calf pens. A few basic concepts regarding colostrum should be understood:

1. Maternal immunoglobulin is concentrated in the mammary gland of the dry cow via an active transport mechanism during the last few weeks of gestation. Although IgG_1 is the major immunoglobulin transferred, IgG_2, IgM, and IgA are found as well. Resultant colostrum contains IgG at much higher concentrations than maternal serum, and transfer of maternal antibody into colostrum temporarily decreases maternal serum IgG_1 levels. Colostrum should be obtained as close to the time of calving as possible; colostrum collected more than 2 hours after calving shows a significant reduction in total IgG concentration.

2. A minimum of 40 dry days and a maximum of 90 dry days result in the best quality colostrum.

3. Assume dry cows that leak milk before parturition or collection of colostrum have lost the "best" colostrum.

4. Holstein calves must ingest at least 100 g of IgG_1 in the first 12 hours of life for adequate passive transfer

of immunoglobulins. The immunoglobulin concentration in colostrum deemed "acceptable" ranges from 30 to 60 g IgG/L; obviously, if larger volumes of more dilute colostrum are fed, adequate immunoglobulin mass would then be provided. However, many dairy calves simply allowed to nurse dairy breed dams to satiety will not voluntarily ingest an adequate volume of colostrum to meet their required immunoglobulin intake.

5. Certain genetic lines of cattle may be prone to low immunoglobulin levels in colostrum. For example, beef cattle tend to have higher levels than Holsteins. This may reflect genetic selection or merely reflect the dilutional effects of the greater milk volume in dairy cattle.

6. A colostrometer (a hydrometer that measures specific gravity of fluid, thereby indirectly measuring solids and, it is hoped, immunoglobulin concentration) is a common on-farm tool used to assess colostrum quality. Colostrometer readings may be affected by the colostrum temperature; whereas higher temperatures underestimate quality, lower temperatures overestimate quality. Therefore, readings should be made when the colostrum is at room temperature (20° to 25°C). That aside, there is considerable overlap in specific gravity readings among colostrums with low and high immunoglobulin concentration. Previous recommendations state the hydrometer should have a colostrum specific gravity reading of 1.050 or greater at room temperature for adequate immunoglobulin levels. However, given the large number of variables that affect colostrum-specific gravity (e.g., protein concentration, lactation number, cow breed, and temperature), use of the 1.050 cutoff value will misclassify many (up to two thirds) poor-quality colostrums as acceptable.

7. Other measures of colostrum quality and immunoglobulin mass are being increasingly deployed on dairy farms. An alternative to the use of a colostrometer is indirect assessment of IgG concentration in colostrum by Brix refractometry. A Brix reading of 21% to 23% correlates with the target value of 50 g IgG/L, and colostrum with a Brix refractometer value less than 18% should be categorized as being of poor quality. Recent research suggests that Brix-refractometry is the most accurate way of identifying colostrum quality (at least in terms of IgG concentration) on farm. Direct measurement of colostrum IgG concentration is also possible using commercially available immunoassays. One of these cow-side immunoassay kits (Colostrum bovine IgG quick test kit, Midlands Bio-Products, Boone, IA) has been demonstrated to identify poor-quality colostrums (those with IgG concentrations <50 g/L) with 93% specificity; in other words, this test appears to be superior to the hydrometer in accurately identifying poor-quality colostrum.

8. Volume or weight of colostrum at first milking. Weighing the colostrum is a simple method of selecting likely higher quality colostrums. In a large study of Holstein cows, first-milking colostrum weighing <8.5 kg (18.7 lb) was shown to have significantly higher colostral IgG$_1$ concentration than colostrums weighing >8.5 kg. By discarding (or feeding to older calves) Holstein colostrums that weigh more than 8.5 kg, a producer might increase the percentage of high-quality colostrum being fed to calves. Not surprisingly however, the weight or volume of colostrum is a less sensitive indicator of IgG content than other methods such as refractometry and so should only be relied on when other methods are unavailable.

9. Pooled colostrum from each cow's first milking may not ensure adequate immunoglobulin content because the poor-quality (dilute) colostrums tend to lower the immunoglobulin concentration of the entire pool. The practice of pooling colostrum also may increase *Mycobacterium avium* subspecies *paratuberculosis* (MAP), *Salmonella* Dublin and leukemia virus infection rates.

10. Microbiologic quality and cleanliness of colostrum. An increasing volume of data suggests that bacterial contamination of colostrum is a substantial problem on farm and that levels of bacteria in excess of 100,000 colony-forming units (CFU) per mL indicate a problem. Not only do high bacterial load colostrums represent an infectious disease risk, but there is also evidence that there is an increased risk of FPT when colostrum with such high levels of contamination is fed, likely linked to the binding of free IgG in the gut lumen by bacteria. The rapid proliferation or doubling time of bacteria at body temperature obligates producers to quickly refrigerate or freeze colostrum that is not to be immediately fed. Preservatives such as potassium sorbate can be added so as to increase safe storage time up to at least 96 hours at 4°C. If colostrum is not to be used within a few days, it should be frozen; more effective and rapid freezing, thereby curtailing bacterial growth, can be achieved by storage in 1- to 2-L bags rather than the conventional gallon jugs. Colostrum can become heavily contaminated with bacteria if good milking hygiene is not practiced at the first milking. Clean teats and udders, clean milking equipment, sanitized storage containers, and sanitized feeding equipment are necessary to limit the possibility of colostrum becoming a culture medium for pathogenic bacteria, including *Salmonella* spp. and virulent strains of *E. coli*. McGuirk and Collins have provided goals for bacterial contamination of colostrum:

• Total bacteria: <100,000 colony forming units (CFU)/ml
• Fecal coliforms: <10,000 CFU/ml
• Other gram-negative bacteria: <50,000 CFU/ml

- Streptococci (non-*Streptococcus agalactiae*): <50,000 CFU/ml
- Coagulase-negative *Staphylococcus*: <50,000 CFU/ml

Increasingly, larger farms are investing in the specialized equipment necessary for pasteurization of colostrum for the removal of infectious pathogens. Given the physical and chemical characteristics of colostrum, it is probable that careful quality control over time will be necessary to ensure that the pasteurization equipment is maintaining its efficacy. Initial data suggest that pasteurization, when performed properly, can be an excellent tool, increasing adequacy of passive transfer rates and reducing preweaning morbidity from diarrhea.

11. Springing heifers' colostrum has traditionally been considered lower quality than older cows. However, based on immunoglobulin concentration, colostrum from heifers is comparable with cows beginning their second lactation. In theory, the younger heifers have less immunologic "experience" than cows, so it is possible that the antibody "spectrum" (the number of different antigens to which antibodies are produced) is less in heifers than cows. However, the impact of this theoretical issue on calf health remains unproven. Until contrary data are made available, heifer colostrum should be evaluated and administered on the same basis as cow colostrum.

Given this current summation of colostral quality research, the following recommendations are made for newborn dairy calves:

1. High-quality colostrum cleanly collected from Johne's disease–negative and BLV-negative cows may be stored for use. If not fed within 2 hours of milking, colostrum should be refrigerated in sanitized 1- or 2-L containers until fed; as mentioned earlier, use of larger containers may limit prompt cooling, thereby promoting bacterial overgrowth. Fresh colostrum may be refrigerated for no more than 1 week and frozen for up to 1 year. If frozen, thawing should be performed slowly in warm water. Microwave thawing, if done carefully, can be used to thaw colostrums without overheating and denaturation of colostral antibodies. However, if microwave thawing is used, thawing for short time periods, periodically pouring off the thawed liquid and using a rotating tray may help to limit overheating.

2. Calves should receive 4 L of high-quality first milking colostrum during the first 12 hours of life (3 L is often sufficient for Jerseys, Shorthorns, and Guernseys). The first 2 L should be fed within 1 to 2 hours after birth, and the second 2 L should be fed before 12 hours of life. Many operations have chosen to feed all 4 L by esophageal feeder in a single feeding to larger calves.

3. The exact means of feeding (nipple vs tube) is less important than the timing of colostrum feeding, the volume fed, and the total immunoglobulin mass contained in that volume of colostrum.

4. Passive transfer status can be tested directly by radial immunodiffusion (RID) or indirectly by measurement of serum total protein levels or Brix refractometry per centage. Between 1 and 7 days of age, adequate passive transfer is indicated by a serum IgG concentration >1000 mg/dl and a serum total protein >5.5 g/dL or a Brix refractometry reading of at least 8.4% and preferably closer to 10%. If the serum sodium sulfite turbidity test is used, use of the 1+ endpoint (turbidity in 18% solution) as an indicator of adequate passive transfer status will maximize the percentage of calves correctly classified by this assay.

5. Regular evaluation of passive transfer status of all newborn calves in a herd allows the veterinarian to objectively monitor colostrum management over time. An on-farm testing method that has been scientifically validated (e.g., serum total protein, immunoassay kit, RID, or sodium sulfite turbidity test) should be used. On a herd basis, producers should aim for greater than 75% (i.e., at least 9 of a sample size of 12) of all calves tested between 2 and 7 days of age to demonstrate a total protein of greater than 5.5 g/dL when maternal colostrum is the means of passive transfer. Periodic quality control checks of conventional or Brix refractometers (against distilled water or sugar solution standards for calibration) is advised.

6. Calves born prematurely or from difficult births may have a variety of physical problems (e.g., swollen tongue) and physiologic disturbances (e.g., hypoxia) that may impact their ability to suckle colostrum or absorb immunoglobulins from the gut. Special attention should be paid to these calves to ensure adequate colostrum ingestion, and subsequent testing of serum is recommended to allow early detection and correction of FPT. For valuable calves believed to be at high risk by virtue of dystocia or phenotype (e.g., large in vitro fertilization calves), IV plasma (where available) or whole-blood transfusion from an appropriately screened donor may be considered in the first day of life. Calves fed colostrum of questionable quality, those not receiving their first colostrum feeding until after 12 hours of life, and calves of exceptional value warrant testing for FPT. Calves found to have FPT should receive a 40-mL/kg dose of commercial plasma or whole bovine blood or plasma from their dam or from a BLV- and BVDV-negative cow.

7. Esophageal feeders and bottles used to feed colostrum must not be used for older or ill calves and must be disinfected and dried between uses.

8. Colostral supplements and replacers are frequently used in place of, or in addition to, colostrum. Some of these products may provide IgG concentrations that are reportedly adequate but do not supply IgA, vitamins, maternal leucocytes, growth factors, and so on, that are normally present in colostrum. Furthermore, these products often do not result in serum protein or immunoglobulin levels equal to that of colostrum-fed calves when used per label. Some of these products, especially those marketed as supplements, contain very low immunoglobulin mass. Although colostrum replacers containing

immunoglobulins derived from serum, milk, colostrum, or eggs provide IgG for newborn calves, none appear to be equal or superior to natural colostrum when used as a replacement. Use of such products has recently been implemented in certain herds as a tool to limit transfer of infectious agents to the calf via colostrum, such as MAP, the causative agent of Johne's disease, the bovine leukosis virus, *S. Dublin*, and *Mycoplasma bovis*. The most commonly used colostrum replacers in the United States will not reliably achieve the total protein or total solids cutoff point of 5.5 g/dL in the serum in a 2- to 7-day-old calf when used per label, so expectations will need to be lowered if a testing policy is in place. Adequate total protein and IgG concentrations can often be achieved when additional doses or bags of such replacement products are used, but with this comes an increased financial cost. Recent research suggests that when 200 g of IgG (two packets) of a common colostrum replacement product is administered to newborn calves, antibody titers to common viral pathogens reach comparable levels and persist for at least as long as those seen with approximately 4 L of maternally derived colostrum. It is our opinion that the mixing of supplements or replacement products with maternal colostrum as a theoretical means of boosting neonatal IgG levels should be avoided. Although unproven, we believe there might be an increased risk of acute *Clostridial* spp. diarrhea when these are fed together.

In addition to the possibility of decreased efficiency of IgG absorption, maternity (calving) pen management practices that predispose to *E. coli* septicemia must be corrected. The importance of maternity pen hygiene cannot be overstated because no level of passive immunoglobulin transfer can protect completely against gross filth in the environment, and conversely, even calves with partial or complete FPT may survive when cleanliness is exceptional. Dry cows should not be kept in filthy environments that allow heavy fecal contamination of the coat and udder. Maternity stalls or calving areas should be cleaned, disinfected, and adequately bedded between uses by different cows.

Newborn calves should be removed from the calving area as soon as possible after birth because they will inevitably incur fecal–oral inoculation as they attempt to stand and nurse. Ideally, calves should be moved from the maternity area into individual hutches without being allowed to contact one another. This may not be feasible on larger dairies with limited manpower. In such situations, a small "safe pen" for calves can be constructed adjacent to the maternity pens. A safe area is a sheltered, fenced-in, well-drained, bedded concrete-floor pen located in or near the maternity area. These typically measure approximately 20 ft by 20 ft. Walls should be constructed to prevent contact with cows or bedding from the maternity area. This small area can be cleaned and disinfected daily with relative ease, and fresh bedding can be added. A large gate to facilitate cleaning with a bucket loader should be installed at one end of the safe pen to facilitate efficient (and therefore regular) removal of all bedding before cleaning and disinfection, which should be rigorous

and regularly scheduled. This pen becomes the holding area for all newborn calves in the maternity area. Personnel on the dairy are made responsible for moving newborn calves into the safe pen as soon as possible after birth; use of gloves and footbaths will aid in the prevention of pathogen spread via boots or clothing. Subsequently, calves are less likely to become rapidly inoculated with pathogens from the maternity area. The calves are kept here until the calf attendant can provide colostrum and move them to hutches. It is critical that the safe pen be disinfected regularly and not be used as a long-term housing area for calves, or accumulation of pathogens is inevitable. On large dairies, particularly those experiencing high calf morbidity and mortality problems in the first 2 weeks of life, it may be cost-effective to dedicate one employee to the maternity pen whose sole responsibility is the prompt removal of newborn calves and near immediate colostrum administration. Only larger dairies will be able to implement this because 24-hour coverage will be necessary to monitor all calvings.

Enterotoxigenic *Escherichia coli*

Etiology

ETEC produce enterotoxins that cause secretory diarrhea in the host intestine. ETEC are characterized by the presence of both specific adhesins and by the production of specific toxins. The adhesins of relevance in farm animal species are all encoded by fimbrial operons and are referred to as F-4, F-5, F-6, F-17, and F-41. Several types of enterotoxins have been identified, and a single ETEC may be capable of producing one or more enterotoxins. Both heat-labile (LT I, LT II) and heat-stable (STa, STb) enterotoxins have been identified in ETEC infections. In calves, ETEC producing the low-molecular-weight STa cause the majority of neonatal diarrhea problems.

Pathogenic ETEC must be able to attach to the host enterocytes to create disease. Once adhered, the organism releases enterotoxin, which induces the intestinal epithelial cell to secrete a fluid rich in chloride ions. Water and sodium, potassium, and bicarbonate ions follow chloride, creating a massive efflux of electrolyte-rich fluid into the intestinal lumen. Although some of this fluid is reabsorbed in the colon, the efflux of secreted fluid exceeds the colonic capacity for fluid absorption, and watery diarrhea results.

Because enterotoxins are nonimmunogenic, efforts to control ETEC in calves have centered on inducing antibody against fimbrial proteins. The fimbrial adhesins that allow pathogenic ETEC to attach to enterocytes are proteins that initially were categorized with the capsular (K) antigens. Currently, classification of fimbrial adhesins as F antigens helps to avoid confusion, but the literature still occasionally refers to K-99, K-88, and so forth rather than the current designation, F-5 and F-4, respectively. In calves, F-5 (K-99) has received the most attention regarding diagnostics and vaccine production for calves. However, ETEC possessing other fimbrial antigens or multiple fimbrial antigen types including F-6, F-17, and F-41 are capable of causing diarrhea in calves. Current literature suggests that F-4 is not associated with diarrhea in calves and that F-17 is found most often in diarrheic calves compared with other fimbrial antigen types, although there is some doubt as to the pathogenic role of F-17, and some sources maintain that it requires other fimbrial antigens to be present to be pathogenic. F-5 and F-41 currently have the strongest association with the presence of diarrhea and are currently considered the most common and significant of the ETEC adhesins. Some ETEC possess several types of fimbriae, and both F-41 and F-5 types may be isolated from an individual diarrheic calf. Colostrum possessing passive antibodies against a specific ETEC fimbrial type will protect newborn calves against that specific F type but will not cross-protect against others. Current and old nomenclature alongside toxin type elaborated for several common ETEC are given in Table 6.1.

As is the situation with nonpathotypic *E. coli* septicemia, ensuring prompt feeding of adequate levels of colostrum is extremely important to protect calves against ETEC. However, because of lack of cross-protection against various fimbrial antigens, even calves with excellent passive transfer are at risk for ETEC with F types other than those against which the dam has provided colostral antibodies. Colostrum containing antibodies against specific F types will prevent attachment of homologous ETEC to calf enterocytes by coating the fimbriae binding sites. Therefore, colostral protection is a local effect of IgG in the gut. To be effective, colostrum containing antibodies against ETEC F antigens must be fed as early in life as possible, lest ETEC colonize the gut before colostrum has been consumed. Although one experimental design showed colostral F-5 antibodies to be effective up to 3 hours after experimental oral challenge with ETEC F-5, it is more practical to assume colostrum should "beat" the ETEC to the gut. Other management factors in addition to colostral feeding are also important in the pathogenesis of ETEC diarrhea. Conditions that allow or encourage buildup of ETEC in the dry cows, in the maternity or neonatal calf facilities, or in stored colostrum increase the risk of ETEC diarrhea, as is true with *E. coli* septicemia. Marrow products in colostrum may also decrease the risk of ETEC by binding to toxin receptors or preventing proliferation of pathogenic bacteria.

Affected calves are usually 1 to 7 days of age, with most cases seen in calves less than 5 days of age. For example, calves are most susceptible to F-5 ETEC during the first 48 hours of life and thereafter begin to build resistance to the organism. Concurrent infection with rotavirus may extend the age of susceptibility to ETEC diarrhea to approximately 10 days of age. In older calves, continued exposure to heavy inocula of pathotypic ETEC may result in intestinal colonization and shedding of the organism in normal or diarrheic stools, thereby facilitating new infections in other neonates.

Clinical Signs

These signs vary from mild diarrhea with resultant spontaneous recovery to peracute syndromes characterized by diarrhea and dehydration that progress to shock and death within 4 to 12 hours.

Because of the multitude of ETEC types and variability in their pathogenicity, as well as the influence of passive transfer, individual farms may have sporadic or endemic problems resulting from ETEC. Mild disease is common on many farms and seldom is brought to a veterinarian's attention. These calves have loose or watery feces but continue to nurse (Fig. 6.4). Spontaneous recovery or apparent response to the farmer's favorite "calf-scour" treatment (usually an oral antibiotic) is the rule. Owners usually call for veterinary assistance only when peracute cases develop, a high morbidity is apparent, calves fail to respond to over-the-counter (OTC) medications, or death in neonatal calves is experienced.

Peracute cases may produce dehydrated, weak, and comatose calves within hours of the onset of the disease.

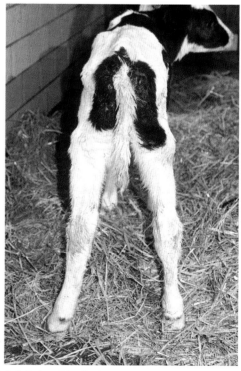

• **Fig. 6.4** A 5-day-old calf with mild "calf scours" caused by enterotoxigenic *Escherichia coli* (ETEC). The perineum, tail, and hocks are stained by watery or soupy diarrhea. This type of diarrhea could be caused by enteric pathogens other than ETEC, and clinical signs are not specific for diagnosis.

TABLE 6.1	Fimbrial Antigens for ETEC	
Designations		
New	**Old**	**Toxin**
F-4	K-88	LT I
F-5	K-99	STa
F-6	987-P	STa
F-41		Sla

Historically, these calves usually have nursed normally and appeared healthy until signs develop. Dehydration and weakness are the predominant signs (Fig. 6.5). Mucous membranes are dry, cool, and sticky. The suckle reflex is weak or absent.

Most peracute cases show evidence of voluminous diarrhea (Fig. 6.6), with watery feces coating the tail, perineum, and hind legs. Some calves with peracute disease may not have diarrhea; however, the pooling of fluid in the intestinal lumen creates abdominal distension, and fluid splashing sounds can often be detected by simultaneous auscultation and ballottement of the right lower abdominal quadrant. Mild, transient colic may be noted early in the disease course. Bradycardia and cardiac arrhythmia accompany the systemic signs in some peracute cases and result from hypoglycemia, hyperkalemia, or both. Atrial standstill has been documented in some bradycardiac calves with hyperkalemia. Rectal temperatures usually are normal or subnormal if the calf is recumbent.

Differentiation of *E. coli* septicemia from peracute ETEC infection often is difficult in the field setting because of several commonalities, including overlap in age at presentation alongside peracute onset and profound depression. In prodromal, peracute ETEC cases, the presence of massive fluid in the intestine, as evidenced by abdominal contour, simultaneous auscultation and ballottement, or abdominal ultrasonography, is a key indicator that the characteristic voluminous diarrhea is impending. Furthermore, on resuscitation with IV fluids, ETEC cases typically break with voluminous diarrhea, and provided the concurrent abnormalities in hydration, electrolyte, acid–base, and glucose status are addressed properly with IV fluids, calves with ETEC typically show rapid clinical improvement. In contrast, calves with *E. coli* septicemia show less voluminous diarrhea, and diarrhea typically develops later in the disease course. Also, in contrast to ETEC cases, calves with *E. coli* septicemia typically fail to demonstrate a dramatic clinical response to fluid resuscitation. Neonatal salmonellosis, especially that associated with *Salmonella* Dublin acquired in the immediate postnatal period, is another important differential.

Acute ETEC cases show obvious watery diarrhea, progressive dehydration, and weakness over 12 to 48 hours. The character and color of the feces vary as well, but feces usually are voluminous, watery, and yellow, white, or green. Such calves may have low-grade fever or normal temperatures and deterioration in the systemic state and suckle response. Continued secretory diarrhea gradually worsens the hydration and electrolyte deficiencies; weight loss is rapidly apparent, especially if fluid intake is decreased by reduced suckling.

Translocation of bacteria from the gut into the systemic circulation is an uncommon event when ETEC is the sole agent involved because these organisms do not invade the deeper layers of the gut wall and they incite minimal intestinal inflammation. Therefore, evidence of localized infection (e.g., hypopyon, arthritis) is uncharacteristic of ETEC infection and more indicative of colisepticemia or septicemia secondary to other enteric diseases, especially salmonellosis.

Clinical Pathology

Peracute infections resulting from ETEC cause severe secretory diarrhea that results in a classic metabolic acidosis

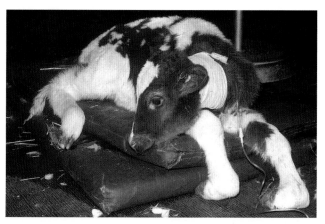

• **Fig. 6.5** Patient with peracute enterotoxigenic *Escherichia coli* diarrhea that is recumbent, extremely dehydrated, and has severe metabolic acidosis.

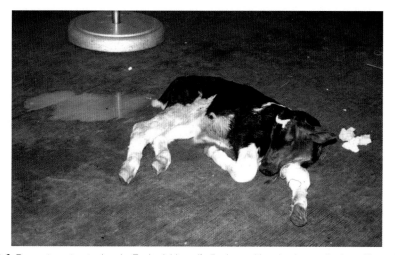

• **Fig. 6.6** Peracute enterotoxigenic *Escherichia coli*) diarrhea with voluminous diarrhea. The calf had a plasma bicarbonate level of 6 mEq/L, a systemic pH of 6.98, and a potassium level of 8.4 mEq/L. After sodium bicarbonate therapy, the calf made a quick recovery.

with low plasma bicarbonate and low venous pH. Hyperkalemia and hypoglycemia also are characteristic. Hyperkalemia results from efflux of K^+ from the intracellular fluid in exchange for excessive hydrogen ions in the extracellular fluid (ECF). Reduced renal perfusion also contributes to retention of K^+ in the ECF. Mild hyponatremia and hypochloremia are inconsistently present. Dehydration is generally greater than 8%, and corresponding elevations in packed cell volume (PCV) and total protein are typical. The WBC count usually is normal, although elevated numbers of WBC may be present because of extreme hemoconcentration, and stress leukograms occasionally are discovered. Leukopenia, left shifts, and toxic cytologic changes in neutrophils are uncommon in ETEC infections, and those findings more likely support *E. coli* septicemia or salmonellosis.

Hypoglycemia is more likely to be present if the interval between feedings is prolonged; this finding is not present in all peracute cases. Blood values for a typical case are shown in Table 6.2. Mild azotemia resulting from prerenal causes (reduced renal perfusion) is common and should be kept in mind when use of potentially nephrotoxic drugs is considered in these patients.

Diagnosis

The diagnosis is suggested by the calf's age, physical signs, and laboratory data. Peracute ETEC may be difficult to differentiate from *E. coli* septicemia and salmonellosis in neonatal calves based on clinical signs alone. Response to appropriate fluid therapy strongly supports ETEC infection, as does confirmation of adequate serum immunoglobulin in the patient.

Definitive diagnosis requires isolation or demonstration of an *E. coli* possessing pathogenic F antigens that allow intestinal attachment in calves having typical clinical signs. When submitting diagnostic samples, the clinician should indicate that ETEC infection is a possibility and should request typing of *E. coli* isolates for F antigens (by immunofluorescence, slide agglutination, or polymerase chain reaction [PCR]) and, if available, for enterotoxin (by PCR or, rarely, by ligated gut loop assays). In fatal cases, ETEC can be cultured from the ileum; a section of ileum should be tied off, placed in a sterile container, and transported on ice packs

to the laboratory. Isolation of ETEC from diarrheic feces of older calves (>5 days of age) is generally considered to merely reflect the presence of the pathogen in the calf population on that particular farm. In such cases, fresh specimens of jejunum and ileum should be examined carefully for histologic evidence of attachment of ETEC to enterocytes. These findings suggest participation in enteric disease by ETEC rather than simple intestinal colonization by the organism. Obtaining samples for culture before antibiotic therapy, particularly when oral antibiotics are being given, is an important factor in the diagnostic workup of a potential ETEC outbreak.

Histologic examination of fresh samples of ileum and jejunum of affected calves greatly aids in confirming the diagnosis of ETEC infection. Sections of ileum should be cut into 2- to 3-cm lengths and then split longitudinally and swirled in 10% neutral buffered formalin solution to aid in rapid fixation of the mucosa. Samples for histology should not be tied off because this delays fixation of the mucosa. In classic ETEC infection, a dense population of gram-negative rods is found adherent to the mucosa of the ileum.

Because mixed infections with combinations of ETEC, rotavirus, coronavirus, and *Cryptosporidium* spp. are common, feces or intestinal contents should also be analyzed for viral and protozoal pathogens. Salmonellosis also must be included in the differential diagnosis because many types of *Salmonella* spp. can cause severe diarrhea, dehydration, shock, and acid–base disturbances similar to ETEC. Fever, neutropenia, and a left shift are more commonly observed in *Salmonella* patients. In addition, enterotoxemia resulting from *Clostridium perfringens* must be considered, especially in peracute cases with abdominal distension but no diarrhea. Calves with clostridial enterotoxemia may be weak, dehydrated, or "shocky" but seldom have as dramatic a metabolic acidosis as that found in ETEC infections.

Treatment

Appropriate replacement and maintenance fluids constitute the primary therapy for ETEC infection in neonatal calves. Correction of metabolic acidosis and hypoglycemia and reestablishment of normal hydration status are imperative. Calves with peracute signs or those that are recumbent require IV therapy. Calves that can stand but show obvious dehydration, have cool and dry mucous membranes, and have a reduced or absent suckle reflex also should initially be given IV therapy. Calves that are ambulatory and have a good suckle response usually can be treated with oral fluids.

Assessment of concentrations of required electrolytes based on subjective clinical parameters rather than objective laboratory tests is empirical but sometimes necessary in field situations. Therefore, rules of thumb include:

Recumbent calves 12% to 15% dehydrated; base deficit 15 to 20 mEq/L

Weak calves 8% to 12% dehydrated; base deficit 10 to 15 mEq/L

Ambulatory calves 5% to 8% dehydrated; base deficit 5 to 10 mEq/L

TABLE 6.2	Laboratory Data from a Typical Peracute Enterotoxigenic *Escherichia coli* Infection in a 3-Day-Old Holstein Calf		
Variable	Measured Value	Reference Range	
Na^+	127	132–150	
K^+	8.1	3.9–5.5	
Cl^-	104	97–106	
HCO_3^-	12	20–30	
Total CO_2	10	26–38	
Ven pH	7.09	7.35–7.50	

These rules of thumb are not absolute, and chronic low-grade bicarbonate loss or increased D-lactate production in the gut may create profound acidosis over a period of days in a calf having only minimal signs of dehydration. A 40-kg calf that is judged 10% dehydrated will need 4 L of fluid simply to address current needs. For all calculations of replacement electrolytes, a 50% ECF will be assumed for neonates. Therefore, a 40-kg calf will be assumed to have 40 x 0.5 = 20 L ECF compartment. If this 40-kg calf has a venous plasma bicarbonate concentration of 10 mEq/L, and 25 to 30 mEq/L is the desired normal level, then 15 to 20 mEq of bicarbonate must be replaced in each liter of ECF. Therefore 20 L x 15 mEq = 300 mEq would be necessary to correct the bicarbonate deficit associated with the metabolic acidosis. Total CO_2 of venous blood also may be used to calculate base deficits in lieu of HCO_3 values.

A great deal of research data as well as strong individual clinical opinion exist as to the most appropriate composition of initial fluid therapy for ETEC infections in calves. An effective solution, first proposed by Dr. R.H. Whitlock, is formulated by adding 150 mEq of $NaHCO_3^-$ to 1 L of 5% glucose. This combination is used for the initial 1 to 3 L of IV therapy, depending on the severity of measured or suspected metabolic acidosis. Glucose corrects hypoglycemia if present, and both bicarbonate and glucose facilitate potassium transport back into cells, thereby lessening the potential cardiotoxicity associated with hyperkalemia. Some reports minimize the importance of hyperkalemia and suggest using IV potassium in the initial fluid. The authors of these papers emphasize that dehydrated calves having severe ETEC-induced secretory diarrhea have a total body K^+ deficit despite having an elevated ECF potassium concentration. Although this may undoubtedly be true, it seems risky to tempt fate by administering K^+-containing solutions as the initial therapy for a patient known to be hyperkalemic. This is especially true for a patient with bradycardia or arrhythmias because death has occasionally occurred when potassium-containing fluids have been given as initial therapy. After plasma K^+ and HCO_3^- levels are quickly improved by the initial 1 to 3 L of 5% dextrose with 150 mEq $NaHCO_3^-$/L, potassium-containing fluids can be safely used. Balanced electrolyte solutions such as lactated Ringer's solution suffice for maintenance fluid needs, but supplemental $NaHCO_3^-$ and dextrose may be required to address continued secretory losses and anorexia. Response to treatment usually is dramatic in calves with secretory ETEC diarrhea. Calves that were initially recumbent usually appear much improved after administration of 2 to 4 L of appropriate IV fluids and usually can stand within 6 hours and begin to nurse within 6 to 24 hours of the initiation of therapy. This type of prompt response strongly suggests a correct diagnosis and tends to rule out septicemia because septicemic calves seldom respond so promptly, if at all. Depending on the setting (field vs clinic), maintenance or intermittent IV fluid therapy may be continued or replaced by oral fluids in those calves that quickly regain a suckle response and are eager to eat.

Antibiotic therapy for peracute ETEC infections remains controversial, with current concerns focused on antimicrobial residues in meat and indiscriminate and unnecessary use of antimicrobials leading to resistance. However, in peracute cases, the overlap of many clinical signs with colisepticemia often prompts the clinician to include antimicrobial treatment in the therapeutic regimen. In a Canadian study, diarrheic calves 5 days of age or younger were found to be at significantly greater risk of bacteremia than older calves; this age range obviously includes calves at risk for ETEC infection. Furthermore, in cases with fever and severe debilitation, the veterinarian is often prompted to consider the possibility of complicating conditions such as bacterial pneumonia. In his thorough reviews of the subject, Constable found published evidence supporting the logic and clinical efficacy of antimicrobial use to all calves that exhibit systemic signs of illness or that have blood or mucosal casts in their stool. Extra-label drug use can be justified because the health and potential survival of the patient is threatened, and there is a paucity of approved, labeled claims for the treatment of neonatal diarrhea. In the United States, however, clinicians must always be mindful of federal law that prohibits extra-label third-generation cephalosporin use and limits the use of fluoroquinolones to specific clinical indications. Because of the challenges in differentiating ETEC, *E. coli* septicemia, and peracute salmonellosis, clinicians are often faced with patients in whom it may be impossible to clinically differentiate true bacteremia from merely lumenally confined enteric bacterial infections when making therapeutic decisions. Parenteral antimicrobials that are bactericidal with a gram-negative spectrum therefore have intuitive appeal for undifferentiated cases. In patients with pure ETEC infections, oral antimicrobial treatment offers the potential benefit of reducing the number of ETEC in the gut, and by reducing the source of enterotoxin, one might also reduce the drive for hypersecretion and ameliorate the metabolic consequences of the enteric infection. Oral amoxicillin trihydrate (10 mg/kg orally every 12 hours) or amoxicillin trihydrate–clavulanate potassium (12.5 mg combined drug/kg orally every 12 hours) for at least 3 days for treatment of such cases is justifiable if the ETEC strain is believed or proven to be susceptible to the antibiotic. Repeated use of these products over the long term is likely to induce resistance and cause further disruption of the intestinal microbiome; therefore, long-term efforts must focus on prevention rather than treatment. Recommended treatments for diarrheic calves with signs of severe systemic illness (e.g., fever and weakness that persist after fluid resuscitation) include ceftiofur, amoxicillin, potentiated sulfonamides (25 mg/kg IV or intramuscularly [IM] every 24 hours) or ampicillin (10 mg/kg IM every 12 hours). Systemic antibiotics usually are continued for 3 to 5 days based on the calf's clinical response, temperature, and character of the feces.

Data from across the world increasingly report that many ETEC cases that result in high calf mortality have limited antibiotic susceptibility, and therefore sensitivity testing or mean inhibitory concentration (MIC) levels should always be determined when the herd history or clinical data suggest high morbidity and mortality from ETEC.

Feces usually remain more watery than normal for 2 to 4 days. If diarrhea persists beyond this time, concurrent infection with other organisms is likely. Other treatments for peracute cases may include flunixin meglumine (1.1–2.2 mg/kg IV every 24 hours) for potential endotoxemia, resolution of fever, and reduction of pain associated with fluid-filled bowel. Repeated dosages of this product carry the risk of renal and GI injury because continued use of flunixin meglumine interferes with vasodilatory prostaglandin synthesis in the gut and kidney.

Milk or milk replacer should be withheld for no more than 24 to 36 hours, during which time a high-quality oral electrolyte energy source may be fed several times (four to six times) daily. Holding ETEC-infected calves off milk or replacer for prolonged times creates weight loss from inadequate energy intake and places calves at risk of starvation. Even though many oral electrolytes are supplemented with dextrose as an energy source, no commercial oral electrolyte solution provides enough energy for maintenance needs, especially for dairy calves in hutches during winter weather. Weight will be lost, and starvation may occur if these electrolyte solutions are fed as the only ration for more than 1 or 2 days. In highly valuable calves undergoing hospitalization, treatment with parenteral nutrition offers an excellent option to at least approximate maintenance calorific needs while the calf is nil per os (NPO). Calves with ETEC are so significantly catabolic that they will still lose weight despite calorific supplementation with IV lipid and amino acids. Careful monitoring of blood glucose for hyperglycemia and strict attention to aseptic technique, as well as catheter and fluid line maintenance, are important when administering parenteral nutrition. Consequently, it is rarely practical outside of a referral hospital.

The alkalinizing potential of oral electrolyte solutions is of great importance, especially when those solutions are used as ongoing therapy for peracute cases after initial IV fluids or when those solutions are used as sole therapy of less severely affected calves having ETEC. Continued HCO_3^- loss accompanying secretory ETEC diarrhea must be anticipated and treated. Therefore, oral electrolyte solutions containing bicarbonate or some other alkalinizing anion are most helpful. The optimal oral electrolyte solutions typically possess 70 to 80 mEq of alkalinizing potential per liter (typically as bicarbonate, propionate or acetate), dextrose, and electrolytes; these should be fed at 4 to 6 L/day. Oral electrolyte solutions that when mixed with water are nearly isotonic are preferred over those that are markedly hypertonic.

Concerns regarding adding oral electrolyte solutions to milk or milk replacers revolve around the alkalinizing solutions' tendency to interfere with abomasal

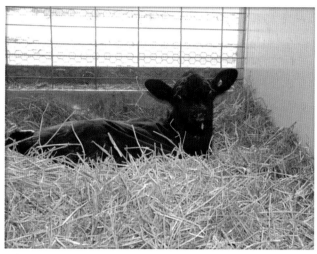

• **Fig. 6.7** A Holstein calf in deep straw bedding. This depth of bedding is appropriate for recovery and normal "nesting" behavior of calves in winter weather. The lower limbs are not visible from outside the pen. (Courtesy of Dr. Sheila McGuirk.)

clot formation. Therefore, oral electrolytes are fed during separate feedings at least 30 minutes before or after a milk feeding. Calves do not digest sucrose effectively, and addition of table sugar to "home remedy" electrolyte mixtures will reliably worsen fluid and electrolyte losses in diarrheic stools. After 24 to 36 hours of oral electrolyte treatment, calves may be fed small volumes of milk or milk replacer. Calves that respond rapidly to initial fluid resuscitation can be started back on small volumes of milk or milk replacer at an earlier time. During recuperation, calves should be deeply bedded in dry straw (Fig. 6.7) or similar bedding material and provided shelter from rain and snow. When milk feedings are resumed, feedings are best performed in small volumes frequently. If this is not possible, whole milk or replacer should be divided into at least two to three daily feedings. Supplemental oral electrolyte solutions can be continued if ongoing fluid and electrolyte losses are assumed to result from continued diarrhea, and these solutions should be fed at intervals between whole milk or replacer feedings. Unless the calf is hypoglycemic or acidotic, isotonic electrolyte solutions are preferred because they allow a more normal abomasal transit than do hypertonic solutions.

Treatment of acute ETEC infections in calves that are ambulatory and still able to suckle may not require IV therapy. Cessation of whole milk or replacer feeding coupled with substitution of oral electrolyte–glucose solutions for 24 to 36 hours may be sufficient. Bicarbonate loss and resulting metabolic acidosis should not be underestimated, however. It is imperative to use highly alkalinizing electrolyte glucose solutions to provide 4 to 6 L of fluids per day. Parenteral antibiotics are indicated if the affected calf is febrile, and oral antibiotics may be administered when the herd medical history indicates involvement of a highly pathogenic ETEC. Milk or replacer should be reinstituted after 24 to 36 hours, and electrolyte feedings can then be used as fluid supplements in the intervals between milk feedings as needed.

Mild ETEC infections seldom require veterinary care. Spontaneous recovery is the rule, and supportive care with oral electrolyte solutions frequently is used by owners in such cases. Use of OTC remedies is widespread among dairy farmers treating mild ETEC infections or nonspecific "calf scours." Although little scientific evidence is found to justify these products, anecdotal testimonials from farmers exist for many oral products and protectants. Oligosaccharides have received increased interest in recent years, the suggested therapeutic rationale being that they provide competitive binding sites within the intestinal lumen for the fimbrial adhesins of ETEC, thereby facilitating intestinal transit and elimination. Although their administration via water has been shown to reduce intestinal coliform counts in experimental ETEC infection, there has yet to be conclusive proof of improved clinical outcomes in challenge studies. OTC calf diarrhea products that contain methscopolamine, atropine, or products that reduce intestinal motility are contraindicated and may cause bloat and ileus if overdosed. Bismuth subsalicylate is palatable and can be used safely in calves. Most recently, an OTC crofelemer extract Neonorm™, a natural product with antisecretory properties, was shown to significantly increase fecal dry matter of neonatal calves with experimentally induced enterotoxigenic *E. coli* diarrhea.

Prevention

Prevention assumes prime importance when a high morbidity rate, significant mortality rate, or both occur on a dairy farm. It is not unusual to encounter 70% to 100% morbidity and mortality when virulent strains of ETEC are present. These strains also tend to be resistant to many antibiotics. The usual situation is that the owner tries multiple OTC products on the first few affected calves and then calls for veterinary assistance to select a "better" antibiotic. One or more calves may die or require intensive therapy before a thorough investigation of the problem ensues.

The veterinarian must avoid the temptation to simply provide or suggest a "newer" or better antibiotic if the problem is to be solved. Feces must be submitted from *more than one* acutely affected calf. If necessary, bull calves should be raised in an identical manner to heifers just to allow them to develop disease and allow early sampling. A qualified diagnostic laboratory must identify the *E. coli* as an ETEC strain with specific attachment antigens and determine antibiotic susceptibility. Diagnostic efforts beyond mere speciation are vitally important.

Management must be meticulously assessed as to the cleanliness of dry cows, colostrum, feeding instruments, maternity areas, and newborn calf facilities. Evidence of successful passive transfer of immunoglobulins must be evaluated in several consecutive calves to rule out *E. coli* septicemia or poor colostral feeding as the major cause of ETEC infection. Culturing of colostrum at milking and from the bucket or bottle immediately before its feeding can be used to assess the cleanliness of colostrum milking

procedures, colostrum storage, and feeding instrument hygiene. Readers are directed to the previous section on colisepticemia for more details on assessment of colostrum management. Evaluation of whole milk or milk replacer feeding and the detailed specifics by which diarrheic calves are being treated become extremely important. Mixing errors leading to hyperosmolality of oral feedings (especially electrolyte solutions) or milk replacer can add a further and compromising degree of nutritional diarrhea in some situations. It is remarkable how many extra supplements can be added to the feeding regimen on problem farms such that the end product becomes a contributor to the persistence and severity of the diarrhea. The osmolality of electrolyte solutions should be in the range of 300 to 600 mOs/L, although some solutions at the high end of this range may be problematic if ad libitum water is not available. The ad libitum provision of palatable fresh water is imperative, hyperosmolality of administered oral fluids being compounded by the lack of water by which the calf can compensate. The two biggest challenges to adequate water intake are the health or severity of illness in the calf and the freezing conditions during northern U.S. winter months. Water intake is maximal immediately after milk feeding, so at the very least fresh, warm unfrozen water should be made available shortly after milk or milk replacer intake. Measuring total solids in milk replacer, as fed, is a highly relevant part of a herd investigation as is checking osmolality of any oral rehydration solutions, again as fed. Total solids of milk replacer solutions should never exceed 18%, and it is always reassuring to be able to demonstrate consistency by virtue of a less than 1% variation from feeding to feeding. Milk replacer hygiene is just as relevant as total solids or osmolality; substantial bacterial contamination of milk, colostrum, or milk replacer because of unsanitary equipment, powder storage, or the use of unpasteurized waste milk has detrimental health consequences for all calves but especially those for whom adequacy of passive transfer was compromised. Targets established by Dr. Sheila McGuirk are a total bacterial count of less than 20,000 CFU/mL, a total coliform count of less than 1000 CFU/mL and a total *E. coli* count of less than 100 CFU/mL for pasteurized waste milk; for milk replacer, the set points are less than 10,000 CFU/mL, less than 1000 CFU/mL, and zero, respectively. Samples for testing should be sampled as fed; for example, they should be taken via the nipple in a group pen situation rather than at the time of mixing.

If an ETEC with attachment antigens such as F-5 is identified in the feces of more than one affected calf, more specific preventive measures can be instituted. Management factors including colostral feeding must be emphasized, lest preventive vaccines are looked on by the farmer as a "silver bullet" that obviates any need for management changes. When specific F antigen ETEC are involved, a commercial bacterin containing these F types can be administered to the dry cows 6 weeks and 3 weeks before freshening or at manufacturer's recommended times. Autogenous bacterin manufacturers should be required to show data on endotoxin levels in bacterins because administration of endotoxin-rich vaccines to adult cattle can cause dramatic production losses or abortion. When vaccines are first used those calves born in the immediate 3-4 weeks following may still not receive adequate specific colostral antibody protection because of insufficient time and may be given commercially available oral monoclonal antibodies against F-5 (K99). This should only work if a commercial product is available and has been confirmed as the attachment factor for the ETEC in question. Monoclonal antibody products must be given immediately after birth before colostrum is fed (Ecolizer, Elanco Animal Health, Greenfield, IN, and First Defense, Immucell, Portland, ME). Valuable calves at risk and born to these same dry cows also may receive oral antibiotics for the first 3 to 5 days of life in an effort to prevent infection with the ETEC identified, and selection of appropriate antibiotics should be based on antibiotic susceptibility testing of the causative organism.

Rarely, a particular serotype of *E. coli* other than the F-5 type is isolated from the small intestine of scouring neonatal calves. If the organism is consistently confirmed as the pathogen (based on samples from multiple affected calves) and commercial dry cow vaccines have not altered the incidence of disease, an autogenous bacterin should be considered. However, the use of autogenous bacterins can only be justified when an absolute diagnosis of a highly pathogenic ETEC has been confirmed by isolates from several affected calves and commercial bacterins fail to stop the disease. Because free endotoxin content may be high in some autogenous vaccines made from gram-negative organisms, the manufacturer should "wash" the preparation to reduce endotoxin content, and data on endotoxin content in the final product should be requested. It is important to resist the temptation to initiate autogenous bacterin production using a nonspecific *E. coli* isolate obtained from one or more calves that merely had colisepticemia as a result of FPT.

Other *Escherichia coli* Diarrhea
Etiology

Although less common than ETEC, other forms of pathotypic *E. coli* have been identified as causes of calf diarrhea. Enteropathogenic strains are defined as those capable of attachment and effacement of intestinal cell microvilli. Attaching and effacing (AEEC) *E. coli* are EPEC that do not produce enterotoxins but may produce cytotoxins of various types. They do not possess *Shigella*-like invasiveness. These organisms have been isolated from calves with diarrhea that have histologic evidence of effacement of microvilli in the cecum, colon, and distal small intestine. Cellular degeneration may ensue if the organisms produce cytotoxins. These histologic changes enable differentiation of AEEC from ETEC that attach to enterocytes but do not cause histologic damage. Because the lesions of EPEC typically involve the large intestine, dysentery and diarrhea may be observed. Malabsorption, maldigestion, and protein loss are characteristic of disease with AEEC or EPEC. Calves from 2 days of age up to 4 months of age may be infected, and other enteric pathogens often are present concurrently.

They can also be identified in the feces of healthy calves such that their role is somewhat controversial. For example, a recent large meta-analysis of the epidemiology of *E. coli* in calves demonstrated that EPEC are twice as likely to be found in healthy calves as diarrheic ones. However, cattle are frequently identified as being an important reservoir for these and other pathotypic *E. coli* in humans.

Shiga toxin-producing *E. coli* (STEC) are another type of *E. coli* that produce hemorrhagic colitis and the hemolytic uremic syndrome in humans. These organisms are often more broadly grouped within the enterohemorrhagic *E. coli* (EHEC) and occasionally have been found in sick calves. Some of these strains invade the mucosa to reside in the lamina propria of the large intestine and produce a severe hemorrhagic colitis. Ulcerative colitis with hemorrhage may be present grossly and microscopically in necropsy specimens. STEC are defined by their ability to produce at least one of the Shiga toxins, Stx1 or Stx2, and the role of these pathogens in cattle has not been conclusively elucidated, although fatal cases have been documented. Approximately 75% of human outbreaks with EHEC have been linked to bovine derived products or cattle, highlighting the importance of public health awareness for this zoonotic pathogen to the dairy industry. Enteroaggregative *E. coli* (EAEC), diffusely adherent *E. coli* (DAEC), and enteroinvasive *E. coli* (EIEC) are yet more groups of pathotypic *E. coli* with characteristic pathogenetic and histologic features that can be linked to specific, different toxins; however they are of uncertain relevance in calf diarrhea. EAEC, for example, have the ability to form mucoid biofilms and secret potent cytotoxins linked genetically to a plasmid that encodes both for fimbriae and toxins. This plasmid may be found in the same strains of *E. coli* responsible for calf diarrhea and septicemia in neonatal farm animals.

Clinical Signs

As observed with ETEC diarrhea, dehydration, depression, and weakness are common signs associated with EPEC, AEEC, and STEC (EHEC) infections in calves. Dysentery or fresh blood in the feces, when present, suggest severe colitis and distinguish the disease from ETEC secretory diarrhea. Fever tends to be more common with AEEC and STEC because of mucosal damage and erosive or ulcerative damage to the intestine. Diarrhea is profuse in some calves and intermittent but blood and mucus tinged in others. Tenesmus may be observed as a result of colonic inflammation. Blood loss in the feces may be negligible with some AEEC or severe enough to cause anemia and hypovolemic shock in some with STEC (EHEC). Dysentery or frank blood in the feces always dictates that *Salmonella* spp. be ruled out as a cause of the diarrhea because clinical signs of AEEC and STEC (EHEC) can closely resemble those found in patients with *Salmonella* infection. Affected calves usually are 4 to 28 days of age, and morbidity and mortality vary greatly.

Laboratory Data

Calves affected with EPEC, AEEC, and STEC have maldigestion and malabsorption and may have protein loss from erosive or ulcerative colonic lesions. Therefore, total protein and the albumin fraction of serum may be low. Anemia may be present because of GI blood loss. Total WBC counts may be normal or low with a left shift. Although shock and lactic acidosis may create a metabolic acidosis in recumbent patients, calves still standing tend not to have a remarkable base deficit because the pathophysiology of their diarrhea is different than the secretory diarrhea of ETEC.

Diagnosis

The emphasis for most veterinary diagnostic laboratories is in the identification of typical ETEC fimbrial antigens when processing diagnostic samples from calf diarrhea cases. The definitive diagnosis of other pathotypic *E. coli* requires more specific analytical methods to demonstrate specific toxins such as Stx1, Stx2, and enterotoxin or to demonstrate specific in vitro adhesion or cytopathic effect. Categorization and typing of these organisms can only be performed by specialized diagnostic laboratories (e.g., Animal Diagnostic Laboratory, Pennsylvania State University, University Park, PA). Because coexisting enteric, bacterial, viral, or protozoan infection is present in most calves with AEEC or STEC, feces should be analyzed for rotavirus, coronavirus, ETEC, *Salmonella* spp., *C. perfringens* type C, and *Cryptosporidium parvum*. If the incidence of diseased calves with diarrhea is found to be high, fecal samples from several acute cases should be evaluated to ensure that the suspected AEEC or STEC is in fact consistently the cause of calf diarrhea on this farm.

Treatment

Therapy is similar to that for ETEC infection except that whole blood transfusions of 1 to 2 L of blood may be necessary in calves with severe dysentery and fecal blood loss. Ceftiofur is the most frequently used parenterally administered antimicrobial for this disease. Broad-spectrum antibiotics such as gentamicin (6.6 mg/kg intramuscular (IM) or IV every 24 hours), amikacin (15 mg/kg SC or IV every 24 hours), or trimethoprim–sulfa combinations (22 mg/kg SC, IM, IV or orally every 12 hours) are also used because of the microvillus or mucosal damage within the intestine, but these represent extra-label drug use in the United States, and aminoglycosides should only be administered after appropriate laboratory diagnostics and understanding of prolonged meat withdrawal. Prognosis is guarded for calves with AEEC or STEC infections unless intensive care is provided. Colonic, cecal, or distal ileal pathology may be so severe as to cause ulceration or perforation of the intestine in some cases. Because of the gross and histologic intestinal pathology, corticosteroids and prostaglandin inhibitors are contraindicated except when used once in conjunction with initial shock therapy because these drugs reduce cytoprotective mechanisms within the bowel.

Because of the maldigestion and malabsorption created by these organisms, oral electrolyte–energy sources may be less useful than in ETEC. These products, however, usually are recommended for at least the first 36 to 48 hours of therapy. Calves continuing to have diarrhea after 48 hours can be returned to milk or replacer feeding but may be candidates for TPN if they are valuable enough to warrant the expense.

Prevention

Because AEEC and STEC do not possess typical F-5 fimbriae, commercial dry cow bacterins and monoclonal antibodies against F-5 are unlikely to prevent future outbreaks. Therefore, management procedures should be examined carefully and corrected when found deficient. If multiple isolates confirm a single AEEC or STEC strain, autogenous bacterins administered twice during the dry period may be considered. Colostral management (hygiene and feeding) and passive transfer of immunoglobulins must be assessed.

If rotavirus, coronavirus, *C. parvum,* or other enteric pathogens are found to be concurrent problems, these should be addressed from a management and preventative standpoint. The frequent association of these pathogens with AEEC and STEC raise concern that these pathogens may be the primary cause of intestinal injury, and the AEEC or STEC in fact may be secondary.

The veterinarian responsible for herd health must consider the public health concerns associated with some AEEC or STEC. Currently, the 0157:H7 strain has caused a great deal of bad publicity for the dairy industry because cattle have been blamed as carriers of this organism that may infect people, causing severe colitis and occasionally hemolytic uremic syndrome. Therefore, sanitation, disinfection, and very careful handling of feces to avoid human infection are indicated.

Rotavirus
Etiology

Rotaviruses are members of the Reoviridae family and are classified further via complicated division into groups (serogroups), serotypes, and subgroups. The rotaviruses cause diarrhea in multiple species, including humans. Although the rotaviruses share certain antigens and cross-infection of species occurs with some strains, in general resistance is specific, and cross-protection against heterologous strains is poor. They are not zoonotic.

Calves usually are infected by group A and less commonly by group B serotypes. Initially identified by Mebus and coworkers, the Nebraska rotavirus isolate was used extensively for study and vaccine production. Other group A serotypes have been identified in the United States and abroad. Exposure to rotaviruses apparently is widespread in the cattle population based on serologic surveys. Older calves and adult cattle serve as carriers of the virus, shedding the virus intermittently in feces. In addition, up to 20% of healthy calves may shed rotavirus. As a rule, rotaviruses coexist with other neonatal enteric pathogens such as ETEC and *C. parvum* in herd calfhood diarrhea outbreaks. Experimental mixed infections of rotavirus with bovine viral diarrhea virus (BVDV) have been shown to result in more severe diarrhea than infection with either of these agents alone, suggesting some synergistic effect in pathogenicity.

Neonatal calves (<14 days of age) are at greatest risk for infection by enteric rotavirus, and most infections occur during the first week of life. Prevalence of infection in neonatal calves born on dairy farms harboring the virus is high, morbidity is high (50% to 100%), and mortality varies greatly. Clinical manifestations of disease and mortality in calves are influenced by several factors, including level of immunity to the virus, magnitude of viral inoculum, viral serotype, concurrent infection of the gastrointestinal tract or other systems, stress, and crowding. Germ-free calves infected by rotavirus have self-limiting diarrhea and rapid recovery. Infected calves in field situations may have inapparent, mild, moderate, or fatal disease. As is true with most enteric pathogens, the younger the patient, the higher the likelihood of severe disease because of losses of water, electrolytes, and body nutrient reserves secondary to diarrhea.

Rotavirus infection is limited to the small intestine and characterized by destruction of villous enterocytes and subsequent replacement of these columnar cells by immature and more cuboidal cells derived from the intestinal crypts. Although these new immature cells are resistant to further viral infection, they are unable to carry out the normal digestive and absorptive tasks necessary for villous enterocytes because of deficient disaccharidase and sodium–potassium ATPase activities. Therefore, rotavirus diarrhea is characterized by maldigestion and malabsorption. To further complicate matters, the intestinal crypt cells continue their normal secretory function, which is no longer balanced by absorptive villous function. Thus, net secretion outweighs absorption and contributes further to diarrhea. Increasing intraluminal osmotic pressure also may draw further water into the bowel as lactose and other undigested nutrients pass through the gut and are fermented in the colon to volatile fatty acids. Bacterial fermentation of undigested lactose creates both D- and L-isomers of lactic acid; in diarrheic calves, absorption of the slowly metabolized D-isomer may result in accumulation of this acid in the systemic circulation, thereby contributing to the development of metabolic acidosis and clinical depression. Water and electrolyte losses of variable severity occur in affected calves.

The level of local passive immunity conferred to calves by colostral intake somewhat determines the risk and relative severity of infection. Colostrum with a high virus-neutralizing antibody titer ($\geq$1:1024) against rotavirus is protective against experimental infection. However, unless colostrum or colostrum–milk combinations with titers this high continue to be fed, this local protection "wears off" within a few days, and the calf becomes susceptible to infection. Colostral rotavirus specific IgA is likely most responsible for protection. Colostrum or colostrum–milk combinations with lower virus neutralizing titers may impart partial protection. Feeding of colostrum having very high levels of IgG_1 antibodies against rotavirus soon after birth may establish high circulating humoral antibodies against rotavirus. Although this humoral protection will not, by itself, protect a calf from infection, a portion of these IgG_1 antibodies is secreted back into the intestine over time and is thought to confer additional local protection against infection.

Data from numerous studies consistently demonstrate that rotavirus is either the most common or second most common infectious agent identified in calf diarrhea investigations.

Clinical Signs

No pathognomonic signs of rotavirus exist in dairy calves that allow differentiation of the disease from ETEC or other enteropathogens. In addition, infections may be subclinical, mild, moderate, or severe based on factors such as inoculum dose and serotype virulence of virus, immunity of the calf, concurrent enteric or other system infections in the calf, and other stressors.

Depression, reduced suckle response, diarrhea, and dehydration comprise the major clinical signs. Fever, hypersalivation, and recumbency may be observed in some patients. Feces usually are watery and yellow in pure rotavirus enteritis. Because mixed infections are common, however, the color, consistency, and composition of the feces vary greatly.

Signs of depression, dehydration, and shock are more likely to occur in the youngest calves (< 5 days of age) and seldom occur in calves more than 2 weeks of age unless D-lactic acid production is high. Recumbent calves usually have profuse watery diarrhea and abdominal distention of the right lower quadrant with fluid-filled small intestine.

Ancillary Data

Laboratory data are not specific enough to aid in the diagnosis of rotavirus enteritis in calves. Severely affected calves will develop a metabolic acidosis with low plasma bicarbonate. Other electrolytes and glucose values tend to be low but vary with the severity and duration of disease.

Diagnosis

Diagnosis requires identification of rotavirus particles or nucleic acid in the feces of acutely infected calves. Feces should be collected within the first 24 hours of illness and diarrhea. Until recently, feces submitted to qualified diagnostic laboratories were examined by electron microscopy (EM) to observe viral particles or subjected to testing using a latex agglutination test or an enzyme-linked immunosorbent assay (ELISA) to detect viral antigen. Fluorescent antibody (FA) stains also are available for tissue analysis from fatal cases. The accuracy of EM and ELISA tests, although high and commonly in agreement in side-by-side studies, is certainly less sensitive than PCR methods, such that the majority of diagnostic laboratories have now moved to PCR as the standard test for the diagnosis of rotavirus infection. Because of the frequency of mixed infections, feces submitted from acute neonatal diarrhea cases should be analyzed for viruses, bacteria, and *C. parvum*. Feces from more than one acute case in the herd must be tested before staking an entire prevention program on one etiologic agent. Affected calves should also be assessed for adequacy of passive transfer of immunoglobulins to rule out FPT.

Treatment

Treatment is nonspecific and generally follows therapy described for ETEC regarding indications and types.

Several differences are noted, however:

1. Because of villous enterocyte pathology, the efficiency of absorption of oral electrolyte and energy sources is likely reduced compared to ETEC infections. Obviously, this comment is relative, not absolute because generally less than 100% of the small intestinal villi are damaged. Therefore, absorption of some proportion of the glucose, electrolytes, and water that comprise the oral fluids will occur, and aggressive oral fluid therapy (4–6 L/day) is still indicated in this disease. Isotonic electrolyte replacements may be preferable unless the calf is hypoglycemic. Electrolyte solutions containing glutamate mixed with yogurt may speed intestinal recovery, although this is not proven in calves.

2. Maldigestion and malabsorption influence the duration of diarrhea and the digestibility of whole milk or milk replacers in patients with viral enteritis. When diarrhea from rotavirus becomes evident, the damage to the intestinal lining has already occurred, and only time and supportive care can allow the intestine to heal. Nutritional support is a critical component of that supportive care, particularly because rotaviral scours may persist for 3 to 7 days. Producers should be counseled that provision of milk or milk replacer is necessary in viral enteritis even though the maldigestion of the milk nutrients may contribute in part to the pathologic process. Denial (for >24 hours) of milk feeding to a calf with viral diarrhea places the calf at significant risk for cachexia and may lower its resistance to opportunistic disease. Death from starvation may occur in such cases, particularly during times of inclement weather (Fig. 6.8). To quote Dr. Chuck Guard, "If a calf scours for a week, and all that the calf is fed is oral electrolyte replacer, then that calf will be well hydrated and will have absolutely perfect blood electrolyte concentrations and acid–base balance on the day it starves to death." Producers should learn to live with the "more-in, more out" rule: The more milk that goes in the front end, the more diarrhea comes out the back end. However, this process is not necessarily harmful because digestion and absorption of some fraction of milk nutrients is likely to occur, and these nutrients are necessary to support the tissue synthesis required to return the intestine to normal.

Any exacerbation of fluid losses and acidosis that may result from maldigestion of milk nutrients can be offset by aggressive fluid and electrolyte replacement. Ideally, the affected calf should be fed small amounts frequently with the addition of lactase-containing tablets. Because maldigestion is part of the pathophysiology, common sense suggests that dividing milk feeding into smaller but more frequent meals would allow improved digestion and lower the amount of carbohydrate reaching

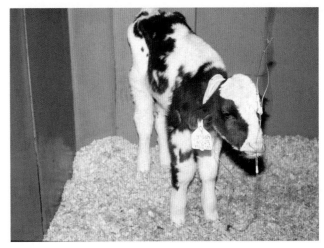

• **Fig. 6.8** A 3-week-old Red and White Holstein calf with chronic diarrhea and emaciation caused by rotavirus and *Cryptosporidium* infection. The calf was normally hydrated and had normal electrolytes but was deteriorating because of malabsorption and maldigestion and cachexia. This is one of the first calves we successfully treated using parenteral nutrition (in 1982).

the colon. Excessive amounts of carbohydrates reaching the colon may worsen diarrhea, systemic metabolic status especially D-lactic acidosis, and the clinical status of the calf.

3. Maturation of immature villous replacement cells of crypt origin will allow the intestinal tract to return to normal within several days to 1 week in most patients that recover.

Intravenous fluid therapy is necessary for recumbent, extremely dehydrated, or "shocky" patients and patients that have lost their suckle reflex. It is best guided by acid–base and electrolyte determinations. If this is not practical or available, however, the most severely affected calves with acute diarrhea should be assumed to have metabolic acidosis, low bicarbonate, high potassium, and low glucose values. Guidelines for fluid therapy are available in the section on treatment of ETEC. Parenteral nutrition may be "lifesaving" in calves with cachexia.

Although there is no need for antibiotic therapy in pure rotaviral enteritis, the likelihood of mixed infections and the pathologic damage to enterocytes that fosters attachment of bacterial pathogens may be reason enough to treat severely affected calves with systemic antibiotics.

Control

Rotavirus is ubiquitous in cattle populations; therefore, management procedures that decrease the magnitude of exposure of neonatal calves to rotavirus must be the focus of preventive efforts. Cleaning maternity pens between calvings, immediately removing the calf from the dam (and thus exposure to feces), placing the calf in an individual hutch that has been cleaned and relocated since removal of the last occupant, and feeding the calf from its own nipple bottle or pail rather than a common feeding device all help reduce spread of viral pathogens. Feces from a clinically diseased calf may contain hundreds of millions of viral particles per gram and can contaminate inanimate objects and workers' feet, clothing, and hands to be passed to a naïve calf. The use of a safe pen can also be considered (see discussion in section on colisepticemia).

Vaccination of newborn calves or dry cows is somewhat controversial because passive humoral immunoglobulins derived from colostrum probably are not as effective as passive local immunoglobulins derived by continued feeding of colostrum or colostrum–milk combinations that contain high antibody levels against rotavirus. Oral modified-live virus (MLV) vaccination of newborn calves before feeding them colostrum has been practiced. However, it is somewhat cumbersome for most management teams and risks bacterial infection and FPT because colostrum is withheld until several hours after the MLV oral vaccination to prevent inactivation of the vaccine by colostral antibodies. Although neonatal calf vaccination can induce cell-mediated immunity and secretory IgA and IgM against rotavirus of vaccine serotype, efficacy in field studies has been questioned. The utility of PCR assays as the favored diagnostic test for the diagnosis of rotaviral diarrhea is also complicated when MLV vaccines have been administered to neonates. Viral nucleic acid of vaccinal origin can give false-positive results for a length of time that likely exceeds false-positive results given by EM or ELISA. The precise length of time that the vaccinated calf will remain fecal PCR positive is unknown, but this eventuality should be considered probable for a minimum of 3 days after vaccination.

Because colostrum, colostrum–milk combinations, or milk containing virus-neutralizing antibodies with a titer of 1:1024 or greater will protect the gut from infection by local means, feeding such material to calves for the first 14 to 30 days of life usually will prevent rotavirus infection. This also requires that the serotype of rotavirus to which the calves are exposed be the same as that from which the colostral antibodies have been derived. It also requires that management prevent overwhelming exposure of neonatal calves to challenge with this or other combined infections.

Boosting the level of rotavirus antibody in colostrum is a potential means to prevent enteric rotavirus infection if calves are fed adequate to large amounts of colostrum to achieve local protection. If colostrum is only fed for 1 or a few days, the local protective effect will "wear off," and the calf will become susceptible to rotavirus enteritis. Continued feeding of colostrum is ideal but often not practical. Initial postnatal ingestion of very high antibody-containing colostrum may in fact create high enough humoral antibody levels to establish high levels of secretory IgG$_1$ antibodies in the gut. Boosting the level of colostral antibodies against rotavirus usually is done by vaccinating the dry cow with MLV or killed vaccines containing rotavirus and coronavirus, sometimes in combination with ETEC antigens. Currently, the killed products generally are recommended, and the dry cow should be vaccinated 6 and 3 weeks before freshening (or according to manufacturer's recommendations)

and subsequently given booster shots each year, no less than 4 weeks before freshening. No vaccine or antibody can overcome massive viral challenge, and conversely, less concern for passive protection is necessary when management excels at reducing risk for the newborn calf. Given the practical limitations and expense and impracticality of continued colostrum (or colostrum supplement) feeding of calves, the producer should focus on initial colostrum administration to newborns, maternity pen and hutch hygiene, dry cow vaccination, and controlling spread by fomites and personnel. Incidence of rotavirus diarrhea has been decreased on some farms and reported in two clinical trials by mixing some colostrum (10%) with milk or replacer for up to 30 days.

Being a nonenveloped virus, rotavirus is stable in the environment (6 months in fecal matter) and relatively resistant to the effects of some disinfectants. Decontamination of hutches and maternity pens requires thorough physical efforts to remove fecal matter and other organic debris because most disinfectants show reduced, even negligible, activity in their presence. Application of appropriately diluted bleach, a phenolic, or a peroxysulfate disinfectant to a thoroughly cleaned solid surface, with provision of long (> 10 minutes) contact time and subsequent sunlight exposure and drying, will effectively reduce the number of infectious rotavirus particles. Heavily soiled areas, such as the ground beneath calf hutches, may need to be stripped down to the packed surface and exposed to sunlight and dry conditions for several days to weeks (depending on weather conditions) before being considered habitable for the next calf.

Coronavirus
Etiology

Based on seroprevalence studies, the bovine coronavirus (BCoV) responsible for calf diarrhea is quite prevalent in U.S. cattle herds, as is rotavirus. There is much debate among researchers at this point as to whether BCoV isolates obtained from calf and adult diarrhea cases are the same virus or distinct from those that have been incriminated in respiratory disease outbreaks in feedlot and dairy calves. Whether or not there are antigenic or genomic differences in BCoV strains that mediate different organ tropism is similarly unclear. Winter dysentery in adult cattle has been associated with BCoV, and the same strain that causes diarrhea in calves has been used to experimentally create winter dysentery in adult cattle. Therefore, the upper age limit of susceptibility to infection by this agent is apparently longer than traditionally thought.

Although not as common as rotavirus as a cause of viral enteritis in dairy calves, coronavirus has been identified in neonatal calf diarrhea outbreaks, especially in the winter months and with mixed infections. A number of studies indicate that clinical disease associated with BCoV in calves is more severe than rotavirus, with higher mortality rates. Affected calves tend to be slightly older than calves infected with pure ETEC or pure rotavirus. They average 7 to 10 days of age at onset, with some observed as late as 3 weeks of age. The virus causes a severe enterocolitis characterized by villous enterocyte destruction in the small intestine and destruction of both ridges and crypts in the large intestine. Maldigestion, malabsorption, and inflammation all contribute to the pathophysiology of coronavirus diarrhea in calves. The virus is cytolytic, and affected villous enterocytes in the small intestine are replaced by cuboidal cells from the crypts, but the colonic lesions leave denuded mucosa in affected areas of the colon. The severity of this damage helps explain why coronavirus enteritis, unlike rotavirus, may cause some flecks of blood to appear in the stool and can kill calves even in a germ-free isolation facility. Thus, in the natural setting, coronavirus enteritis creates a severe clinical diarrhea and can also be associated with > 50% mortality when combined with other viral, bacterial and *C. parvum* infections.

Clinical Signs

Acute, severe diarrhea, as well as dehydration, reduced appetite or suckle reflex, and progressive depression and weakness are typical, albeit nonspecific, signs of coronavirus infection in calves. Because of the colonic pathology, mucus and flecks of blood may be quite apparent in feces. Coronavirus is also commonly found in the respiratory tract of young calves, and a pneumonia–enteritis complex may occur in these individuals.

Ancillary Data

Coronavirus enterocolitis causes variably severe changes in acid–base and electrolyte status that are also common to *E. coli* and rotavirus. In severe coronavirus infections or mixed infections that include coronavirus, metabolic acidosis and low plasma bicarbonate are the rule. Potassium values vary with the severity and duration of the diarrhea and acidosis. Hemoconcentration secondary to the diarrhea elevates PCV and total protein values. Leukograms are variable. Although nonspecific, the acid–base and electrolyte assessments are of greatest value for individual patient management.

Diagnosis

Submission of feces from calves with acute or peracute diarrhea provides the best diagnostic approach for live patients. Feces collected during the first 24 hours of diarrhea are best. Electron microscopy, ELISA, or PCR may be used to detect virus. As with rotavirus, PCR testing has generally superseded antigen or electron microscopy as the diagnostic test of choice. FA testing of tissue samples obtained from both the small and large intestines is advised for necropsy specimens, principally because one is usually uncertain of the etiologic cause at the time. The spiral colon has, however, been demonstrated to be the best diagnostic sample source at postmortem for specific identification of coronavirus infection. Because of the cytolytic nature of coronavirus, the virus can disappear rapidly from tissue. Therefore, chronically affected calves are not good candidates for etiologic diagnostic sampling.

Treatment

Treatment principles are the same as those previously listed under ETEC and rotavirus treatment. As with rotavirus, oral electrolyte–energy sources may be less efficiently absorbed in coronavirus infections because of enterocyte loss. However, even given these limitations, oral electrolyte–energy sources may contribute to the patient's well-being during the time of intestinal repair. Diarrhea is likely to persist to some degree for 1 week with coronavirus because of the severe enterocolitis. Systemic antibiotics are often indicated to help affected calves cope with secondary bacterial infection of the lung, gut, and other systems.

Control

Every effort should be made to control management factors that predispose calves to infection. These are described in the control of rotavirus. Because coronavirus is an enveloped virus, its persistence in the environment and resistance to disinfectants are considerably lower than those of rotavirus. Dry cows should be vaccinated at 6 and 3 weeks before calving with a killed rotavirus and coronavirus vaccine and boosted each year thereafter at 4 weeks prepartum. Because it is assumed that local antibody is more important than humoral antibody, the feeding of colostrum containing high antibody levels against coronavirus is advantageous, and when possible, prolonged feeding of such colostrum during the first 30 days of life might confer greater protection for problem farms. Active immunization of calves at birth with multivalent products containing coronavirus (usually in combination with *E. coli* and rotavirus) is also quite commonly practiced but should be considered a less reliable and effective method of protecting calves compared with the absorption of high IgG$_1$ concentration colostrum from immunized dams. Specific antibody products are available and can be administered to newborn calves at birth. One such product contains K-99 antibodies and coronavirus antibodies (First Defense, ImmuCell Corp., Portland, ME) derived from hyperimmune bovine colostrum. In an experimental challenge study with BoCV, dairy calves fed a commercial product containing spray-dried bovine serum showed increased feed intake and higher scores for certain clinical parameters as compared with control calves. The expense of such products is considerable, and discussion of the cost and therapeutic benefit is often warranted before use. Most recently, a modified-live coronavirus vaccine (Bovilis Coronavirus, Merck Animal Health, Madison, NJ) for intranasal administration to calves was shown to decrease the incidence and severity of scours.

Cryptosporidium Infection
Etiology

Cryptosporidiosis is an important cause of diarrhea in neonatal calves that occurs most commonly from 5 to 28 days of age. Cryptosporidiidae are a family of coccidian protozoans grouped with the Sarcocystidae and Eimeriidae families in the suborder Eimeriina. Similar to other coccidia, members of the Cryptosporidiidae family have both sexual and asexual components to their life cycle but differ from other coccidia in having less host specificity. *Cryptosporidium* spp. are much smaller than *Eimeria* spp. and are therefore difficult to detect in fecal flotation. Laboratory techniques that use acid-fast stains or immunologic techniques greatly aid detection. The true prevalence and pathogenicity of cryptosporidiosis in calves have only recently been appreciated.

At the time of the original description of the parasite in a calf, cryptosporidiosis was thought to be a novel or sporadic infection that most likely affected immunocompromised calves. During the 1980s, it became apparent that the organism was much more prevalent, epidemic to endemic on many farms, and a primary or component cause of neonatal calf diarrhea.

There are currently 30 named species of *Cryptosporidium* in humans and animals, but their taxonomy and nomenclature are confusing. Recent molecular methods rely heavily on single-stranded ribosomal RNA (ssrRNA) sequencing for species identification, but one can still find genotype assignments as a form of taxonomic nomenclature in the literature. Molecular and experimental evidence suggests that humans and cattle are hosts for 14 and 13 of these species, respectively, although there will likely be increases in these numbers in the future (the number of new species identified is growing at about 1 per year). However, not all of these potentially infective species are frequent parasites of clinical importance in either host species. In cattle, the majority of infections are associated with *C. parvum, C. bovis, and C. andersoni.* Zoonotic transmission from cattle to people is most commonly caused by *C. parvum,* and neither *C. bovis* nor *C. andersoni* are considered as major a human health risk as *C. parvum. C. parvum* can infect calves, lambs, young pigs, foals, humans, and other species such as suckling rodents. Public health concerns regarding spread of *C. parvum* from animals to people are real and require diligence in the diagnosis and management of this parasite.

C. parvum is an intestinal pathogen of preweaned calves, but both *C. andersoni* and *C. bovis* are more likely to be found in the feces of calves postweaning (highest prevalence is in calves from weanling age to yearlings). However, neither of these two species is typically associated with clinical disease in cattle. *C. andersoni* is located within the peptic glands of the abomasum rather than the intestine, where, at least histologically, it can cause thickening of the abomasal folds. *C. pestis, C. ubiquitum, C. suis, C. hominis,* and *C. ryanae* are all species that have been identified in cattle by ssrRNA methods, but their relevance as bovine pathogens is uncertain.

In cattle, neonates are at greatest risk of infection and disease because age-related resistance seems to be strong; this trend is less evident in humans. Veterinarians, students, technicians, and other individuals involved in handling affected calves, feeding equipment, bedding, or even clothing from in-contact individuals may develop clinical disease if strict hygienic measures are not followed. Immunocompetent hosts usually develop self-limiting diarrhea. However, the organism causes a particularly devastating disease in immunocompromised hosts, in whom persistent infections can occur.

The organism usually infects via the fecal–oral route, but contaminated ground water, improperly treated municipal water, and contaminated feedstuffs can induce infection. The infective dose of *Cryptosporidium* likely varies among individual animals and humans, but the infective dose in a susceptible individual may be less than 100 oocysts. Given that infected calves may shed millions of infective oocysts in each gram of diarrheic stool, there is strong potential on many farms for accumulation of massive infectious challenge. *C. parvum* is the most common species seen in calves up to 1 month of age and the only species typically found in calves younger than 3 weeks of age. Large epidemiologic surveys from diagnostic laboratories in the United States demonstrate that more than one third of submissions from diarrheic calves in the first month of life have detectable cryptosporidial oocysts.

Sporulated oocysts are readily infective to neonatal calves and release sporozoites that infect primarily the small intestinal (but some colonic) enterocytes by infecting the microvillus brush border. A parasitophorous vacuole that resides adherent to the cell but outside the cytoplasm is formed. The life cycle phases of *C. parvum* then result in destruction of cells as the parasitophorous vacuoles break to release merozoites that infect other host cells. The subsequent sexual life cycle phase results in formation of oocysts infective to susceptible hosts. Villous atrophy, villous fusion, and inflammation of intestinal crypts ensue. Autoinfection within the intestine occurs, wherein specialized oocysts are released to infect other enterocytes without exiting the host. Clinical signs of diarrhea reflect a mixed pathophysiology of maldigestion, malabsorption, and osmotic effects with or without secretory and inflammatory factors. The autoinfection process has been hypothesized to account for occasional protracted or relapsing cases that can result in cachexia. The prepatent period for *C. parvum* is 3 to 4 days, although the majority of clinical cases are not detected until at least 7 days of age unless there is massive, immediate postpartum exposure. Damage to the microvilli appears to predispose the calf to combined infections with *E. coli,* viruses, or *Salmonella* spp. Therefore, it is unusual in dairy calves to find only *C. parvum* when investigating endemic calf diarrhea. However, because oocyst shedding typically begins with the onset of clinical signs and persists until several days after diarrhea resolves, fecal testing may tend to reveal this pathogen more consistently than rotavirus or coronavirus, which are shed early in the disease course and for a shorter period of time than *C. parvum.* This reiterates the importance of testing affected calves early in the disease course when investigating the etiology of calf diarrhea. Combinations of enteric pathogens in neonatal calves complicate treatment, worsen the clinical signs and prognosis, tend to result in higher mortality, and predispose to malnutrition.

C. parvum may by itself produce severe diarrhea in immunocompromised calves and those exposed to inclement weather or poor nutrition.

Clinical Signs

Diarrhea, dehydration, and reduced appetite are the major clinical signs and thus do not differentiate *C. parvum* infection from bacterial and viral enteropathogens in neonatal calves. Morbidity tends to be greater than 50% in calves less than 3 weeks of age, but the mortality rate is low unless mixed infections occur or supportive treatment is less than adequate. When *C. parvum* is the only pathogen, diarrhea usually persists for up to 7 days, but most calves do not lose their ability to nurse or their interest in nursing during this time. When mixed infections occur, dehydration, acid–base and electrolyte abnormalities, and dysentery are possible. Malnutrition is a possible sequela to *C. parvum* infections when poor supportive therapy and poor nutritional quality coexist with the rather chronic diarrhea. Malnutrition is quite common in *C. parvum*–infected calves raised outside in hutches during winter weather extremes in northern climates. Because these calves normally have greatly increased caloric needs over calves raised at moderate temperatures, maldigestion, malabsorption, and fluid losses greatly compromise their well-being.

Diagnosis

Microscopic identification of *C. parvum* oocysts has been relied on historically for positive diagnosis but may require a trained microscopist! In most instances, standard flotation on feces from acutely affected calves is performed, but very fresh necropsy tissue samples of the ileum and colon also may be examined after tissue preparation and staining. Acid-fast stains are commonly used to assist in the identification of *C. parvum*. Immunofluorescence, ELISA, and PCR are all believed to be more sensitive and specific than microscopy. The antigen-based techniques probably detect all of the species documented to be infectious in calves, as do the immunofluorescence tests, but do not discriminate among species. PCR methods detect lower levels of infection than antigen-based tests, the former being sensitive to as low as 50 oocysts per gram of feces. Fecal flotation and acid-fast staining probably are only sensitive down to 10^3 to 10^6 oocysts per gram. This latter fact is not too problematic diagnostically because many clinically affected animals are shedding very high numbers ($\geq 10^6$). Because they are of similar size, microscopy cannot distinguish oocysts of *C. parvum* from *C. andersoni* or *C. bovis*. Genetic analysis of bovine or human isolates may be performed to aid in epidemiologic investigations, particularly when zoonotic cases are suspected. Even when *C. parvum* is suspected and confirmed, mixed infections should be considered likely and feces submitted for bacteriologic and virologic evaluation.

Treatment

Treatment is almost always merely supportive and consists of fluids by whatever route indicated by the severity of clinical dehydration. In addition, a high-quality source of nutrients such as whole milk or a quality milk replacer should be continued to be fed if at all possible. Mixed infections with other primary enteropathogens may necessitate a short period of feed withdrawal. If oral electrolyte energy sources are fed during the acute phase of diarrhea, they should not remain the only source of nutrients for more than 24 hours. Thereafter, milk or replacer should be fed at least twice daily and oral electrolyte–energy sources fed between milk feedings to compensate for the fluid losses caused by *C. parvum* diarrhea. During cold or extreme winter weather, hutch-sheltered or neonatal calves left outside should receive milk or high-quality replacer at least three times daily if twice-daily feeding fails to maintain body condition or *C. parvum* diarrhea, maldigestion, and malabsorption interfere with efficient utilization of nutrients.

Antibiotics are not necessary, although they may be indicated in mixed infections that include bacterial pathogens. Many drugs have been tested for efficacy against *Cryptosporidium* spp., but none has been found to be completely effective or economically justifiable. Standard coccidiostats are ineffective with the exception of lasalocid at doses so high as to be toxic to calves. Recent work in Europe and Canada has demonstrated that treatment with halofuginone lactate will reduce oocyst shedding and delay the onset of diarrhea in calves, but similar to many other investigated therapies, it does not significantly impact the incidence or severity of diarrhea in treated calves compared with control animals. Paromomycin, nitazoxanide, azithromycin, and a few other drugs have shown some activity against *C. parvum*, and ongoing research to benefit human patients with AIDS might drive future discoveries in this area. These drugs could potentially be used in valuable calves with cryptosporidiosis. Halofuginone (100 μg/kg) for 7 days is approved in several countries for the preventive treatment of cryptosporidiosis in calves, and although this will decrease oocyst shedding, it may not reduce diarrhea. In a report by Dr. Ollivett, treatment of *C. parvum*–infected calves with nitazoxanide reduced the duration of oocyst shedding and improved fecal consistency. Considerable research effort toward the development of effective vaccines over the past decade has yet to prove successful. Egg yolk antibody products for passive protection of new born calves, as well as recombinant subunit *C. parvum* vaccines for active immunization of dry cows have been closely examined but with inconsistent results. There is no currently available passive or active immunization protocol for this disease.

Control

Because specific treatment is not possible, prevention assumes supreme importance. Unfortunately, many dairy farms fail to effectively control *C. parvum* when environmental contamination becomes extreme. Although diseased calves serve as the primary source of environmental contamination, oocysts are also spread by movement of laborers, equipment, and animals. Given the low dose of oocysts necessary to cause disease in susceptible animals, the morbidity rate can become unacceptably high. Therefore, control requires a careful, open-minded reexamination of all management practices related to calf rearing, including maternity pen hygiene; colostrum management; cleaning of feeding equipment, hutches, and the ground surrounding hutches; labor allocation; and the order by which laborers feed and handle calves.

First, calf facilities should include individual calf housing rather than grouping. Ideally, newborn calves should be separated from the dam at birth and moved to a cleaned and disinfected calf hutch on new dry ground or concrete. Placing a calf in a hutch on the same ground as that used for the previous occupant will not work because *C. parvum* oocysts can persist for months in such areas, and the ground beneath used calf hutches is often heavily contaminated. Bedding from within and around hutches should be completely removed and disposed of, the ground stripped bare, and the bare ground allowed several days to weeks of sunlight exposure under dry conditions before being considered habitable for another calf. Extremes of temperature can more rapidly inactivate the oocysts, such that infectivity is lost at 40°C and at −22°C. Moving cleaned hutches to new ground or placing them on concrete slabs that can be cleaned, disinfected, and allowed to dry between calves is the best technique. Because *Cryptosporidium* oocysts are highly resistant to the effects of almost all disinfectants, hutches and feeding equipment must be vigorously and thoroughly scrubbed with soap and water and rinsed well with hot water to physically dislodge oocysts. Drying and ultraviolet light are relatively effective against the oocysts; therefore, more hutches should be made available than would be occupied at any given time; a 20% vacancy rate for newly scrubbed hutches will often allow ample time for sun exposure and drying of recently emptied hutches. The role that moisture can play in encouraging oocyst persistence has been further demonstrated by epidemiologic studies that find that a slope of 5% to 10% in the calf housing area will diminish risks of infection, but rainfall will increase shedding rates. A peroxygen-based disinfectant (Virkon-S, Antec International, Sudbury, Suffolk, United Kingdom) has been shown to reduce the infectivity of *Cryptosporidium* oocysts under experimental conditions and is currently used in some veterinary hospitals to disinfect thoroughly cleaned surfaces. Newer generation, peroxygen-based compounds have also shown promise for reduction of oocyst viability.

Calves should have individual feeding implements, and removal of manure from the hutch should be done in such a way that calves are not exposed to manure from neighboring calves or hutches. When doing chores, laborers should move from young calves to older calves and from healthy to sick calves to limit spread of oocysts. It should also be remembered that calves raised in inclement weather, those kept on wet bedding, or calves receiving inadequate nutrition causing failure to gain weight or even loss of weight in the first week of life are more susceptible to having clinical disease after *C. parvum* infection.

Salmonellosis (Calves)
Etiology

Salmonella is a genus of gram-negative, facultative anaerobic, rod-shaped bacteria belonging to the family Enterobacteriaceae. Two species are recognized: *Salmonella enterica*, which is further divided into six subspecies, and *Salmonella bongori*. More than 2600 *Salmonella* serovars, differentiated by their antigenic composition, have been identified to date. Serovar classification is based on O (somatic), H (flagellar), and Vi (capsular) antigens. Most current serogroups are divided by O antigens and listed by capital letters (e.g., A, B, C, D and E). The majority of cattle isolates are *Salmonella* of types B, C, and E, which are non–host specific, or *Salmonella* Dublin (type D), which is host-adapted to cattle. The vast majority of serovars with veterinary and human medical significance belong to *Salmonella enterica* subsp. *enterica* and are typically referred to by their serovar classification for convenience (e.g., *Salmonella enterica* subsp. *enterica* serovar Newport, is conventionally abbreviated to *Salmonella* Newport). Despite the diversity of serovars, relatively few are responsible for a large proportion of clinical infections among cattle and other mammals. Many of these serovars are capable of causing clinical disease in a broad range of host species (e.g., Enteritidis, Typhimurium, and Newport). However, others are almost exclusively associated with a single host species (host-restricted serovars, such as Abortus ovis in sheep) or have a predilection for a particular host species but can also cause disease in other hosts (host-adapted serovars, such as *S.* Dublin in cattle).

Although many infections remain subclinical, *Salmonella* is an important cause of disease among calves and adult dairy cattle. Salmonellosis is costly for dairy producers because of treatment and labor expenses, mortality, reduced milk yield, and increased cull rates. Salmonellosis as a sporadic cause of diarrhea has been long recognized in cattle, but intensive management systems have contributed to endemic disease in dairy calves, veal calves, and adult dairy cattle. Currently, salmonellosis ranks as one of the two most important bacterial causes of diarrhea in adult dairy cattle (MAP being the other) and has surpassed *E. coli* in this respect in calves on many operations. *Salmonella* spp. also pose a formidable threat to human health, causing approximately 1.2 million illnesses, 20,000 hospitalizations, and 400 deaths annually in the United States alone. Antimicrobial resistance among *Salmonella* isolates magnifies the problem, limiting treatment options and increasing the risk of therapeutic failure. In humans, infection with resistant *Salmonella* strains has been associated with adverse patient outcomes. Such human health relevance continues to heighten and accentuate the scrutiny of antimicrobial use in food-producing animals.

Some broad characterization of the clinical syndromes associated with certain serotypes can be made. With group B infections such as *S.* Typhimurium, as well as with many group E infections, a herd outbreak of diarrhea and septicemia may occur in adults and calves. Abortion or early embryonic death may occur as a result of acute endotoxemia and shock. However, as the population develops immunity to the agent, clinical signs often dissipate within 1 to 2 months. Infections with group C *Salmonella* are more difficult to characterize because infection and clinical disease may persist in the herd for variable periods of time. Infection may also be perpetuated over the long term by environmental contamination or by group C *Salmonella* cycling through rodents, birds, or insects. Infection with the host-adapted *S.* Dublin (the most common group D isolate from cattle) is characterized by establishment of a higher percentage of carrier animals in the population. When *S.* Dublin is established in a population, some adults experience asymptomatic infection and may serve as shedders (even in milk and colostrum), and pneumonia, septicemia, and acute death become the primary manifestations of disease in calves. Some calves that develop infection and survive will become long-term carriers. Sporadic abortions may also occur with *S.* Dublin.

Calves with acute, chronic, or carrier intestinal infections shed the organism to varying degrees in their feces; this serves as the major source of infection to other naive calves via fecal–oral transmission. Calves with peracute or acute disease often are septicemic and may shed organisms from other secretions such as saliva and urine. Fecal–oral transmission is the norm for types B, C, and E *Salmonella*; infection of the distal small intestine, cecum, and colon ensues. Mucosal injury causes maldigestion, malabsorption, and loss of protein and fluid. A secretory component to the diarrhea also is thought to contribute to further electrolyte and fluid depletion. *S.* Dublin is unique in that respiratory signs may predominate, and transmission may occur via several secretions as well as feces. Adult dairy cattle may be carriers and harbor *S.* Dublin in the intestine or mammary gland. Milk, colostrum, or feces from infected or carrier *S.* Dublin cows can be infective to calves. Clinical epidemics of many *Salmonella* types, including *S.* Dublin, are common in calves in the northeastern United States and other parts of the country. Geographic differences in serogroup prevalence do occur, but widespread transport of calves or adult cows and assembly of herds from distant locations has tended to negate geographic limits for various *Salmonella* serogroups.

Factors that adversely affect the normal enteric flora tend to favor growth of *Salmonella*, which are common, albeit low in number components of the GI flora of carrier or "normal" cattle. Parturition, transport, concurrent disease, anesthesia, and withholding of feed and water are just a few of the stresses that cause intestinal ileus, reduced host immunity, or shifts in enteric bacterial populations that induce proliferation of *Salmonella*. In calves, antibiotics that alter the intestinal flora may also favor the growth of *Salmonella*. When shedding of large numbers of organisms occurs in a carrier animal, naive calves are at increased risk if crowding, poor sanitation, use of common feeding implements, or

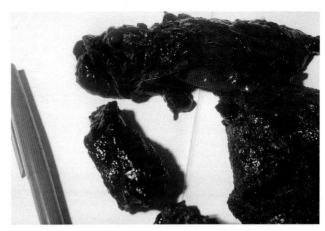

• **Fig. 6.9** Blood in the stool from a calf with salmonellosis.

comingling, concurrent diseases, or stress are present. Both humoral and cellular immune mechanisms are involved in resistance to *Salmonella*. Calves persistently infected (PI) with BVDV are at high risk for developing acute salmonellosis following exposure to the organism.

Clinical Signs

Fever and diarrhea are the hallmark signs of clinical salmonellosis in dairy calves. Fever may precede clinical signs of diarrhea but seldom is detected before calves begin to show diarrhea and appear ill. Fresh blood and mucus in the feces (some calves may have blood in feces before diarrhea) also are common with *Salmonella* enteritis (Fig. 6.9). Blood-stained mucus or whole blood clots may be apparent based on the severity of infection and *Salmonella* type. Clinical signs associated with septic physitis, arthritis, meningitis, and pneumonia may be seen in some calves. Sporadic or endemic disease may occur, and although calves from 2 weeks to 2 months are most commonly affected, those of any age may develop the disease. Newborn calves can develop severe disease in the first few days of life when either the maternity area or calf housing facility into which they are born or moved is massively contaminated. This can be a feature of herd outbreaks of clinical salmonellosis when parturient adult and sick fresh cows are shedding excessive numbers of organisms into the environment or when calf housing and common use equipment becomes heavily contaminated due to a large number of clinical cases. Because of the true carrier status and the ability to pass the organism via colostrum and milk from asymptomatic dams, special consideration should be given to *S.* Dublin as a differential when clinical signs suggestive of salmonellosis occur in calves during the first week of life on a farm. Tremendous variation in clinical severity of disease exists based on the virulence and infecting dose of the *Salmonella* serotype in question, and the age, immune status, and existence of concurrent disease in the calf. Type E *Salmonella,* such as *S.* Anatum, tend to cause mild signs of diarrhea and fever with variable morbidity and low mortality, but types B and C are

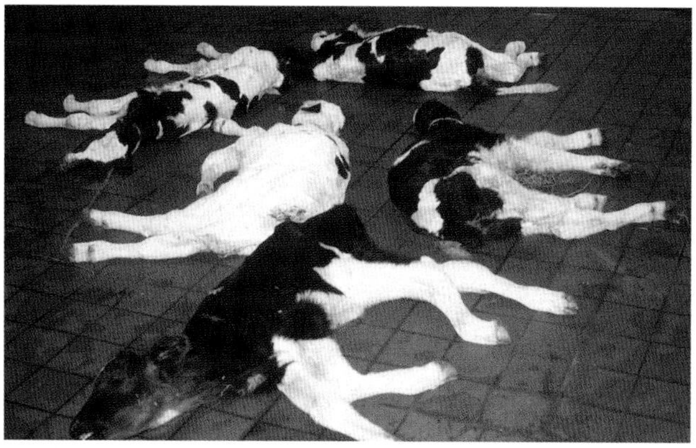

• **Fig. 6.10** One day's death toll of neonatal calves from a dairy farm suffering high mortality in cattle of all ages during an epidemic caused by a highly virulent *Salmonella* Typhimurium strain.

more likely to cause high morbidity and variable mortality based on strain, exposure dosage of organisms and the immunologic status of the calf. Neonatal calves have a greater risk of death caused by *Salmonella* spp. because of septicemia and fluid losses leading to severe dehydration and electrolyte imbalances (Fig. 6.10).

Peracute septicemia resulting from *Salmonella* types B, C, and D may cause death before diarrhea becomes obvious. These calves rapidly dehydrate into their intestinal tract, have abdominal distension as a result of filling of the small and large intestine and sometimes forestomach. They may die secondary to bacteremia or endotoxemia induced by release of cell wall products of this gram-negative infective agent. Bacteremic calves shed large numbers of *Salmonella* organisms in other bodily secretions and feces and quickly contaminate premises. Acute cases caused by types B, C, and E show classical acute diarrhea, often with fresh blood and mucus in the feces, as well as fever and dehydration. Feces are foul smelling (septic tank odor) and vary in color and consistency, with the most virulent strains causing profuse watery diarrhea with whole blood clots present. The infected calves are frequently bacteremic, and pneumonia, arthritis, physitis, and meningitis may occur.

Acute disease in calves usually is associated with high morbidity and variable mortality that is dictated by the interaction of strain virulence and calf immunology. Fecal contamination of the environment is especially problematic when calves are housed in group housing, raised slatted stalls, or crowded areas, or when born in a stall used both as a maternity pen and sick cow area. Milk and feces from adult cows shedding *Salmonella* and contaminated feeds or feeding devices are all potential sources of *Salmonella*. Chronic infection leads to long standing or intermittent diarrhea, weight loss, hypoproteinemia, and failure to thrive. Some chronically infected calves typically evolve from epidemics of acute salmonellosis in dairy calves and thus enhance the risk of exposure for naive herdmates.

Acute infection associated with *S.* Dublin may be much harder to diagnose because diarrhea may not be the principal sign. Fever, depression, and respiratory signs may be most obvious in acute *S.* Dublin infections in calves. Although diarrhea may be present, it is seldom the predominant clinical sign, which may lead to the erroneous assumption that a calf pneumonia problem exists on the farm. Fever and depression unresponsive to antibiotics may be observed. Abortions may also occur on the premises. Calves infected with *S.* Dublin are typically 4 to 8 weeks of age although it can also be seen in neonatal calves and group-housed calves postweaning. Clinical signs of acute salmonellosis caused by *S.* Dublin in 4-week or older calves are most commonly respiratory in nature combined with depression caused by acute bacteremia, hematogenous pneumonia and septic shock.

Laboratory Data

Peracute or acute infection with *Salmonella* has variable effects on the patient's leukogram. A degenerative left shift with neutropenia and band neutrophilia is considered typical for severely affected animals, but it is not consistent, and many patients have neutrophilia or normal leukograms. Although blood may be present in the feces, hemoconcentration tends to mask mild anemia resulting from any blood loss. PCV is normal or elevated because of dehydration. Total protein and albumin concentrations are usually normal or low because of protein loss into the gut and malabsorption. Renal function may be compromised by dehydration, reduced renal perfusion, endotoxemia, or nephritis secondary to bacteremia with renal infection. Peracute and acute infections cause inflammatory, secretory, and malabsorption–maldigestion types of diarrhea and result in metabolic acidosis and hyponatremia and hypochloremia. These electrolyte changes are particularly common in instances when the calf loses electrolytes and water in the diarrheic stool but is only allowed access to water for rehydration. Potassium may range from high (peracute) to low (subacute, chronic) depending on severity and duration of diarrhea, subsequent fluid losses, and acid–base status.

The leukogram in *S.* Dublin–infected calves is extremely variable and reflects duration of infection. Acute cases may be neutropenic with a left shift, severely neutropenic, or have normal WBC counts. Subacute or chronic *S.* Dublin infections have a mild to moderate neutrophilia or stress leukogram.

Diagnosis

Regardless of the type or strain of *Salmonella,* isolation of the organism, coupled with history and clinical signs, confirms the diagnosis. Fecal cultures are the standard test necessary to identify serotypes other than *S.* Dublin, but fecal, blood, transtracheal wash, or lung tissue samples may be necessary to identify *S.* Dublin. Fecal samples submitted from suspect calves should be sent to qualified diagnostic laboratories equipped to culture enteric pathogens. When neonatal calves are involved, the laboratory should be forewarned that

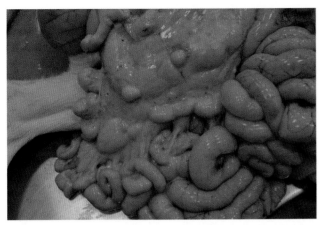

• **Fig. 6.11** Marked mesenteric lymphadenopathy at postmortem in a 10-week-old ill-thriven Holstein calf in association with chronic *Salmonella* Dublin infection (see also Video Clip 6.1).

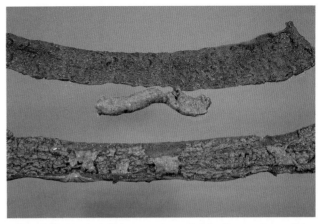

• **Fig. 6.12** Classical fibrinonecrotic or diphtheritic membrane lining the intestine of a calf that died from subacute *Salmonella* Typhimurium enterocolitis.

Salmonella and *E. coli* are suspected. When affected calves vary in age from neonatal to several months old, *Salmonella* is more likely than *E. coli* because the latter tends to more commonly affect only neonates. Sample handling is pivotal in reaching a definitive diagnosis, and practitioners should familiarize themselves with their local diagnostic laboratory requirements and recommendations for maximizing the chances of a positive culture from feces, environmental samples, or postmortem tissues. *Salmonella* spp. are quickly overgrown by many other fecal organisms, and pre-enrichment or the use of specific selective transport media may be indicated for samples obtained in the field.

Calves that die peracutely should be necropsied and cultures obtained from the ileum, cecum, or colon. In addition, the mesenteric lymph nodes (Fig. 6.11 and see Video Clip 6.1), gallbladder, and heart blood should be cultured. Calves that die after respiratory and enteric signs should have lung and intestinal samples cultured for *S.* Dublin.

Although pathologists associate salmonellosis with gross enteric lesions such as diphtheritic membranes in the distal small or large intestines, it must be emphasized that peracute *Salmonella* types B or C and acute *S.* Dublin infections often cause minimal demonstrable gross lesions. This fact has been borne out by observing necropsy specimens from many calf mortality epidemics and dictates bacteriologic investigation rather than empiric gross determination of etiology.

Subacute or chronic cases may have fibrinonecrotic or diphtheritic membranes scattered throughout the large and distal small intestine (Fig. 6.12). Petechial hemorrhages and edematous mesenteric lymph nodes are other gross pathologic findings in some cases.

Treatment

Fluid and antibiotic therapy are the cornerstones of treatment for calves with salmonellosis. Decisions as to route of fluid administration are based on physical signs, severity of the diarrhea, and economic considerations. As with

E. coli infections, calves that are "shocky," unable to rise, and severely dehydrated and those that have no suckle response should be given IV fluids. Calves that are ambulatory, able to suckle, and only moderately dehydrated usually can be managed with oral and possibly SC fluids. Peracute and acute salmonellosis caused by types B, C, D or E may result in a metabolic acidosis similar to that found in ETEC infections. However, losses of Na^+ and Cl^- tend to be more severe in salmonellosis than those found in ETEC-infected calves. Bicarbonate-rich solutions are indicated in peracute *Salmonella* infections and should be considered when profound depression or shocklike signs accompany peracute diarrhea. After correction of metabolic acidosis, balanced electrolytes may be used IV or oral fluids substituted (see section discussing treatment of ETEC). Oral electrolyte–energy solutions are helpful but limited by the maldigestion, malabsorption, and inflammatory lesions in the patient's intestinal tract. Diarrhea tends to persist longer in *Salmonella* infections than ETEC infections and may become chronic if the intestine is permanently damaged.

Whole blood transfusion occasionally is necessary because of fecal blood losses, and colloids are commonly indicated as a result of severe hypoproteinemia associated with albumin loss from the inflamed intestine. Whole blood (free of BLV and BVDV) is sometimes more economical than plasma for calves having severe hypoproteinemia. Hetastarch is currently a reasonably priced alternative to plasma, but it only augments colloidal pressure, lacking globulins and other homologous proteins that can be more specifically therapeutic in septic or inflammatory conditions.

Severe peracute infections that result in shock may necessitate one-time administration of corticosteroids or flunixin meglumine in conjunction with IV fluids. Continued or repeated use of full dosages of either of these products warrants caution because their side effects on the gastric mucosa and renal vasculature appear to be augmented by volume depletion.

Antibiotic therapy for calves having salmonellosis is somewhat controversial and deserves comment.

Reasons not to use antibiotics include:

1. Fear of creating antibiotic-resistant strains that may present a risk to humans and animals in the future.
2. Although antibiotic therapy may aid clinical recovery, it does not stop fecal shedding or positively affect the duration of fecal shedding.
3. *Salmonellae* are facultative intracellular organisms, and antimicrobial penetration into the infected host cell is often limited even for antimicrobials that show in vitro efficacy against the organism.

Reasons to use antibiotics include:

1. Bacteremia is common with salmonellosis of any type in neonates and is very common with *S. Dublin*.
2. Veterinarians cannot always predict which calves are septicemic and which are only endotoxemic when faced with signs of shock and severe diarrhea.
3. Although intracellular penetration of infected host cells by antibiotics may be limited, adequate blood concentrations of an effective antibiotic may limit spread of infection from the gut to other tissues by acting on the organisms that are free in the blood and ECF.
4. Clinical impressions suggest a shorter course of disease and higher recovery rate when antibiotics are used.
5. Secondary infections (e.g., septic meningitis, arthritis) are possible in severely ill calves with salmonellosis.

Antibiotic therapy is justified for calves with peracute or acute signs that suggest overwhelming infection. Calves having mild signs, that are asymptomatic, and with chronic disease do not appear to benefit from antibiotic therapy. Given the characteristically unpredictable nature of antibiotic susceptibility exhibited by *Salmonella* spp., selection should be based on culture and sensitivity. Currently, some strains are resistant to beta-lactam antibiotics, macrolides, and tetracyclines but are frequently sensitive to aminoglycosides, fluoroquinolones, and trimethoprim–sulfas. Antibiotic therapy should be maintained at least 5 to 7 days for peracute and acute salmonellosis and is more likely to be necessary in type B, C, and D infections than with type E. A decision not to use antibiotics for calves with salmonellosis is easier to enforce when the mortality rate is low or nonexistent. This same decision is impossible to enforce when a high mortality rate occurs because owners will not tolerate such losses and will demand antibiotics or change veterinarians in the hope of saving sick calves. Ultimately, decisions on antibiotic use must be based on humane considerations weighed against the public health concerns related to induction of resistance in an organism with demonstrated zoonotic potential. Wholesale treatment of calves at risk and the use of oral antibiotics such as tetracycline for all calves in a group are contraindicated because these techniques are more likely to be ineffective or lead to antibiotic resistance. Antibiotics should be considered as potential components of the treatment regimen, with aggressive fluid and electrolyte replacement, good nursing care, and maintenance of adequate nutrition as primary considerations. Experience suggests that resolution of a salmonellosis problem on a dairy requires far more critical and influential decisions than antibiotic selection for individual cases.

Control

Although an individual calf sporadically becomes infected with *Salmonella* spp. as a result of stress or FPT, endemic infection is increasingly the rule in dairy and veal operations. Infected calves shed large numbers of organisms into the environment, and contamination is worsened by the fluid characteristic of feces in diarrheic calves. Infection spreads quickly when calves are grouped in confinement or crowded into pens. Fecal contamination of feed, water, or feeding devices is common, and septicemic calves may shed organisms in other body secretions as well as feces. *S. Dublin*–infected calves may shed organisms from body secretions, feces, or the respiratory tract. Inapparent or subclinical infections are common and represent a constant source of environmental contamination.

Cleanliness and disinfection of housing units are extremely important to the control of salmonellosis because a primary determinant of the severity of infection appears to be the magnitude of challenge or infective dose. Many severe outbreaks have resulted from contamination of feed, and this area deserves particular scrutiny in any herd investigation because this route serves as a very efficient means of oral inoculation for new hosts.

Detection of previous infection with *S. Dublin* can be achieved through a well-established ELISA assay currently available through the New York State Diagnostic Laboratory. Both milk samples (group or bulk tank samples for example) and serum can be used in this assay, providing a much more sensitive test than traditional culture methods. In other parts of the world, this assay is being used for surveillance and control of *S. Dublin* on a national level through screening of herds every 3 months. It seems unlikely at this point in time that a national program of this nature will come into effect in the United States, but it is worth remembering that *S. Dublin* tends to be more pathogenic in human patients than many other serovars and that its prevalence is undoubtedly on the increase in this country. One has to be careful when interpreting a positive ELISA result in young calves because of the possibility of passively derived antibody rather than naturally acquired titers. It is probable that passively derived antibody for *S. Dublin* wanes along the same time frame as other colostrally derived antibodies, hence calves might be expected to be negative by early postweaning and certainly before breeding age unless true postnatal exposure has occurred. Detection of carrier animals by culture is very difficult because of inapparent infections, variable patterns of shedding, and the failure of negative cultures to completely rule out a carrier state. In the case of non-Dublin serovars recovered animals continue to shed type B, C, and E organisms for 3 to 6 months or more in some instances. Therefore, control measures based on detection and elimination of infected animals or carriers are more easily instituted when small groups are infected; they can be impractical and unlikely to succeed in very large free-stall herds where animal movement, comingling of heifers from multiple source farms, and new purchases are the norm.

Vaccination against *Salmonella* spp. is controversial. Because cell-mediated immunity is a major factor in host resistance, killed bacterins that stimulate only humoral immunity give questionable protection. Vaccination of dry cows with specific *Salmonella* bacterins may protect neonatal calves somewhat for the first 2 to 3 weeks of life but probably not thereafter. Autogenous bacterins developed from the specific *Salmonella* serotype involved in an epidemic may be more helpful in this regard. Advances in on-farm efficacy in vaccines for the protection of cattle against *Salmonella* spp. has been challenged by the numerous serotypes encountered on many farms over time and the fact that cross protection between serotypes is notoriously poor, especially with killed products. Killed vaccines administered to neonatal calves have not performed well in research trials, primarily because calves appear to respond poorly to the oligosaccharide side chain antigens that comprise the protective antigens. Both commercial and autogenous bacterins must be used with caution because anaphylactic or endotoxic reactions are possible and are thought to represent an inherited hypersensitivity to endotoxin or other mediators. Aromatic-dependent *S.* Typhimurium and *S.* Dublin strains have been used as MLVs in calves and appear promising because they stimulate both cellular and humoral immune responses. One such product is available commercially in the United States for protection against *S.* Dublin (Entervene-D, Boehringer Ingelheim Vetmedica, St. Joseph, MO); it is labeled for use in calves older than 2 weeks of age and has enjoyed quite widespread use as a component of *S.* Dublin control efforts on many farms. A word of caution, however, is indicated with the product because it can be associated with life-threatening anaphylactoid reactions, and producers and veterinarians need to discuss this risk and be prepared for this eventuality when administering it to calves preweaning. The use of this vaccine will, of course, interfere with serologic testing efforts to identify individuals previously naturally infected with the organism. This product has also been demonstrated to inspire a serologic increase in antibody titers against *S.* Dublin when administered to dry cows, and this can result in increased antibody levels in calves by passive transfer. The health benefits of this increase in *S.* Dublin antibody titer in either the dam or calves are not known however at this time.

The use of a commercially available subunit vaccine has become quite commonplace in adult cattle within the U.S. dairy industry, but the product (*Salmonella* Newport Bacterial Extract [SRP], Zoetis, Florham Park, NJ) is not labeled for use in calves. Recent research has demonstrated that this product can elicit specific IgG antibody against *S.* Newport in colostrum when administered at dry off and 4 weeks later and that this can be transferred passively to new born calves after ingestion of colostrum. Unfortunately, at this point in time, what is unknown is whether this passive antibody will confer a protective effect for calves against natural challenge to either the vaccinal serotype or other strains in a farm environment. This subunit vaccine utilizes siderophore receptors and porins as antigens from *S.* Newport to stimulate an immune response against iron acquiring mechanisms employed by the bacterium (as well as other serotypes of *Salmonella* and other gram-negative species) during rapid bacterial growth. By "starving" the bacteria of iron, there will hopefully be attenuation and reduction in the severity of any subsequent infection; possibly conferring cross protection against multiple serotypes, even with other gram-negative species. There are philosophical similarities with the use of gram-negative core mutant products such as J5 and Endovac-Bovi as a component of *Salmonella* control in calves in that these products raise antibody against conserved epitopes of the gram-negative bacterial cell wall to hopefully ameliorate the pathogenic effects of endotoxin or lipopolysaccharide (LPS), but similarly do not entirely prevent infection. The use of these gram-negative core mutant products as a means of inspiring passive protection through dry cow immunization and colostral transfer, or by active immunization of preweaned calves also continues to enjoy some acceptance within the dairy industry, but there is relatively little scientific evidence to support either approach. For example, although immunization of calves with commercial J-5 vaccines has been shown to reduce mortality from salmonellosis in an experimental challenge study, in a large field trial, J-5 immunization of calves did not affect survival to 100 days.

Control of epidemic salmonellosis in dairy calves entails the basic principles of infectious disease control. Isolation of active cases, hygiene, disinfection, education of handlers, and perhaps culling or depopulation may be required. Whole-herd epidemics are frightening experiences that lead to tremendous public health concern. It is critical that the producer understands that after an outbreak is well established, control measures may mitigate the severity of the outbreak but often fail to immediately bring resolution. Patience, persistence, and communication are important. The reality for many farms, and commercial heifer rearers in particular, is that salmonellosis has become an endemic issue that requires persistent management efforts to position calves for health rather than disease when inevitable challenge with the pathogen occurs.

Methods of *Salmonella* control in calves include:
- Establish diagnosis via culture and sensitivity or serology (in older calves, >3months old) for *S.* Dublin; conduct investigation of the premises.
  A. Several affected animals should be cultured in epidemics to confirm a common pathogen, although some clinically ill animals will be culture positive on a single sample.
  B. Cultures of feces must always be performed.
  C. Colonic contents, bile, and mesenteric lymph nodes may be cultured from necropsy submissions.

D. If *S.* Dublin infection is suspected, blood, tracheal wash, or lung tissue samples may be cultured in addition to feces. Serology can be used after waning of any colostrally derived antibody by 3 months of age for evidence of *S.* Dublin in older calves also.

E. Carefully examine herd medical records and conduct an inspection of the premises to characterize the spatial and temporal characteristics of the problem. Is there a common sick cow pen or maternity stall, for example?

F. Critique flush water flow patterns and traffic patterns for personnel and vehicles.

G. Trace feedstuffs (including colostrum, whole milk, milk replacer, and water, as well as solid feeds) from their storage, preparation, transport to the animals, and delivery to the individual. Consider the possibility of contaminated feed, feed storage areas and transport equipment, feeding utensils, feed bunks, or buckets as potential sources of oral inoculation of healthy animals. Culture and then disinfect accordingly.

H. It is often useful to culture milk or milk replacer, water, and dry feeds for *Salmonella* spp. at the time of preparation or initial storage, during transport in containers, and after they are placed in the final container and presented to the calf (i.e., in a bucket or nipple feeder). This helps to identify potential sites of contamination and amplification of the organism. Producers often forget that milk and milk replacer are excellent culture media for *Salmonella* spp., and initially small inocula can become tremendous pathogen loads as the organisms replicate in feeds.

- *Isolate* infected animals:

A. This measure is relative and imperfect because some infected animals may not appear ill. However, calves with fluid feces, fever, dehydration, or other related signs should be isolated because they are shedding billions of organisms into the environment.

B. *Salmonella* control is often a numbers game, and reduction in pathogen load requires evaluation of all facets of calf handling and colostrum and milk feeding. Carefully scrutinize each and every step of the process of calf handling from parturition (maternity area hygiene) through placement in the hutch or pen. Often the first material ingested by the newborn calf is directly from the maternity environment, immediately after birth, and before consuming colostrum. In an outbreak on a Colorado dairy, a colleague of the authors, Dr. Rob Callan, isolated *Salmonella* Infantis from the nose and mouth of a newborn calf less than 5 minutes after being born. This calf had been pulled several yards across the ground of the maternity pen to a separate area where calves were then fed colostrum. In this situation, *Salmonella* was likely ingested well before consuming colostrum, greatly increasing the risk of infection. Although maternity pen hygiene is essential for minimizing exposure in calves, prompt removal of calves to individual calf hutches can also be

pivotal in control. Washable industrial wheelbarrows and wheeled bins make for excellent transfer vehicles for moving calves from the maternity area to designated calf housing. Alternatively, a calf "safe pen" can be considered (see previous section on colisepticemia).

C. All feeding and cleaning implements for sick calves should be scrubbed with soap and hot water and then disinfected between uses and never used on healthy calves.

D. Distance can be an effective buffer for reducing pathogen load to calves. When possible, calves should be moved to new, well-protected ground that is well removed and upwind from adult cows and protected from water flow from the main operation.

E. If labor is spread thin, it may be easiest for the producer to hire additional labor or reallocate personnel such that certain people are solely dedicated to the husbandry of calves. Disinfection and good hygiene take time, and personnel with multiple time demands often fail to fully and persistently implement good sanitation practices when handling calves. Epidemiologic studies from Europe have suggested that a single dedicated employee whose sole responsibility is the timely and hygienic collection and administration of colostrum to neonates is a significant positive factor in the control of *S.* Dublin.

F. Identify and remove all animals PI with BVDV from the herd.

- Therapy for infected animals:

A. Fluids to maintain hydration, acid–base balance, and serum electrolyte concentrations.

B. Additional protection from weather stress.

C. Maintain adequate nutrition.

D. Treat with appropriate antibiotics when indicated.

- Physically clean environment, improve hygiene, and disinfect premises.

A. Separate calves from adult cattle in every way possible (particularly critique flush water flow patterns and maternity pen hygiene because these are common means of spread of infection from adults to calves).

B. Clear maternity stalls and disinfect between calvings. Consider use of a "safe pen" for calves (see previous section on colisepticemia) and cleanable, plastic wheeled bins or wheelbarrows for transfer of calves out of the maternity area.

C. Do not house preweaned calves in a group, especially during an outbreak. If group housing is the preferred husbandry system for nursing calves, then endemicity is inevitable; it can still be a consequence when calves are individually housed.

D. Disinfect with a disinfectant approved to kill *Salmonella* spp. after physically cleaning organic debris from surfaces.

E. Being an opportunist, *Salmonella* spp. often flourish and cause disease in cattle populations under conditions of suboptimal nutrition or reduced immune function. Poor transition cow management, a high prevalence of animals PI with BVDV, and alterations in feed intake brought about by temperature extremes or poor bunk management are examples of the "intangibles" that often determine whether *Salmonella* infection becomes problematic on a given operation. With respect to calves, the same stressors of nutrition and climate can contribute to higher morbidity and mortality rates.

- Educate the farm owner and workers regarding public health concerns:
  A. Farm workers, calf handlers, and their families frequently become infected by *Salmonella* spp. during calf epidemics, and workers must be educated on how to minimize this risk.
  B. Insist on handlers wearing separate footwear and coveralls when handling infected calves. Allocate labor to prevent cross-infection from diseased calves to healthy calves. If certain personnel are responsible for all calves, have these individuals handle healthy calves first. Disinfect boots, hands, and implements. Be very careful about personal hygiene.
  C. Do not drink raw milk from adult cows if any signs of enteric disease or abortion have been observed in the herd.
- Recognize that recovered animals will shed intermittently or constantly for some time and thus represent significant risk to uninfected animals and people. Therefore, ongoing hygiene, disinfection, and surveillance are necessary.
- Immunization with modified-live (preferred) or killed vaccines (commercially available or autogenous) should be considered as an adjunct measure to be used only when the aforementioned management changes do not result in satisfactory abatement of the problem. Producers should be reminded that immunity is finite, and increased herd-level immunity brought about by the use of a vaccine is unlikely to succeed over the long term if initiated without meaningful changes in husbandry and hygiene.
- Feeding prebiotics or oligosaccharides may be beneficial.

Clostridium perfringens Type C Enterotoxemia.
Etiology

Enterotoxemia caused by *C. perfringens* type C is a commonly fatal disease that occurs in dairy and beef calves. Enteric disease caused by types A, B, and D has been reported in calves but is far less common. Neonates are most commonly affected, although disease losses in older calves (usually ≤3 months of age) can be significant. *C. perfringens* type A is a gram-positive anaerobic bacterium that is part of the normal intestinal flora of vertebrates. Intake of large quantities of soluble carbohydrate or protein is considered a risk factor for the development of type C enterotoxemia; the organism undergoes explosive growth under such conditions, creating a "superinfection" of the enteric lumen and producing exotoxins (termed *major lethal toxins*) that cause the majority of damage to host tissues. The exact reason for

clinical disease is often difficult to determine in sporadic cases but usually can be linked to "pushing" calves nutritionally when endemic problems are observed in a herd. Feeding of large volumes of milk or milk replacer, especially in the form of large meals, appears to be a common triggering factor. Heavy grain feeding, foraging on grain crops, sudden access to high-quality forage, or overfeeding after a period of hunger are also considered risks.

Beta toxin (CPB) is the principal major lethal toxin of type C, although variable amounts of alpha toxin (CPA) are produced by this organism too. The contribution of CPA to the pathogenicity of *C. perfringens* type C infections is considered minimal. CPB is a necrotizing toxin that forms membrane pores in susceptible cells such as those of the intestinal epithelium and thereby induces necrosis of enterocytes in the small intestine. This induced intestinal damage allows toxin access to the deeper layers of the gut wall, which creates extensive submucosal necrosis and intraluminal hemorrhage. Alpha toxin is a phospholipase that destroys lecithin within host cell membranes and membranous organelles. Terminally, multisystemic signs of disease can result from absorption of the major lethal toxins and from other gut-origin toxins or organisms gaining entry to the bloodstream via the damaged gut epithelium.

Beta toxin is a protein that is inactivated by exposure to trypsin. Thus, the lethal effects of CPB may be exacerbated in neonates because of either low pancreatic trypsin production or the presence of trypsin inhibitors in colostrum. When calves ingest large volumes of milk or concentrate, the calf's pancreatic enzymes may be sufficiently diluted to prevent inactivation of CPB; alternatively, the organism may proliferate to such a degree that the massive amounts of toxin released simply exceed the limited volume of trypsin available luminally in the gut. Similarly, feedstuffs such as sweet potatoes and soy beans that contain natural trypsin inhibitors may occasionally be associated with clinical disease due to this organism in more mature animals. We have also observed severe *C. perfringens* diarrhea in neonatal calves that were fed a normal feeding of colostrum or milk but that had a large amount of colostral supplements or replacers added to the meal.

Clinical Signs

Signs of enterotoxemia are acute or peracute and consist of colic, abdominal distension, dehydration, depression, and diarrhea. Sudden death or at least such rapid progression of signs that the calf is not observed to be ill for long before death can occur in peracute infections. Colic and abdominal distension usually precede diarrhea, and although the feces are loose, they are never as voluminous or watery as those found in calves with ETEC or salmonellosis. Feces in some enterotoxemia calves contain obvious blood and mucus (Fig. 6.13). Acute cases characterized by abdominal distension and colic may mimic intestinal obstructions unless diarrhea develops to rule out this out. Ballottement of the right lower quadrant reveals increased fluid in the small intestine. Progressive dehydration, depression, abdominal

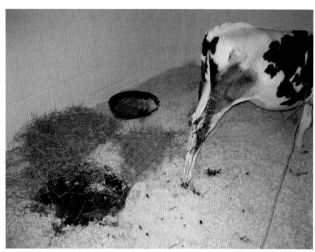

• **Fig. 6.13** A 5-week-old Holstein with acute and severe hemorrhagic enteritis caused by *Clostridium perfringens* type C. The calf recovered after intensive therapy with intravenously (IV) administered antibiotics (penicillin and ceftiofur), IV fluids, clostridium antitoxin, blood transfusion, flunixin meglumine, gastroprotectants, and transfaunation.

distension, and shock ensue unless intensive therapy is instituted. Neurologic signs are observed occasionally in the terminal stages of fatal cases of type C enterotoxemia. Affected calves usually have been in excellent condition and are often reported to have been vigorous eaters.

Ancillary Data

Blood work seldom is helpful or specific in enterotoxemia patients. Hemoconcentration is a given, but the leukogram and serum chemistry may be normal. In subacute cases, the serum albumin may be low because of intestinal losses and some loss into the peritoneal cavity. Hyperglycemia and glycosuria have been purported to be diagnostic but are more indicative of *C. perfringens* type D in lambs, not enteric clostridiosis in cattle. Any stressful disease may result in hyperglycemia and glycosuria in neonatal ruminants, and these findings are not pathognomonic for enterotoxemia in calves.

Acid–base and electrolyte data are not dramatically abnormal. Enterotoxemia calves *do not* usually have as severe a metabolic acidosis as calves severely affected with acute ETEC or *Salmonella*.

Diagnosis

Other than the physical signs, there are few clues to assist in the diagnosis of enterotoxemia. For fatal cases, necropsy findings often are quoted as diagnostic. However, they seldom are, and necropsy is used primarily to rule out other diseases. In field situations, it may be impossible to obtain meaningful samples and have them reach a diagnostic laboratory in time to be helpful. Recent pathologic description of confirmed cases has detailed that hemorrhagic, coagulative intestinal necrosis is common, especially affecting the jejunum and ileum and that hemorrhagic stool is more common than nonhemorrhagic stool but not invariant. Pathologic lesions can also be found outside the small intestine, with the abomasum, spiral colon, and cecum often

demonstrating extensive hemorrhagic necrosis. All dead animals have some *C. perfringens* in their intestines, so the relative numbers, types and toxins present must be assessed to accurately diagnose the type of *C. perfringens* involved and attach significance to the organism. Intestinal enzymes tend to break down alpha and beta toxins within hours of death. Commensal *C. perfringens* type A may proliferate in the gut and invade tissues within a short period after death, especially in warm weather. In fact, postmortem enteric proliferation of *C. perfringens* type A may be so extensive that it masks the presence of type C when luminal contents are cultured. The absolute diagnosis of enterotoxemia caused by type C organisms requires culturing *C. perfringens* from the gut; genotyping by PCR to determine that the isolate is type C; demonstration of gross or histologic lesions; and, if available, testing to identify beta toxin from the intestine of fatal cases (usually by ELISA). In the less common type B and type D enterotoxemias in cattle, absolute diagnosis requires identification of the organism by culture and genotyping in addition to demonstration of the epsilon toxin in the case of type D. Genotypic analysis is usually performed by multiplex PCR (mPCR), although mouse protection testing can also be used.

Calves with acute enterotoxemia may be diagnosed primarily based on clinical signs of colic, abdominal distension due to increased fluid within the small intestine, dehydration, diarrhea, and a rapidly progressive course. Ancillary data, if available, can help rule out other differential diseases. Progressive shock secondary to abomasal perforation with diffuse peritonitis can be ruled out by transabdominal ultrasonography and paracentesis. Acid–base and electrolyte determinations on venous blood and fecal cultures help rule out ETEC and acute salmonellosis because enterotoxemia calves seldom have a profound metabolic acidosis.

Feces or enteric contents may be cultured and assayed for toxins. Toxin identification is laborious and difficult because the toxins are labile and may be rapidly degraded. Proper sampling, storage, and shipment to a qualified laboratory are essential.

Treatment

Supportive treatment requires IV fluids (crystalloids and colloids such as plasma or Hetastarch; 5–10 mL/kg) with appropriate electrolytes and glucose to rehydrate the calf. Ideally, IV potassium or sodium penicillin (44,000 U/kg IV every 6 hours) should be given for the first 24 to 48 hours of therapy but can then be replaced by procaine penicillin (44,000 U/kg IM every 12 hours) if the calf is improved. Calves that are in shock may also be given dexamethasone or flunixin meglumine (0.5–1.1 mg/kg IV) as one-time treatments.

Resolution of clinical signs is gradual and slow. Abdominal distension sometimes takes days to resolve, and diarrhea becomes sporadic rather than voluminous. Recovering calves have variable appetites primarily based on their degree of abdominal distension and hydration status. Recovery in successful cases may require fluid and antibiotic support for up to 7 days. Progressive intestinal ulceration and subsequent perforation with peritonitis have been observed as an occasional complication in recovering calves. Therefore, repeated use of nonsteroidal and steroidal drugs is contraindicated to avoid further damage to the intestinal tract. Prolonged ileus and failure of abomasal emptying may evolve as a problem in recovering calves. If conservative therapy with IV fluid support and antibiotics fails to resolve this problem and the patient becomes more distended after drinking milk or electrolytes, metoclopramide (0.1–0.25 mg/kg SC every 8 to 12 hours or as a continual infusion) may be helpful to increase abomasal emptying and relieve abdominal distension. Administration of proton pump inhibitors or histamine antagonists may also be considered as described by Ahmed et al in calves with poor abomasal emptying as a means of trying to increase luminal pH and lessen the chances of mucosal ulceration (cimetidine 50–100 mg/kg orally every 8 hours, ranitidine 10–50 mg/kg orally every 8 hours, or preferably, ranitidine 1.5 mg/kg IV every 8 hours). Antitoxins are available commercially, and although they may be of use early in the course of the disease, efficacy of these products is difficult to determine. Blood or plasma transfusions may be needed because of intestinal damage and protein loss.

Control

Presentation of excessive amounts of starch, sugar, or soluble protein into the abomasum or intestine is considered pivotal in the development of enterotoxemia; thus, all potential influences on this critical pathogenic event must be considered when formulating a preventive plan. Evaluation of ration net energy, fiber content and forage length, bunk space, animal hierarchy within a pen, feeding frequency, the rate and magnitude of changes in ration between successive production groups, and feed mixing practices are essential to identify and correct problems with carbohydrate overload or slug feeding in older calves and adults. For pasture-fed animals, turnout onto a new pasture should be very gradual (e.g., day 1, 15 minutes of grazing; day 2, 30 minutes; day 3, 1 hour; day 4, 2 hours, and so on). Prevention of enterotoxemia in nursing calves requires consideration of environmental or management factors that may trigger ingestion of larger than normal volumes of milk or replacer. Decreasing the volume of milk fed per feeding by increasing the frequency of feedings has met with some success. Milk and milk replacer should be fed at or near body temperature to prevent induction of ileus or esophageal dysfunction.

Vaccination with *C. perfringens* toxoids is indicated for herds that have experienced sporadic or endemic enterotoxemia. When successful diagnostic tests confirm a specific type, toxoids obviously should contain that type. When specific types have not been identified, types C and D toxoid usually are suggested because type C is most commonly identified in calf enterotoxemia.

All dry cows and heifers should be vaccinated twice, 2 to 4 weeks apart (or according to manufacturer's recommendations); thereafter yearly boosters should be given 1 month before calving, and calves should be vaccinated with the same vaccine at 8 and 12 weeks of age. Immunization of neonatal calves has been used for enterotoxemia control in problem herds. However, no change in antibody titers to *C. perfringens* toxins has been demonstrated in immunized calves (immunized at ~7 weeks of age) or lambs (immunized twice up to 6 weeks of age) that received colostrum from vaccinated dams.

Clostridium perfringens Enterotoxemia and Abomasitis

Etiology

Sporadic cases of enterotoxemia associated with *C. perfringens* type A have been reported in calves. Abomasitis, abomasal tympany and bloat, and ulceration of the abomasum have also been linked to *C. perfringens* type A. It is uncertain whether the *Clostridium* organism is always the sole cause of this condition, and *C. septicum*, *C. fallax*, *Salmonella* spp., and *Sarcina* spp. have also been implicated in the condition in calves and other ruminants.

Abomasitis is a sporadic disorder of neonatal to weanling age calves, lambs, and kids. This disease is characterized by diffuse, hemorrhagic to necrotizing inflammation of the abomasal mucosa, frequently involving the deeper layers of the abomasal wall in severe or chronic cases. Intramural emphysema and edema of the abomasal wall may be present. Abomasal ulceration and perforation may occur in a subset of affected animals.

A variety of putative etiologies for this form of abomasitis existed historically, including primary bacterial or fungal infection, immunosuppression, and pica; trauma from coarse feed or trichobezoars; and vitamin or mineral deficiencies. In 1987, investigators at Kansas State University detected *C. perfringens* types A and E in stomach contents of affected calves and the following year reproduced the disease experimentally by intraruminal inoculation of *C. perfringens* type A in calves. The ability of this organism to produce gas is considered to contribute to the abomasal dilation and intramural emphysema evident in affected animals. More recently, *S.* Typhimurium DT104 was isolated from the abomasal wall of midwestern veal calves with abomasitis. Although authors of earlier case reports associated copper deficiency with abomasitis and abomasal ulcers in beef calves, Roeder and colleagues demonstrated that, in the absence of copper deficiency, abomasitis could occur spontaneously and be induced experimentally. Thus, although copper deficiency may act as a contributory factor for abomasitis and enteric disease of calves, it does not appear to be a requisite factor for either condition. Abomasal stasis and ruminal accumulation of milk have also been proposed as risk factors for the abomasitis/ulceration and the disease is further discussed in Chapter 5.

Diagnostic studies indicate that *C. perfringens* type A is now the most common bacterial isolate in cases of dairy calf clostridial enteritis and that affected calves typically exhibit tympany, hemorrhagic abomasitis, and abomasal ulceration. The presence of the organism as a member of the normal flora of all mammals has clouded its definitive etiologic role, but because inoculation with the organism can reproduce the disease experimentally, much interest has focused on this organism, particularly in herds that experience repeated cases, or outbreaks, of peracute abomasitis, tympany, and death in nursing calves.

Clinical Signs

Clinical signs include lethargy, abdominal tympany, colic, bruxism, fluid distension of the abomasum, diarrhea, and death. Although the number of case studies concerning abomasitis is few, on review of the available literature, the case fatality rate appears to be very high (75%–100%). Typically, significant signs of tympany and colic precede diarrhea, which is usually low in volume. Appropriate diagnostics are described in the previous section.

Treatment

Treatment of enterotoxemia caused by *C. perfringens* type A is similar to that used for types C or D. Unfortunately, antitoxin for types C and D has unknown efficacy in the treatment of type A cases. For abomasal tympany or abomasitis, IV fluid therapy, plasma therapy, parenteral antibiotic therapy, and antitoxin administration as described in the previous section are warranted in the initial medical management. Orogastric tube passage and decompression may be helpful in some cases; elevation of the calf's forequarters while the tube is placed may be helpful in releasing gas; however, because the predominant site of tympany is the abomasum, not the rumen, the therapeutic benefit of orogastric intubation is often minimal. Oral antibiotics such as penicillin or tetracycline may be helpful in reducing the rate of intraluminal gas production. Decompression of the abomasum via percutaneous ventral abomasocentesis has been described, and intraluminal injection of antibiotics could be performed after decompression. The blind trocharization of the left paralumbar fossa of tympanitic calves in the field is to be avoided. It is understandably tempting to attempt to decompress what can be a massively distended abdomen in this more typical anatomic location on the mistaken belief that it is the rumen that is causing the distension, but we have seen several lacerated abomasums when a 14-gauge needle is placed dorsally in this way—as the thin, distended abomasum deflates, the needle continues to cut into the organ like cheesewire. In cases that become progressively distended or in valuable calves, a laparotomy to drain the abomasal contents and oversew severe abomasal ulcers is often lifesaving. Laxatives appear to be of limited benefit in affected individuals, and large doses of magnesium oxide–hydroxide laxatives are likely contraindicated because they may exacerbate metabolic alkalosis seen in early stages of the disease, induce hypermagnesemia, and simply pull more fluid into the gut lumen.

A large, right-sided tympanic resonance in an ill calf may be a case of abomasal or cecal volvulus, and surgical exploration is indicated if initial medical management does not quickly result in resolution of tympany. Similarly, a left-sided tympanic resonance may reflect left displacement of the abomasum (LDA), and given the apparent high rate of ulceration of the abomasum associated with LDA in calves, surgical exploration is similarly warranted in those cases that

do not respond to medical management. Abomasotomy may be indicated for refractory cases of abomasal tympany. Abomasotomy allows for removal of luminal foreign bodies such as hairballs and putrefying milk, both of which may prevent a satisfactory response to medical management.

Prevention

In dairy calves, poor milk hygiene, intermittent feeding of large volumes of milk, and feeding cold milk or milk replacer, often via bucket, have been empirically incriminated as potential contributory factors for abomasal tympany, ulceration, and abomasitis. Anecdotal reports indicate that changing from bucket to bottle feeding, increasing the frequency of milk or milk replacer feeding and decreasing the volume fed at each feeding, as well as maintaining milk or replacer at body temperature until it is fed, may reduce the incidence and severity of this condition. A vaccine (*C. perfringens* type A toxoid, Novartis Animal Health, Larchwood, IA) that induces high antibody titers against alpha toxin, a primary virulence factor of *C. perfringens* type A, is available in the United States for prevention of diseases in cattle caused by this organism. As a dry cow vaccine, this product may increase colostral titers against alpha toxin, but the efficacy of this product in reducing calfhood diseases caused by *C. perfringens* type A is currently undetermined. A small proportion of *C. perfringens* type A strains associated with abomasal tympany and abomasitis in dairy calves are also CPB2 positive (the beta2 toxin encoding gene), so there may be some occasional therapeutic benefit to the administration of antitoxin to *C. perfringens* type C or the prophylactic use of toxoids against type C.

Giardiasis

Giardia duodenalis (also referred to as *G. lamblia* or *G. intestinalis*) is a common protozoal parasite of mammals, and the increased diagnostic sensitivity of PCR over previous immunofluorescence techniques has allowed prevalence investigations in a number of dairying areas worldwide. There are seven major genotypes (called Assemblages) of *G. duodenalis*, three of which have been demonstrated in cattle, specifically assemblages A, B, and E. Some of the specific interest in giardiasis relates to its zoonotic potential, although of the 3 genotypes identified in cattle in the United States, only assemblages A and B are considered zoonotic. Studies in the United States have revealed that the nonzoonotic assemblage E is the most common genotype in dairy calves and calves in cow and calf beef operations. Longitudinal studies have revealed that preweaning calves are more likely to be infected compared with postweaning or breeding-age heifers. The prevalence of infection in adult dairy cows in the United States appears to vary significantly from farm to farm, ranging from 0% to as high as 25%. Prevalence rates in replacement stock vary among studies but are commonly in the 40% to 70% range for preweaning-age calves and in the 25% to 40% range postweaning. A number of studies have revealed a low prevalence of zoonotic assemblage A, either in isolation, or in mixed infections with assemblage E in dairy calves, so dairy heifers must still be considered a zoonotic risk.

The clinical relevance of *G. duodenalis* is uncertain, prevalence studies in the literature tending to be based on fecal sampling of healthy, nondiarrheic calves or the sampling of diarrheic calves when other likely and well-known pathogens were not investigated extensively. Caution should therefore be taken when the organism is identified in either preweaned or group-housed calves because Koch's postulates have not been fulfilled for this protozoan in cattle, and it is a common finding in healthy calves, especially if modern, highly sensitive molecular techniques are used diagnostically. Fenbendazole at 15 mg/kg for 3 days has been a recommended treatment when practitioners are convinced that giardiasis is a clinical issue, specifically when other etiologic causes of loose stool, with or without blood, have been ruled out by appropriate sampling.

Campylobacteriosis

Much of the interest in *Campylobacter jejuni,* alongside other non-*jejuni* species such as *C. coli* and *C. faecalis,* stems not from their proven role as agents of calf diarrhea but because of the zoonotic risk that meat and dairy products contaminated with these organisms pose to human health. Furthermore, increased attention to antimicrobial resistance patterns among food animal–derived isolates of *Campylobacter* spp. heightens awareness of antimicrobial use in the dairy and beef industry and the potential role that both therapeutic and nontherapeutic drug use may play in increasing the public health threat of these foodborne pathogens. *C. jejuni* and *C. coli* can commonly be found in the feces of healthy calves (especially *C. jejuni*), and several studies have demonstrated that the prevalence of culture-positive fecal samples in dairy calves preweaning is in the range of about 15% of all calves on farm and that this rate is similar when diarrheic calves and normal calves are sampled. There has been an increasing level of tetracycline resistance among *C. jejuni* isolates from dairy animals in the United States in recent years, with some studies reporting up to 50% of strains being resistant. Worldwide, both fluoroquinolone and macrolide resistance are also becoming equally threatening problems.

Clostridium difficile

Rather similarly to campylobacteriosis, the predominant reason for recent interest in *C. difficile* comes not from an established role as a causative pathogen of calf diarrhea but because of the human health implications of the organism. Numerous studies across the world, including the United States, have demonstrated that the feces of dairy and veal calves as well as adult cows can contain toxigenic strains of *C. difficile*, albeit at low prevalence rates. Experimental inoculation of neonatal dairy calves with a highly toxigenic strain of the organism did not cause diarrhea or produce detectable toxin in their feces.

Other Possible Infectious Causes of Calf Diarrhea

With the advent of PCR, reverse transcriptase PCR (RT-PCR), and next-generation sequencing, molecular diagnostic techniques have become increasingly more sensitive and versatile in the past decade, and there has been an increase in the identification of novel viral agents in the feces of neonatal calves with diarrhea. Multiplex PCR assays for example enable screening for an array of different agents simultaneously, and there are several publications from diagnostic laboratories identifying bovine enterovirus, bovine norovirus, bovine torovirus, nebovirus, aichivirus, and bovine astrovirus in fecal samples obtained from dairy calves in the United States, South America, Africa, and the Far East. It is important to point out that many of these agents can also be found in the feces of normal calves and that for each of the viral agents listed, there has as yet been no successful recreation of enteritis experimentally in well-designed studies. In many cases, these agents have been identified along with more traditional viral, bacterial, and protozoal infections as part of a mixed infection in diarrheic calves. Control and prevention methods for viral diarrhea, specifically for what are all contagious, feco-orally spread organisms, would not deviate markedly from those listed earlier in this chapter.

Diarrhea and Emaciation Caused by Milk Replacer Feeding

Etiology

There has been a great deal of change in composition and formulation of modern-day milk replacers compared with early milk replacers produced during the 1950s and 1960s. Similar to adult cow rations, milk replacers may be formulated on a least-cost basis for ingredients, especially those comprising the crude protein fraction because this is the most expensive component. Since diarrhea and emaciation caused by inadequate milk replacer feeding is often initially considered to be an infectious diarrhea it is discussed here.

Milk proteins have been the preferred protein source for milk replacers, and pasteurized skim milk powder (low heat prepared and then spray dried) is ideal. Unfortunately, the price of skim milk has risen to a point where it is no longer economically possible to include it as the total source of protein in most milk replacers. Most milk replacer proteins are now derived from whey protein concentrate, dried whole whey, dried whey products that are byproducts of cheese manufacturing with casein and fat extracted, or spray-dried plasma (often from other species, e.g., porcine).

Other protein sources such as modified soy protein, soy protein concentrate, soy protein isolate, and special processed soy flour also have been used. Special processing of these soy protein sources chemically or by heat is necessary to deter allergic gastroenteritis in calves that ingest them. Such processing reduces antinutritional factors in soy proteins and allows for a soluble product. Moreover, soy proteins seldom are fed as the entire protein source and often comprise less than 50% of total protein, thus allowing their inclusion and successful use for milk replacer protein sources.

The total protein content of a milk replacer should be a minimum of 20%, with most current minimal recommendations suggesting at least 22%. Milk proteins should make up as much of the protein as possible, and processing of the proteins should not damage the nutrient by subjecting it to high temperatures or other factors.

Fat content of milk replacers is another source of controversy between feed companies and nutritionists. Countless feeding trials have been conducted to show that each company's product is the perfect feed. However, in northern climates, there is no question that a 20% or higher fat content is best based on field observations.

The fiber level in milk replacers roughly correlates with plant origin sources of protein in some instances. With the advent of acceptable soy protein sources, however, fiber levels cannot be the sole means of evaluation. Early milk replacers with soy flour or another soy source added could be judged somewhat by crude fiber because each 0.1% crude fiber suggested 10% of the protein to be of plant origin. Inclusion of modified soy protein, soy protein concentrate, and soy protein isolate, however, does not increase the fiber content significantly. Therefore, crude fiber is not of great correlative value when evaluating current milk replacer protein content.

Yet another controversial aspect of milk replacer feeding involves physiologic "clotting" in the calf abomasum. Milk fed by conventional means causes reflex esophageal groove closure and diversion into the abomasum rather than forestomach. In the abomasum, milk quickly is separated into a casein and milk fat coagulum and a liquid component; whey. Chymosin (rennin) and pepsin in the presence of calcium and hydrochloric acid assist this separation. The whey, which contains lactose, protein, immunoglobulins, and minerals, passes into the duodenum for digestion, but the casein or fat coagulum is digested slowly. For many years, it was thought that milk replacers had to "clot" in the abomasum or else they were inferior and caused diarrhea and poor growth. Because only milk or skim milk feeds have casein and whey components, tests for clotting were most applicable to milk replacers with skim milk as the source of protein. In essence, tests for clotting were designed to detect skim milk-origin whey proteins that had been heat denatured by excessive temperatures during processing or drying and therefore would not clot. Because most current milk replacers have a high composition of whey protein or soy-origin protein, they do not clot, yet they appear to be well digested.

In addition to the composition of milk replacers, practitioners should be familiar with the common errors associated with milk replacer feeding. The amount of milk replacer fed may or may not be enough for maintenance and growth of suckling calves. Similarly, the dilution may be too great or the owner may be skimping because of economic pressures. Replacer should be reconstituted at approximately 12.5% solids (similar to whole milk) and fed at least twice daily for a total of *at least* 10% to 12% body weight. Cold weather extremes and northern winter housing necessitate higher volumes or

a third or fourth feeding each day. Some manufacturers do not recommend enough milk replacer to meet maintenance *and* growth requirements under these conditions. Therefore, recommended total amounts may be erroneous.

Another problem with some milk replacers is the high sodium content, which may cause neurologic signs if free water is unavailable for whatever reason! Fresh water consumption being most consistent immediately after milk ingestion, it is imperative that fresh, palatable, unfrozen water is available to all calves immediately after milk feeding. The issue of malnutrition related to inadequate calorific intake of lower quantity or lower quality protein and fat content milk replacers is significantly compounded when calves have illnesses during the first month of life. The calorific needs of calves with, or recovering from, enteritis or pneumonia are multiples of normal maintenance requirements; the lower the fat and protein content, the greater the necessary volume to be ingested will be. This phenomenon is predictable and repeatable during the winter months in the northern United States when endemic scours and respiratory disease problems are often at their worst.

In the past, it was more commonplace for newborn calves to receive colostrum until 3 to 4 days of age and then be switched to replacer or whole milk. This is no longer as frequently practiced, and milk replacer may be fed as early as day 2 of life in most settings. Yet another common feeding error for farmers using milk replacer is not increasing the amount fed as the calf ages. In other words, the calf receives 1 cup of milk replacer in 2 quarts of water twice daily at 4 days of age and is still being fed the same amount at 4 weeks of age. Only through a step-by-step discussion with the owner and by careful observation can the veterinarian detect and correct some calf feeding problems.

High-quality calf starter grains can mask the effect of a poor-quality milk replacer; some authors believe that up to 50% to 75% of calf weight gain before weaning may result from high-quality calf starter intake. Milk replacers containing antibiotics or decoquinate are advertised widely, but their value is difficult to assess because studies have yielded contradictory results.

Calf diarrhea, emaciation, or both can result from errors in milk replacer feeding. The preceding discussion lists some of the common problems in milk replacer composition and feeding. The true "etiology" of milk replacer-related calf mortality varies but includes;
- Poor-quality milk replacer (i.e., one with <22% protein, 20% fat, or a poor-quality or over-processed protein source)
- Feeding at the wrong dilution
- Feeding the wrong amount (usually not enough; see later section on feeding for disease or during cold stress)

Clinical Signs

Calves with malnutrition from poor-quality milk replacer appear thin; have dull hair coats with patchy alopecia; usually have diarrhea that coats their perineum, tail, and hind legs; and are hungry. Affected calves have a normal or subnormal temperature unless an opportunistic infection (e.g., pneumonia) causes a fever in the terminal stages. Calves have no body fat and are weak. Owners complain about calf death that usually occurs at 3 to 6 weeks of age and attribute death to chronic diarrhea or pneumonia. Calves may die suddenly but often remain hungry and willing to nurse even if recumbent 1 to 2 days before death. All calves in the preweaning group look thin. The owner may report that the calves look good for the first week but then seem to deteriorate. Calves that survive to weaning often do well on high-quality solid feeds and regain condition.

Ancillary Aids

If calves are dying as early as 3 weeks of age, enteric pathogens and parasites must be ruled out by submission of either fecal samples from live animals or feces and gut samples from necropsy samples. It may be necessary to assess blood selenium and vitamin E values from calves that become recumbent. Total protein values may be low because of persistent low protein intake or fecal losses associated with enteritis, a result of poor-quality protein sources. Blood work results are normal unless a stress leukogram exists. Assessment of adequacy of passive transfer is also prudent.

Necropsy confirms malnutrition based on serous atrophy of fat in the epicardial grooves, omentum, and perirenal areas. Gut contents are often fluid, reflecting either poor digestion of nutrients in the cachectic state or opportunistic, secondary enteric infections of the compromised host. Pneumonia may be present as a concurrent condition.

Diagnosis

Diagnosis usually can be made by inspection of the calves coupled with a careful history and evaluation of the milk replacer and feeding procedures. Differential diagnoses include infectious causes of neonatal diarrhea, coccidiosis, and selenium deficiency. Whereas calves that are younger than 3 weeks of age require careful consideration of infectious enteric bacterial, viral, or protozoan pathogens, older calves between 3 weeks of age and weaning require consideration of coccidiosis and salmonellosis. The owner will be adamant that an infectious disease is responsible because so many calves appear to be affected by ill thrift and looser than normal stool.

Improper preparation and mixing are occasional factors that augment malnutrition. Careful reading of the instructions on milk replacers or consultation with a nutritionist affiliated with the manufacturer may reveal that mixing at hot temperatures (104° to 106°F) is required for complete solubilization of fat in the replacer; subsequent cooling to body temperature is necessary for acceptance by calves. In such cases, greasy residue may be detected in the mixing vessel as well as in the bottles or buckets following ingestion by the calves.

Inspection of the whole group of calves is very helpful, especially when the veterinarian routinely observes the calves at monthly visits. The sight of a whole group of malnourished but hungry and bright nursing calves in a barn that usually has well-conditioned calves almost guarantees that the owner has switched to a new (cheaper) milk replacer. Calves "eat until they die" and appear hungry even though they are in poor condition. Necropsy of fatal cases confirms serous atrophy of fat and allows other diseases to be ruled out after submission of appropriate samples.

Prevention

Correction and prevention merely require the feeding of a high-quality milk replacer at proper dilution and in proper quantities. The owner must be convinced that milk replacer is not the place to save pennies. In fact, given the increased costs associated with calf losses in such cases, it can be stated that the most expensive milk replacer a producer can buy is often the cheapest one. Milk replacer is never as good as whole milk for calves; therefore, whenever possible, owners should be encouraged to feed calves whole milk that is at least 22% crude protein and 20% crude fat (dry matter basis) unless there is a problem with Johne's disease, *Salmonella, Mycoplasma,* or leukosis in the herd. Milk discarded because of antibiotic residues is not ideal and should not be fed to group-housed calves. It carries an increased risk for transmission of several contagious infectious diseases unless pasteurization is performed. Many owners need to reassess the costs of feeding milk versus milk replacer because feeding proper quantities of high-quality milk replacer may be nearly as expensive as whole milk and can never be as good a diet. Use of a pasteurizer for feeding waste milk to calves has been shown to be of economic benefit on larger dairies. Pasteurization of waste milk is worthy of consideration for operations that routinely produce calves for sale as replacement stock because milk-borne transmission of infectious agents of concern (e.g., *Mycoplasma* spp.) may be reduced.

Soured colostrum and pickled colostrum can be excellent sources of feed for calves, but their storage problems and an increased potential for spreading pathogens frequently discourage farmers from using them.

If the veterinarian has made a diagnosis of diarrhea and emaciation caused by milk replacer issues and feeding of pasteurized whole milk cannot be done, the following instructions can be followed:

1. Ensure adequate colostral feeding to ensure passive transfer of immunoglobulins during the first 12 hours of life. Quality control for proof of adequacy of passive transfer is advisable; total protein measurement by handheld refractometer to confirm that more than 75% of all calves between 1 and 7 days of age have total protein levels of 5.5 g/dL or higher is recommended. If a Brix refractometer is used, the reading should be greater than 8.5%.
2. Feed colostrum for the first 3 days of the calf's life at 10% to 12% body weight but only if sure the cow is not shedding *M. paratuberculosis* or *M. bovis*. On larger dairies, consider colostrum pasteurization.
3. Begin feeding a high-quality milk replacer on day 4 at 10% body weight:
   - Minimum 22% protein—most or all of milk origin if possible
   - Minimum 20% fat
   - Minimal crude fiber
4. After the first week, quantity can gradually be increased to maintain at least 10% to 12% body weight intake.

5. Be sure dilution factors for milk replacer are correct to mimic the total solids of milk.
6. All calves should have fresh water and a high-quality calf starter available at all times. Feed starter in small amounts initially until the calf begins to eat well enough that the starter does not spoil in the feeder. High-quality hay can be available in small quantities starting at 2 weeks of age.
7. Regularly monitor the preparation and feeding temperature of the milk replacer.

An excellent calf starter, adequate feed intake, and good management may mask the effects of a poor-quality milk replacer. This is why some farms seem to have "starving" calves on a specific milk replacer but others seem to achieve acceptable growth with the same product.

Feeding Dairy Calves Milk Replacer for Cold, Illness, or Stress

Because calves are born with little to no body fat that can be mobilized for energy, nutrition becomes a critical element of health management, welfare, and future performance. Nutritional management of the young dairy calf is very dynamic, with requirements for protein and energy increasing each week so that calves can double their birth weight by 56 to 60 days of age. Accomplishing an optimal rate of gain is made more complex in cold weather, hot weather, or for any calves living in conditions outside of their thermoneutral zone (58° to 72°F). It is also significantly complicated by concurrent disease and convalescence. Although the National Research Council (NRC) provides excellent guidelines for feeding calves under a wide range of environmental temperatures, it does not offer specific guidance for feeding calves under conditions of heat stress, disease, immune challenge, vaccination, or other environmental or management stressors. Most veterinary practitioners and academicians are in agreement that the protein and energy requirements for calves are increased under these conditions, but unfortunately, precise feeding guidelines are not available for each situation.

To provide the calf with the ability to meet increased nutritional demands, whether it is attributed to cold weather, hot weather, stress, illness, pain, or immune challenge, it is important to provide more milk or milk replacer. To encourage intake and prevent digestive problems caused by dietary inconsistency, it is optimal to simply feed a greater daily volume of the same milk or milk replacer mix to which calves are already accustomed. Optimally, the increased volume is delivered by providing at least one additional daily feeding to calves. Alternatively, a concentrated energy source is added to the regular liquid diet or a higher concentration of dried milk replacer powder is fed at the same number of daily feedings. When changes are made in the concentration of milk replacer being fed then this should be done gradually; total solids of liquid feed should not increase by more than 1% at a time (per day) and must never exceed a maximum of 17%. Hyperosmolality and hypernatremia are not issues provided fresh water is available to calves at all times and incremental changes to total solids are made gradually. Table 6.3 shows how the

TABLE 6.3	Increasing Requirement for Whole Milk in the Diet of a Dairy Calf in Cold Weather[*]	
	Cold: Temperature <50°F	Warm: Temperature 50° to 75°F
4 quarts/day	0–3 days	0–7 days
6 quarts/day	4–10 days	8–14 days
8 quarts/day	11–49 days	15–49 days

[*]Assuming colostrum administration at a minimum of 10% of calf's bodyweight within first 12 hours of life.

NRC predicts an increasing requirement for the volume of whole milk fed by calf age under cold and warm environmental conditions for an 80 lb birthweight calf. As ambient temperature drops still further into the temperature ranges experienced in the northern US in winter the amount of whole milk being fed would need to be adjusted higher from the volumes detailed in Table 6.3.

Many use the NRC calculator available online to predict the allowable daily gain from energy and protein for different dairy calf diets. In Table 6.4, the NRC calculator has been used to predict the average daily gain (ADG) of a 2-week-old, 95-lb Holstein calf being fed 6 quarts daily (30 oz of milk replacer powder) using different milk replacer formulations and different environmental temperatures.

By week 3 of age, a Holstein calf on-target to double birth weight by day 56 should be gaining 1.6 lb/day. Table 6.4 shows that neither a 20:20 nor a 22:20 milk replacer is predicted to meet that expectation. At cold temperatures (20° and 40°F), a 6-quart per day diet is both protein and energy deficient, but at the warmer temperatures of 60° and 80°F, the 6 quart per day diet is only protein deficient. With the higher protein milk replacers (24:18 and 28:20), the 6-quart diet is limited by energy intake at colder temperatures. At 20°F, both the 24:18 and 28:20 milk replacers are too low in energy, but at 40°F, only the 24:18 milk replacer is limiting ADG because of lack of energy. If the same 2-week-old, 95-lb Holstein calf is fed 8 quarts of milk replacer per day (40 oz of milk replacer powder), all of the milk replacers shown in Table 6.4 would meet energy and protein requirements to achieve at least an ADG of 1.6 lb/day. Although the tables are focused on NRC predictions for feeding milk or milk replacer at different temperatures, they are useful to guide clinicians in feeding sick, stressed, or immune-challenged calves. It is still recommended to feed sick calves for expected ADG. One can provide more frequent feedings of the typical milk or milk replacer diet to which the calf is accustomed to achieve adequate intake. Milk, milk replacer, and water should be delivered at the temperature to which the calf has been accustomed but it is important to offer it at a temperature of at least 93°F. To encourage feed intake under conditions of illness or stress, it is imperative to provide continuous access to fresh, clean, warm (especially in cold weather) water along with a high quality texturized calf starter with a crude protein content of at least 18%.

TABLE 6.4   National Research Council Predictions of Average Daily Gain (lb/day) for a 2-Week-Old, 95-lb Holstein Calf Fed 6 Quarts of Milk Replacer (30 oz of Milk Replacer Powder) Per Day

Temperature (°F)	Milk Replacer Crude Protein to Fat Ratio			
	20:20	22:20	24:18	28:20
20	1.2	1.2	1.2	1.3
40	1.4	1.5	1.5	1.6
60	1.4	1.5	1.6	1.9
80	1.4	1.5	1.6	1.9

TABLE 6.5   Diagnostic Plan for Workup of Herd Neonatal Diarrhea Problems (<14 Days of Age)

Management	Patient

I. Assess success of passive transfer on at least two or three consecutive affected calves
    A. TP, TS, or Brix refractometry
    B. Specific immunoglobulin level on serum from affected calves
II. Discuss management of dry cow
    A. Vaccines
    B. Housing
    C. Calving area (cleanliness and so forth)
    D. Colostrum quality, quantity and feeding
    E. Are affected calves from primiparous or multiparous dams or both?
III. Statistics on morbidity and mortality in calves
IV. What are calves fed after initial colostrum?
	I. Feces collected immediately after onset of diarrhea to diagnostic laboratory on at least two or three consecutive affected calves
	    A. Bacterial
	        • *Escherichia coli* (type, toxin identification and antibiotic sensitivity) *Salmonella* spp. (type and antibiotic sensitivity)
	        • *Clostridium perfringens* (relative numbers, type and toxin identification)
	    B. Viral—PCR, EM, ELISA
	        • Isolation possibly
	        • Rule out BVDV by buffy coat isolation from blood
	    C. Parasitic—*Cryptosporidium*
	II. CBC, total protein, whole blood selenium
	III. Acid–base and serum/plasma chemistries
	IV. Hydration status
	V. Body condition

Generalities

1. If FPT, ignore *Escherichia coli* unless same organism confirmed also on non-FPT calves.
2. Whenever possible, more than one calf should be sampled before blaming the whole herd problem on a single isolate.
3. Only fresh cases are worth sampling.
4. If patient older than 2 weeks, consider poor replacer rather than infectious diseases.

BVDV, Bovine viral diarrhea virus; *ELISA,* enzyme-linked immunosorbent assay; *EM,* electron microscopy; *FPT,* failure of passive transfer; *GGT,* γ-glutamyl transferase; *PCR,* polymerase chain reaction; *TP,* total protein; *TS,* total solids.

Summary Diagnostic Protocol for Investigation of Neonatal Calf Diarrhea

Table 6.5 gives a diagnostic plan for herd neonatal diarrhea problems. Also see Table 18.2.

Coccidiosis

Etiology

Coccidiosis has become one of the more serious problems encountered in raising dairy calves when the calves are grouped housed either pre- or postweaning. Traditionally, it has been considered a problem in group-housed weaned calves, but the prepatent period is such that clinical disease can be seen before weaning in modern group-reared nursing calf management systems. This style of management currently is very popular because it decreases the labor requirements for many large dairies and is convenient in colder climates.

Although up to 20 species of *Eimeria* may infect cattle, *E. bovis* and *E. zuernii* are considered the major pathogenic species. Sporulated oocysts that are infective for calves and older cattle arise from oocysts passed in the feces of cattle with patent infections. Whereas moisture and cool conditions are conducive to sporulation, extreme heat and dryness are detrimental. Oocysts can remain viable for more than 1 year in favorable conditions that include moisture and absence of temperature extremes. Fecal contamination of feedstuffs, water, or hair coats allows ingestion of infective oocysts by other cattle. Conditions favoring fecal contamination of feed and water exist when calves are grouped in mini free stalls, bedded packs, or other group housing systems such as is becoming increasingly popular with automated milk feeding of calves. Calves may ingest feces containing oocysts from feed bunks that become contaminated when calves come running up to the bunk to be fed and then splash manure into the bunk or waterers, from calves licking themselves and ingesting feces or fecal-stained hair, or from browsing on contaminated bedding in a housing unit.

Coccidia are quite host-specific intracellular parasites that complete both the asexual and sexual phases of reproduction within the host, but as mentioned previously, sporulation occurs outside the host. Ingested sporulated oocysts excyst in the host, release sporozoites that invade host cells (central lacteals of ileal villi for *E. bovis*, connective tissue cells of ileal lamina propria for *E. zuernii*), and grow to schizonts (meronts) that release merozoites that then infect epithelial cells in the cecum and colon. Second-generation schizonts then form in these cells and subsequently release merozoites that begin the sexual phase of the reproductive cycle by invading yet another host epithelial cell and become microgamonts (male) or macrogamonts (female). Microgamonts release microgametes that seek host cells containing macrogametes (matured macrogamont), fertilization takes place, and a zygote forms and matures to an oocyst that then is released by rupture of the host cell. Invasion of cells and subsequent release of merozoites and oocysts incite varying degrees of pathology within the epithelium of the cecum and colon of affected calves. The magnitude of enteric pathology appears to be related to the dose of oocysts ingested. Small doses of ingested oocysts may result in inapparent infection and eventual induction of immunity. Large doses are more likely to result in clinical disease.

Oocysts are observed in feces (patent infection) approximately 17 to 20 days after infection with *E. bovis* and 16 to 17 days with *E. zuernii*. The numbers of oocysts in the feces do not always correspond with the degree of enteric pathology or clinical signs because even asymptomatic animals may shed fairly large numbers of oocysts. Conversely, some calves become severely ill before the majority of protozoa complete their life cycle and produce oocysts; therefore, fecal oocyst counts may be relatively low despite the serious pathology present in the large intestine.

Recovered calves are thought to be relatively immune to reinfection by the same species of *Eimeria* but at risk for infection by other species. Factors that have a negative influence on the calves' immune competence enhance the pathogenicity of coccidia. Therefore, calves exposed to coccidia oocysts and simultaneously subjected to climatic stress, poor nutrition, exogenous corticosteroids, concurrent inflammatory diseases, or acute or persistent BVDV infection would likely show severe signs of coccidiosis.

Clinical Signs

Classical textbook signs of acute coccidiosis in calves include diarrhea containing mucus and blood, tenesmus, depression, and reduced appetite. Rectal prolapse may occur secondary

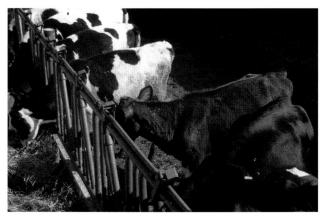

• **Fig. 6.14** Typical signs of coccidiosis in dairy calves. Some of the calves are well grown and have normal hair coats, but others (especially the heifer that is not in a lock-in stanchion) are undergrown; have a rough, dry, unshed hair coat; and are thin. Many have looser feces than normal for their diet, and the hindquarters are stained by loose manure.

to proctitis and prolonged tenesmus. Affected calves appear dehydrated and thin and have poor hair coats. Milder cases merely show mild diarrhea without systemic signs and many cases are subclinical.

In fact, these textbook signs of acute coccidiosis seldom occur in dairy calves. The predominant signs of coccidiosis in group-raised dairy calves are loose manure, poor condition, poor growth rates, and poor hair coats (Fig. 6.14). The feces seldom contain blood or mucus and tend to have a pea soup consistency. Feces stain the perineum, tail, and hocks of typical cases. Although most calves in the group are infected, only those with severe infection show dramatic signs. Coccidiosis is a perfect example of the "weak sister" law in parasitology; this law states that when a group of animals are parasitized, the most seriously affected bring attention to the problem and act as a signal that the entire group needs treatment. Dairy calves and heifers occasionally show textbook signs of blood- and mucus-stained feces, tenesmus, and inappetence. Tenesmus can be severe and sufficient to prevent the patient from concentrating on eating or drinking.

Coccidiosis is a major disease in group-raised dairy calves and heifers. Heifers raised in confinement groups require prophylactic treatment for coccidiosis, or growth rates can be severely compromised. The age of onset for clinical signs varies. Theoretically, it is possible that calves will show signs by 3 weeks of age based on life cycles of *E. zuernii* and *E. bovis*. Fortunately, this seldom occurs unless newborn calves are put in heavily contaminated environments such as group housing arrangements or hutches that have not been cleaned since previous occupancy by infected calves. In general, coccidiosis becomes a problem for dairy calves at weaning when they are grouped. Weaning and grouping of calves that were previously housed individually induce stress. This stress, combined with an environment that more commonly fosters fecal contamination of feedstuffs, water sources, and hair coats, creates an ideal situation for coccidiosis. Therefore, clinical signs of coccidiosis are most commonly seen in 8- to 16-week-old calves raised in mini free-stall or automatic lock-in facilities. Occasional outbreaks have been observed in 12- to 18-month-old heifers as well but only very rarely in milking age animals. It would be assumed that older animals showing signs of coccidiosis had not previously developed resistance to the *Eimeria* spp. involved.

Morbidity is often higher than expected because many infected animals remain subclinical or show only mild signs such as diminished weight gain. The mortality rate is low unless the problem is neglected, a severe oocyst loads exist, or if concurrent disease affects the coccidiosis patients.

Nervous coccidiosis has been well described in Canada and the northern United States. Although this form has been observed primarily in beef calves, it may occur in dairy calves as well. Heavy loads of coccidia coupled with severe winter weather seem to be contributing factors to nervous coccidiosis. Affected calves can show a variety of neurologic signs, including (but not limited to) severe tremors, nystagmus, and recumbency. Opisthotonos may be observed and confuse the diagnosis with that of polioencephalomalacia. The mortality rate is high for calves with nervous coccidiosis.

Diagnosis

Clinical signs coupled with fecal flotation (standard flotation or McMaster's flotation) to confirm high numbers of coccidia allow a positive diagnosis. The diagnostic limitations of fecal oocyst counts must be kept in mind:

1. Diarrhea may precede the highest oocyst counts by a few days in acute cases because merozoite damage to the colonic epithelium may cause diarrhea before full patency and maximal oocyst shedding occur. In other words, an animal severely affected by coccidiosis may have a relatively low or even zero oocyst count on a given fecal sample. Necropsy and histopathology may be necessary to confirm the diagnosis in such cases.
2. Nonpathogenic species of coccidia may artificially elevate oocyst counts as they traverse the intestinal tract.
3. Healthy animals may have oocysts in their feces.

In general, oocyst counts of > 5000/g of feces are considered significant when coupled with clinical signs. Several calves should be sampled to confirm the diagnosis because severely affected groups of calves tend to show higher oocyst counts as a population.

The major differential diagnoses are salmonellosis, BVDV infection, endoparasitism as a result of nematodes, and poor nutrition. These diseases should be ruled out when response to treatment for coccidiosis fails to correct the problem. Nervous coccidiosis dictates a much broader differential diagnosis, including polioencephalomalacia, *Histophilus somni* meningoencephalomyelitis, salt poisoning, lead poisoning, and many other neurologic diseases. A CSF tap is a valuable test to rule in or out some of these differential diagnoses.

Calves that die from acute, severe coccidiosis may or may not have gross pathologic lesions in the cecum and colon. Severe infections may cause a diphtheritic membrane from sloughed mucosa, blood, and fibrin. Whole blood clots occasionally are found in the colon, and the mucosa of the cecum, colon, and rectum may be thickened. Small white spots (schizonts) may be apparent on close inspection of the mucosa of the ileum or colon. Microscopic lesions mainly reflect colonic damage secondary to second-generation schizonts and sexual phases of the parasite life cycle. Inflammation, sloughing of epithelial cells, cellular infiltrates, and alteration of the appearance of infected epithelial cells to a less columnar shape may be observed. Whereas schizonts of *E. bovis* tend to be located in the villous tips, *E. zuernii* schizonts are located adjacent to the muscularis layer.

Treatment and Prevention

Treatment and prevention of coccidiosis in calves entail orally administered coccidiostatic or coccidiocidal agents. It is commonplace within the U.S. dairy industry to medicate calves prophylactically because exposure of calves to coccidia is likely. Amprolium, monensin, lasalocid, and decoquinate are the drugs used most commonly to treat groups of affected or at-risk calves. These drugs are added to feed or water at the rates listed in Table 6.6.

Ionophores such as monensin and lasalocid are fed continuously in many calf-raising operations where coccidiosis is known to exist; the same is true for decoquinate. Manufacturers' warnings, dosages, and withdrawal times must be observed and are subject to change. Decoquinate is not toxic to young calves, but ionophores may be. Although various sulfa drugs were the first treatments for coccidiosis in animals, they are not used at present except to treat small groups or individual calves so sick they may not be eating or drinking well enough to ingest therapeutic dosages of drugs added to their feed or water. When sulfa drugs are used for treatment, it is beneficial to treat simultaneously with amprolium at therapeutic levels.

Although parasitologists question the efficacy of the aforementioned drugs in treating clinical coccidiosis, sulfaquinoxaline (13.2 mg/kg orally once daily) in combination with amprolium (10 mg/kg daily) for 5 days appears to provide a good clinical response. Strict adherence to recommended meat withdrawal is required when sulfonamides are used. Individual calves that are severely dehydrated may require supportive fluids; colloids; and, rarely, blood transfusions if colonic hemorrhage has been severe. Tenesmus may be so severe and persistent as to require epidural anesthesia to allow the calf or heifer to rest, eat, and drink.

Although the aforementioned drugs are used widely for prophylaxis in calves at risk for coccidiosis, they should not be thought of as the only means of control. Management practices that allow dirty environments, manure buildup, feeding on ground level, feed and water contamination by

TABLE 6.6 Drugs that Aid in Prevention and Treatment of Coccidiosis

Drug	Name	Use	Dose
Amprolium	Corid*	Prophylactic	5 mg/kg bwt for 21 days
		Therapeutic	10 mg/kg bwt for 5 days
Monensin	Rumensin†	Prophylactic	16.5–33.0 g/ton feed continuously or 1.0 mg/kg bwt for 28 days
Lasalocid	Bovatec‡	Prophylactic	1 mg/kg bwt continuously
Decoquinate	Deccox§	Prophylactic	0.5 mg/kg bwt for 30 days
Sulfamethazine	Several products available	Therapeutic	140 mg/kg bwt loading dose; then 70 mg/kg bwt for 5–7 days
Sulfadimethoxine		Therapeutic	55 mg/kg bwt loading dose; then 27.5 mg/kg bwt for 5–7 days
Sulfaquinoxaline		Therapeutic	13.2 mg/kg orally once daily for 3–5 days

*Corid (amprolium), Merial, Duluth, GA.
†Rumensin 60 (monensin sodium), Elanco Animal Health, Greenfield, IN.
‡Bovatec (lasalocid), Zoetis, Parsippany, NJ.
§Deccox (decoquinate), Zoetis, Parsippany, NJ.
Bwt, Body weight.

manure, and crowding should be corrected. If calves are kept in a clean environment, manure should be scraped away daily to prevent "splashing" of feces into bunks, troughs, waterers, and all over calves' bodies. If premises are cleaned and disinfected between consecutive groups of calves, the risk of coccidiosis is lowered tremendously. Unfortunately, many farmers would rather rely on a drug placed in the feed than do the required cleaning. Many of the coccidiostats are only effective for as long as fed, so calves become at risk if medicated feed is discontinued or there is an interruption in medicated feed or water consumption for some other reason. Therefore, anticoccidial drugs usually are included in the ration for extended periods such as from weaning through breeding age rather than based on manufacturer's recommendations (e.g., 30 days). Increasingly, calf starters and milk replacers including coccidiostats are being marketed for dairy calves. Although these drugs may not be necessary in preweaned calves, it is possible that clinical coccidiosis could occur as early as 2 to 3 weeks of age. Although the rumen is poorly developed in neonatal calves, lasalocid fed from day 1 improves gain and counterbalances coccidial infection (experimentally induced) before weaning. Careful attention to accurate dosing of ionophores in preweaned calves is especially important because this age of animal seems rather prone to toxicity, typically manifested as neurologic signs reminiscent of meningitis or salt poisoning. Certainly, if management conditions allow preweaning coccidiosis, mixed infections of the GI tract would be possible in 2- to 4-week-old calves. *C. parvum,* rotavirus, coronavirus, *E. coli,* or *Salmonella* spp. could also be involved. Obviously mixed infections could worsen the pathology.

Nematodes

Etiology

Intestinal nematodes are an important concern for pastured calves and growing heifers. Although current trends make pasturing of young dairy calves and heifers uncommon, consideration of intestinal parasite burdens is still worthwhile for confined heifers and essential for growing heifers on pasture. A basic understanding of parasites' life cycles and the geographic incidence of the various intestinal parasites is essential when making recommendations to owners. Pastured heifers require planned parasite control programs that include both management and anthelmintic components.

The major nematode parasites of the abomasum include *Ostertagia ostertagi, Trichostrongylus axei,* and *Haemonchus placei. O. ostertagi* (brown stomach worm) is the most important nematode in cattle because of its ability to undergo hypobiosis or arrested development of the L4 stage within the abomasum of infected young cattle. Arrested larvae reside in the lumen of gastric glands during seasons of the year that would likely interfere with the parasites' existence outside the host. Therefore, larvae acquired during late fall and early winter at temperatures found in northern climates persist in the host as inhibited larvae for weeks to months before maturing in late winter and spring. In southern temperate zones, larvae acquired during the spring become inhibited and finally mature in late summer or early fall. The biologic purpose of *O. ostertagi* hypobiosis is to avoid exposure of eggs and larval stages to weather not conducive to survival of the parasite. Therefore, harsh winters are avoided in the north, as are hot dry summers in southern zones. In the abomasal wall, hypobiotic larvae are apparently not targeted by the immune system for elimination, even in previously exposed adult cattle. When arrested larvae emerge from the abomasal glands, they tend to do so with a vengeance that creates severe abomasal pathology and illness known as ostertagiasis type II. Maturation and emergence of large numbers of inhibited L4 larvae cause acute anorexia, weight loss, hypoproteinemia, and severe diarrhea as a result of abomasal mucosal injury, increased abomasal pH because of parietal cell dysfunction, and hyperplasia. The mortality rate is high with this form, although prevalence usually is low. The resultant greatly thickened and nodular abomasal wall has caused pathologists to describe the gross lesion as "Moroccan leather" in appearance. Because ostertagiasis type II occurs in the late winter and spring in northern zones and late summer or fall in southern areas, parasites may not be considered as the cause of illness in affected heifers. Inhibited larvae also are resistant to many commonly used anthelmintics. Ostertagiasis type I is more classically typical of nematode infections because pastured heifers acquire significant loads of larvae that mature to adults over approximately 3 weeks. Type I infections occur during peak pasture seasons and can result in diarrhea, weight loss, hypoproteinemia, or simply poor weight gain.

H. placei and other species found less commonly in cattle also possess the ability to undergo hypobiosis to avoid temperature extremes detrimental to survival outside the host. *H. placei* is pathogenic as a result of blood sucking that can lead to severe anemia.

T. axei may cause injury to the abomasal mucosa that leads to hypoproteinemia, altered digestion and intestinal defense mechanisms, and diarrhea. *Gongylonema* spp. also live in the abomasum and forestomach but are not thought to be major pathogens. Small intestinal nematodes include other *Trichostrongylus* spp., *Cooperia* spp., *Nematodirus helvetianus*, *Bunostomum phlebotomum*, *Toxocara vitulorum*, and several other parasites. *Bunostomum phlebotomum* and *Cooperia* spp. are bloodsuckers that damage the intestinal mucosa and create anemia. *N. helvetianus* is an extremely hardy, weather-resistant parasite that causes diarrhea in cattle when present in great numbers.

Large intestinal nematodes include *Oesophagostomum radiatum*, *Chabertia ovina*, *Trichuris discolor*, and *Trichuris ovis*. *O. radiatum* causes diffuse inflammatory reactions in the cecum and colon of cattle. This inflammation, subsequent nodule formation, and hemorrhage cause inflammatory bowel disease that results in diarrhea, weight loss, and hypoproteinemia in heavily parasitized animals. Subsequent long-term pathology and full or partial immunity allow *O. radiatum* nodules to become necrotic or calcified. These chronic lesions are grossly apparent in the bowel serosa and are responsible for the parasite being labeled the "nodular worm." Intussusceptions sometimes occur at the site of chronic *O. radiatum* lesions; therefore, pathologists theorize that the lesions may disrupt or alter normal intestinal motility.

Trichuris spp. occasionally are identified as the cause of severe diarrhea in heifers. *Trichuris* spp. are known as "whipworms" and concentrate in the cecum of cattle hosts.

The aforementioned nematodes all possess pathogenicity of varying degrees in either young or mature animals not previously exposed to parasites. Pastured animals, especially those pastured on lands that are grazed every year, are at risk. The first pasture season of an animal's life presents the greatest risk. Thereafter, partial or full immunity may be present in animals during their adult years. Fortunately, anthelmintics are available to counteract these parasites. Anthelmintics used appropriately, combined with pasture management, allow dairy heifers to be pastured successfully. All authorities agree that parasites are detrimental to calves and heifers, especially those on pasture. Much controversy exists, however, when the topic of worming adult dairy cattle is discussed.

Natural immunity (at least for cows that grazed pasture and acquired exposure to parasites as heifers) should protect adult cattle previously exposed to parasites. Attempts to demonstrate milk yield difference between wormed and nonwormed dairy cattle have given mixed results, and much debate exists as to the relative merits of adult cow deworming, particularly under current confinement housing management systems.

Clinical Signs

As with any parasitic infestation or infection, overt clinical signs may be present only in a few animals within a group. However, all animals in the group will harbor parasite loads. Mild nematode levels simply deter normal growth and gain rates in heifers without causing clinical signs of disease. Moderate levels of nematodes cause some animals in the group to show variable amounts of diarrhea, weight loss, poor hair coats, decreased appetite, hypoproteinemia, and anemia. Heavy nematode levels cause acute appearance of these signs and a greater prevalence of animals showing signs within the group. Appetite depression is consistent and contributory to weight loss or lack of weight gain and, as yet, is unexplained. The predominant types of nematodes in each herd will dictate the signs observed. For example, in type II ostertagiasis, acute hypoproteinemia, severe diarrhea, and inappetence would be observed in some animals within the group, and the time of year would not coincide with a typical pasture associated parasitic problem. If *Haemonchus* spp., *Bunostomum* spp., or *Cooperia* spp. predominate, anemia could be the major sign.

Ancillary Data

Anemia caused by blood loss and hypoproteinemia characterized by hypoalbuminemia are the major abnormalities detected on complete blood count and serum biochemistry. Abomasal pH increases as acid production decreases secondary to parietal cell dysfunction. Pepsinogen is not activated completely to pepsin, a proteolytic enzyme, because this activation requires a low abomasal pH. Therefore, increased plasma pepsinogen levels may be demonstrated when severe abomasal pathology exists as a result of *O. ostertagi* or less commonly *T. axei*. Few, if any, veterinary diagnostic laboratories in North America routinely offer serum pepsinogen analysis on a commercial basis, however. Eosinophilia may or may not be present in WBC differentials and is not an essential or accurate aid to diagnosis. Fecal flotation and larval culture provide the definitive diagnostic tools. Very severe, acute infections with profuse diarrhea may be associated with electrolyte losses of Na^+, Cl^-, $HCO3^-$, and K^+.

Diagnosis

A definitive diagnosis requires identification of worm eggs or larvae in the feces of cattle having signs consistent with nematodiasis and ruling out other infectious or toxic diseases. When diarrhea is a major sign, salmonellosis, BVDV infection, coccidiosis, and toxicities that result in diarrhea must be ruled out.

Treatment and Control

Minimizing pasture contamination by parasite eggs and larvae is a major component of parasite control for dairy heifers. Heifers should be wormed before turnout and then at 3 and 6 weeks after turnout (or 3 and 8 weeks after turnout if ivermectin is used). This schedule helps to reduce recently ingested worm burdens before mature females begin to contaminate pastures with eggs, and the second treatment should kill ingested overwintered larvae that contaminate the pasture. The two-treatment program helps prevent the dramatic L3 load that generally occurs in northern climate pastures during late summer and early fall. Migration of L3 from manure to herbage occurs earlier during wet summers than dry ones, but L3 loads tend to peak in the fall in northern climates.

Although it may be ideal to select an anthelmintic specifically directed against the major nematodes present on each farm, it is more practical to select broad-spectrum anthelmintics that kill most types of nematodes. Available anthelmintics for nonlactating or nonbreeding-age dairy cattle are listed in Table 6.7. Label recommendations and changes in status of approval may occur with any of the drugs listed in this table. Therefore, practitioners should always verify that label approval exists for dairy animals. Pasture rotation with worming before movement to new pasture is another management tool seldom practiced with dairy operations because of limited acreage.

Although worming and parasite control are definitely beneficial to pastured heifers, the economic benefits of worming adult lactating dairy cows are controversial. Worming programs for lactating cattle may be justified if the cattle are pastured for a significant time each year. Worming would primarily benefit first calf heifers and newly acquired cattle that perhaps had not been pastured as heifers and thus are not likely to have parasite resistance. Dairy herds with a high percentage of first calf heifers and using pasture for a portion of the year probably can justify anthelmintic treatment of lactating cattle.

Economic justification may be lacking for use of anthelmintics in lactating cows in totally confined herds whose heifers never are pastured. Available anthelmintics for lactating dairy cattle are listed in Table 6.8.

TABLE 6.7	Anthelmintics Approved for Nonlactating Dairy Animals (Data Assembled from Information Given on Manufacturer's Labels)			
Drug	**Dose**	**Slaughter Withdrawal Time (days)**	**Spectrum and Comments**	
Albendazole	10 mg/kg PO	27	GI nematodes, including hypobiotic *Ostertagia* L4, lungworms, *Moniezia* (tapeworms), adult liver flukes (*Fasciola* spp.) Not for use in female dairy cattle of breeding age; potentially teratogenic if administered in early pregnancy	
Doramectin injectable	200 µg/kg SC	35	GI nematodes, including hypobiotic *Ostertagia* L4, lungworms, grubs, sucking lice, mites Not for use in female dairy cattle of breeding age or in veal calves	
Doramectin (pour-on)	500 µg/kg topically	45	GI nematodes, including hypobiotic *Ostertagia* L4, lungworms, grubs, sucking and biting lice, mites Not for use in female dairy cattle of breeding age or in veal calves	
Eprinomectin (pour-on)	500 µg/kg topically	0	GI nematodes, including hypobiotic *Ostertagia* L4, lungworms, grubs *(Hypoderma)*, sucking and biting lice, mites, and horn flies Effective when applied to wet cattle	
Eprinomectin (injectable)	1 mg/kg SC 5 mg/kg PO	8–13 (depending on product)	GI nematodes, including hypobiotic *Ostertagia* L4, lungworms Not for use in female dairy cattle 20 months or older or in veal calves	
Fenbendazole	10–15 mg/kg PO	8–13 (depending on product)	GI nematodes, including hypobiotic *Ostertagia* L4, lungworms, tapeworms; on rare occasion, fenbendazole may cause bone marrow suppression in calves younger than 1 month of age	

TABLE 6.7   Anthelmintics Approved for Nonlactating Dairy Animals (Data Assembled from Information Given on Manufacturer's Labels)—cont'd

Drug	Dose	Slaughter Withdrawal Time (days)	Spectrum and Comments
Ivermectin (injectable)	200 µg/kg SC	35	GI nematodes (adult and larvae), including hypobiotic *Ostertagia* L4, *Dictyocaulus* (lungworm), grubs *(Hypoderma)*, sucking lice, and mites Not for use in female dairy cattle of breeding age or in veal calves
Ivermectin (pour-on)	500 µg/kg topically	48	GI nematodes, including hypobiotic *Ostertagia* L4, *Dictyocaulus* (lungworm), grubs *(Hypoderma)*, sucking and biting lice, mites, and horn flies Not for use in female dairy cattle of breeding age or in veal calves
Levamisole	Varies with formulation	7	GI nematodes (adult), lungworms Not for use in female dairy cattle of breeding age
Moxidectin (injectable)	200 µg/kg SC	21	GI nematodes (adult and larvae), including hypobiotic *Ostertagia* L4, *Dictyocaulus* (lungworm), grubs *(Hypoderma)*, sucking lice, and mites Not for use in female dairy cattle of breeding age or in veal calves <3 months of age
Moxidectin (pour-on)	500 µg/kg topically	0	GI nematodes, including hypobiotic *Ostertagia* L4, *Dictyocaulus* (lungworm), grubs *(Hypoderma)*, sucking and biting lice, mites, and horn flies Not for use in veal calves
Morantel tartrate	0.44 g/100 lb PO	14	GI nematodes (adult)
Oxfendazole	4.5 mg/kg PO	7	GI nematodes, including hypobiotic *Ostertagia* L4, lungworms, tapeworms Not for use in female dairy cattle of breeding age
Clorsulon	7 mg/kg	8	*Fasciola hepatica* adults and late immature larvae
Clorsulon and ivermectin	1 mL/110 lb SC	49	GI nematodes (adult and larvae), including hypobiotic *Ostertagia* L4, lungworms, *F. hepatica* adults, grubs *(Hypoderma)*, sucking lice, and mites Not for use in female dairy cattle of breeding age or in veal calves

GI, Gastrointestinal; *PO,* oral; *SC,* subcutaneous;

TABLE 6.8   Anthelmintics Approved for Lactating Dairy Cattle (Assembled from Manufacturers' Labels)

Drug	Dose	Withdrawal Period for Slaughter and Milk (days)	Spectrum
Eprinomectin (pour-on as Ivomec Eprinex)	500 µg/kg topically	Meat = 0 Milk = 0	GI nematodes, including hypobiotic *Ostertagia* L4, lungworms, grubs *(Hypoderma)*, sucking and biting lice, mites, and horn flies Effective when applied to wet cattle
Fenbendazole	5 mg/kg PO	Meat: 8-13 (depending on product) Milk: 0	GI nematodes (adult), lungworms
Morantel tartrate	0.44 g/100 lb PO	Meat = 14 Milk = 0	GI nematodes (adult)
Moxidectin (pour-on)	0.5 mg/kg topically	Meat = 0 Milk = 0	GI nematodes, including hypobiotic *Ostertagia* L4, lungworms, grubs *(Hypoderma)*, sucking and biting lice, mites, and horn flies

GI, Gastrointestinal; *PO,* oral.

Trematodes

Etiology and Clinical Signs

Liver flukes are a greater problem in beef than dairy cattle, but certain geographic areas harbor flukes and their intermediate hosts, thereby representing risks for pastured dairy heifers and cows. *Fasciola hepatica* is found most commonly in certain areas along the Gulf Coast and western United States; it is rare in the northern United States. Cattle, along with sheep, are the primary definitive hosts of *F. hepatica* and shed eggs in feces. Eggs require a moist environment to hatch miracidia, which find a snail intermediate host. After a complicated reproductive cycle in the snail, the parasite eventually produces metacercariae, which are ingested by grazing animals. Metacercariae invade the duodenum, and immature flukes then penetrate the gut and seek out the liver, where they penetrate the capsule, migrate in the parenchyma, and eventually reside in the bile ducts. This wandering through the gut and liver parenchyma creates a great deal of pathology, which in heavy infestations may cause hypoproteinemia, anemia, reduced appetite, peritonitis, and importantly, predispose to clostridial diseases such as bacillary hemoglobinuria *(C. hemolyticum)*, or black disease *(C. novyi)*.

Fascioloides magna, the deer liver fluke, is a large fluke that can infect cattle and sheep. The fluke is found along the Gulf Coast, the Great Lakes region, and the northwestern United States. Although cattle can be infected, the resulting parenchymal cyst does not allow egg release, thus making cattle dead-end hosts. In deer, the natural host, thin-walled parenchymal cysts are formed that allow eggs to emerge into bile ducts. *F. magna* is particularly vicious in sheep because continued migration without encystment is the rule. Because infections are not patent in cattle, liver condemnation or gross postmortem lesions are the major consequences of *F. magna* infection.

Dicrocoelium dendriticum occurs in many geographic regions around the world and in a few areas in the northeastern United States (including the central New York region) and Canada. The life cycle is complex, with both the land snail *(Cionella lubrica)* and the black ant *(Formica fusca)* necessary for transmission back to a definitive host, such as cattle, sheep, goats, horses, pigs, and people. Metacercariae (in ants) ingested by host cattle penetrate the duodenum and directly enter the bile ducts, where they usually cause little detectable illness. However, heavy infestations can occasionally inflame or obstruct biliary ductules and the gallbladder. Most cases are self-limiting.

Fasciola gigantica is limited to tropical regions and will not be discussed here.

Paramphistomum, the rumen fluke, is thought not to be highly pathogenic in the United States but can cause illness in tropical zones. Ingested metacercariae may encyst in the duodenum or migrate to the duodenum wall, where they stay for weeks before migrating upstream to become adults in the rumen and reticulum. Acute paramphistomiasis, which is rare in the United States, refers to duodenal pathology created by large populations of wandering and invading immature flukes.

Diagnosis

Identification of fluke eggs in the feces is possible for *F. hepatica* and *D. dendriticum*. *Paramphistomum* spp. eggs can be confused with *F. hepatica*, especially because both are operculated, but *F. hepatica* eggs are slightly smaller and stained yellow. Routine sampling of feces from 10 to 15 at-risk animals is indicated when *F. hepatica* is suspected. An ELISA serologic test also has been developed to diagnose *F. hepatica* infections. Necropsy specimens are very helpful whenever fluke infestations are suspected.

Treatment

Table 6.7 also lists the available drugs to counteract fluke infestation in nonlactating dairy heifers. Albendazole, clorsulon, and clorsulon–ivermectin are effective against adult and late immature *F. hepatica*. Albendazole is effective against *F. magna* and *D. dendriticum*. Control measures include avoidance of pastures harboring intermediate hosts or killing intermediate hosts such as snails with molluscicides. Veterinarians practicing in endemic fluke regions should be familiar with diagnosis and control measures if their clients pasture heifers. Vaccination against clostridial conditions such as bacillary hemoglobinuria and black disease is prudent in endemic areas.

Cestodiasis

Moniezia benedeni is the small intestinal tapeworm of cattle and is thought to be nonpathogenic. Oribatid mites are the intermediate hosts, and after ingestion of infective cysticercoids by cattle, the worms mature over 2 months and then are shed spontaneously several months later. Treatment with albendazole is effective when necessary. Other tapeworms such as *Taenia saginata,* the beef tapeworm of humans; *Taenia hydatigena* (adults in dogs); and *Echinococcus granulosus* are not major parasites of dairy cattle in the United States and will not be discussed here.

Papular Stomatitis

Etiology

Bovine popular stomatitis virus (BPSV) is a member of the *Parapox* virus genus, within the Pox virus family, and is very closely related, and therefore hard to distinguish from other species members of this genus, including the virus of pseudocowpox and contagious ecthyma virus of sheep and goats. The application of modern molecular diagnostic techniques for more sensitive and specific differentiation of these different species of *Parapox* viruses has been prompted by not just altruistic scientific advance but also by the desire to rapidly identify the precise viral agent causing suspicious vesicular lesions of ruminants and to trace the cause of skin lesions in humans because

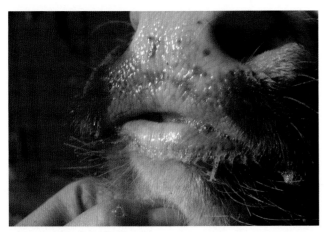

• **Fig. 6.15** Typical raised circular lesions of papular stomatitis on the muzzle and lips of a calf.

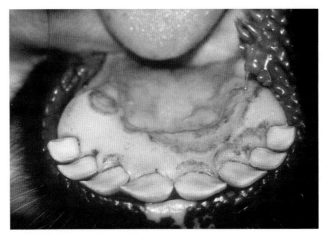

• **Fig. 6.17** Papular stomatitis lesions caudal to the incisor teeth and ventral to the tongue in a calf. The lesions are brownish-yellow in color, are slightly raised, and have rough edges.

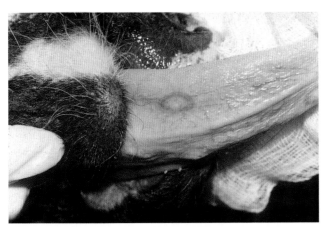

• **Fig. 6.16** Circular papular stomatitis lesions on the ventrum of a calf's tongue.

all of these agents are zoonotic. Such differentiation is now possible using quantitative PCR (qPCR) techniques. In cattle, the disease is spread by contact between infected and noninfected calves or via common feeding devices or containers. The virus is quite contagious in young calves, and it is worth remembering that it also can cause lesions on the skin of humans working with calves. Such zoonotic infection creates lesions similar to the milker's nodules of pseudocowpox in people. Papular stomatitis virus lesions on the muzzle and in the oral cavity of calves frequently are confused with erosions caused by BVDV or potentially other vesicular diseases such as foot and mouth, vesicular stomatitis, or epizootic hemorrhagic disease. It was first described in the United States in 1960.

Clinical Signs

A raised papule on the muzzle or nares is the most commonly observed lesion because of the external nature of the lesion (Fig. 6.15). Papules on the palate, tongue, or lips probably are more common but are less likely to be observed (Fig. 6.16). Although red and raised on the external mucosa, the lesions may appear crusty or brownish-yellow in the oral cavity and have roughened edges (Fig. 6.17). Oral cavity lesions may be flat and therefore confused with erosions. Some papules develop a necrotic white center that sloughs, leaving an ulcerated area within the raised papule. Papular stomatitis lesions may cause an affected calf to show mild salivation and reluctance to nurse or eat, although most calves show no clinical signs associated with the lesions. Such signs usually lead to examination of the oral cavity and subsequent diagnosis. Many, if not most, cases are asymptomatic and go undiagnosed.

Calves from several weeks to several months of age are most commonly affected, but the disease has also been observed in older growing cattle. Lesions also occur in the esophagus and forestomach mucosa but are only detected in those locations during necropsy examination. Such lower alimentary lesions may be confused with infectious bovine rhinotracheitis (IBR)– or BVDV-induced lesions.

Severe illnesses or immunodeficiencies frequently allow extensive proliferation of papular stomatitis virus and subsequently more advanced lesions may be seen. When such severe lesions occur, they are clinically suspected to be BVDV related. In fact, concurrent BVDV infection in immunocompetent calves or poor-doing BVDV-PI calves greatly accentuates papular stomatitis lesions when both viruses are present. Similarly, IBR virus and chronic bacterial infections predispose to worsening of existing papular stomatitis virus lesions. Clinical errors are most common, however, when BVDV-PI calves with a superinfection with cytopathic (CP)-BVDV or chronic concurrent diseases develop amplification of papular stomatitis lesions. Most spontaneous, uncomplicated papular stomatitis lesions resolve within several weeks in immunocompetent animals and are diagnosed by inspection. Severe cases may require biopsy and viral isolation, immunohistochemistry, or PCR to differentiate the lesions from BVDV. Intracytoplasmic, eosinophilic inclusions are typical in the cytoplasm of degenerating cells.

Although the disease may be fatal, most early reports that cited extensive lesions and fatalities probably represented concurrent BVDV infections.

Treatment and Prevention

No specific treatment or method of prevention exists other than to minimize spread by housing calves separately and not using common feeding devices or buckets.

Infectious Diseases Of The Gastrointestinal Tract—Adults

Actinobacillosis

Etiology

Actinobacillus lignieresii, a gram-negative pleomorphic rod, is a normal commensal organism in the oral flora of cattle. Injuries to the oral mucosa or skin that become contaminated with *A. lignieresii* may develop soft tissue infection characterized by an initial cellulitis that evolves into a classical pyogranulomatous infection that can be confused with neoplasia or actinomycosis. Sulfur granules, which are yellow-white cheesy accumulations containing the organism, develop within pus or pyogranulomatous soft tissue lesions associated with *A. lignieresii* infection.

"Wooden tongue," a soft tissue infection of the tongue, is the classical example of *A. lignieresii* infection in cattle, but soft tissue granulomas developing around the head, neck, or other body areas are common as well.

Granulomas of the esophagus, forestomach, and occasionally other visceral locations also are possible. Lymphadenitis, lymph node abscesses, and infectious granulomas originating from lymph nodes may follow soft tissue infections of the oral cavity or pharynx. Extremely fibrous feed material has been incriminated as the cause of mucosal injury that allowed opportunistic *A. lignieresii* infection as a herd problem in dairy heifers. Direct inoculation of the organism into mucosal wounds can occur in the oral cavity, esophagus, and forestomach. Inoculation probably occurs from oral secretions or saliva when soft tissue wounds of the skin are infected at sites distant from the oral cavity.

Clinical Signs

A textbook case of acute wooden tongue in cattle appears as a diffusely swollen, firm tongue that fills the oral cavity. Firm or fluctuant intermandibular swelling usually accompanies the inflammatory enlargement of the tongue (Fig. 6.18). Excessive salivation is observed, and the swollen tongue may protrude from the oral cavity. Anorexia is relative or complete because the tongue has reduced mobility and may be injured by the teeth if chewing is attempted. Fever is present in acute infections but frequently absent in subacute or chronic cases. Distended salivary ducts appearing as ranulae may be observed ventral to the tongue. Although this is the typical "textbook" *A. lignieresii* clinical description, many cases do not involve the tongue but instead cause soft tissue infection in the pharynx or other regions of the mouth. The specific location of the disease is likely associated with an injury to the mucosa in that area. Historically, poor-quality hay containing sticks or briars has been associated with the disease in heifers.

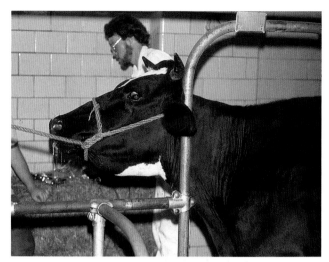

• **Fig. 6.18** Acute wooden tongue with intermandibular cellulitis and salivation.

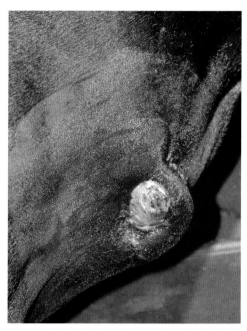

• **Fig. 6.19** Atypical actinobacillosis granuloma in the jugular furrow of a cow secondary to a perivascular administration of concentrated dextrose solution.

Chronic wooden tongue lesions consist of pyogranulomatous masses and fibrosis of the tongue or other soft tissue sites that are infected. Weight loss and marked salivation are common in chronically infected cattle.

Atypical *A. lignieresii* infection is characterized by granulomas, pyogranulomas, or lymph node abscesses. Serous or mucoid nonodorous pus may drain from abscessed infections. Granulomas are raised, red, fleshy to firm in consistency, and contain sulfur granules. Granulomas may occur in the oral cavity, esophagus, forestomach, or other visceral locations. In addition, external granulomas have been observed in the nares, eyelids, face, pharyngeal region, neck, limbs, and abdomen (Fig. 6.19). Infection of abomasopexy toggles or sharp incision sites also has produced these granulomas (Fig. 6.20).

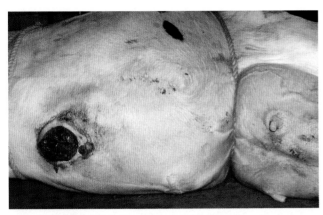

• **Fig. 6.20** Actinobacillosis granuloma at the site of an abomasopexy incision.

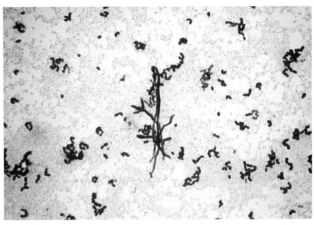

• **Fig. 6.21** Gram stain of aspirate from lumpy jaw lesion. Gram-positive branching filamentous rods are characteristic of *Actinomyces bovis*.

Diagnosis

Excision or biopsy of granulomas to provide material for bacterial culture and histopathology is the only means to confirm a diagnosis of *A. lignieresii* infection. Clinical appearances and the presence of sulfur granules are suggestive of diagnosis but not specific because the masses must be differentiated from actinomycoses, botryomycosis, neoplasia, parasitic or foreign body granuloma, and exuberant granulation tissue. Acute wooden tongue can be diagnosed by aspiration of fluid-distended salivary ranulae, the tongue itself, or intermandibular phlegmon when present. Aspirates are submitted for cytology and culture. Chronic wooden tongue lesions are best diagnosed by biopsies submitted for both culture and histopathology.

Treatment

Wooden tongue and other lesions of *A. lignieresii* infection often respond to systemic sodium iodide therapy. Intravenous sodium iodide (20% solution) is an extremely irritating preparation that should be administered IV only by a veterinarian. It is administered at a dose of 70 mg/kg body weight. This dose is repeated at 2- to 3-day intervals until iodism occurs. Alternatively, oral organic iodide can be fed (1 oz/450 kg body weight, daily) after initial IV therapy until iodism occurs. Unfortunately, parenteral iodide preparations are not currently permitted for use in lactating dairy cattle in the US. Signs of iodism include serous lacrimation, seromucoid nasal discharge, and scaly dandruff-like skin appearing on the face and neck of treated cattle. For acute wooden tongue lesions, response to iodine therapy is usually dramatic. Subacute lesions respond more slowly, and chronic lesions carry a guarded prognosis. In calves chronic lesions of the tongue often prevent the patient from eating and starvation may ensue. Sulfonamides, tetracycline, or beta-lactam antibiotics also may be useful and can be used alone or in conjunction with iodine therapy for severe *A. lignieresii* infections of the tongue.

Treatment of *A. lignieresii* granulomas consists of debridement or debulking (if the involved anatomic area allows surgical intervention), coupled with medical therapy as outlined previously. Recurrent or severe lesions can be treated with combined antimicrobial therapy as discussed previously. Cryosurgical treatment has been combined with surgical debulking of some *A. lignieresii* granulomas and appears most effective when mushrooming granulomas attached to a narrow skin base are selected for therapy.

The exact reason that iodides are effective in *A. lignieresii* infection is not known. Suggested mechanisms include penetrance into granulation tissue and destruction of organisms, simple decrease in the granulomatous response, and combinations of activity against *A. lignieresii* and the granulomatous inflammatory response. Iodides are unlikely to cause abortion in cattle, although some commercially available preparations of injectable sodium iodide are labeled with a warning that forbids their use in pregnant cattle. Prevention is best accomplished by feeding hay or other forage that does not contain sticks or other foreign bodies that may damage the oral mucosa.

Actinomycosis

Actinomyces bovis, a gram-positive filamentous organism (Fig. 6.21) that can assume many forms, is the cause of lumpy jaw in cattle and occasionally causes granulomatous infection in other areas of the body. In young cultures, diphtheroid organisms are observed, but in older cultures and crushed preparations of sulfur granules obtained from pus, the organism may be filamentous, branching, coccoid, club-shaped, or diphtheroid. Infection with *A. bovis* typically results in formation of "sulfur granules" in pus or infected tissue. These so-called sulfur granules contain large numbers of the organism. In older literature, the term *actinomycosis* implied granulomatous infections containing sulfur granules and did not differentiate *A. lignieresii* or staphylococcal infections from those caused by *A. bovis*.

The organism is difficult to culture to the degree necessary for bacterial susceptibility testing. This fact contributes to the dearth of scientific information regarding the appropriate therapy for lumpy jaw in cattle. Many other species of *Actinomyces* have been studied in humans, and comparative information from these studies suggests that *A. bovis* is much more resistant to antibiotic therapy than human isolates such as *Actinomyces israeli*.

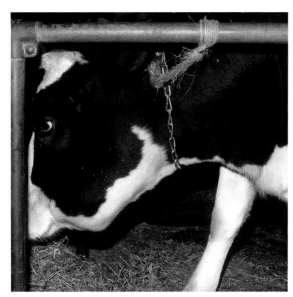

• **Fig. 6.22** Early lumpy jaw lesion consisting of an edematous soft tissue swelling overlying a painful, firm, bony swelling on the mandible.

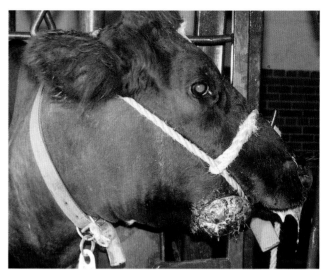

• **Fig. 6.23** Severe *Actinomyces bovis* infection of the mandible with ulceration of the skin and granulomatous proliferation.

Lumpy jaw is a debilitating disease of cattle resulting from infection of the mandible or maxilla by *A. bovis*. The organism has been described as a normal inhabitant of the oral flora and digestive tract of cattle. It is assumed that infection of bones and teeth occurs after injury to the oral mucosa by fibrous feeds or dental eruption (this may be a reason that lumpy jaw seems most common in young adult cattle) and subsequent inoculation of *A. bovis*. The organism also may penetrate around the alveoli of the teeth or contaminate skin wounds via common feed and water troughs. Dr. Rebhun observed one herd with an epidemic of lumpy jaw, with 7 of 60 cows affected. The point source cow had a large, draining, lumpy jaw lesion, and all cows ate silage twice daily from a feed bunk made of coarse boards. Discharge of the organism from the point source cow certainly contaminated the sideboards and bunk. Whether the organism had gained access through the oral cavity, injury to the oral cavity by wood splinters, or skin puncture from wood slivers on the sideboards could not be ascertained. Lumpy jaw usually is a sporadic infection, but as in the aforementioned herd, can be an epidemic or endemic herd problem.

Rarely, *A. bovis* causes infectious granulomas on soft tissues similar to those caused by *A. lignieresii*. Granulomas caused by *A. bovis* have been identified in the trachea, testes, and digestive tract.

Clinical Signs

Early *A. bovis* infections of the mandible or maxilla appear as warm, painful swellings consisting of distinct edema overlapping a firm, painful, bony swelling (Fig. 6.22). Such early infections easily could be confused with a traumatic injury. Over a period of weeks, however, bone enlargement becomes obvious and soft tissue edema much less apparent. Salivation and some difficulty in eating may be observed, but inappetence and weight loss seldom are a problem in early cases. After the infection is established in bone, the swelling becomes hard and often painful (Figs. 6.23 to 6.25). Severe cases will

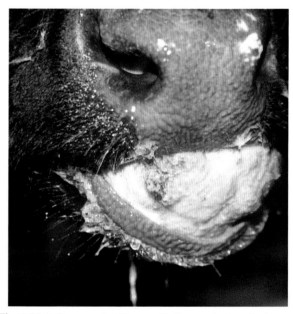

• **Fig. 6.24** Actinomycosis of the mandibular symphysis region in a cow.

have distortion of the teeth anchored in the affected bone when the mouth is examined. External swelling is merely the "tip of the iceberg" as established by skull radiographs that confirm severe osteomyelitis with multifocal radiolucencies caused by rarefaction of bone. Pyogranulomatous infection of bone and associated soft tissues evolves in untreated cases, and these animals will have granulomas develop at the site of draining tracts through the skin or into the oral cavity (Fig. 6.26). Because of distortion, malocclusion, or loss of teeth, eating becomes more difficult for severely affected cows. Salivation, reduced appetite, hesitant attempts to chew, and dropping food from the mouth may be observed. Oral mucosal or tongue lacerations may be apparent. Draining tracts discharge copious quantities of serous or mucopurulent pus that should be considered infectious to other cows.

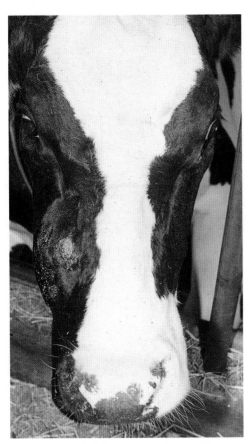

• **Fig. 6.25** Actinomycosis of the maxilla.

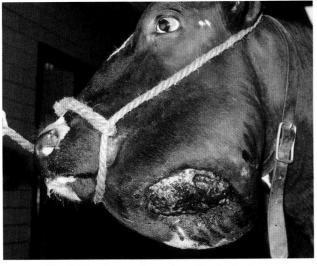

• **Fig. 6.26** Advanced lumpy jaw with draining tracts.

Diagnosis

Absolute diagnosis requires a tissue core biopsy or fluid aspirate to identify the causative organism. Core biopsies also allow histologic confirmation. Radiographs confirm osteomyelitis with multiple radiolucent zones and proliferation of periosteal bone (Figs. 6.27 and 6.28). Radiographs also help differentiate lumpy jaw from bony neoplasia; tooth root infections; fractures; sequestra, and when the maxilla is involved, sinusitis.

Treatment

Recommended treatment for lumpy jaw usually includes sodium iodide, but this treatment is often ineffective and should be considered an adjunct, at best, to appropriate antibiotic therapy.

Any discussion of treatment also must allow for the tremendous variation in the severity of osteomyelitis caused by *A. bovis*. Basketball-sized lesions are unlikely to respond to any therapy, but early lesions may be resolved successfully by several protocols. Therefore, treatment is best instituted early. Long-term antibiotic therapy is necessary for well-established infections, and this fact makes owners reluctant to treat cows that do not appear ill and that are still producing well. Ironically, when this same untreated cow eventually becomes ill as the lesion enlarges, many owners will then want something to be done.

Streptomycin or penicillin–streptomycin combinations have been the drugs of choice for lumpy jaw; unfortunately, streptomycin and penicillin–streptomycin combinations no longer are available for use in cattle in North America. Therefore, other treatments will need to be considered. In one comparative study, erythromycin was active in vitro against *A. bovis* when an MIC of 0.06 to 0.12 was achieved. Therefore, erythromycin may be a good choice. Isoniazid can be used at 10 to 20 mg/kg orally every 24 hours for 30 days, and rifampin can be used at 20 mg/kg orally every 24 hours for 30 days or used at 5 to 10 mg/kg orally every 24 hours and combined with procaine penicillin at 22,000 U/kg SC every 24 hours for 30 days. Isoniazid may cause abortion, should be used with caution in pregnant cattle, and both isoniazid and rifampin represent inappropriate extra-label drug use in the United States. Because antibiotic therapy necessitates prolonged administration and may involve extra-label use of drugs, the implications of such therapy should be discussed with owners before treatment is begun. Use of rifampin in the US currently requires the owner to guarantee that neither milk nor meat from that individual will be sold commercially.

Current recommendations include penicillin 22,000 U/kg once daily and sodium iodide IV (30 g/450 kg) administered once or repeated at 2- to 3-day intervals until iodism occurs. Parenteral iodide preparations are not currently permitted in lactating dairy cattle in the US. Alternatively, organic iodides can be fed at 30 g/450 kg body weight once daily until iodism occurs. Duration of therapy is dependent on the severity of the lesion and response to therapy. We have also had some success in chronic cases, even some with substantial bony involvement via the placement of antibiotic-coated (penicillin or erythromycin) beads into the lesion. Long-term antibiotic therapy has resulted in a surprising cure in a few advanced cases.

Surgery has been suggested and still is used by some as treatment for lumpy jaw of the maxillae. Surgical debulking or removal of large pyogranulomas projecting from the skin of advanced cases may reduce the size of the lesion. Surgical debulking may incite severe hemorrhage. In addition, the affected bone may be further compromised or

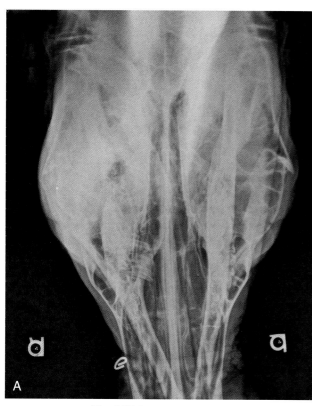
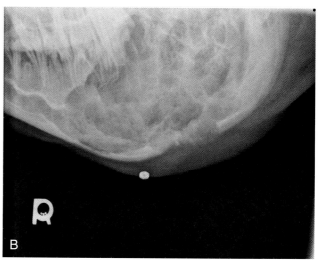

• **Fig. 6.27** Dorsoventral (**A**) and lateral (**B**) and skull radiographs of a mature Holstein cow affected with advanced lumpy jaw of the right mandible. Osteomyelitis and characteristic multifocal radiolucencies are present. A draining tract was present at the ventral mandibular margin.

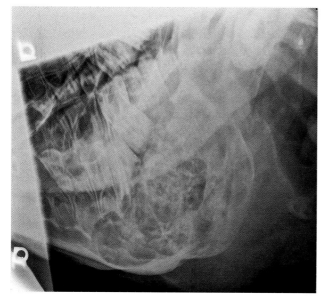

• **Fig. 6.28** Lateral oblique radiograph of 6-year old Brown Swiss cow with an advanced lumpy jaw lesion. Note the bony resorption around the mandibular cheek tooth; oblique views can help "skyline" dental alveoli to assess tooth root involvement.

fractured if overzealous debridement and curettage are performed. Again, the external swelling or masses are just the tip of the iceberg. Loose teeth may require extraction, and fistulous tracts may be flushed with iodine solution as ancillary aids.

Vesicular Stomatitis

Etiology

Vesicular stomatitis virus (VSV) causes lesions that may be indistinguishable from those of foot-and-mouth disease (FMD) in cattle and pigs. Horses also may be infected with VSV, but FMD does not occur in horses. The causative virus of VSV is a member of the genus *Vesiculovirus* in the family Rhabdoviridae, and two distinct serotype groups—Indiana and New Jersey types—are recognized. Each of these major types may be further subdivided into subtypes. The New Jersey VSV type tends to be more pathogenic in cattle. VSV is considered endemic in parts of South America, Central America, and the southwestern United States. In recent years, many livestock operations in the intermountain West have been quarantined after detection of VSV infection in cattle and horses. VSV usually occurs during the summer and fall, but one large epidemic developed during the late fall and early winter in California during 1982 and 1983. In more recent outbreaks, the disease has sporadically occurred in Texas, New Mexico, and Arizona in spring and early summer and then proceeded to spread northward into Colorado, Idaho, Montana, Idaho, Utah, and as far north and west as Nebraska. The general trend for cases to occur in the summer and fall is suggestive of an arthropod vector. Attention has focused on a species of midge, *Culicoides sonorensis,* as a likely vector for VSV because viral replication in multiple tissues of this insect has been documented following experimental VSV infection. Ingestion of infected grasshoppers has also been shown to induce infection in cattle. Other insects, such as blackflies and sandflies, may act as mechanical vectors for transmission among animals. Many different animals can be infected by VSV, including sheep, goats, wildlife, birds, and insects.

During outbreaks, the virus spreads rapidly from infected animals through secretions and aerosol transmission. Intact skin is not penetrated by VSV, but abrasions or injuries allow infection through the skin and may explain the spread of teat lesions through infected herds by milking machines. When epidemics occur, morbidity is high—especially in dense populations of animals—but mortality usually is low.

Clinical Signs

After VSV is introduced to susceptible animals, clinical signs of varying intensity occur. Classical signs include salivation, fever, lameness, and teat lesions. Fever may precede the more obvious signs because viremia is short-lived. Blanched lesions of the oral mucosa, coronary band, and teats evolve into vesicles that rupture and then slough the involved mucosa to leave denuded surfaces. Within the oral cavity, the lips, tongue, gums, or other areas may be involved. Obvious problems with mastitis occur when teat lesions are widespread. Many animals in some outbreaks have minimal or subclinical lesions that escape detection. When the disease is signaled by a few animals with obvious lesions, physical examination of other animals on the premises frequently will reveal small erosions or ulcers resulting from earlier infection. As with many diseases, the severity of disease varies greatly based on serotype of VSV, density of the population infected, concurrent diseases, and other factors. Many of these signs cannot be distinguished from FMD lesions.

People working with VSV-infected animals or with VSV in laboratories can become infected asymptomatically or develop signs of fever, muscular aches and pains, and possibly lip blisters.

Infected cattle usually recover; mortality rates are low. However, economic losses resulting from decreased production are profound. Oral lesions cause infected cows to eat less, thereby affecting production. Lameness, if present, further deters appetite and access to feed. Teat lesions represent the most disastrous consequence of VSV because mastitis can easily follow incomplete "milk-out" as a consequence of the teats being painful. Therefore, although the mortality rate of the natural disease is low, the cull rate and economic losses can be catastrophic to dairy farmers.

Diagnosis

Whenever a diagnosis of vesicular stomatitis is possible, state and federal regulatory veterinarians should be alerted for help in diagnosis and ruling out FMD. Currently, the diagnosis is definitively arrived at either via serologic tests or identification of virus in tissue samples.

Treatment and Control

Common sense measures such as milking cows with teat lesions last, using aggressive disinfection practices in the milking parlor, reducing animal density, attempting isolation of clinical cases, and reducing stress are the only means of treatment. Softened feeds may be more easily ingested by affected animals. Secondary bacterial infections of lesions may necessitate occasional use of antibiotics.

Control measures and containment must be left to regulatory veterinarians. On Colorado dairies that experienced repeated annual outbreaks, the rate and scope of spread on infected dairies have been curtailed when aggressive insect control measures were initiated soon after detection of the disease. Humans working with infected cattle should wear gloves and perhaps masks.

Bluetongue

Etiology

Bluetongue virus (BTV) is an *Orbivirus* transmitted by *Culicoides* gnats from infected to noninfected ruminants. BTV is almost uniformly asymptomatic in cattle. Cattle and wild ruminants are thought to be reservoirs of BTV, but sheep suffer a more apparent clinical disease characterized by fever, edema, excessive salivation, frothing, and hyperemia of the nasal and buccal mucous membranes. These acute signs in sheep progress to crusting, erosions, and ulcers of the mucous membranes. In addition, affected sheep are lame, resulting from both coronitis and myositis. Pregnant ewes infected with BTV may abort, resorb, or subsequently give birth to lambs with congenital anomalies such as hydranencephaly, cerebellar lesions, spinal cord lesions, retinal dysplasia, and other ocular anomalies or skeletal malformations. The aforementioned clinical signs for sheep summarize a "classical" case, but BTV can be subclinical in sheep as well as in cattle.

In fact, tremendous variation in clinical manifestations and consequences is possible after BTV infection. One reason for this variation worldwide is the multitude of BTV serotypes (at least 24) that have been identified. In addition, there are at least seven serotypes of epizootic hemorrhagic disease virus—a similar *Orbivirus* that primarily affects whitetail deer but can affect cattle causing BTV-like signs—that have been identified. In the United States, 15 BTV serotypes and 3 epizootic hemorrhagic diarrhea virus (EHDV) serotypes have been identified. BTV-positive cattle have not been found in the northeastern United States nor in the upper Midwest states of Wisconsin, Michigan, and Minnesota unless the cows were transported from other regions. Canada remains free of BTV with the exception of southern British Columbia.

Control of the disease is difficult for several reasons:
1. The biologic vector, *Culicoides* spp., is difficult to control, and the virus may overwinter in the larval form of these insects.
2. Infection in cattle, goats, and possibly other wild ruminants can remain subclinical, but infected hosts can act as reservoirs of disease. Sheep are the major species to show clinical signs of disease.
3. Multiple serotypes require specific testing rather than group antigen testing for best detection.

4. Some strains of BTV may cause only subclinical infections in cattle, thereby not arousing clinical suspicion of disease.

Transmission of virus from infected to susceptible animals by *Culicoides* spp. has been studied and results in seroconversion. Transmission of BTV in the United States is predominantly thought to occur via *C. sonorensis* and *C. insignis*, species of midge with a proven role in the epidemiology of the disease; however, there are other species, specifically *C. stellifer* and *C. debilipalpis* that are suspected to play a role in the transmission of both BTV and EHDV. Laboratory or experimental infections in cattle usually do not result in clinical illness, but some reports of field outbreaks describe obvious clinical illness with signs similar to those in sheep with BTV (see also Chapter 16). Therefore, even though most BTV in cattle is thought to be subclinical, certain husbandry or environmental conditions or strains of BTV in field outbreaks appear capable of causing clinical disease. Sunlight may enhance and worsen the clinical signs when sheep are infected with BTV.

Clinical Signs

Most cattle infected with BTV are asymptomatic. When clinical signs are observed in field outbreaks, mucosal and skin lesions predominate. Hyperemia and oral vesicles that ulcerate may involve the mucous membranes of the mouth or tongue. The muzzle may undergo similar vesicular changes that lead to a "burnt" appearance with a dry cracked skin that may slough. Salivation is common, and swelling of lips may occur. Fever is present. Stiffness or lameness is common as a result of both myositis and coronitis. Coronary band hyperemia, ulceration, necrosis, exudates, or sloughing may occur. The skin of the neck and withers may become thickened, exudative, and painful. Therefore, depending on the clinical signs demonstrated, the differential diagnosis for a bovine case of BTV infection might include BVDV, vesicular stomatitis, FMD, malignant catarrhal fever (MCF), IBR, rinderpest, and bovine papular stomatitis. Obviously given the overlap of clinical signs of some BTV infections in cattle with important foreign animal diseases, regulatory officials must be contacted after detection of such lesions.

Reproductive consequences are rare in infected cattle but include fetal death, fetal resorption, abortion, persistent infection of immunotolerant fetuses, and congenital defects such as hydranencephaly, skin disorders, ocular disorders, and skeletal lesions. Infected bulls may become temporarily sterile.

Most cattle with clinical signs recover but may carry the virus for prolonged periods, and others have prolonged lameness or poor condition.

Diagnosis

Clinical signs aid diagnosis and require differentiation from photosensitization, BVDV, MCF, IBR, VSV, EHDV, and FMD. If sheep reside on the premises,

clinical signs may be obvious in this species. Regulatory veterinarians should be consulted immediately when BTV is suspected because the differential diagnosis includes exotic diseases.

Absolute diagnosis can be achieved by a variety of diagnostic techniques that include virus isolation or detection of viral antigen, nucleic acid, or antibody. Currently, in many diagnostic laboratories, samples are first screened by conventional or RT-PCR before virus isolation. BTV isolation can be performed on heparinized blood, fetal specimens, spleen, or bone marrow. Samples should not be frozen. In an experimental challenge study BTV could be isolated from the blood of infected cattle for up to 49 days postinoculation; however, infected cattle maintained a level of viremia infective for *Culicoides* spp. for a maximal duration of 3 weeks. Because different strains of BTV may behave differently in cattle, monoclonal FA, virus neutralization, or molecular assays may help further characterize serotypes of virus isolated from blood or tissues. The blood of infected cattle remains positive for viral nucleic acids by RT-PCR for a much longer duration (nearly 4 months) than for virus isolation.

An outer-coat protein, VP2, is responsible for causing virus-neutralizing antibody against BTV in infected animals. Inner-core protein VP7 is a serogroup-specific antigen as are the nonstructural proteins NS1 and NS2. The older complement fixation tests and serum neutralization antibody tests primarily detected group antigens. An immunodiffusion test has also been used, but currently a competitive ELISA is recommended. The ELISA test is quantitative and is serotype-specific through incorporation of monoclonal antibody.

In utero infection resulting in persistent infection of immunotolerant animals can be confirmed only by viral isolation or nucleic acid assays, probably best performed by collecting precolostral blood so that maternal passive antibody in colostrum does not confuse the situation. Precolostral blood for ELISA testing may allow diagnosis of in utero infection and seroconversion of immunocompetent fetuses with or without congenital anomalies. For adult cattle, virus isolation, positive PCR tests, or paired ELISA tests on serum to confirm an increasing titer are required for diagnosis.

Treatment

If clinical cases occur, treatment should be symptomatic. Affected cattle should be kept out of sunlight if possible because sunlight exacerbates skin lesions.

Control

As previously mentioned, control is extremely difficult. Regulatory veterinarians should be consulted. Although a stable positive serum antibody titer only indicates past infection, the economic implications of a positive titer are profound. Export markets, embryo transfer potential, sale of bulls to bull studs, and sale of semen to various markets are negated by positive BTV antibodies in healthy cattle. Geographic incidence of BTV antibodies varies greatly, with serologic evidence of infection in the Northeast and upper Midwest being rare but relatively common in the southern states, Great Plains, and West.

Epizootic Hemorrhagic Disease

Etiology

Epizootic hemorrhagic disease virus (EHDV), similar to BTV, is an *Orbivirus* from the Reoviridae family that is transmitted between ruminants and maintained in nature via a *Culicoides* vector. Worldwide the virus exists in many tropical and temperate climates and of the seven proposed serotypes of the virus that are identified globally, EHDV-1 and EHDV-2 have been responsible for the majority of cyclical epidemics of the disease in the United States. Over the past decade, a novel EHDV serotype, EHDV-6, which represents a reassortment of endemic EHDV-2 and an exotic EHDV-6 strain, has been repeatedly demonstrated in ruminants in the United States. White tailed deer are the most common hosts for EHDV in North America and the disease can be severe in this species. EHDV has been spreading east and northward in the past few years and has been responsible for high-mortality outbreaks in deer in several midwestern and northeastern states since 2014. *C. sonorensis* is the only confirmed vector of EHDV in the United States but other insect vectors are likely, especially given the fact that the virus has been moving recently into areas of the nation that are not considered part of the natural range of this arthropod species.

Clinical Signs

Clinical disease in cattle has been reported from several midwestern states since 2013, but fortunately, it is a low-morbidity, low-mortality disease in domestic cattle. The primary outcome in cattle is subclinical infection or a mild to moderate transient febrile illness. Occasional cases in the midwestern United States in the past 3 years have demonstrated more obvious systemic illness with inappetence, oral erosions and hypersalivation, diminished milk yield, coronitis, and lameness, in addition to fever. We have seen quite marked dysphagia that has persisted for several days accompanied by fairly severe esophagitis and upper GI erosions. The majority of cattle recover with supportive care (see Chapter 16).

Diagnosis

Exactly the same comments regarding diagnostic testing made in the section on BTV apply for EHDV diagnosis; such are the similarities between the viruses that comparable, but virus specific, serologic, and nucleic acid tests are used by most diagnostic laboratories.

Control

As with BTV, control is very difficult, made even more complicated by white-tailed deer, the natural reservoir of infection in the United States, being so ubiquitous.

Pharyngeal Trauma

Etiology

Natural or iatrogenic pharyngeal trauma commonly results in GI and respiratory consequences in affected cattle. Coarse or fibrous feeds, awns, and metallic foreign bodies occasionally cause pharyngeal punctures or lacerations, but the most common cause of pharyngeal trauma in dairy calves and cattle is iatrogenic injury. Inappropriate, rough, or malicious use of balling guns, paste guns, esophageal feeders, magnet retrievers, Frick speculums, and stomach tubes are the usual causative instruments. Failure of laypeople to lubricate implements, judge appropriate depth of the oral cavity, or hold the animal's head and neck straight when administering oral medication are the most common errors. Purely rough or sadistic treatment also is common.

Acute pharyngeal injury or trauma can have many sequelae. Small punctures may have few acute consequences but eventually result in cellulitis or pharyngeal abscesses. Most acute injuries result in both local and systemic effects. Local effects include pain, reluctance or inability to swallow, salivation, and cellulitis. Systemic effects reflect damage to vagus nerve branches in the pharynx. Such nerve damage can affect rumen motility, eructation, and swallowing, and predisposes to inhalation pneumonia. Bloat resulting from failure of eructation reflects direct or inflammatory injury to vagus nerve branches controlling the complex act of eructation, which requires coordinated activity of larynx, pharynx, and proximal esophageal muscle.

Often cattle that sustain pharyngeal injuries had primary illnesses, the treatment of which included administration of oral medications. Therefore, early clinical signs of pharyngeal injury may be thought to represent failure of response or worsening of the primary condition. Pharyngeal trauma is common in dairy cattle and is underdiagnosed as a cause of illness.

Clinical Signs

The chief complaint in cattle with pharyngeal trauma is anorexia and a suspected abdominal disorder that has not responded to medication (including orally administered medications). Direct tissue trauma is quickly complicated by cellulitis or phlegmon of the retropharyngeal tissue. Clinical signs usually include salivation, a "sore throat" as evidenced by an extended head and neck, fever, fetid breath, soft tissue swelling in the throat latch, and localized or diffuse pharyngeal pain (Fig. 6.29). Most cattle are unable or unwilling to eat. Dysphagia may be present in severe cases and may lead to dehydration because of an inability to drink. Other GI signs caused by varying amounts of direct or indirect damage to vagus nerve branches may occur; these include bloat, rumen stasis, or signs of vagal indigestion. Megaesophagus is an infrequent complication. Respiratory complications include nasal discharge associated with dysphagia, inspiratory stridor, and inhalation pneumonia. Subcutaneous

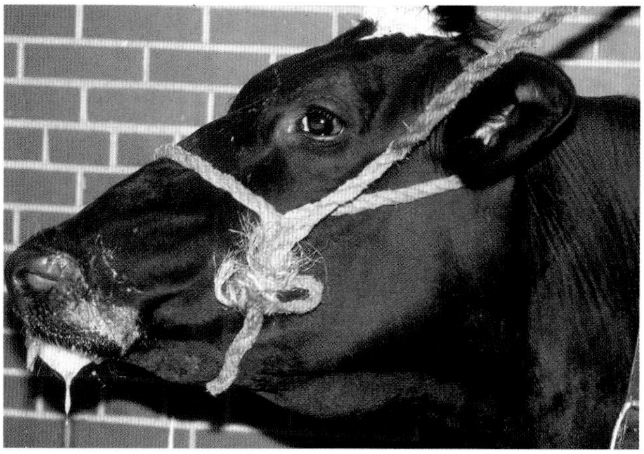

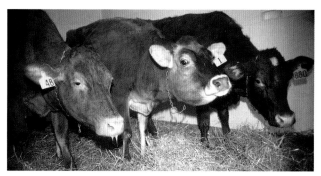

• **Fig. 6.29** Anxious expression, extended head and neck, salivation, and soft tissue swelling in the throat latch region of a cow with pharyngeal trauma.

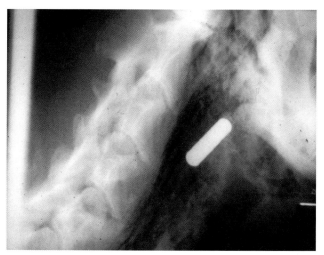

• **Fig. 6.31** Radiograph of a cow showing a magnet embedded within the retropharyngeal tissues after iatrogenic injury during administration using a balling gun; note evidence of soft tissue swelling and cellulitis in pharyngeal region around the foreign body.

• **Fig. 6.30** Three representative Jersey cows from a herd with an epidemic of pharyngeal trauma associated with mass medication delivered by an owner. Salivation, extended heads and necks because of sore throats, anxious or depressed appearance, dyspnea, inhalation pneumonia, bloat, and subcutaneous emphysema occurred to varying degrees in the affected cattle.

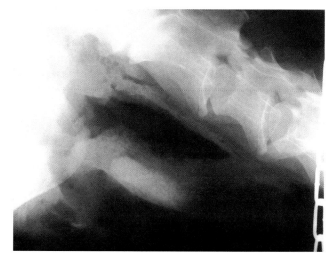

• **Fig. 6.32** Radiograph of the pharyngeal region of a cow that sustained pharyngeal trauma, laceration, and foreign body deposition of a sulfa bolus delivered with a balling gun. A large radiolucent area and tissue emphysema are apparent ventral to the cervical vertebrae, and the bolus can be seen embedded between the air density dorsally and the trachea.

emphysema is present in some patients as air is sucked into the retropharyngeal area and dissects subcutaneously. Although SC emphysema sometimes is limited to the retropharyngeal area, usually air dissects down the neck and reaches the thorax or locations further caudal.

Pharyngeal trauma usually only occurs in one animal in the herd, but herd epidemics have been associated with mass medication (Fig. 6.30).

Diagnosis

Frequently, the clinical signs, coupled with a manual examination of the oral cavity to palpate the pharyngeal laceration, are sufficient for diagnosis. Most injuries are in the caudal pharyngeal region dorsal to the larynx. Severe lacerations also may damage the soft palate or proximal esophagus. Administered boluses or magnets may still be embedded in the retropharyngeal tissues in some cases (Fig. 6.31). An oral speculum and focal light examination also may allow a view of pharyngeal injuries. Manual examination of the oral cavity in affected adult cows can often detect lacerations or abnormal soft tissue swellings.

Endoscopy and radiology are very helpful ancillary aids, especially when a manual examination of the oral cavity is inconclusive or when the size of the animal—as with a calf—precludes manual examination. Endoscopy usually allows a view of pharyngeal injuries, but diffuse swelling of the pharynx, larynx, and soft palate sometimes interferes with this procedure. Radiographs are diagnostic of pharyngeal trauma in most cases because air densities and radiolucent retropharyngeal tissues are readily apparent. Pharyngeal foreign bodies and embedded boluses or magnets also are apparent with radiographs (Figs. 6.31 and 6.32).

Treatment

Broad-spectrum antibiotics, analgesics, and supportive measures such as IV fluids are the major components of therapy for pharyngeal trauma. If an abscess has formed in the pharynx, manual examination and rupture of the abscess into the pharynx is indicated. Whenever possible, it is best to avoid any oral medications until the injury heals. However, sometimes gentle passage of a stomach tube to provide an economical means to hydrate a patient with dysphagia is necessary. Most small pharyngeal lacerations respond to antibiotics such as ceftiofur, tetracycline (9 mg/kg IV every 24 hours), ampicillin (6.6–11.0 mg/kg IM or SC every 12 hours), or other broad-spectrum combinations. Penicillin is not a good initial choice on its own because it seldom is able to control the expected mixed infection. Judicious use of analgesics such as flunixin meglumine (0.5–1.1 mg/kg IV every 24 hours) aids patient comfort, relieves the "sore throat," and may allow an earlier return of appetite. Resolution of dysphagia, when present, is an important positive prognostic sign because the patient can now drink effectively and hydrate herself. Resolution of fever is another positive prognostic sign but may be misleading if the temperature decreased because of concurrent therapy with nonsteroidal antiinflammatory drugs (NSAIDs).

Nursing procedures and ensuring access to fresh clean water and soft feeds such as silage or gruels of soaked alfalfa pellets are helpful. In severe cases, placement of a rumen fistula may be necessary to allow for placement of mashes or liquids directly into the rumen, thereby bypassing the damaged and painful tissues. Antibiotic therapy should be continued 7 to 14 days or longer depending on response to treatment and healing of the pharyngeal wound. Foreign bodies, boluses, or magnets embedded in retropharyngeal locations must be removed.

The prognosis is good for most cases but is guarded for cattle having large lacerations, soft palate lacerations, proximal esophageal lacerations, inhalation pneumonia, or vagal indigestion.

Prevention

Veterinarians should educate laypeople on how to safely administer oral medications. Stomach tubes, specula, esophageal feeder tubes, and balling guns should be inspected after each use to identify any sharp edges or "burrs" that may incite future injury. Proper size specula, tubes, and so on should be based on the animal's size and not "one size fits all."

Alimentary Warts

Etiology

Papillomas and fibropapillomas are observed sporadically in the oral cavity, esophagus, and forestomach of dairy cattle. Oral lesions may occur on the hard palate, soft palate, or tongue. Bovine papilloma viruses (BPV), of which there are currently 14 types recognized, are the suspected cause of these lesions. Because BPV types can be found in normal skin as well as cutaneous papillomas and fibropapillomas, it is uncertain which BPV types actually cause

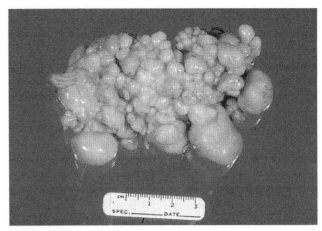

• **Fig. 6.33** A fibropapilloma that was surgically removed via rumenotomy from a 2-year-old cow with chronic bloat.

the lesions. Recent studies have identified the DNA of several different BPV types in many cutaneous papilloma and fibropapilloma lesions. Experimentally, cutaneous papillomas can be induced by the inoculation of BPV-1 or BPV-2, but the upper alimentary tract lesions are often histologically classified as squamous papillomas and are thought to be associated with BPV-4 infection. The prevalence of upper GI papillomas can be increased by exposure to bracken fern, which is believed to be immunosuppressive. Bracken fern exposure is not, however, necessary for the development of upper GI squamous papillomas because they occur in the absence of this plant. Squamous fibropapillomas of the upper GI tract are thought due to BPV-2 infection. BPV-2 has also been demonstrated in association with urinary bladder carcinomas in cows with chronic enzootic hematuria. The E5 oncoprotein produced by Deltapapilloma viruses, the group to which BPV-2 belongs, is thought important in the development of these neoplastic bladder lesions.

Signs

Papillomas and fibropapillomas of the mouth, esophagus, and forestomach create no clinical signs unless they interfere with eructation. Lesions sometimes occur as clusters or along a line in the esophagus, suggesting that trauma from fibrous feed material may facilitate mucosal inoculation of the inciting BPV type. Occasional warts at the cardia or distal esophagus act as a ball valve to interfere with eructation and cause chronic or recurrent bloat, leading to signs of vagal indigestion (Fig. 6.33). Such lesions may be precursors for carcinomas, but this has not been proven except when associated with the ingestion of bracken fern.

Diagnosis

Inspection, endoscopic biopsy, and histopathology are the means of diagnosis. Rumenotomy may be necessary to confirm lesions at the cardia.

Treatment

Lesions are not treated except when discovered during rumenotomy in cattle with failure of eructation. In such cases, removal is curative. In the majority of immunocompetent cattle, upper alimentary papillomas spontaneously resolve within a year of development.

Salmonellosis

Etiology

Much of the discussion regarding salmonellosis has been addressed in the section on calf diarrhea. *Salmonella* spp. cause enterocolitis that varies tremendously in severity in adult cattle. Septicemic salmonellosis may also result in abortion or shedding of the causative organism into milk and colostrum. The organism also may be found in milk secondary to environmental contamination and subsequent mastitis. This latter route appears to be typical of *S.* Dublin mastitis and possibly to lesser degrees for other types.

Salmonella spp. are facultative intracellular organisms that can hide in macrophages, be distributed along with these cells, and occasionally cause bacteremia after invasion of the intestine. Fecal–oral infection is the most common route of infection, but other mucous membranes can be invaded by some serotypes. After ingestion of *Salmonella* organisms, a cow may or may not become clinically ill. Factors that determine pathogenicity include:

1. Virulence of the serotype.
2. Dose of inoculum.
3. Degree of immunity or previous exposure of host to this serotype.
4. Other stressors currently affecting the host.

Given the variability in factors 1 through 4 for most adult dairy cows, it is not perhaps surprising that such a spectrum of clinical signs, prevalence, morbidity, and mortality can be seen. Because *Salmonella* spp. often act as opportunistic pathogens, management, nutritional, and environmental factors that adversely impact the cow's defenses are often at play when the disease becomes problematic on a given operation.

Salmonellosis was primarily a sporadic disease in dairy cattle in the northeastern United States until the 1970s. A single cow within a herd might develop the disease secondary to septic metritis, septic mastitis, BVDV, or other periparturient disorders. Infection seldom spread to other cows. However, in recent decades, larger herds and increased use of free stall housing have changed the clinical epidemiology of salmonellosis, such that herd outbreaks with subsequent endemicity and variable morbidity and mortality are now the rule. Free-stall housing creates a nightmarish setting for diseases such as salmonellosis that are spread by fecal–oral transmission. Stressors include such things as concurrent infection with other bacterial or viral pathogens, transportation, parturition, poor transition cow management, GI stasis or disturbance of the GI flora by recent feed changes, heat or cold, and recent anesthesia or surgery.

S. Dublin is host adapted to cattle, but other types are non–host adapted. A particularly frightening characteristic of *S.* Dublin infection is that infected cows may remain carriers for a long time or even forever. Some shed consistently, others intermittently, and others are "latent" carriers that shed only when stressed. *S.* Dublin also causes mastitis, which tends to be subclinical and persistent. Clinical mastitis caused by *S.* Dublin is thought to originate from environmental contamination of the udder by feces from infected cattle rather than septicemic spread to the udder. Infected calves shed large numbers of organisms, frequently are septicemic, and have respiratory signs coupled with fever that confound the diagnosis and mislead veterinarians unfamiliar with this disease. Other than *S.* Dublin–infected cattle, most cattle infected with non–host adapted serotypes such as *S.* Typhimurium are thought to shed the organism for less than 6 months. However, latent carriers or chronic infection may occur occasionally, and chronic *S.* Typhimurium mastitis has been documented after an enteric epidemic.

Another contributing factor to herd infections is contaminated ration components fed to dairy cattle. Protein source supplements and animal by-product components may be contaminated with *Salmonella*. Improperly ensiled forages that fail to reach a pH <4.5 can also harbor *Salmonella* spp. Birds shedding *Salmonella* can contaminate cut forages or feed bunks to infect adult cattle. This latter pathogenesis has been suspected in several herd outbreaks with type E serotypes, but birds also could transmit other types of *Salmonella* by acting as either biological or mechanical vectors. Farm implements used to handle manure or haul sick or dead animals can be a very efficient means of spreading *Salmonella* if they are used to haul feed, bedding, or apparently healthy animals. The spreading of liquid manure on fields in addition to no-plow planting of crops has caused an increase in forage contamination.

Herd epidemics with an acute onset and high morbidity should be investigated as point source outbreaks of feed or water contamination. Chronic, endemic problems may represent spread of infection by carrier cattle to susceptible or stressed herdmates who then propagate the herd problem by shedding large numbers of organisms in feces during acute disease. It is not unusual to have a herd outbreak in lactating cows without an outbreak in young calves or vice versa.

Salmonella spp. are capable of attachment to, and destruction of, enterocytes. Pathogenic serotypes gain access to the submucosal region of the distal small intestine and colon where their facultative intracellular characteristics guard them against normal defense mechanisms of naive cattle. From this location, the organisms enter lymphatics and may commonly create bacteremia in calves. As with most facultative intracellular bacteria, the host's cell-mediated immune system is essential for effective defense. Diarrhea caused by *Salmonella* spp. is primarily of inflammatory origin with lesser contributions (in some serotypes) by secretory mechanisms. Because mucosal destruction occurs, maldigestion and malabsorption contribute to the diarrhea, and protein loss into the bowel is significant when virulent strains infect cattle. Severe inflammation of the colon is common with resultant fresh blood in the feces or dysentery.

Epidemiology

Domestic and wild animals serve as reservoirs for *Salmonella* spp. Thus, *Salmonella* spp. can be found in the GI tract of a wide range of hosts, often without evidence of clinical disease; humans, cattle, horses, pigs, goats, sheep, poultry, wild birds, dogs, cats, rodents and other mammalian wildlife, reptiles, amphibians, and fish As a result, introduction of *Salmonella* spp. onto a dairy farm can occur through a variety of routes, including purchased cattle, heifers returning to the home farm from off-site raising facilities, wild animals such as birds and rodents, contaminated feed or water, human traffic, and even insects. The presence of *Salmonella* spp. on a dairy farm is therefore not an unexpected finding, and transmission to cattle is primarily via ingestion. The United States Department of Agriculture (USDA) National Animal Health Monitoring System (NAHMS) Dairy 2007 study, based on a single sampling visit to dairy operations in 17 major dairy states, showed that 40% of herds included had at least one cow that was *Salmonella* positive by fecal culture.

In a comprehensive study of more than 800 dairy operations in the northeastern United States, the herd-level incidence rate for laboratory-confirmed salmonellosis was estimated to be 8.6 positive herds per 100 herd-years. However, fewer than 20% of the positive herds accounted for more than 70% of the clinical *Salmonella* cases. Clustering of disease among dairy herds suggests a need for focused efforts to improve bovine health and safeguard public health. The most efficient approach for controlling *Salmonella* at the farm level might be to address prevention and control strategies (e.g., biosecurity and hygiene practices) among the relatively few herds with high frequency of disease, as well as striving to prevent pathogen spread from such herds to those that remain uninfected. In the same study of more than 800 herds, the animal-level incidence rate for salmonellosis among preweaned female calves was estimated to be 8.1 cases per 1000 animal-years compared with 1.8 cases per 1000 animal-years among adult cows. Older heifers rarely developed salmonellosis over the course of the study. Because the mortality rate has been found to be higher among calves than adults with salmonellosis, dairy herd outbreaks that involve calves are an especially important economic concern for herd owners.

Dairy cattle with salmonellosis shed *Salmonella* organisms in the feces while ill and after clinical recovery, and the duration and magnitude of shedding are important determinants of transmission dynamics. The Kaplan-Meier median duration of fecal *Salmonella* shedding among dairy cattle after clinical disease was found to be 50 days, which is well beyond the typical period of clinical signs in cattle with salmonellosis. However, the duration of fecal *Salmonella* shedding exceeded 1 year in some animals. Adult cattle with salmonellosis tend to shed *Salmonella* organisms in their feces longer than calves do, in part because calves often die early in the course of disease. Infected cattle shed copious numbers of *Salmonella* organisms in their feces; the concentration of *Salmonella* within the manure of an infected cow ranges from 10^2 to 10^7 organisms per gram of fresh feces. As adult dairy cattle generate approximately 70 kg of manure per day, this translates into a daily environmental contamination of between 7×10^6 and 7×10^{11} *Salmonella* organisms per cow. This undoubtedly leads to widespread and rapid contamination of the dairy farm environment, and *Salmonella* organisms can survive for prolonged periods in suitable conditions outside the host. Thus, fecal *Salmonella* shedding increases the risk of within-herd transmission and inadvertent spread to other herds. Importantly, in addition to impacting the health and productivity of dairy cattle, these factors lead to an increased risk of zoonotic transmission.

Many *Salmonella* infections in dairy cattle remain subclinical. According to the USDA NAHMS Dairy 2007 study, 14% of cows designated as healthy were *Salmonella* positive based on fecal culture results. As with clinical salmonellosis cases, there is an uneven distribution of subclinical *Salmonella* shedding among dairy herds: about 15% of sampled dairy operations yielded 75% of the positive samples from healthy cows. The prevalence of fecal *Salmonella* shedding among healthy cattle appears to be higher in dairy herds with cases of laboratory-confirmed salmonellosis, as opposed to herds with subclinical *Salmonella* infections only. Multiple studies have shown that the prevalence of fecal *Salmonella* shedding among dairy cattle is highest in summer and fall.

This seasonal association is presumably related to temperature and moisture conditions that prevail in the summer and fall months, but whether these conditions are impacting the bacteria, host species, or both is unclear. The ability of *Salmonella* to thrive in warm, moist environments likely increases the probability of cattle exposure and infection. The effect of heat stress is another potential explanation because such physiologic stress could predispose cattle to intestinal colonization by *Salmonella*. Observations from previous studies also demonstrate variations in the regional prevalence of *Salmonella* burden among dairy cattle in the United States, specifically that there is an increase along a southerly gradient. For example, 33% of more than 700 cows culled from Texas dairy farms were *Salmonella*-positive based on fecal culture results, but only 13% of sampled dairy cows scheduled for culling across the entire the United States were found to be culture-positive for *Salmonella* spp. The underlying mechanisms for this and the seasonal trend are likely similar.

Salmonella spp. have also been isolated from the lymph nodes of dairy cattle, including the superficial cervical and subiliac lymph nodes. Lymph nodes located in fat tissue are not generally removed during carcass processing and thus may be ground with trimmings to produce ground beef. Therefore, superficial cervical and subiliac lymph nodes may be a source of *Salmonella* contamination of ground beef. However, it is unknown whether the presence of *Salmonella* in these lymph nodes has clinical implications for dairy cattle.

Clustering of clinical salmonellosis and subclinical *Salmonella* shedding among dairy farms implies that management practices and other herd-level factors may be associated with increased risk of pathogen introduction, survival, and dissemination. Several studies have reported an association between herd size and fecal *Salmonella* shedding. Herds with at least 400 dairy cows have a higher incidence of clinical salmonellosis than smaller herds. Similarly, herds with more than 500 cows have higher odds of having at least one *Salmonella*-positive cow, relative to smaller herds. Larger herds may have a greater likelihood of purchasing cattle from various outside sources, with the accompanying risk of introducing *Salmonella* via a subclinical shedder that has been stressed by transport. High cattle density may also be a feature of larger herds and could promote *Salmonella* transmission; animal crowding not only enhances contact among cattle but may also emphasize the immunologic and clinical impact of stressful group dynamics. Additionally, larger herds are likely to be characterized by management practices that play a role in increasing the probability of feco-orally transmitted diseases such as *Salmonella*. Unfortunately, herd size is a risk factor that does not easily lend itself to practical intervention because of the management trends and economic constraints that prevail in the modern dairy industry.

Use of free-stall housing may be associated with increased odds of fecal *Salmonella* shedding. Free-stall housing, associated primarily with large herds, presents considerable challenges when combating manure-transmitted pathogens. Freedom of movement in free-stall barns allows cattle to have direct contact with manure from other members of the herd, and it facilitates fecal contamination of common feed and water sources. Disposal of manure in liquid form by irrigation or application of slurry (as opposed to use of a broadcast or solid spreader to discard manure) has also been associated with *Salmonella* shedding. Manure in liquid form may be conducive to *Salmonella* persistence and can be dispersed broadly into the environment, increasing the likelihood of cattle exposure to the organism. Use of sprinklers or misters for heat abatement during the warmer months has also been associated with *Salmonella*-positive herd status. It is possible that this is related to the ability of *Salmonella* to thrive in moist environmental conditions. Alternatively, use of heat abatement practices may simply be a proxy for warmer geographic regions where *Salmonella* prevalence tends to be higher. Other herd-level risk factors for *Salmonella* shedding include lack of an enclosed building for feed storage and cow access to surface water such as ponds and streams, underscoring the importance of biosecurity measures. Finally, feeding anionic salts to cows near the time of parturition was found to be a risk factor for *Salmonella*-positive herd status, although the mechanism underlying this association is unclear. Obviously, some of these herd-level risk factors for *Salmonella* shedding are more amenable to intervention than others.

S. Newport and *S.* Typhimurium are two of the predominant serovars among dairy cattle in the United States.

Together, they accounted for 60% (346 of 576) of laboratory-confirmed cases in the Northeast, and both serovars were widespread among dairy farms. Nearly 90% of the *S.* Newport and *S.* Typhimurium isolates were resistant to five or more antimicrobial agents. Similarly, these two serovars accounted for 64% (32 of 50) of salmonellosis cases among hospitalized dairy cattle drawn from the same geographic area of the United States during a similar time frame.

Recent evidence suggests that *Salmonella* Cerro (serotype K) is an emerging pathogen among dairy cattle in the United States. Although rarely detected among clinically ill cattle prior to 2007, *S.* Cerro was isolated from nearly 60% (71 of 120) of the dairy cattle with clinical evidence of salmonellosis in a New York field study. Furthermore, *S.* Cerro is currently the leading serovar among *Salmonella* isolates from clinical bovine samples submitted to veterinary diagnostic laboratories in the northeastern United States. Dairy herd outbreaks of salmonellosis with *S.* Cerro have also recently been reported from the Midwest. To date, antimicrobial resistance has been uncommon among *S.* Cerro isolates from dairy cattle. Isolation of *S.* Newport from dairy cattle with salmonellosis appears to have decreased coincident with the rise in *S.* Cerro. The emergence of *S.* Cerro as a pathogen is particularly noteworthy because previously published reports on this serovar suggested a lack of disease association in cattle.

Similar to serovar Cerro, *S.* Dublin is increasingly being isolated from dairy cattle with salmonellosis in the United States, with a high frequency of multidrug resistance among isolates. *S.* Dublin is a cattle-adapted serovar and thus has unique epidemiologic aspects. Illness occurs primarily in calves younger than 3 months of age, and the predominant clinical manifestation is febrile respiratory illness rather than GI disease. This serovar is particularly challenging because of its tendency to yield chronic, subclinical carriers that continuously or intermittently shed high numbers of organisms into the environment. These carrier animals play a key role in maintaining infection in dairy herds via shedding of *S.* Dublin in feces, milk, and colostrum. Some cattle remain carriers for life. Mature cattle at highest risk for becoming *S.* Dublin carriers include heifers infected between 1 year of age and first calving as well as cows infected near the time of calving. The association between infection around the time of calving and becoming a carrier underscores the potential role of physiologic stress in the pathogenesis of the carrier status. Occurrence of an outbreak of clinical disease has also been reported to be a herd-level risk factor for carrier development. Among dairy herds with a history of previous *S.* Dublin infection, successful control has been associated with avoidance of purchasing cattle from herds identified as *S.* Dublin positive and use of appropriate management strategies in the calving area, such as applying suitable hygiene measures and refraining from placing sick cattle in this area. *S.* Dublin also poses a particular threat to public health, as this serovar has a well-documented predilection for causing invasive disease with relatively high case fatality among human patients.

Trends in antimicrobial resistance among *Salmonella* isolates from clinical dairy cattle samples submitted over an 8-year period in the northeastern United States were recently evaluated by Cummings et al in 2013. The prevalence of resistance to several commonly used veterinary antimicrobial agents (including ampicillin, ceftiofur, florfenicol, neomycin, and various sulfonamides and tetracyclines) decreased significantly over the course of the study period and no increasing trends in antimicrobial resistance were noted. Two antimicrobial agents of particular interest are ciprofloxacin and ceftriaxone because of their importance in treating severe *Salmonella* infections among adults and children, respectively. Resistance to ciprofloxacin among bovine *Salmonella* isolates was not detected during the study period. Nalidixic acid resistance, which is correlated with decreased susceptibility to ciprofloxacin, was also absent among study isolates. In contrast, nearly 40% of bovine *Salmonella* isolates displayed phenotypic resistance to ceftriaxone.

As a leading cause of acute bacterial enteritis in people, *Salmonella* remains a major public health challenge. Disease manifestations may include diarrhea, fever, anorexia, abdominal pain, vomiting, and malaise. Although clinical disease generally resolves within 3 to 7 days, *Salmonella* can also produce invasive infections that may be fatal. Children younger than 5 years of age, elderly adults, and immunocompromised persons are especially susceptible to severe, extraintestinal disease. Foodborne transmission is the most common route and can occur via a variety of sources, including undercooked meat and eggs, raw produce, and unpasteurized dairy products. Bulk-tank milk or milk filter samples from 28% of sampled dairy operations throughout the United States were PCR-positive for *Salmonella* in a study published in 2011, and consumption of unpasteurized milk is reported to be common among dairy farmers and their families. *Salmonella* spp. can also be transmitted by direct contact with the feces of infected dairy cattle, as some veterinarians and farm employees can attest, underscoring the relevance of occupational and environmental exposure for veterinarians, dairy farmers, and those who interact with dairy cattle in public settings.

Clinical Signs

As in calves with salmonellosis, adult cattle infected with *Salmonella* spp. may have enteric disease of greatly varying severity. Type E organisms usually cause mild diarrhea, dehydration, fever for 1 to 7 days, and a clinical situation that resembles winter dysentery in that affected cattle appear neither severely dehydrated nor toxic. As a rule, fresh blood is seen less commonly in the feces of type E infections than in types B and C infections. However, the same type E organisms may overwhelm cattle stressed by concurrent infections or metabolic disease due to altered defense mechanisms or those with preexisting acid–base and electrolyte abnormalities.

Fever and diarrhea are consistently expected in salmonellosis, although at the time diarrhea is evident, fever may be

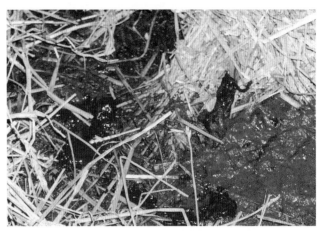

• **Fig. 6.34** Fresh blood clots mixed with feces of a cow that had a type C *Salmonella* enterocolitis.

absent or have preceded the onset of diarrhea by 24 to 48 hours. This prodromal fever has been confirmed in hospitalized animals that acquired nosocomial salmonellosis. These patients were found to have fever without any signs of illness 24 to 48 hours before developing diarrhea subsequently confirmed as being associated with *Salmonella* types B or C. Fever ranges from 103.0 to 107.0°F (39.4° to 41.7°C) and correlates poorly with other clinical signs as regards severity of illness. However, detection of fever in sick or apparently healthy cows during a herd outbreak is an extremely important aid to diagnosis of an infectious disease rather than a dietary indigestion. Diarrhea is consistent, at least in adult cattle with clinical disease, and may appear as loose manure, watery manure, loose manure with blood clots, or dysentery (Fig. 6.34). Endotoxemia and dehydration accompany diarrhea when virulent strains are encountered or when enteric invasion and bacteremia exist. Anorexia usually accompanies the onset of diarrhea and may be transient in mild cases or prolonged in patients with severe diarrhea and endotoxemia. Feces from cows with type B or C salmonellosis often are foul smelling, containing blood and mucus. Whenever diarrhea with fresh blood and mucus is observed in cattle, salmonellosis should be considered. Recently fresh cows are very susceptible to infection during herd epidemics, and errors in transition cow management often amplify the impact of disease on these cows. Cows with clinical salmonellosis and concurrent abomasal displacements may have a less favorable prognosis after surgical correction of the displacement than surgically repaired cows without salmonellosis. Cows with severe hepatic lipidosis and salmonellosis have an unfavorable prognosis in one author's (TJD) experience. Environmental factors such as heat stress tend to amplify the clinical signs and increase morbidity and mortality. Recording temperatures in apparently healthy cows during a herd outbreak may confirm fevers in some that are about to develop diarrhea or may represent subclinical infections.

Concurrent infection with *Salmonella* spp. and BVDV after the purchase of herd additions can lead to devastating mortality rates. Dr. Rebhun observed one herd with this combination of acute infections that lost 35 of 130

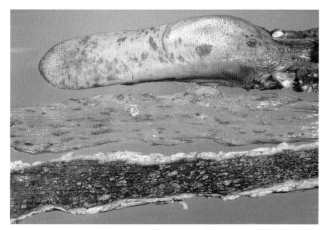

• **Fig. 6.35** Necropsy specimens from a cow having concurrent bovine viral diarrhea virus (BVDV) and salmonellosis. The tongue *(top)* shows multiple BVDV erosions, the esophagus *(middle)* shows multifocal linear BVDV erosions, and the colon *(bottom)* shows severe inflammatory colitis with mucosal necrosis caused by salmonellosis. (Courtesy of Dr. John M. King.)

adult cattle within 7 days (Fig. 6.35). By comparison, the reported mortality rate in herd outbreaks of *S.* Typhimurium, for example, is approximately 5% to 10%.

Abortions are common, especially when serotypes B, C, or D cause infection and can occur for several reasons:
1. Septicemia with seeding of the fetus and uterus causing fetal infection and death.
2. Endotoxin and other mediator release that cause luteolysis via prostaglandins and apparent alteration in hormonal regulation of pregnancy.
3. High fever or hyperthermia brought about by concurrent fever and heat stress during hot weather.

Cows may abort at any stage of gestation, but as with many causes of abortion, expulsion of 5- to 9-month fetuses is most likely to be observed by dairy personnel.

Salmonella spp. may be found in the milk of infected cattle. With types B, C, and E organisms, this contamination of milk may represent septicemic spread of the organism to the mammary gland, environmental fecal contamination of the milk and milking equipment, or both. Herds infected with *S.* Dublin have chronic mastitis in a percentage of cows infected by this organism. Mastitis caused by *S.* Dublin may be subclinical, and environmental contamination of quarters has been shown to be a more likely cause than septicemic spread to the udder. Occasional cows have chronic mastitis with *Salmonella* serotypes other than *S.* Dublin. Quarters that shed organisms and feces from infected cows create major public health concerns for farm workers and milk consumers. Contaminated milk is a major risk for the entire dairy industry and reason enough to investigate every herd outbreak of diarrhea in dairy cattle with appropriate diagnostic tests. Whereas proper pasteurization reliably eliminates the organism from milk, raw milk should not be consumed.

Diarrhea and illness caused by salmonellosis are common in farm workers and families whenever herd outbreaks occur. It is the veterinarian's obligation to inform clients and workers regarding the public health dangers of salmonellosis and to direct sick farm workers or family members to physicians for treatment.

Ancillary Aids and Diagnosis

Hematology and acid–base electrolyte values are valuable ancillary aids for individual or valuable cattle but are not diagnostic because of the great variation in clinical illness. Fecal cultures are the "gold standard" for diagnosis, and samples from several patients in the early stages of the disease should be submitted to a qualified diagnostic laboratory. Isolates should be typed and antibiotic susceptibility determined. Unlike salmonellosis in horses, *Salmonella* spp. can often be cultured from even a "watery" fecal sample from cattle with salmonellosis. As discussed under the section on calves, serologic confirmation of infection with *S.* Dublin is also available in some European countries and the United States.

Peracute salmonellosis associated with virulent serotypes tends to create a neutropenia with degenerative left shift in the leukogram and metabolic acidosis with Na^+, K^+, and Cl^- values all lowered in affected adult cattle. Elevations in PCV, blood urea nitrogen (BUN), and creatinine can be anticipated in patients with severe diarrhea. Total protein values initially may be elevated because of severe dehydration but are just as likely to be normal or low in time because albumin values decrease quickly as a result of the severe protein-losing enteropathy. BUN and creatinine may be elevated simply because of prerenal azotemia or because of acute nephrosis resulting from septicemia/endotoxemia.

Just as fever precedes the onset of diarrhea in some patients, so may the expected neutropenia with left shift. This has been documented in some cattle that acquire nosocomial hospital infections, although it is unlikely to be detected in field outbreaks because cattle yet unaffected with diarrhea seldom are sampled. Cattle with less than overwhelming acute salmonellosis may have neutropenia, normal WBC numbers, or neutrophilia. Recovering cattle tend to have a neutrophilia.

Sodium, potassium, and chloride tend to be low in most cattle having severe or prolonged diarrhea. As mentioned, peracute severe salmonellosis will result in metabolic acidosis as a result of massive fluid loss and endotoxic shock, but most adult cattle with nonfatal diarrhea do not develop significant acidosis.

The differential diagnosis of salmonellosis in adult cattle is brief if limited to diseases causing fever and diarrhea. BVDV infection and winter dysentery are the primary differentials. Herds with serotypes such as type E or K causing relatively mild signs of fever and diarrhea require differentiation from winter dysentery (depending on the time of year), BVDV infection, and indigestions. Herds with deaths associated with very virulent type B, C or D infections must be differentiated from BVDV infection or toxicities that cause intestinal disease and death. The differential list for cases of more chronic diarrhea includes subacute ruminal acidosis, internal parasites, Johne's disease, eosinophilic enteritis, lymphosarcoma, chronic peritonitis, and copper deficiency (see Chapters 17 and 18). PCR assays for BVDV should be requested from feces, blood samples, or necropsy specimens to rule out BVDV infection and fecal cultures from multiple patients or necropsy samples evaluated for presence of *Salmonella* spp. Infections caused by *Campylobacter* spp. and *Yersinia* spp. occasionally have been reported in adult cows with fever and diarrhea. The significance and disease incidence associated with these organisms are unknown.

Classical gross necropsy lesions of diffuse or multifocal diphtheritic membranes lining a region of mucosal necrosis in the distal small bowel and colon are present in subacute and chronic cases. In peracute cases, however, minimal gross lesions other than hemorrhage and edema may exist within the involved bowel and enlarged mesenteric lymph nodes. The more acute the death, the less likely gross lesions will be observed. Fibrin casts sometimes are found in the gallbladder and are considered pathognomonic for salmonellosis by some pathologists; bile can be a worthwhile diagnostic sample to submit for culture from necropsy cases if there is a suspicion of salmonellosis.

Treatment

Supportive treatment with IV fluids is necessary for patients that have anorexia, depression, and significant dehydration. Individual patients may be treated aggressively after acid–base and electrolyte assessment. However, outbreaks in field settings seldom allow extensive ancillary workup, and fluid therapy is administered empirically. Use of balanced electrolyte solutions such as lactated Ringer's solution is sufficient for most cattle. Cattle having severe acute diarrhea and >10% dehydration are likely to have metabolic acidosis and may require supplemental bicarbonate therapy. For example, a 600-kg patient judged to be 10% dehydrated and mildly acidotic (base excess = -5.0 mEq/L) should receive 60 L of balanced fluids for correction of dehydration. Rehydration alone may decrease the lactic acid and correct the metabolic acidosis. (The only times that IV bicarbonate therapy is absolutely needed for correction of acidosis in dairy cattle are in the treatment of severe rumen acidosis, enterotoxigenic *E. coli*, or other enteric infections causing excessive production of D-lactate.) If balanced electrolyte fluid therapy does not correct the metabolic acidosis, the cow may however benefit from the administration of bicarbonate. The hypothetical 600 kg cow has 200 kg or L of ECF (0.3 [ECF] X 600), and the base deficit of -5.0 mEq/L implies that each liter of her ECF is in need of 5.0 mEq/L HCO_3^-. Thus 1000 mEq $NaHCO_3$ (0.3 X 600 X 5 mEq) could be added just to make up the existing deficit, and more $NaHCO_3$ would likely be necessary to compensate for anticipated continued losses. This example readily highlights the feeling of helplessness that veterinarians and herd owners experience when a virulent serotype causes serious dehydration in more than a few cows.

Jugular vein catheter placement may allow for repeated administration of IV fluids and repeated IV administration of flunixin meglumine. Hypertonic saline (7.5 times normal) administered at 3 to 5 mL/kg followed by 10 to 20 gallons of oral electrolyte solution, either consumed voluntarily or given by orogastric tube, is a highly practical method of fluid resuscitation in a field setting. This method has become commonplace and is a time- and labor-efficient way of addressing dehydration in grade cattle. Placement of a catheter in an auricular vein may prevent catheter damage from head catches, a common problem with jugular catheters on dairies. Administration of hypertonic saline into smaller diameter veins, such as the auricular vein, may result in phlebitis and catheter failure. When multiple animals merit oral fluid administration during an outbreak of salmonellosis or any other contagious enteric disease or if the same equipment is to be used for drenching of other cattle, laypeople should be aggressively educated as to the possibility of cross-contamination and the need for disinfection between uses. As a crude rule of thumb, cattle that show no voluntary interest in drinking after rapid IV administration of 3 to 5 mL/kg of 7.5 times normal saline solution should provisionally be given at best a guarded prognosis and are mandatory candidates for large-volume oral fluid drenching.

Oral fluids and electrolytes may be somewhat helpful and much cheaper than IV fluids for cattle deemed to be mildly or moderately dehydrated. The effectiveness of oral fluids may be somewhat compromised by malabsorption and maldigestion in patients with salmonellosis but still should be considered useful. Cattle that are willing to drink can have specific electrolytes (NaCl, KCl) added to drinking water to help correct electrolyte deficiencies.

Antibiotic therapy is controversial. Its opponents warn of the potential for emergence of resistant strains that may present great risk for people and animals in the future. Evidence for this phenomenon is sparse except for long-term feed additive antibiotics, and one could argue that antimicrobial use in other species, including humans, represents similar risks. Further opposition states that systemic antibiotics prolong the excretion of *Salmonella* spp. in the feces and may not shorten the clinical course of purely enteric disease. However, discerning animals with infection limited to the gut wall from those animals with gut wall *and* systemic infection is never easy.

Proponents of antibiotic therapy remind us that salmonellosis frequently induces bacteremia (although this is most common in calves), thereby risking septicemic spread of the organism. Clinical differentiation of septicemia versus endotoxemia without septicemia is not easy unless localized infection appears in a joint, eye, the meninges, or lungs. In other words, clinicians can seldom accurately predict which patients with salmonellosis are truly septicemic. In addition, appropriate antibiotic therapy may reduce the total number of organisms shed into the environment by counteracting septicemic spread that allows all bodily secretions, not just feces, to harbor the organism. These points should be considered by veterinarians and probably dictate against the use of antibiotics in patients with salmonellosis having mild to moderate signs (e.g., low-grade fever, diarrhea, and mild dehydration). Except for valuable cattle that are seriously ill with salmonellosis, systemic antibiotics are seldom administered to adult cows with salmonellosis in the Cornell University or University of Wisconsin Teaching Hospitals.

Therefore, antibiotics are sometimes used when patients appear moderately to severely ill and show signs of fever, dehydration, and have profuse diarrhea or dysentery. These patients usually have elevated heart and respiratory rates, are weak, and appear endotoxemic or septicemic. Given the unpredictable antimicrobial susceptibility patterns for *Salmonella spp.*, antimicrobial therapy should always be guided by culture and susceptibility results. Withdrawal periods should be observed for any nonlabel usage of antibiotics and the Animal Medicinal Drug Use Clarification Act (AMDUCA) guidelines followed at all times. Antibiotics should be continued for 4 to 7 days in patients that are improving.

NSAIDs, especially flunixin meglumine, may be helpful for "antiendotoxic" effects and blockage of various mediators of inflammation and shock. Cattle may be started on 1.1 mg/kg body weight IV every 24 hours and then tapered to 0.5 mg/kg body weight every 24 hours, or the medication may be discontinued after 1 to 2 days. In the United States, this medication must be given intravenously, not intramuscularly or subcutaneously, in dairy cattle. Overdosage or administration of repeated doses of flunixin may cause abomasal or renal pathology and may inhibit intestinal repair. Corticosteroids are contraindicated except as a *one-time* dose of water-soluble corticosteroid for a gravely ill patient in shock. Prednisolone sodium succinate is preferred in this instance.

Isolation of patients with salmonellosis is ideal, albeit difficult, in field settings. Whenever possible, cattle with diarrhea should be confined to an area of the barn away from the rest of the herd. Workers must be educated regarding mechanical transmission of infected feces and other discharges from infected to uninfected cattle. Workers should also be educated regarding the zoonotic implications inherent with salmonellosis.

Prevention and Control

Herd epidemics appear to be increasing in frequency based on confirmed isolations from multiple cow outbreaks identified in New York and the rest of the northeastern United States. Conditions that contribute to an increasing incidence of epidemic salmonellosis include larger herd size; more intensive and crowded husbandry; and the trend for free-stall barns with loose housing, which contributes to fecal contamination of the entire premises. Other major contributing factors include the use of feedstuffs that may be contaminated with *Salmonella* spp. and spreading contaminated manure on unplowed fields.

Outbreaks caused by types C and E *Salmonella* spp. have been caused by contaminated feed components, and type E also has been spread by birds that are carriers of the organism.

When salmonellosis has been confirmed in a herd, the following control measures should be considered:
1. Conduct an epidemiologic investigation to help determine the source.
   - Commodities barn or feed storage and handling: Inspect and document source(s) and obtain samples of commodities for culture. Are there other dairies in the area with similar problems? Who hauls the feed onto the farm, and in what? Is this vehicle or trailer used solely for feed transport (not animals, bedding, or manure)? On the farm, how is the feed handled? Is the feed-hauling equipment used for other purposes (e.g., carcass hauling, bedding removal)? Are there other animals or a large population of birds with exposure to the feeds?
   - Water sources: Is there likely fecal contamination? What are the containers used to haul water to pastured cattle, and how/by whom are they transported?
   - Manure handling: Equipment used and destination? What is the flow pattern of flush water? Are the personnel involved in manure handling later handling animals or their feed? Is the manure being spread on unplowed crop fields? Flow patterns of labor, vehicles, water, bedding, and movement of sick and healthy cattle on the dairy should be critiqued. Is there potential cross contamination of feedbunks or feed alleys with contaminated manure by equipment, people or animal movement?
   - Introduction of new animals: Are newly purchased animals quarantined, cultured or serologically investigated for *S.* Dublin infection? How are cattle taken to shows handled on return? Has bulk tank milk been tested for BVDV?
   - Management of cows in the sick pen and maternity pen: Too often, these two sets of cattle are managed and housed together, creating ideal circumstances for infection of fresh cows and heifers! Physical separation and careful allocation of personnel and equipment to each group should be reviewed.
2. Isolate obviously affected animals to one separate group or location if possible.
3. Treat severely affected animals.
4. Institute measures to minimize public health concerns.
   - No raw milk should be consumed.
   - Workers and milkers should wear coveralls, disposable or rubber boots, gloves, and perhaps masks when milking or cleaning barns. Workers and milkers should be encouraged to wash well after work and before eating. Disinfectant footbaths should be placed at exits and entrances to the barn and parlor (for humans and animals), and these footbaths should be maintained diligently.
5. Physically clean the environment, improve hygiene, and disinfect premises (see also the section on calf

salmonellosis). Pressure spraying to physically remove organic matter may seem helpful before disinfection but can be a means of aerosolizing infectious organisms so that both humans and cattle still in that air space at the time of cleaning could be at risk. Because removal of organic debris is incomplete on some surfaces, use of a disinfectant that retains its activity in organic debris and that has documented efficacy against *Salmonella* spp. is optimal. Because shedding is likely to occur from recovered cattle for some time, ongoing efforts at improved hygiene are in order. In particular, protect dry cows and disinfect maternity areas.

6. After resolution of the outbreak or crisis period, a mastitis survey should be conducted that includes bulk tank surveillance. If any *Salmonella* organisms are recovered, culture of the whole herd is indicated to identify carrier cows that should be culled immediately. For *S.* Dublin outbreaks, all cattle should be screened by milk culture, and, if available, serologic testing performed to detect carriers that should be culled, although high prevalence rates in some herds might make immediate culling impractical.

If an epidemic continues despite all of these guidelines, autogenous bacterins may be considered. Although the efficacy and safety of autogenous bacterins are (justifiably) questioned, many practitioners have claimed excellent results when all other measures fail to stop ongoing endemic infections when freshening cows become ill, abortions continue to appear, or calves continue to become ill because of salmonellosis. The siderophore receptor/porin vaccine derived from *S.* Newport (*Salmonella* Newport Bacterial Extract, Zoetis Inc., Kalamazoo, MI) is used by many dairies as a component of *Salmonella* control. The product is typically administered to dry cows as an initial two injection primary series and then boostered annually, although it can be given at any stage of lactation, or to heifers. Although it does not prevent infection, it is often associated with amelioration of disease severity and clinical impact after an outbreak or on endemic farms. The efficacy of J-5 vaccines in salmonellosis control in adult cattle is unknown. Unfortunately, it is difficult to evaluate the efficacy of vaccines used to control endemic salmonellosis in field settings because improvement may be attributed to the vaccine but influenced by herd immunity or alterations in management. (For a further discussion of vaccinations for salmonellosis, see the section on calf salmonellosis.)

Prevention in adults is best accomplished by maintaining a closed herd and maintaining good general health and nutritional management of the late dry period and early lactation cattle. It is inevitable that dairy cattle will be exposed to multiple serotypes of *Salmonella* on many dairies, and the highest risk population for clinical disease are cattle in the late transition period through the first few weeks of lactation. Excellent husbandry, augmented by facilities and practices that allow identification and separation of affected individuals, will position producers to minimize the health and economic impacts of the disease.

Hemorrhagic Bowel Syndrome (Jejunal Hemorrhage Syndrome)

Hemorrhagic bowel syndrome (HBS) is an emerging, often fatal intestinal disease that has been recognized most frequently in adult dairy cows in the United States. Recently, reports of HBS in Canadian dairy and beef cattle have been published, and the condition has also been sporadically identified in dairy cattle from Europe and the Middle East. Other names given to HBS include jejunal hemorrhage syndrome, bloody gut, dead gut, and clostridial enteritis. HBS is characterized by sudden, progressive, and occasionally massive hemorrhage into the jejunum, with subsequent formation of clots within the intestine that create obstruction. Affected areas of the intestine can become necrotic, and affected cows appear to suffer from the combined effects of blood loss, intestinal obstruction, and devitalization of bowel. The disease is seen most commonly in adult dairy cows in the first 4 months of lactation, although cases occasionally occur in late lactation or the dry period. In the United States, the disease is reported to be more common in Brown Swiss cattle.

Etiology

The cause of HBS is currently unknown, and no proven, consistent predisposing factor or factors have been identified. The majority of HBS cases occur during the first 5 months postpartum. In a large survey of American dairy producers, the median parity for cows affected by HBS was reported to be the third lactation, and the median number of days in milk for affected cows was 104 days. During this period, dairy cows experience physiologic stress associated with peak milk yield. In addition, the rations fed during this stage of production are rich in energy and protein and fiber-depleted relative to rations fed later in lactation. These factors have been proposed to place cows at greater risk for HBS, but the events that lead up to the development of this disease remain undetermined. The disease is sporadic, although undoubtedly some "problem" farms experience clusters of cases over relatively short periods followed by quiescent periods of variable duration when no new cases may occur for many months. Identifying potential risk factors that prompt each "outbreak" of new cases can be immensely frustrating for both producers and veterinarians.

The gross and histologic features of HBS have been described in a few reports. Gross lesions are usually segmental or multifocal in distribution in the small intestine, primarily in the jejunum with occasional involvement of the duodenum or ileum. Affected segments show purple or red discoloration of the intestinal wall, with distension of affected segments caused by intraluminal casts or clots of blood (Figs. 6.36 and 6.37). The intestine orad to these lesions may be distended with fluid and gas, indicating obstruction of affected segments. Fibrin accumulation on the serosal surface of affected intestine may be evident, and affected segments may rupture antemortem or postmortem. The blood clot in affected segments is often tenaciously

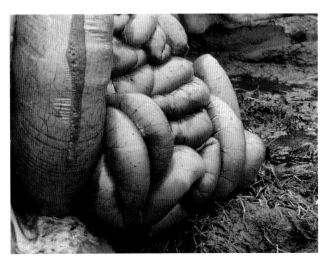

• **Fig. 6.36** Fresh field autopsy performed within minutes of death on a mature Holstein cow with hemorrhagic bowel syndrome. Note the purplish discoloration and gas production throughout the small intestine. There was diffuse jejunal involvement.

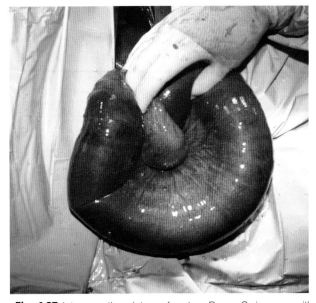

• **Fig. 6.37** Intraoperative picture of mature Brown Swiss cow with hemorrhagic bowel syndrome. In contrast to the cow in Fig. 6.36, this animal demonstrated the rather more common involvement of just a segment of jejunum with a blood clot obstructing an approximately 12-inch section of bowel. (Courtesy of Dr. Liz Santschi.)

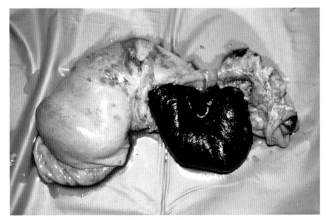

• **Fig. 6.38** Resected section of jejunum cut open to show tenacious intraluminal blood clot from an adult Holstein with hemorrhagic bowel syndrome.

attached to the mucosa, and manual removal of the clot often results in "peeling off" of the surrounding mucosa (Fig. 6.38). On histologic examination of affected bowel, HBS often appears to be a segmental, necrohemorrhagic enteritis, with submucosal edema, mucosal ulceration, transmural hemorrhage, and neutrophil accumulation evident in affected areas. Sloughing of mucosa in affected areas may also be present. A recent retrospective pathologic report demonstrated consistent splitting of the muscularis mucosae or lamina propria from the muscularis layer in the jejunum by hematoma formation without significant inflammation, suggesting that the hemorrhage begins in the lamina propria

secondary to a disturbance in blood or lymphatic flow. As with much of the observational data on this condition, the inability to prospectively reproduce the condition, means that it is hard to draw accurate scientific conclusions about both its the etiology and pathogenesis.

Several reports indicate an association between *C. perfringens* type A and HBS. This association is based on the following observations; (1) affected cows frequently have positive fecal cultures for this organism; (2) *C. perfringens* type A can be readily isolated in heavy growth from blood clots in the jejunum of affected cows; (3) there can be microscopic evidence of intestinal necrosis associated with a dense intraluminal population of large, gram-positive bacteria; and (4) other enteric pathogens associated with hemorrhagic enteritis are rarely identified in tissues or enteric contents of affected cows. In addition, based on anecdotal evidence, reduced monthly incidence of HBS has occurred after administration of autogenous *C. perfringens* vaccines to adult cows on certain dairies. At present, data from controlled studies are not available for evaluation of the effect of such vaccines on the incidence of this disease.

C. perfringens is a large, gram-positive, anaerobic bacillus that is considered to be ubiquitous in the environment and in the GI tracts of most mammals. The rate of isolation of the organism from the GI tracts of cattle may be enhanced by high grain diets. Genetic classification of *C. perfringens* can be performed by real-time PCR. Type A usually produces alpha toxin, although different isolates may produce different quantities of this toxin. Alpha toxin is a calcium-dependent phospholipase that is capable of cleaving phosphatidylcholine in eukaryotic cell membranes. Additionally, the recently discovered beta2 toxin may also be produced by *C. perfringens* type A. Beta2 toxin is also a lethal toxin, and strains of *C. perfringens* with the *cpb2* gene produce variable amounts of beta2 toxin in vitro.

In two studies, *C. perfringens* type A and/or type A + beta2 toxin was isolated from feces and/or intestinal contents of 28 of 32 cows with HBS. These bacteriologic findings are concordant with those of other reports. In the past, veterinary microbiologists have been reluctant to consider

C. perfringens type A as an important disease-causing pathogen of livestock because this organism is part of the normal flora of the cow's intestine. Furthermore, this organism proliferates rapidly in the intestine after death, making isolation from necropsy specimens of questionable diagnostic significance. Because *C. perfringens* type A , with or without beta2 toxin, can be isolated from the gastrointestinal tract of apparently healthy animals, the diagnostic significance of isolation of these organisms from animals with enteric disease is increased if the corresponding toxins can be detected in gastrointestinal contents or blood. In one study, *C. perfringens* types A and A + beta2 toxin were isolated from multiple sites of the intestinal tract of HBS cows at a significantly higher rate than unaffected herdmates (cows with LDA). In addition, intraluminal toxin production was demonstrated in the intestine of HBS cows but not in the intestine of control herdmates with LDA.

It is unclear at present whether enteric proliferation of, and intraluminal toxin production by, *C. perfringens* type A occur as part of the primary insult to the intestine or if these processes occur secondary to another disease or triggering factor. Attempts to reproduce the disease by the experimental inoculation of *C. perfringens* type A into the bowel of early lactation, intensively fed cows have so far failed. Hemorrhage into the intestine from another cause could, in theory, initiate secondary proliferation of the ubiquitous *C. perfringens* because this organism is likely to rapidly multiply when large quantities of soluble protein or carbohydrate is presented to the intestine. In other words, blood certainly could act as a very rich culture medium for this organism. When the organism proliferates, however, the toxins that it releases during rapid growth could contribute to the degradation of the intestinal wall that is characteristic of HBS.

Investigators at Oregon State University at the turn of the century focused on characterizing the potential role of *Aspergillus fumigatus,* a fungus that can be found in livestock feeds. Genetic material of this fungal agent can be detected in the blood and intestine of affected cattle but not in unaffected cattle. Two major hypotheses can be presented regarding the possible participation of *A. fumigatus* in HBS; (1) it acts as a primary contributor to the intestinal lesion or (2) it is involved as an agent that impairs the cow's immune system, thereby facilitating or inciting whatever disease process triggers HBS in the first place. It is also perhaps feasible that DNA of *A. fumigatus* is present both locally and systemically as an opportunist, proliferating and disseminating subsequent to marked intestinal damage associated with some other primary pathology. More recently, Baines et al were able to demonstrate the presence of Shiga toxin producing *E. coli* and mycotoxigenic fungi, including *A. fumigatus,* in the intestinal mucosa and feed respectively, of beef cattle with HBS in Western Canada. There is no classic confirmatory literature fulfilling Koch's postulates to provide definitive proof of a role for any of the theorized etiologic causes at this point in time; rather, observational and retrospective studies provide inconsistent associations between infectious organisms and clinical cases of HBS.

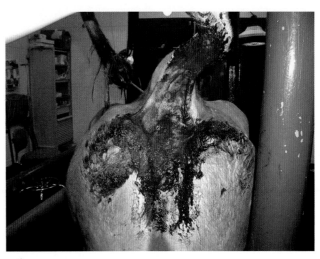

• **Fig. 6.39** Perineum of mature Brown Swiss cow demonstrating the admixture of fresh and digested blood clots typical of hemorrhagic bowel syndrome.

One study worthy of mention attempted to reproduce the condition using a toxigenic isolate of *C. perfringens* type A obtained from a clinical bovine case of HBS in dairy cattle but with no disease noted.

Clinical Signs

Cattle with HBS are typically first noted by owners to be colicky with a rapid pulse and elevated respiratory rate consistent with abdominal pain. The onset is classically peracute, many cattle having been normal, appetent, and high producing at the previous milking. The severity of the colic can be variable from bruxism with kicking at the abdomen through to recumbency and rolling. The cow's extremities are often cool, and the rectal temperature is often below normal. The most significant initial differentials are simple indigestion or obstructive conditions of the small intestine. Retrospective studies have highlighted that this condition tends to be seen during midlactation, affected dairy cows often being between the third and fifth months of lactation. Fecal production and character in affected cattle is very helpful; in the early stages, cattle often have scant to absent manure, but over the following hours, feces become dark and tarlike and may contain dark red to black clots of digested blood (Fig. 6.39). The admixture of fresh, as well as digested blood, distinguishes the condition from bleeding of purely abomasal origin. As clots form in the affected segments of the intestine, the intestine often becomes obstructed, causing some cows to show abdominal distension and subsequently, reduced fecal output. Even in cattle that do continue to pass some feces, bilateral abdominal distension and sucussible fluid in the right ventral quadrant are consistently seen in association with ileus and rumen hypomotility. When viewed from behind, the abdominal contour is typically round or pear shaped in the standing animal. Progressive distension is often appreciated in the lower right abdomen, resulting from accumulation of multiple loops of blood-filled small intestine and ileus in the

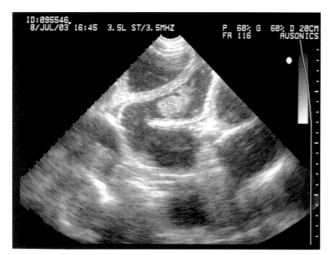

• **Fig. 6.40** Transabdominal ultrasound image of lower right quadrant of a cow with hemorrhagic bowel syndrome, demonstrating variably distended loops of small intestine and one small, nonadherent, hyperechoic intraluminal blood clot.

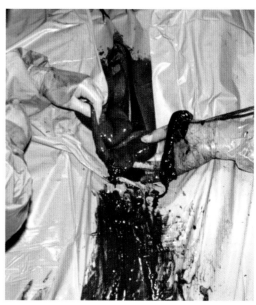

• **Fig. 6.41** Intraoperative image of enterotomy site being used to manually remove and massage obstructing blood clots out of the jejunum in a cow with hemorrhagic bowel syndrome. (Courtesy of Dr. Ryland Edwards.)

ventral abdominal cavity. Scattered, low-pitched "pings" may be evident in the lower right abdomen. In our experience, rectal examination often does not reveal distended loops of intestine because the blood-filled segments of intestine seem to sink to the ventral abdomen, thereby becoming beyond the reach of the examiner. However, small intestinal distension was palpable per rectum in six of eight cows in a Canadian study. Cows with HBS generally have elevated heart rate, normal or subnormal rectal temperature, and little or no interest in feed, but these findings are similar in most diseases that cause small intestinal obstruction. Blood work on affected cattle is neither specific nor prognostically helpful. It is unusual for affected cattle to bleed sufficiently to become anemic, and electrolyte and acid–base changes are usually only mild and typical of other proximal GI conditions in cattle.

Ultrasonography can be used to visualize intestinal distension and clot formation within loops of affected bowel. A 3.5 or 5.0 MHz, sector- or linear-array probe is placed on the abdominal wall at the lower aspect of the right side. Dilated loops of intestine can often be seen stacked on top of one another, and on occasion, material consistent with the appearance of clotted blood can be seen within the distended loops (Fig. 6.40). Some motility is usually retained in these dilated segments when viewed ultrasonographically even if the individual is no longer producing feces.

Differential diagnoses include indigestion, intussusception, intestinal volvulus, enteritis, and abomasal ulcer. Cows with an abomasal ulcer may show melena and shock but do not have the combination of fresher blood with the melena and rarely develop the progressive abdominal distension characteristic of HBS. Indigestion does not progress to feces with melena and blood and does not cause systemic signs associated with shock. Cattle with enteritis continue to pass significant quantities of feces, particularly after treatment with fluids and calcium salts, but cattle

with HBS usually do not. Furthermore, when hydration, electrolyte balance, and normocalcemia are restored by fluid therapy, cattle with enteritis typically show resolution of any mild abdominal distension that might have developed as a result of ileus. Differentiation of HBS from intussusception and intestinal volvulus requires exploratory laparotomy.

Treatment

Successful treatment of this disease is difficult. Occasional anecdotal reports exist of successful treatment with fluids, laxatives, antiinflammatory drugs, and antibiotics; however, it appears that such treatment successes with purely medical therapy are quite rare. Cows treated with medical support alone almost inevitably develop ileus, intestinal necrosis with subsequent peritonitis, and shock. Death of affected cattle occurs within several hours to 1 to 2 days after the onset of clinical signs.

The best chances for recovery are offered by a combination of medical treatment and surgery. At surgery, intraoperative findings depend on the extent of clot formation within the intestine and duration of the condition. The serosal surface of affected segments is often dark red, to purple, to black in color, depending on the degree to which the bowel has become compromised. In long-standing cases the affected segments of intestine may be very turgid with luminal blood and highly friable, with the serosal surface already coated with fibrin. The casts of clotted blood within the lumen of the intestine impart a gelatin-like feel to the affected bowel (Fig. 6.41). When there is extensive involvement of multiple segments of jejunum or if extension into the ileum or duodenum has occurred, there will be no opportunity for intestinal resection and anastomosis. Other earlier cases may have fluid filled jejunum proximal to a short segment of intraluminal clot within bowel that looks much healthier. Techniques for surgical management of HBS cases to date include manipulation of the affected intestine to break down the obstructing clots, enterotomy and removal of the offending clots, and resection and anastomosis of affected segments. At the University of Wisconsin, we routinely attempt manual reduction of the clot(s) without enterotomy at initial surgical exploration and caution owners about the challenges and much poorer outcomes experienced with resection and anastomosis. With manual massage alone, we have a success rate of about 60% to discharge from the hospital, although it should be noted that of these short-term survivors, there is a recurrence rate that approximates 25% over the future life of the cow. Surgical therapy is combined with high-dose penicillin, one to two treatments with flunixin meglumine at 1.1 mg/kg, IV crystalloids, and oral cathartic laxatives. Common reasons for poor surgical outcome include discovery of multiple segments of nonviable bowel, septic peritonitis, and bowel rupture during intestinal manipulation.

Other retrospective studies have not documented such good outcomes, although it is worth noting that these studies examined animals that had been treated by medical therapy alone in some cases or likely those that had been referred after lengthier attempts at treatment on farm than would be typical at our institution. Many Brown Swiss producers, the breed in which this condition has been particularly problematic, have become very adept at recognizing the early signs through hard-won experience and seek veterinary attention promptly.

Prevention

Preventive strategies for HBS remain somewhat speculative at present, given the lack of understanding about the etiopathogenesis of this disease. In addition, controlled studies on the clinical efficacy and economic impact of particular preventive measures have not been completed. Nonetheless, potential risk factors for clostridial overgrowth in the intestine of ruminants have been identified in previous studies, and strategies to reduce those risks might, at least in theory, provide benefits in HBS control. Similarly, the potential role of pathogenic fungi in HBS warrants careful consideration when designing preventive strategies. In short, until more defined information regarding the cause of HBS is published, it may be best to first consider all proposed causes or risk factors (e.g., anaerobic bacteria, fungi, and reduced host disease resistance) and take measures to mitigate these potential risk factors. In so doing, one should consider (1) identifying and correcting management and environmental factors that might impair cow immunity, (2) performing a careful partial budget analysis of the cost of specific preventive measures, and (3) deciding on which specific corrective measure(s) might be most justified for a particular dairy.

To begin with a thorough analysis of transition and fresh cow management should be performed to identify problems with cow comfort, hygiene, nutrition, and disease control that might impact disease resistance during the apparent period of greatest risk for HBS, which is the first 3 to 4 months of lactation. Ration formulation and mixing should be reviewed as well, with due consideration given to such issues as effective fiber and soluble carbohydrate content and their potential dietary influences on gut flora. Feed bunk and pen management should be carefully critiqued to ensure that feed intake is consistent; efforts should focus on identifying and correcting management problems that cause "slug feeding" (e.g., pen overcrowding, poor parlor throughput, and infrequent feeding) and that predispose to subacute rumen acidosis. Silage management, commodity storage, and feed preparation should be examined to determine whether spoilage and mold formation are problematic. Because these critical areas impact numerous facets of cow health other than HBS, identification and correction of problems in these areas will likely provide an overall benefit to cow health. Finally, potential use of feed additives or vaccines directed against specific, potential contributory pathogens should be considered carefully, with the costs of the proposed interventions and their potential efficacy weighed against the prevalence and costs of the disease.

Currently, it is common on farms that have experienced multiple individual cases or occasional sporadic clusters of cases to use either autogenous *C. perfringens* type A vaccines or a commercially available product licensed in the United States (*Clostridium perfringens* type A toxoid, Novartis Animal Health US Inc, Greensboro, NC). There is no reason to believe that commercial toxoids directed against *C. perfringens* types C and D would be helpful in controlling this disease. When autogenous products are used, it is advisable for the manufacturers to use a strain that is both alpha and beta2 toxin producing and to verify that a combination bacterin-toxoid is provided to the client. Anecdotal reports suggest that the incidence of HBS can be reduced on dairies following the introduction of a feed supplement (Omnigen AF, Phibro Animal Health Corporation, Teaneck, NJ) into the ration. This supplement inhibits mold growth and may confer a wider benefit against other mycotoxicoses in dairy cattle to whom it is administered. Other potential supplements that might more generally improve intestinal health such as prebiotics and probiotics may also be considered. There have been no controlled studies to confirm the protective value of any of these immunologic or feed additive approaches to HBS control; very often the enthusiasm for using them is driven by the impact the disease is making currently and the price of milk at the time.

Bovine Viral Diarrhea Virus

Etiology and Background

The disease commonly referred to as bovine virus diarrhea (BVD) was first described by Olafson and Dr. Francis Fox et al in 1946. This initial disease was highly infectious and contagious and imparted high mortality. The causative organism was later isolated and so began the prolific long-term research into this pathogen of cattle. The initial clinical descriptions of BVD by Fox were of a severe disease characterized by high fever, diarrhea, mucosal lesions, and leukopenia. However, throughout the period from 1950 to 1975, the disease was largely disregarded in parts of the United States—including the northeast—because serologic surveys suggested that most adult cows had serum neutralization titers against BVDV. These results were interpreted to mean that BVDV frequently infected cattle as a subclinical or mild infection and was of little clinical significance. A direct consequence of this thinking was a nearly complete lack of interest in vaccination of dairy cattle against BVDV. The major clinical evidence of BVDV during the years 1950 to 1975 was sporadic subacute or chronic infection in one or more heifers on a farm. These affected animals usually were between 6 and 24 months of age; they developed diarrhea, typical mucosal lesions, fever, and weight loss and survived in poor condition for a variable time before death. Because of the sporadic appearance of such cases, these animals were thought to be immunodeficient and therefore susceptible to BVDV. This theory was tenable for single-case infections but became less believable when four to six heifers on one farm developed similar signs because the likelihood of multiple immunodeficient animals on one farm seemed small.

During that time, the use of modified-live BVDV (ML-BVDV) vaccines occasionally preceded the development of signs of BVD in a group of heifers by 1 to 4 weeks. Although this further discouraged the use of BVDV vaccines, it was explained as an unfortunate circumstance and likely that the heifers had already been incubating field virus. These subacute or chronic cases—usually in heifers—were often called "mucosal disease" because of the easily observable oral erosions and GI lesions found at necropsy, as well as the characteristic clinical signs of fever, weight loss, and diarrhea. Virologic limitations at many diagnostic laboratories during this period added further confusion to the disease clinically referred to as BVD or mucosal disease. Diagnosis was based primarily on serum neutralization titers and FA procedures on tissue samples rather than viral isolation. Current knowledge helps explain why so many of these clinically obvious BVD patients had low or nonexistent serum neutralization (SN) titers against BVDV. Furthermore, the FA techniques used were poor tests that gave erratic results. Therefore, in many cases over this time period, a textbook example of clinical BVD could not be confirmed as BVDV infection.

Reproductive and fetal consequences of infections with the virus were studied during these years (1950–1975), and the implications of BVDV in reproductive failure were suggested clinically but seldom confirmed. The virus was shown to be a potential cause of abortion and congenital anomalies such as cerebellar hypoplasia and ocular defects. Absolute diagnosis of BVDV infection as a cause of clinical reproductive, GI, or other system disease was made difficult by limited laboratory capabilities.

The past 40 years have brought both a wealth of research regarding the virus and the reemergence of BVDV as a major pathogen in cattle. The virus had been classified as a pestivirus within the Togaviridae family because of similarities with hog cholera virus and the virus of Border disease. Recent reclassification finds BVDV as a member of the genus *Pestivirus* within the family Flaviviridae. BVDV is classified in vitro into one of two "biotypes," cytopathic (CP-BVDV) or noncytopathic (NCP-BVDV) based on how each biotype affects cell cultures. Whereas CP-BVDV causes vacuolation and death of certain cell lines within days of inoculation into cell culture, NCP-BVDV inoculation into cell culture results in inapparent infection. NCP-BVDV is the more prevalent biotype in cattle. It serves as the parent virus from which, after genetic recombination, CP-BVDV arises.

In addition, a multitude of "strains" or heterologous isolates exist within each of the BVDV biotypes. The exact number of strains or genetic variation in the virus is not known, but the implications regarding clinical presentations and effective immunization against these multiple strains constitute the major current concerns for BVDV. Furthermore, the strain of virus used to complete a research study may or may not have implications for cattle exposed to a heterologous strain in the "real world." Some strains may be capable of causing congenital anomalies, but others cause severe GI injury. Therefore, the strain chosen for study may have a profound outcome on the study results.

Through genetic sequencing, BVDV can be further classified according to one of two major genotypes (commonly called "types" and sometimes referred to as "species"): 1 and 2. Type 1 strains are considered the classic genotypes banked since the 1950s. Type 2 BVDV was first detected by genetic sequencing of isolates from severe clinical cases in adult cattle and calves in the northeastern United States and eastern Canadian provinces in 1993 to 1994. There are currently 17 recognized subgenotypes of BVDV type 1 (designated 1a–1q) and 3 subgenotypes of type 2 (designated 2a–2c). Viral isolates within a given subgenotype are closely related in nucleotide sequence, sharing > 90% sequence homology. In the United States, three major subtypes have predominated, namely types 1a, 1b, and 2a, although in the past 20 years, the emphasis has shifted from 1a to 1b in terms of prevalence in field cases. On those occasions that type 2 subgenotypes have been identified in the United States, they have been mainly type 2a. In 2014, 3 U.S. isolates of type 2c were identified for the first time. Although severe clinical disease was characteristic of the outbreak of type 2 BVDV in the early 1990s, it should be emphasized that virulent strains of type 1 exist.

Perhaps the most important discovery about BVDV has been the identification and explanation for cattle PI with BVDV. Animals that are BVDV-PI and that have little or no SN antibody against the homologous strain were recognized and later produced experimentally by infecting fetuses between 40 and 120 days of gestation with NCP-BVDV. These researchers were able to cause the PI state by directly infecting fetuses in seropositive dams (58–125 days) or infecting seronegative dams carrying fetuses (42–114 days) with NCP-BVDV. For unknown reasons, PI cannot be caused by experimental challenge with CP-BVDV.

A brief review of the PI condition is warranted here. Fetuses that are exposed to NCP-BVDV between the approximate ages of 40 and 125 days of gestation may become PI with this strain of virus. These animals are immunotolerant of that NCP strain because immunologically speaking they consider the viral antigens to be self. Such PI fetuses have several potential outcomes; being born normal and growing to adulthood normally; being born apparently normal but succumbing to disease before 1 year of age; or being born weak, small, or dead. However, if a PI animal is challenged by a heterologous CP-BVDV, severe disease may ensue, and in such instances, PI animals usually succumb with signs of acute, subacute, or chronic BVD. Apparently the immunotolerance of the PI animal to its homologous NCP-BVDV renders it unable to mount functional immunologic defenses against certain CP-BVDV strains. This scenario of de novo infection by CP-BVDV in NCP-BVDV-PI animals was assumed by many previous researchers to be the only way animals could get the characteristic "mucosal disease" or fatal clinical BVD. Furthermore, this "superinfection" of PI animals by CP-BVDV strains appeared to explain the outbreaks of BVD that followed use of ML-BVDV vaccines.

More recent studies have shown that animals that develop naturally occurring BVDV-PI often harbor antigenically similar CP and NCP viruses. Genetic studies of these viruses have revealed that insertion of novel RNA into the NCP-BVDV can cause conversion into the CP-BVDV biotype. In other words, a PI animal may develop fulminant CP-BVDV infection from genetic reassortment of its own virus, from transfer of genetic material from a heterologous strain to its own virus, or from exposure to an entirely novel CP or NCP strain. In each of these instances, classic "mucosal disease" may develop in the PI animal.

"Mucosal disease" is often considered as a separate entity from "BVD" by clinicians and researchers. Dr. Rebhun believed strongly that mucosal lesions do not dictate a separate, uniformly fatal entity that is necessarily distinct from BVD and that signs of BVD follow the biologic bell-shaped curve. True, it has been proven that certain CP-BVDV strains can cause superinfection of PI animals, resulting in fatal disease. This fatal disease may follow an acute, subacute, or chronic course and is frequently characterized by fever, diarrhea, weight loss, mucosal ulcerations of the GI tract, digital lesions, or dermatologic lesions. However, clinical experience has shown that naive non BVDV-PI cattle can have mucosal lesions caused by NCP-BVDV infection, yet subsequently survive and form SN titers against this strain. Clinical experience also has shown that fatal BVD has occurred solely as a result of virulent strains of NCP-BVDV and that PI animals are not the only animals that die when exposed to certain CP- or NCP-BVDV. In short, the presence of mucosal lesions is not predictive of death or

survival, nor of the PI status. Although the signs of BVD may be more obvious or more profound in superinfected PI than in non-PI animals, the same disease is present.

Similarly, it has been tempting to be "clear-cut" when explaining temporal variation in consequences of fetal exposure to BVDV. Exposure to infected semen may prevent implantation or result in embryonic failure (for reasons that are unclear) until the dam develops immunity against the virus. Infection of the fetus before day 40 may or may not result in fetal death or infertility. Some work suggests embryonic death is likely during this time, but some cattle (or some cattle infected with some strains of virus) can conceive despite acute infection created by oral or IV routes.

Fetuses that are infected with NCP-BVDV before 125 days of gestation are at risk for PI. Fetuses exposed to NCP-BVDV strains between 80 and 150 days may also develop congenital anomalies such as cerebellar hypoplasia, ocular lesions, and many other problems. Because of the overlap between possible PI and congenital lesions, a calf born with a congenital lesion caused by BVD may be either PI or possess a precolostral titer against the BVDV depending upon the gestational age when in utero infection occurred. Experience suggests that the latter (antibody positive, virus negative) is rather more common than the former in calves with congenital lesions. Fetuses exposed to NCP-BVDV after 180 days of gestation are thought to either form antibodies against the virus and survive or be aborted. CP-BVDV strains apparently do not cause PI when pregnant seronegative cows are infected before fetal immunocompetence. Fetal infection by CP-BVDV may cause fetal death, abortion, or the subsequent birth of healthy calves having precolostral antibodies against the infecting CP-BVDV. Congenital lesions may also result from in utero CP-BVDV infections.

The major concern raised by PI animals is constant dissemination of virus because these animals remain a reservoir of BVDV within the herd and shed large amounts of virus in secretions and excretions. Although non-PI herdmates can be vaccinated against BVDV, potential risk to fetuses and young calves remains a concern for herds harboring PI animals. Put simply, PI animals may shed so much virus that the finite immunity in herdmates can be overwhelmed, resulting in infection of non-PI, immunocompetent, and previously exposed or immunized herdmates. Exposure of pregnant herdmates to asymptomatic PI animals is a well-established means of perpetuating endemic BVDV infection in both dairy and beef herds.

Animals being PI explains many heretofore confusing aspects of clinical problems created by BVDV but does not explain the profound variations and patterns of clinical disease caused by BVDV. This variation is more likely explained by multiple strains of NCP-BVDV and CP-BVDV, some of which appear to have a degree of organ specificity. Obviously, previous exposure of cattle to BVDV through natural exposure or vaccination, other diseases that exist concurrent to BVDV exposure, the age and genetics of the cattle, and the strain of BVDV all have a great influence on the clinical picture created when a group or herd of cattle is exposed. There is no question, however, that within each herd having detectable clinical disease associated with BVDV, the specific clinical signs of disease are repeatable. For example, herds with abortions as a common finding will continue to see abortion, and herds with calves affected with congenital lesions will continue to see such calves without necessarily having cows affected with high fever and diarrhea. Thus, it is unusual to see multiple clinical scenarios within a single herd experiencing disease caused by BVDV. A specific "set" or pattern of signs is more typical, and clinicians never should underestimate the ability of BVDV infection to assume multiple appearances. Future research may allow further distinction of BVDV strains capable of producing specific clinical signs such as thrombocytopenia, specific congenital anomalies, abortions, or GI disease. The disturbing implications of multiple BVDV strains—each possibly possessing individual pathogenicity—center on the consequential need for vaccines that can protect cattle and their fetuses against the heterogenous array of BVD viruses.

The immunosuppressive effects of BVDV infection in cattle are complex and likely contribute significantly to the clinical impact not only of primary BVDV infection but also the clinical outcome for concurrent exposure to other infectious agents, particularly those of the respiratory and GI tract. Immunosuppression that follows BVDV infection occurs because of a combination of lymphocyte depletion and impairment of both innate and acquired immune responses. Highly virulent strains of BVDV are often associated with profound suppression of T helper cell responses alongside increased apoptosis of both B and T cells through downregulation of major histocompatibility complex II and interleukin-2. These effects help explain the enhanced morbidity and mortality seen when herds experience concurrent exposure to other pathogens such as *Mannheimia* and *Salmonella* spp. Immunosuppression may also be an explanation as to why PI animals suddenly develop pneumonia or other infectious diseases when in contact cattle remain normal.

Clinical Signs

A multitude of clinical signs are possible in cattle exposed to BVDV. Frequently, it is emphasized that most naïve cattle or calves experimentally infected with BVDV show little if any evidence of illness yet seroconvert and develop neutralizing antibodies against the infecting strain of BVDV. Such subclinical infection and absence of overt disease also may occur in field situations. However, many other factors such as the age of the animal, concurrent diseases or stresses, relative exposure, dosage, strain and biotype of BVDV, herd and individual cow immune status from previous exposure to BVDV via natural or vaccination means, and presence or absence of PI cattle in the herd must be considered in field situations. As discussed previously, herds experiencing clinical disease because of BVDV will tend to establish a specific pattern of signs rather than variable signs. Clinicians

must keep an open mind when considering BVDV as a cause of disease because the signs may be so variable. New signs of BVDV may emerge as more strains evolve. Much of the available experimental data with BVDV has been generated using a limited number of strains. These strains may or may not cause signs similar to wild or field strains. Certain field strains seem capable of causing specific clinical signs. For example, a field strain of NCP-BVDV (genotype 2) found to cause thrombocytopenia clinically was able to create thrombocytopenia in experimentally infected cattle. However, it is obvious that not all strains of BVDV cause thrombocytopenia.

The reported dearth of clinical signs in cattle acutely infected with BVDV is further questioned now that many references to support this theory are quite dated. In addition, the strains responsible for subclinical infections as evidenced by these serologic surveys may not be as prevalent currently as they were 20 to 30 years ago. Clinical signs will be described based on field outbreaks that have been confirmed as BVDV infections.

Acute Illness

Classical signs of fever and diarrhea are possible in naive but immunocompetent calves or adult cattle infected with certain strains of BVDV. Fever and depression usually precede the onset of diarrhea by 2 to 7 days, and fever is frequently biphasic. This biphasic fever starts high (105.0° to 108.0°F [40.6° to 42.2°C]) and diminishes over several days only to recur 5 to 10 days after the onset of the original fever. Diarrhea and GI erosions may be observed during or after the second fever spike, or the patient may recover without showing further signs. Oral erosions will be present in only 30% to 50% of the infected cattle, so absence of oral erosions does not rule out BVDV. Outbreaks of BVDV are most common in 6- to 10-month-old heifers but could occur at any age in naïve populations. A high incidence of clinical disease (mostly high fever) can sometimes be seen in recently fresh cows that are exposed to a new PI animal.

Initial clinical signs in addition to fever include slight to moderate depression and reduced appetite and production. Cattle with a very high initial fever often show tachypnea and may be erroneously diagnosed as having a "viral pneumonia." The tachypnea usually is simply a physiologic response to allow loss of heat caused by fever. If a second fever wave occurs, the clinical signs tend to worsen as appetite and milk production plummet. If GI lesions develop, the cow's appetite is completely suppressed. Few diseases cause the severe degree of anorexia apparent in acute BVDV patients with the severest combination of fever, diarrhea, and GI lesions.

Oral erosions and digital lesions (described later) may be the only "lesions" of BVDV visible to clinicians seeking signs of the disease. Because many, if not most, acutely infected cattle show lesions in neither area, clinicians must maintain an index of suspicion based on other signs (e.g., fever, diarrhea) and examine as many affected animals as possible. In some herds having this form of BVDV, only recently fresh cows develop signs,

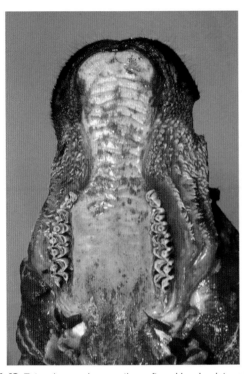

• **Fig. 6.42** Extensive erosions on the soft and hard palate regions of a heifer that died from chronic bovine viral diarrhea virus (BVDV) infection. This heifer was persistently infected with BVDV. Oral erosions in most field cases of BVDV infection involving naïve cattle are not this dramatic or extensive. (Courtesy of Dr. John M. King.)

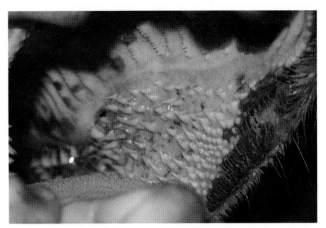

• **Fig. 6.43** Hyperemia and erosion of the mucosa of the papillae near the lip commissures of an acutely infected naïve cow. The papillae in the middle of the region are eroded, inflamed, and more pink or red than unaffected papillae. Such papillae may or may not appear "blunted."

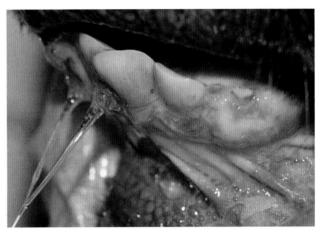

• **Fig. 6.44** Distinct erosions of the mucosa adjacent to the incisor teeth of an acutely infected cow from a herd outbreak of bovine viral diarrhea virus.

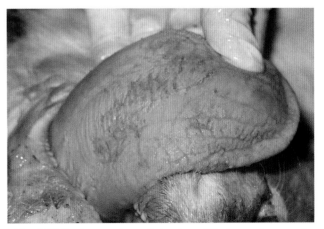

• **Fig. 6.45** Erosions on the ventral surface of the tongue in a superinfected bovine viral diarrhea virus persistently infected heifer.

and these affected fresh cows are observed sporadically rather than as an epidemic. Morbidity and mortality levels vary with the classical acute illness but both usually range from 10% to 30%. Occasional catastrophic outbreaks with much higher mortality rates are still encountered in naïve or highly stressed groups of cattle. When present, oral erosions are much less obvious than those observed in pathology texts or in chronic or classic mucosal disease (Fig. 6.42). Focal or multifocal erosions can occur anywhere in the oral cavity and are most common on the hard or soft palates. Hyperemia and erosive changes on the papillae near the lip commissures are sometimes apparent. The papillae may be blunted, shortened, or simply have erosions on the apical portion, causing these areas to appear much more pink or red than the bases (Fig. 6.43). Erosions at the gingival area adjacent to the incisor teeth may occur but sometimes are difficult to interpret because of the natural pink appearance of the gingiva adjacent to the teeth. Close inspection of this area will distinguish sloughing epithelium and erosions from the normal healthy pink mucosa (Fig. 6.44). Both the dorsal and ventral surfaces of the tongue should be examined carefully for ulcers (Fig. 6.45). Slight to moderate salivation may be observed in cattle with oral erosions, and grinding of the teeth may indicate pain caused by other GI lesions. Digital lesions are infrequent in adult cattle experiencing acute BVDV infection, but when present, they appear as coronary band hyperemia, exudation and erosion, or interdigital erosions. Lameness is a distinct sequela to such lesions. The character of the feces in BVDV patients with diarrhea varies from simply loose to watery, and blood or mucus may be apparent in severe cases or in those having thrombocytopenia. Tenesmus may develop secondary to profuse diarrhea and rectal irritation and may be confused with signs of coccidiosis. Leg edema and dermatitis may be noticeable in some PI animals. Ocular discharge may occur in some severely affected cattle.

Immunocompetent seronegative cows exposed to strains of BVDV capable of causing classical acute signs usually seroconvert and survive. However, some seronegative non-PI cows exposed to these viruses become seriously ill and may die. Some NCP-BVDV strains possess sufficient pathogenicity to kill adult, immunocompetent, seronegative cattle. This fact was highlighted by the 1994 epidemic of BVD in Ontario and the northeastern United States. Therefore, a cow or calf does not have to be PI to be killed by a field strain of BVDV. Fatal consequences of BVDV (other than superinfection of PI animals) can occur directly as a result of BVDV-induced thrombocytopenia with subsequent hemorrhage; electrolyte, fluid, and protein losses caused by severe diarrhea; and other causes. Most commonly, however, fatal consequences of BVDV are secondary to opportunistic pathogens creating concurrent infection during BVDV viremia. Even immunocompetent healthy cattle suffer profound alterations in innate and acquired immune defense mechanisms during the time between the onset of BVDV infection and humoral antibody production or recovery. Most healthy cattle exposed to BVDV infection survive this time uneventfully, but less fortunate ones may develop pneumonia, mastitis, metritis, or other bacterial infections while viremic. Temporarily altered cellular immunity affects lymphocytes, neutrophils and macrophages and may predispose to bacteremia or interfere with clearance of circulating microbes. The clinical consequence of this temporary lapse in cellular defenses is an inability of such patients to overcome routine infections. Cattle infected with BVDV experimentally may or may not be exposed to other routine infections, but cattle naturally infected with BVDV are subject to multiple stresses and infections. During the period of viremia and altered cellular defense, dairy calves and cows may succumb to IBR virus, other enteric pathogens (especially *Salmonella* spp.), bacterial mastitis, bacterial pneumonia, and other infections. High mortality rates have been observed when BVDV and *Salmonella* spp. concurrently infect groups of calves or cows. Recently assembled herds or purchased groups of replacement heifers may trigger severe disease by introducing a new strain of BVDV to a resident herd. Immune responsiveness returns to normal as BVDV infection wanes and serum neutralization titers against the virus increase. Therefore, seronegative immunocompetent cattle infected with BVDV do not have any residual or permanent immunodeficiency after resolution of the infection and seroconversion. Both increased severity of concurrent disease and lack of responsiveness to conventional therapy for that disease may be seen during the window of time that

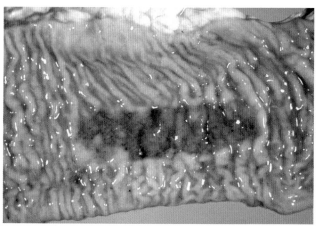

• **Fig. 6.46** Necrosis of Peyer's patch in necropsy specimen of fatal bovine viral diarrhea virus infection. (Courtesy of Dr. John M. King.)

a patient is viremic with BVDV. Concurrent infections such as IBR or pneumonia caused by *Mannheimia haemolytica* in animals viremic with BVDV may be so severe as to mask the underlying BVDV because signs of illness or postmortem lesions incriminate respiratory pathogens as the cause of illness. Failure of these more obvious infections to respond to conventional therapy should raise the index of suspicion regarding BVDV infection. For example, a severe outbreak of *M. haemolytica* pneumonia masked underlying BVDV in a herd that had recently added 20 replacement heifers. Cultures obtained from affected cattle via tracheal washes and necropsy, confirmed *M. haemolytica* sensitive to several antibiotics. The indicated antibiotics had been used to treat affected animals, but the expected clinical response was not obtained. Mucosal lesions subsequently were found in a few of the fatal cases, and an NCP-BVDV was isolated from the buffy coat of several affected animals.

In addition to altered cellular immune responsiveness, acute BVDV usually causes a leukopenia characterized by lymphopenia and sometimes neutropenia. Therefore, not only are WBC functions diminished but their absolute numbers are as well. Leukopenia increases the risk of opportunistic bacterial infection, and neutropenia seems to be associated with increased severity of concurrent diseases.

BVDV also attacks lymphoid tissues such as the spleen, lymph node germinal centers, and Peyer patches and can infect lymphocytes and macrophages (Fig. 6.46).

Combining all the aforementioned negative effects on host immunity helps explain why some non-PI cattle die during acute BVDV infection. Some would argue that these cattle in fact die from *Mannheimia* spp., *Salmonella* spp., or whatever secondary infection overwhelms the animal during the period of transient altered immunity caused by acute BVDV infection rather than from BVDV itself. The net effect, however, is death, and some BVDV strains can kill or contribute to the death of seronegative, immunocompetent adult cattle.

Thrombocytopenia associated with type 2 acute BVDV infection has been observed in adult dairy cattle,

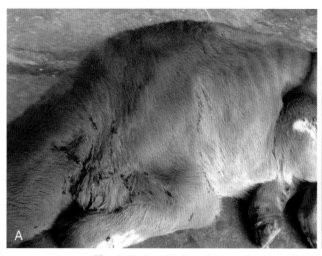

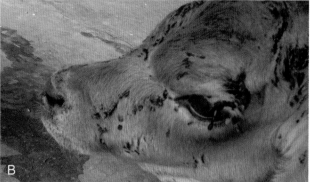

• **Fig. 6.47** **A** and **B,** Two Jersey calves from the same farm affected by type 2 bovine viral diarrhea virus infection causing thrombocytopenia and hemorrhage from trivial trauma such as insect bites during the summer.

dairy calves, and veal calves. Although platelet counts <100,000/μL are considered abnormal, clinical evidence of bleeding seldom is observed unless the platelet count is <50,000/μL. Conditions such as stress, injections, trauma, or insect bites that may contribute to clinical signs of bleeding in thrombocytopenic clinical patients may not be present in experimental models. Thrombocytopenia associated with bleeding causes blood loss anemia, and is commonly fatal unless treated with fresh whole blood transfusions. Thrombocytopenia occurs as a result of viral infection and destruction of megakaryocytes in bone marrow. Dysfunction of circulating platelets may contribute to clinical signs of impaired coagulation. Field outbreaks of acute BVDV with thrombocytopenia are characterized by one or more of the affected cattle having signs of epistaxis, bloody diarrhea, bleeding from injection or insect bite sites, ecchymoses and petechial hemorrhages on mucous membranes, or hematoma formation (Figs. 6.47 and 6.48). Not all infected cattle show signs of bleeding, and the magnitude of thrombocytopenia varies greatly. In addition, inapparent infection with subsequent seroconversion may occur in some herdmates. However, when bleeding is associated with other clinical signs such as diarrhea, fever unresponsive to antibiotics, GI ulceration, and leukopenia, then BVDV should be strongly suspected. Platelet counts and identification of BVDV by RT- PCR, virus isolation from mononuclear cells in whole blood, or antigen detection by ELISA confirm the diagnosis. Other causes of bleeding can be ruled out by coagulation panels, including assessment of fibrin degradation products.

Acute BVDV infection of naïve, non-PI calves may cause inapparent infection with seroconversion or clinical signs that include fever and diarrhea of varying severity. The greatest risk for calves with acute BVDV infection is concurrent infection with other enteric or respiratory pathogens. Transient reduction of cellular immune

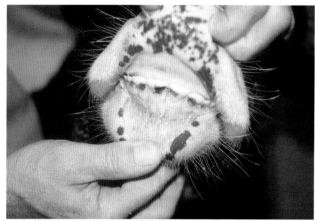

• **Fig. 6.48** Petechiation and severe intestinal bleeding (packed cell volume, 10%) in an 8-month-old heifer having thrombocytopenia associated with acute bovine viral diarrhea virus infection. After a blood transfusion, the heifer recovered.

function and defense mechanisms during BVDV viremia predispose to, and worsen, concurrent infection. Therefore, diarrheic neonatal calves (< 2 to 3 weeks of age) can have acute BVDV infection masked by identification of encapsulated *E. coli, Salmonella* spp., rotavirus, coronavirus, or *C. parvum* (Fig. 6.49). Similarly, calves up to several months of age may have overt respiratory disease caused by *Mannheimia* spp., *H. somni,* or respiratory viruses that are isolated from tracheal wash or necropsy specimens. In all of these situations, concurrent BVDV should be suspected when the severity of disease, morbidity, and mortality seem excessive for the identified pathogens. Naïve, non-PI calves born to seropositive cows should acquire passive antibody protection against homologous strains for at least 3 months and in some cases as much as 12 months. However, this passive protection may or may not protect against heterologous strains and may not be protective if calves receive less than adequate amounts of colostrum. In addition, overwhelming exposure to BVDV may override

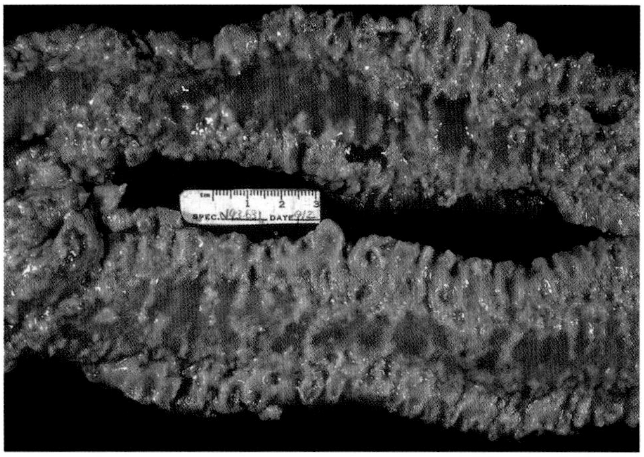

• **Fig. 6.49** Concurrent *Salmonella* Typhimurium and bovine viral diarrhea virus–induced intestinal lesions in a neonatal calf. (Courtesy of Dr. John M. King.)

any passive protection in some instances. Seronegative calves are at risk at all times. Whenever severe calf mortality associated with enteric or respiratory pathogens occurs, BVDV should be considered and ruled in or out by viral isolation or PCR from blood, necropsy tissue samples, or tracheal wash samples.

Persistent Infection

During the first 18 days of pregnancy, while the bovine embryo is still unattached, if a dam develops viremia because of BVDV infection, no infection of the embryo will typically occur because the zona pellucida prevents viral penetration. Between 30 and approximately 45 days of gestation, it is more likely that embryonic infection will lead to embryonic death; however, between about day 30 and day 125, PI can arise because of fetal infection, but only if the infecting strain is a NCP-BVDV. Such calves are typically born seronegative and PI if the dam is PI. The ability of NCP-BVDV to inhibit the induction of a normal interferon type 1 response by the fetus to viral infection is what gives rise to the PI status. Calves born to a PI dam are always PI themselves, a phenomenon that may be explained by recent research that has identified that BVDV can localize to the oocytes of PI females. Alternatively, a PI calf can be born to a non-PI, immunocompetent dam—the sole requirement is NCP-BVDV infection that creates viremia in the dam of sufficient magnitude to cause transplacental infection at the appropriate time of gestation. PI calves may be transiently seropositive if the dam (PI or not) was infected during pregnancy and passed antibodies to the calf through colostrum; PI dams may generate colostral antibody titers to heterologous strains of BVDV. Surprisingly, many immunocompetent dams that are carrying PI calves actually have very high antibody titers by mid- to late pregnancy because of continual antigenic challenge.

PI calves may appear normal at birth, grow normally, and become productive members of the herd. This situation is perhaps the most frightening because such PI cattle are not easily detected and continue to harbor and shed

homologous BVDV through body secretions. Recent data suggest that up to approximately one quarter of PI animals will survive to adulthood (2 years or older), and if one uses an estimate of 1% PI animals in an untested cattle population, it is easy to see how destructive and threatening the PI status can be in both the dairy and beef industries. Apparently healthy PI cattle also reliably reproduce PI offspring that subsequently act as reservoirs of infection for herdmates. PI calves or cattle that are clinically normal may develop signs of acute or chronic ("mucosal disease") BVD if exposed to heterologous strains of CP-BVDV through natural exposure, administration of ML-BVDV vaccines, or genetic recombination of their homologous BVDV strain. In fact, the conversion to CP from NCP biotype probably most commonly occurs by insertions, deletions, and single nucleotide changes of the PI animal's own original strain.

At one time, it was assumed that all heterologous strains of BVDV would cause fatal infections in PI cattle because such cattle would not recognize these strains as foreign. It also was assumed that CP-BVDV strains were necessary to cause disease in PI animals because many workers found both CP- and NCP-BVDV in cattle having chronic or mucosal disease. Not all heterologous strains of BVDV cause PI animals to develop illness, however. Experimental inoculation of PI cattle with certain CP-BVDV strains not only may fail to produce disease but also may be associated with seroconversion against the heterologous CP-BVDV and continued failure of seroconversion against the homologous NCP-BVDV. This situation and that of the PI calf that attains passive-colostrum origin antibodies from its dam constitute two reasons why a PI animal could have serum-neutralizing antibodies against BVDV.

Apparently healthy PI animals often remain in the herd, produce PI offspring, and represent significant sources of perpetuating infection for herdmates and fetuses. Some PI calves are born weak, or small, or die shortly after birth. Weak calves that survive generally succumb to conventional enteric or respiratory pathogens within the first few weeks of life. Clinical signs and gross necropsy findings may not suggest BVDV infection, and death is attributed to enteritis or pneumonia of varying causes. This clinical scenario allows BVDV to escape detection unless blood or tissue samples are submitted for PCR, viral isolation, or antigen detection. Some workers have observed domed skulls and finer-than-normal maxillary shape ("deer noses") in PI calves that are weak, small at birth, and often do not thrive (Fig. 6.50).

The intermediate clinical presentation for PI calves falls somewhere between the apparently healthy PI calf that remains healthy, and the calf that is obviously weak, small, or nonviable at birth. This intermediate type is apparently normal at birth but usually dies before 2 years of age. The cause of death in such PI animals is variable. Recurrent or chronic infections are the hallmark of these calves. Enteritis, pneumonia, ringworm, pinkeye, ectoparasites, or endoparasites may affect such calves, and they may persist or respond

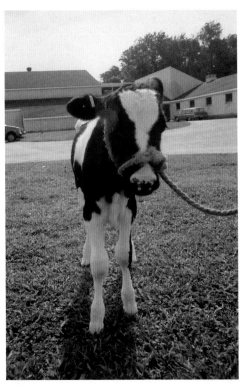

• **Fig. 6.50** A 6-week-old bovine viral diarrhea virus persistently infected calf with poor growth and an abnormally developed skull.

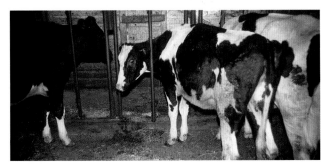

• **Fig. 6.51** A bovine viral diarrhea virus persistently infected yearling heifer that is stunted and has not grown well. The heifer is stanchioned between two healthy herdmates of the same age.

poorly to therapy. Unexplained pneumonia or diarrhea in a single growing heifer on a farm should arouse a suspicion of PI in that animal. Poor growth and stunting compared with herdmates is obvious in these PI animals (Fig. 6.51). Because chronic bacterial, parasitic, or fungal infections typify many of the PI calves in this category, the integrity of immune responses must be questioned. Although PI animals initially were thought to have complete immunocompetence except for the "self" BVDV that they harbor, complete immunocompetence seems unlikely in all cases. There may be a variable expression of cellular or secretory immunity, and other factors, such as the exact time of in utero infection and the strain of NCP-BVDV, may play roles in relative immunocompetence. At least some PI animals appear to have reduced lymphocyte and neutrophil function.

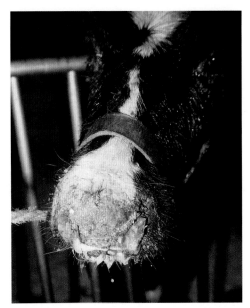

• **Fig. 6.52** "Classic" mucosal disease in a 6-month-old heifer. After contact with "outside" cattle, an entire group of replacement heifers developed fever, diarrhea, and dermatitis, but this heifer that was a persistently infected animal was the only one that died.

In addition to apparently heightened susceptibility to a variety of opportunistic pathogens, PI animals in this category can succumb to superinfection with CP-BVDV (Fig. 6.52), as discussed previously for classical mucosal disease. In fact, PI animals in this category (e.g., chronic disease, poor-doers, less than 2 years of age) compose the majority of "classic BVD," "chronic BVD," or "mucosal disease" cases. Signs of BVD tend to be profound with diarrhea, poor condition, dehydration, mucosal lesions, and sometimes leg edema (Fig. 6.53), and skin and digital lesions. The course of disease is highly variable—some cases die rapidly, but others linger on as poor-doers. The major differential diagnoses for chronic poor-doer BVDV-PI animals are bovine leukocyte adhesive deficiency (BLAD) and chronic internal abscessation because all of these conditions yield similar gross clinical appearances.

Congenital Lesions

Some BVDV herd infections may only become apparent after the birth of calves with congenital lesions. The teratogenic effects of BVDV are typically manifest after fetal exposure between 80 and 150 days of pregnancy. Again, the individual pattern of disease or set of signs within a specific herd may be unique to that herd. Pregnant adult cattle may experience subclinical infection that results in abortion or the subsequent birth of calves with congenital anomalies such as cerebellar hypoplasia, cataracts, retinal and optic nerve degeneration, hydranencephaly, hypomyelinogenesis, brachygnathism, varying degrees of hairlessness, and other congenital lesions (Figs. 6.54 to 6.56). It must be mentioned here that BVDV is not responsible for all congenital cataracts; there are many other causes. Although a plethora of types of congenital lesions are

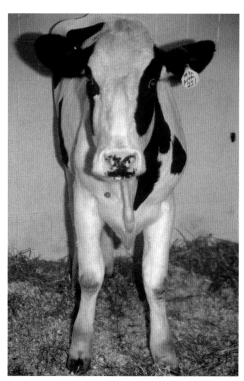

• **Fig. 6.53** A 12-month-old heifer with recurrent fever and edema of all four legs caused by vasculitis and persistent infection with bovine viral diarrhea virus.

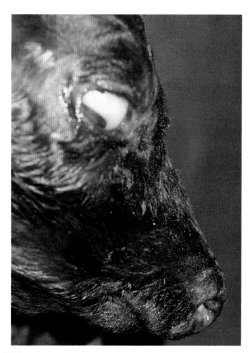

• **Fig. 6.54** Brachygnathism in a calf associated with in utero bovine viral diarrhea virus infection.

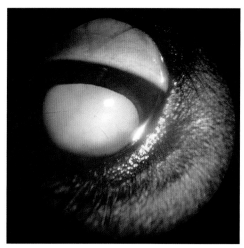

• **Fig. 6.55** Diffuse cataract (bilateral) in a calf that was infected by bovine viral diarrhea virus during the midtrimester of gestation.

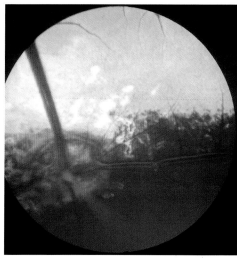

• **Fig. 6.56** Optic nerve degeneration and chorioretinal scarring apparent as hyperreflective zones dorsal to the optic disc in a calf infected by bovine viral diarrhea virus during the midtrimester of gestation.

possible, only one or two may appear in a single herd and will be repeated in affected calves born over a period of weeks to months. Usually several consecutive calves are affected with the same type of congenital lesion. For example, in a herd that Dr. Rebhun investigated, brachygnathism and cataracts typified the congenital lesions, but in other herds, other ocular lesions or cerebellar hypoplasia may predominate. The strain of infecting BVDV certainly may play a role in determining the anatomic area of congenital malformation because some strains seem to possess a degree of organ specificity. Both CP and NCP strains are capable of inducing fetal anomalies. Most congenital lesions are thought to indicate in utero infection between days 80 to 150 of gestation. Overlap between this time and the period for persistent infection (40–125 days) exists. Therefore, calves born with congenital lesions may be PI or may be seropositive in precolostral blood samples depending on exactly when the in utero infection occurred and whether NCP or CP BVDV caused the congenital lesion. Calves with congenital lesions should be tested to determine whether they are PI, especially if the congenital lesions are not life threatening and the owner would like to keep the animal.

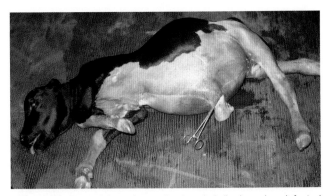

• **Fig. 6.57** Aborted fetus from a bovine viral diarrhea virus–infected cow.

Reproductive Signs

In addition to fetal congenital defects, BVDV may be associated with a variety of reproductive consequences. Abortion always is a possibility when in utero BVDV infection occurs (Fig. 6.57). Abortion has been observed or caused (experimental infections) at most stages of gestation with CP-BVDV and is possible in the midtrimester or last trimester as a result of NCP-BVDV. Fetuses may be infected several weeks or months before abortion in some instances. Mummification also is possible after in utero BVDV infection.

Perhaps the greatest concerns for future BVDV research revolve around effective protection of fetuses from BVDV. The temporal relationships among PI, congenital lesions, and, to a lesser degree, abortion or mummification seem to have been worked out. However, the consequences of early in utero fetal infection (0–40 days) are not as well known, nor is the degree to which current immunoprophylaxis prevents fetal infection at each stage of pregnancy. The latter becomes vitally important when one remembers that the biggest threat within cattle populations remains PI animals, and the ability to prevent this from happening by vaccination would be a significant step forward in the control of the disease.

Acutely infected immunocompetent bulls and PI bulls shed BVDV in semen. Insemination with infected semen causes infection and subsequent seroconversion in seronegative female cattle. Cattle infected by such semen tend not to conceive until establishing immunity and seroconversion. Oophoritis has been detected several weeks after experimental infection, and ovarian dysfunction may be responsible for the impaired fertility seen in some infected cow populations. Semen is a possible source of infection and probably has been the occasional cause of reduced fertility and other BVDV related problems in some herds. Frozen semen also has been shown to be capable of BVDV transmission to susceptible cattle. Although PI bulls may have detectable semen abnormalities, these are not consistent, and standard semen testing should not be used in lieu of nucleic acid amplification, viral isolation, or antigen detection to identify infected bulls. Some immunocompetent (non-PI) bulls may also shed the virus in their semen for an extended time after infection. Most commercial bull studs now routinely screen incoming bulls for the PI status, positive serology, or virus shedding before semen collection for AI purposes.

Intrauterine infusion of BVDV at the time of insemination was shown to cause susceptible cows to have early reproductive failure, low pregnancy rates, high return rates, and seroconversion. Reproductive failure occurred as a result of failure of fertilization. However, when either seronegative or seropositive cattle were infected orally or nasally rather than intrauterine, conception was not affected. Thus, the consequences of maternal exposure to BVDV at the times of breeding, fertilization, implantation, or early gestation remain somewhat unknown when infection by routes other than intrauterine occur.

Fluids containing BVDV-contaminated fetal bovine serum used for embryo transfer also can serve as a source of infection in susceptible cattle and be associated with reproductive failure. The potential consequences of PI embryo donors or PI recipients currently dictate rigorous testing of animals to be used for these purposes in embryo transfer.

Diagnosis

In classic cases with fever, diarrhea, mucosal lesions, and digital lesions, diagnosis may be made with some confidence based on the clinical signs, although one should always bear in mind the possibility of other, often notifiable, vesicular diseases depending on location and circumstance. Unfortunately, this represents a distinct minority of the cases. Clinicians must remember that even in epidemic acute disease < 50% of infected cattle may have detectable lesions on clinical examination. In addition, because most cattle infected by strains of BVDV have subclinical or mild infections, signs suggestive of BVDV may be absent. Specific physical examination findings are limited to oral mucosal lesions and digital lesions. Such lesions may be obvious in superinfected PI animals having all of the signs of severe BVD ("mucosal disease") but may be subtle or absent in seronegative animals experiencing acute BVDV infection. Mucosal lesions also may lag behind nonspecific early signs of fever, depression, and reduced milk production. Whenever BVDV infection is suspected, a methodical examination of the oral cavity—aided by focal light illumination—is essential if subtle erosions are to be found. Lesions can be in any area of the oral cavity, but focal erosions of the hard and soft palates, tongue erosions, erosions at gingival border of the incisor teeth, and blunted hyperemic papillae that are eroded at the tip are most commonly seen. Digital lesions are even less common than oral mucosal lesions in field outbreaks of BVDV. When present, coronitis and interdigital erosions are most common. Laminitis usually is observed only secondary to chronic coronitis in PI animals with superinfection. Although not widely practiced, endoscopy to see the esophageal mucosa might allow detection of typical linear erosions that are quite common in both acute and chronic infections (Fig. 6.58).

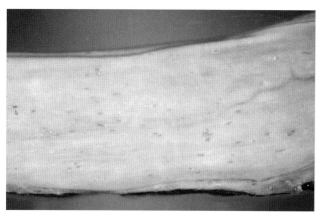

• **Fig. 6.58** Multifocal linear erosions of the esophageal mucosa caused by acute bovine viral diarrhea virus infection.

Persistence of high fever or biphasic high fever occurring over more than 7 days is found in many acute BVDV infections. Initially, the affected animal may not appear seriously ill and may be thought to have a "respiratory virus." If, however, fever persists and is unresponsive to antibiotics, these same cattle may show more overt anorexia, depression, and dehydration after several days. Diarrhea and mucosal lesions are more common at this time. Few diseases of dairy cattle cause the profound and complete anorexia observed in BVDV-infected cattle having mucosal GI lesions. Oral erosions, esophageal erosions, forestomach erosions, and lower GI lesions contribute to patient pain, discomfort, and subsequent anorexia. Salivation and bruxism also may be observed in these patients.

Bleeding associated with fever and diarrhea in several calves or cows should raise the suspicion of thrombocytopenia associated with acute BVDV infection; it necessitates confirmation of both BVDV infection through appropriate diagnostic tests and thrombocytopenia through taking platelet counts. Similarly, herd reproductive problems such as abortions, mummified fetuses, or dramatically reduced conception rates should be grounds for ruling BVDV in or out as a potential cause. Congenital malformations or lesions in one or a series of calves born within a few weeks or months also should suggest BVDV becomes part of the differential diagnosis.

Routine hematology may suggest BVDV infection but is not reliable as a sole diagnostic aid. For example, leukopenia characterized by lymphopenia is present in most calves and cattle with acute infection with BVDV. Many of these animals are neutropenic as well. Fever of unknown origin coexisting with persistent leukopenia should raise suspicion of acute BVDV but could be mimicked by other diseases such as salmonellosis.

Without question, the most clinically and diagnostically challenging outbreaks of BVDV infection occur with concurrent illness due to *Mannheimia haemolytica* spp. pneumonia, *Salmonella* spp. enterocolitis, or viral

respiratory infections such as IBR or BRSV. In such outbreaks, morbidity and mortality may be exceedingly high, and physical findings and lesions at necropsy are predominated by the non-BVDV diseases. Cattle with acute BVDV infection may have had little time to develop pathognomonic gross lesions consistent with BVDV before dying from their concurrent diseases because of the transient immune suppression of cellular defense mechanisms during acute BVDV infection. Necropsy findings in such cases identify overwhelming bronchopneumonia due to *Mannheimia haemolytica*, respiratory pathology consistent with IBR or BRSV, or severe enterocolitis caused by *Salmonella* spp. Lesions consistent with BVDV infection may be absent or only present in a minority of the fatal cases. The temptation for the clinician and pathologist is to accept these gross lesions as sufficient evidence of the primary cause and thus fail to submit samples for appropriate BVDV testing. Many diagnostic laboratories now include BVDV tests, usually in the form of PCR assays, as part of a broader etiologic "panel" when enteric and respiratory disease investigations are carried out using either ante- or postmortem samples.

Similarly, some PI calves or yearlings that are chronic poor-doers and have chronic pneumonia, ringworm lesions, chronic or intermittent diarrhea, chronic parasitism, chronic pinkeye, or other lesions that have not responded to conventional therapy may be written off as having illness caused by the other more obvious infectious diseases if viral lesions are not present or missed. Again, diagnostic testing to demonstrate the presence of BVDV in the animal is essential for positive diagnosis.

Although high mortality calf diarrhea outbreaks are more typically caused by *E. coli,* rotavirus, coronavirus, *Cryptosporidium,* and *Salmonella* spp., occasional outbreaks may have concurrent BVDV infection, and viral isolation should be a part of the diagnostic material submitted from both live and necropsied calves in such cases (see Chapter 18). The differential diagnosis for BVDV infection is lengthy and depends somewhat on the clinical signs present in the affected herd. Acute infections characterized by diarrhea and fever must be differentiated from salmonellosis and other causes of enteritis by bacterial fecal cultures and blood cultures. Abortion epidemics must be differentiated from other bacterial, viral, and protozoan causes of abortion. When hemorrhages are present along with signs of fever and diarrhea, BVDV must be differentiated from bracken fern intoxication, disseminated intravascular coagulation (DIC), other coagulopathies and certain mycotoxicoses.

Other mucosal diseases such as BTV, EHDV and vesicular diseases—both endemic and exotic—must be considered in unusual cases and may necessitate consultation with federal regulatory veterinarians if confusion exists as to the definitive diagnosis.

Concurrent bacterial, viral, or parasitic diseases may confuse or mask the presence of BVDV infection. Whenever multiple animals fail to respond to conventional therapy for suspected or confirmed bacterial infection, the possibility of BVDV infection should be investigated. Weak or unthrifty PI calves must be differentiated from animals affected by bacterial septicemia, selenium deficiency, and enteric pathogens. The source of illness in chronic "poor-doers" or unthrifty PI calves or yearlings with multiple problems must be differentiated from BLAD, chronic internal abscesses, malnutrition, parasitism, and chronic pneumonia or enteritis.

Because of the variability in clinical signs of BVDV infection, the only absolute proof of BVDV infection is diagnostic testing to demonstrate the presence of virus in tissues or blood. Tracheal wash samples may contain virus in some live calves, and tissues such as intestine, lymph nodes, spleen, and lung may demonstrate virus on necropsy specimens. The presence of virus in blood can be confirmed through submission of whole blood samples for viral isolation from the buffy coat or for detection of viral genetic material through PCR. Virus isolation is still considered the gold standard, but the use of RT-PCR has largely superseded virus isolation as the modern, accurate, and rapid test of choice. PCR is inexpensive, is not restricted to laboratories with cell culture expertise, and is highly sensitive. A variety of samples including whole blood, serum, milk, semen, tracheal fluid, follicular fluid and tissue samples can be tested successfully by RT-PCR. Primers from the 5′ untranslated region of the viral genome allow for identification of either type 1 or type 2 BVDV strains and the test is applicable to either PI or acute infections. A repeat test at least 4 weeks after an initial positive PCR result confirms a PI infection; an acutely infected immunocompetent animal would be expected to have seroconverted and cleared virus by 2 weeks postinfection. A quantitatively high viremia on a single time point sample is however highly suggestive of PI.

RT-PCR can also be used on bulk tank milk samples or pooled serum samples as a means of identifying PI animals within a group of animals. It has been theorized that the maximum herd size that can be tested by bulk tank sampling to identify just one infected animal is 500, although by comparison, it is believed that the pool size for identification of a single positive animal by serum testing is much smaller, probably in the order of 50 individuals. A positive PCR test result from a pooled sample should then direct smaller group testing to identify the infected individual(s). It should be remembered that this positive test result will not distinguish between acute and PI infection and that further repeat testing will be needed to establish the number of infected individuals and specific type of infection present.

Antigen-capture ELISA (AC-ELISA) can also be used in adults and calves older than 6 months of age to detect virus. There are currently AC-ELISA tests available commercially that use serum, milk, or tissue samples. It can be a reliable test for the identification of PI animals but does not have the same sensitivity as RT-PCR when both are compared with the gold standard of virus isolation.

AC-ELISA cannot be used with pooled serum samples. AC-ELISA is also considered less reliable in younger calves because colostral antibody may bind to the virus in the blood and limit the ability of antibodies on the ELISA plate to bind to, and therefore detect, the virus. Furthermore, AC-ELISA may not be able to detect the low levels of viremia in some acute infections, so this test may lack sensitivity relative to other viral detection methods for acute cases.

In young calves with colostral antibodies against BVDV, PCR on whole blood is the preferred diagnostic test. Alternatively, skin biopsy (usually ear notches) in formalin or kept cold in saline (check with the diagnostic laboratory) can be submitted for immunohistochemical (IHC) staining, virus isolation, AC-ELISA, or PCR. Ear notch testing has become a very popular test in the United States for the identification of PI animals because virus antigen is consistently found in the ear skin of these animals at any age. Occasionally, acutely infected animals will also show a positive result by ear notch IHC, and this positivity can last for long periods of time, so it is advised that positive animals have a repeat test approximately 4 weeks after a positive IHC ear notch to confirm that they are PI. Because the only appropriate choice is to cull PI animals, it is prudent to run this confirmatory second test, probably a PCR test, particularly in the case of valuable calves. In acute infection of immunocompetent adults, detectable viremia persists for up to 2 weeks. On rare occasions, acutely infected, immunocompetent animals may remain viremic up to 30 to 40 days. The period of viremia tends to be much shorter in subclinically infected animals.

Serology, despite limitations in PI animals, may be helpful when seroconversion can be demonstrated after illness; many animals possess titers > 1:512 following a recent herd epidemic. Paired sera can be obtained at a 14-day interval from animals with clinical signs and/or their penmates; serologic testing for both type 1 and type 2 BVDV should be performed. Obviously, serum titers representing neutralizing antibody levels may be greatly influenced by vaccinations and natural infection. Antibody titers from recently infected, immunocompetent animals are often indistinguishable from vaccination-induced titers.

Positive viral identification coupled with low or nonexistent neutralizing antibody levels suggests acute infection (immunocompetent animal) or persistent infection with BVDV (immunotolerant animal). Generally, immunocompetent animals seroconvert and clear viremia within 2 to 4 weeks, but PI animals remain viremic with low or nonexistent titers to the homologous strain.

Persistently infected animals can be detected by virus isolation or PCR performed on whole blood, and skin biopsies can be submitted for immunohistochemistry, virus isolation, AC-ELISA, or PCR. A positive result on any of these tests may simply reflect acute infection in a normal animal, so PI status is technically confirmed by repeat testing and detection of the virus at least 3 to 4 weeks after the initial positive result. Animals confirmed as PI should be culled or well isolated from the remainder of the herd because they serve as a constant source of high viral challenge for their herdmates. Again, on occasion, acutely infected, immuno-competent (non-PI) animals can remain viremic for 30 to 40 days. Delaying the second test for 6 weeks may be preferred if the tested animals are of particularly high value; in such cases, false incrimination of an animal as PI would result in significant financial loss. Such animals should be considered PI until proven otherwise by the second test and well isolated from their herdmates. Methods for screening the herd for PI animals are discussed further below in the section on prevention.

Treatment

Cattle with mild clinical disease associated with acute BVDV infection do not require specific therapy but should be offered fresh feed and water and not be subjected to any exogenous stress, transport, or vaccinations. Cattle with specific problems such as diarrhea may require oral or IV fluid therapy if continued diarrhea coupled with relative or absolute anorexia causes dehydration. Clinically ill animals (i.e., those with fever, depression, diarrhea, and dehydra-tion) should not be subjected to any extraneous stress and may benefit from prophylactic bactericidal antibiotics to minimize the potential for opportunistic bacterial infections such as those known to cause pneumonia. Calves with acute BVDV infection are more likely to require supplemental fluids and electrolytes.

In cattle with clinical evidence of bleeding caused by thrombocytopenia, benefit may be derived from fresh whole blood transfusions. Usually 4 L of whole fresh blood collected from a BLV-negative, non-PI-BVDV donor is adequate in an adult unless blood loss has caused life-threatening anemia. In recent years, we have seen this con-dition more often in calves rather than adults and hence the volume of blood to transfuse will be less; typically, 1 to 2 L is sufficient. Other affected cattle in these herds with thrombocytopenic strains of BVDV may merely be observed if clinical bleeding is not apparent. Such cattle should not be subjected to surgical procedures, parenteral injections, or crowding and should have insect popula-tions controlled to avoid multiple insults that could cause clinical bleeding. Clinical bleeding seldom occurs unless platelet counts are <50,000/µL and trauma to skin or tis-sues is excessive. Diarrhea may become bloody in some patients in these herds because inflammatory GI lesions may sufficiently irritate the colon to cause bleeding.

Even though most acute BVDV infections are subclini-cal, this does not hold true for all field epidemics, and some immunocompetent animals do develop severe illness as a result of acute infection with various BVDV strains and thus may benefit from symptomatic therapy. Acute BVDV can be fatal to immunocompetent calves and adult cattle that are naïve to the infecting strain, particularly if other concurrent stressors such as transportation, processing or overcrowding occur. Death caused by BVDV does not implicitly confirm superinfection of PI animals. This is especially true when complications such as thrombocytopenia or secondary bac-terial or viral infections befall an immunocompetent indi-vidual with transiently depressed cellular immune responses resulting from acute BVDV infection.

Corticosteroids and NSAIDs are contraindicated in cattle with acute BVDV infection because both categories of drug further predispose to digestive tract erosion and ulceration. Animals that are ingesting feed and water are sometimes treated with judicious doses of aspirin as an antipyretic, but aspirin will reduce cytoprotective prosta-glandins in the GI tract and kidney. Meloxicam might be a reasonable choice because it is a more selective cyclooxy-genase-2 inhibitor with fewer side effects than other com-monly used NSAIDs.

Prevention

The currently available diagnostic tests for BVDV facilitate successful BVDV control and possibly even eradication. Test and cull practices in recent years in a growing number of European countries have proven that eradication is achiev-able but needs central or federal coordination and consistent producer and veterinarian attention to be successful. Even if eradication is not achieved, several countries have been able to reduce the prevalence of PI animals to less than 0.5% from prior levels that were 5 five 10 times as high by using rigorous herd level testing and removal of positive, proven PI animals. Undoubtedly there are now a large number of U.S. dairy herds that individually and informally have some form of PI screening, but it should be part of every herd's biosecurity protocol, independent of cow numbers. Large dairies that use heifer rearers or purchase replacement stock through markets have particular challenges in appropri-ately screening and "protecting" all pregnant animals from exposure to BVDV during early gestation. The incidence of acute BVDV clinical disease appears to have noticeably decreased over the past 2 decades, presumably because of better vaccination programs and both early detection and elimination of PI calves.

Effective control of BVDV infection in dairy cattle requires four fundamental steps.
1. Improvement of herd immunity through immunization.
2. Identification and removal of PI animals within the herd.
3. Screening of new animals for PI status before introduc-tion into the herd.
4. Implementation of biosecurity practices to prevent fetal exposure to BVDV; in other words, prevention of future PI animals.

Each of these items is detailed in the following section.
1. Improvement of herd immunity through immunization.

The goals of a BVDV immunization program on dairies include; (1) prevention or reduction in severity of acute disease in adults and young stock, (2) prevention or reduc-tion in the rate of fetal infection in pregnant heifers and cows, and (3) enhancement of colostral immunity for protection of newborns. Two fundamental challenges to effective vaccination for BVDV have existed historically. First, the broad antigenic diversity of BVDV makes it difficult to create a vaccine that induces immunity to all of the potential strains that a herd may encounter over time. Second, the massive amounts of virus shed by PI animals may result in infection even in immunized cattle. The importance of this second issue cannot be overemphasized. Exposure to viremic animals compromises any effort at complete protection of a herd through immunization, and elimination of PI animals from the herd is *the vital step* in BVDV control.

At any one time, there are a plethora of U.S. Department of Agriculture (USDA)-licensed BVDV vaccines commercially available. The practitioner must choose between modified-live and inactivated (killed products). Both have advantages and disadvantages, summarized below:

MLVs—advantages:
- Activation of cellular and humoral immunity
- Long duration of immunity
- Good, albeit incomplete, fetal protection; greater than inactivated vaccines

MLVs—disadvantages:
- Potential for transient immunosuppression
- Potentially unsafe for administration to pregnant cattle (not for all products; some have documented safety for use in pregnant animals)
- Colostrum-derived antibodies may block immune response in calves
- Potential for transient ovarian infection and transient impairment of fertility (not to be used in cattle immediately before breeding)
- May induce acute disease in PI cattle—this should not be a deterrent to use, however

Inactivated (killed) vaccines—advantages:
- Not immunosuppressive
- No risk of fetal or ovarian infection (safe for administration to pregnant cattle and immediately before breeding)

Inactivated (killed) vaccines—disadvantages:
- Primarily activate the humoral immune response (less cell-mediated immunity)
- Require more frequent administration (boostering)
- Shorter duration of immunity
- Variable fetal protection (field versus vaccine strain heterogeneity may limit efficacy)

In the past, MLV vaccines were suspected of inducing clinical disease, including persistent infection, because of insufficient attenuation of the virus used in the product or live virus contamination of vaccine reagents. With greater testing procedures available for extraneous virus testing, as well as higher standards for reagents such as fetal bovine serum for cell culture systems, the risk of live virus contamination of MLV has been greatly reduced compared to the past. To ensure that these precautions are used for a given product, safety data and quality control procedures for vaccine production should be requested from manufacturers of MLV vaccines. There is no doubt that the addition of safer, highly immunogenic MLV vaccines against BVDV in recent years has been a major step forward in the control of acute BVDV infection and the protection of fetuses against in utero exposure and PI. The evolution of BVDV vaccines in the United States has closely followed the antigenic changes in natural infection in the country. In the early 1990s when type 2 BVDV appeared for the first time, there was incorporation of type 2a strains along with the traditional type 1a strains already present into both killed and MLV products. Unfortunately, in recent years, there has been an increase in the prevalence of BVDV type 1b in the United States from natural cases. Although there is good experimental evidence to support cross protection against heterologous strains, one company (Elanco) has now produced a vaccine that contains type 1b BVDV. A recent, thorough meta-analysis examining the effectiveness of currently available BVDV vaccines to prevent reproductive disease concluded that polyvalent vaccines offered greater effective prevention against abortion and fetal infection compared to monovalent products and that the relative risk for abortion and fetal infection was lower with MLV compared with killed products. It is worth pointing out that the beneficial effect of the killed multivalent products was still significant, and it is very important to use MLV products according to label instructions regarding prior vaccination in particular.

A single recommendation for vaccination for dairy herds is unlikely to be uniformly accepted as optimal. This likely reflects different practitioners having varying experiences with a variety of different vaccines. It is likely that this variation in professional opinion occurs because practitioners have been observing a spectrum of BVDV strains challenging a variety of herds over time. The following guidelines are recommended by us and others.

- Replacement heifers (separated from pregnant cows and heifers): Immunize with a MLV product, ideally containing type 1 and type 2 strains at 5 to 6 months of age and again 60 days before breeding. This schedule allows replacement heifers to receive two doses of vaccine before they become pregnant and limits potential problems caused by transient ovarian infection by vaccine virus.
- Adult cows: Administer a MLV vaccine with a label claim for safety in pregnant cattle, once annually 2 to 4 weeks before breeding.

Immunosuppression after MLV BVDV vaccination has been documented, so immunization should be timed to occur during periods of relatively low stress and low pathogen challenge.

If killed products are to be used, the manufacturer's recommendations should be followed regarding the timing of the priming and booster immunization; the interval for these immunizations is typically 2 to 3 weeks. To maximize antibody spectrum, a product containing inactivated type 1 and type 2 virus should be used, or at least one giving demonstrative cross protection against both. Cows and heifers should receive a booster immunization before breeding, in midgestation or midlactation, and for lactating animals, again at dry-off. Killed products may be optimal for administration to newly purchased, pregnant heifers and cows of unknown previous vaccination status.

Adequately vaccinated dams should impart passive antibody protection to calves through colostrum—at least against homologous strains of BVDV. This passive protection probably dissipates between 3 and 8 months of age in most instances. Therefore, the timing of initial active immunization of calves against BVDV is somewhat controversial. If killed products are used, calves born to vaccinated cows should probably be vaccinated three times—at 12, 14, and 18 weeks of age. Manufacturer's recommendations as regards appropriate intervals between dosing should be followed, but all calves or older cattle of questionable immune status must be vaccinated at least twice to establish primary immunity. Semiannual boosters are then recommended.

Modified-live vaccines are more likely to be blocked by maternal-derived (colostral) antibody in calves, so delaying administration of the first dose until 5 to 6 months is recommended. If protection of younger calves is desired, killed products may be administered at an interval determined by the label.

A common error in vaccination programs is to give only a single killed vaccine to first-calf heifers that have never received previous adequate primary immunization. Management deficiencies allow this mistake to occur more commonly than we realize. Do not assume that dairy farmers have "done it right" and always make directions for use clear-cut when selling vaccine to owners. With more widespread use of computerized records, documentation of proper timing of immunization can be implemented by making BVDV vaccination a recorded "health event" for all cattle.

As dairies become larger, the gap between management and cow-side workers has widened. What the manager perceives to be the standard operating procedure for vaccination and what occurs when cows and calves are vaccinated may be vastly different. Therefore, it is imperative the veterinarian take an active role in training workers on proper vaccine storage, handling, and administration. Personal observation of immunization practices often allows the veterinarian to detect and quickly correct problems. Incomplete protection against BVDV has been documented due to inappropriate storage and handling of vaccines; it is important that farm employees who are responsible for immunization are informed about the correct way to do these tasks. Because labor forces on dairies may turn over rapidly, repeated training sessions on this topic are often required. When necessary, the veterinarian should be willing to assume the role of long-term educator of the workforce.

A mistake we have observed in individually valuable cattle, who are repeatedly used for embryo transfer or oocyte recovery work, is that of linking vaccination to stages in the adult cow's lifecycle; many of these cattle may have very long intervals between dry periods. Consequently, the timing of boosters according to dry off may result in that individual going 18 months or more between boosters and thus being inadequately protected. This can be disastrous when it results in a PI calf but it is also of concern with respect to protection against other antigens frequently combined with BVDV in multivalent vaccines such as BRSV and IBR. A similar phenomenon may present itself in grade cattle that have experienced illness or delayed conception for some other reason. This level of fine detail may escape busy farm managers.

2. Identification and removal of PI animals from the herd.

The prevalence of PI animals is thought to vary greatly from dairy to dairy. Data from a few large prevalence studies indicate that PI dairy cattle typically represent less than 2% of the cattle population. Because the virus may be transmitted vertically, even closed herds may have PI animals.

In the past, serologic screening of the herd after immunization was used to attempt to identify PI animals; the concept was that these animals, being immunotolerant to BVDV, would tend to have low titers, and low-titered animals could then be targeted for testing by virus isolation to confirm PI status. However, in light of the fact that PI animals may mount an immune response to heterologous field or vaccine strains, this method is unlikely to accurately identify all PI animals and is not endorsed.

Tests that detect the presence of virus in the live animal are considered necessary for accurate identification of the PI state. Initially, all animals in the herd, regardless of age or apparent health status, should be included for testing. Tests include virus isolation on whole blood; PCR on whole blood, serum, milk, or tissue; AC-ELISA on blood or milk; and IHC on skin biopsies. AC-ELISA should not be used on calves younger than 6 months of age, owing to potential problems with colostrum-derived antibody interference with viral detection. To prevent confusion between acutely viremic immunocompetent animals and PI animals, it may be necessary to repeat testing on any positive animal a minimum of 3 to 4 weeks (or, for valuable animals, 30–40 days) after the first positive test result. A high level of viremia determined by RT-PCR on an initial blood sample would be suggestive of PI, alternatively BVD antigen positive samples from skin or blood taken prior to colostrum administration in the newborn calf would also be strongly supportive of PI.

To reduce testing costs on large numbers of animals, certain laboratories offer testing on pooled samples; for example, skin biopsies from multiple animals can be placed together in saline, and PCR can be run on the pooled sample to detect the presence of BVDV. Alternatively, composite milk samples can be pooled together and checked for the presence of virus by PCR or virus isolation. Bulk tank samples or string samples can also be used to screen large numbers of lactating cows. Current recommendations state that pooled milk samples should represent fewer than 400 animals to optimize chances of detection of PIs. It is best to check with the regional veterinary diagnostic laboratory for the preferred number of samples to be pooled, shipment requirements, and so on. Obviously, a positive result on a pooled sample would require follow-up testing of the constituent individuals to identify the viremic or PI animal(s).

On rare occasions, infected bulls may shed virus only in the semen. Therefore, to cover this rare yet complication-rich scenario, bulls that test negative for virus in blood or skin biopsy should ideally have their semen screened by virus isolation or PCR.

Ethical considerations regarding the fate of PI animals are worthy of mention. Sale of animals known to be PI at livestock auctions is simply unethical because these animals serve as virus-producing machines that expose many other animals, causing potentially devastating disease on the farms of the unknowing purchasers. The most ethical practice is to euthanize these animals on the premises, although otherwise healthy animals may be considered for slaughter. To our knowledge, no studies currently exist on the persistence of BVDV in properly composted carcasses, but data on the survivability of viruses related to BVDV indicate that long-term environmental persistence is unlikely. Alternatively, carcasses of PI animals can be removed from the premises for rendering.

After all animals in the herd have been tested and PI animals removed, testing should focus on the calves born to gestating, non-PI females. After these calves have been tested and PIs removed, testing should focus on new introductions, show animals, semen and embryos, and heifers raised off-site (see numbers 3 and 4 below). The producer must understand, however, that introduction of a novel strain of BVDV onto a farm may result in fetal infection in non-PI, pregnant females, warranting eventual testing of their offspring.

3. Screening of new animals for PI status before introduction into the herd.

Reducing risk of introduction of BVDV is best accomplished by avoiding the purchase of untested cattle. Without question, the greatest disasters resulting from acute BVDV have followed the purchase of assembled cattle from sales to increase herd size. These purchased animals may be PI. Alternatively, they may be acutely infected—in either case, they represent sources of new virus for the herd. In addition, if newly purchased cows or heifers were exposed to BVDV and became viremic in early pregnancy, they may be carrying PI fetuses. Dr. Joe Brownlie in the United Kingdom, a world-renowned expert on BVDV, aptly refers to these individuals as the "Trojan cow" of BVDV transmission. Therefore, for optimal herd protection, purchased adults should be tested before introduction into the herd; later, the offspring that they were carrying at the time of purchase should be tested for PI status too because PI calves can be born to immuno-competent dams. Whenever possible, new herd introductions should be tested and well isolated from the remainder of the herd for 4 to 6 weeks. During this period, any PI animals in the group of new introductions can be identified and removed, and any acutely infected animals can be given adequate time to recover. Any contact between isolated new introductions and the remainder of the herd, even at fence lines, should be avoided during this period.

Tests to detect virus should be used on newly purchased cattle. Virus isolation, PCR, immunohistochemistry, or AC-ELISA on blood or skin biopsies can be used. Pooling of samples can be considered when large numbers of animals are to be introduced (see number 2). Collection of samples for testing for other diseases in newly purchased stock (e.g., Johne's disease, *Mycoplasma* spp. mastitis) can be performed at the same time.

4. Implementation of biosecurity practices to prevent fetal exposure to BVDV.

Fetal infection leading to the PI state is a critical control point because PI animals represent a massive source of viral challenge for the herd. Even with good vaccination practices, all immunity is finite, and overwhelming viral challenge could theoretically lead to transplacental passage of virus even in immunized, pregnant females. Therefore, protection of pregnant cows and heifers from exposure to high viral challenge is a critical goal of BVDV control within a herd biosecurity program.

Contact with cattle outside the herd should be eliminated or minimized, even at fence lines. Cows and heifers in the first trimester of pregnancy should be considered the most susceptible to creation of the fetal PI state. These animals should be located on the farm in the area that is most protected from contact with outside cattle, new introductions, and show cattle. Pen allocation and pen milking sequence should be critiqued and, if necessary, changed to maximize protection of these animals. Contact of these animals with ill cattle should be minimized whenever possible. The possibility of transmission from wild ruminant species exists, such as white-tailed deer, but this probably represents a very unlikely method of acquiring new infection for most commercial U.S. dairies.

Heifers raised and bred at heifer-raising operations warrant particularly careful scrutiny in a BVDV control program. Heifers from multiple herds are often raised on such operations, and viral challenge from PI animals or acute BVDV infections on that operation could easily induce fetal infection in pregnant heifers. Therefore, young heifers should be tested before transport to heifer-raising operations; if this is not feasible, prompt testing after arrival on such operations is warranted. In addition, all calves born to heifers raised offsite should be considered potential PI animals and tested after birth.

Cattle taken to shows should be considered another source of novel virus on a farm. In the ideal world, show cattle should be tested and confirmed to be non-PI before being taken to shows or sales; this is simply a good ethical practice intended to protect other animals and producers. Show cattle should also be well immunized to limit the likelihood of them developing acute infection while off the premises. Given the shortcomings of vaccines in protecting against the tremendous number of strains of BVDV, even well-vaccinated show cattle should be considered potentially exposed to novel BVDV at shows or sales and ideally kept isolated from the home herd for 4 to 6 weeks on return. If exposed at shows, pregnant show cows and heifers may experience viremia of sufficient magnitude to induce fetal infection, and their calves should be subsequently tested for PI status.

Most reputable sources of semen, embryos, and fetal calf serum have BVDV testing strategies in place. However, nothing should be taken for granted, and the individuals or companies providing bull semen or embryos should be requested to provide documentation of their current control programs and quality control measures for reagents. Control of BVDV in embryo and semen production operations has been recently reviewed. In short, acutely or PI bulls, embryo donors, and embryo recipients are potential animal sources of BVDV. Animals within these populations that shed large amounts of virus may cause fetal infection in others, so BVDV testing of all animals with which bulls, embryo donors, and embryo recipients come in contact during semen or embryo collection, transfer, and pregnancy is necessary. Rarely, infected bulls may shed virus only in semen (i.e., test negative on blood or skin IHC), and semen testing by PCR or virus isolation is considered optimal. All animal-origin reagents used in embryo transfer or in vitro fertilization (including semen and oocytes) should be screened for the presence of BVDV.

Winter Dysentery

Etiology

The etiologic agent responsible for winter dysentery has remained elusive for as long as the disease has existed. In the northern hemisphere, the disease is characterized by explosive herd outbreaks of diarrhea between the months of October and April. *Campylobacter fetus jejuni* long was suspected as a cause, but Koch's postulates never were confirmed. MacPherson, however, was able to infect susceptible cattle using filtered feces from infected cows and therefore believed a virus was involved. Bovine coronavirus has been demonstrated in feces and colonic epithelium of affected cattle, and the same strain that causes diarrhea in calves has been used to experimentally create winter dysentery in adult cows. In Europe, Breda virus (*Torovirus* genus) has been associated with winter dysentery outbreaks. In North America, bovine coronavirus is likely responsible for most outbreaks. It may be introduced into the herd by carrier animals or alternatively an established herd member may be a carrier. Virus shedding in the manure during winter months is thought to allow propagation of the virus and may result in infection and clinical signs in susceptible adult cattle and heifers.

Winter dysentery is of economic importance primarily because of production losses both during the acute outbreak and because some cows do not return to previous production levels for the remainder of the lactation. Death losses are minimal but do occur—almost always in first-calf heifers that develop hemorrhagic diarrhea.

The disease is highly contagious and can spread easily from an affected herd to unaffected herds via fomites—both inanimate and animate. Veterinarians, milk tank drivers, inseminators, salespeople, and other farm visitors frequently are blamed for spreading the disease. Newly purchased cattle and cattle attending shows during the fall, winter, or early spring also can be infected and instigate a herd outbreak. Herds experiencing winter dysentery subsequently appear immune for 2 to 3 years, based on clinical impressions that many herds have an outbreak every third year. Relative age-related resistance is observed, but this protection is incomplete. Cattle infected for the first time tend to have more severe clinical signs than those previously affected.

Clinical Signs

Signs include acute diarrhea in 10% to 30% of the cows within a herd followed by similar signs in another 20% to 70% of the animals within the ensuing 7 to 10 days. The diarrhea is explosive and appears semifluid, dark brown in color, has a pea-soup consistency, is malodorous, and forms bubbles as puddles of manure are formed. Most affected cows have decreased appetite, production losses of 10% to 50%, and become mildly to moderately dehydrated. Some develop cool peripheral parts and sluggish rumen motility suggestive of hypocalcemia. Severely affected animals—especially first lactation cattle experiencing the disease for the first time—have hemorrhagic enterocolitis with dysentery and fresh blood clots in the feces. Tenesmus may be present in these animals, and blood loss anemia may develop. A soft, moist cough is often apparent in several of the affected animals, but the lungs auscult normally in these cattle. Fever usually precedes clinical signs by 24 to 48 hours, and experienced clinicians will detect fever in apparently healthy herdmates that have not yet developed diarrhea. Some cattle have mild fever 103.0° to 104.0°F (39.44° to 40.0°C) accompanying the onset of diarrhea. Herd production decreases commensurate with incidence and severity of disease. Affected cows, especially those in mid or late lactation, may not return to previous production levels for the remainder of their current lactation.

Diagnosis

Winter dysentery must be differentiated from dietary diarrhea, coccidiosis, BVDV, and salmonellosis. Dietary indiscretions that induce diarrhea seldom cause fever and are usually associated with feed changes. Coccidiosis can cause diarrhea, dysentery, whole blood clots, and tenesmus in heifers and on very rare occasions in first lactation animals but does not affect multiparous cows. Fecal smears and flotation allow a diagnosis of coccidiosis. Usually BVDV infection causes leukopenia, higher fever, more prolonged disease, and could be ruled out by PCR or viral isolation. The most likely differential diagnosis is salmonellosis caused by types E, K or mildly pathogenic types of B or C *Salmonella* spp. Salmonellosis of these types can cause fever—frequently preceding the onset of diarrhea—and a variable number of animals may develop diarrhea that contains blood, fibrin strands, or mucus. A neutropenia with left shift in the leukogram would suggest acute salmonellosis but is not a consistent finding. Fecal culture obtained from several acute cases is the only way to rule out salmonellosis.

Confirmation of the presumptive diagnosis requires demonstration of bovine coronavirus in feces by electron microscopy, ELISA, or PCR. IHC staining of colonic tissue may be used on necropsy specimens in acute cases. Outbreaks of diarrhea in North American adult cattle that occur outside the October to April time period are unlikely to be winter dysentery.

Treatment

For most affected cattle, supportive treatment with oral astringents remains the time-tested mode of therapy. Occasional high-producing cattle require parenteral calcium solutions to counteract secondary hypocalcemia or treatment of ketosis secondary to reduced appetite. Oral fluids and electrolytes may be necessary for moderately dehydrated cattle. All cattle should have access to salt and to fresh water.

Severely dehydrated cows occasionally require IV fluid therapy, and first-calf heifers that become anemic because of blood loss require fresh whole blood transfusions in some rare instances. Cattle with tenesmus may necessitate epidural anesthesia to allow rest and reduce rectal and colonic irritation.

Treatment usually is only necessary for 1 to 5 days, by which time most affected cows have recovered their appetites and normal manure consistency. Unfortunately, the disease often dwindles through the herd for 7 to 14 days, such that new cases are still appearing at a time when most cattle are recovered. Although there is no proven efficacy to preventive measures, practicing sound herd biosecurity regarding new herd introductions and show cattle may reduce the likelihood of outbreaks (see descriptions in section on BVDV). Furthermore, disinfected boots and equipment should be required for all visitors to a dairy, as well as clean outer garments. The efficacy of immunization with commercially available coronavirus vaccines is currently unknown.

Campylobacter jejuni

Etiology

Campylobacter jejuni, formerly *Vibrio jejuni*, is a gram-negative, curved to spiral, motile rod capable of causing enterocolitis in many species, including humans, in whom the organism is one of the major causes of bacterial enterocolitis. *C. jejuni* may be present in the normal intestinal flora of many domestic animals and people but is found with greater incidence in diarrhea patients. Because of its ubiquitous nature, the significance of isolation of *C. jejuni* from diarrheic feces of cattle is hard to interpret. However, isolation of *C. jejuni* coupled with failure to isolate other pathogens such as *Salmonella* spp., *Clostridium* spp., or enteric viruses should be considered significant.

Diarrhea and other clinical signs vary from inapparent or mild to fulminant and may be influenced by concurrent diseases, stress, inoculum, strain of *C. jejuni*, other enteric pathogens, and other factors. This variation is highlighted by the reported profound differences observed between experimental infection of gnotobiotic calves and experimental infections of calves with normal GI flora. Gnotobiotic calves had mild catarrhal enteritis with minimal clinical signs, but fever, chronic diarrhea for up to 2 weeks, and some degree of dysentery were observed in nongnotobiotic calves. Although most experimental infections have been conducted in calves, adult cattle are thought to be susceptible as well. Infection in people can occur at any age.

The strain of *C. jejuni* and other factors may influence the site of colonization within the intestine, but most strains affect both the small intestine and colon. *C. jejuni* produces a cholera-like enterotoxin that is an important component of pathogenicity. The organism is mucosa associated but does not appear to be invasive, at least in experimental studies.

Clinical Signs and Diagnosis

Mild or inapparent cases yield little or no detectable signs. Clinical patients with severe signs of diarrhea, fever, dehydration, anorexia, cessation of milk production, and dysentery tend to be sporadic or only represent a low percentage of cattle within a herd. Both adult cows and calves are at risk.

The signs are nonspecific and require differentiation from those indicating salmonellosis, coccidiosis, BVDV infection, and other enteric pathogens. Isolation of *C. jejuni* from diarrheic feces and ruling out other enteric pathogens are essential for diagnosis. Enterocolitis resulting from *C. jejuni* seldom is confused with winter dysentery because of low morbidity in the former contrasted with high morbidity in the latter. Salmonellosis represents the primary differential diagnosis.

Treatment

Calves or cattle with severe diarrhea or dysentery may require 7 to 14 days for recovery. Some diarrhea may persist despite improved vital signs in recovering patients. Oral or IV fluids may be required, and it is best to select fluids following blood acid–base and electrolyte analysis. In humans, antibiotics such as erythromycin, tetracycline, fluoroquinolones, and aminoglycosides are often effective, but penicillin, ampicillin, cephalosporins, and trimethoprim–sulfa combinations appear ineffective. Increasing concern exists regarding *C. jejuni* isolates obtained from human cases of campylobacteriosis and antibiotic resistance (see section on calf diarrhea). Antibiotic susceptibilities are not known for *C. jejuni* infections in cattle and would be best determined by fecal culture and susceptibility results.

Control

Because animals and animal products, such as unpasteurized milk and improperly cooked meat, usually are blamed for *C. jejuni* enterocolitis in humans, a positive diagnosis of *C. jejuni* diarrhea in cattle justifies public health concerns. Infected cattle may recover from the infection over several weeks or may remain carriers. Obviously, many cattle (and people) are asymptomatic carriers, so wide-scale herd testing serves little purpose. However, veterinarians should advise caution in handling infected cattle and avoidance of unpasteurized milk on farms where the problem is confirmed. *C. jejuni* will grow in milk and may arrive in milk from septicemic spread but is more likely to contaminate milk because of environmental contact.

Enterotoxemia in Adult Dairy Cattle

Etiology

Enterotoxemia thought to be caused by *C. perfringens* has been observed as a sporadic cause of acute death in adult dairy cattle. Some herds have had endemic problems with more than one cow being found dead or agonal over a few months. Premonitory signs are not observed, and, as in calves, the condition is believed to be related to diets exceptionally rich in protein and energy. *C. perfringens* organisms of multiple types that are present in the intestinal tract take advantage of such rich diets and proliferate to produce excessive exotoxins, especially beta-toxin in the case of *C. perfringens* type C. Two recent reports have identified *C. perfringens* type E associated with hemorrhagic enteritis and abomasitis in adult cattle from both North and South America, suggesting a role for the iota toxin elaborated by this particular organism. Because more than one *C. perfringens* type and toxin have been identified from acute necropsy specimens in adult cattle, it is not known which and how many strains of the organism might be responsible for the adult cow disease.

Clinical Signs

Signs are minimal, and most affected cows are found down, agonal, or already dead. Diarrhea may be observed or the animal simply may have abdominal distension, colic, and depression. Another clinical syndrome is one that causes fever, anorexia, small-volume diarrhea, and death, with severe abomasal edema found at necropsy.

Diagnosis

Fresh necropsy specimens must be obtained if *C. perfringens* is suspected as a cause of acute death. Necropsy lesions, as in calves infected by *C. perfringens* type C, may be minimal but might include small intestinal fluid distension, serosal hemorrhages, and an edematous mesentery. Feces and small intestinal content should be cultured for *C. perfringens*; if possible, luminal contents should be tested for the presence of toxins. Samples should be transported in a cooled but unfrozen state. A complete necropsy to rule out other causes of acute death is imperative because the diagnosis of *C. perfringens* enterotoxemia is suggested by exclusion of other diseases such as peracute, virulent salmonellosis.

Treatment and Control

Treatment is seldom possible, but if a specific *C. perfringens* organism and toxins are identified, vaccination with appropriate toxoids would be indicated for potential control. Nutritional management to prevent "slug" feeding is also prudent, especially with high crude protein diets.

Malignant Catarrhal Fever

Etiology

Malignant catarrhal fever has been observed in domestic and wild ruminants worldwide and is caused by a group of gamma herpesviruses. It is a severe lymphoproliferative disease characterized by high fever, corneal edema, mucosal erosions, and lymph node enlargement in clinically affected animals. Lymphocytic vasculitis of a variety of tissues is the classic microscopic lesion. Many ruminant species and pigs are susceptible to MCF viruses, and losses have been incurred on dairies, feed lots, ranches, game farms, zoos, and deer meat–raising facilities. It also causes high mortality rates in bison. Several epidemiologic forms of MCF exist, and they are classically defined by their reservoir ruminant species. In Africa, the causative agent has been isolated and identified as Alcelaphine herpesvirus-1 (AHV1). The term Alcelaphine relates to the subfamily of Bovidae, Alcelaphinae, in which wildebeest, hartebeest, and topi are classified. These species are thought to be the reservoir. The virus apparently is highly cell associated but can be spread during times of stress such as parturition or shipment and may be free in fetal fluids or the young of wildebeest. At times when the virus is released, it becomes infectious for cattle.

In other parts of the world, including the United States, MCF is termed "sheep associated" because sheep appear to be the most likely reservoir of infection. Ovine herpesvirus type 2 (OvHV2) has been identified from ruminants with MCF using PCR, and seroconversion of cattle with MCF to OvHV2 can be demonstrated using competitive inhibition ELISA (CI-ELISA). Recent molecular studies have identified no significant difference in the genome of OvHV2 from sheep and a cow clinically affected by MCF. This suggests that the pathogenesis of sheep associated MCF is not associated with any genomic rearrangement as had been previously theorized. Even though OvHV2 cannot be cultured in vitro, its genome has been sequenced, allowing an increase in the amount and variety of research on the disease and potentially accelerating progress toward a vaccine. In North America, sheep-associated MCF occurs in cattle, bison, pigs, deer, elk, and moose.

Most sporadic or epidemic MCF in cattle has been associated with proximity to sheep. Outbreaks have most frequently occurred when both sheep and cattle were housed on the same farm or cattle were exposed to sheep at fairs. Infection is widespread in North American sheep, and ovine infection is almost always asymptomatic. Cattle and sheep do not have to interact or be in common pastures for the disease to appear. In cattle, cases can be observed at any time of year, although in bison it has tended to be a late winter or early spring disease. In addition, some cattle that develop MCF have no historical direct or indirect exposure to sheep. Asymptomatic, persistent infections with OvHV2 in cattle may occur, and these infections may or may not develop into clinical MCF. Hence, the incubation period for this disease has been difficult to ascertain, with infected cattle developing disease weeks to months after exposure. This may explain why some cases do not seem linked to exposure to sheep. In one study, most dairy cattle exposed to OvHV2 under natural conditions (close proximity to a sheep feed lot) developed asymptomatic infection rather than overt signs of MCF.

OvHV2 is carried as a lifelong subclinical infection in sheep, and under most husbandry conditions, lambs are not infected as true neonates but after 2 months of age. Rearing sheep from a young age in the absence of adults is a management practice that has proven successful in the reduction of infection prevalence. Nasal shedding by adult sheep is the predominant means of transmission and it is suggested that adolescent sheep (6–9 months of age) shed the most infectious virions; indeed, adult ewes only shed intermittently and at lower amounts then these younger animals. Shedding occurs all year round and contrary to what was often thought there is no association between parturition and increased shedding in ewes.

Clinical Signs

Most cattle affected with MCF have dramatic clinical signs of multisystemic inflammatory disease. Profound pathologic changes can be seen associated with lymphocyte infiltration, diffuse vasculitis, and necrosis throughout the body. Many studies in cattle, bison, and experimental animal infections in rabbits have revealed that CD8 lymphocytes are the predominant cell type associated with vasculitic lesions as well as lymphoid hyperplasia. A great deal of clinical variation is possible, possibly related to the marked variation in tissue tropism demonstrated by OvHV2 at different times in its replication cycle (hence the reason for such difficulty in propagating it in cell culture), and this has caused many authors to categorize MCF based on the predominant organ system involved clinically (i.e., head and eye, enteric, skin). Such categorization is difficult because significant overlap and intermediate clinical situations occur frequently. Sporadic cases are most common in cattle, but herd epidemics have been described in several areas of the United States.

Fever is common in all cases and is high (105.0° to 108.0°F [40.56° to 42.2°C]). Peracute, acute, chronic persistent, and chronic intermittent cases all have fever that usually persists as long as signs are observed. Lymphadenopathy is another finding that is common to most cases. All other signs result from a severe vasculitis that affects many organs but may affect some organs more than others in individual patients. Vasculitis is profound and histologically associated with lymphocytic infiltrates that occasionally can be so extensive as to suggest lymphoreticular neoplasia. Vasculitis affects the GI tract, central nervous system (CNS), eyes, urinary system, liver, skin, upper respiratory tract, and other areas. Hematuria is a common finding if the kidneys and bladder are involved.

Peracute cases may die within 1 to 2 days because of overwhelming viremia and vasculitis of all major organs and yet have minimal clinical signs other than fever, lymphadenopathy, depression, and prostration. Terminal neurologic signs are possible as a result of CNS vasculitis.

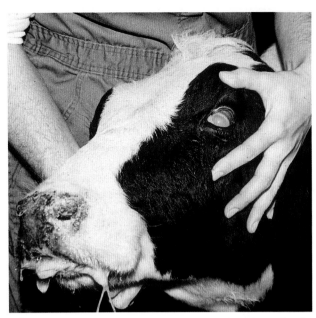

• **Fig. 6.59** Adult Holstein cow with the head and eye form of malignant catarrhal fever.

The classical "head and eye" form of MCF is most common in sporadic cases. This form is characterized by persistent high fever (105.0° to 108.0°F [40.56° to 42.22°C]), lymphadenopathy, severe nasal and oral mucosal lesions, ocular lesions, and remarkable depression (Fig. 6.59). In acute cases, extensive mucosal lesions may make it appear as though the animal has had its mucous membranes burned. Frequently, the muzzle and large regions of the oral mucosa appear hyperemic and have a blanched necrotic epithelium that sloughs to leave erosions and ulcers if the patient survives long enough for this to occur. The muzzle may appear dried or sunburned, and the superficial epithelium subsequently may slough away. Sloughing of the nasal mucosa may result in diphtheritic crusts that occlude the airways. Salivation and copious nasal discharge are typical findings. On occasion, oral and nasal lesions are present in the caudal aspect of the mucosal surfaces, out of visual range during physical examination.

Bilateral ophthalmitis results from vasculitis throughout the eyes that spares only the choroid in most cases. Corneal edema is the most common lesion and occurs because of inflammatory changes and exudative cellular deposits on the corneal endothelium that disrupt this layer, thereby allowing overhydration of the corneal stroma. The corneal edema typically begins at the limbus within 2 to 5 days after the onset of fever. The corneal edema then rapidly spreads to the center of the cornea. This centripetal spread of edema distinguishes the ocular features of MCF from contagious keratoconjunctivitis (pinkeye). A severe anterior uveitis, scleritis, conjunctivitis, and retinitis usually coexist. As in other regions of the body, mononuclear cell infiltrates appear in the eyes. Depression is profound because of CNS vasculitis, and CSF confirms a dramatic inflammation characterized by increased protein values and mononuclear cell pleocytosis. Other neurologic signs are possible. Skin lesions and inflammation of the coronary bands and horn basal epithelium also are possible in those patients that survive more than a few days. The clinical course for most "head and eye" MCF cattle is 48 to 96 hours, although some cases may survive for a longer time, and a few have even been reported to survive.

Acute MCF also may cause severe enterocolitis with diarrhea being a predominant sign. Such cases also are febrile and can have some degree of mucosal lesions, ocular lesions, and other organ involvement. This "enteric form" is again a relative designation because patients frequently have other detectable lesions in addition to diarrhea. However, severe diarrhea may be the most apparent sign and thus may confuse the diagnosis of MCF with BVDV, rinderpest, or other enteric diseases. In bison, enteric signs tend to predominate in acute cases.

Mild forms of MCF also have been observed. The broad spectrum of potential and observed clinical signs in MCF also makes it likely that some cattle have subclinical mild disease such as enteritis, recover, and respond immunologically to the causative virus. Although previously considered to be a highly fatal disease, up to 50% of MCF cases may survive the acute disease to either recover or become chronic cases.

A rare acute form of the disease presents as a severe hemorrhagic cystitis with hematuria, stranguria, and polyuria. Cattle having this form of acute infection have high fever and only survive 1 to 4 days. Although the most striking clinical signs are limited to the urinary system, histologic evidence of vasculitis and lymphocytic infiltration are generalized on necropsy study.

Chronic MCF is characterized by a long clinical course—usually weeks—of high fever, erosive and ulcerative mucosal lesions, bilateral uveitis, papular or hyperkeratotic skin lesions, lymphadenopathy, and digital lesions (Figs. 6.60 and 6.61). Mucosal lesions tend to be severe, slough tissue, and cause salivation and inappetence (Fig. 6.62). Some chronic cases recover only to relapse weeks to months later. Such cases appear healthy between episodes, but recurrence of fever and mucosal, ocular, and skin lesions is debilitating. It is rare for chronic MCF cattle to recover completely and survive.

Diagnosis

Given the wide variability of possible clinical signs of MCF in cattle, the differential diagnosis could include many diseases. Head and eye lesions could be confused with severe IBR associated respiratory and conjunctival infections because corneal edema can occur in some severely affected IBR conjunctivitis cases. However, IBR usually is epidemic and affected animals have characteristic mucosal plaques present on the palpebral conjunctiva and nasal mucosa. Many mucosal diseases such as BVDV, BTV, VSV, EHDV, and FMD may need to be considered depending on the duration, geographic location, and severity of signs. Cattle having severe diarrhea but minimal mucosal lesions could be confused with BVDV infection (see Chapter 16).

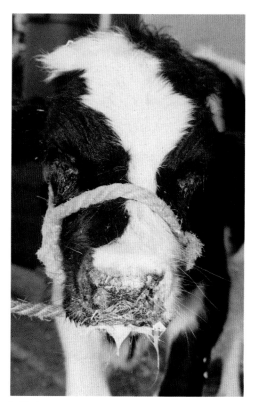

• **Fig. 6.60** A 6-month-old Holstein bull with chronic malignant catarrhal fever.

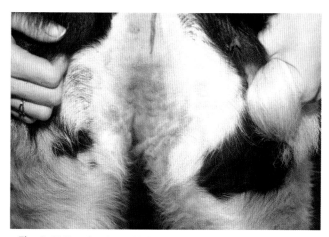

• **Fig. 6.61** Papular dermatitis in the escutcheon region in a calf with chronic malignant catarrhal fever.

Acute bracken fern intoxications, bacillary hemoglobinuria, and other causes of hematuria may be considered in acute MCF characterized by hemorrhagic cystitis. Acute or subacute mucosal lesions that cause sloughing of muzzle epithelium could be confused with primary or secondary (hepatic) photosensitization.

When ocular lesions are present in MCF patients, the diagnosis is made easier because none of the other mucosal diseases cause severe uveitis and such profound panophthalmitis. As mentioned, IBR conjunctivitis can have corneal edema in severe cases, but intraocular inflammation does not occur with IBR. There are no ocular lesions in acute or chronic postnatal BVDV infections.

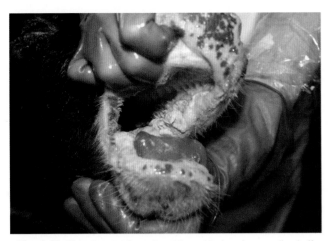

• **Fig. 6.62** Chronic necrotic oral and lingual lesions in a yearling heifer with chronic recurrent malignant catarrhal fever.

The acute mucosal lesions of MCF also are unique in classic cases. The oral mucosa is diffusely inflamed and appears as though the patient drank boiling water. The muzzle mucosa appears burnt, crusty, or eroded in these same patients. Unfortunately, these classic mucosal lesions do not occur in all MCF patients, and patients with multifocal erosions or ulcers can be more difficult to differentiate from those with BVDV and other mucosal diseases.

High fever (105.0° to 108.0°F [40.56° to 42.22°C]) that persists through the entire clinical course is characteristic of most acute MCF cases. Chronic MCF cases also have persistent fever that may or may not be as high as that found in acute cases.

Nervous signs suggest a diagnosis of MCF because CNS involvement is rare with other mucosal diseases. However, high fever and terminal prostration are common in fatal cases of most mucosal diseases and could be confused with neurologic signs.

Clinical diagnosis of MCF can be supported by CSF analysis. The characteristic CSF mononuclear cell pleocytosis and elevated protein value found in MCF patients is useful whenever the patient's clinical signs dictate consideration of differential diagnoses. Confirmation of sheep-associated MCF requires demonstration of the viral genome in the blood through PCR analysis of white cells obtained from a whole blood (ethylenediaminetetraacetic acid [EDTA]) sample. Depending on the primers used, PCR for OvHV2 can be specific for that virus and will not detect the genome of AHV1. Alternatively, CI-ELISA can be used to detect MCF antibodies, but this test may not be positive at the time of initial clinical signs. CI-ELISA detects antibodies to either OvHV2 or AHV1 and cannot currently distinguish between wildebeest-and sheep-associated MCF.

Histopathology allows detection of pathognomonic diffuse vasculitis with lymphocytic infiltrates in many organs, including the GI tract, urinary tract, liver, adrenals, CNS, skin, and eyes. Necrotizing vasculitis is present in lymphoid tissues.

Prevention

Prevention of MCF centers on limiting exposure to infected wildebeest and sheep. Airborne transfer of OvHV2 is suspected to occur over a distance of more than 70 m, so segregation of cattle from sheep by greater distances may be protective. This should be considered when housing cattle and sheep at fairs. For cattle and bison herds, Callan recommends a separation distance of 1 mile from sheep. Carrier (asymptomatically infected) cattle may be identified by CI-ELISA on serum and PCR on whole blood. The CI-ELISA test detects seroconversion in exposed individuals that may, owing to varying viral loads in blood, be intermittently negative by PCR on whole blood. Alternatively, acutely infected animals may be positive on PCR but negative on CI-ELISA owing to the delays inherent in generation of an immune response. Therefore, application of both tests may provide optimal sensitivity for detecting infected cattle. Although OvHV2 DNA can be detected in milk, nasal secretions, and ocular secretions of asymptomatic and clinically affected cattle, this viral DNA appears to be cell associated and does not pose a significant risk for horizontal transmission. Transmission from cattle or bison to other animals has not been demonstrated and is considered likely to be a rare event, if it occurs at all.

Johne's Disease (Paratuberculosis)

Etiology

Paratuberculosis (Johne's disease) is a chronic intestinal infection of cattle and other ruminants, caused by *Mycobacterium avium* subsp. *paratuberculosis* (MAP). The disease has a worldwide distribution, and in the United States, recent surveys conducted by the National Animal Health Monitoring system have demonstrated that 70% to 90% of all U.S. dairies have MAP-infected animals.

The etiologic agent is an acid-fast organism that has fastidious in vitro growth requirements requiring special media and may require up to 16 weeks to cultivate from fecal samples. It survives well in farm environments and can survive for 1 year or more in soil and water. The organism is an intracellular pathogen that survives within macrophages. Although regarded as primarily an enteric infection, as the infection progresses MAP may spread via macrophages in blood or lymph to other important sites such as supramammary lymph nodes, mammary gland, (and milk), and uterus (and fetus). Regional surveillance of Pennsylvania and, indirectly, other areas of the northeastern United States confirmed a dairy cow prevalence of up to 7.3% in many areas. With ever increasing dairy herd size, largely the consequence of purchase of cows of unknown status, the herd prevalence will continue to increase. In the United States, MAP-related average costs have been estimated to lie between $22 and $27 per cow per year, but the economic impact of the disease in positive herds versus confirmed negative herds is much higher and may exceed $100 per cow per year when infection progresses to clinical signs of disease. Without question, this disease is of tremendous economic importance to the entire cattle industry and especially to the dairy industry.

Transmission

The most important means of transmission of MAP is by the fecal–oral route. The MAP organisms are shed in the feces of infected cattle and ingested by susceptible animals. Resistance to infection increases with age, so important sites for exposure include maternity pens, cows' udders, colostrum (especially pooled colostrum), milk or milk replacer feeding implements, calf housing areas, and anywhere young calves can be exposed to feces from adult cows. Direct contact is not necessary because studies have shown that in heavily contaminated farm environments, MAP may aerosolize with dust and contaminate surfaces located short distances from adult cow housing areas. Infected cows can also shed MAP directly in milk, and transplacental transmission has been documented in 20% of subclinically infected pregnant cows and up to 40% of cows with clinical signs of Johne's disease.

Older calves have a more variable outcome after infection, and larger doses of MAP are required to cause infections that lead to later onset of clinical signs. Furthermore, young adult or adult cattle seem to have even greater age-related resistance. However, this resistance is relative rather than absolute, and some experimental infections of older calves and adults have been reported. Factors including concurrent diseases, genetics, environment, and other stressors may contribute to increased susceptibility to infection. Semen and reproductive tracts from infected bulls also have yielded *M. paratuberculosis,* but semen rarely appears to be a source of infection, although of course infected bulls will potentially shed the organism in their feces.

Pathogenesis and Progression

After oral ingestion, MAP organisms invade intestinal epithelial cells, most notably through specialized cells within ileal Peyer patches (M cells), which deliver the organisms to submucosal macrophages. The subsequent course of infection is determined by numerous factors, including the dose of MAP organisms ingested and the animal's individual susceptibility to MAP, which in turn is determined by the age of the animal and the ability of its innate and adaptive immune responses to control MAP. Resistance to MAP infection is estimated to have approximately 10% heritability. Thus, in some exposed animals, MAP organisms will be contained or eliminated by macrophages, and infection will not become established, but in others, the infection will ultimately progress. In the early stages of infection, macrophages are activated by interferon-γ produced by Th1 helper lymphocytes and limit proliferation of the MAP and thereby its spread to other sites. However, the immune response to control MAP results in "collateral damage," inciting a granulomatous response within the intestinal mucosa. This is characterized by progressive infiltration by epithelioid cells, multinucleate giant cells, and lymphocytes surrounding MAP-laden macrophages. In this early stage of infection ("eclipse phase"), during which MAP organisms are slowly proliferating and the inflammatory process is slowly progressing, no clinical signs are observed. The animals are outwardly healthy, fecal shedding of MAP rarely occurs, and serum antibodies are not produced. This makes it very difficult to diagnose the infection at this stage.

Gradually, the ability of the cow to contain the infection wanes, as a Th2 type immune response begins to predominate. Cows remain asymptomatic, but fecal shedding at low levels will begin, and detectable serum antibodies will be produced soon after fecal shedding. Milk production and reproductive performance are not generally affected in these asymptomatic, low-shedding cattle, which can thus serve as a source of MAP for environmental contamination.

Ultimately, spread of the infection accelerates. Fecal shedding at high levels begins, even though there are no clinical signs, and MAP organisms may spread systemically to the mammary gland and fetus. Studies have indicated a 16% reduction in milk production in later stages of asymptomatic infection (i.e., the lactation immediately before culling). Finally, the granulomatous infiltration of the bowel progresses to a severity that results in malabsorption and protein-losing enteropathy, and the cow begins to show the characteristic clinical signs associated with Johne's disease. The entire length of the incubation period before outward signs of illness can be long, often requiring at least 2 to 3 years but up to 10 years in some cases from time of initial infection.

Several points deserve emphasis.

1. Most infected cattle never develop clinical signs before being culled from the herd. Factors that contribute to clinical disease versus asymptomatic infection are not known but probably include organism dose, age at infection, nutrition, concurrent diseases, stresses, and genetics. Infected cattle shed MAP in their manure and transmit the disease to herdmates by MAP contamination of the environment. Herd infection prevalence varies from 20% to 100% in heavily infected herds. Despite this rather high incidence of infection, it is unusual to see clinical signs in more than 5% to 10% of adult cows in the herd per year. Johne's disease has been shown to persist in some herds for more than 10 years with no overt clinical signs of infection.

2. It is widely accepted that cattle that develop clinical signs shed large numbers of organisms and represent the greatest threat to contaminate the environment. Super-shedders may shed MAP in higher concentrations (1–5 million CFU/g of manure) than cattle with clinical disease. Potentially, these animals represent the greatest source of environmental contamination and reservoir for possible transmission to herdmates. Most super-shedders are asymptomatic with no evidence of diarrhea or weight loss yet excrete huge numbers of MAP organisms into the environment.

3. Passive shedding of MAP may occur when noninfected cattle ingest manure contaminated forage or water. With a super-shedder in the herd, ingestion of as little

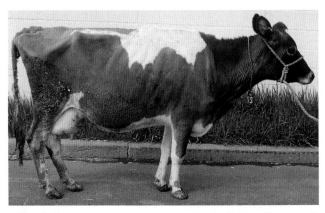

• **Fig. 6.63** Jersey cow affected with Johne's disease. Poor condition, a dry hair coat, and fecal staining of the hind quarters and tail are apparent.

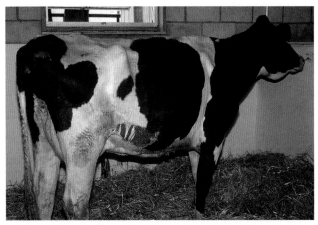

• **Fig. 6.64** Four-year-old Holstein cow with submandibular edema (bottle jaw) and weight loss caused by Johne's disease. Diarrhea was minimal. The diagnosis was confirmed by right flank laparotomy and ileal lymph node biopsy.

as 5 mL of manure contamination in forage may result in passive shedding and give rise to a positive fecal culture for a previously uninfected cow. The risk of misclassification of such cattle must be considered when control programs include fecal cultures of all adult animals and culling decisions are based on the results. It is possible that this phenomenon may represent 50% of all culture-positive cattle in the herd when a super-shedder is present.

Clinical Signs

The hallmark clinical sign of Johne's Disease is watery, projectile diarrhea. It has been described as pea soup in consistency and often forms bubbles because of the rather liquid consistency. In advanced cases, the diarrhea stains the tail, perineum, and hind limbs. It will stain the rear quarters if the tail switches liquid feces onto the quarters, flanks, and gluteal region. There is typically no blood or mucus present, and the animal is afebrile and does not exhibit tenesmus. However, given today's laxative diets, the diarrhea observed in a patient with Johne's disease is best described as looser compared with herdmates. The animal maintains a good appetite and remains well hydrated but has a significant decline in milk production and rapid loss of body condition. As well as temperature, other vital signs are normal. Moderate to advanced clinical cases have obvious weight loss characterized by muscle wasting, a poor dry hair coat, significant production losses, dehydration, and reduced feed intake, particularly high-energy feedstuffs (Fig. 6.63). Protein-losing enteropathy leads to hypoproteinemia with submandibular and brisket edema. Ventral edema is apparent but may vary in the anatomic area involved. Intermandibular, brisket, ventral, udder, and lower limb edema all are possible (Fig. 6.64). Clinical laboratory tests reveal hypoalbuminemia and possibly anemia of chronic disease. Although most cattle infected with MAP remain asymptomatic, cattle with clinical signs signal the diagnosis and alert both veterinarian and herd owner to the possibility of a herdwide problem.

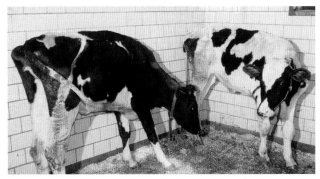

• **Fig. 6.65** A pair of 18-month-old Holstein heifers with advanced Johne's disease. These heifers were representative of an age-grouped epidemic involving 12- to 24-month-old heifers on a single farm. This would imply extremely heavy environmental contamination with *Mycobacterium avium* subspecies *paratuberculosis*.

Despite loose manure, loss of body condition, and diminished milk production, cows with Johne's disease do not appear seriously ill until the terminal stages when finally the appetite is markedly reduced. Occasionally, cattle have diarrhea intermittently rather than continually, but this is unusual. We have also observed cows with Johne's disease with obvious diarrhea that spontaneously reverted to apparently normal manure after shipment to our hospital for diagnosis. Whether stress associated with shipment or a change in diet is responsible for this temporary improvement in fecal consistency is unknown. However, if the animal is not culled, the disease will progress to the point that the animal becomes inappetent, weak, and cachectic, and ultimately death will follow.

Clinical signs develop only after a prolonged incubation period and usually appear between 2 and 5 years of age. However, signs have been observed in heifers younger than 12 months of age and in mature cows up to 8 to 10 years of age (Fig. 6.65). If several 2-year-old heifers in a herd develop clinical signs of diarrhea, it suggests a rather heavy dose of MAP at an early age, but clinical signs in 5- to 7-year-old cows suggest a much lower dose of MAP or older age at the time of exposure. Thus, the age of onset of clinical signs will assist an astute clinician as to the severity of the herd problem. Age of onset is probably affected by many factors, such as dose and duration of exposure to infectious organisms, nutrition, genetics, concurrent diseases or stresses, and other factors. The clinical impression that signs frequently develop after the onset of lactation in the first, second, or third lactations suggests lactational stress may be sufficient to amplify subclinical signs and hypoproteinemia to a clinical state. It also is possible that this observation is simply a reflection of closer monitoring of appetite, production, and body condition in lactating animals as opposed to heifers or dry cows. Lactation stress is not a prerequisite to the development of clinical signs, as proven by bulls and steers having clinical Johne's disease. Interestingly, some severely affected bulls and steers with Johne's disease have developed abomasal displacements during the advanced stages of disease.

Many cattle with signs of Johne's disease are culled because of poor production before the diagnosis is confirmed or suspected. This is especially common in free-stall operations in which an individual cow's manure consistency may not be as obvious as it would be in conventional housing and individual stalls. Dairy cattle with confirmed MAP infection have been shown to have higher cull rates than uninfected herdmates because of weight loss and reduced milk yield when clinical disease is evident and decreased production and mastitis when the infection is still, as yet, subclinical. Subclinical infections have also been associated with infertility. Increased mastitis and reproductive failure may be partially explained by hypoproteinemia, negative energy and protein balance, stress, and poor condition. A recent study on two large Minnesota dairy farms identified a threefold increase in the relative risk for culling in MAP fecal culture–positive cattle compared with fecal culture–negative cows. This study is noteworthy in that these herds were typical upper midwestern free stall dairies with an approximately 8% prevalence for MAP fecal culture positive animals. The calculated costs for lost production alongside diminished cull value associated with being fecal culture positive in this study were substantial, in fact greater than $400 per cow.

Diagnosis

Cattle with advanced signs of Johne's disease are easily suspected of having the disease because of diarrhea, hypoproteinemia, production loss, weight loss, and overall deterioration of condition. The only abnormalities detected routinely in serum biochemistry are hypoalbuminemia, hypoproteinemia, and occasionally hyperphosphatemia (>7 mg/dl). Clinical Johne's disease must be differentiated from chronic gastrointestinal parasitism, chronic salmonellosis, toxicities, intestinal neoplasia, copper deficiency, heart failure, glomerulonephropathies, renal amyloidosis, eosinophilic enteritis, and chronic BVDV infections. Postmortem examination of clinically advanced cases reveals grossly visible thickening and increased corrugation of the

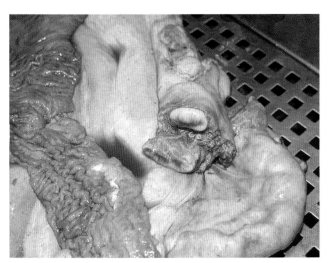

• **Fig. 6.66** Necropsy view of thickened ileum and edematous (cut) ileocecal lymph node from a cow with advanced Johne's disease.

ileal mucosa (Fig. 6.66), and enlargement of the ileocecal lymph nodes. Histopathology confirms a granulomatous enterocolitis with macrophages and epithelioid cells in the submucosa and lower mucosa. Ziehl-Neelsen staining confirms the presence of MAP in the intestine and lymphatics. However, culture of these same tissues has a much greater sensitivity to detect MAP than does histopathology. Lesions may be present in the cecum and colon of advanced clinical cases and can extend orad from the ileum to more proximal regions of the small intestine. Although MAP may be isolated from other organs such as the liver, uterus, or fetus in some advanced cases, gross lesions consisting of granuloma formation are rare in these organs, and truly disseminated infections having gross lesions are very rare. However, disseminated infections as detected by culture of MAP from lymphatic fluid and lymph nodes such as the prescapular, prefemoral, supramammary, or popliteal lymph nodes do occur in cattle with clinical disease. Aortic calcification has been observed in advanced cases. Mild clinical cases may have a thickened edematous ileum with distended lymphatics on the serosal surface (Fig 6.67). Thickening of the mucosal surface and a raised corrugated appearance is typical. Lymphatic distension is obvious on the serosal surface of the ileum, and the ileocecal lymph nodes, as well as other mesenteric lymph nodes, are enlarged and edematous on cut sections.

Available confirmatory antemortem diagnostic tests include those that directly detect the organism in feces or those that detect the animal's immune response to MAP infection. Organism detection methods include culture on solid media (Herrold's Egg Yolk Media [HEYM]), culture on liquid media, or detection by PCR. Organism detection tests have the advantage of detection earlier in the course of disease (compared with ELISA) in most cases because fecal shedding usually precedes the development of antibody production. These tests also have the ability to determine the quantity of MAP organisms being shed and thus are helpful for prioritizing animals for culling based on relative impact on environmental contamination. Culture methods require 4 to 16 weeks for results, depending on the technique used.

Antibody tests used most frequently are serum ELISA or milk ELISA. The complement fixation test and agar gel immunodiffusion tests are inferior in performance, but some nations may still list these tests as being required before importation. The ELISAs have a lower sensitivity to detect asymptomatic fecal shedders (15%) but are often used because they are considerably less expensive and for heavy shedding or clinically affected animals the sensitivity is higher (90%–100% for clinically affected animals).

When presented with an adult animal for which clinical Johne's disease is considered likely, the presence of projectile watery diarrhea, lack of fever, and low plasma protein should raise the index of suspicion, especially if the animal originates from a herd known to harbor the infection. In this situation, a diagnostic test with a rapid turnaround time is essential to aid in clinical decision making. Either ELISA or fecal PCR perform well for this purpose because both have high sensitivity and specificity in evaluation of clinically affected cattle. In contrast, when screening asymptomatic cows in infected herds to assist with culling decisions or biosecurity issues such as maternity pen and colostrum management, organism detection tests are more sensitive than ELISA but may be cost prohibitive and may be positive in passively shedding, noninfected cattle. A cost effective approach is to use milk ELISA, using not just the dichotomous results (i.e., "positive" or "negative") but using the quantitative result (optical density (OD) value or sample to positive (S/P) ratio), recognizing that the strongest reactors are most likely to be heavy fecal shedders and pose the greatest risk for contaminating the environment with MAP. Unfortunately, neither organism detection tests nor antibody tests are useful in screening asymptomatic young cattle (<3 years of age) as herd replacements or for use as embryo transfer recipients because cattle at this age are usually in the "eclipse" phase of infection and will be test negative even if infected. Surgical biopsy of the ileum and ileocecal lymph node could detect MAP infection in these animals but is generally not practical for this screening purpose. The most effective way to prevent introduction of MAP is to purchase animals from herds known to be free of MAP, such as herds that have achieved status 4 level or above in the Voluntary Johne's Disease Control Program.

The gold standard for diagnosis has long been considered culture of ileum, ileocecal lymph nodes, or other mesenteric lymph nodes for cattle with clinical Johne's disease. This technique has been used to identify Johne's disease–infected cattle at slaughterhouses and to gather epidemiologic data regarding prevalence of the disease. Although harvesting ileocecal lymph nodes constitutes an invasive procedure for clinical patients, extremely valuable or individually purchased cows suspected of having Johne's disease may warrant this invasive technique to diagnose the condition definitively, especially when the herd has not been known to have Johne's disease in the past. A right flank exploratory laparotomy is performed to harvest a full-thickness 1.0-cm wedge of ileum and an ileocecal lymph node. The

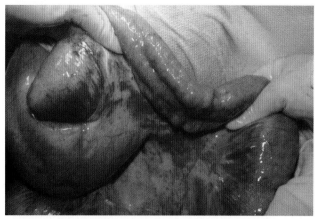

• **Fig. 6.67** Thickened, edematous ileum and visibly distended lymphatics on the serosal surface in a cow showing early signs of Johne's disease. A rapid definitive diagnosis was established by biopsy of the ileum and ileocecal lymph node.

ileal biopsy and half of the lymph node are submitted for culture and histopathology, including a Ziehl-Neelsen stain. The remaining half of the lymph node is used for impression smears that are stained for acid-fast organisms. An absolute diagnosis usually is possible from the impression smears, but if this fails or is questionable, the histopathology generally confirms or denies the diagnosis without the prolonged delay associated with cultures.

Treatment

Cattle with clinical Johne's disease are rarely treated. Occasionally, valuable animals may be treated to allow for salvage of genetic material by embryo transfer or to prolong the life of "pet" cattle. Treatment should not be undertaken to salvage the fetus of a pregnant cow with Johne's disease because in utero infection is likely. Uninfected embryos can be obtained from infected cows, via conventional embryo transfer provided proper embryo washing steps are followed, or after in vitro fertilization subsequent to oocyte pickup.

Owners that wish to undertake treatment should be advised that daily, lifelong treatment is required; treated animals may continue to shed MAP in their feces even if clinical signs are reversed; and relapse will ensue when treatment is stopped. Treatment involves extra-label use of antimicrobial medications for an extended period, which in the United States must comply with regulations set forth in the AMDUCA. Thus, owners should be advised that the treated animal or its products must not enter the human food supply chain.

Monensin is an ionophore antibiotic shown to have activity against MAP and have a beneficial effect in infected cattle. Monensin, approved in the United States as a feed additive, may not be used in an extra-label fashion according to the dictates of AMDUCA. However, if the drug can be legally prescribed for its other indications (coccidiostat, rumen digestion efficiency), it might be used. Clofazimine is an antileprosy drug that has been successfully used to treat Johne's disease at a dose of 2 mg/kg, orally every 24 hours, alone or in combination with other antimicrobials. Resolution of diarrhea and improvement in plasma total protein can be observed within 2 weeks of starting treatment, although fecal shedding may continue. The drug is no longer available from commercial sources in the United States, so alternative antimycobacterial medications such as isoniazid (10–20 mg/kg orally every 24 hours) combined with rifampin (10 mg/kg orally every 24 hours) are often used. Rifampin usage in the United States currently requires a commitment from the producer that neither milk nor meat from that individual will ever be sold for human consumption, further diminishing the likelihood of dairy cattle ever being treated for this condition.

Control

Herds that are free of MAP can best prevent introduction of the disease by maintaining a closed herd. Purchase of replacement cattle from herds of unknown status poses a great risk for introducing asymptomatic but MAP-infected animals. If herd additions must be purchased, they should be purchased from herds participating in the Voluntary Johne's Disease Control Program that have achieved status level 4 or higher. If this cannot be done, then depending on the age of replacement animals, prepurchase testing for MAP infection may not be a foolproof method of screening new additions (see earlier).

Control of the disease in infected herds will depend in part on the objectives of the herd. Large production herds with no interest in selling replacement cattle may perceive little financial incentive to spend money on controlling the disease because they believe that culling for other reasons will often occur before MAP infection affects production. At the opposite end of the spectrum, eradication may be the goal for a herd from which genetic seed stock will be sold, requiring an aggressive, prolonged, and potentially impressive strategy, including test-and-cull strategies using organism detection tests, with management changes to prevent transmission. Although difficult, eradication of the infection from a herd will require intensive and repeated use of fecal cultures on all animals older than 24 months of age for many years.

Calves should be born in disinfected, cleaned maternity areas and removed from the dam immediately. Calves should be raised completely separately—preferably on a separate farm—from the adult cattle. All calves should be fed colostrum from ELISA-negative, or better, fecal culture–negative cows. Pooled colostrum feeding to calves should be avoided in herds with infected cattle. Colostral replacements could be used as a substitute for colostrum in herds with a high MAP incidence, but their use as a replacement for colostrum may lead to an increased incidence of other diseases in calves such as septicemia or diarrhea. Colostrum that is properly heat treated (60 min at 60°C and with constant stirring) will reduce the number of MAP but might not eliminate the organism completely from the colostrum. If whole milk is fed to calves in known infected herds, pasteurization should be considered. The purchase of replacement animals from herds of unknown Johne's disease status continues to represent the greatest risk to introduce or reintroduce MAP to such herds. Minimizing fecal contamination of feedstuffs, water, pastures, and exposure of calves to adult cow feces

are essential and must be evaluated on an individual herd basis. Equipment used for manure removal or that could be contaminated by manure must remain separate from feeding implements and the calf environment. Although these principles for eradication are seemingly straightforward, they may not be practical or affordable in many instances. In between these two extremes, production herds that wish to "contain" the disease, to prevent the prevalence of MAP infection from increasing on the farm, and to reduce the risk of losing animals or milk production to clinical Johne's disease may use an intermediate approach. This may include identifying heavily infected animals through interpretation of milk or serum ELISA alongside management steps to reduce exposure of calves to MAP from feces of adult cows that are potentially shedding the organism. Additionally, these same herds may choose to sell heavy shedders (based on ELISA serology results) or clinical cases immediately, and moderate shedders would be culled at the end of their current lactation.

In the United States, the only licensed vaccine (Mycopar, Boehringer Ingelheim Vetmedica, St. Joseph, MO) is a suspension of heat-killed organisms in an oil adjuvant. Vaccination is shown to prevent or reduce losses from the development of clinical Johne's disease in vaccinated animals. However, it does not prevent infection with MAP, and vaccinated cattle can become infected and shed MAP in feces, although importantly the vaccine does prevent clinical disease in almost all recipients. Any protection from vaccination may be overcome by failure to implement other management changes to reduce exposure to the organism. Vaccination is normally only used in herds experiencing significant losses caused by Johne's disease and should be combined with management changes designed to reduce the spread of infection between cattle. Permission from the state veterinarian is required, and a complete herd tuberculosis (TB) test must be performed before implementation. The vaccine is administered SC in the brisket and frequently predisposes to a local abscess over the next few months or years. Vaccination can result in false-positives on the caudal tail fold test for TB and will also result in positive serology for paratuberculosis. Accidental self-injection of the vaccine can result in a severe painful granulomatous inflammatory response at the site of injection.

Foreign Animal Diseases

Mucosal diseases such as BVDV, BTV, EHDV, MCF, and VSV require differentiation from foreign animal diseases that threaten livestock in the United States (Table 6.9). Extreme vigilance is necessary to prevent entrance of these diseases to this country, and consultation with regulatory state or federal veterinarians is imperative whenever confusion exists. Because a great deal of overlap is possible for the clinical signs present in domestic and foreign mucosal diseases, positive diagnosis including appropriate serologic and virologic confirmation is essential. A description of rinderpest is included in the table for completeness although the World Health Organization declared that it had been completely eradicated globally in 2011.

TABLE 6.9	Foreign or Exotic Animal Diseases Affecting the Gastrointestinal Tract				
Disease	Cause	Clinical Signs	Major Differential Diagnosis	Diagnosis	Reference
Foot-and-mouth disease (Aftosa)	FMDV = genus *Aphthovirus*, family Picornaviridae	Fever, salivation, lip smacking, lameness, teat lesions	Vesicular stomatitis	Call regulatory veterinarians	Kahrs (1981)
(Aphthous fever)	Seven distinct serotypes with multiple subtypes	Vesicles progressing to erosions and ulcers of oral mucosa, nasal mucosa, interdigital space, coronary band, teats Abortion	BVDV Bluetongue MCF Rinderpest	Fluid from vesicles Oropharyngeal fluid Tissues Paired sera	Sutmoller (1992)
Rinderpest (cattle plague) (Peste bovine)	RV=genus *Morbillivirus*, family Paramyxoviridae	Peracute—high fever, death	BVDV	Call regulatory veterinarians	Kahrs (1981)
	One major serotype with field strains possessing variable pathogenicity	Classic fever, mucous membrane congestion, necrosis, and subsequent erosion	MCF Vesicular stomatitis Foot-and-mouth disease	Samples best obtained from febrile animals with mucosal lesions (early cases)	
		Mucous membrane lesions cause salivation, ocular discharge	Salmonellosis Bluetongue	Serologic testing Viral isolation	Seek and Cook (1992)
		Severe hemorrhagic diarrhea and tenesmus start several days after mucosal lesions	Arsenic poisoning		
		Dehydration, death Subacute or atypical; lower mortality, greater difficulty in distinguishing from differential diagnosis			

BVDV, bovine viral diarrhea virus; *FMDV,* foot and mouth disease virus; *MCF,* malignant catarrhal fever

Liver Abscess

Etiology

Abscesses of the liver occur in all ages of cattle. In calves, liver abscesses are often the result of omphalophlebitis; in older cattle, they most often are secondary to reticulorumenitis. In feedlot cattle, it is well recognized that the change from pasture to a high-concentrate ration causes a rapid increase in rumen fermentation and organic acid production, which may result in erosion and inflammation of the rumen epithelium. Metastasis of bacteria from the inflamed and necrotic rumen wall to the liver occurs via the portal vein. In dairy cattle, similar failure of adaptation of rumen fermentation may occur at the onset of lactation when there is an abrupt increase in the energy content of the diet. Liver abscesses are therefore common potential sequelae to acute or subacute rumen acidosis; indeed, their presence in several cows within a herd should raise concern about nutritional management and the likelihood of subacute rumen acidosis as a herd problem. Liver abscesses also may occur as a result

of traumatic reticulitis, where they tend to be an individual cow problem. The most common organisms isolated from hepatic abscesses are *Fusobacterium necrophorum, Bacteroides nodosus,* and *Trueperella pyogenes.* Streptococci and staphylococci also may be isolated from mixed cultures.

Clinical Signs

Local, circumscribed liver abscesses are characteristically silent clinically and are not associated with systemic abnormalities or with hepatic dysfunction. Such abscesses are found incidentally during the postmortem examination of slaughtered cattle or during abdominal ultrasound examination but are often only of importance economically because of the condemnation of affected livers. As mentioned earlier, the repeated identification of such abscesses either postmortem or by ultrasonography should serve as a sentinel warning regarding nutritional management.

Liver abscesses, when located adjacent to the vena cava, may distort the vessel wall and cause phlebitis and

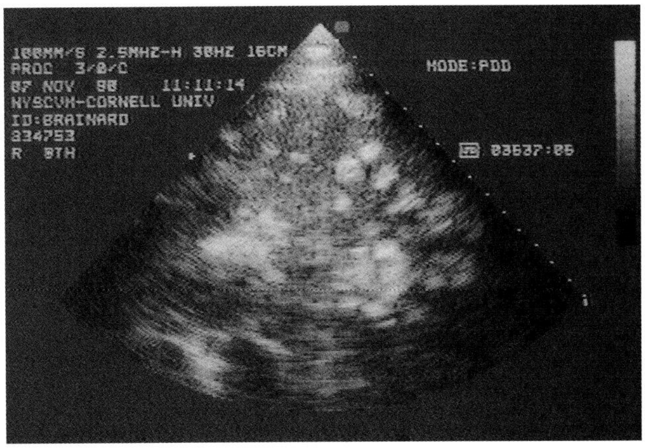

• **Fig. 6.68** Transabdominal sonogram of the liver in a mature cow with multiple hyperechoic abscesses. The hyperechoic appearance suggests dense purulent exudate, decreasing the chances of successful treatment.

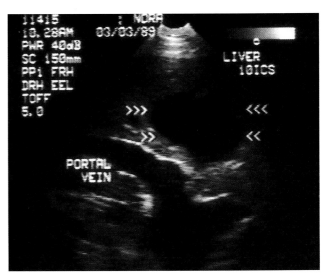

• **Fig. 6.69** Transabdominal sonogram of the liver in a 3-year-old Holstein cow with weight loss and diminished production. A single large hypoechoic abscess can be seen, and the cow recovered after 1 month of systemically administered penicillin treatment.

thrombosis. Septic thromboembolism from the vena cava may cause a respiratory syndrome, referred to as caudal vena caval thrombosis syndrome, characterized by cough, dyspnea, or pulmonary hemorrhage that is described in Chapter 4. In a postmortem series of 6337 slaughtered cattle, liver abscesses were found in 368 (5.8%), and of these, 24% were located in the craniodorsal aspect of the liver with the potential for causing vena caval thrombosis.

Liver abscesses may be associated with constitutional abnormalities that include fever, anorexia, weight loss, and reduced milk production. Neutrophilic leukocytosis and significant increases in serum globulin and fibrinogen are characteristic. Hepatic derived enzymes may not be elevated in the serum of affected cattle, although GGT values may be increased with large abscesses. Growth of a liver abscess near the common bile duct may obstruct bile flow and may result in clinical signs and laboratory abnormalities associated with impeded flow of bile (see below). Liver abscessation also has been recognized as a cause of vagal indigestion.

Ultrasonographic examination of the liver is a valuable diagnostic procedure for determining the location of the abscess(es) and for evaluating prognosis and response to therapy (Figs. 6.68 and 6.69). The lesions may vary in diameter from a few centimeters to more than 20 cm. Characteristically, they may be visualized in three or four adjacent intercostal spaces, and needle aspiration may not be necessary for diagnosis. On rare occasion a large liver abscess can be seen on radiographs displacing the diaphragm (Fig. 6.70).

Treatment

When liver abscesses are recognized clinically and their location identified, it is possible to consider antibiotic therapy, surgical drainage, or both. The decision regarding drainage of liver abscesses depends on the size, location, and the condition of the cow. Penicillin treatment can be successful in some cows with smaller, hypoechoic abscesses, but relapses often occur unless treatment is for 4 or more weeks. Even with surgical drainage, relapses may occur. The prognosis for treatment of liver abscesses that have caused clinical signs is guarded and is least favorable for large and hyperechoic

abscesses. Successful surgical treatment of a liver abscess that caused vagal indigestion has been described.

Bile Duct Obstruction and Cholangitis

Intrahepatic cholestasis is observed in lactating cattle with severe fatty liver during the periparturient period and is described in Chapter 15. Intrahepatic cholestasis may also occur from "sludge" or stones within hepatic ducts (see Video Clip 6.2). Extrahepatic cholestasis is caused by obstruction of bile flow from choleliths within the common bile duct or by obstruction of flow in the common bile duct as a result of external mechanical pressure exerted on the common bile duct by liver abscesses, by extensive adhesions in the area of the cystic and common bile ducts, or by smaller inflammatory lesions of the common duct near the hilus or the duodenal papilla.

The characteristic sterility of the biliary tract is maintained by the continued production and flow of bile into the intestine. Partial or complete obstruction of bile flow predisposes to ascending infection of the biliary tract by intestinal microorganisms. Infection of the biliary tree causes cholangitis and may result in significant alterations in the physical characteristics of bile, including the accumulation of inspissated products of inflammation and of precipitated bile constituents (bile acids, cholesterol, and even stone formation) (Fig. 6.71), which further impedes the flow of bile.

The clinical signs of extrahepatic bile duct obstruction and cholangitis include malaise, colic, fever, icterus with orange-colored urine (Fig. 6.72), and, in some cases photodermatitis (Fig 6.73) secondary to retention of phylloerythrin. Abnormal laboratory findings consist of leukocytosis, hyperfibrinogenemia, hyperbilirubinemia, bilirubinuria, and elevations in serum globulin and the activities of sorbitol dehydrogenase (SDH), aspartate aminotransferase (AST), alkaline phosphatase (AP), and gamma glutamyltransferase (GGT). Ultrasonographic

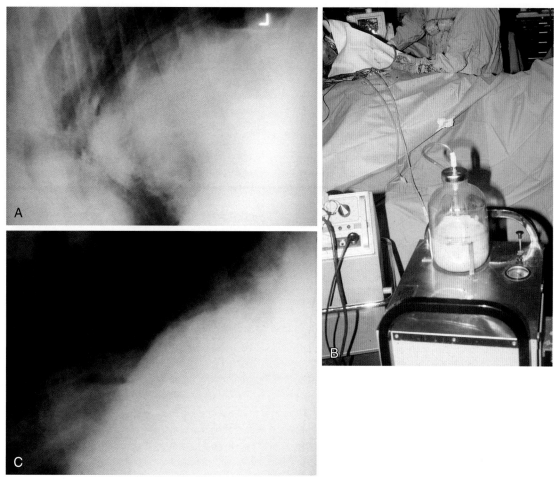

• **Fig. 6.70 A,** Thoracic radiographs of a 14-month-old Holstein heifer showing a very large mass (liver abscess) displacing the diaphragm. **B,** The liver abscess was drained surgically. **C,** Radiographs repeated after drainage.

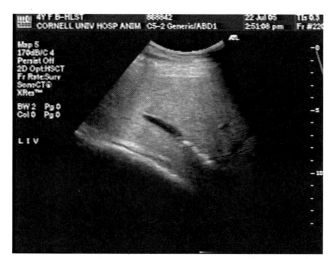

• **Fig. 6.71** Abdominal sonogram of an adult Holstein cow hospitalized because of anorexia and mild colic. The cow's γ-glutamyl transferase level was 1500 U/L. Stones are observed in the intrahepatic ducts. There was a marked clinical improvement within 3 days of initiating therapy with penicillin, intravenous fluids, flunixin meglumine, and forced feeding.

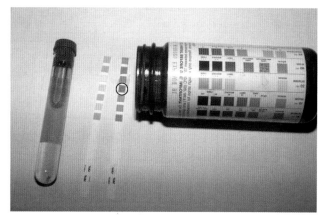

• **Fig. 6.72** A sample of urine collected from an adult cow with icteric membranes, fever, anorexia, depression, and hepatogenous photosensitization of the muzzle. The cow responded well to symptomatic treatment similar to the patient described in Fig. 6.71. The urine is orange and positive on multistrip examination for bilirubin. The *circled square* is a positive test result. There is an untested strip to the left.

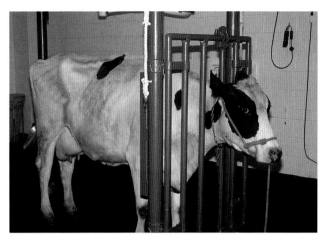

• **Fig. 6.73** The cow described in Fig. 6.72 with pronounced hyperemia (photosensitive dermatitis) of the muzzle.

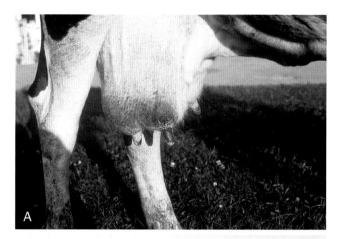

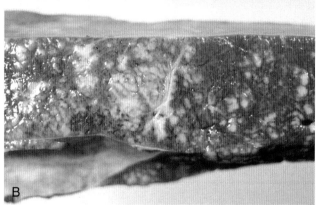

• **Fig. 6.74** **A,** An 8-year-old Holstein cow with weight loss, inappetence, and photosensitization, which is best seen on the teats and udder. **B,** The cow had a cholangiocarcinoma.

findings in cows with extrahepatic cholestasis include severe dilatation of the gallbladder, the cystic and common duct, and other major intrahepatic bile ducts. Dilatation of the gallbladder is not specific because in all anorectic cows, the gallbladder may be distended. The diagnostic findings for extrahepatic cholestasis, however, are dilatation of the cystic and common bile ducts and of the major intrahepatic bile ducts (see Video Clip 6.3).

A case of cholelithiasis with cholestasis has been reported by Drs. Rebhun and Cable that was clinically similar to those in which bile duct obstruction is caused by external mechanical pressure on the common bile duct. A laparotomy was performed, and concretions 1 to 3 cm in diameter were palpated in the gallbladder. The choleliths in the gallbladder were crushed manually, and the material was massaged through the distended cystic and common ducts, into the duodenum, and on into the jejunum. After the procedure, there was significant improvement in clinical condition and in liver function test results, although the improvement was transient.

A syndrome of unknown etiology has been observed that is clinically similar to that of extrahepatic obstruction to the flow of bile but in which there is no ultrasonographic or laparotomy evidence of extrahepatic cholestasis. The clinical signs and laboratory test results are similar. When force fed for a few days and treated with penicillin for at least 1 month, there has been gradual improvement in clinical signs and laboratory abnormalities return to normal (see Figs 6.72 and 6.73).

Primary hepatic neoplasms are unusual in cattle but could cause obstruction of bile flow and should be considered in cows with both icterus and photosensitization. In a necropsy series of 66 primary bovine hepatic neoplasms, 40 were classified as hepatocellular carcinomas, 10 as hepatocellular adenomas, and 10 as cholangiocellular tumors. Less frequently observed primary tumors of the liver in this series included hemangiosarcoma, hemangioma, fibroma, and Schwannoma. In the postmortem examination of the livers of 24,169 slaughtered cattle, primary liver tumors of hepatocellular

origin were identified in 22 (0.09%). In a third series of 1.3 million livers of cattle examined at slaughter, 36 had primary liver tumors of which 13 were classified as primary hepatocellular neoplasms and 21 as cholangiocarcinomas.

The clinical signs of cattle associated with primary hepatic neoplasms have not been extensively described. The expected clinical signs would be those associated with the growth of an expanding hepatic mass or with metastasis to the lung or to the spleen, both of which have been observed at necropsy. If the tumor obstructs bile flow, then icterus and photosensitization would be expected (Fig. 6.74). One of the authors (SP) has also seen hyperammonemic hepatic encephalopathy associated with an extensive cholangiocarcinoma and complete biliary obstruction in an aged cow. Dermatitis caused by photosensitization is frequently most severe on the teats and muzzle, although it may be more generalized (Fig. 6.75). Ultrasonography should be of value in locating, guiding biopsy, and otherwise assessing the location and prognosis of primary liver tumors.

Hepatic Insufficiency Associated with Sepsis

A syndrome of hepatic insufficiency has been described in lactating cattle after acute septic mastitis or metritis

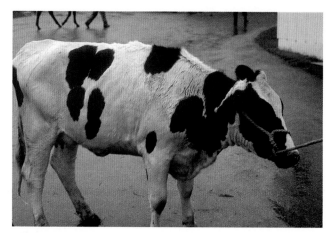

• **Fig. 6.75** Hepatogenous photosensitization caused by a suspected hepatotoxin.

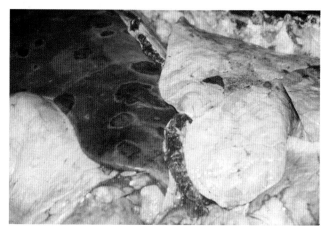

• **Fig. 6.76** The liver from a 6-year-old Holstein that had intestinal (forestomach and abomasum) and hepatic aspergillosis secondary to generalized sepsis and treatment with broad-spectrum antibiotics.

in which the initial clinical signs were compatible with endotoxemia. Subsequent clinical signs included anorexia; weight loss; reduced milk production; and, in one case, photodermatitis. In addition to increased serum activities of liver enzymes, the cows had remarkable delays in the sulfobromophthalein (BSP) plasma clearance test. Liver biopsies showed hepatocellular vacuolization or necrosis that was attributed to the effects of endotoxemia associated with acute systemic infection. Similar hepatic injury has been reported in humans after endotoxic shock. Five such cases were treated by force feeding and with other symptomatic support. Three of the cows responded satisfactorily to therapy, one failed to respond, and the fifth cow was lost to follow-up evaluation. Based on these observations, it is important to consider the possibility of hepatic injury in the initial management of cows with postpartum sepsis and in their longer term management when there is a sluggish response to therapy of the acute disease. If there is a history of prolonged antimicrobial therapy, intestinal and hepatic mycosis must also be considered (Fig. 6.76). Cows with persistent fever, complete anorexia and elevation of hepatic origin enzymes in the serum after prolonged

antimicrobial treatment for diseases such as mastitis or rumenitis may have intestinal and hepatic mycosis. This is usually a fatal disease.

Acknowledgment

We would like to thank Dr. Dave Van Metre, Professor at Colorado State University, Dr. Robert Whitlock, Emeritus Professor at the University of Pennsylvania, and Dr. Bud Tennant*, Emeritus Professor at the New York State College of Veterinary Medicine at Cornell University for their contributions in the previous edition of Diseases of Dairy Cattle.

Recommended Readings

Abeywardena, H., Jex, A. R., & Gasser, R. B. (2015). A perspective on *Cryptosporidium* and *Giardia* with an emphasis on bovines and recent epidemiological findings. *Adv Parasit, 88,* 244–283.

Abutarbush, S. M., Carmalt, J. L., Wilson, D. G., et al. (2004). Jejunal hemorrhage syndrome in 2 Canadian beef cows. *Can Vet J, 45,* 48–50.

Abutarbush, S. M., & Radostits, O. M. (2005). Jejunal hemorrhage syndrome in dairy and beef cattle: 11 cases (2001 to 2003). *Can Vet J, 46,* 711–715.

Acres, S. D. (1985). Enterotoxigenic Escherichia coli infections in newborn calves: a review. *J Dairy Sci, 68,* 229–256.

Adaska, J. M., Aly, S. S., Moeller, R. B., et al. (2014). Jejunal hematoma in cattle: a retrospective case analysis. *J Vet Diag Invest, 26,* 96–103.

Adhikari, B., Besser, T. E., Gay, J. M., et al. (2009). The role of animal movement, including off-farm rearing of heifers, in the interherd transmission of multidrug-resistant *Salmonella. J Dairy Sci, 92,* 4229–4238.

Ahmed, A. F., Constable, P. D., & Misk, N. A. (2001). Effect of orally administered cimetidine and ranitidine on abomasal luminal pH in clinically normal milk-fed calves. *Am J Vet Res, 62,* 1531–1538.

Alcaine, S. D., Sukhnanand, S. S., Warnick, L. D., et al. (2005). Ceftiofur-resistant Salmonella strains isolated from dairy farms represent multiple widely distributed subtypes that evolved by independent horizontal gene transfer. *Antimicrob Agents Chemother, 49,* 4061–4067.

Al-Mashat, R. R., & Taylor, D. R. (1980). Production of diarrhoea and dysentery in experimental calves by feeding pure cultures of Campylobacter fetus subspecies jejuni. *Vet Rec, 107,* 459–464.

Almawly, J., Prattley, D., French, N. P., et al. (2013). Utility of halofuginone lactate for the prevention of natural cryptosporidiosis of calves, in the presence of co-infection with rotavirus and *Salmonella typhimurium. Vet Parasit, 197,* 59–67.

Anderson, B. C. (1988). Gastric cryptosporidiosis of feeder cattle beef and dairy cows. *Bov Pract, 23,* 99–101.

Ares-Mazas, E., Lorenzo, M. J., Casal, J. A., et al. (1997). Effect of a commercial disinfectant ('Virkon') on mouse experimental infection by Cryptosporidium parvum. *J Hosp Infect, 36,* 141–145.

Arthington, J. D., Jaynes, C. A., Tyler, H. D., et al. (2002). The use of bovine serum protein as an oral support therapy following coronavirus challenge in calves. *J Dairy Sci, 85,* 1249–1254.

Audet, S., Crim, R., & Beeler, J. (2000). Evaluation of vaccines, interferons, and cell substrates for pestivirus contamination. *Biologicals, 28*, 41–46.

Baines, D., Erb, S., Turkington, K., et al. (2011). Mouldy feed, mycotoxins and Shiga toxin – producing *Escherichia coli* colonization associated with jejunal hemorrhage syndrome in beef cattle. *BMC Veterinary Research, 7*, 24–33.

Bartier, A.L., Windemeyer, M. C., & Doepel, L. (2015). Evaluation of on-farm tools for colostrum quality measurement. *J Dairy Sci, 98*, 1878–1884.

Bellamy, J., & Acres, S. D. (1983). A comparison of histopathological changes in calves associated with K99- and K99+ strains of enterotoxigenic *E. coli. Can J Comp Med, 47*, 143–149.

Berchtold, J. F., Constable, P. D., Smith, G. W., et al. (2005). Effects of intravenous hyperosmotic sodium bicarbonate on arterial and cerebrospinal fluid acid-base status and cardiovascular function in calves with experimentally induced respiratory and strong ion acidosis. *J Vet Intern Med, 19*, 240–251.

Berghaus, R. D., McCluskey, B. J., & Callan, R. J. (2005). Risk factors associated with hemorrhagic bowel syndrome in dairy cattle. *J Am Vet Med Assoc, 226*, 1700–1706.

Bertone, A., & Rebhun, W. C. (1984). Tracheal actinomycosis in a cow. *J Am Vet Med Assoc, 185*, 221–222.

Besser, T. E., & Gay, C. C. (1985). Septicemic colibacillosis and failure of passive transfer of colostral immunoglobulin in calves. *Vet Clin N Am Food Anim Pract, 1*, 445–459.

Besser, T. E., Gay, C. C., & Pritchett, L. (1991). Comparison of three methods of feeding colostrum to dairy calves. *J Am Vet Med Assoc, 198*, 419–422.

Besser, T. E., Lejeune, J. T., Rice, D. H., et al. (2005). Increasing prevalence of Campylobacter jejuni in feedlot cattle through the feeding period. *Appl Environ Microbiol, 71*, 5752–5758.

Besser, T. E., McGuire, T. C., Gay, C. C., et al. (1988). Transfer of functional immunoglobulin G (IgG) antibody into the gastrointestinal tract accounts for IgG clearance in calves. *J Virol, 62*, 2234–2237.

Bettini, G., & Marcato, P. S. (1992). Primary hepatic tumours in cattle. A classification of 66 cases. *J Comp Pathol, 107*, 19–34.

Bezek, D. M., & Mechor, G. D. (1992). Identification and eradication of bovine viral diarrhea virus in a persistently infected dairy herd. *J Am Vet Med Assoc, 201*, 580–586.

Bistner, S. I., Rubin, L. F., & Saunders, L. Z. (1970). The ocular lesions of bovine viral diarrhea-mucosal disease. *Pathol Vet, 7*, 275–285.

Blanchard, P. C. (2012). Diagnostics of dairy and beef cattle diarrhea. *Vet Clin N Am Food Anim Pract, 28*, 443–464.

Boileau, M. J., & Kapil, S. (2010). Bovine coronavirus associated syndromes. *Vet Clin N Am Food Anim Pract, 26*, 123–146.

Bolin, S. R., & Grooms, D. L. (2004). Origination and consequences of bovine viral diarrhea virus diversity. *Vet Clin N Am Food Anim Pract, 20*, 51–68.

Bolin, S. R., McClurkin, A. W., Cutlip, R. C., et al. (1985). Severe clinical disease induced in cattle persistently infected with noncytopathic bovine viral diarrhea virus by superinfection with cytopathic bovine viral diarrhea virus. *Am J Vet Res, 46*, 573–576.

Bonneau, K. R., DeMaula, C. D., Mullens, B. A., et al. (2002). Duration of viraemia infectious to *Culicoides sonorensis* in bluetongue virus-infected cattle and sheep. *Vet Microbiol, 88*, 115–125.

Booth, A. J., & Naylor, J. M. (1987). Correction of metabolic acidosis in diarrheal calves by oral administration of electrolyte solutions with or without bicarbonate. *J Am Vet Med Assoc, 191*, 62–68.

Borzacchiello, G., Iovane, G., Marcante, M. L., et al. (2003). Presence of bovine papillomavirus type 2 DNA and expression of the viral oncoprotein E5 in naturally occurring urinary bladder tumours in cows. *J Gen Virol, 84*(Pt II), 2921–2926.

Braun, U. (2005). Ultrasound as a decision-making tool in abdominal surgery in cows. *Vet Clin North Am Food Anim Pract, 21*, 33–35.

Braun, U., Gotz, M., & Guscetti, F. (1994). Ultrasonographic findings in a cow with extrahepatic cholestasis and cholangitis. *Schweiz Arch Tierheilkd, 136*, 275–279.

Braun, U., Pospischil, A., Pusterla, N., et al. (1995). Ultrasonographic findings in cows with cholestasis. *Vet Rec, 137*, 537–543.

Braun, U., Pusterla, N., & Wild, K. (1995). Ultrasonographic findings in 11 cows with a hepatic abscess. *Vet Rec, 137*, 284–290.

Brodersen, B. W. (2014). Bovine viral diarrhea virus infections, manifestations of infection and recent advances in understanding pathogenesis and control. *Vet Pathol, 51*, 453–464.

Brownlie, J. (May 19, 1990). The pathogenesis of mucosal disease. A dual role for bovine viral diarrhea virus. In *Proceedings 2nd University of Nebraska Mini-Symposium on Veterinary Infectious Diseases— Bovine Viral Diarrhea Virus: New Challenges for the New Decade* Lincoln, NE.

Brownlie, J., Clarke, M. C., & Howard, C. J. (1984). Experimental production of fatal mucosal disease in cattle. *Vet Rec, 114*, 535–536.

Bruer, A. N. (1955). Actinomycosis of the digestive tract in cattle. *Vet J, 3*, 121–122.

Bruner, D. W., & Gillespie, J. H. (1988). *Hagan's infectious diseases of domestic animals* (8th ed.). Ithaca, NY: Comstock Publishing Associates.

Buczinski, S., & Vandewaard, J. M. (2016). Diagnostic accuracy of refractometry for assessing bovine colostrum quality. A systematic review and meta-analysis. *J Dairy Sci, 99*, 7381–7394.

Bueschel, D. M., Jost, B. H., Billington, S. J., et al. (2003). Prevalence of cpb2, encoding beta2 toxin, in *Clostridium perfringens* field isolates: correlation of genotypee with phenotype. *Vet Microbiol, 94*, 121–129.

Cable, C. S., Rebhun, W. C., & Fortier, L. A. (1997). Cholelithiasis and cholecystitis in a dairy cow. *J Am Vet Med Assoc, 211*, 899–900.

Callan, R. J. (2001). Malignant catarrhal fever: recent findings. Proceedings 19th Annual Forum. *Amer Coll Vet Int Med, 19*, 336–338.

Callan, R. J. (2006). *Unpublished data*. Fort Collins, CO.

Campbell, S. G., & Cookingham, C. A. (1978). The enigma of winter dysentery. *Cornell Vet, 68*, 423–441.

Campbell, S. G., Whitlock, R. H., Timoney, J. F., et al. (1975). An unusual epizootic of actinobacillosis in dairy heifers. *J Am Vet Med Assoc, 166*, 604–606.

Carlson, S. A., Stoffregen, W. C., & Bolin, S. R. (2002). Abomasitis associated with multiple antibiotic resistant *Salmonella enterica* serotype *typhimurium* phagetype DT104. *Vet Microbiol, 85*, 233–240.

Castrucci, G., Frigeri, F., Ferrari, M., et al. (1984). The efficacy of colostrum from cows vaccinated with rotavirus in protecting calves against experimentally induced rotavirus infection. *Comp Immun Microbiol Infect Dis, 7*, 11–18.

Centers for Disease Control and Prevention (CDC). (2014). *National Salmonella Surveillance Annual Report, 2012*. Atlanta, GA: U.S. Department of Health and Human Services, CDC.

Chamorro, M. F., Walz, P. H., Haines, D. M., et al. (2014). Comparison of levels and duration of detection of antibodies to bovine virus diarrhea virus type 1, bovine virus diarrhea virus type 2, bovine respiratory syncytial virus, bovine herpes virus 1 and bovine parainfluenza virus 3, in calves fed maternal colostrum or a colostrum replacement product. *Can Vet J Res, 78*, 81–88.

Chigerwe, M., Dawes, M. E., Tyler, J. W., et al. (2005). Evaluation of a cow-side immunoassay kit for assessing IgG concentration in colostrum. *J Am Vet Med Assoc, 227*, 129–131.

Cho, K. O., Halbur, P. G., Bruna, J. D., et al. (2000). Detection and isolation of coronavirus from feces of three herds of feedlot cattle during outbreaks of winter dysentery-like disease. *J Am Vet Med Assoc, 217,* 1191–1194.

Cho, K. O., Hasoksuz, M., Nielsen, P. R., et al. (2001). Cross-protection studies between resporatory and calf diarrhea and winter dysentery coronavirus strains in calves and RT-PCR and nested PCR for their detection. *Arch Virol, 146,* 2401–2419.

Cho, Y., Han, J., Wang, C., et al. (2013). Case-control study of microbiological etiology associated with calf diarrhea. *Vet Microbiol, 166,* 375–385.

Clark, M. A. (1993). Bovine coronavirus. *Br Vet J, 149,* 51–70.

Cobbold, R. N., Rice, D. H., Davis, M. A., et al. (2006). Long-term persistence of multi-drug-resistant Salmonella enterica serovar Newport in two dairy herds. *J Am Vet Med Assoc, 228,* 686–692.

Constable, P. D. (2004). Antimicrobial use in the treatment of calf diarrhea. *J Vet Intern Med, 18,* 8–17.

Constable, P. D. (2009). Treatment of calf diarrhea: antimicrobial and ancillary treatments. *Vet Clin N Am Food Anim Pract, 25,* 101–120.

Corapi, W. C., French, T. W., & Dubovi, E. J. (1989). Severe thrombocytopenia in young calves experimentally infected with noncytopathic bovine viral diarrhea virus. *J Virol, 63,* 3934–3943.

Coria, M. F., & McClurkin, A. W. (1978). Specific immune tolerance in an apparently healthy bull persistently infected with bovine viral diarrhea virus. *J Am Vet Med Assoc, 172,* 449–451.

Craig, T. M. (2003). Treatment of external and internal parasites of cattle. *Vet Clin N Am Food Anim Pract, 19,* 661–678.

Cummings, K. J., Divers, T. J., McDonough, P. L., et al. (2009). Fecal shedding of Salmonella spp among cattle admitted to a veterinary medical teaching hospital. *J Am Vet Med Assoc, 234,* 1578–1585.

Cummings, K. J., Perkins, G. A., Khatibzadeh, S. M., et al. (2013). Antimicrobial resistance trends among Salmonella isolates obtained from dairy cattle in the northeastern United States, 2004-2011. *Foodborne Pathog Dis, 10,* 353–361.

Cummings, K. J., Warnick, L. D., Alexander, K. A., et al. (2009). The duration of fecal Salmonella shedding following clinical diseaseamong dairy cattle in the northeastern USA. *Prev Vet Med, 92,* 134–139.

Cummings, K. J., Warnick, L. D., Alexander, K. A., et al. (2009). The incidence of salmonellosis among dairy herds in the northeastern United States. *J Dairy Sci, 92,* 3766–3774.

Cummings, K. J., Warnick, L. D., Davis, M. A., et al. (2012). Farm animal contact as risk factor for transmission of bovine-associated Salmonella subtypes. *Emerg Infect Dis, 18,* 1929–1936.

Cummings, K. J., Warnick, L. D., Elton, M., et al. (2010). The effect of clinical outbreaks of salmonellosis on the prevalence of fecal Salmonella shedding among dairy cattle in New York. *Foodborne Pathog Dis, 7,* 815–823.

Cummings, K. J., Warnick, L. D., Elton, M., et al. (2010). Salmonella enterica serotype Cerro among dairy cattle in New York: an emerging pathogen? *Foodborne Pathog Dis, 7,* 659–665.

Davidson, H. P., Rebhun, W. C., & Habel, R. E. (1981). Pharyngeal trauma in cattle. *Cornell Vet, 71,* 15–25.

de Graaf, D. C., Vanopdenbosch, E., Ortega-Mora, L. M., et al. (1999). A review of the importance of cryptosporidiosis in farm animals. *Int J Parasitol, 29,* 1269–1287.

de la Rosa, C., Hogue, D. E., & Thonney, M. L. (1997). Vaccination schedules to raise antibody concentrations against epsilon toxin of *Clostridium perfringens* in ewes and their triplet lambs. *J Anim Sci, 75,* 2328–2334.

Dennison, A. C., Van Metre, D. C., Callan, R. J., et al. (2002). Hemorrhagic bowel syndrome in adult dairy cattle: 22 cases (1997-2000). *J Am Vet Med Assoc, 221,* 686–689 erratum 221:1149.

Dennison, A. C., Van Metre, D. C., Morley, P. S., et al. (2005). Comparison of the odds of isolation, genotypes, and in vivo production of major toxins by *Clostridium perfringens* obtained from the gastrointestinal tract of dairy cows with hemorrhagic bowel syndrome or left displaced abomasum. *J Am Vet Med Assoc, 227,* 132–138.

de Verdier, K. K. (2000). Enhancement of clinical signs in experimentally rotavirus infected calves by combined viral infections. *Vet Rec, 147,* 717–719.

Donis, R. O. (1988). Bovine viral diarrhea: the unraveling of a complex of clinical presentations. *Bov Proc, 20,* 16–22.

Drolet, B. S., Campbell, C. L., Stuart, M. A., et al. (2005). Vector competence of *Culicoides sonorensis* (Diptera: Ceratopogonidae) for vesicular stomatitis virus. *J Med Entomol, 42,* 409–418.

Dubovi, E. J. (1993). *Personal communication [to W.C. Rebhun].* Ithaca, NY.

Elhanafy, M. M., French, D. D., & Braun, U. (2013). Understanding jejunal hemorrhage syndrome. *J Am Vet Med Assoc, 243,* 352–358.

Elitok, B., Elitok, O. M., & Pulat, H. (2005). Efficacy of azithromycin dihydrate in treatment of cryptosporidiosis in naturally infected dairy calves. *J Vet Intern Med, 19,* 590–593.

Embury-Hyatt, C. K., Wobeser, G., Simko, E., et al. (2005). Investigation of a syndrome of sudden death, splenomegaly, and small intestinal hemorrhage in farmed deer. *Can Vet J, 46,* 702–708.

Englen, M. D., Hill, A. E., Dargatz, D. A., et al. (2007). Prevalence and antimicrobial resistance of Campylobacter in US dairy cattle. *J Appl Microbiol, 102,* 1570–1577.

Ernst, J. V., & Benz, G. W. (1986). Intestinal coccidiosis in cattle. *Vet Clin North Am Food Anim Pract, 2,* 283–291.

Espinasse, J., Viso, M., Laval, A., et al. (1982). Winter dysentery: a coronavirus-like agent in the faeces of beef and dairy cattle with diarrhoea. *Vet Rec, 11,* 385.

Ewaschuk, J. B., Naylor, J. M., Palmer, R., et al. (2004). D-lactate production and excretion in diarrheic calves. *J Vet Intern Med, 18,* 744–747.

Ewoldt, J. M., & Anderson, D. E. (2005). Determination of the effect of single abomasal or jejunal inoculation of *Clostridium perfringens* type A in dairy cows. *Can Vet J, 46,* 821–824.

Farrell, C. J., Shen, D. T., Wescott, R. B., et al. (1981). An enzyme-linked immunosorbent assay for diagnosis of *Fasciola hepatica* infection in cattle. *Am J Vet Res, 42,* 237–240.

Fayer, R., Morgan, U., & Upton, S. J. (2000). Epidemiology of *Cryptosporidium*: transmission, detection, and identification. *Int J Parasitol, 30,* 1305–1322.

Fayer, R., Santin, M., & Xiao, L. (2005). *Cryptosporidium bovis* n. sp. (Apicomplexa: Cryptosporidiiae) in cattle (*Bos taurus*). *J Parasitol, 91,* 624–629.

Fidler, A. P., Hilley, M. L., & Smith, G. W. (2011). Serum immunoglobulin G and total protein concentrations in dairy calves fed a colostrum replacement product. *J Dairy Sci, 94,* 3609–3612.

Firehammer, B. D., & Myers, L. L. (1981). *Campylobacter fetus* subspecies *jejuni*: its possible significance in enteric disease of calves and lambs. *Am J Vet Res, 42,* 918–922.

Fleenor, W. A., & Stott, G. H. (1980). Hydrometer test for estimation of immunoglobulin concentration in bovine colostrum. *J Dairy Sci, 63,* 973–977.

Fossler, C. P., Wells, S. J., Kaneene, J. B., et al. (2005). Herd-level factors associated with isolation of Salmonella in a multi-state study of conventional and organic dairy farms I. Salmonella shedding in cows. *Prev Vet Med, 70,* 257–277.

Fossler, C. P., Wells, S. J., Kaneene, J. B., et al. (2005). Cattle and environmental sample-level factors associated with the presence of Salmonella in a multi-state study of conventional and organic dairy farms. *Prev Vet Med, 67,* 39–53.

Fowler, M. E. (1992). Recent calf milk replacer research update. In *Proceedings: American Association Bovine Practitioners Convention* (Vol. 2) (pp. 168–175).

Fubini, S. L., Ducharme, N. G., Murphy, J. P., et al. (1985). Vagus indigestion syndrome resulting from a liver abscess in dairy cows. *J Am Vet Med Assoc, 186*, 1297–1300.

Garcia, A, & Shalloo, L. (2015). The economic impact and control of paratuberculosis in cattle. *J Dairy Sci, 98*, 5019–5039.

Garcia, J. P., Anderson, M., Blanchard, P., et al. (2013). The pathology of *Clostridium perfringens* type C in calves. *J Vet Diag Invest, 25*, 438–442.

Garmory, H. S., Chanter, N., French, N. P., et al. (2000). Occurrence of *Clostridium perfringens* beta2-toxin amongst animals, determined by using genotyping and subtyping PCR assays. *Epidemiol Infect, 124*, 61–67.

Georgi, J. R. (1985). *Parasitology for veterinarians* (4th ed.). Philadelphia: WB Saunders, 62–72.

Gibbs, E. P. J. (1983). Bluetongue—an analysis of current problems, with particular reference to importation of ruminants to the United States. *J Am Vet Med Assoc, 182*, 1190–1194.

Gibbs, E. P. J. (1983). Bluetongue disease. *Agri-Practice, 4*, 31–38.

Gibbs, H. C., & Herd, R. P. (1986). Nematodiasis in cattle: importance, species involved immunity, and resistance. *Vet Clin North Am Food Anim Pract, 2*, 211–224.

Gibert, M., Jolivet–Reynaud, C., & Popoff, M. (1997). Beta2 toxin, a novel toxin produced by *Clostridium perfringens. Gene, 203*, 65–73.

Giles, N., Hopper, S. A., & Wray, C. (1989). Persistence of Salmonella typhimurium in a large dairy herd. *Epidemiol Infect, 103*, 235–242.

Gillespie, J. H., Bartholomew, P. T., Thomson, R. G., et al. (1967). The isolation of non-cytopathic virus diarrhea from two aborted fetuses. *Cornell Vet, 57*, 564–571.

Givens, M. D., & Waldrop, J. G. (2004). Bovine viral diarrhea virus in embryo and semen production systems. *Vet Clin N Am Food Anim Pract, 20*, 21–38.

Godden, S., Frank, R., & Ames, T. (2001). Survey of Minnesota veterinarians on the occurrence of and potential risk factors for jejunal hemorrhage syndrome in adult dairy cows. *Bov Pract, 35*, 97–103.

Godden, S. M., Smolenski, D. J., Donahue, M., et al. (2012). Heat treated colostrum and reduced morbidity in preweaned dairy calves: Results of a randomized trial and examination of mechanisms of effectiveness. *J Dairy Sci, 95*, 4029–4040.

Goldman, L., & Ausiello, D. (2004). Campylobacter enteritis. In J. B. Wyngaarden, & L. H. Smith, Jr. (Eds.), *Cecil textbook of medicine* (22nd ed.). Philadelphia: WB Saunders.

Goodger, W. J., Thurmond, M., Nehay, J., et al. (1985). Economic impact of an epizootic of bovine vesicular stomatitis in California. *J Am Vet Med Assoc, 186*, 370–373.

Gragg, S. E., Loneragan, G. H., Brashears, M. M., et al. (2013). Cross-sectional study examining Salmonella enterica carriage in subiliac lymph nodes of cull and feedlot cattle at harvest. *Foodborne Pathog Dis, 10*, 368–374.

Grahn, T. C., Fahning, M. L., & Zemjanis, R. (1984). Nature of early reproductive failure caused by bovine viral diarrhea virus. *J Am Vet Med Assoc, 185*, 429–432.

Griesemer, R. A., & Cole, C. R. (1960). Bovine papular stomatitis. *J Am Vet Med Assoc, 137*, 404–410.

Grooms, D., Baker, J. C., & Ames, T. R. (2002). Diseases caused by bovine virus diarrhea virus. In B. P. Smith (Ed.), *Large animal internal medicine* (3rd ed.) (pp. 707–714). St. Louis: Mosby.

Grooms, D. L. (2004). Reproductive consequences of infection with bovine viral diarrhea virus. *Vet Clin N Am Food Anim Pract, 20*, 5–19.

Grooms, D. L., Brock, K. V., & Ward, L. A. (1998). Detection of bovine viral diarrhea virus in the ovaries of cattle acutely infected with bovine viral diarrhea virus. *J Vet Diagn Invest, 10*, 125–129.

Guerrant, R. L., Van Gilder, T., Steiner, T. S., et al. (2001). Infectious Diseases Society of America. Practice guidelines for the management of infectious diarrhea. *Clin Infect Dis, 32*, 331–351.

Habing, G. G., Lombard, J. E., Kopral, C. A., et al. Farm-level associations with the shedding of Salmonella and antimicrobial-resistant Salmonella in U.S. dairy cattle. *Foodborne Pathog Dis, 9*, 815–821.

Haggard, D. L. (1985). Bovine enteric colibacillosis. *Vet Clin North Am Food Anim Pract, 1*, 495–508.

Haines, D. M., Chelck, B. J., & Naylor, J. M. (1990). Immunoglobulin concentrations in commercially available colostrum supplements for calves. *Can Vet J, 31*, 36–37.

Haley, B. J., Allard, M., Brown, E., et al. (2015). Molecular detection of the index case of a subclinical Salmonella Kentucky epidemic on a dairy farm. *Epidemiol Infect, 143*, 682–686.

Hammerberg, B. (1986). Pathophysiology of nematodiasis in cattle. *Vet Clin North Am Food Anim Pract, 2*, 225–234.

Hand, M. S., Hunt, E., & Phillips, R. W. (1985). Milk replacers for the neonatal calf. *Vet Clin North Am Food Anim Pract, 1*, 589–609.

Hansen, D. E., Thurmond, M. C., & Thorburn, M. (1985). Factors associated with the spread of clinical vesicular stomatitis in California dairy cattle. *Am J Vet Res, 46*, 789–795.

Hasoksuz, M., Hoet, A. E., Loersch, S. C., et al. (2002). Detection of respiratory and enteric shedding of bovine coronaviruses in cattle in an Ohio feedlot. *J Vet Diagn Invest, 14*, 308–313.

Hebeller, H. F., Linton, A. H., & Osborne, A. D. (1961). Atypical actinobacillosis in a dairy herd. *Vet Rec, 73*, 517–521.

Hendrick, S. H., Kelton, D. F., Leslie, K. E., et al. (2006). Efficacy of monensin sodium for the reduction of fecal shedding of *Mycobacterium avium* subsp. *paratuberculosis* in infected dairy cattle. *Prev Vet Med, 75*, 206–220.

Herd, R. P., & Heider, L. E. (1980). Control of internal parasites in dairy replacement heifers by two treatments in the spring. *J Am Vet Med Assoc, 177*, 51–54.

Herd, K. P., & Heider, L. E. (1985). Control of nematodes in dairy heifers by prophylactic treatments with albendazole in the spring. *J Am Vet Med Assoc, 186*, 1071–1074.

Hernandez, D., Nydam, D. V., Godden, S. M., et al. (2016). Brix refractometry in serum as a measure of failure of passive transfer compared to measured immunoglobulin G and total protein by refractometry in serum from dairy calves. *Vet J, 211*, 82–87.

Heuschele, W. P. (1992). Malignant catarrhal fever. In Committee on Foreign Animal Diseases (Ed.), *Foreign animal diseases*. Richmond, VA: United States Animal Health Association.

Hoelzer, K., Moreno Switt, A. I. Wiedmann, M., et al. (2011). Animal contact as a source of human non-typhoidal salmonellosis. *Vet Res, 42*, 34–42.

Hogan, I., Doherty, M., Fagan, J., et al. (2015). Comparison of rapid laboratory tests for failure of passive transfer in the bovine. *Ir Vet J, 68*, 18–23.

Holloway, N. M., Tyler, J. W., Lakritz, J., et al. (2002). Serum immunoglobulin G concentrations in calves fed fresh colostrum or a colostrum supplement. *J Vet Intern Med, 16*, 187–191.

Holmberg, S. D., Osterholm, M. T., Senger, K. A., et al. (1984). Drug-resistant Salmonella from animals fed antimicrobials. *N Engl J Med, 311*, 617–622.

Howard, T. H., Bean, B., Hillman, R., et al. (1990). Surveillance for persistent bovine viral diarrhea virus infection in four artificial insemination centers. *J Am Vet Med Assoc, 196,* 1951–1955.

Jamaluddin, A. A., Carpenter, T. E., Hird, D. W., et al. (1996). Economics of feeding pasteurized colostrum and pasteurized waste milk to dairy calves. *J Am Vet Med Assoc, 209,* 751–756.

Jarrett, W. F. H., Campo, M. S., Blaxter, M. L., et al. (1984). Alimentary fibropapilloma in cattle. A spontaneous tumor, nonpermissive for papillomavirus replication. *J Nat Cancer Inst, 73,* 499–504.

Jarrett, W. F. H., et al. (1980). Papilloma viruses in benign and malignant tumors of cattle. *Cold Spring Harbor Conference on Cell Proliferation,* 215–222.

Jeong, W. I., Do, S. H., Sohn, M. H., et al. (2005). Hepatocellular carcinoma with metastasis to the spleen in a Holstein cow. *Vet Pathol, 42,* 230–232.

Jones, T. F., Ingram, L. A., Cieslak, P. R., et al. (2008). Salmonellosis outcomes differ substantially by serotype. *J Infect Dis, 198,* 109–114.

Kahrs, R. F. (1981). *Viral diseases of cattle.* Ames, IA: Iowa State University Press.

Kahrs, R. (1973). Effect of bovine viral diarrhea on the developing fetus. *J Am Vet Med Assoc, 163,* 877–878.

Kahrs, R., Atkinson, G., Baker, J. A., et al. (1964). Serological studies on the incidence of bovine virus diarrhea, infectious bovine rhinotracheitis, bovine myxovirus, parainfluenza-3, and Leptospira pomona in New York State. *Cornell Vet, 54,* 360–369.

Kahrs, R. F. (2001). Rotavirus associated with neonatal diarrhea. In R. F. Kahrs (Ed.), *Viral diseases of cattle* (2nd ed.) (pp. 239–246). Ames, IA: Iowa State University Press.

Kahrs, R. F., Scott, F. W., & de Lahunte, A. (1970). Congenital cerebellar hypoplasia and ocular defects in calves following bovine viral diarrhea-mucosal disease infection in pregnant cattle. *J Am Vet Med Assoc, 156,* 1443–1450.

Katayama, S. I., Matsushita, O., Minami, J., et al. (1993). Comparison of the alpha-toxin genes of *Clostridium perfringens* type A and C strains: evidence for extragenic regulation of transcription. *Infect Immun, 61,* 457–463.

Kelling, C. L., Steffen, D. J., Cooper, V. L., et al. (2002). Effect of infection with bovine viral diarrhea virus alone, bovine rotavirus alone, or concurrent infection with both on enteric disease in gnotobiotic calves. *Am J Vet Res, 63,* 1179–1186.

Kelling, C. W. (2004). Evolution of bovine viral diarrhea virus vaccines. *Vet Clin N Am Food Anim Pract, 20,* 115–129.

Kendrick, J. W., & Franti, C. E. (1974). Bovine viral diarrhea: decay of colostrum-conferred antibody in the calf. *Am J Vet Res, 35,* 589–591.

Kenney, D. G., Weldon, A. D., & Rebhun, W. C. (1993). Oropharyngeal abscessation in two cows secondary to administration of an oral calcium preparation. *Cornell Vet, 83,* 61–65.

Ketelsen, A. T., Johnson, D. W., & Muscoplat, C. C. (1979). Depression of bovine monocyte chemotactic responses by bovine viral diarrhea virus. *Infect Immun, 25,* 565–568.

Kimball, A., Twiehaus, M. J., & Frank, E. R. (1954). *Actinomyces bovis* isolated from six cases of bovine orchitis: a preliminary report. *Am J Vet Res, 15,* 551–553.

Kingman, H. E., & Paven, J. S. (1951). Streptomycin in the treatment of actinomycosis. *J Am Vet Med Assoc, 118,* 28–30.

Kirkpatrick, M. A., Kersting, K. W., & Kinyon, J. M. (2001). Case report—Jejunal hemorrhage syndrome of dairy cattle. *Bov Pract, 35,* 104–116.

Knight, A. P., & Messer, N. T. (1983). Vesicular stomatitis. *Compend Contin Educ Pract Vet, 5,* S517–S534.

Kolenda, R., Burdukiewicz, M., & Schierack, P. (2015). A systematic review and meta-analysis of the epidemiology of pathogenic Escherichia coli of calves and the role of calves as reservoirs for human pathogenic E. coli. *Front Cell Infect Microbiol, 5,* 1–12.

Koohmaraie, M., Scanga, J. A., De La Zerda, M. J., et al. (2012). Tracking the sources of Salmonella in ground beef produced from nonfed cattle. *J Food Prot, 75,* 1464–1468.

Koopmans, M., van Wuijckhuise-Sjouke, L., Schukken, Y. M., et al. (1991). Association of diarrhea in cattle with torovirus infections on farms. *Am J Vet Res, 52,* 1769–1773.

Kumper, H. (1995). A new treatment for abomasal bloat in calves. *Bov Pract, 29,* 80–82.

Lanyon, S. R., Hill, F. I., Reichel, M. P., et al. (2014). Bovine viral diarrhea: pathogenesis and diagnosis. *Vet J, 199,* 201–209.

Lechtenberg, K. F., & Nagaraja, T. G. (1991). Hepatic ultrasonography and blood changes in cattle with experimentally induced hepatic abscesses. *Am J Vet Res, 52,* 803–809.

Lee, K. M., & Gillespie, J. H. (1957). Propagation of virus diarrhea virus of cattle in tissue culture. *Am J Vet Res, 18,* 952–953.

Lerner, P. I. (1974). Susceptibility of pathogenic actinomycetes to antimicrobial compounds. *Antimicrob Agents Chemother, 5,* 302–309.

Li, H., Cunha, C. W., Taus, N. S., et al. (2014). Malignant catarrhal fever: inching towards understanding. *Annu. Rev Anim Biosci, 2,* 209–233.

Li, H., Shen, D. T., O'Toole, D., et al. (1995). Investigation of sheep-associated malignant catarrhal fever virus infection in ruminants by PCR and competitive inhibition enzyme-linked immunosorbent assay. *J Clin Microbiol, 33,* 2048–2053.

Lilley, C. W., Hamar, D. W., Gerlach, M., et al. (1985). Linking copper deficiency with abomasal ulcers in beef calves. *Vet Med, 80,* 85–88.

Lofstedt, J., Dohoo, I. R., & Duizer, G. (1999). Model to predict septicemia in diarrheic calves. *J Vet Intern Med, 13,* 81–88.

Loneragan, G. H., Thomson, D. U., McCarthy, R. M., et al. (2012). Salmonella diversity and burden in cows on and culled from dairy farms in the Texas High Plains. *Foodborne Pathog Dis, 9,* 549–555.

Lorenz, I. (2004). Influence of D-lactate on metabolic acidosis and on prognosis in neonatal calves with diarrhoea. *J Vet Med A Physiol Pathol Clin Med, 51,* 425–428.

Lucchelli, A., Lance, S. E., Bartlett, P. B., et al. (1992). Prevalence of bovine group A rotavirus shedding among dairy calves in Ohio. *Am J Vet Res, 53,* 169–174.

Luedke, A. J., Jones, R. H., & Jochim, M. M. (1967). Transmission of bluetongue between sheep and cattle by *Culicoides variipennis, Am J Vet Res, 28,* 457–460.

MacPherson, L. W. (1957). Bovine virus enteritis (winter dysentery). *Can J Comp Med, 21,* 184–192.

Maddox, C., Hattel, A., Drake, T., et al. (1999). Clostridium perfringens type A strains recovered from acute hemorrhagic enteritis of adult lactating dairy cattle (abstract). San Diego: Proceedings of the 42nd Annual Meeting, American Association of Veterinary Laboratory Diagnosticians, 51.

Malone, J. B., Jr. (1986). Fascioliasis and cestodiasis in cattle. *Vet Clin North Am Food Anim Pract, 2,* 261–275.

Manteca, C., Daube, G., Pirson, V., et al. (2001). Bacterial intestinal flora associated with enterotoxaemia in Belgian Blue calves. *Vet Microbiol, 81,* 21–32.

Manteca, C., Jauniaux, T., Daube, G., et al. (2001). Isolation of *Clostridium perfringens* from three calves with hemorrhagic abomasitis. *Rev Med Vet, 152*, 637–639.

Markham, R. J. F., & Ramnaraine, M. L. (1985). Release of immunosuppressive substances from tissue culture cells infected with bovine viral diarrhea virus. *Am J Vet Res, 46*, 879–883.

McAloon, C. G., Whyte, P., More, S. J., et al. (2015). The effect of paratuberculosis on milk yield – A systematic review and meta-analysis. *J Dairy Sci, 99*, 1449–1460.

McClurkin, A. W., Bolin, S. R., & Coria, M. F. (1985). Isolation of cytopathic and noncytopathic bovine viral diarrhea virus from the spleen of cattle acutely and chronically affected with bovine viral diarrhea. *J Am Vet Med Assoc, 186*, 568–569.

McClurkin, A. W., Coria, M. F., & Cutlip, R. C. (1979). Reproductive performance of apparently healthy cattle persistently infected with bovine viral diarrhea virus. *J Am Vet Med Assoc, 174*, 1116–1119.

McClurkin, A. W., Littledike, E. T., Cutlip, R. C., et al. (1984). Production of cattle immunotolerant to bovine viral diarrhea virus. *Can J Comp Med, 48*, 156–161.

McCluskey, B. J., Petzel-McCluskey, A. M., Creekmore, L., et al. (2013). Vesicular stomatitis outbreak in the southwestern United States, 2012. *J Vet Diag Invest, 25*, 608–613.

McDonough, P. L. (1985). Epidemiology of bovine salmonellosis. In *Proceedings of the 18th Annual Convention of American Association Bovine Practitioners* (pp. 169–173).

McGuirk, S. M. (1992). Colostrum: quality and quantity. In *Proceedings of the XVII World Buiatrics Congress* (Vol. 2) (pp. 162–167).

McGuirk, S. M., & Collins, M. (2004). Managing the production, storage, and delivery of colostrum. *Vet Clin N Am Food Anim Pract, 20*, 593–603.

McLauchlin, J., Amar, C., Pedraza-Diaz, S., et al. (2000). Molecular epidemiological analysis of *Cryptosporidium* spp. in the United Kingdom: results of genotyping *Cryptosporidium* spp. in 1,705 fecal samples from humans and 105 fecal samples from livestock animals. *J Clin Microbiol, 38*, 3984–3990.

Mebus, C. A., Newman, L. E., & Stair, E. L. (1975). Scanning, electron, light and immunofluorescent microscopy of intestine of gnotobiotic calf infected with calf diarrhea coronavirus. *Am J Vet Res, 36*, 1719–1725.

Mebus, C. A., Underdahl, N. R., Rhodes, M. B., et al. (1969). Calf diarrhea (scours): reproduced with a virus from a field outbreak. *Univ Nebr Res Bull, 233*, 2–15.

Mechor, G. D., Gröhn, Y. T., & VanSaun, R. J. (1991). Effect of temperature on colostrometer readings for estimation of immunoglobulin concentration in bovine colostrum. *J Dairy Sci, 74*, 3940–3943.

Meer, R., & Songer, J. G. (1997). Multiplex polymerase chain reaction assay for genotyping Clostridium perfringens. *Am J Vet Res, 58*, 702–705.

Megarick, V., Holfack, G., & Opsomer, G. (2014). Advances in prevention and therapy of neonatal calf diarrhea: a systematical review with emphasis on colostrum management and fluid therapy. *Acta Veterinaria Scandanavica, 56*, 75–83.

Meyling, A., & Jensen, A. M. (1988). Transmission of bovine virus diarrhoea virus (BVDV) by artificial insemination (AI) with semen from a persistently infected bull. *Vet Microbiol, 17*, 97–105.

Miller, H. V., & Drost, M. (1978). Failure to cause abortion in cows with intravenous sodium iodide treatment. *J Am Vet Med Assoc, 172*, 466–467.

Milne, M. H., Barrett, D. C., Mellor, D. J., et al. (2001). Clinical recognition and treatment of bovine cutaneous actinobacillosis. *Vet Rec, 148*, 273–274.

Moon, H. W., McClurkin, A. W., Isaacson, R. E., et al. (1978). Pathogenic relationship of rotavirus, *Escherichia coli,* and other agents in mixed infections in calves. *J Am Vet Med Assoc, 173*, 577–583.

Morley, P. S., Morris, N., Hyatt, D. R., et al. (2005). Evaluation of the efficacy of disinfectant footbaths as used in veterinary hospitals. *J Am Vet Med Assoc, 226*, 2053–2058.

Mortier, R. A., Barkema, H. W., & De Buck, J. (2015). Susceptibility to and diagnosis of Mycobacterium avium subspecies paratuberculosis infection in dairy calves: a review. *Prev Vet Med, 121*, 189–198.

Motiwala, A. S., Li, L., Kapur, V., et al. (2006). Current understanding of the genetic diversity of *Mycobacterium avium* subsp. *paratuberculosis. Microbes Infect, 8*, 1406–1418.

Muller-Doblies, U. U., Li, H., Hauser, B., et al. (1998). Field validation of laboratory tests for clinical diagnosis of sheep-associated malignant catarrhal fever. *J Clin Microbiol, 36*, 2970–2972.

Munday, J. S. (2014). Bovine and human papillomaviruses: a comparative review. *Vet Pathol, 51*, 1063–1075.

Nagarja, T. G., & Chengappa, M. M. (1998). Liver abscesses in feedlot cattle: a review. *Anim Sci, 76*, 287–298.

Naylor, J. M. (2002). Neonatal ruminant diarrhea. In B. P. Smith (Ed.), *Large animal internal medicine* (3rd ed.) (pp. 352–381). St. Louis: Mosby, Inc.

Naylor, J. M. (1987). Severity and nature of acidosis in diarrheic calves over and under one week of age. *Can Vet J, 28*, 168–173.

Neitz, W. O., & Riemerschmid, G. (1944). The influence of solar radiation on the course of bluetongue. *Onderstepoort J Vet Res, 20*, 29–55.

Newcomer, B. W., Walz, P. H., Daniel Givens, M., et al. (2015). Efficacy of bovine viral diarrhea virus vaccination to prevent reproductive disease. *Theriogenology, 83*, 360–365.

Nielsen, L. R., Schukken, Y. H., Grohn, Y. T., et al. (2004). Salmonella Dublin infection in dairy cattle: risk factors for becoming a carrier. *Prev Vet Med, 65*, 47–62.

Nielsen, L. R., Warnick, L. D., & Greiner, M. (2007). Risk factors for changing test classification in the Danish surveillance program for Salmonella in dairy herds. *J Dairy Sci, 90*, 2815–2825.

Nielsen, T. D., Vesterbaek, I. L., Kudahl, A. B., et al. (2012). Effect of management on prevention of Salmonella Dublin exposure of calves during a one-year control programme in 84 Danish dairy herds. *Prev Vet Med, 105*, 101–109.

Niilo, L. (1980). *Clostridium perfringens* in animal disease: a review of current knowledge. *Can Vet J, 21*, 141–148.

Niilo, L. (1988). *Clostridium perfringens* type C enterotoxemia. *Can Vet J, 29*, 658–664.

Norman, L. M., Hohenboken, W. D., & Kelley, K. W. (1981). Genetic differences in concentration of immunoglobulin G1 and M in serum and colostrum of cows in serum of neonatal calves. *J Anim Sci, 53*, 1465–1472.

Nunamaker, R. A., Lockwood, J. A., Stith, C. E., et al. (2003). Grasshoppers (Orthoptera: Acrididea) could serve as reservoirs and vectors of vesicular stomatitis virus. *J Med Entomol, 40*, 957–963.

Nydam, D. V., & Mohammed, H. O. (2005). Quantitative risk assessment of Cryptosporidium species infection in dairy calves. *J Dairy Sci, 88*, 3932–3943.

Ogilvie, T. H. (1986). The persistent isolation of *Salmonella typhimurium* from the mammary gland of a dairy cow. *Can Vet J, 27*, 329–331.

Olafson, P., MacCallum, A. D., & Fox, F. H. (1946). An apparently new transmissible disease of cattle. *Cornell Vet, 36*, 205–213.

Olivett, T. L., Nydam, D. V., Bowman, D. W., et al. (2009). Effect of nitazoxanide on cryptosporidiosis in experimentally infected neonatal dairy calves. *J Dairy Sci, 92*, 1643–1648.

Oma, V. S., Traven, M., Alenius, S., et al. (2016). Bovine corona-virus in naturally and experimentally exposed calves; viral shedding and the potential for transmission. *Virology Journal, 13,* 100–111.

Omidian, Z., Ebrahimzadeh, E., Shahbazi, P., et al. (2014). Application of recombinant Cryptosporidium parvum P23 for isolation and prevention. *Parasitol Res, 113,* 229–237.

O'Sullivan, E. N. (1999). Two-year study of bovine hepatic abscessation in 10 abattoirs in County Cork, Ireland. *Vet Rec, 145,* 389–393.

Palotay, J. L. (1951). Actinobacillosis in cattle. *Vet Med Feb,* 52–54.

Panciera, R. J., Thomas, R. W., & Garner, F. M. (1971). Cryptosporidial infection in a calf. *Vet Pathol, 8,* 479–484.

Pangloli, P., Dje, Y., Ahmed, O., et al. (2008). Seasonal incidence and molecular characterization of Salmonella from dairy cows, calves, and farm environment. *Foodborne Pathog Dis, 5,* 87–96.

Parish, S. M., Evermann, J. F., Olcott, B., et al. (1982). A bluetongue epizootic in northwestern United States. *J Am Vet Med Assoc, 181,* 589–591.

Parreno, V., Bejar, C., Vagnozzi, A., et al. (2004). Modulation by colostrum-acquired antibodies of systemic and mucosal antibody responses to rotavirus in calves experimentally challenged with bovine rotavirus. *Vet Immunol Immunopathol, 100,* 7–24.

Peek, S. F., Hartmann, F. A., Thomas, C. B., et al. (2004). Isolation of Salmonella spp from the environment of dairies without any history of clinical salmonellosis. *J Am Vet Med Assoc, 225,* 574–577.

Peek, S. F., Santschi, E. M., Livesey, M. A., et al. (2009). Surgical findings and outcome for dairy cattle with jejunal hemorrhage syndrome, 31 cases, 2000-2007. *J Am Vet Med Assoc, 234,* 1307–1312.

Pellerin, C., van den Hurk, J., Lecompte, J., et al. (1994). Identification of a new group of bovine viral diarrhea virus strains associated with severe outbreaks and high mortalities. *Virology, 203,* 260–268.

Perdrizet, J. A., Rebhun, W. C., Dubovi, E. J., et al. (1987). Bovine virus diarrhea—clinical syndromes in dairy herds. *Cornell Vet, 77,* 46–74.

Perino, L. J., Sutherland, R. L., & Woollen, N. E. (1993). Serum gamma-glutamyltransferase activity and protein concentration at birth and after suckling in calves with adequate and inadequate passive transfer of immunoglobulin G. *Am J Vet Res, 54*(1), 56–59.

Perry, G. H., Vivanco, H., Holmes, I., et al. (2006). No evidence of *Mycobacterium avium* subsp. *paratuberculosis* in *in vitro* produced cryopreserved embryos derived from subclinically infected cows. *Theriogenology, 66,* 1267–1273.

Perryman, L. E., Kapil, S. J., Jones, M. L., et al. (1999). Protection of calves against cryptosporidiosis with immune bovine colostrum induced by a *Cryptosporidium parvum* recombinant protein. *Vaccine, 17,* 2142–2149.

Petit, L., Gibert, M., & Popoff, M. (1999). Clostridium perfringens: toxinotype and genotype. *Trend Microbiol, 7,* 104–110.

Phillips, R. W. (1985). Fluid therapy for diarrheic calves: what, how, and how much. *Vet Clin North Am Food Anim Pract, 1,* 541–562.

Plowright, W. (1968). Malignant catarrhal fever. *J Am Vet Med Assoc, 152,* 795–806.

Pohlenz, J., Moon, H. W., Cheville, N. F., et al. (1978). Cryptosporidiosis as a probable factor in neonatal diarrhea in calves. *J Am Vet Med Assoc, 172,* 452–457.

Popísil, Z., et al. (1975). Decline in the phytohaemagglutinin responsiveness of lymphocytes from calves infected experimentally with bovine viral diarrhoea-mucosal disease virus and parainfluenza 3 virus. *Acta Vet Brno, 44,* 360–375.

Potgieter, L. N. D., McCracken, M. D., Hopkins, F. M., et al. (1985). Comparison of the pneumopathogenicity of two strains of bovine viral diarrhea virus. *Am J Vet Res, 46,* 151–153.

Powers, J. G., Van Metre, D. C., Collins, J. K., et al. (2005). Evaluation of ovine herpesvirus-2 infections, as detected by competitive inhibition ELISA and polymerase chain reaction assay, in dairy cattle without signs of malignant catarrhal fever. *J Am Vet Med Assoc, 227,* 606–611.

Pritchett, L. C., Gay, C. C., Besser, T. E., et al. (1991). Management and production factors influencing immunoglobulin G1 concentration in colostrum from Holstein cows. *J Dairy Sci, 74,* 2336–2341.

Pritchett, L. C., Gay, C. C., Hancock, D. D., et al. (1994). Evaluation of the hydrometer for testing immunoglobulin G1 in Holstein colostrum. *J Dairy Sci, 77,* 1761–1767.

Puntenney, S. B., Wang, Y., & Forsberg, N. E. (2003). Mycotic infections in livestock: recent insights and studies on etiology, diagnostics, and prevention of hemorrhagic bowel syndrome. Tucson, AZ: Proceedings, Southwest Animal Nutrition Conference, University of Arizona, Department of Animal Science, 49–63.

Pyorala, S., Laurila, T., Lehtonen, S., et al. (1999). Local tissue damage in cows after administration of preparations containing phenylbutazone, flunixin, ketoprofen, and metamizole. *Acta Vet Scand, 40,* 145–150.

Qi, F., Ridpath, J. F., & Berry, E. S. (1998). Insertion of a bovine SMT3B gene in NS4B and duplication of NS3 in a bovine viral diarrhea virus genome correlate with the cytopathogenicity of the virus. *Virus Res, 57,* 1–9.

Quilez, J., Sanchez-Acedo, C., Avendano, C., et al. (2005). Efficacy of two peroxygen-based disinfectants for inactivation of *Cryptosporidium parvum* oocysts. *Appl Environ Microbiol, 71,* 2479–2483.

Radostits, O. M. (2000). Clinical examination of the alimentary system—ruminants. In O. M. Radostits, I. G. Mayhew, & D. M. Houston (Eds.), *Veterinary clinical examination and diagnosis* (pp. 409–468). London: WB Saunders.

Radostits, O. M., Gay, C., Blood, D. C., et al. (1989). Veterinary medicine. A textbook of the diseases of cattle, sheep, pigs, goats and horses (7th ed.). Philadelphia: Bailliere Tindall [with contributions by Arundel JH, Gay CC]. (The latest edition is the 9th edition.).

Radostits, O. M., & Stockdale, P. H. (1980). A brief review of bovine coccidiosis in Western Canada. *Can Vet J, 21,* 227–230.

Raizman, E. A., Fetrow, J. P., & Wells, S. J. (2009). Loss of income from cows shedding Mycobacterium avium subspecies paratuberculosis prior to calving compared with cows not shedding the organism on two Minnesota dairy farms. *J Dairy Sci, 92,* 4929–4936.

Ramsey, H. A. (1982). Non-milk protein in milk replacers with special emphasis on soy products. Presented at the Annual Meeting American Dairy Science Association.

Rebhun, W. C., French, T. W., Perdrizet, J. A., et al. (1989). Thrombocytopenia associated with acute bovine virus diarrhea infection in cattle. *J Vet Intern Med, 3,* 42–46.

Rebhun, W. C., King, J. M., & Hillman, R. B. (1988). Atypical actinobacillosis granulomas in cattle. *Cornell Vet, 78,* 125–130.

Reggiardo, C., & Kaeberle, M. L. (1981). Detection of bacteremia in cattle inoculated with bovine viral diarrhea virus. *Am J Vet Res, 42,* 218–221.

Ridpath, J., & Bolin, S. (1998). Differentiation of types Ia, Ib, and 2, bovine viral diarrhea virus (BVDV) by PCR. *Mol Cell Probes, 12,* 101–106.

Roberts, S. J. (1957). Winter dysentery in dairy cattle. *Cornell Vet, 47,* 372–388.

Rodak, L., Babiuk, L. A., & Acres, S. D. (1982). Detection by radioimmunoassay and enzyme-linked immunosorbent assay of coronavirus antibodies in bovine serum and lacteal secretions. *J Clin Microbiol, 16,* 34–40.

Roden, L. D., Smith, B. P., Spier, S. J., et al. (1992). Effect of calf age and *Salmonella* bacterin type on ability to produce immunoglobulins directed against *Salmonella* whole cells or lipopolysaccaride. *Am J Vet Res, 53,* 1895–1899.

Rodriguez-Palacios, A., Stampfli, H. R., Stalker, H. R., et al. (2007). Natural and experimental infection of neonatal calves with Clostridium difficile. *Vet Microbiol124,* 166–172.

Roeder, B. L., Chengappa, M. M., Nagaraja, T. G., et al. (1988). Experimental induction of abomasal tympany and abomasal ulceration by intraruminal inoculation of *Clostridium perfringens* type A in neonatal calves. *Am J Vet Res, 49,* 201–207.

Roeder, B. L., Chengappa, M. M., Nagaraja, T. G., et al. (1987). Isolation of *Clostridium perfringens* type A from neonatal calves with ruminal and abomasal tympany, abomasitis, and abomasal ulceration. *J Am Vet Med Assoc, 190,* 1550–1555.

Rood, J., & McClane, B. (1997). *The Clostridia, molecular biology and pathogenesis.* San Diego: Academic Press, 153–160.

Ross, C. E., Dubovi, E. J., & Donis, R. O. (1986). Herd problems of abortions and malformed calves attributed to bovine viral diarrhea. *J Am Vet Med Assoc, 185,* 429–432.

Ross, C. E., & Rebhun, W. C. (1986). Megaesophagus in a cow. *J Am Vet Med Assoc, 188,* 623–624.

Roth, J. A., Bolin, S. R., & Frank, D. E. (1986). Lymphocyte blastogenesis and neutrophil function in cattle persistently infected with bovine viral diarrhea virus. *Am J Vet Res, 47,* 1139–1141.

Ruder, M. G., Lysyk, T. J., Stallknecht, D. E., et al. (2015). Transmission and epidemiology of blue tongue and epizootic hemorrhagic disease in North America: current perspectives, research gaps, and future directions. *Vector Borne and Zoonotic Dis, 15,* 348–363.

Runnels, P. L., Moon, H. W., Matthews, P. J., et al. (1986). Effects of microbial and host variables on the interaction of rotavirus and *Escherichia coli* infections in gnotobiotic calves. *Am J Vet Res, 47,* 1542–1550.

Sahal, M., Karaer, Z., Yasa Duru, S., et al. (2005). Cryptosporidiosis in newborn calves in Ankara region: clinical, haematological findings and treatment with lasalocid (article in German). *Dtsch Tierarztl Wochenschr, 112,* 203–210.

Saif, L. J., Redman, D. R., Smith, K. L., et al. (1983). Passive immunity to bovine rotavirus in newborn calves fed colostrum supplements from immunized or nonimmunized cows. *Infect Immun, 41,* 1118–1131.

Saif, L. J., & Smith, L. (1985). Enteric viral infections of calves and passive immunity. *J Dairy Sci, 68,* 206–228.

Saliki, J. T., & Dubovi, E. J. (2004). Laboratory diagnosis of bovine viral diarrhea virus infections. *Vet Clin N Am Food Anim Pract, 20,* 69–83.

Sanchez, J., Dohoo, I., Leslie, K., et al. (2005). The use of an indirect Ostertagia ostertagi ELISA to predict milk production response after anthelmintic treatment in confined and semi-confined dairy herds. *Vet Parasitol, 130,* 115–124.

Santin, M., Trout, J. M., & Fayer, R. (2009). A longitudinal study of Giardia duodenalis genotypes in dairy cows from birth to 2 years of age. *Vet Parasitol, 162,* 40–45.

Sattar, S. A., Jacobsen, H., Rahman, H., et al. (1994). Interruption of rotavirus spread through chemical disinfection. *Infect Control Hosp Epidemiol, 15,* 751–756.

Scallan, E., Hoekstra, R. M., Angulo, F. J., et al. (2011). Foodborne illness acquired in the United States-major pathogens. *Emerg Infect Dis, 17,* 7–15.

Schlafer, D. H., & Scott, F. W. (1979). Prevalence of neutralizing antibody to the calf rotavirus in New York cattle. *Cornell Vet, 69,* 262–271.

Scott, F. W., Kahrs, R. F., De Lahunta, A., et al. (1973). Virus induced congenital anomalies of the bovine fetus: I. cerebellar degeneration (hypoplasia), ocular lesions and fetal mummification following experimental infection with bovine viral diarrhea-mucosal disease virus. *Cornell Vet, 63,* 536–560.

Seek, B., & Cook, R. (1992). Rinderpest. In Committee on Foreign Animal Diseases (Ed.), Foreign animal diseases. Richmond, VA: United States Animal Health Association.

Selim, S. A., Cullor, J. S., Smith, B. P., et al. (1995). The effect of *Escherichia coli* J5 and modified live *Salmonella* Dublin vaccines in artificially reared neonatal calves. *Vaccine, 13,* 381–390.

Silverlas, C., Bjorkman, C., & Egenvall, A. (2009). Systematic review and meta-analyses of the effects of halofuginone against calf cryptosporidiosis. *Prev Vet Med, 91,* 73–84.

Sinks, G. D., Quigley JD III, & Reinemeyer, C. R. (1992). Effects of lasalocid on coccidial infection and growth in young dairy calves. *J Am Vet Med Assoc, 200,* 1947–1951.

Slapeta, J. (2013). Cryptosporidiosis and Cryptosporidium species in animals and humans: A thirty colour rainbow? *Int J Parasit, 43,* 957–970.

Smith, B. P. (2002). Salmonellosis in ruminants. In *Large animal internal medicine* (3rd ed.) (pp. 775–779). St. Louis: Mosby.

Smith, B. P. (1986). Understanding the role of endotoxins in gram-negative septicemia. *Vet Med, 81,* 1148–1161.

Smith, B. P., Dilling, G. W., Roden, L. D., et al. (1984). Aromatic-dependent *Salmonella dublin* as a parenteral modified live vaccine for calves. *Am J Vet Res, 45,* 2231–2235.

Smith, B. P., Oliver, D. G., Singh, P., et al. (1989). Detection of *Salmonella dublin* mammary gland infection in carrier cows using an ELISA for antibody in milk or serum. *Am J Vet Res, 50,* 1352–1360.

Smith, B. P., Reina-Guerra, M., Hoiseth, S. K., et al. (1984). Aromatic-dependent *Salmonella typhimurium* as modified live vaccines for calves. *Am J Vet Res, 45,* 59–66.

Smith, G. W., Alley, M. L., Foster, D. M., et al. (2014). Passive immunity stimulated by immunization of dry cows with a Salmonella Bacterial Extract. *J Vet Intern Med, 28,* 1602–1605.

Smith, G. W., Smith, F., Zuidhof, S., et al. (2015). Characterization of the serologic response induced by vaccination of late gestation dry cows with a Salmonella Dublin vaccine. *J Dairy Sci, 98,* 2529–2532.

Smith, H. W. (1951). A laboratory consideration of the treatment of *Actinobacillus lignieresii* infection. *Vet Rec, 63,* 674–675.

Smith, R. H., & Wynn, C. F. (1971). Effects of feeding soya products to preruminant calves. *Proc Nutr Soc (London), 30,* 75A.

Smithlie, L. K., & Modderman, E. (1975). BVD virus in commercial fetal calf serum and normal and aborted fetuses. In *Proceedings: 18th Annual Meeting American Association Veterinary Laboratory Diagnosis,* 113–119.

Snodgrass, D. R., Fahey, K. J., Wells, P. W., et al. (1980). Passive immunity in calf rotavirus infections: maternal vaccination increases and prolongs immunoglobulin G_1 antibody secretion in milk. *Infect Immun, 28,* 344–349.

Snodgrass, D. R., Stewart, J., Taylor, J., et al. (1982). Diarrhea in dairy calves reduced by feeding colostrum from cows vaccinated with rotavirus. *Res Vet Sci, 32,* 70–73.

Snodgrass, D. R., Terzolo, H. R., Sherwood, D., et al. (1986). Aetiology of diarrhea in young calves. *Vet Rec, 119,* 31–34.

Snyder, D. E., Floyd, J. G., & DiPietro, J. A. (1991). Use of anthelmintics and anticoccidial compounds in cattle. *Compend Contin Educ Pract Vet, 13,* 1847–1860.

Sockett, D. C., Brower, A. I., Porter, R. E., et al. (2004). Hemorrhagic bowel syndrome in dairy cattle: preliminary results from a case control study. In *Proceedings, 47th Annual Conference* (p. 37). Greensboro, NC: American Association of Veterinary Laboratory Diagnosticians.

Songer, J. G. (1998). Clostridial diseases of small ruminants. *Vet Res, 29,* 219–232.

Songer, J. G. (1996). Clostridial enteric diseases of domestic animals. *Clin Microbiol Rev, 9,* 216–234.

Songer, J. G. (1999). *Clostridium perfringens* type A infection in cattle. In *Proceedings, 32nd Annual Convention* (pp. 40–44). American Association of Bovine Practitioners.

Songer, J. G., & Miskimins, D. W. (2005). Clostridial abomasitis in calves: Case report and review of the literature. *Anaerobe, 11,* 290–294.

Speer, C. A., Scott, M. C., Bannantine, J. P., et al. (2006). A novel enzyme-linked immunosorbent assay for diagnosis of *Mycobacterium avium* subsp. *paratuberculosis* infections (Johne's disease) in cattle. *Clin Vaccine Immunol, 13,* 535–540.

Spier, S. J., Smith, B. P., Cullor, J. S., et al. (1991). Persistent experimental Salmonella dublin intramammary infection in dairy cows. *J Vet Intern Med, 5,* 341–350.

Stockdale, P. H., & Niilo, L. (1976). Production of bovine coccidiosis with *Eimeria zuernii, Can Vet J, 17,* 35–37.

Stott, J. L. (1992). Bluetongue and epizootic hemorrhagic disease. In Committee on Foreign Animal Diseases (Ed.), Foreign animal diseases. Richmond, VA: United States Animal Health Association.

Sulaiman, I. M., Xiao, L., Yang, C., et al. (1998). Differentiating human from animal isolates of Cryptosporidium parvum. *Emerg Inf Dis, 4,* 681–685.

Sutmoller, P. (1992). Vesicular diseases. In Committee on Foreign Animal Diseases (Ed.), Foreign animal diseases. Richmond, VA: United States Animal Health Association.

Swarbrick, O. (1967). Atypical actinobacillosis in three cows. *Br Vet J, 123,* 70–75.

Sweeney, R. W., Divers, T. J., Whitlock, R. H., et al. (1988). Hepatic failure in dairy cattle following mastitis or metritis. *J Vet Intern Med, 2,* 80–84.

Sweeney, R. W., Uzonna, J., Whitlock, R. H., et al. (2006). Tissue predilection sites and effect of dose on *Mycobacterium avium* subs. *paratuberculosis* organism recovery in a short-term bovine experimental oral infection model. *Res Vet Sci, 80,* 253–259.

Sweeney, R. W., Whitlock, R. H., McAdams, S., et al. (2006). Londitudinal study of ELISA seroreactivity to *Mycobacterium avium* subsp. *paratuberculosis* in infected cattle and culture-negative herd mates. *J Vet Diagn Invest, 18,* 2–6.

Takahashi, E., et al. (1980). Epizootic diarrhoea of adult cattle associated with a corona-like agent. *Vet Microbiol, 5,* 151–154.

Teixeira, A. G., Stephens, L., Divers, T. J., et al. (2015). Effect of crofelemer extract on severity and consistency of experimentally induced enterotoxigenic Escherichia coli diarrhea in newborn Holstein calves. *J Dairy Sci, 98*(11), 8035–8043.

Tennant, B., Ward, D. E., Braun, R. K., et al. (1978). Clinical management and control of neonatal enteric infections of calves. *J Am Vet Med Assoc, 173,* 654–660.

Terzolo, H. R., Lawson, G. H. K., Angus, K. W., et al. (1987). Enteric campylobacter infection in gnotobiotic calves and lambs. *Res Vet Sci, 43,* 72–77.

Tewari, D., Sandt, C. H., Miller, D. M., et al. (2012). Prevalence of Salmonella Cerro in laboratory-based submissions of cattle and comparison with human infections in Pennsylvania, 2005-2010. *Foodborne Pathog Dis, 9,* 928–933.

Thornhill, J. B., Krebs, G. L., & Petzel, C. E. (2015). Evaluation of the Brix refractometer as an on-farm tool for the detection of

passive transfer of immunity in dairy calves. *Aust Vet J, 93*(1–2), 26–30.

Timoney, J. F., Gillespie, J. H., Scott, F. W., et al. (1988). *Hagan and Bruner's microbiology and infectious diseases of domestic animals* (8th ed.). New York: Cornell University Press.

Tompkins, T. (1993). Milk replacer options. *Large Anim Vet January,* 24–29.

Tompkins, T., & Drackley, J. K. (1992). Clotting factor in bovine pre-ruminant nutrition. In *Proceedings: XVII World Buiatrics Congress* (Vol. 2) (pp. 176–181).

Tompkins, T., & Jaster, E. H. (1991). Preruminant calf nutrition. *Vet Clin North Am Food Anim Pract, 7,* 557–576.

Toth, J. D., Aceto, H. W., Rankin, S. C., et al. (2011). Survival characteristics of Salmonella enterica serovar Newport in the dairy farm environment. *J Dairy Sci, 94,* 5238–5246.

Torres-Medina, A., Schlafer, D. H., & Mebus, C. A. (1985). Rotaviral and coronaviral diarrhea. *Vet Clin North Am Food Anim Pract, 1,* 471–493.

Trainin, Z., et al. (1980). Oral immunization of young calves against enteropathogenic *E. coli.* In *Proceedings: XI International Congress on Diseases of Cattle* (p. 1313).

Traven, M., Naslund, K., Linde, N., et al. (2001). Experimental reproduction of winter dysentery in lactating cows using BCV—comparison with BCV infection in milk-fed calves. *Vet Microbiol, 81,* 127–151.

Troxel, T. R., Gadberry, M. S., Wallace, W. T., et al. (2001). Clostridial antibody response from injection-site lesions in beef cattle, long-term antibody response to single or multiple doses, and response in newborn beef calves. *J Anim Sci, 79,* 2558–2564.

Tsunemitsu, H., Smith, D. R., & Saif, L. J. (1999). Experimental inoculation of adult dairy cows with bovine coronavirus and detection of coronavirus by RT-PCR. *Arch Virol, 144,* 167–175.

Tyler, J. W., Hancock, D. D., Wilson, L., et al. (1999). Effect of passive transfer status and vaccination with Escherichia coli (J5) on mortality in commingled dairy calves. *J Vet Intern Med, 13,* 36–39.

Tyler, J. W., Parish, S. M., Besser, T. E., et al. (1999). Detection of low serum immunoglobulin concentrations in clinically ill calves. *J Vet Intern Med, 12,* 40–43.

Tyler, J. W., Steevens, B. J., Hostetler, D. E., et al. (1999). Colostral IgG concentrations in Holstein and Guernsey cows. *Am J Vet Res, 60,* 1136–1139.

Udall, D. H. (1954). *The practice of veterinary medicine* (6th ed.). Ithaca, NY: published by the author, 624.

Underdahl, N. R., Grace, O. D., & Hoerlein, A. B. (1957). Cultivation in tissue culture of a cytopathogenic agent from bovine mucosal disease. *Proc Soc Exp Biol Med, 94,* 795–797.

United States Department of Agriculture (USDA). (2011). *Salmonella, Listeria, and Campylobacter on U.S. Dairy Operations, 1996-2007.* Fort Collins, CO: USDA-APHIS-VS, CEAH.

Uzal, F. A., Blanchard, P., Songer, G., et al. (2000). Studies on the so-called "clostridial enteritis" of cattle (abstract). In *Proceedings, 43rd Annual Meeting* (p. 15). Birmingham, AL: American Association of Veterinary Laboratory Diagnosticians.

Van Campen, H. (2006). *personal communication.* Fort Collins, CO.

Van Kessel, J. A., Karns, J. S., Lombard, J. E., et al. (2011). Prevalence of Salmonella enterica, Listeria monocytogenes, and Escherichia coli virulence factors in bulk tank milk and in-line filters from U.S. dairies. *J Food Prot, 74,* 759–768.

Van Kessel, J. S., Karns, J. S., Wolfgang, D. R., et al. (2007). Longitudinal study of a clonal, subclinical outbreak of Salmonella enterica subsp. enterica serovar Cerro in a U.S. dairy herd. *Foodborne Pathog Dis, 4,* 449–461.

van Schaik, G., Stehman, S. M., Jacobson, R. H., et al. (2005). Cow-level evaluation of a kinetics ELISA with multiple cutoff values to detect fecal shedding of *Mycobacterium avium* subspecies *paratuberculosis* in New York State dairy cows. *Prev Vet Med, 73*, 221–236.

Vance, H. N. (1967). A survey of the alimentary tract of cattle for Clostridium perfringens. *Can J Comp Med Vet Sci, 31*, 260–264.

Voges, J., Horner, G. W., Rowe, S., et al. (1998). Persistent bovine pestivirus infection localized in the testes of an immunocompetent, non-viraemic bull. *Vet Microbiol, 61*, 165–175.

Walz, P. H., Bell, T. G., Steficek, B. A., et al. (1999). Experimental model of type II bovine viral diarrhea virus-induced thrombocytopenia in neonatal calves. *J Vet Diagn Invest, 11*, 505–514.

Walz, P. H., Steficek, B. A., Baker, J. C., et al. (1999). Effect of experimentally induced type II bovine viral diarrhea virus infection on platelet function in calves. *Am J Vet Res, 60*, 1396–1401.

Wang, Y. Q., Puntenney, S. B., & Forsberg, N. E. (2004). Identification of the mechanisms by which OmniGen-AF, a nutritional supplement, augments immune function in ruminant livestock. In *Proceedings* (p. 55). Western Section, American Association of Animal Science.

Ward, G. M., Roberts, S. J., McEntee, K., et al. (1969). A study of experimentally induced bovine viral diarrhea-mucosal disease in pregnant cows and their progeny. *Cornell Vet, 59*, 525–539.

Warnick, L. D., Kanistanon, K., McDonough, P. L., et al. (2003). Effect of previous antimicrobial treatment on fecal shedding of *Salmonella enterica* subsp. *enterica* serogroup B in New York dairy herds with recent clinical salmonellosis. *Prev Vet Med, 56*, 285–297.

Warnick, L. D., Nielsen, L. R., Nielsen, J., et al. (2006). Simulation model estimates of test accuracy and predictive values for the Danish Salmonella surveillance program in dairy herds. *Prev Vet Med, 77*, 284–303.

Washburn, K. E., Step, D. L., Kirkpatrick, J. F., et al. (2000). Bluetongue and persistent bovine viral diarrhea virus infection causing generalized edema in an adult bull. *J Vet Intern Med, 14*, 468–469.

Watts, T. C., Olsoh, S. M., & Rhodes, C. S. (1973). Treatment of bovine actinomycosis with isoniazid. *Can Vet J, 14*, 223–224.

Weaver, D. M., Tyler, J. W., Barrington, G. M., et al. (2000). Passive transfer of colostral immunoglobulins in calves. *J Vet Intern Med, 14*, 569–577.

Weaver, L. D. (1979). Malignant catarrhal fever in two California dairy herds. *Bov Pract, 14*, 121–127.

Weldon, A. D., Moise, N. S., & Rebhun, W. C. (1992). Hyperkalemic atrial standstill in neonatal calf diarrhea. *J Vet Intern Med, 6*, 294–297.

White, D. M., Wilson, W. C., Blair, C. D., et al. (2005). Studies on overwintering of bluetongue viruses in insects. *J Gen Virol, 2*, 453–462.

Whitmore, H. L., Zemjanis, R., & Olson, J. (1981). Effect of bovine viral diarrhea virus on conception in cattle. *J Am Vet Med Assoc, 178*, 1065–1067.

Williams, J. C., Corwin, R. M., Craig, T. M., et al. (1986). Control strategies for nematodiasis in cattle. *Vet Clin North Am Food Anim Pract, 2*, 247–260.

Williams, J. C., Knox, J. W., Marbury, K. S., et al. (1985). *Osterlagia ostertagi*: a continuing problem of recognition and control. *Anim Nutr Health March*, 42–45.

Wilson, W. C., Daniels, P., Ostlund, E. N., et al. (2015). Diagnostic tools for Bluetongue and Epizootic Hemorrhagic Disease viruses applicable to North American veterinary diagnosticians. *Vector Borne Zoonotic Dis, 15*, 364–373.

Yim, L., Sasias, S., Martinez, A., et al. (2014). Repression of flagella is a common trait in field isolates of Salmonella enterica serovar Dublin and is associated with invasive human infections. *Infect Immun, 82*, 146 5-1476.

You, Y., Rankin, S. C., Aceto, H. W., et al. (2006). Survival of Salmonella enterica serovar Newport in manure and manure-amended soils. *Appl Environ Microbiol, 72*, 5777–5783.

Zhao, H., Wilkins, K., Damon, I. K., et al. (2013). Specific qPCR assays for the detection of orf virus, pseudocowpox virus and bovine popular stomatitis virus. *J Virol Methods, 194*, 229–234.

7

Skin Diseases

DANNY W. SCOTT

Infectious Diseases

Papillomatosis (Fibropapillomas, "Warts")

Etiology

Papillomas are the most common tumors in dairy cattle; fortunately, most papillomas are benign and self-limiting. Animals between 6 and 24 months of age seem most at risk for warts, and previous incidence of the tumors gives an individual a degree of immunity. Papillomas are well documented to be caused by bovine papillomavirus (BPV) types 1 through 14. These viruses have some common antigenic components but do not have good immunologic cross-reactivity. BPV1, and especially BPV2, cause typical warts on the head, neck, trunk, and legs of young cattle (Fig. 7.1). A "typical" wart means that a true fibropapilloma exists histopathologically. These masses usually are cauliflower-like, rough, or crusty-surfaced skin lesions that are colored white to gray. Some appear flatter, more gray, and have a broad-based skin attachment. Others have a pedunculated base. The virus infects the basal cells of the epithelium; as these cells eventually reach the surface, large quantities of virus are available to contaminate fomites and the environment. Therefore, warts tend to become endemic rather than occur sporadically. Stanchions, feed bunks, neck straps, brushes, halters, pens, and back rubs all become coated with virus. Abrasions of the skin caused by mild trauma from sharp objects (e.g., nails, splintered wood, barbed wire, and bolt ends) allow inoculation of the virus into skin and increase the incidence in a group of calves. Epidemic and endemic situations have also been associated with dehorning (Fig. 7.2), ear tagging, and the use of tattooing devices or emasculatomes when disinfection of a common instrument has not been performed. This is especially true when laypeople perform the aforementioned procedures. Insects also have been suspected of spreading or inoculating the virus into skin, but this remains difficult to prove.

Cattle with large multiple warts that do not regress probably have concurrent deficient cell-mediated immunity (Fig. 7.3) or some other immunodeficiency such as persistent infection with bovine viral diarrhea virus (BVDV) or bovine leukocyte adhesion deficiency (BLAD). Genital fibropapillomas caused by BPV1 are commonly found on the penis of young bulls (Fig. 7.4), on the teats, and occasionally in the vagina of heifers.

Atypical warts that tend to persist for years have been associated with BPV3 infections. Young and mature animals may be affected; the lesions are multiple, low, flat, and annular, with fingerlike or frondlike projections that are composed of epithelial proliferation without dermal fibrosis. These lesions are not raised as noticeably as BPV1 or BPV2 warts and may simply be interspersed with normal-haired skin.

Alimentary warts involving the esophagus, forestomach, and oral cavity are thought to be associated with BPV4. Although cattle with alimentary fibropapillomas are usually asymptomatic, occasionally fibropapillomas interfere with effective eructation and result in signs associated with vagal indigestion. Malignant transformation of BPV4-induced

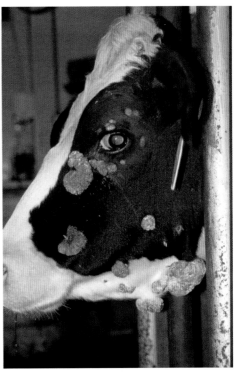

• **Fig. 7.1** Holstein heifer with multiple small- to medium-sized fibropapillomas on the eyelids and masseter and mandibular regions.

alimentary lesions to carcinomas is also possible and is a much greater risk when carcinogens such as bracken fern make up a major portion of the diet.

BPV4, as well as BPV1 and BPV2, may contribute to urinary bladder tumors in cattle consuming bracken fern at pasture. This condition, known as enzootic hematuria, can be life-threatening to affected cattle.

BPV5 causes so-called "rice-grain" teat fibropapillomas, probably the most common form of teat wart seen in dairy cattle in the United States. (This virus is discussed further in Chapter 8.) It is spread by milking procedures and machines that predispose to teat chapping or minor teat abrasions. Similarly, BPV6 through BPV12 have been shown to cause

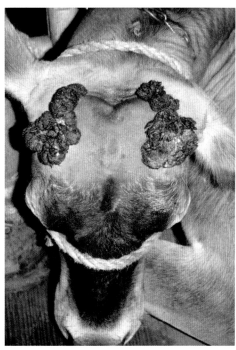

• **Fig. 7.2** Large bilateral fibropapillomas in a Jersey calf representative of an epidemic occurrence following dehorning by a layperson.

papillomatous frondlike lesions on the skin of the teats and udder.

Signs

Signs usually are obvious for skin papillomas, but flat, wide-based, gray warts occasionally may be misdiagnosed as crusty ringworm lesions. Lesions tend to be multiple and mainly occur in facial, neck, shoulder, and trunk locations. Lesions limited to a common anatomic area in most infected animals may help identify the cause of infection. This is especially easy for eartag and dehorning wounds, for example. Fly irritation, myiasis, and bleeding are common problems associated with large cauliflower-like warts that appear during warm weather. Hemorrhage may be life-threatening in rare cases with huge, multiple warts over a large portion of the individual's body.

Penile warts in young bulls may interfere with breeding, and can spread the virus to cows naturally serviced or to other bulls from artificial vaginas that are not routinely disinfected. Bleeding from the penis or sheath after collection or service is the usual owner complaint concerning affected bulls. Heifers with vaginal fibropapillomas frequently go undetected unless the mass becomes large and protrudes from the vulva.

Alimentary warts seldom are observed clinically except during oral examination, esophageal endoscopy, or rumenotomy. The lesions commonly are observed during gross postmortem examination.

Enzootic hematuria leads to obvious hematuria and dysuria or stranguria in affected cattle on pastures containing bracken fern.

Although teat lesions of fibropapillomas (BPV1, BPV2), rice-grain lesions (BPV5), or papillomas (BPV6) may be observed in individual cattle, they frequently become endemic in a herd. Warts may interfere with effective milking or be irritated by milking, but seldom cause serious problems unless they occur at the teat end. Cattle that have teat end warts are at increased risk for interference with milkout and mastitis.

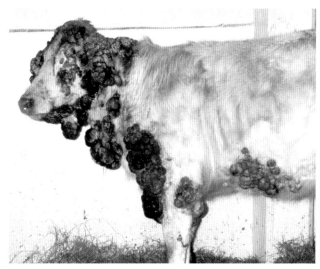

• **Fig. 7.3** Multiple large warts that failed to regress over a 6-month period in a heifer.

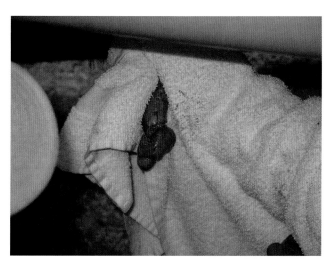

• **Fig. 7.4** Large genital fibropapilloma on the penis of a yearling Holstein bull associated with bovine papillomavirus type 1 infection.

Diagnosis

Clinical signs are sufficient for diagnosis in most instances. Atypical lesions may require biopsy and histopathologic study. Gross sectioning of surgically excised fibropapillomas also is suggestive because epidermal proliferation over dermal fibroplasia is obvious on cut sections.

Treatment

Because skin warts usually are self-limiting within 1 to 12 months, treatment seldom is necessary. However, the variable duration of warts (up to 12 months) before self-cure causes owners to request treatment, particularly in young show cattle. In addition, various treatments, vaccines, and quack medications have gained acceptance because owners attribute eventual resolution of warts to treatment with these products rather than to a spontaneous immunologic cure. Commercial or autogenous vaccines have been used extensively. Unfortunately, they suffer from some major deficiencies:

1. Vaccines tend to be used for treatment rather than prevention.
2. The strains of virus used in commercial products may not be homologous with those causing the clinical warts in specific anatomic locations.
3. When used as treatment, no way exists to prove the vaccines more efficacious than a time-related natural cure.

Vaccination may be helpful when used as a preventive measure to decrease the risk of penile warts for bull calves assembled in bull studs, or in herds with a high incidence of warts.

"Emergency treatment" is a frequent owner request during the summer months when heifers compete in cattle shows. This frustrating situation results from regulations forbidding animals with warts from being shown for fear of contagion. Veterinarians are pressured into doing "something" to resolve lesions quickly, which may be impossible.

Many treatments, such as surgical removal or crushing of individual warts, have been tried in an effort to stimulate the cell-mediated immunity that is essential to eventual resolution of the problem. In addition, autogenous vaccines injected intradermally or subcutaneously (SC), levamisole, and other products have been tried. The success of these techniques is not known. Cryosurgery on selected tumors may be used both to destroy the tumor and to stimulate cell-mediated immunity to cause rejection of other tumors in the same animal. The author has found this technique most useful in severe epidemics of warts after dehorning by laypeople in which each affected heifer has bilateral warts overlying the skin of the dehorning wounds.

Prevention is the best form of treatment, and includes identification of likely fomites, husbandry errors and contaminated or sharp structural devices that can be removed or corrected. In addition, surgical instruments, tattooing implements, and dehorners should be sterilized or disinfected with virucidal solutions between uses.

Penile fibropapillomas in bulls require careful surgical dissection followed by cryosurgery of the base of the wart. A double freeze–thaw–freeze cycle can give excellent results. Although the tumor base should be frozen to at least −30.0°C, it is difficult to use thermocouples to monitor temperature in this tissue, so subjectively ensuring adequate freezing by viewing the ice ball may be necessary. Pedunculated penile warts are much easier to treat and less likely to recur than those with a broad base. Electrocautery, surgical excision, and laser techniques are all possible treatment modalities, as described in Chapter 10. Vaginal fibropapillomas requiring treatment are rare. When necessary, excision at the base or cryosurgery may be successful. Vaginal warts may have extremely vascular stalks, and ligatures are sometimes necessary to prevent severe hemorrhage during removal.

Flat or rice-grain teat warts seldom are removed, but raised fibropapillomas or papillomas on the teat or teat end that mechanically interfere with milking may have to be removed flush with the skin by scissors (see Chapter 8).

Individual cattle with large multiple warts that persist indefinitely probably have deficient cell-mediated immunity. This may be a genetic fault, or be associated with medical problems such as persistent infection with BVDV or BLAD. This problem, when unrelated to either persistent infection with BVDV or BLAD, seems more common in beef cattle (especially Herefords) than in the dairy breeds.

Dermatophytosis ("Ringworm")

Etiology

Dermatophytosis, or ringworm, is extremely common in dairy calves and may also occur in adult cows. *Trichophyton verrucosum* is the most common pathogen, with less frequent instances of *Trichophyton mentagrophytes* and other dermatophytes. Calves older than 2 months of age through yearling stage are most commonly affected. This coincides with the ages of young dairy animals that are grouped rather than managed individually. The causative organisms are extremely hardy and survive on inanimate objects, bedding, and soil for months after cattle have been removed. Concentration or grouping of young cattle—especially during the winter months—leads to an increased incidence in herds that have the problem. It is not unusual to find yearly epidemics in heifers on farms that have had ringworm in the past. Conversely, herds that do not have clinical ringworm seem to remain free of the problem unless new animals that are infected are introduced. Adult cattle may experience severe infections as well. These outbreaks tend to occur during the winter months, and frequently follow infected freshening heifers being introduced into the milking herd. Although adult cows that had ringworm as calves have been assumed to be "immune for life," the existence of outbreaks in adult cattle raises serious questions as to the longevity of immunity after natural exposure.

Dermatophytes affect the keratinized layers of skin and hair, thanks to toxins and allergens, with resultant exudation, crusting, and alopecia. Fungal organisms themselves do not invade tissue, but survive best when they provoke little host inflammatory reaction. Lesions tend to be oval or

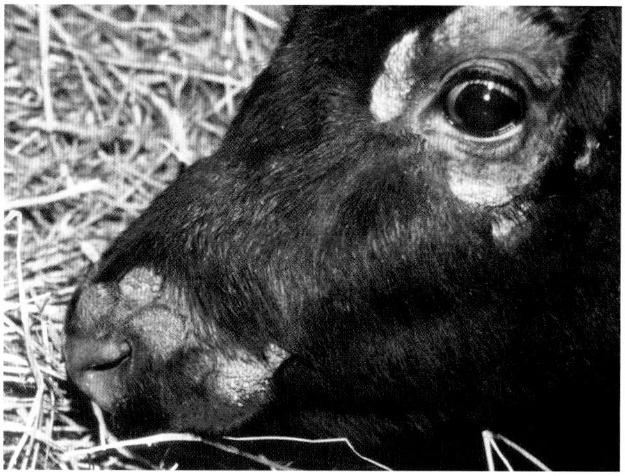

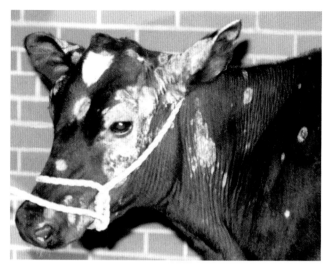

• **Fig. 7.5** Raised, crusted lesions of ringworm involving the facial and periocular region of a Holstein calf.

• **Fig. 7.6** Multifocal ringworm lesions that appear as dry, crusted areas of alopecia of the head, neck, and shoulders in a Holstein heifer.

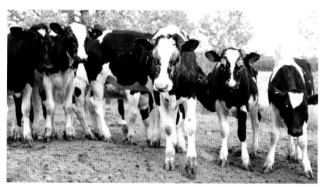

• **Fig. 7.7** Epidemic ringworm in a group of Holstein yearlings. (Courtesy of Dr. Pam Powers.)

circular, and are often multifocal. Incubation requires 1 to 4 weeks, and lesions persist for 1 to 3 months in most circumstances. Infection by contact is accelerated by mechanical irritation of the skin by contaminated objects. Stanchions, neck straps, halters, milking straps for old-fashioned bucket milking machines, brushes or currycombs, chutes, and other devices may spread infection through a group of cattle. Chronically ill, unthrifty, poorly nourished, or acutely ill cattle will show diffuse or rapidly progressive lesions compared with herdmates. This may imply either cellular or humoral factors that contribute to worsening of dermatophytosis. Calves persistently infected with BVDV and calves with BLAD are examples of animals that frequently have severe ringworm lesions; healthy herdmates remain either unaffected or have only mild lesions. Adult cows or heifers with typical ringworm lesions may progress to diffuse lesions when stressed by acute severe infections such as pneumonia or peritonitis. Exogenous corticosteroids worsen existing ringworm lesions.

Lack of sunlight also has been proposed as a contributing cause because animals penned indoors seem to have a higher incidence. This theory also led many veterinarians to administer vitamins A and D as a treatment. However, the appearance of ringworm in both calves and adult cows during the summer months seems to diminish the importance of sunlight in prevention or cure.

Signs

Round or oval areas of crusting and alopecia that range from 1.0 to 5.0 cm in diameter are typical for ringworm in calves. Early lesions may appear raised because of serum oozing from, or secondary bacterial pyoderma underlying, the crust (Fig. 7.5). In calves, the periocular region, ears, muzzle, neck, and trunk are most commonly affected, but lesions may occur anywhere (Figs. 7.6 and 7.7). Head and neck lesions are common because lock-ins, stanchions, or neck straps become contaminated and help spread the disease. Posts or beams that are used for scratching by a group of heifers may provide the means by which the trunk becomes infected. The escutcheon

is another area that frequently is affected with one or more lesions. Skin lesions may be painful but are rarely pruritic.

In adult cattle, the lesions may be anywhere on the body but often appear on the trunk and neck, with fewer cows showing the typical facial lesions found in calves. In addition to oval and circular lesions, larger geographic lesions of ringworm occasionally appear in adult cattle.

During ringworm outbreaks in adult cattle, individual cows that experience unassociated systemic illness may show dramatic worsening of their ringworm lesions. Ketotic cattle treated with corticosteroids may also show worsening of the ringworm condition. Adult cattle also may have lesions on the udder, skin of the flank, or hind limbs that increase the risk of zoonotic disease because these lesions occur where milkers come into contact with the animals. Lesions of ringworm in milkers or handlers of infected cattle are a common occurrence, and ringworm is the most common example of a zoonosis in cattle practice.

Diagnosis

Cultures of hair from the peripheral zone of a lesion on selective media, scrapings of lesions, plucking of hairs for mineral oil or potassium hydroxide preps, or skin biopsies can be used to confirm the diagnosis, but clinical signs usually suffice. Early lesions may be sufficiently raised in appearance to mimic warts or other lesions, but careful examination will differentiate them.

Treatment

Although hundreds of products have been used to treat ringworm in cattle, few have been shown to be efficacious. The self-limiting nature of ringworm infection in most cattle that are otherwise healthy makes it difficult to assess how much, if at all, the treatment helped natural healing. Controlled studies are essential for any product to be proven as efficacious against ringworm.

Treatment often is requested because of zoonotic potential or because an affected heifer or cow has been selected to go to a show or a sale. Animals with ringworm, as with warts, are ineligible for admission to shows or sales. This latter situation often leads to the sudden "emergency" status of ringworm, even though it has been present on the animals for months.

Before discussing various treatments, one must realize the magnitude of the labor required to treat hundreds of ringworm lesions in a group of calves, heifers, or cows. The failure of treatment and lack of owner interest in it are simply based on the sometimes impossible task of catching, restraining, and treating groups of heifers. Treatment more often involves selected animals that need to be "cured" so they can enter a fair or a show. Owners who are willing to treat their calves also should be educated about disinfection, prevention and zoonotic risks.

Topical treatments that probably are efficacious when applied as a spray or dip daily for 5 days then once weekly until resolution include:
1. Lime sulfur 2% to 5%
2. 0.5% sodium hypochlorite
3. 0.02% enilconazole; not currently available in the United States nor labeled for use in dairy cattle
Topical treatments that may be effective for limited lesions or selective treatment of a few animals include:
1. Miconazole or clotrimazole or terbinafine cream once or twice daily; not approved for use in dairy cattle
Systemic treatment that probably is efficacious:
1. Griseofulvin 20 to 60 mg/kg orally for 7 or more days. Griseofulvin is not approved for use in cattle
Systemic treatments that may be efficacious:
1. Sodium iodide 20% solution: 150 cc per 450 kg intravenously (IV), repeated in 3 to 4 days
2. Vitamins A and D: only indicated if animals have been kept completely out of sunlight; efficacy not proven
For best results, animals that are treated with any of the aforementioned products should first have their lesions scraped or brushed to remove the infective crusts. Clipping also may be helpful, but risks spread of the infection. Remember that brushes, currycombs, and clippers used on infected animals should be cleaned and disinfected. Workers handling the cattle should wear gloves or wash thoroughly with an iodophor or tincture of green soap following handling of the animals.

Disinfection of premises and fomites offers the best opportunity to avoid future outbreaks. Physical cleansing and pressure spraying can be followed with lime sulfur or sodium hypochlorite disinfection. Premises should be allowed to dry and supplied with new bedding. Only animals without detectable lesions should be reintroduced.

Vaccines have been developed in some parts of the world and have been reported to be efficacious; however, they are not available in the United States.

Dermatophilosis ("Rain Scald")
Etiology

Dermatophilosis, also called Streptothricosis, rain rot, or rain scald, is a common skin infection of cattle and other large animals caused by *Dermatophilus congolensis*. Moist environmental conditions predispose to contagious infection by *D. congolensis*. Heifers that are housed outside and herds of adult cattle that have access to outdoor environments each day are most at risk for dermatophilosis. Rain and snow that wet hair coats and cause matting present the greatest opportunity for infection. In addition to moisture, physical damage to the skin is necessary because *D. congolensis* is thought not to be able to invade healthy skin. Depending on the region and time of year, external parasites such as flies and lice may sufficiently injure skin and help spread the infection. Other sources of skin injury include abrasions from scratching, rubbing, or licking, and moist dermatitis that develops under wet matted hair.

D. congolensis probably is part of the normal skin flora in some cattle, and is known to proliferate in a moist environment. Cattle that are highly stressed by illness, transient or long-standing alterations of their immune status, or treated with corticosteroids may develop severe lesions.

Signs

In animals housed outdoors, a crusty dermatitis along the topline represents the classical distribution of dermatophilosis. Animals with short hair coats may have a folliculitis with mildly raised crusts and tufts of hair, whereas more classical cases with long hair coats have thick tufts of matted hair and crusts that can be plucked off to expose a thick, yellow-green pus on the skin and attachment areas of crust. Pink areas of dermis may be apparent after removal of crusted tufts of hair (Fig. 7.8).

Cattle that have access to farm ponds, deep mud, or lush wet pastures may develop lesions on the lower limbs and muzzle rather than the classical dorsal distribution. Bulls may develop the lesions on the skin of the scrotum, and occasionally cows develop lesions on the udder and/or teats.

Dermatophilosis that becomes widespread or covers more than 50% of the body surface may be fatal. Fortunately, severe dermatophilosis is rare in the United States, but this disease remains a serious cause of cattle mortality in tropical climates, where greater heat and humidity, coupled with more profound insect and tick loads, exist (Fig. 7.9). Death may occur in severe cases as a result of debility, discomfort, protein loss, and septicemia.

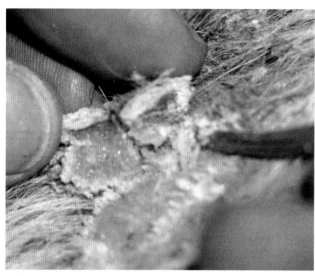

• **Fig. 7.8** A crusted tuft of hair being removed from a cow infected with dermatophilosis. Although the underside of this tuft appears somewhat dry, more typical cases have a thick pus evident.

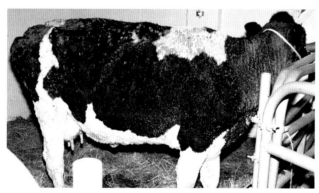

• **Fig. 7.9** Unusually severe dermatophilosis in a single Holstein cow from a New York herd. A heavy summer fly load apparently contributed to the diffuse spread of the organism in this cow. That no other herd-mates were affected and that the disease occurred during July both were unusual in this case.

Animals with long hair coats; crusts of matted hair with underlying pus; and a dorsal distribution, especially over the gluteals, loin, and withers, are easily diagnosed by physical examination. Animals with short hair coats that have signs of folliculitis or lesions on the extremities may present a difficult differential diagnosis that includes staphylococcal folliculitis, viral infections, zinc-responsive dermatoses, dermatophytosis, and immune-mediated dermatoses.

Diagnosis

When pus can be found underneath plucked tufts of hair or on the bottom of the detached tuft, it provides an excellent diagnostic specimen for direct microscopic examination. Smears may be examined with Gram stain, new methylene blue, or Diff-Quik to look for chains of branching and multiseptate coccoid bacteria resembling hyphae, and clumps of gram-positive coccoid cells arranged in characteristic parallel rows ("railroad tracks"). When pus cannot be found, the diagnosis is made more difficult. Crusts

may be ground up and made into smears for microscopic examination, but the most helpful techniques remain skin biopsy and culture. Histopathology may show folliculitis, intracellular edema of keratinocytes, and surface crusts with alternating layers of keratin and leukocytic debris (palisading crusts); the organisms are observed in crusts or other locations. Gram stain used on sections may highlight the organisms more so than standard hematoxylin and eosin.

Treatment

Treatment is difficult and time consuming. In wet or damp, cold environments, the thought of bathing large numbers of cows to treat the condition is dismissed quickly by most owners. Infections often resolve spontaneously over several weeks if affected animals can be kept dry and cutaneous injury (insects, and so forth) can be controlled. In addition to keeping the animals dry, it is helpful to remove tufts of crusted hair or to clip matted hair to reduce the numbers of organisms present. Whenever possible, combining grooming with an iodine or chlorhexidine shampoo is an excellent treatment. Unlike ringworm, dermatophilosis lesions seldom are focal enough to be treated individually. Therefore, overall grooming or clipping usually is necessary. Clippers, combs, and other grooming equipment must be thoroughly disinfected with chlorhexidine, iodophors, or bleach before reuse, to prevent cross-contamination. The rational treatment of this disease also is complicated by the fact that, in the winter, animals may need as much hair as possible to survive outdoors. Unless there is an opportunity for indoor housing, owners are reluctant to clip hair. Systemic therapy with penicillin or oxytetracycline is highly efficacious, and can be life saving for animals with diffuse disease. Therefore, standard treatment recommendations include:

1. Topical—whichever of the following that is practical:
   Grooming to remove crusts is very helpful
   Clipping long hair, if possible
   Iodine or chlorhexidine shampoos, or lime sulfur rinses, if possible
2. Systemic—intramuscular (IM) penicillin twice daily dosed at 20,000 U/kg twice daily for 5 to 7 days, or SC long-acting oxytetracycline dosed at 20 mg/kg once

Human infections with *D. congolensis*, although rare, are possible, and veterinarians should advise handlers to wear gloves and wash themselves with iodophor soaps after handling or treating affected cattle.

Other Cutaneous Diseases Caused by Infectious Agents

Numerous bacterial, fungal, viral, and protozoal infections may produce dermatologic lesions. An in-depth discussion of these diseases, especially their noncutaneous manifestations, is beyond the scope of this chapter, but a listing of these disorders is provided in Table 7.1.

TABLE 7.1 Miscellaneous Bacterial, Fungal, Viral, and Protozoal Disorders of the Skin

Disorder	Signs
Bacterial Disorders	
Abscess	Any age; anywhere on the body; fluctuant, subcutaneous, often painful; especially *Trueperella pyogenes*
Actinobacillosis ("wooden tongue")	Adults; single or multiple nodules and abscesses; especially face, head, and neck; *Actinobacillus lignieresii*
Actinomycosis ("lumpy jaw")	Adults; firm, variably painful, immovable swellings with nodules, abscesses, and draining tracts; especially mandible and maxilla; *Actinomyces bovis* and *A. israelii*
Bacterial pseudomycetoma ("botryomycosis")	Adults; single or multiple crusted nodules and ulcers on udder; *Pseudomonas aeruginosa*
Cellulitis	Any age; marked swelling and pain with variable exudation and draining tracts; especially leg (*Staphylococcus aureus*, *T. pyogenes*, or *Streptococcus dysgalactiae*) or face, neck, and brisket (*Fusobacterium necrophorum*, *Bacteroides* spp., *Pasteurella septica*)
Clostridial cellulitis	Any age; acute onset and rapidly fatal; poorly circumscribed, painful, warm, pitting, deep swellings progressing to necrosis and slough with variable crepitus; especially leg (*Clostridium chauvoei*; "black leg") or head, neck, shoulder, abdomen, groin, and following tail docking (*C. septicum*, *C. sordelli*, *C. perfringens*; "malignant edema")
Corynebacterium pseudotuberculosis granuloma	Adults; single or multiple subcutaneous abscesses and ulcerated nodules; anywhere on body (especially head, neck, shoulder, flank, and thigh)
Farcy	Adults; firm, painless subcutaneous nodules with enlarged and palpable lymphatics; anywhere on body (especially head, neck, shoulder, legs); *Mycobacterium senegalense*
Impetigo	Adults; pustules, erosions, and crusts on udder, teats, ventral abdomen, medial thighs, vulva, perineum, and ventral tail; nonpruritic and nonpainful; *S. aureus*
Necrotic vulvovaginitis	Postparturient first lactation; erythema, edema, hemorrhage and necrosis of vulva, vagina and perineum; *Porphyromonas levii*
Necrobacillosis	Adults; moist, necrotic, ulcerative, and foul-smelling lesions anywhere on body (especially axillae, groin, udder, between digits); *F. necrophorum*
Nodular thelitis	Adults; painful papules, plaques, nodules, and ulcers on teats and udder; *Mycobacterium terrae* and *M. gordonae*
Opportunistic mycobacterial granuloma	Adults; single or multiple nodules, often in chains with enlarged and palpable lymphatics; especially distal leg; *Mycobacterium kansasii*
Staphylococcal folliculitis and furunculosis	Adults; tufted papules, crusts, and alopecia; anywhere on body (especially rump, tail, perineum, distal legs, neck, face); nonpruritic; *S. aureus*, occasionally *S. hyicus*
Ulcerative lymphangitis	Adults; firm to fluctuant nodules, often with enlarged and palpable lymphatics, usually unilateral on distal leg, shoulder, neck, or flank; especially *T. pyogenes*, *C. pseudotuberculosis*, and *S. aureus*
Ulcerative mammary dermatitis	Adults; moist ulceration, foul odor on anterior udder; *Treponema* spp.
Fungal Disorders	
Phaeohyphomycosis	Multiple ulcerated, oozing nodules over rump and thighs (*Dreschlera rostrata*) or pinnae, tail, vulva, and thighs (*Bipolaris spicifera*)
Malassezia otitis externa	Ceruminous to suppurative otitis externa; predominantly *Malassezia sympodialis* in summer and *M. globosa* in winter; organism may also cause udder dermatitis
Viral Disorders	
Cowpox (orthopoxvirus)	Adults; typical pox lesions and thick, red crusts; usually confined to teats and udder, but occasionally medial thighs, perineum, vulva, and scrotum
Pseudocowpox (parapoxvirus)	Adults; edema, pain, orange papules, dark red crusts (especially in "ring" or "horseshoe" shape); usually teats and udder but occasionally medial thighs, perineum, and scrotum
Bovine popular stomatitis (parapoxvirus)	Calves, rarely adults; typical pox lesions on muzzle, nostrils, and lips, especially on calves; occasionally flanks, abdomen, hind legs, scrotum, prepuce, and teats

Continued

TABLE 7.1 Miscellaneous Bacterial, Fungal, Viral, and Protozoal Disorders of the Skin—cont'd

Disorder	Signs
Viral Disorders, continued	
Bovine lumpy skin disease (capripoxvirus)	Adults; acute onset of papules and nodules, progressing to necrosis, slough, ulcer, and scar; especially tail, head, neck, legs, perineum, udder, and scrotum
Infectious bovine rhinotracheitis (bovine herpesvirus 1)	Any age; erythema, pustules, necrosis, and ulceration of muzzle, vulva, and rarely perineum and scrotum
Herpes mammillitis (bovine herpesvirus 2)	First lactation heifers, rarely adults; acute swollen, tender teats, and udder skin progressing to vesicles, sloughing, and ulceration and crusting
Pseudolumpy skin disease (bovine herpesvirus 3)	Adults; similar in appearance and distribution to true lumpy skin disease, but more superficial
Herpes mammary pustular dermatitis (bovine herpesvirus 4)	First lactation heifers, rarely adults; vesicle and pustules on lateral and ventral aspects of udder
Malignant catarrhal fever (alcelaphine herpesvirus 1, wildebeest; ovine herpesvirus 2, sheep)	Adults; erythema, scaling, necrosis, ulceration, and crusting of muzzle and face, and occasionally udder, teats, vulva, and scrotum; variable coronitis
Pseudorabies (porcine herpesvirus 1)	Adults; intense, localized, unilateral pruritus; especially head, neck, thorax, flank, and perineum
Bovine viral diarrhea virus (pestivirus)	Any age; erosions of muzzle, lips, and nostrils, and occasionally vulva, prepuce, coronet, and interdigital space; rarely crusts, scales, and alopecia on perineum, medial thighs, and neck
Foot-and-mouth disease (aphthovirus)	Any age; vesicles and bullae, painful erosions and ulcers in mouth and on muzzle, nostrils, coronet, interdigital space, udder, and teats
Vesicular stomatitis (vesiculovirus)	Any age; vesicles, painful erosions and ulcers in mouth and on lips, muzzle, feet, and occasionally prepuce, udder, and teats
Rinderpest (morbillivirus)	Any age; erythema, papules, oozing, crusts, and alopecia over perineum, flanks, medial thighs, neck, scrotum, udder, and teats
Bluetongue (orbivirus)	Any age; edema, dryness, cracking, and peeling of muzzle and lips; ulcers and crusts may be seen on udder and teats
Protozoal Disorders	
Sarcocystosis	Any age; loss of tail switch; variable alopecia of pinnae and distal legs
Besnoitiosis	Adults; warm, painful swellings on distal legs and ventrum, skin then becomes thickened, lichenified, alopecic, and may fissure, ooze, scale, and crust

Neoplastic Diseases

Lymphosarcoma (Lymphoma)

Etiology

Lymphosarcoma may involve the skin in the classic "skin form" of lymphosarcoma, wherein affected cattle usually are serologically negative for antibodies against the bovine leukemia virus (BLV), or present as sporadic skin tumors associated with lymphadenopathy and other organ involvement with the adult form of lymphosarcoma that occurs in BLV-positive animals.

The skin form of lymphosarcoma usually occurs in cattle 6 to 24 months of age and is a progressive disease causing multifocal skin tumors. Lymphadenopathy may accompany the skin lesions. The skin form of lymphosarcoma is observed in all breeds, but is most common in Holsteins. This may simply reflect the number of Holsteins in the United States.

Genetic predisposition has not been demonstrated, and there does not appear to be an association between cutaneous lymphosarcoma and BLV. Therefore, this is considered a sporadic form of lymphosarcoma. Skin tumors caused by lymphosarcoma in adult cattle are uncommon compared with tumors in more typical target organs (e.g., abomasum, heart, uterus, retrobulbar area, and lymph nodes).

Signs

Diffuse nodular skin masses (1.0–10.0 cm in diameter) develop over the neck and trunk of young cattle with the skin form of lymphosarcoma. Lesions are initially dermal or subcutaneous, and the overlying skin appears normal. However, alopecia, crusting, hyperkeratosis, and ulceration develop with time (Fig. 7.10). The tumors may become numerous enough to obliterate any normal skin spaces between them (Fig. 7.11). Tumors may occur on

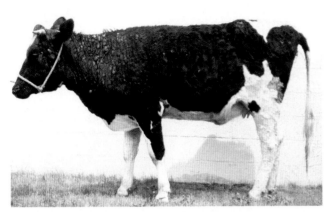

• **Fig. 7.10** The skin form of lymphosarcoma in an 18-month-old Holstein heifer.

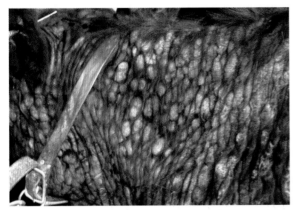

• **Fig. 7.11** Cutaneous lymphosarcoma. Multiple plaques and nodules exhibiting variable hair loss, scaling, and crusting.

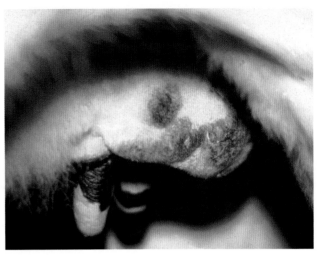

• **Fig. 7.12** A 4-year-old Holstein cow with the cutaneous form of lymphosarcoma involving the udder.

the skin over any portion of the body. Peripheral lymph nodes are usually enlarged. The heifer or young cow seems otherwise healthy at the onset. However, over a period of 6 to 12 months, affected animals become uncomfortable because of the tumor burden, and visceral masses may develop. Fly and other insect irritation can be intense during warm weather, causing bleeding from the enlarging nodular tumors, which may have become alopecic. Most cases are BLV negative and the disease is not caused by BLV infection.

In adult cattle with lymphosarcoma, singular or multiple skin tumors may appear along with typical signs of lymph node enlargement and target organ lesions. Skin tumors in this form are larger, often plaquelike, and may be on the neck, chest or trunk, udder (Fig. 7.12), or eyelids. Physical examination usually identifies other lesions or locations of lymphosarcoma.

Fine-needle aspirates or skin biopsies are both possible means of diagnosis for cutaneous lymphosarcoma. Punch or small surgical biopsies are the most reliable means of obtaining a definitive diagnosis. Although advanced cases of the skin form are unlikely to require diagnostics, early cases with fewer lesions may require differentiation from other neoplasms and diseases such as urticaria and infectious or sterile granulomas.

Treatment

Although corticosteroids may reduce the size of tumors or result in short-term remission, it is impractical to treat cattle with lymphosarcoma because the tumors can never be fully controlled, and the animal will suffer a prolonged course or complications as a result of the medication.

Angiomatosis

Angiomatosis, although uncommon, is a cause for concern to owners of affected cattle because of the friable nature of the skin masses that predisposes to repeated bouts of hemorrhage that are dramatic given the small size (1.0–2.5 cm) of the tumors. Affected cattle tend to be mature with the average age reported to be 5.5 years.

The soft, pink, or reddish masses are located on the dorsum over the withers, back, and loin. They may be singular or multiple, and are always fragile. Treatment is by surgical removal. The author has seen one Holstein cow with angiomatosis in which the lesion spontaneously resolved over 12 months, but generally it is better to remove the masses, lest insect irritation during the summer cause repeated hemorrhage.

Lipomatosis (Infiltrative Lipoma)

A rare condition in dairy cattle that may represent a hamartoma involving fat, lipomatosis appears as enlarging masses in the facial area or heavy muscles of the hind limbs (Fig. 7.13). The masses may be so large as to interfere with function (e.g., mastication or respiration). They are fluctuant and soft on palpation, but attempts at fluid aspiration often yield nothing. Fine-needle aspirates or biopsy provides the diagnosis. No treatment exists because surgical removal is impossible as a result of infiltration of the fatty mass into musculature.

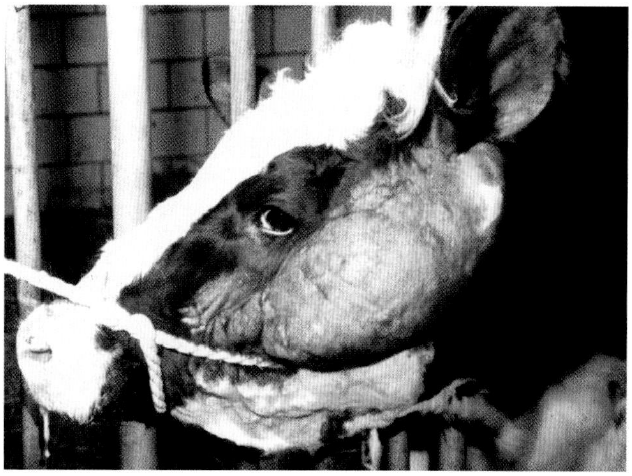

• **Fig. 7.13** Lipomatosis of the facial muscles in a yearling Holstein heifer.

Squamous Cell Carcinomas

Squamous cell carcinomas are the most common malignant skin tumors of dairy cattle. Skin at mucocutaneous junctions, such as the eyelids and vulva, in cattle lacking pigment in these locations are at greatest risk. Cows that are mostly white, or any cows with nonpigmented, mucocutaneous regions may be affected. Holsteins are the most common dairy breed the author has observed to have squamous cell carcinomas, but this probably is because of the larger numbers of Holsteins in the United States compared with other breeds. Ayrshires, Guernseys, and Milking Shorthorn cattle also may be at risk, depending on pigment patterns. There are two major reasons the overall incidence of squamous cell carcinoma in dairy cattle is less than in beef cattle:

1. Dairy cattle in the United States seldom experience as much sunlight as pastured beef cattle.
2. Fewer dairy cattle reach or exceed the age of greatest risk (7–9 years) because of culling for other reasons.

Sunlight, age, genetics, and infections with BPV are all factors in the occurrence of squamous cell carcinoma in cattle.

In addition to mucocutaneous junctional areas, squamous cell carcinoma occasionally may arise from chronically irritated skin wounds via tissue metaplasia. Brand keratomas occasionally transform into squamous cell carcinomas. Aged cattle with squamous cell carcinoma of the udder or ear tips also have been observed.

Signs

Clinical signs of a pink, cobblestone, raised or ulcerated mass arising from a depigmented area of skin are pathognomonic for squamous cell carcinoma (Fig. 7.14). Frequently, a white or yellow "cake frosting" of necrotic material covers the pink, highly vascular tumor surface, and an anaerobic or necrotic odor is detectable. Heavy purulent discharges make the tumors greatly attractive to flies and maggots. Biopsies provide definitive diagnosis.

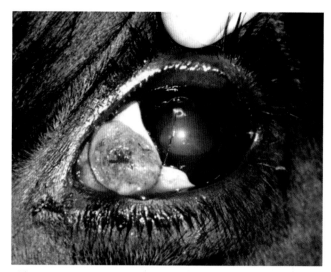

• **Fig. 7.14** Squamous cell carcinoma of the nictitans in a Holstein cow.

Treatment

Treatment may be easy or may be impossible based on the size of the tumor, its anatomic location, and the presence or absence of obvious metastases to regional lymph nodes.

Small squamous cell carcinomas are amenable to many treatment modes such as cryosurgery, radiofrequency hyperthermia, radiation, immunotherapy, or even sharp surgery. Each tumor must be evaluated by anatomic location, how much tissue may be destroyed without loss of tissue function (e.g., an eyelid), and expense of treatment. Treatment for ocular squamous cell carcinoma is addressed in detail in Chapter 14. In general, cryosurgery, radiofrequency hyperthermia, and radiation are the best treatments for small tumors and allow preservation of critical normal structures. Immunotherapy, especially with intratumor injections of Bacillus Calmette Guérin (BCG) or other mycobacterial cell wall products, will risk false positive tests for tuberculosis in the future and should not be used. Other topical or intralesional treatments that are used in horses for sarcoids could be beneficial, but no reports are available and some drug treatments would not be legal in cattle. Regional lymph nodes should be palpated and biopsied if they appear enlarged or firm, thus possibly indicating metastasis. Metastases have been reported to occur in about 10% of bovine squamous cell carcinomas, but clinically, obviously neglected or large tumors are more likely to metastasize than early or small lesions. Local tissue invasion and local lymph node involvement are more frequently a clinical problem than distant metastasis.

Other Cutaneous Neoplasms and Nonneoplastic Growths

A number of neoplastic and nonneoplastic growths occur in the skin of cattle. A listing of these uncommon to very rare disorders is provided in Table 7.2.

TABLE 7.2   Miscellaneous Neoplastic and Nonneoplastic Growths

Disorder	Signs
Basal cell tumor	Adult to aged animals; solitary firm to fluctuant nodule; often alopecic and ulcerated; anywhere on body; benign
Trichoepithelioma	Adult to aged animals; solitary firm to fluctuant nodule; often alopecic and ulcerated; anywhere on body; benign
Sebaceous adenoma	Adult to aged animals; solitary nodule; anywhere on body (especially eyelid); benign
Sebaceous adenocarcinoma	Adult to aged animals; solitary nodule; anywhere on body (especially jaw); malignant
Epitrichial (apocrine) adenoma	Adult to aged animals; solitary nodule; tail; benign
Fibroma	Adult to aged animals; solitary, firm or soft, dermal or subcutaneous nodule; anywhere on body (especially head, neck, shoulder); benign
Fibrosarcoma	Adult to aged animals; solitary, firm or soft, dermal or subcutaneous nodule; anywhere on body (especially head, neck); malignant
Hemangioma	Adult to aged animals; develop solitary, firm to soft, red to blue to black dermal nodules; anywhere on body (especially head, legs); benign; when multiple lesions occur congenitally or in animals younger than 1 year old these may be accompanied by widespread internal lesions
Hemangiosarcoma	Adult to aged animals; solitary nodule, often necrotic, ulcerated, and bleeding; anywhere on body (especially leg); malignant
Hemangiopericytoma	Adult to aged animals; solitary nodule, anywhere on body (especially jaw); benign
Lymphangioma	Congenital or animals younger than 1 year old; solitary soft nodule; anywhere on body (especially leg, brisket); benign
Myxoma	Congenital to aged; solitary soft nodule; anywhere on body (especially pinna, leg); benign
Myxosarcoma	Adult to aged animals; solitary nodule; anywhere on body; malignant
Neurofibroma (Schwannoma; neurofibromatosis)	Congenital to adults; usually multiple firm papules and nodules; unilateral or bilateral; anywhere on body (especially muzzle, face, eyelids, neck, brisket); benign
Lipoma	Adult to aged animals; solitary subcutaneous nodule; anywhere on body (especially trunk); benign
Mast cell tumor	Adult to aged animals; solitary or multiple papules and nodules that are often alopecic, erythematous, and ulcerated; anywhere on body; multiple lesions can be present congenitally on calves; 60% of animals with widespread lesions have metastases
Melanocytic neoplasms	All ages (>50% of cases in cattle <18 months old); about 80% of lesions are benign (melanocytoma), and 20% are malignant (melanoma); usually solitary dermal to subcutaneous nodules, gray to black in color, firm to fluctuant; anywhere on body (especially leg)
Dermoid cyst	Congenital; solitary nodule; especially dorsal midline of neck, eyelid, and periocular area; benign
Branchial cyst	Congenital; solitary firm to fluctuant swelling in ventral neck area; benign
Cutaneous horn	Adult to aged animals; hornlike hyperkeratosis, usually overlies squamous cell carcinoma or papilloma

Allergic or Immune-Mediated Diseases

Urticaria, Angioedema, and Anaphylaxis

Etiology

Urticaria, angioedema, and anaphylaxis are the most obvious clinical consequences of hypersensitivity reactions or "allergic" reactions. Urticaria ("hives") appears as skin wheals or mucous membrane swellings as a result of dermal edema (Fig. 7.15). Angioedema tends to imply larger swelling or plaques of edema that involve subcutaneous tissue. Anaphylaxis is the life-threatening extreme manifestation of these hypersensitivity reactions, and its rapid onset causes severe respiratory and cardiovascular signs resulting from smooth muscle contraction and vascular alteration. Anaphylaxis usually is fatal

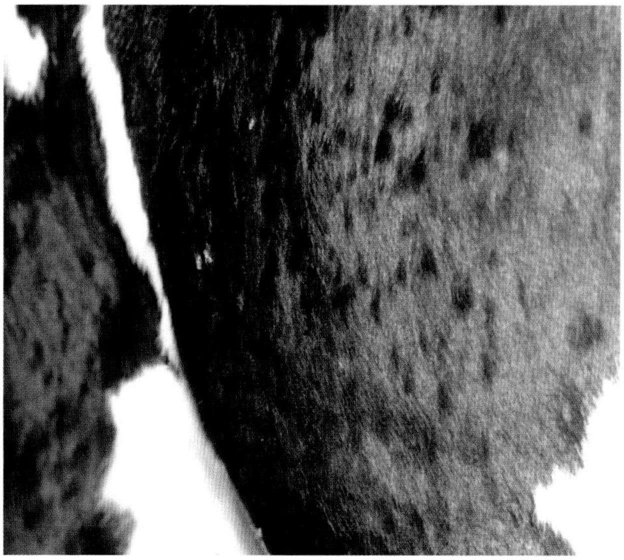

• **Fig. 7.15** Urticaria on the thorax and flank of an adult Holstein cow. Raised tufts of hair appear over painful areas of dermal edema. These lesions appeared within 20 minutes after an intramuscular injection of ampicillin.

unless attended immediately, and may or may not have urticaria and angioedema associated with it. A plethora of drugs, biologics, feeds, and other stimuli may evoke hypersensitivity reactions in calves and adult cattle. The exact immunologic phenomenon or type of hypersensitivity reaction (types I–IV) is sometimes difficult to determine, but most commonly represents type I or type III hypersensitivity reactions. Type I hypersensitivities are IgE mediated, but type III are associated with immune complexes. Type I hypersensitivities cause mast cell and basophil degranulation with subsequent release of histamine, leukotrienes, prostaglandins, and other mediators. Type I reactions probably provoke most ruminant causes of urticaria, angioedema, and anaphylaxis. Type III reactions may include some drug-induced causes, but this conclusion is largely speculative.

In dairy cattle, most cases of urticaria, angioedema, and anaphylaxis result from injections of various products, including antibiotics, vaccines, whole blood, lidocaine, and IV fluids. Insect bites occasionally cause urticaria and angioedema, but seldom anaphylaxis. Milk allergy is another important cause of urticaria, angioedema, and anaphylaxis that ranges from mild to severe in individual patients. Milk allergy is observed in cattle (any breed, but more commonly Channel Islands' breeds) at drying off or when delays in milking occur either accidentally or intentionally when showing or selling cattle. Alpha-casein appears to be the milk protein that causes type I hypersensitivity in these cows.

Virtually any antibiotic can cause sporadic hypersensitivity reactions. Penicillin, tetracycline, ampicillin, various sulfonamides, and streptomycin have been incriminated. It is important to differentiate procaine reactions from true hypersensitivity to penicillin when procaine penicillin has been given. Many owners and veterinarians interpret the relatively common procaine reactions as penicillin hypersensitivity, but this is wrong. Cattle with procaine reactions

may still be safely given penicillin, provided good injection technique is maintained to prevent intravascular administration of the drug.

Vaccines are the most common cause of anaphylaxis in cattle. Although serum origin products are used less frequently, many "antisera" are still available on the market; these are especially dangerous as they can cause both immediate and delayed manifestations of hypersensitivity reactions. Polyvaccines have gained favor in the cattle industry, and it is not unusual to give a single injection that contains antigens of four viruses, five serotypes of leptospirosis, and a vehicle. Reactions to such polyvaccines make determining the causative antigen difficult. Strain 19 Brucella vaccine occasionally caused either immediate or delayed hypersensitivity reactions, but this appears to be less common with its replacement biologic, RB51. A rare reaction involves the larynx, causing severe laryngeal edema within 24 hours of Strain 19 vaccine.

Although some vaccines are more notorious than others as causes of anaphylaxis, any vaccine may cause an occasional reaction. Various gram-negative bacterins containing slight amounts of bacterial-origin endotoxin can induce reactions that mimic anaphylaxis through a genetic sensitivity, especially in Holsteins. This theory may explain why reactions are seen in some herds but not in others.

Whole blood or plasma may cause skin hypersensitivity reactions when administered IV. Transfusion reactions are possible because of genetic blood types or too rapid administration. Intravenous fluids, especially formulated fluids, occasionally cause hives and angioedema. This is most likely a result of white or red blood cell antigens in whole blood or contaminants and cleaning chemicals incompletely rinsed from large fluid jugs, or from endotoxin.

Hypoderma larvae that are killed in situ have caused anaphylactic reactions or reactions to toxins that mimic anaphylactic reactions. Feeds certainly may cause hypersensitivity reactions in individual cattle.

Signs

With urticaria, skin wheals or "hives" appear in variable numbers anywhere on the body within minutes to hours of the antigenic stimulus. Most commonly, these 1.0- to 10.0-cm raised areas of skin appear round or oval, but smaller urticarial swellings may resemble multiple fly bites or areas of raised hair. In cattle, concurrent swelling of mucous membranes and mucocutaneous junctions is very common, so that marked swelling of the eyelids, lips, vulva, or anus may appear. On occasion, the wheals or areas of edema may become erythematous, especially in areas of hairless skin as the urticaria resolves (Fig. 7.16). Some cows have swelling in only one location, but others have multicentric skin lesions and mucocutaneous junctional swellings. Other signs include trembling, salivation, mild rumen tympany, and diarrhea. Abortion or renal failure may occasionally occur within 1 week after a severe hypersensitivity reaction. Although animals with urticaria may be anxious and painful, they are not in a life-threatening situation unless pulmonary or laryngeal

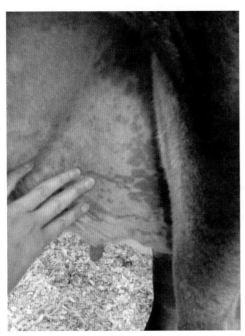

• **Fig. 7.16** Multiple erythematous and edematous areas over the hairless skin of the udder on an adult Jersey cow shortly after generalized urticaria developed during a blood transfusion. Spontaneous resolution was observed of all lesions over 12 hours. (Courtesy of Dr. Chelsea Holschbach.)

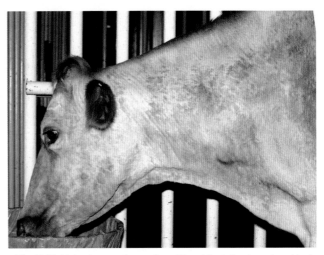

• **Fig. 7.17** Urticaria over the neck and head that developed suddenly in an excellent Guernsey cow that had been dried-off the night before (milk allergy). The cow was treated with subcutaneously administered antihistamines, and the hives resolved. The cow was 7.5 months pregnant, and steroid administration would have been contraindicated!

edema develops. With anaphylaxis, however, life-threatening vascular and smooth muscle effects occur rapidly, often before urticaria or angioedema even appear on the skin. Depression, dyspnea, anxiety, and hair coat standing on end are early signs of anaphylaxis. Later signs include salivation, pulmonary froth at the muzzle, severe dyspnea, and collapse.

Treatment

Removal of the offending antigen or subsequent avoidance is the long-term goal of treatment, but of more immediate concern is stopping the hypersensitivity reaction from injuring the host. When urticaria or angioedema is present but the animal displays no dyspnea, antihistamines and nonsteroidal antiinflammatory agents with or without corticosteroids are indicated for treatment. If the animal is pregnant or has an infectious medical problem, however, corticosteroids should be avoided. When corticosteroids are used, 100 to 500 mg of methylprednisolone sodium succinate or 40 mg of dexamethasone is adequate for adult, nonpregnant cattle. Antihistamines and flunixin meglumine should be used at standard dosages. Treatment may need to be repeated at 8- to 12-hour intervals for one or two additional treatments. In pregnant cattle, isoflupredone acetate could be used as a nonabortifacent alternative.

Adult cattle with dyspnea or any sign of respiratory distress should receive epinephrine (1–5 mL at 1:1000 dilution IV or 4 to 8 mL IM or SC) in addition to the aforementioned drugs. If laryngeal edema is judged to be life-threatening to the patient, a tracheostomy may be required; if pulmonary edema is severe, furosemide (0.5–1.0 mg/kg IV) may be indicated.

Because cattle with milk allergy should be milked out immediately, they may not be able to be immediately dried off (Fig. 7.17). This is variable because some cattle only show one or a few bouts of milk allergy, but others can be very difficult to dry off. Some cows with milk allergy are culled out of frustration with the problem.

Allergies to feeds or feed components are difficult to diagnose specifically, and tend to be sporadic rather than endemic. Individual cows may show urticaria and angioedema (especially of the vulva and anus) when exposed to high levels of corn or wheat (this must be differentiated from "estrogenic mycotoxins"). However, today's dairy cattle feeds are so complex that determination of the exact antigen would be similar to searching for a needle in the haystack.

Prevention is difficult when vaccines are causative because all avoidance of vaccines would be disastrous to cattle health. However, certain vaccines and hyperimmune sera products that seem to cause a high incidence of anaphylactic reaction should be avoided, and a safe product sought through discussion with colleagues. Calves younger than 6 months of age seem most susceptible to anaphylaxis from polyantigen vaccines. A particular concern currently exists in the United States for young calves receiving a commercially available live *Salmonella* Dublin vaccine, such that it is prudent to discuss this risk with the producer and be prepared to treat symptoms of acute anaphylaxis whenever this product is used. Whether this propensity for vaccine reactions in calves represents residual passive immunity, direct antigenic reaction, genetically mediated sensitivity to small amounts of endotoxin in bacterins, or reaction to vehicles is not known. Veterinarians vaccinating cattle always should have epinephrine and other treatments for anaphylaxis available. Veterinarians who sell cattle vaccines for owner administration may consider selling epinephrine with strict instructions regarding indication and use to avoid medicolegal entanglements if anaphylaxis occurs in one or more of the cattle.

Contact Dermatitis

Contact dermatitis may be irritant-induced, resulting from extreme concentration of a contacting agent, or allergic, wherein even small concentrations incite a hypersensitivity reaction. Irritant causes include chemicals added to bedding (such as coarse limestone) and disinfectants or teat dips used on teats and udders. Strong iodine solutions, concentrated chlorine bleach, concentrated chlorhexidine, and teat dips that have separated into layers because of freezing all have caused irritant contact dermatitis. Certain light-skinned cows appear to develop contact dermatitis when at pasture, but this may be difficult to differentiate from sunburn in some instances. Soaps or disinfectants that are not thoroughly rinsed off after preparation of the perineum during dystocia or vaginal examination are another source of contact dermatitis to the skin of the perineum, tail, and mucous membranes of the vulva and rectum. Fly sprays and other chemicals may evoke a contact dermatitis if applied in excess or if applied under a bandage.

Calves frequently develop an irritant contact dermatitis when fed milk replacer from a bucket. Alopecia develops at the muzzle, nose area, and ears, but the skin itself does not seem to be inflamed beyond occasional erythema. Some cases may have concurrent *Dermatophilus* infections at this site. Urine and fecal scalding are very common in calves that are kept in poorly cleaned pens or have prolonged recumbency because of systemic illness or musculoskeletal disease. The perineum, ventrum, and hind legs show alopecia and a pink-red erythematous skin within the areas of alopecia. Calves with chronic diarrhea may show scalding of the tail, perineum, and medial hind limbs. Adult cows with prolonged recumbency may develop urine and fecal scalding as well.

Allergic contact dermatitis is less common than irritant contact dermatitis and may be seen in response to plants, bedding, and chemicals. Whereas allergic contact dermatitis usually is limited to one animal, irritant contact dermatitis frequently affects multiple cows in the herd. Avoidance, dilution, or replacement of causes of irritant contact dermatitis constitutes the treatment. For cattle with allergic contact dermatitis, a careful history may give the most useful insight into possible causes in the form of new bedding or recent exposure to pasture, among other sources. If a cause can be determined, avoidance is the only practical treatment.

Damage from Physical Agents

Thermal Injury

Sunburn

Etiology. Ultraviolet rays, a form of shortwave radiation, may cause thermal injury to the skin of lightly pigmented cattle exposed to intense or prolonged sunlight. The skin of the teats and udder may become sufficiently burned to make milking painful to the cow. Resultant difficulty in milking, failure to milk out completely, and mastitis

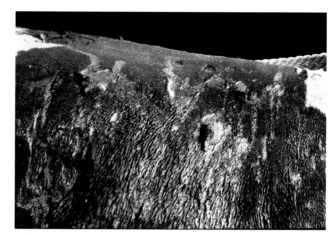

• **Fig. 7.18** Acute second- and third-degree burns on the dorsum of a yearling Holstein bull that had been in a barn fire.

are all clinical consequences. Teat skin, being hairless, is most at risk. Burning may be worse on the lateral teat surfaces in cows with well-conformed udders, but is generalized in cows with pendulous udders. Maximal burning occurs when cows are recumbent. Once burned, blisters, chafing, peeling, and dryness of the affected skin will be present for 1 to 2 weeks. During this time, other irritants such as teat dips may slow healing. Colonization of the dry cracked teat skin by environmental organisms increases the risk of clinical mastitis outbreaks as well. Lightly pigmented haired skin on the dorsum also will be erythematous, but is seldom burned.

Treatment. Avoidance of direct sunlight by turning cows out in the early morning or evening is one alternative. Topical treatment with lanolin or aloe-based emollient ointments may soothe affected skin. Severely burned cows, such as down cows exposed to prolonged periods of direct sunlight, may require more intensive therapy.

Fire Injuries (Barn, Brush)

Thermal injury caused by flames is long-wave radiation damage classified based on the depth of the skin injury. First-degree burns involve only the superficial layers of the epidermis, whereas second-degree burns involve the entire epidermis. Blisters resulting from fluid accumulations between the stratum corneum and basal layers are common in second-degree burns. Eschars are produced by severe second- and third-degree burns. Third-degree burns damage dermis and epidermis and also destroy hair follicles. Fourth-degree burns extend through skin to destroy fascia, muscle, tendons, and other tissues deep to the skin.

Burns tend to be most severe on the dorsum in barn fires (Fig. 7.18) and on the ventrum in brush fires. Depending on the animals' surroundings, facial burns also are common.

Thermal injuries caused by fire are associated with much more than skin pathology. Shock, dehydration, respiratory distress, elevated catecholamine levels from extreme stress, electrolyte shifts caused by cellular destruction, smoke inhalation, and decreased resistance to local and systemic

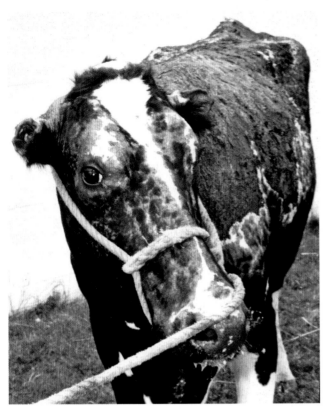

• **Fig. 7.19** Adult Holstein cow that had been burned in a barn fire 1 month earlier. Skin sloughing was caused by third-degree burns over the dorsum.

infections are only a few of the potential medical problems in burn patients. The profound anxiety, fear, and stress associated with fire itself affect surviving cattle. They may be apprehensive in addition to being in pain from burns.

The full extent of thermal injury often is impossible to predict immediately. Large areas of skin on the dorsum may appear warm with hair loss but apparently remain intact peracutely; later full-thickness skin may slough off the back (Fig. 7.19). The development of blisters, fluid separation of epidermis and dermis, and eschars may not appear until several days after the injury. Eschars feel leathery, firm, and taut and often are seen in cattle with underlying fluid that is subject to infection by opportunistic bacteria. Eschars eventually slough.

Wound or burn infection is common in cattle, and *Pseudomonas aeruginosa* is the most common organism to establish infection. The normal skin defense mechanisms (e.g., epidermis, sebum) are injured or destroyed following second-degree or worse burns. Thus, opportunistic bacteria from the normal skin flora or environment may be able to colonize the skin, fluid in blisters, or tissue and fluid under eschars. Infection under eschars is a common problem in cattle in which large areas of dorsal skin are burned.

Signs. The signs are dramatic and along with the history suffice for diagnosis. The odor of burnt hair lingers around affected animals and the whole area of the fire. Individual surviving animals should be assessed as to extent of skin

injury, degree of other injury or smoke inhalation, and likelihood of survival. Pain may be minimal or absent in deeper burns because of loss of innervation, but this is a poor means of assessment because simple edema may also cause reduced sensation.

Burns that involve large areas of skin on the dorsum and sides are likely to heal poorly and require lengthy treatment. Facial burns, muzzle encrustation, and dyspnea should alert the clinician to upper and lower airway damage by heat and smoke. Burnt teats that will not withstand milking indicate a grave prognosis because mastitis is inevitable regardless of other skin damage. Badly burned feet may slough claws. Facial burns involving the cornea may lead to permanent stromal opacities even after re-epithelialization.

Unfortunately, emotionalism makes it difficult for the veterinarian to be objective and predict which, if any, surviving animals have a reasonable prognosis. Many times, owners want to "do everything" to save survivors only to complain weeks later when ongoing complications and wound care require immense effort despite the prognosis for the animals remaining poor. It is imperative to warn clients during the highly emotional aftermath of fire that badly burned survivors will not only look worse later (after the skin sloughs) but also that they may never again be productive.

Treatment. Immediate treatment consists of assessing surviving cattle for systemic needs, burn needs, and likelihood of survival and future productivity. By circumstance, this must be done in a chaotic, emotion-filled environment. Immediate treatment includes:

1. Overall assessment of survivors: Recumbent, obviously badly burned, suffering animals should be euthanized.
2. Individual surviving cattle may benefit from mild sedation that allows better evaluation of systemic and local injuries.
3. Cool water can be run through a hose to cool all burned cattle in the immediate phase of treatment.
4. Treat for shock, smoke inhalation, and dehydration if necessary.

After the immediate treatment, individual cattle that are to be treated for burns should again be gently hosed with running water to remove charred hair, crusts, and debris. First-degree burns can be coated with 1% silver sulfadiazine cream in regions where this treatment is permitted; currently in the United States this would be illegal in a lactating dairy cow. Initial blisters should be allowed to remain in place for 1 to 2 days on second-degree burns. Ruptured blisters should be debrided, the underlying tissue gently cleansed with iodophor or chlorhexidine, and silver sulfadiazine ointment applied under loosely applied moist gauze, again if permitted.

Second- and third-degree burns may be managed by occlusive dressings (closed) or by eschar, which is Mother Nature's coating of burnt tissue overlying the wound. In cattle and other large animals, it is difficult for either of these techniques to be used. Closed treatment with dressings may be impossible because of the anatomic location and size of skin burns. Eschars seldom stay in place long enough to allow complete epithelialization, or remain intact enough that bacteria do not invade the underlying tissue. The environment of large animals is not conducive to good burn management because of the constant potential for contamination of wounds. Loosely woven gauze and petroleum jelly are a good combination for either occlusive dressings or dressings laid over large areas of burns to prevent desiccation and continued fluid loss from the tissue. Heat loss and fluid loss are ongoing problems for animals with large areas of thermal injury. This also is true even when an eschar covers the injured area.

Eschars over large second- or third-degree burns should be left undisturbed unless separation of the healthy skin–eschar border becomes apparent or if infection is likely under the eschar. Infection of fluid under the eschar leads to fever and malaise, as well as a detectable fluctuation in the area of the burn.

Regardless of the treatment method used, the goal is epithelialization. Complete epithelialization should be possible with mild second-degree burns but may require skin grafts for severe second-degree and virtually all third-degree burns. If permitted, silver sulfadiazine treatment to protect the wounds against opportunistic bacteria (especially *Pseudomonas* spp.), gentle washing, and moisture-holding occlusive or semiocclusive dressings are indicated until such time as skin grafting is possible. Lanolin or aloe-based products also may be helpful when incorporated into wound care to prevent drying of the skin or epithelial edges. Fragile layers of epithelium bridging large skin burns may be subject to cracking because of desiccation or excessive motion. Scratching or licking at burns can lead to delayed healing or self-mutilation in some cows. In one case, the author treated a Holstein cow injured in a barn fire in which pruritus and consequent licking became so intense that sedation was necessary.

Supportive therapy includes analgesics, daily nursing care, as clean an environment as possible, and adequate nutrition. Corticosteroids are never indicated unless used during the immediate postfire treatment for smoke inhalation. Systemic antibiotics are not as effective as topical dressings for most burn wounds. However, large areas of eschar formation over the dorsum that present a high risk of infection may benefit from systemic antibiotics in large animals. Broad-spectrum coverage is indicated if systemic antibiotics are deemed necessary. The negative side effect is further patient discomfort caused by injections.

Skin grafting can be performed for third-degree burns when a healthy bed of granulation tissue covers the wound. Pinch grafts are most commonly used, and success rates vary because of difficulties encountered in aftercare of the grafts. Problems include physical and bacterial contamination of the graft site–especially on large dorsal burns–failure of graft to take, and self-induced trauma or scratching. Skin for grafts may be obtained from healthy areas of loose skin elsewhere on the patient.

Frostbite

Etiology. Excessive exposure of tissue to cold or windchill may cause frostbite. Mild frostbite leads to blanching of the tissue and reduced sensation, followed by painful erythema, scaling, and alopecia. Severe frostbite leads to dry gangrene, anesthesia, and eventual sloughing. The most commonly affected areas are the extremities such as ear tips, tails, teats, scrotum, and lower limbs. Neonates and animals whose peripheral circulation is reduced because of systemic illness are at much greater risk for frostbite.

Extremities that become wet and are then subjected to severe environmental cold are at risk of frostbite. This is especially true for cows milked in milking parlors that are discharged to the free-stall environment before teat dip solutions have dried on the teats. Similarly, neonatal calves housed in hutches may show superficial muzzle sloughing from frostbite caused by the rapid freezing of milk or milk replacers on the muzzle following feedings. Frostbite seldom is encountered in healthy animals when environmental temperatures are greater than 10.0°F (−12.22°C). Frostbite is not unusual when temperatures reach 0°F (−17.78°C) or windchill lowers the cold level to less than 0°F (−17.78°C). Unhealthy animals that are suffering decreased perfusion to extremities are at greater risk of frostbite even at higher environmental temperatures. Heifers with severe periparturient udder edema and subsequent reduced perfusion to the teats are at great risk of frostbitten teats when temperatures are less than 0°F (−17.78°C).

Treatment. If the condition is noticed promptly, the animal should be moved to an area where refreezing is not possible, and the frostbitten tissues should be thawed rapidly using water at a temperature of 105.0° to 111.0°F (40.5° to 43.9°C). Rapid warming is more painful than slow warming but leads to less cellular destruction in the affected tissue. Lanolin or aloe ointments should be applied and the animal kept protected from subnormal temperatures until healing occurs. Tissue having suffered frostbite once is more susceptible to the problem in the future.

Severe frostbite leads to dry gangrene and sloughing of tissue. The edges of healthy and gangrenous tissue should be kept clean, protected, and allowed to slough naturally. Daily checks for infection under the sloughing skin should be performed. Systemic antibiotics and tetanus immunization may be indicated for cattle with extensive frostbite.

Gangrene

Etiology

Gangrene implies necrosis and sloughing of tissue. Moist gangrene is found when lymph and venous vessels are obstructed. Dry gangrene occurs when arterial blood supply is lost but venous and lymph vessels remain intact. Whereas moist gangrene usually is associated with infection, dry gangrene is sterile. Classical examples of toxic causes of dry gangrene include ergotism and fescue foot. Ingestion of the sclerotium of the fungus *Claviceps purpurea*, which can contaminate seed grains, is the cause of ergotism. Chronic ingestion of contaminated grain and the toxic alkaloids

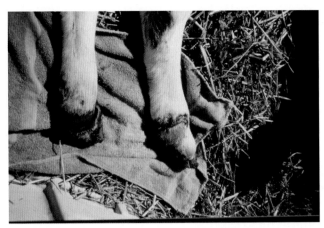

• **Fig. 7.20** Gangrenous skin on distal hind limbs of a calf that had survived acute *Salmonella* Dublin septicemia. Note the line of sharp demarcation and skin sloughing between the fetlock and coronet on both feet. Deeper tissues were still viable.

associated with this fungus lead to small arterial dysfunction and decreased arterial blood supply to extremities. Similarly, toxins from molds contaminating tall fescue grass are thought to be responsible for "fescue foot," a dry gangrene of the extremities observed in cattle, –mostly calves, –that have chronic access to tall fescue pasture or hay.

These classic examples of toxic causes of gangrene are rare in dairy cattle because of modern management systems. More common causes of gangrene in dairy cattle include:

1. Pressure necrosis—encircling bands, wires, strings, or adhesive tape may cause necrosis in extremities. A common example is the intentional application of elastrator bands to the tails of dairy cattle to dock tails. Far more common, however, is local pressure over bony prominences that results in decubital (pressure) sores. These are areas of moist gangrene that become infected and slough after chronic impingement on venous and lymphatic return. Decubital sores are the most common cause of spontaneous gangrene in calves and cows. Prolonged recumbency, musculoskeletal lesions that cause extended periods in recumbency, and poor bedding of concrete surfaces increase the likelihood of decubital sores. Internal pressure caused by severe cellulitis occasionally may cause gangrene of skin, and internal pressure (edema) plus chafing are responsible for udder sores in adult cattle.
2. Thermal injury—burns of all types and frostbite.
3. Snake bite—regional problems associated with vascular pathology due to envenomation.
4. Vasculitis—an unusual cause in cattle.
5. Infectious diseases that cause thrombosis, septic thrombosis, or thromboemboli. Most commonly, young calves with septicemia may slough extremities as a result of gram-negative organisms such as *Salmonella* spp. (Fig. 7.20). Cattle with clostridial myositis certainly have skin gangrene at the site of muscular infection if they survive long enough for this to be detected (Fig. 7.21). Septic mastitis that results in gangrenous mastitis with sloughing of skin plus the teat and gland occasionally occurs as a result of *Staphylococcus aureus*, anaerobes, *Bacillus cereus* (Fig. 7.22), or *Escherichia coli* infections.

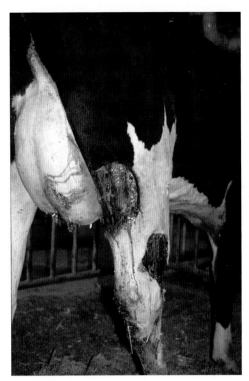

• **Fig. 7.21** Skin sloughing caused by gangrene associated with clostridial infection in the hind limb of a first-lactation heifer. An inappropriately distal parenteral injection with prostaglandin in the affected limb was the likely cause.

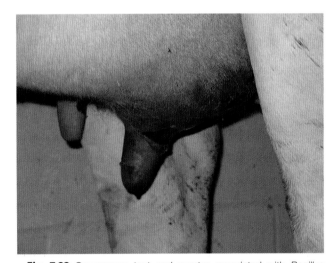

• **Fig. 7.22** Gangrenous teat and quarter associated with *Bacillus cereus* mastitis. Aggressive systemic treatment allowed recovery, but the affected gland sloughed over the next 10 days.

Herpes mammillitis infections frequently cause geographic necrosis of the skin of the udder or teats, and it is not unusual for an entire teat to slough because of dry gangrene.

Signs

With moist gangrene, the area that eventually will slough becomes swollen, discolored, edematous, and infected. A necrotic odor is apparent. Moist gangrene occurs in pressure or decubital sores, and following septic infarction of venous return in systemic states. The latter condition is

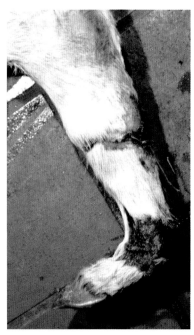

• **Fig. 7.23** Dry gangrene of the distal hind limb in a calf.

most common in calves and causes a moist, fetid swelling close to the coronary band before sloughing of the hoof or digit. Moist gangrene also has been observed with gauze or adhesive tape tail wraps inadvertently left on tails after surgery. Although dry gangrene is expected with encircling pressure, the tape or gauze appears to exert lesser but sufficient pressure to cause moist gangrene. Gangrene caused by encircling band pressure is best exemplified by elastrator bands placed on scrotums or tails. Accidental encircling bands such as rubber jar rings, washers, strings, wires, or twine occasionally are found in encircling areas of necrosis on an extremity.

Gangrenous mastitis first appears as a red or reddish-blue cool discoloration of a teat and the adjacent skin over the gland. Within hours, a blue or blue-black hue predominates, and the skin may become moist as necrosis proceeds.

Ergotism and fescue toxicosis cause dry gangrene of the lower limbs, tail, ear tips, teats, and scrotum (Fig. 7.23). Antecedent blue or blue-red alopecic skin appears before the lesions dry; it becomes leathery, insensitive, cold, and mummified and shows sloughing. Frostbite appears in a similar manner, and teats that slough secondary to herpes mammillitis also appear as dry gangrene.

Treatment

Gangrene implies irreversible necrosis of the involved skin. However, in some instances, the core of tissue in an extremity has not lost its blood supply, even though the skin has. If diagnosed early, some encircling bands may be removed in time to save the extremity. Gangrenous mastitis requires rapid action to amputate or incise the teat and allow escape of secretions, organisms, and toxins. The prognosis for life remains guarded. Treatment of frostbite has been discussed. When moist gangrene is present, necrotic tissue should be allowed to drain and slough naturally. Similarly, dry gangrene establishes its own plane of dissection and is best left to separate naturally. Systemic antibiotics may be more indicated for those with severe moist gangrene than dry. Tetanus prophylaxis always is indicated, and 2 doses of tetanus toxoid 2 weeks apart are the best means of protecting the individual during sloughing of tissue. Fly control is necessary to avoid myiasis in patients with gangrenous wounds.

Lameness and neurologic signs may be observed in some cattle with ergotism before the appearance of sloughing digits or extremities. When dry gangrene appears, it may already be too late to save the animal, but the obvious treatment is to discontinue feeding the toxin-containing feed whenever ergotism or fescue toxicosis is diagnosed or strongly suspected.

Photosensitization

Photosensitization occurs when a photodynamic substance enters the skin and is acted upon by sufficient ultraviolet light to activate inflammation or create a photochemical reaction that releases energy, causing subsequent skin damage (Box 7.1). The absorption of ultraviolet light of specific wavelengths and sufficient duration to activate photodynamic substances primarily occurs in light or nonpigmented regions of skin and is especially noticeable where the skin is both nonpigmented and has few hairs. Areas of mucocutaneous junctions and patches of white hair are the most common sites of photosensitization in cattle.

Primary photosensitization implies that a photodynamic agent or metabolite reaches the skin, usually through the circulation following ingestion or parenteral administration. Other primary photodynamic agents merely require contact with the skin.

Most causes of primary photosensitization are plants such as St. John's wort (Hypericum perforatum); buckwheat (Fagopyrum esculentum); and various types of rape, trefoil, and clover. Chemical causes of primary photosensitization also exist, with phenothiazine being the classic example. Tetracyclines, sulfonamides, and other drugs also have been incriminated as chemicals capable of causing primary photosensitization.

Photosensitization also may occur secondary to liver disease (hepatogenous) and aberrant pigment synthesis as occurs in porphyria. In hepatogenous photosensitization, liver function has been reduced to such a degree that phylloerythrin levels in the blood are exceedingly high, allowing this metabolite to act as a photodynamic agent. Phylloerythrin, a metabolite of chlorophyll, is normally conjugated within the liver and excreted in the bile. Liver or biliary pathology interferes with this normal metabolism and excretion to varying degrees. As blood levels of phylloerythrin increase, dermal levels of phylloerythrin eventually increase to a threshold level necessary for photosensitization.

Although severe hepatobiliary pathology predisposes all large animals to secondary photosensitization, many cattle with severe hepatic or biliary and hepatic pathology do not show photosensitization. This probably results from

• BOX 7.1 Causes of Photosensitization

Primary photosensitization
Plants
    St. John's wort (*Hypericum perforatum*)
    Buckwheat (*Fagopyrum esculentum, Polygonum fagopyrum*)
    Bishop's weed (*Ammi majus*)
    Dutchman's breeches (*Thamnosma texana*)
    Wild carrot (*Daucus carota*)
    Spring parsley (*Cymopterus watsonii*)
    Prairie lily (*Cooperia pedunculata*)
    Smartweeds (*Polygonum* spp.)
    Perennial ryegrass (*Lolium perenne*)
    Burr trefoil (*Medicago denticulata*)
    Alfalfa silage
Chemicals
    Phenothiazines, thiazides, acriflavines, rose Bengal, methylene blue, sulfonamides, and tetracyclines
Hepatogenous photosensitization
Plants
    Burning bush, fireweed (*Kochia scoparia*)
    Ngaio tree (*Myoporum* spp.)
    Lechuguilla (*Agave lechuguilla*)
    Rape, kale (*Brassica* spp.)
    Coal oil brush, spineless horsebrush (*Tetradynia* spp.)
    Moldy alfalfa hay
    Sacahuiste (*Nolina texana*)
    Salvation Jane (*Echium lycopsis*)
    Lanta (*Lantana camara*)
    Heliotrope (*Heliotropium europaeum*)
    Ragworts, groundsels (*Senecio* spp.)
    Tarweed, fiddleneck (*Amsinckia* spp.)
    Crotalaria, rattleweed (*Crotalaria* spp.)
    Millet, panic grass (*Panicum* spp.)
    Ganskweed (*Lasiopermum bipinnatum*)
    Verrain (*Lippia rehmanni*)
    Bog asphodel (*Narthecium ossifragum*)
    Alecrim (*Holocalyx glaziovii*)
    Vuusiektebossie (*Nidorella foetida*)
    Athanasia trifurcata
    Asaemia axillaris
Fungi
    Pithomyces chartarum (especially rye)
    Anacystis spp. (blue-green algae in water)
    Periconia spp. (Bermuda grass)
    Phomopsis leptostromiformis (lupins)
    Fusarium spp. (moldy corn)
    Aspergillus spp. (stored feeds)
Infections
    Leptospirosis
    Liver abscess
    Parasitic liver cysts (flukes, hydatids)
    Rift Valley fever
Neoplasia
    Lymphosarcoma
    Hepatocellular carcinoma
    Cholangiocarcinoma
Chemicals
    Copper, phosphorus, carbon tetrachloride, and phenanthridium
Aberrant pigment synthesis photosensitization
    Erythropoietic porphyria
    Protoporphyria

confinement away from sunlight. Hepatotoxic plants are the most common cause of hepatogenous photosensitization in cattle. Pyrrolizidine alkaloids (*Senecio* spp., *Crotalaria* spp.), blue-green algae, *Panicum* spp., some *Brassica* spp., and many other plants have the potential to cause hepatic injury. Molds such as *Aspergillus* spp., *Fusarium* spp., and *Pithomyces* spp. produce hepatotoxic mycotoxins and thereby predispose to photosensitization as well.

Diffuse infection or neoplasia of the liver also may predispose to hepatogenous photosensitization, but these causes are rare in dairy cattle. Liver flukes, a hepatic abscess that obstructs bile flow, leptospirosis, or necrotic hepatitis after bacterial toxemia may result in hepatogenous photosensitization. It is very rare for hepatic lipidosis to cause photosensitization in dairy cattle!

Bovine erythropoietic porphyria (bovine congenital porphyria), also known as "pink tooth," is an autosomal recessive trait in many breeds of cattle and is a disease to be remembered when cattle are sold or sent to bull studs. It is of primary concern in Holsteins, but cases have been observed in Ayrshires and Shorthorns. The basic defect concerns the porphyrin structure of hemoglobin. Affected cattle are deficient in uroporphyrin III cosynthetase, a necessary enzyme for proper formation of hemoglobin. Therefore, uroporphyrin and coproporphyrin accumulate and are deposited in bones, teeth, skin, urine, and other tissues. Accumulations of these porphyrin metabolites in the skin predispose to photosensitization. Affected animals also have an anemia as a result of a variety of red blood cell problems, such as reduced life span, delayed maturation in bone marrow, and hemolysis.

Bovine protoporphyria is an autosomal recessive trait associated with decreased heme synthetase (ferrochelatase) levels. Increased levels of protoporphyrin accumulate in blood and tissues. Protoporphyria is distinguished clinically from erythropoietic porphyria by the absence of anemia and discoloration of teeth and urine.

In addition to the aforementioned primary and secondary causes of photosensitization, occasional sporadic cases of photosensitization are observed in individual cattle having none of the known primary or secondary causes. Usually these cattle have been on pasture of clover or alfalfa, but the exact cause is never known and liver function is normal (Fig. 7.24).

Signs

Signs of photosensitization include edema, erythema, vesicles, dermal effusions, and skin necrosis. These are quickly followed by crusting; ulcerations; and sloughing of leathery, necrotic patches of skin. Lesions are generally confined to nonpigmented regions of the body, and are more severe on those areas receiving the most sunshine and ultraviolet light. Affected cattle are uncomfortable because of the pain associated with photosensitization, and pruritus may be a prominent sign.

Cattle with severe hepatic diseases and hepatogenous photosensitization also may show jaundice, but this is neither specific nor pathognomonic. Cattle with advanced

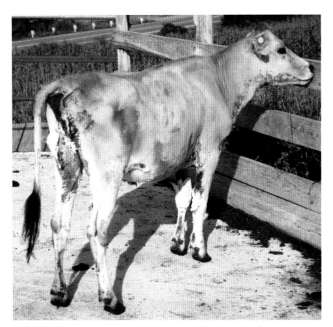

• **Fig. 7.24** Jersey heifer with photosensitization of unknown cause. The heifer had been on pasture, was the only animal affected, recovered fully after confinement, and subsequently became a productive cow.

hepatic diseases usually are very ill with inappetence, decreased milk production, and weight loss.

Cattle affected with bovine erythropoietic porphyria show photosensitization, red or brownish-red urine, brownish-red or pink teeth, anemia, and stunting or poor growth rates. Ultraviolet examination of teeth and urine with a Wood's lamp reveals an obvious orange or red fluorescence.

Diagnosis

Clinical signs usually suffice for diagnosis of photosensitization, but establishing the cause of photosensitization may be difficult. Serum biochemistry with specific requests for tests for liver disease such as gamma glutamyl transferase, aspartate aminotransferase, and sorbitol dehydrogenase, as well as function tests (e.g., conjugated bilirubin) should be requested on all animals showing photosensitization unless the etiology is quickly established to be a primary photosensitization or porphyria. Liver or biliary disease and porphyria should be ruled out in this way for all cases suspected to be primary photosensitization, and the causative primary agent should be sought. In hepatogenous photosensitization, hepatotoxic plants must be searched for and identified in pastures or forage; ultrasound and liver biopsies may be helpful in categorizing the type of hepatobiliary disease.

Confinement of dairy cattle limits both the risk for, and the clinical signs associated with, primary photosensitization and many of the hepatogenous causes. However, farm ponds (blue-green algae) and pastures still exist on many farms, and forages also may be contaminated with potentially causative agents.

Cattle with erythropoietic porphyria have greatly elevated blood and urine levels of uroporphyrin I and

coproporphyrin I. Cattle with protoporphyria have greatly elevated blood levels of protoporphyrin.

Treatment

Treatment of primary photosensitization includes removing the animals from exposure to sunlight, and avoidance or removal of the causative plant or chemical from the environment. If secondary bacterial dermatitis develops in areas of photosensitized skin, systemic antibiotics may be necessary. Sloughing skin may need to be debrided, and surveillance for myiasis is indicated. The prognosis is fair to good unless extensive skin loss has occurred.

Treatment of hepatogenous photosensitization requires specific and supportive measures to counter, to reverse, and ameliorate the hepatobiliary disease combined with removal of affected animals from sunlight. When multiple animals are affected because of toxins or poisonous plants, identification of the causative agent and avoidance is necessary to reduce further incidence of disease. The prognosis is poor for hepatogenous photosensitization patients because most have severe hepatic or hepatobiliary disease. No treatment exists for bovine erythropoietic porphyria or protoporphyria other than keeping affected animals out of sunlight. However, affected animals should be culled and specific recommendations made to breed organizations regarding the carrier status of both dams and sires of affected cattle.

Congenital and Inherited Skin Diseases

Numerous congenital and inherited skin conditions have been described in cattle. Because of the relative infrequency of these diseases and the excessive number of them, only a brief description of those diseases most likely to be found in dairy herds is included in Table 7.3.

Miscellaneous Diseases of Cattle

Anagen Defluxion (Effluvium)

Widespread loss of hair over the neck, trunk, limbs, and – to a lesser degree – the head, that leaves healthy skin underneath occasionally develops in calves and adults that have recently been severely ill with high fever resulting from pneumonia, septicemia, or severe diarrhea (Figs. 7.25 and 7.26). This condition in the past has been called telogen defluxion (effluvium); however, telogen defluxion describes a delayed shedding of hair 2 to 3 months after a stressful disease or incident. Anagen defluxion occurs within days of the calf's illness as a result of injury to the anagen portion of hair growth. Frequently, it coincides with clinical improvement of the primary condition, but causes great concern in the owner as to the calf's prognosis. The skin remains healthy, assuming the calf is provided good nursing care and bedding. Stubbled hairs can be felt at the skin surface. Hair growth recommences within weeks, and recovery is complete if the primary disease fully resolves.

TABLE 7.3 Congenital and Inherited Disorders of the Skin

Disorder	Inheritance and Signs
Anhidrotic ectodermal dysplasia	Holstein; X-linked recessive; hypotrichosis; hypodontia; decreased atrichial (eccrine) sweat glands
Lethal hypotrichosis	Holstein-Friesians; autosomal recessive; sparse hair coat present only on muzzle, eyelids, pinnae, tail, and pasterns
Semi-hairlessness	Ayrshires; autosomal recessive; sparse hair coat of coarse, wiry hairs
Viable hypotrichosis	Guernseys, Jerseys, Holsteins; autosomal recessive; hair present only on legs, tail, eyelids, and pinnae
Hypotrichosis and missing incisors	Holstein-Friesians; autosomal dominant; hypotrichosis on face and neck; lack 4 to 6 incisors Friesian crosses; X-linked, incomplete penetrance; generalized hypotrichosis and absent incisors
Streaked hypotrichosis	Holstein-Friesians; sex-linked dominant in females; hypotrichosis in vertical streaks over hips and sometimes sides and legs
Tardive hypotrichosis	Friesians; sex-linked recessive in females; hypotrichosis of face, neck, and legs begins at 6 weeks to 6 months of age
Inherited epidermal dysplasia ("baldy calf syndrome")	Holstein-Friesians; autosomal recessive; absent horn buds and elongated, narrow, pointed hooves; generalized thinning of hair coat and patchy areas of scale, crust, and thickened and wrinkled skin; begins at 1 to 2 months of age; tips of pinnae curl medially; ulcers and crusts on carpi, hocks, and stifles
Color-related follicular dysplasias	Black and white or tan ("buckskin") and white Holsteins; normal at birth, but hypotrichosis and scaling develop in the black or tan areas
Ichthyosis	Mild form in Holsteins and Jerseys; autosomal recessive; generalized hyperkeratosis and hypotrichosis at birth or within a few weeks. Severe form in Friesians and Brown Swiss; autosomal recessive; generalized alopecia, hyperkeratosis, thickening, and fissuring at birth; ectropion and eclabium; dead at birth or within a few days
Cutaneous asthenia ("dermatosparaxis", "Ehlers-Danlos syndrome")	Holstein-Friesians; autosomal recessive; variable degrees of loose skin, cutaneous fragility and hyperextensibility
Epidermolysis bullosa ("epitheliogenesis imperfecta")	Holsteins, Jerseys, Ayrshires; autosomal recessive; vesicles, bullae, and ulcers in oral cavity, distal legs, pressure points, and pinnae; at birth or within a few days
Hereditary zinc deficiency ("inherited parakeratosis", "Adema disease", "lethal trait A46")	Holstein-Friesians; autosomal recessive; erythema, scale, crust, and alopecia of face, distal legs, and mucocutaneous areas begin at 4 to 8 weeks of age; dark hair coat often fades, especially periocularly ("spectacles")
Lymphedema	Ayrshires; autosomal recessive; variable degrees of edema of hind legs, and sometimes the front legs, tail, prepuce, pinnae, and face

The condition needs to be differentiated from vitamin C-responsive dermatosis (Fig. 7.27), urine and fecal scalding, and inherited hypotrichoses (see Table 7.3).

Urine or Fecal Scalding

Although most accurately discussed within the context of a contact irritant dermatitis, urine and fecal scalding occasionally leads to large areas of alopecia that are confused with inherited hypotrichoses, anagen defluxion, and nutritional dermatoses. Calves or cows that are forced to lie in filthy or urine-drenched stalls for prolonged periods because of protracted recumbency, musculoskeletal diseases, metabolic diseases, severe systemic illness or simply poor husbandry are at risk for urine and fecal scalding. Large areas of skin over pressure points, the hind limbs, and the ventrum may lose hair and appear pink or pink-red as a result of chemical irritation by urine and feces. This skin remains intact and non-ulcerated unless inadvertent trauma or pressure necrosis associated with prolonged recumbency ensues. Similarly, many calves and occasionally adult cattle with severe diarrhea develop alopecia and pink-red irritated skin around the perineum, tail, and caudal aspect of the hind limbs from fecal-contact irritant dermatitis. Adult cattle with tail paralysis secondary to sacral or coccygeal injury also are at risk because they cannot effectively raise their tails when defecating or urinating.

Treatment consists of gently washing and cleaning affected areas with mild soap, drying, and providing dry bedding. Recumbent animals should be moved several times daily to allow dry bedding to be placed beneath them. Soothing and drying ointments, such as zinc oxide, may be applied to denuded areas of skin. Recovery is complete if the

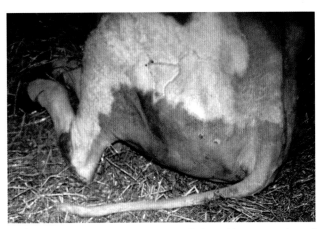

• **Fig. 7.25** Anagen defluxion in association with pneumonia and pyrexia. Marked alopecia over the rump, thighs, and tail is present.

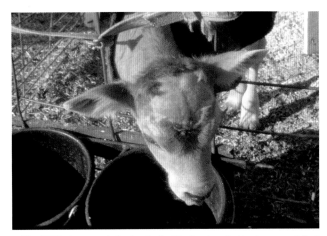

• **Fig. 7.26** Anagen defluxion limited to the head of a Jersey calf that had recovered from peracute *Salmonella* enteritis.

primary condition resolves. Cattle with sacral nerve injuries causing permanent tail paresis or paralysis may require continual care or tail amputation.

Leukotrichia and Leukoderma

Leukotrichia and leukoderma are acquired depigmentations of hair and skin, respectively, that develop after traumatic or inflammatory insults to the skin. In cattle, leukotrichia is commonly observed in the neck region corresponding to pressure and irritation from calves being tied with baling twine or tight neck straps of any type. Management systems that keep young calves and heifers tied with baling twine have a high incidence of this lesion appearing as a rather circumferential ring of white hair in the midcervical region. Leukotrichia appears during calfhood and may remain in the adult, depending on the degree of damage to melanocytes in the area. Leukotrichia also may appear in areas of skin previously injured by decubital sores, lacerations, thermal injuries, and tumors (usually large papillomas). Leukoderma probably implies such a drastic reduction in melanocytes that the skin remains depigmented. Burns, freeze brands, cryosurgery scars, deep full-thickness wounds, and other

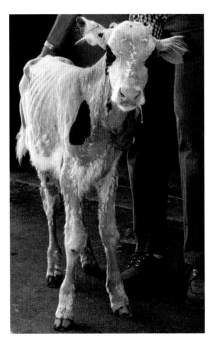

• **Fig. 7.27** A 6-week-old Holstein calf with vitamin C–responsive dermatosis.

skin injuries may result in leukoderma in cattle. No practical treatment exists, and tattooing seldom is indicated for leukoderma because cosmetics rarely are of concern.

Alopecia Areata

Alopecia areata is a rare autoimmune dermatosis. Anagen hair follicle antigens are the targets of cell-mediated and humoral autoimmune responses. There are no apparent age, sex, or breed predilections.

Lesions may be solitary or multiple and consist of annular-to-oval areas of alopecia (Fig. 7.28). The exposed skin appears normal. Lesions most commonly occur on the face, neck, brisket, and shoulder. Darkly pigmented hairs are preferentially targeted. Spontaneous regrowth of hair often features hairs that are lighter in color and smaller in size than normal. Affected cattle are healthy otherwise.

The diagnosis is confirmed by skin biopsy. Animals with one or just a few lesions may spontaneously recover over the course of a year. Animals with widespread lesions usually do not recover. Successful treatment has not been reported.

Parasitic Diseases

Hypodermiasis (Warbles) (Grubs)
Etiology

The warble or heel flies of cattle are *Hypoderma lineatum* and *Hypoderma bovis*. Whereas *H. lineatum* lay eggs on the heels of the forelegs and dewlap, *H. bovis* lay eggs on the hindquarters and loin area. The adult flies of *H. bovis* frighten cattle because of a bumblebee-like noise they make. Cattle may become extremely anxious and frightened when beset by these flies. Cattle frequently run wildly

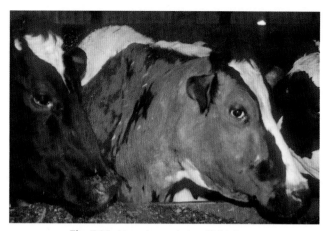

• **Fig. 7.28** Alopecia areata in a Holstein cow.

("gadding") from the flies and may injure themselves or run through fences during this panic. This behavior can be observed in pastured cattle during the late spring and early summer in the northeastern United States. Geographic and climatic conditions cause the life cycle of these parasites to vary as to specific time of year for the appearance of various stages.

Eggs hatch within 1 week, and first instar larvae burrow through the skin, aided by proteolytic enzymes. Further migration ensues with *H. lineatum* larvae eventually reaching the submucosa of the caudal third of the esophagus and *H. bovis* larvae reaching the epidural adipose tissue between the dura mater and periosteum of the thoracolumbar vertebrae. The esophagus and spinal canal usually are reached by the larvae in approximately 4 weeks, and are known as the "winter resting sites" where the larvae spend 2 to 4 months. Mature first instar larvae of *H. bovis* and *H. lineatum* arrive at their "spring resting site" in the subcutaneous tissue of the back during the late winter or spring. Again, the precise timing will vary based on climatic and latitude conditions. At this site, they establish a breathing hole and molt to a second instar phase. During this molting, the visible subcutaneous swellings in the back of affected cattle appear. A second molt to the third instar larvae occurs within 1 month after completion of the first molt. The third instar larvae eventually leave the warble, drop to the ground, pupate in the soil for 1 to 2 months, and finally emerge as adult flies that live less than 1 week.

Warbles are more common in first-calf heifers than older cows because of age-related resistance to the parasite.

Economic losses as a result of hypodermiasis occur for several reasons:
1. Frightened cattle on pasture cannot eat or gain weight at normal rates when being attacked by adult flies.
2. Major economic losses occur because of hide injury and meat trim from warbles. This is a major economic loss in beef cattle more than dairy cattle.
3. Occasional complications occur including; esophageal and spinal injuries from larvae killed too late in the life cycle by insecticides (see Treatment section); toxic or

anaphylactic reactions caused by grubs being killed inside a warble; and cosmetic defects associated with warbles in show or sale animals.

Signs

Clinical signs of adult fly activity can be observed when pastured cattle run wildly about the pasture. Some even bellow in fright as they try to escape *H. bovis* adults. The only other obvious clinical sign is the "warble" itself on the back of affected cattle. Individual cattle may have only one swelling or as many as several hundred. Air holes are visible and further clarify the diagnosis.

Treatment

Treatment starts with fly control measures to minimize the environmental factors that propagate fly numbers. Heifers at pasture should be treated with fly repellents (e.g., dust bags) to minimize the irritation of flies. Specific treatment with systemic insecticides should be performed routinely on dairy heifers. The exact time of year for treatment varies with climate and latitude, but this information is readily available from regional extension agencies. In the northeastern United States, for example, treatment for early *Hypoderma* spp. larvae occurs between October 15 and November 15, after frosts have usually ended the fly season but before the larvae have reached a large size. Adult lactating cows should not be treated because they have a lower incidence of infestation as a result of age-acquired immunity and to avoid the entire issue of milk residues. Heifers may be treated during routine fall handling for vaccinations. Heifers due to freshen within several months should not be treated.

Because chemical formulations and approvals change constantly, recommendations must be based on currently available products that are allowed for dairy cattle. Always read the label! Pour-on products such as eprinomectin and moxidectin currently are approved for dairy cattle with no milk discard time issues when used according to the labels.

Local reactions at the sites of first instar larvae occasionally are observed after treatment. These reactions are much more likely if treatment is delayed beyond the proper time within a geographic area because the larvae are larger. Adverse reactions to *H. lineatum* larvae include esophageal inflammation that may result in choke-like signs of salivation, bloat, and an inability to eat. Adverse reactions with *H. bovis* larvae include temporary or permanent paralysis caused by aberrant migration or simple inflammation in the extradural region of the thoracolumbar spinal cord. Reports of "paralysis" are widely debated, and very few factual references exist as to the pathology that causes signs of paralysis. Many of these reactions may have been caused by drug toxicities rather than host–parasite interactions. The use of larvicidal insecticides late in the first instar life cycle may cause reactions to the dying larvae that appear as severe swelling along the topline. The same reaction has occurred when larvae in warbles have been accidentally killed by crushing or by owners attempting to "squeeze" the larvae out of an airhole. Such reactions may result from larval toxins and proteases, or may be an immune-mediated reaction caused by both cellular and humoral immune responses that have evolved as the parasite migrates through the host. Occasional "anaphylactic" reactions with toxemia or death of the cow have occurred after crushing of a larva in a warble. No reference specifically and factually explains whether such reactions are anaphylactic or are caused by the release of potent toxins from the dead larvae. In either event, owners should be warned not to interfere with the natural life cycle of *Hypoderma* spp. after subcutaneous lesions in the back appear.

Although vaccination against *Hypoderma* spp. has been attempted, no commercially available vaccines are currently available in the United States.

Louse Infestation (Pediculosis)

Etiology

Louse infestation in cattle seldom is thought of as a significant deterrent to weight gain or production, but this has not been the author's experience. Sucking lice, such as *Haematopinus eurysternus; Solenopotes capillatus;* and *Linognathus vituli,* and biting lice, such as *Bovicola bovis (Damalinia bovis),* can reach high levels of infestation during winter in northern climates. Longer hair coats, cooler skin and environmental temperatures, and confinement aid in propagation of lice during winter. Lice are host specific, spending their entire life cycle on the host; moreover, each species of louse has a favorite location on the host's body. Sunlight and heat are great deterrents to reproduction and survival of lice. Thus, shorter hair coats, exposure to direct sunlight, and high environmental temperatures in summer tend to depress the louse population naturally. Age-specific resistance does not appear significant in cattle in response to louse infestation. Biting lice feed on skin debris and prefer the dorsum and flank region. Sucking lice prefer the head, neck, withers, axillae, and ventrum. However, when louse populations are extensive, the parasites can be found anywhere on the body. Lice, as is true of many parasites, are likely to have the greatest negative effect on animals subjected to poor nutrition, systemic illnesses, overcrowding, and other stresses, all of which may be more common in calves. Severe infestation with fleas (*Ctenocephalides felis* [cat flea]) may occur in calves, but anemia, weakness, and weight loss are the predominant clinical signs.

Signs

Pruritus, restlessness, and excessive licking are the major signs of louse infestation in cattle (Fig. 7.29). Mild infestations are not likely to result in clinical signs that owners observe, but large numbers of lice definitely interfere with growth of calves and production in dairy cattle. Cattle with heavy infestations are made uncomfortable or irritable by the parasites and spend a great deal of time rubbing against inanimate objects and licking themselves. Heavy infestation of sucking lice in young calves or animals kept under poor husbandry conditions may result in blood loss anemia. Louse infestations often are detected by the "weak sister" principle of parasitology. That is, one or

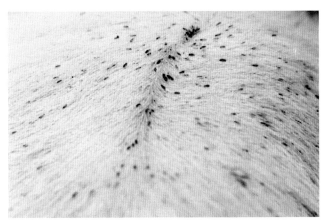

• **Fig. 7.29** Heavy louse infestation in a Holstein calf. The calf was hypothermic, causing the lice to move from the skin surface and become more obvious in the hair coat than normal.

a few animals will show obvious clinical signs caused by severe infestation when in fact a herd problem exists. Signs are most apparent in the winter when longer hair coats and lower environmental temperatures contribute to heavy louse infestation.

Lick marks created by the tongue in response to pruritus that resemble the marks left by a wet paintbrush are classic on calves and cows with louse infestations (Fig. 7.30). Lick marks are present over the sides, flanks, dorsum, hindquarters, and wherever the animal can reach if not confined (Fig. 7.31). Stanchioned cattle are very restless because their restraint limits their ability to lick or scratch. They tend to "rattle" the stanchions and rub vigorously back and forth or up and down in the stanchion, causing areas of hair loss on the neck and shoulders. Dr. Francis Fox described excessive "rattling" of stanchions as one of the cardinal signs of heavy louse infestation in stanchioned cattle. Self-induced alopecia and excoriations are common, and generalized scaling may be observed. Hairballs may be more common in calves with louse infestation as a result of chronic licking.

Diagnosis

The diagnosis is made by observing clinical signs and finding lice during the physical examination. Usually a penlight and careful separation of the hair is sufficient for identification. Areas that appear most disturbed by licking or rubbing are excellent locations to examine. The neck, dorsum, and gluteal regions frequently harbor sufficient numbers of lice to allow early diagnosis. Another tremendous aid to diagnosis is clipping hair. The author has found this to be a dramatic means by which to demonstrate lice in our hospital, and also in the field when cattle are clipped in preparation for abdominal surgery. Lice are apparent as brown "dots" that do not wash away easily. Hundreds or thousands may be observed in some heavily infested cattle when the abdomen is clipped before paramedian or flank surgery.

Cattle that have died or are hypothermic as a result of shock may have lice leave the skin and appear in large numbers on the external hair coat. This abandonment of the host has been compared with rats leaving the sinking ship.

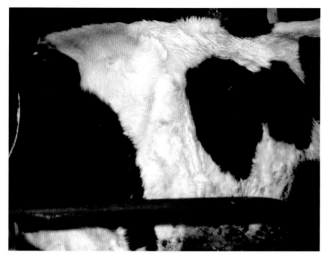

• **Fig. 7.30** Lick marks on the dorsum, thorax, and flank of a Holstein cow infested with lice.

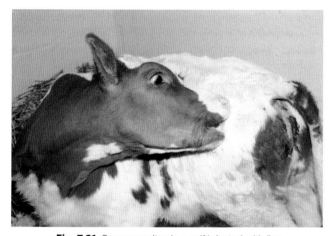

• **Fig. 7.31** Severe pruritus in a calf infested with lice.

Treatment

Purely individual treatment seldom is warranted because heavy infestation in one or a few cattle indicates a herd problem. Treatment of all animals and the environment is indicated whenever significant numbers of lice are identified. Only products approved for dairy cattle should be used. Eprinomectin and moxidectin pour-ons are approved, effective, and have no milk or meat withdrawal issues when used according to the label. Several pyrethrin or permethrin preparations and coumaphos products are available for appropriate use in dairy cattle and calves. These products may be used as sprays or powders. All bedding should be cleared away, the barn sprayed, and all animals treated as a blitz treatment. Repeat treatment in 2 to 4 weeks, or as indicated by manufacturers of selected products, should follow. Herds having annual problems should be treated in the fall before peak louse numbers. Housed cattle should be clipped whenever possible to prevent excessively long hair coats that foster increased numbers of lice.

Flies

Fly control contributes greatly to cow comfort and production. Excessive numbers of flies not only irritate cows and farm workers but may represent vectors of infectious keratoconjunctivitis, environmental causes of mastitis through teat end injury, dermatophilosis, papillomatosis, and other infectious diseases. Mosquitoes, *Culicoides* spp., tabanids, horn flies *(Haematobia* spp.), blackflies *(Simulium* spp.), stable flies *(Stomoxys calcitrans)*, and others are all capable of being annoying and causing painful bites and skin injury to cattle. *Phormia regina* (black blowflies) are blowflies that lay eggs in wounds, causing subsequent maggot infestation. Calliphorids (blue blowflies) may lay eggs on dead animal or plant material and cause fly strike in some geographic areas of the world. *Cochliomyia hominivorax,* the true screw worm that feeds on living flesh, requires regulatory vigilance to prevent return of this parasite to the United States from Mexico. *Musca domestica,* a filth fly, may mechanically transmit pathogens but does not bite. Mosquitoes, blackflies, tabanids, and *Culicoides* spp. reproduce prolifically when nearby water allows fertile breeding grounds. Stable flies, horn flies, and *Musca* spp. lay eggs in manure, so poor husbandry or dirty yards contribute to increased numbers of these pests. All of these insects reach peak numbers during the summer months.

Every farm has fly problems to some degree, and control is frequently frustrated by limited labor and management procedures to deter excessive fly numbers. However, the brevity of this section should not be interpreted as a lack of significance regarding the importance of flies as an irritant to cattle. Flies create a tremendous negative impact on cow comfort and subsequent productivity.

Signs

The clinical signs of excessive flies and other biting insects in cattle include restlessness; irritability; decreased feed intake; decreased production; and painful skin papules, wheals, or crusts. One simply has to enter the cows' environment to appreciate and experience the problem. On a warm summer day, it may be impossible to perform a thorough physical examination on a cow that is being bitten by large numbers of flies because of her discomfort and irritability.

The diagnosis is made by observation of the cattle and their environment.

Treatment

Management practices that reduce fly breeding areas are of primary concern in prevention and treatment of excessive fly numbers. Draining swamps, stagnant water, and ponds may reduce mosquitoes, tabanids, and *Culicoides* spp. Blackflies usually require moving water or fast-flowing streams as breeding grounds. Stable flies, *Musca* spp., and horn flies can be reduced by cleaning away manure from barns, barnyards, and collection or feeding areas. Dead animals, placentas, and surgically removed tissue should be discarded rather than left for blowflies, and wounds should be attended daily to avoid blowflies and subsequent maggots.

Insecticides and larvicides comprise the treatment options that most owners use—sometimes in lieu of management procedures—to reduce fly numbers. Sprays for premises and insecticides to be used on cattle should be labeled specifically for use on dairy cattle and on dairy premises. Some premise sprays are designed for use in barns when the cattle are not present. Chemical toxicities are possible if cattle are sprayed directly with sprays intended only for use on the premises. Barns should be sprayed early in the season rather than at the peak of fly populations.

Self-applicating dust bags for dairy cattle should contain only approved substances for lactating cows. Fly baits should be placed in areas where cattle cannot ingest them. Feed-additive insecticides such as stirofos may reduce filth flies (*Musca* spp., *Stomoxys calcitrans,* and blowflies) by killing fly larvae in manure, but should not be used unless specifically labeled and approved for use in dairy cattle.

Insecticide-impregnated ear tags may be used in heifers or nonlactating animals as a deterrent to face flies (*Musca autumnalis*), which are the major vectors of infectious bovine keratoconjunctivitis. These same ear tags may also help control horn flies (*Haematobia irritans)*, and thereby reduce "fly worry" and irritation caused by these pests. Eprinomectin and moxidectin pour-ons are approved and effective for horn fly control and have no milk discard time issues.

Tick-Borne Diseases

Ticks represent important vectors of infectious disease that can also cause parasitic irritation, damage to hides, and great economic loss in some cattle-raising areas of the world. Seldom are cattle the only host for the ticks that will be discussed; each species of tick varies in life cycle, host range, and time periods for blood feeding. Various soft-bodied ticks (*Argasidae* spp.) and hard-bodied ticks (*Ixodidae* spp.) parasitize cattle. Ticks tend to be less host-specific than lice. Specific ticks that are disease vectors for cattle in North America are discussed further in Chapter 16.

Signs

In addition to systemic illness related to tick-borne parasitemia, painful bites that heal poorly or become secondarily infected are a major problem for cattle infested with ticks. Damage to hides is an economic concern when beef cattle are affected with large numbers of ticks. Irritation, anxiety, and decreased feed consumption and growth rates are symptomatic of painful infestation with ticks and other ectoparasites.

In addition to these localized signs, diseases such as anaplasmosis and babesiosis can be spread easily by ticks. Because ticks are not highly host specific, ticks in cattle may additionally represent a threat to human health because of the many infectious diseases they carry.

Diagnosis

Identification of ticks on cattle or confirmation of tick-borne disease in cattle suffices for diagnosis.

Treatment

Treatment is difficult and expensive because it is labor intensive. In addition, various stages of the life cycle of some ticks may not occur on the animal. Chemical dips, sprays, pour-on and spot-on products, and ivermectin products have been used to control ticks. Ticks have developed resistance to many acaricides, and new products with regulatory approval will hopefully continue to appear on the market. Dips have provided the most reliable means of post application control in the past, but newer chemicals and innovative delivery systems (e.g., slow-release, spot-on formulations) may reduce the labor necessary for treatment. Obviously, tick infestations are more likely in pastured and range cattle than confined dairy cattle. However, in many areas of the United States, dairy cattle are at risk for tick infestation and subsequent tick-borne problems. Products selected for acaricides must be approved for use in dairy cattle. In the United States, the avermectins (ivermectin and eprinomectin) and milbemycins (moxidectin) pour-on treatments represent the most likely effective, and approved, treatments for the control of cattle ticks.

Genetic resistance to ticks appears in Zebu cattle *(Bos indicus)* and Zebu-cross cattle. This fact has allowed the beef industry in regions with heavy tick populations to breed cattle requiring less tick treatment.

Mange
Chorioptic Mange

Etiology. *Chorioptic* mange is the most common mange to cause clinical signs in dairy cattle. *Chorioptes bovis* feeds primarily on epidermal debris and is host adapted. The mite has a life cycle that requires 2 to 3 weeks and is completed on the host. The length of time that *C. bovis* mites can survive off the host has been debated, but this seldom is of major concern if adequate treatment is provided.

The major problems observed in dairy cattle affected with clinically apparent chorioptic mange are discomfort, pruritus, agitation, and subsequent interference with feed intake and maximal production. Calves seldom are affected clinically, and the disease tends to occur in mature milking cows in affected herds. Sporadic cases may be observed, but it is more common to have 10% to 20% of the herd showing mild lesions. The greater the percentage of clinically apparent lesions, the greater the effect is on herd milk production.

Chorioptic mange appears to be more common during the winter months. This may reflect biologic activity of the mites, environmental factors, longer hair coats, confinement causing increased density of cattle during winter, or other factors. The disease may regress spontaneously during warmer months, and residual mite populations are thought to concentrate in the pastern, tail head, perineum, or lower digital skin during this time.

Signs. Pruritus characterized by restlessness, treading, violent swishing of the tail, and rubbing of the tail and perineum against stationary objects is prominent in moderate to severe

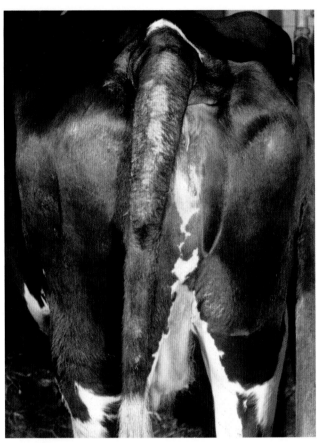

• **Fig. 7.32** Chorioptic mange lesions on the tail head, tail, perineum, medial thigh, and udder.

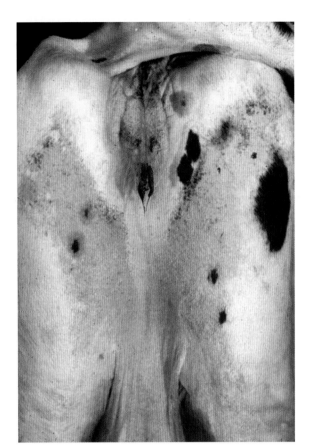

• **Fig. 7.33** Chorioptic mange in a Holstein cow. Erythema, papules, crusts, and traumatic alopecia can be seen.

cases. Skin lesions with alopecia and crusting may be apparent in the ischiatic fossa, tail head, perineum, caudal udder, medial thigh, or scrotum (Figs. 7.32 and 7.33). Papules and erythema of the infested skin may be prominent, especially if the cow has been scratching against solid objects. Very heavy crusts on the tail head or between the tail head and pin bones are common with mild to moderate infestations, and frequently are observed during routine rectal palpations for reproductive purposes. Similar lesions of the skin of the digit also may be observed, but are less common than the aforementioned lesions of the perineum and hind end in dairy cattle.

Diagnosis. The clinical signs are highly suggestive, but definitive diagnosis requires skin scrapings to identify *C. bovis* mites specifically. Important differentials include lice infestation and the reportable manges—sarcoptic and psoroptic.

Treatment. As with other ectoparasites, many insecticides are available to kill *C. bovis*, but few are approved for dairy cattle. Coumaphos (0.03%) applied as a spray at approved concentrations for dairy cattle is very effective when 2 applications at 2-week intervals are completed. Lime sulfur (2%) applied once weekly for 4 treatments also is effective. Eprinomectin and moxidectin pour-ons are approved and effective, and have no milk discard time

issues when used according to the label. All cattle in the herd should be treated rather than just those showing obvious dermatologic signs. It also is helpful to use a curry comb to remove heavy crusts before the insecticide treatment, although this increases the labor necessary for herd control. Treatment should be coordinated with complete removal of bedding and cleaning of the environment for best results.

Demodectic Mange

Demodectic mites are considered normal inhabitants of hair follicles and sebaceous glands of cattle, and seldom cause clinical signs of disease. The *Demodex* mites of cattle are host-specific and require no time off the host to complete their life cycle. Demodectic mite infestation of calves is thought to occur naturally through contact with the dam during the first few days of life. Currently, dairy calves often have very little exposure to the dam after birth, and this may decrease transmission. Because most cattle with demodectic mites are asymptomatic, those with symptoms may have genetic or immunologic defects allowing the host–parasite relationship to be altered.

Signs. Palpable nodules and papules over the neck, withers, shoulder, and flank regions characterize the infestation. The number and size of these lesions vary, but most are 0.5 to 1.0 cm in diameter and covered with normal

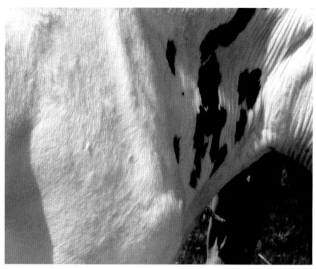

• **Fig. 7.34** Demodectic mange in a Holstein cow. Small raised hair tufts are apparent on the shoulder region and thorax.

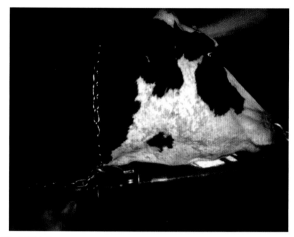

• **Fig. 7.35** Sarcoptic mange on the face of a Holstein cow. Erythema, papules, crusts, and traumatic alopecia are seen.

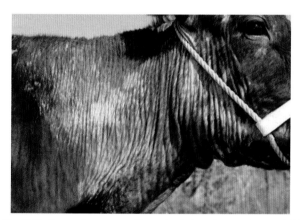

• **Fig. 7.36** Sarcoptic mange with marked alopecia, crusting, and skin thickening over the face and neck.

hair (Fig. 7.34). Pruritus and other clinical signs are not apparent. Clinical signs of crusting, folliculitis, drainage, or ulceration constitute possible advanced lesions with secondary bacterial infection, and occasionally are observed. *Demodex bovis* and an unclassified species are found around the eyelids and body skin. *Demodex ghanensis* has been found primarily around the eyelids in cattle.

Diagnosis. The diagnosis can be confirmed by deep skin scrapings or by expressing exudate harboring mites from lesions for microscopic examination. Because of the follicular location of demodectic mites, other causes of folliculitis (e.g., dermatophytes, staphylococci, and *Dermatophilus*) must be considered. Asymptomatic cases also may appear similar to insect bites.

Treatment. Treatment usually is not necessary. This is fortunate because control of clinical demodectic mange always is difficult at best and would be more so in dairy cattle, given the limited insecticides approved for lactating cows. Individual cattle with overt dermatologic disease caused by *Demodex* spp. should be assessed for immunologic compromise or genetic predisposition.

Sarcoptic Mange

Etiology. A reportable disease in dairy cattle, sarcoptic mange causes dramatic clinical signs and production losses when introduced into a dairy herd. *Sarcoptes* spp. mites burrow in the upper skin layers and feed on fluids and debris, and females reproduce to worsen the condition. The life cycle requires approximately 2 weeks and is completed on the host. Cattle may acquire the disease by direct contact with infested cattle or contact with inanimate objects that have been used for rubbing by infested cattle. *Sarcoptes* spp. mites can only survive for several days off the host and are susceptible to dryness.

Although *Sarcoptes* spp. affecting various domestic species closely resemble each other, parasitologists debate the idea of a common species with adaptation to various hosts versus separate *Sarcoptes* spp. for each host species. Regardless, when examined microscopically, the sarcoptic mites from cattle (*Sarcoptes scabiei* var. *bovis*) appear very similar to those found on other species. Transient, superficial sarcoptic mite infestations may occur in humans working with cattle affected with sarcoptic mange.

Signs. Profound pruritus characterizes sarcoptic mange. Lesions may appear anywhere, but the tail, neck, brisket, shoulders, rump, and inner thighs are common sites (Figs. 7.35 and 7.36). Papules, crusts, alopecia, abrasions, and thickening of the skin are observed in affected areas. Pruritus causes biting, licking, and excessive rubbing on inanimate objects. Self-induced lacerations and skin abrasions are common because cattle occasionally will rub on sharp objects or persist in rubbing until abrasions occur. Dr. Francis Fox was consulted, and diagnosed sarcoptic mange in a free-stall herd in which affected cattle bowed gates so badly through rubbing that all divider gates had been irreparably damaged.

The obvious effects of this intense pruritus are decreased productivity (because affected cattle have reduced feed intake), failure to show heats, and loss of weight. The reduction in milk yield can be dramatic. Untreated animals may become debilitated, and death as a result of secondary diseases and overall debility is possible.

Diagnosis. Clinical signs and deep skin scrapings that identify mites, eggs, and parasitic fecal debris are required for diagnosis. Sarcoptic mites are notorious for being difficult to find, but multiple deep scrapes and persistence usually permit a positive diagnosis.

Treatment. It is important to call regulatory veterinarians since this is a reportable disease. For lactating cattle, 2% lime sulfur heated to between 95.0° and 105.0°F (35.0° to 40.5°C) is used as a dip or spray. No withdrawals are required when this product is used on dairy cattle, but treatment may need to be repeated at 10- to 14-day intervals. Eprinomectin pour-on is approved and effective and has no milk discard time issues. Doramectin is approved and effective but cannot be used in female dairy cattle older than 20 months of age.

Psoroptic Mange

Etiology. Another reportable disease of dairy cattle, psoroptic mange is similar to sarcoptic mange in that severe pruritus characterizes the disease. Psoroptic mites live on the skin surface, feed on serum and lymph fluids, and require 2 to 3 weeks for a complete life cycle from egg to egg-laying female. Psoroptic mites live off the host better than sarcoptic mites and may survive 1 month or more in the environment under certain conditions. The mites survive best off the host during winter and worst during hot, dry summer periods. Similar to sarcoptic mange, psoroptic mange may be spread by both direct and indirect means—that is, contaminated common scratching posts and other inanimate objects in the environment.

Signs. Intensive and overwhelming pruritus that accompanies generalized skin lesions with papules, crusts, abrasions, and alopecia are the main signs. Although skin lesions may appear anywhere, the withers and tail head and then later the back and sides are typical locations. The skin becomes thickened and appears wrinkled with time. Pruritus is so severe that affected cattle can think of little else. Therefore, weight and production losses are profound. Neglected cattle become weak, emaciated, often develop secondary infections, and may die.

Diagnosis. The clinical signs and skin scraping to identify the causative mites, *Psoroptes ovis*, constitute proof of diagnosis.

Treatment. As with sarcoptic mange, once the diagnosis has been made, one should contact regulatory veterinarians; this is a reportable disease. Available treatments are as described for sarcoptic mange. Lime sulfur 2% heated to between 95.0° and 105.0°F (35.0° to 40.5°C) is an approved dip or spray for lactating dairy cattle. Moxidectin pour-on is approved and effective and has no milk discard time issues when used according to the label. Doramectin pour-on is approved and effective but cannot be used on female dairy cattle older than 20 months of age.

Stephanofilariasis

Etiology

Stephanofilaria stilesi is the common cause of a filarial dermatitis on the ventral midline of cattle in the United States. Adults live in the dermis, and microfilariae are ingested by the horn fly, *H. irritans*. Microfilariae develop into infective larvae during a 2- to 3-week time period spent in the fly, and then are injected into the skin of cattle when the fly feeds.

Signs

Dermatitis on the ventral midline consists initially of serous exudate, crusts, and papules. Chronicity leads to alopecia, skin thickening, and hyperkeratosis. The usual site is between the brisket and umbilicus, but extensive lesions may extend more cranially or caudally. Lesions occasionally are observed on the udder. Pruritus causes affected cows to attempt to scratch their bellies while they are partially recumbent. Cows may rise to their knees and rock the brisket and ventral abdomen fore and aft in an effort to relieve the itching sensation associated with dermatitis.

Diagnosis

Clinical signs coupled with skin biopsies provide the best means of establishing a definitive diagnosis. Cross-sections of adult worms are observed in hair follicles when biopsies are examined histologically. Microfilariae and eosinophils are found in the dermis.

Treatment

Approved treatments for stephanofilariasis are not available for lactating cattle. However, both the avermectin and milbemycin families of ectoparasiticides will likely be useful against this parasite. Topical ivermectin and eprinomectin can be used in lactating cattle, as can moxidectin, but doramectin can only be used in female dairy cattle younger than 20 months of age.

Fly-Strike from Maggots (Calliphorine myiasis, Blowflies)

Etiology

Many species of blowflies are capable of causing fly-strike in domestic animals. Several species of calliphorids (blue blowflies) and *Phormia regina* (black blowfly) are the major blowflies in North America. The flies are at peak numbers during spring, early summer, and fall. Adult flies may travel several miles in search of food and egg-laying sites. Dead carcasses, rotten meat or plant material, and necrotic wounds attract adult flies. *P. regina* probably is the primary blowfly to cause fly strike in cattle wounds in the United States, but different calliphorids predominate in other regions of the world.

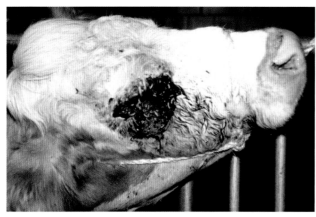

• **Fig. 7.37** Maggots in the orbital region of a cow with a neglected orbital squamous cell carcinoma.

Females lay eggs in wounds such as those caused by dehorning, castration, or trauma. Occasionally, fly strike occurs in exposed retained placentas, the umbilicus of newborn calves, and necrotic or lacerated vulvas following dystocia. Recumbent calves with diarrhea are at risk for fly strike around the diarrhea-soaked anus, perineum, and tail. Calves or cattle that have had corneal perforations, sunken eyes, periocular neoplasia and phthisis bulbi secondary to pinkeye may have fly strike in the affected orbit (Fig. 7.37).

In warm weather, blowfly eggs hatch to maggots in 1 to 3 days. If both warmth and moisture are present, eggs may hatch in less than 12 hours. The maggots persist, and the odor of the wound attracts more blowflies.

Toxemia secondary to myiasis seems to occur more commonly in young calves, but also may develop in adult cattle. Although many animals infested with maggots also have primary diseases, maggots seem to contribute to anorexia, depression, and debility. The exact pathophysiology for this "toxemia" or depressant effect of maggots on the host is not understood. The true screw worm, *Cochliomyia hominivorax*, had been eradicated from the United States but was found in 2016 in Key deer in Florida and remains a constant threat to the southern regions of the United States. True screw worms penetrate and feed on living flesh in wounds. Calliphorine maggots secrete proteolytic enzymes to digest and liquefy host tissue (usually necrotic), but do not feed on living tissue. If maggots are found in living flesh, true screw worm infestation should be ruled out by laboratory identification of the maggot species.

Signs

Signs are grossly obvious to the eyes and nose of the examiner. A sickening, necrotic odor accompanies the disturbing sign of maggots moving within the wound. Secondary bacterial infections of the wounds may add to the odor and probably contribute further to attraction of blowflies. Sometimes it is difficult to assess the degree of illness associated with the primary problem of the animal versus the degree of illness associated with the maggots. Neonatal calves are at greatest risk of death because the precipitant primary diseases (e.g., diarrhea, white muscle disease, and septicemia) that weaken the calf usually are very serious, and maggots add an additional "toxic" component.

Treatment

The wound must be clipped, cleaned, and debrided if necessary, and the maggots must be killed. Clipping the hair is very important for wounds on haired tissue because this procedure will greatly deter future fly strike; moist matted hair creates an ideal fly-strike environment. The wound may be lavaged with warm water and pine oil (1 oz pine oil/32 oz water), or an insecticide may be sprayed on to destroy the maggots. Coumaphos 0.25% may be sprayed locally on the maggots, but application should not be overdone in calves, lest organophosphate toxicity occur. Wounds in nonlactating animals and calves should be treated with topical insecticide sprays or ointments. These products also should be used prophylactically to protect fresh wounds at risk for fly strike.

Lactating cattle require careful selection of insecticides such that only approved products are used. Prevention of maggots is much easier than treatment; therefore, fly control and diligent cleaning and protection of cattle wounds during the fly season are imperative. Wound ointments containing fly repellents or insecticides should be used routinely during the fly season. Fly smears are applied in a circle around the wound rather than to open tissue to minimize the potential for chemical absorption and toxicity, especially in calves.

Miscellaneous Parasitic Causes of Dermatologic Disease

Other parasites are occasional causes of skin lesions in cattle in the United States and abroad (Table 7.4).

Miscellaneous Physical, Chemical, and Nutritional Causes of Dermatologic Disease

Many physical insults, chemical toxicoses, and nutritional imbalances involving minerals and vitamins may directly or indirectly cause skin lesions. Although most of these conditions are rare in dairy cattle because of confinement and ration surveillance, some of the major toxicoses and deficiencies are listed in Tables 7.5 and 7.6. Details of these conditions—particularly their noncutaneous features—are beyond the scope of this chapter, and Tables 7.5 and 7.6 only include their dermatologic features. Several plants and toxins causing photosensitization and gangrene already have been discussed in other sections of this chapter.

TABLE 7.4 Miscellaneous Parasitic Skin Disorders

Disorder	Signs
Psorergatic mange	Subtle degrees of patchy alopecia and scaling with little or no pruritus, especially over dorsum; *Psorergates bos*
Onchocerciasis	Asymptomatic subcutaneous nodules over brisket, hip, and stifle *(Onchocerca gibsoni)*; shoulder, stifle, hip *(O. gutturosa)*; udder, scrotum *(O. ochengi)*
Parafilariasis	Nodules that discharge a bloody exudate; especially neck, shoulder, trunk; *Parafilaria bovicola*; spring and summer
Pelodera dermatitis	Pruritic, papular dermatitis of ventral abdomen and thorax, medial and lateral thighs, udder, and teats; *Pelodera strongyloides*
Rhabditic otitis externa	Bilateral, painful, odoriferous, suppurative otitis externa; *Rhabditis bovis*
Raillietia otitis externa	Bilateral suppurative, painful otitis externa; *Raillietia auris*
Trombiculidiasis	Adults; papules and crusts on legs, face, pinnae, axillae, and groin; variable pruritus; *Trombicula alfreddugesi, T. autumnalis*
Flea infestation	Variable degrees of pruritus and papulocrustous dermatitis, especially legs and trunk; *Ctenocephalides felis*
Louse-fly infestation	Variable dermatitis and pruritus, especially perineum and groin; *Hippobosca equina*

TABLE 7.5 Miscellaneous Physical and Chemical Disorders of the Skin

Disorder	Description
Amanita toxicosis	Eating mushroom *Amanita verna*; papules, vesicles, and necrotic foci around tail base and perineum
Arsenic toxicosis	Dry, dull, easily epilated hair coat progresses to alopecia and exfoliative dermatitis
Chlorinated naphthalene toxicoses	Progressive scaling, hyperkeratosis, thickening, fissuring, and alopecia beginning on the withers and neck
Dermatitis, pyrexia, and hemorrhage syndrome	Pruritic, papulocrustous dermatitis on head, neck, tail head, perineum, and udder
Foreign bodies	Papules, nodules, abscesses and draining tracts; especially legs, hips, muzzle, and ventrum
Hairy vetch toxicosis	Pruritic papules, plaques, oozing, crusts, and alopecia; begins on tail head, udder, and neck, and progresses to face, trunk, and legs
Hematoma	Acute onset, fluctuant, subcutaneous; especially stifle, ischial tuberosity, tuber coxae, perineum, ventral abdomen, lateral thorax, and point of shoulder
Hyalomma toxicosis ("sweating sickness")	Erythema, edema, oozing, foul smell on pinnae, face, neck, axillae, flank, and groin; lesions are painful; matted hair coat is easily epilated leaving erosions and ulcers
Intertrigo	Variable degrees of erythema, edema, and oozing; junction of lateral aspect of udder and medial thigh
Iodism	Scaling—with or without alopecia—especially dorsum, neck, head, and shoulders
Mercurialism	Progressive, generalized alopecia
Mimosine toxicosis	Gradual loss of long hairs (e.g., tail switch) and variable hoof dysplasias
Oat straw toxicosis	Papules, plaques, and fissures on udder, hindquarters, lips, muzzle, and vulva
Polybrominated biphenyl toxicosis	Abscesses and hematomas over back, abdomen, and hind legs; alopecia and lichenification over lateral thorax, neck, and shoulders; hoof dysplasias
Selenium toxicosis	Progressive loss of long hairs, coronitis, and hoof dysplasias
Snake bite	Progressive edema, pain, and discoloration with variable necrosis and sloughing; especially nose, head, and legs
Stachybotryotoxicosis	Necrotic ulcers in mouth and on lips and nostrils
Subcutaneous emphysema	Soft, fluctuant, crepitant, subcutaneous swelling; especially neck and trunk
Vampire bat bite	Multiple bleeding, crusted ulcers; especially dorsum and legs

Continued

TABLE 7.6	Miscellaneous Nutritional Disorders of the Skin
Disorder	**Signs**
Cobalt deficiency	Rough, brittle, faded hair coat
Copper deficiency	Rough, brittle, faded hair coat with variable excessive licking; periocular hair coat fade and hair loss ("spectacles")
High-fat milk replacer dermatosis	Alopecia and scaling of muzzle, periocular area, base of pinnae, and legs
Iodine deficiency	Newborn calves; generalized alopecia and thick, puffy skin (myxedema)
Riboflavin deficiency	Generalized alopecia and rough, brittle, faded hair coat
Selenium deficiency	Dermatitis over rump and tail base
Vitamin A deficiency	Rough, dry, faded hair coat and generalized seborrhea
Vitamin C–responsive dermatosis	Calves; scaling, alopecia, erythema, petechiae and ecchymoses beginning on the head or legs
Zinc–responsive dermatitis	Scaling and erythema progress to crusting and alopecia; face, pinnae, mucocutaneous junctions, pressure points, distal legs, flanks, and tail head; pruritus may be intense or absent

Suggested Readings

Blum, S., Mazuz, M., Brenner, J., et al. (2008). Effects of bovine necrotic vulvovaginitis on productivity in a dairy herd in Israel. *Vet J, 176*, 245–247.

Caron, Y., Groignet, S., Saegerman, C., et al. (2013). Three cases of Parafilaria bovicola infection in Belgium, and a few recent epidemiological observations on this emergent disease. *Vet Rec, 172*, 129.

Chénier, S., Leclère, M., Messier, S., et al. (2008). Streptococcus dysgalactiae cellulitis and toxic shock-like syndrome in a Brown Swiss cow. *J Vet Diagn Invest, 20*, 99–103.

Foster, A. P. (2012). Staphylococcal skin disease in livestock. *Vet Dermatol, 23*, 342–351.

Liénard, E., Salem, A., Grisez, C., et al. (2011). A longitudinal study of Besnoitia besnoiti infections and seasonal abundance of Stomoxys calcitrans in a dairy cattle farm of southwest France. *Vet Parasitol, 177*, 20–27.

Munday, J. S. (2014). Bovine and human papillomaviruses: a comparative review. *Vet Pathol, 51*, 1063–1075.

Rostaher, A., Mueller, R. S., Majzoub, M., et al. (2010). Bovine besnoitiosis in Germany. *Vet Dermatol, 21*, 329–334.

Scott, D. W. (2007). *Color atlas of farm animal dermatology*. Ames, IA: Blackwell Publishing.

Seeliger, F., Drögemüller, C., Tegtmeier, P., et al. (2005). Ectodysplasin-1 deficiency in a German Holstein bull associated with loss of respiratory mucous glands and chronic rhinotracheitis. *J Comp Pathol, 132*, 346–349.

Stamm, L. V., Walker, R. L., & Read, D. H. (2009). Genetic diversity of bovine mammary dermatitis-associated Treponema. *Vet Microbiol, 136*, 192–196.

Timm, K., Rüfenacht, S., von Tscharner, C., et al. (2010). Alopecia areata in Eringer cows. *Vet Dermatol, 21*, 545–553.

Yeruham, I., Tiomkin, D., Freidgut, O., et al. (2007). Necrotic vulvovaginitis in dairy cattle in Israel. *Vet Rec, 160*, 164–166.

8

Diseases of the Teats and Udder

PAOLO MORONI, DARYL V. NYDAM, PAULA A. OSPINA, JESSICA C. SCILLIERI-SMITH, PAUL D. VIRKLER, RICK D. WATTERS, FRANCIS L. WELCOME, MICHAEL J. ZURAKOWSKI, NORM G. DUCHARME AND AMY E. YEAGER

The udder of a dairy cow consists of four separate glands suspended by medial and lateral collagenous laminae. The medial laminae are more elastic, especially cranially, than the lateral laminae and are paired. Caudally, the medial laminae are more collagenous and originate from the subpelvic tendon. The lateral laminae are multiple, inserting at various levels of mammary tissue, and originate from the subpelvic tendon caudally and external oblique aponeurosis cranially. The medial and lateral laminae provide udder support, which is essential for udder conformation and for solid attachment to the ventral body wall. The external pudendal artery constitutes the major blood supply to the udder; the artery courses through the inguinal canal along with the pudendal vein and lymph vessels to supply the craniolateral portion of the mammary gland. Caudally, the internal pudendal artery branches into the ventral perineal artery at the level of the ischiatic arch and courses caudally to the vulva, along the perineum to the base of the rear quarters. The caudal superficial epigastric vein (subcutaneous abdominal vein or milk vein) is the major venous return from the mammary gland. Located superficially along the ventral abdomen, it courses cranially to the "milk well," where it enters the abdomen to join the internal thoracic vein, draining first into the subclavian vein and finally into the cranial vena cava. Lymph drainage moves dorsally and caudally to the superficial inguinal (mammary, supramammary) lymph nodes, which can be palpated by following the rear quarter dorsally until it ends and then palpating deep just above the gland along the lateral laminae. Although the prefemoral (subiliac) lymph nodes that are located in the aponeurosis of the external abdominal oblique muscle, approximately 15 cm dorsal to the patella, are not strictly drainage lymph nodes of the udder, they should be palpated as part of the routine physical examination of cattle. Because of their regional proximity and combined lymphatic drainage with the supramammary lymph nodes into the medial iliac lymph nodes, many cows with mastitis have obvious lymphadenopathy of the prefemoral lymph nodes, and they are easily palpable.

Udder Conditions

Premature Development

Premature symmetric development of the udder in calves and heifers has been associated with chronic estrogenic stimulation resulting from cystic ovaries, feedstuffs containing excessive estrogens, and the mycotoxin zearalenone. In some cases, udder development is accompanied by vulvar swelling. When the more common etiology of ingesting feed containing estrogenic substances has occurred, multiple heifers within a group are typically affected, and successful resolution of the mammary development requires removal of the contributing feed material. Idiopathic symmetric udder development in individual heifers is occasionally encountered when no obvious endocrinologic or intoxicant cause can be elucidated. Asymmetric gland enlargement in group-reared heifers should always raise suspicion of mastitis secondary to cross-sucking. Precocious mammary development may rarely occur in non-lactating cows secondary to ovarian, pituitary or placental disease.

Breakdown or Loss of Support Apparatus

Breakdown of either the lateral or the medial udder supports can occur. Medial laminae breakdown causes the medial longitudinal groove between the left and right halves of the udder to disappear and causes the teats to project laterally. Loss of lateral support laminae causes the halves of the udder to project ventrally to the level of the hocks, or lower. Occasionally, cows lose fore-udder support such that the forequarters appear detached from the ventral abdominal wall, and a hand may be inserted between the skin covering the glandular tissue and the ventral body wall. Similarly, loss of rear udder attachment tends to make the rear udder pendulous, without clearly defined udder attachment alongside obvious stretching of the skin in the escutcheon region. In the latter condition, the rear quarters no longer appear to curve up to the escutcheon but simply hang.

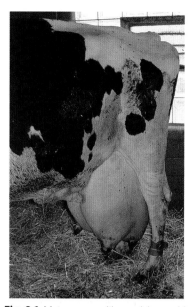

• **Fig. 8.1** Mature cow with pendulous udder.

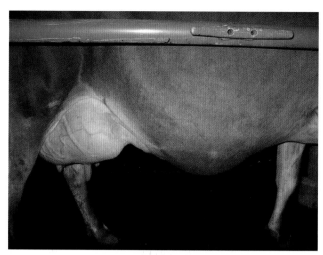

• **Fig. 8.2** Jersey cow with hematoma of both the right front quarter and milk vein following trauma (no injections were given). There was also hyphema in the right eye (not shown).

All of these various deficiencies in udder support predispose to udder edema, teat and udder injuries, and mastitis. Edema is worsened by the pendulous nature of the udder, reduced venous and lymphatic return, and trauma. Injuries to the teat and udder in cows with pendulous udders (Fig. 8.1) result from environmental trauma that includes contact of the udder with flooring when the cow is recumbent and direct damage from claws and dewclaws or from being stepped on by neighboring cows. Mastitis is predisposed to by environmental contamination of the teats and udder, teat injuries that affect milkout, and imperfect milkout caused by persistent edema in the floor of the udder. In some cows—especially those with severe loss of median support—it may not be possible to attach a milking machine claw simultaneously to seriously deviated teats. The result often is mastitis or culling because of milking difficulties. In addition, purebred cattle that are classified are discriminated against during classification scoring if these undesirable mammary characteristics are present.

The etiology of udder breakdown is complex and consists of genetic, nutritional, and management factors. Although udder breakdown is largely thought of as a problem in multiparous cows, in herds that approach an average of 25,000 lb per lactation, breakdown of the udder may occur at earlier ages. Udder breakdown may also be accelerated in show cows because the udder is allowed to become repeatedly enlarged.

No treatments exist for ligament ruptures. Prevention of the condition is also problematic because other than genetic selection and control, and prompt treatment of excessive parturient edema, little else can be done. Udder supports can be used in show cows that maintain a very full udder.

Hematomas

Etiology

Self-induced trauma as a result of awkward efforts to rise or lie down and external trauma from butting or kicking by other cows are theorized as the causes of udder hematomas, but injuries from these sources are seldom witnessed (Fig. 8.2). Caudal udder hematomas originating in the escutcheon region may represent thrombosis or rupture of the perineal vein because they tend to occur during the dry period. Udder hematomas, regardless of cause, are dangerous because blood accumulates subcutaneously and sometimes represent massive, even life-threatening, blood loss. In addition, the exact location of the bleeding often is impossible to determine clinically because of the extensive venous plexus and the rapid development of diffuse swelling. Surgical attempts at finding the bleeding vessel are often futile and may lead to further excessive blood loss and death. Mammary vein hematomas may occur due to vein injury during attempted administration of a drug (e.g., oxytocin) into the mammary vessel.

Signs

Soft tissue swellings immediately cranial to the udder are the most common signs in lactating dairy cattle (Fig. 8.3), but extreme swelling in the escutcheon region ventral to the vulva and dorsal to the rear quarters is more common in dry cows (Fig. 8.4). The swelling may be fluctuant, soft, or firm, depending on the amount of blood causing the distention; usually it is painless and cool. Rare instances of hematomas between the base of the udder and ventral body wall also have been encountered.

Progressive enlargement of the swelling coupled with worsening anemia signal a guarded prognosis for cattle affected with udder hematomas. Signs of anemia include pallor of the mucous membranes and teats (if nonpigmented skin), elevated heart and respiratory rates, and weakness. Cattle with udder hematomas that progressively enlarge may die over 2 to 7 days.

Diagnosis

Progressive fluctuant swelling adjacent to the udder coupled with progressive anemia and absence of fever usually is sufficient for diagnosis. Ultrasonography may be used to confirm

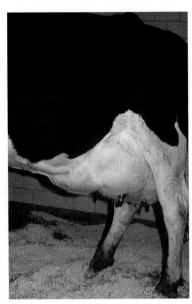

• **Fig. 8.3** Udder hematoma apparent as soft tissue swelling cranial to the udder. The hematoma also has infiltrated the medial laminae to pathologically separate the forequarters.

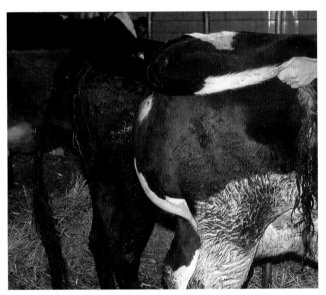

• **Fig. 8.4** Udder hematoma caudodorsal to the rear quarters in a dry cow.

the presence of a fluid-filled mass but does not always make a definitive diagnosis on its own. Ultrasonographic distinction between an abscess and a hematoma can be valuable because clinical experience suggests that aspiration of a hematoma, even under controlled and aseptic conditions, will frequently be associated with subsequent abscess formation. Ultrasonographic evidence of gas shadowing within an encapsulated mass should be taken as proof of an abscess, but mixed echogenicity images can be obtained with both abscesses and hematomas. Abscesses tend to be warm and painful and may cause fever in the affected cow. Seromas are unusual adjacent to the udder but would give similar signs of swelling. However, seromas usually do not enlarge

as much as a hematoma in this location, and progressive anemia would not be expected with a seroma.

In confusing cases, an aspirate under sterile conditions may be needed to differentiate a hematoma from an abscess or seroma. Clinicians should be reluctant to aspirate known hematomas for fear of introducing infection or disturbing pressure equilibrium that might allow further bleeding!

Treatment

For management of mammary gland hematomas, box stall rest and close monitoring of the animal at 12- to 24-hour intervals are important components of therapy. Complete blood counts (CBCs) and coagulation panels may be indicated to rule out bleeding disorders. Flunixin and other nonsteroidal antiinflammatory drugs (NSAIDs) should be withheld during the period of active hemorrhage.

In general, bleeding disorders of cattle are rare and are unlikely causes of udder hematomas. Occasionally, consumptive thrombocytopenia may occur in cows with udder hematomas. Cows that experience hemorrhage sufficient to reduce packed cell volumes (PCVs) to 10% to 12% and have a heart rate exceeding 100 beats/min and a respiratory rate in excess of 60 breaths/min require a whole-blood transfusion of 5 to 8 L. Platelet-rich whole blood from a healthy donor (negative for bovine leukemia virus [BLV], bovine viral diarrhea virus [BVDV], bluetongue virus, anaplasmosis, and Johne's disease) is important if anemia becomes severe.

Whereas stabilization in the size of the hematoma and other clinical signs are positive prognostic indicators, progressive anemia and enlargement of the hematoma despite therapy are negative indicators. Affected cows should be separated from herdmates to avoid further trauma. Incision of udder hematomas to arrest bleeding is unrewarding and may exacerbate hemorrhage; it is therefore contraindicated. Stabilized udder hematomas eventually resorb, but some may abscess and drain over the ensuing weeks because of pressure necrosis of overlying skin. When drainage occurs in the first few weeks large necrotic clots of blood and serosanguineous fluid drain from the area. Surgical debridement of naturally draining hematomas is not indicated except in chronic cases (>4 weeks) with abscessation, in which case ultrasound guidance should be considered. The condition does not recur after it has fully resolved. Udder asymmetry, abnormal teat deviation, and persistent residual edema are common sequelae to udder hematoma and abscess resolution, and although these are of limited economic impact in a grade cow, they may be a considerable frustration for the owners of show and pedigree cows.

Abscesses

Etiology

Udder abscesses may appear anywhere in the mammary tissue or adjacent to the glands. Frequently, skin puncture with subsequent abscessation is suspected when obvious abscesses appear in quarters having completely normal secretion and no evidence of mastitis. These may occur in "springing" heifers or mature cows without mastitis,

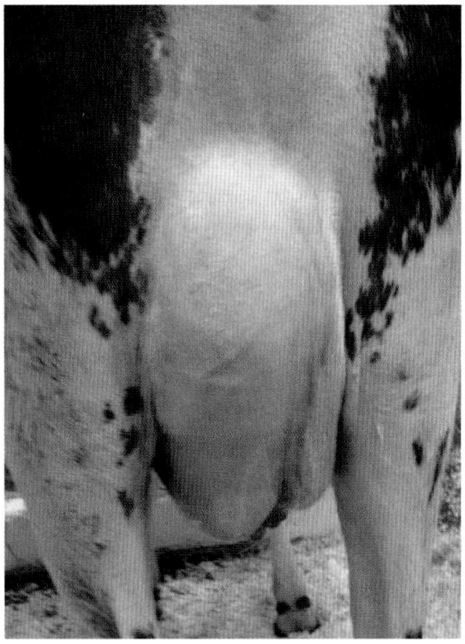

• **Fig. 8.5** Udder abscess with normal milk in a 3-year-old dry Ayrshire cow. *Fusobacterium* spp., *Prevotella* spp., and *Trueperella pyogenes* were cultured from the abscess, which was drained by incision. Interestingly, several cows in this geographic area had similar abscesses that summer.

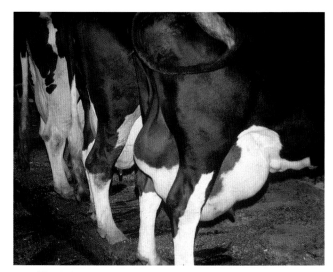

• **Fig. 8.6** Udder abscess associated with the left rear quarter.

and more than one heifer from the farm may be affected. Insect transmission has also been suspected but not proven (Fig. 8.5). Endogenous abscesses can form secondary to mastitis, as is typical of mastitis caused by *Trueperella pyogenes*. However, this discussion will be confined to udder abscesses requiring percutaneous drainage, and discussion of mastitis-origin abscesses will be addressed in the mastitis section.

Most udder abscesses harbor typical contaminants such as *T. pyogenes* or staphylococci, but occasionally other organisms such as *Fusobacterium* spp., *Prevotella* (previously *Bacteroides melaninogenicus*), and *Peptostreptococcus indolicus* may be involved.

Abscesses appear as firm, warm swellings that may be either distinct or indistinct from the gland parenchyma (Fig. 8.6). Palpation of the swelling may be painful to the affected cow. Milk from the affected quarter usually is normal, and the abscesses tend to be well encapsulated.

Diagnosis

Physical signs usually are sufficient for diagnosis, but ultrasonography or aspiration may be indicated if the owner is impatient regarding diagnosis and therapy. Ultrasonography may be beneficial to diagnosis and treatment of udder abscesses because flocculent material with or without gas shadowing may be observed, and major vessels overlying the lesion may be located if aspiration and drainage are necessary. A thick capsule around the abscess is usually observed.

Treatment

A conservative approach usually is rewarded by eventual natural rupture and drainage of the abscess in 2 to 8 weeks.

This has been standard treatment because practitioners understandably fear lancing anything in the udder because of the extensive blood supply to the entire organ. Conservative treatment probably still is the safest. The only risk from conservative therapy is the same as for neglected abscessation in other tissues—that is, chronic antigenic stimuli that may predispose to glomerulonephritis, amyloidosis, or bacteremia, which may cause endocarditis or other embolic sequelae.

Therefore the practitioner may be pressured by owners of valuable or show cattle to establish early drainage. Ultrasonography and aspiration are indicated before draining, as discussed previously.

After natural or surgical drainage, the abscess cavity should be flushed daily with dilute antiseptics or saline, and the drainage hole should be kept open, lest premature closure allow the abscess to re-form. Usually systemic antibiotic treatments are unnecessary.

Thrombophlebitis and Abscessation of the Milk Vein

Thrombophlebitis of the mammary vein is an occasional complication of venipuncture at this site (Fig. 8.7). This vessel seems attractive for the intravenous (IV) administration of pharmaceuticals, particularly in pit parlors and for producers for whom its size and accessibility make it a less challenging alternative compared with the jugular or coccygeal veins. However, the consequences of mammary thrombophlebitis with respect to udder symmetry and future production are sinister enough that it should never be used in show or valuable individual cows. It should only be used under considerable duress even in grade cattle. Abscesses may develop secondary to phlebitis from the use of contaminated needles or subsequent to hematoma formation when vascular damage and perivascular leakage occur as the cow resists the procedure. As with all cases of thrombophlebitis, there is a risk of embolic spread, potentially causing endocarditis or nephritis. If treatment is initiated immediately after the inciting attempt at venipuncture, then

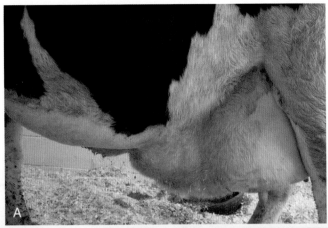

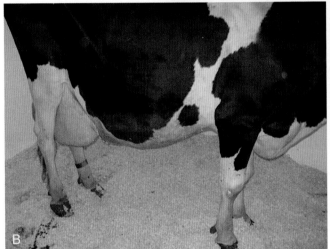

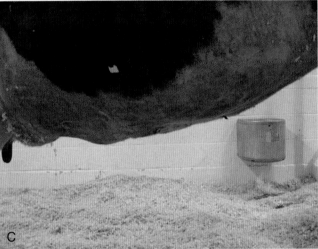

• **Fig. 8.7 A,** Mature Holstein cow with mammary thrombophlebitis subsequent to repeated oxytocin injection to facilitate milk letdown. Note edema cranial to forequarters. **B** and **C,** Mature Holstein cow with septic thrombophlebitis after calcium administration. *Trueperella pyogenes* and *Escherichia coli* were cultured from the vein.

antiinflammatory and antimicrobial therapy is indicated. However, veterinary attention is often only sought after abscessation has already occurred, at which time the goal of therapy should be surgical drainage followed by antimicrobial therapy. It can be challenging to avoid significant blood loss when lancing such abscesses because of the highly vascular nature of the region, and ideally, the procedure should be performed under ultrasound guidance. The bacterial species implicated include the common pyogenic anaerobes, and antimicrobial therapy should reflect this and include β-lactam antibiotics.

Udder Cleft Dermatitis

Etiology

Udder sores are foul-smelling areas of moist dermatitis that most commonly occur between the medial thigh and dorsal attachment of the lateral udder (historically most common in first-calf heifers), on the ventral midline immediately adjacent to the median septum of the foreudder, and on the median septum of the udder—either between the forequarters or in the fold that is centered between the four quarters. The predisposing and etiologic causes for the

disease are not proven. Periparturient udder edema, especially in first-calf heifers in warm months of the year, has historically been blamed, but recent studies suggest the disease is actually most frequent in high-producing dairy cows in the second or later lactations and that the disease is also common in mid to late lactation. Udder conformation (poor fore-quarter attachment), internal milk pressure, udder edema, or compromised local immune defense mechanisms may all be associated with the disease. Pressure necrosis associated with udder edema is enhanced by frictional injury and chafing with limb and udder movement. The abraded skin oozes serum, which, coupled with the omnipresent skin hair, leads to moist dermatitis and progression of the lesion. Finally, opportunistic anaerobic bacteria such as *Fusobacterium necrophorum* and *T. pyogenes* invade and propagate under crusts, scabs, and necrotic skin. These organisms cause the smell that distresses milkers each time they get close to the udder, hence the name "udder rot." Polymicrobial infections are common and include not only the forementioned organisms but also treponemes or even sarcoptic mites. The disease is not associated with mastitis or increased somatic cell counts (SCCs).

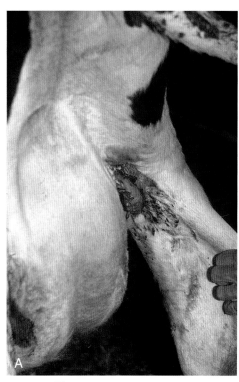
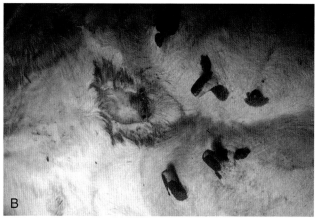

• **Fig. 8.8 A,** Necrotic udder sore in the right inguinal area of a first-calf heifer that had bilateral lesions. **B,** Necrotic udder sore between the forequarters of a cow positioned in dorsal recumbency in preparation for abomasopexy.

Signs

A fetid odor similar to that found in septic metritis or retained placenta emanates from areas of moist dermatitis in the groin area or more commonly the ventral median region of the udder. Skin necrosis may be mild or severe. In the worst cases, large patches of skin (10–30 cm in length) may be peeled off. Matted hair, scabs, and necrotic skin are present (see Fig. 8.8, *A* and *B*). Myiasis may occur in warm weather. In some first-calf heifers, groin infections can be so severe that obvious lameness may occur. Chronic lesions developing into cellulitis and abscessation have been reported to impinge on or invade the milk vein, with subsequent hematogenous spread to the lungs and heart.

Diagnosis

The combination of necrotizing fold dermatitis and malodorous discharge in a postpartum cow is sufficient for the diagnosis of udder cleft dermatitis.

Treatment

There is no evidence-based literature confirming that one particular treatment is more effective than another. For dairies that request therapy, a topically applied astringent such as Granulex Aerosol Spray, which contains castor oil, balsam Peru, and trypsin, or a disinfectant, would be recommended. Keeping the high-risk areas of the udder dry and clean, and early treatment of the disease are recommended. Treatment of udder edema in first-calf heifers may also be helpful in decreasing udder dermatitis. Although systemic β-lactam antibiotics are typically

effective against the organisms involved, their use is rarely justified due to practical economic concerns alongside the perception that the condition rarely if ever reduces appetite or milk production. If the inguinal lesions are causing severe lameness, surgical debridement can speed healing.

The prognosis in cases of udder cleft dermatitis is excellent, but healing time may be prolonged for months in untreated cases.

Udder Dermatitis

Etiology

Udder dermatitis may be associated with a multitude of chemical, physical, and microbiologic causes. Chemical causes of udder dermatitis include irritants in bedding such as hydrated lime, ammonia from urine, copper sulfate, or formaldehyde from foot baths. Physical causes of udder skin inflammation include sunburn, frostbite, and pressure necrosis caused by decubitus. Lesions of photosensitization may appear on the sun-exposed, nonpigmented skin of the teats and udder.

Staphylococci and streptococci occasionally cause a diffuse miliary folliculitis or pustular dermatitis named "udder impetigo." Rarely, *Dermatophilus congolensis* affects the skin of the udder, but this tends to occur as part of a severe generalized infection. Disseminated infections of *Trichophyton verrucosum* may affect the skin of the udder. Viral lesions of the skin of the udder include herpes mammillitis (see the discussion of teat skin infections), BVDV, bovine bluetongue virus infection, epizootic hemorrhagic disease, and malignant catarrhal fever (MCF).

Signs

Signs vary with specific etiology of the lesions. Chemical and physical teat skin dermatitis is characterized by extreme erythema, swelling, and evidence of pain. Vesicles may be present in severe cases associated with irritant chemicals. The skin of both the teats and the udder may be involved. Serum oozing and slight matting of the hair may be apparent.

Sunburned teat skin of dairy cattle has a similar appearance to that found in other species, and the cow may show evidence of sunburn in other locations. The affected skin is warm, painful, and may have vesicles or bullae caused by burns on nonhaired skin near the teat–udder junction. Multiple cows in the herd may show signs simultaneously and resent milking procedures because of painfully burned skin. Signs may be present on only one side of the udder if the cow preferentially lies on one side. Frostbite occurs during extreme winter cold, mostly in free-stall barns and mostly in periparturient cows with udder edema that already compromises tissue circulation. Patchy areas of skin on the teats and udder become cool, discolored, and swollen, and then turn leathery and completely cold. Frostbite must be differentiated from herpes mammillitis.

Other physical causes of udder dermatitis include photosensitization, which again would be apparent because of signs in other depigmented regions of skin and known exposure to sunshine.

Pressure necrosis or decubital sores from extended periods of recumbency occur mostly in cattle with very pendulous udders but may also occur in downer cattle or lame cows that lie down more than normal. Such sores often are located where the medial hock makes contact with the udder. Lesions initially are reddened, ooze serum, and then slough, leaving a necrotic crater-like lesion in the udder.

The clinical signs of infectious dermatitis vary with the causative agent. Staphylococcal dermatitis causes a diffuse folliculitis with small raised tufts of hair joined with dry or moist exudate. Pustules may be apparent in the worst cases. Usually only one or a few cows in the herd are affected, but occasionally, outbreaks of pustular dermatitis have been observed. *D. congolensis* may appear as larger confluent areas of folliculitis with dry or moist crusts that hold tufts of hair together. Plucking these tufts of hair or crusts may reveal purulent material on the underside of the crust or adjacent skin. Cows with dermatophilosis on the skin of the udder usually have other obvious *Dermatophilus* lesions elsewhere.

T. verrucosum lesions on the udder are circular or patchy alopecic areas that are 1.0 to 10.0 cm in diameter. Most lesions have crusts as observed in ringworm lesions in other locations, but some may appear as moist alopecic regions as a result of the paucity of hair in certain areas of the udder. Other ringworm lesions are usually identified during inspection of the cow. Herpes mammillitis lesions typically coexist on the skin of both the teats and udder. Recognition of bullae or vesicles in early cases is imperative to diagnosis.

Herpes mammillitis (bovine herpes virus 2 [BHV2]) most often occurs in first-calf heifers, and usually more than one animal is affected. Another herpesvirus, BHV4, the DN599 strain of BHV that has been isolated from the respiratory tract of cattle, may be capable of causing pustular mammary dermatitis. Multiple vesicles and pustules from 1.0 to 10.0 mm in diameter have been observed on the udder of lactating cows, and lesions have been observed in farm workers.

Treatment

Treatment for chemical dermatitis only requires gentle washing of the udder with warm water and removal of the offending agent from the cow's skin. Individual cows may be sensitive to a chemical despite the majority of cows in the herd being exposed to the same agent yet remaining unaffected. Warm water cleansing of the udder to remove residual chemical followed by application of aloe or lanolin products are recommended.

Physical causes of dermatitis are best treated by preventing further exposure to the specific physical cause and by symptomatic therapy. Sunburned cows must be kept inside or provided shade if at pasture. Cool water compresses followed by aloe or lanolin ointments to deter skin cracking and peeling caused by dryness are helpful. Udder supports may help prevent sunburn by covering vulnerable areas. Frostbite is best prevented by therapy for excessive udder edema and keeping periparturient cows well bedded for warmth. Periparturient cows in free stalls during extreme cold are at greatest risk because free-stall beds usually are poorly bedded for warmth. After frostbite has occurred, careful sharp debridement of necrotic tissue and protection against further injury are the only potentially effective treatments.

Pressure necrosis or decubital sores are treated by providing soft bedding for cows that spend more time in recumbency than normal and minimizing udder edema. Extremely pendulous udders are at greater risk for decubital sores. Treatment of decubital sores requires gentle cleansing and debridement following by the application of Granulex spray. Decubital sores may require weeks or months to heal.

Photosensitization must be treated by avoiding further sunlight, applying cleansing lesions, debriding necrotic skin, and determining the cause of photosensitization (primary or hepatopathic).

Microbiologic causes of udder skin dermatitis are managed according to the specific cause. Staphylococcal folliculitis is treated by clipping the hair on the udder, washing gently with povidone-iodine scrub solutions, rinsing with water, and drying. Washing and rinsing should be done once or twice daily. Antibiotics generally are not necessary. Filthy environmental contributing factors should be eliminated.

D. congolensis infections should be treated by clipping the hair of the udder followed by removal of all crusts through gentle washing with povidone-iodine scrubs and drying. In those with severe or generalized dermatophilosis, penicillin (22,000 U/kg body weight, once or twice daily, intramuscularly [IM]) may be necessary for 5 to 7 days in addition to local therapy.

Ringworm lesions can be managed by clipping the hair on the udder (especially if it is long or filthy) followed by topical application of chlorine bleach diluted 50:50 with water. Care should be taken such that antifungal medications, if used, do not contaminate milk during milking procedures or irritate healthy skin.

No specific treatment exists for udder lesions resulting from herpes mammillitis or other dermatopathic viruses.

Edema

Etiology

Udder edema, also known as "cake," may be physiologic or pathologic. Physiologic udder edema begins several weeks before calving and is more prominent in older first-calf heifers. Many questions remain unanswered regarding the etiology of udder edema. Genetic factors certainly exist, and bull stud services sometimes grade production sires by the probability of udder edema in their female offspring. Obesity, lack of exercise, and high-sodium and high-potassium diets may be risk factors. Individual cows with severe or pathologic edema should be examined to rule out medical considerations that could contribute to ventral or udder edema. Some conditions to consider include cardiac conditions, caudal vena caval thrombosis, mammary vein thrombosis, and hypoproteinemia resulting from any one of a number of diseases. Physical examination and serum chemistry screens may be helpful in the evaluation of such individuals.

Over bagging of show cows to gain a competitive edge is unfortunately common and can result in edema of the udder and discomfort to the cow. The ultrasound appearance of subcutaneous edema due to over bagging appears as alternating hyperechoic and hypoechoic parallel lines in the subcutaneous space and may be distinguishable from physiologic causes of edema. Over bagging of show cows should be discouraged.

Postparturient metritis has been associated with persistence of physiologic or pathologic udder edema by some owners and veterinarians. The pathophysiology of this relationship is unknown.

When many cows in a herd have either severe physiologic udder edema or pathologic udder edema, herd-based causes must be considered. Although feeding excessive grain to dry cows and early lactation cows has long been discussed as a cause of such endemic udder edema problems, feeding trials do not support this theory. Similarly, high-protein diets do not seem to be directly involved. Currently, excessive total dietary potassium and sodium are considered possible culprits in herdwide udder edema problems. Total intake of potassium may be excessive in some instances when high-quality alfalfa haylage constitutes a major portion of the ration. Forages harvested from land that is fertilized repeatedly with manure are becoming an increasing problem because of their high potassium content. One article recommends no more than 227 g/day/head of potassium in heifers. Similarly, sodium levels may be excessive when considering total available sodium in the basic ration, water, and mineral additives plus or minus free-choice salt.

Hypoproteinemia and especially low albumin fractions in affected cows also may contribute to udder edema. Metabolic profiles need to be performed to assess this possibility and determine the origin.

Signs

Physiologic udder edema may start in the rear udder, fore udder, left or right half of the udder, or symmetrically in

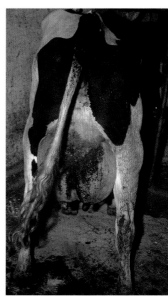

• **Fig. 8.9** Forced abduction of the hind limbs is obvious because of severe udder edema in this first-calf heifer.

all four quarters. Edema tends to be most prominent in the rear quarters and floor of the udder (Fig. 8.9). Cows with moderate to severe udder edema usually have a variable degree of ventral edema extending from the fore udder toward the brisket.

Udder edema pits and associated ventral edema may be soft and fluctuant or firm and pitting. Physiologic edema increases up to calving and then begins to gradually resolve over 2 to 4 weeks.

Pathologic edema persists longer than physiologic edema. Pathologic edema may be present for months after parturition or even for the entire lactation. The tendency for pathologic edema is increased in cows with breakdown of udder support structures, and conversely, pathologic udder edema may contribute to breakdown of udder support structures. Therefore severe edema may affect a cow's longevity and classification in some instances.

Pronounced udder edema interferes with complete milkout because it causes the affected cow discomfort, and milking may accentuate that discomfort. In addition, interstitial edema in the mammary glands may cause pressure differentials that interfere with normal production and letdown of milk. Therefore chronic or pathologic edema may have a negative effect on the lactation potential because cattle never reach their projected production. Interference with complete milkout resulting from pain, as well as mechanical or pressure influences, also may lead to postmilking leakage of milk in cows with severe udder edema. This translates into an increased risk of mastitis.

Cows with udder edema do not act ill but may be uncomfortable or painful because of the swollen, edematous udder swinging as they move or from the udder constantly being irritated by limb movement as they walk. Severe udder edema may also increase the risk of udder cleft dermatitis, a common cause of further discomfort if lesions occur between the udder and hind legs. When resting, the cow may tend to lie in lateral recumbency with the hind limbs extended to reduce body pressure on the udder.

Diagnosis

The diagnosis is based on inspection, palpation, evaluation of milk secretions to rule out mastitis, and ruling out conditions such as udder abscess or hematoma. Pitting edema should be present, especially on the floor of the udder. Pitting edema may also be evident over the entire udder in severe cases, and ventral edema frequently coexists in these instances.

Treatment

Treatment of preparturient or postparturient individuals is indicated when edema has the potential to break down the udder support structure. Treatment also is indicated for preparturient cows having severe udder edema associated with leakage of milk from one or more teats.

Diuretics constitute the principal treatment for udder edema. Preparturient treatment of cattle with furosemide (0.5–1.0 mg/kg body weight) as an initial treatment followed by decreasing dosages once or twice daily for 2 to 4 days is commonly used. Salt restriction should also be considered. Premilking may be indicated in preparturient cows with severe udder edema that are leaking milk. This must be an individual decision based on the owner's experience with premilking. Obviously, if the option of premilking is selected, the newborn calf will require colostrum from another cow. Although premilking is controversial, some owners of show cattle swear by the technique to preserve udder conformation. Udder supports also may be helpful if fitted properly. A word of warning about furosemide: Urinary losses of calcium may be sufficient to increase the risk of periparturient hypocalcemia, and this should be anticipated in multiparous cows receiving multiple doses of the drug!

Parturient and postparturient cows judged to need treatment for udder edema may receive either furosemide or dexamethasone–diuretic combinations orally. Individual cows may respond to one product better than the other, but this is impossible to predict. Furosemide seems to work well in some herds, but the dexamethasone–diuretic combination is superior in others. When considering dexamethasone–diuretic combinations, the veterinarian should first rule out contraindications to corticosteroid use (dexamethasone containing preparations should not be used in late pregnancy for example for fear of inducing labor). Udder supports and salt restriction may or may not be practical but should be considered. Nursing procedures, including udder massage, hot compresses, more frequent milking, and mild exercise, are helpful but labor intensive. Metritis should be ruled out or treated.

In herds with endemic udder edema, nutritional consultations are imperative to evaluate anion–cation balance. Total sodium and potassium amount in the feed and serum chemistry values in affected and nonaffected cows should also be analyzed. Diets with anionic salt supplementation and those with added antioxidants may show some tendency to diminish udder edema in affected herds. Access to water and availability of free-choice salt or salt–mineral combinations should be included in the nutritional evaluation.

Hemorrhage into a Gland

Etiology

Hemorrhage into one or more glands is common at parturition in cows with severe udder edema or pendulous udders that have been traumatized by hind limb movement and awkward posture during recumbency. Milk from one or more quarters contains blood and may appear as pink, red, or reddish-brown with blood clots. Generally, this condition clears within four to eight milkings and is not a major problem. Cows with bloody milk should be watched closely for mastitis because blood provides an excellent growth medium for bacteria.

As opposed to the usually innocuous parturient hemorrhage described previously, severe hemorrhage involving one or more quarters occasionally is observed in dairy cattle during lactation. The cause is unknown, but nonspecific trauma usually is suspected. It is also occasionally encountered in show cattle that have been "overbagged". Thrombocytopenia has been confirmed in some but not all of these cows, and when it is identified, it is not known whether it represents cause or effect.

Signs

The chief complaint for a cow with intramammary hemorrhage is persistent blood-stained milk from one or more quarters. Anemia may develop if extensive bleeding continues to occur over several milkings. The milk usually is red rather than pink, and blood clots are obvious. Large intraluminal clots occasionally plug the papillary duct, causing difficulty in milkout.

Diagnosis

The clinical signs of intramammary hemorrhage are sufficiently diagnostic, but laboratory work should be performed to assess thrombocyte numbers and the severity of anemia. Coagulation profiles that may be used to incriminate specific bleeding disorders in other species are frequently unreliable in cattle. Specific causes of intramammary hemorrhage are seldom identified. Intramammary hemorrhage may increase the risk for mastitis.

Treatment

Decisions regarding appropriate therapy are difficult because of the likelihood of iatrogenic complications. An apparently obvious solution is to stop milking the affected quarters, thereby stopping further blood loss and allowing pressure to build up in the gland to deter further bleeding. However, this approach may provoke such severe blood clotting in the ductules, gland cistern, and teat cistern that future milking is impossible. On the other hand, once- or twice-a-day milking usually allows blood clots to be stripped out but causes more blood loss and may allow continued bleeding from whatever vessel is leaking. Generally speaking, reduction of milking frequency (usually to once daily) has been considered to be the optimal management for intramammary hemorrhage. Blood clots that form may be stripped out and hence will not ruin future milking potential. If this

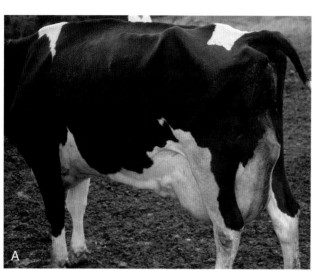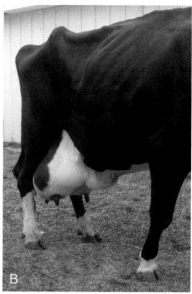

• **Fig. 8.10 A,** A mature Holstein cow affected with lymphosarcoma. The right supramammary lymph node is markedly enlarged and appears as a firm swelling in the dorsal aspect of the right rear mammary gland. The cow also had diffuse infiltration of the mammary gland as well as cardiac neoplasia. **B,** A 14-year-old Holstein cow with mammary gland adenocarcinoma. There was diffuse neoplastic involvement of the gland. Courtesy of R.H. Whitlock.

approach does not resolve the problem within several days, a decision to stop milking and risk severe cisternal clots must be considered to save the cow.

Thrombocytopenia and other coagulation defects should be excluded as causes of the hemorrhage. When thrombocytopenia or severe anemia (PCV <10%) exists, an immediate fresh whole-blood transfusion from a donor that is uninfected by BLV, BVDV, bluetongue virus, anaplasmosis, and Johne's disease should be administered. Approximately 4 to 6 L of blood should be transfused at a single time.

Mammary Tumors

Except for fibropapillomas (warts), mammary tumors in dairy cattle are rare. Lymphosarcoma is by far the most common neoplasm affecting the udder. Relatively few dairy cows live to an old age, but those that do still have a very low incidence of mammary tumors. Both squamous cell carcinomas and mammary gland adenocarcinomas have been observed in older dairy cattle (>15 years). Fibropapillomas are more common on the skin of the teats but also may appear on the skin of the udder. Many other sporadic tumors, including fibromas, fibrosarcomas, and papillary adenomas, have been reported. One case of mammary gland adenocarcinoma occurred in an aged nonlactating rumen donor cow whose clinical signs included anorexia and acute (equine-like) laminitis with extreme reluctance to move.

Lymphosarcoma is the most common tumor to appear within the gland and associated lymph nodes in dairy cattle (Fig. 8.10, *A*). Focal and diffuse infiltration of the gland with lymphosarcoma have been observed. Diffuse involvement of the gland has also been seen with mammary adenocarcinoma (Fig. 8.10, *B*). The mammary gland is hardly ever the only site of lymphosarcoma infiltration, however. Usually tumor masses in other target organs or lymph nodes supersede mammary involvement. Affected glands may merely appear edematous rather than firm, and secretions may appear normal. Diffuse lymphocytic infiltration of the udder may appear similar to the diffuse mild edema that develops in hypoproteinemic cattle. The mammary lymph nodes (superficial inguinal) may be enlarged because of lymphosarcoma or chronic inflammation and should routinely be palpated during physical examination.

Juvenile tumors of the mammary gland have been observed in two heifers referred to our clinic. Surgical extirpation of these masses was performed before udder development. Juvenile tumors found to be fibromas associated with the teat also have been recognized in two yearling heifers.

Signs

Cows affected by mammary lymphosarcoma have a varied clinical presentation ranging from focal to diffuse and massive udder enlargement. Some squamous cell carcinomas are ulcerated, firm, and pink with a malodorous smell. Precursor papilloma or epithelioma masses may have been observed by the owner. Fibropapillomas are obvious, wartlike in appearance, and are of little concern.

Juvenile tumors of the gland cause an obvious enlargement that may be confused with mastitis in the undeveloped udder.

Diagnosis

Biopsy or aspirate of a suspicious mass is essential for diagnosis. Biopsy of the gland may be performed if diffuse

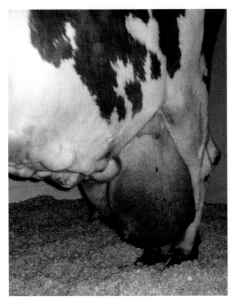

• **Fig. 8.11** Red and White Holstein cow with a severely "dropped" udder that subsequently underwent successful amputation.

lymphosarcoma is suspected, and ultrasound guidance is suggested for more focal masses without cutaneous involvement. Commercial Tru-Cut biopsy needles work very well for mammary gland biopsies, and the procedure is safe.

Treatment

Juvenile tumors of the gland may be excised, but the prognosis for production in the affected gland must be guarded. However, in the two juvenile gland tumors observed by Dr. Rebhun and in the two reported teat skin fibromas in yearlings, long-term follow-up evaluation indicated that all glands that had undergone surgery were functional at first calving. Squamous cell carcinomas may be treated according to their severity. Cryosurgery may suffice in early stages of the disease, but udder amputation may be required in advanced cases. Treatment for lymphosarcoma is rarely undertaken and generally of limited success.

Udder Amputation

Hemimastectomy or radical mastectomy is rarely performed in cattle. Indications for this in valuable or pet cattle are neoplasia, chronic incurable mastitis or persistent precocious udder, and suspensory apparatus failure that causes the udder to sag and become persistently traumatized (Fig. 8.11). Individual animals that undergo udder amputation must be in good general condition. Significant blood loss can occur with udder amputation because of the vascularity of the mammary gland. Cattle with septic mastitis or in poor physical condition should not undergo udder amputation until their physical condition is significantly improved.

The cow must be placed in dorsal recumbency and preferably under general anesthesia. A fusiform skin incision is made to facilitate subsequent skin closure. Therefore the lateral incisions must extend to the junction between the middle and dorsal thirds of the udder to allow sufficient skin for closure under minimal tension. After skin incision, the dissection is first directed toward the inguinal canal, where the pudendal arteries and then veins are ligated. The procedure is repeated on the contralateral side. Using curved Mayo scissors, the loose fascia on the proximal aspect of both lateral laminae is incised starting cranially and extending caudally until the left and right perineal arteries and veins are located and double ligated. To minimize systemic blood loss (through retention in the amputated mammary gland), the caudal superficial epigastric veins are ligated last. The lateral laminae are then sharply transected, and the dissection is extended on the dorsal aspect of the mammary gland to complete the excision.

Before closure, one should attempt to control the extent of postoperative seroma formation by placing two 2.5-cm Penrose drains in the space between the ventral abdominal fascia and the subcutaneous tissues on either side of the midline along the ventral abdomen. Stab incisions are used to create portals for the drains to exit on either side of the incision and they are secured to the skin, using a single interrupted suture to avoid accidental drain removal.

Closure is performed in three layers. The subcutaneous tissue is closed in two layers using no. 2 absorbable suture material (such as poliglecaprone 25 or polyglactin 910) in a simple continuous pattern. Every 2 or 3 cm, the subcutaneous sutures should penetrate the abdominal fascia to reduce dead space. The skin is closed in a forward interlocking pattern with a non-absorbable material (e.g., polyamide), and a stent is sutured over the incision to help diminish tension.

Teat Disease

The tissue layers in the teats of dairy cattle include skin, an inner fibrous layer, stroma, and mucosa. The stroma is a vascular and muscular layer containing veins that drain to the large subcutaneous venous plexus at the juncture of teat and udder. The inner fibrous layer is a thin membrane that is interposed between the mucosa and the stroma (Fig. 8.12).

The papillary duct (teat canal) or streak canal is the exit for milk from the teat sinus or cistern and is surrounded by the teat sphincter muscle. The papillary duct and sphincter muscle represent a significant component of the defense mechanism against mastitis, and they are the most frequently injured portions of the teat.

The streak canal in the healthy state acts both as a valvular obstruction to milk flow and as a unique deterrent to ascending infection of the gland. The canal is lined with keratin as a result of a specialized stratified squamous epithelium arranged longitudinally. Keratin in the papillary duct binds bacteria and then desquamates to form a plug with antimicrobial activities that may deter bacterial entrance.

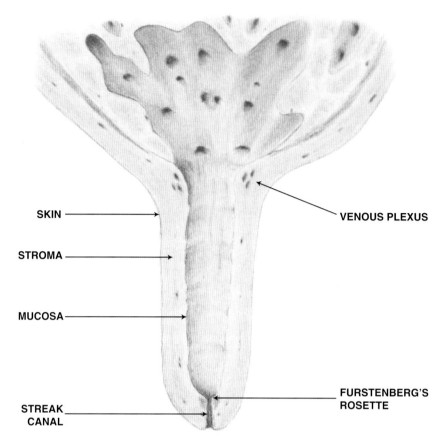

SKIN

STROMA

MUCOSA

STREAK
CANAL

VENOUS PLEXUS

FURSTENBERG'S
ROSETTE

• **Fig. 8.12** Schematic of the bovine teat to illustrate the basic anatomic terms used in this chapter. Image courtesy of Dr. Laurie Peek.

Congenital Anomalies

Etiology and Signs

Supernumerary teats are the most common congenital abnormality and the condition is likely heritable in dairy cattle. There has been little genetic selection away from this trait in heifers simply because it is not reported back to artificial insemination stud services and because the problem is so easily treated. Supernumerary teats are extremely common in certain lines of cattle, especially Guernseys. Usually one to four extra teats are observed, although more can occur. Generally, the supernumerary teats are located caudal to the rear quarter teats or between the rear and forequarter teats. These "extra" teats require removal, lest functional glands evolve that would likely become infected because they cannot be milked effectively. Such infections provide a chronic source of mastitis organisms for other quarters in the herd.

Supernumerary teats that are joined to one of the four major teats have been called webbed or "Siamese" teats. These may appear as distinctly separate teats or only as small raised areas on the wall of one of the major teats (Fig. 8.13). These teats frequently have a separate gland of their own, although they may communicate with the teat or gland cistern of the major teat (Fig. 8.14). In either case, these joined teats require special treatment and careful differentiation from simple supernumerary teats, lest future production of the gland be compromised.

Keratinized corns or keratomas on the teats of heifers have been recognized. These structures are tightly adherent to the teat end and as they progressively enlarge their physical weight stretches and elongates the affected teat (Fig. 8.15).

Juvenile tumors of the skin adjacent to the teats of two heifers have been described and were found to be a fibroma and a fibrosarcoma.

Diagnosis

The diagnosis of supernumerary teats, webbed teats, and keratinized corns simply requires inspection. Supernumerary teats conjoined to a major teat require more careful consideration and treatment, but if identified in calfhood, the treatment is the same. Tumors associated with the teat require biopsy to allow definitive diagnosis.

Treatment

Heifer calves should be examined for the presence of supernumerary teats at a routine time during the first 8 months of life. Most veterinarians perform this examination when vaccinating 4- to 8-month-old calves for brucellosis. After restraint of the heifer, the supernumerary teats are grasped and cut off with scissors at the point where the skin of the

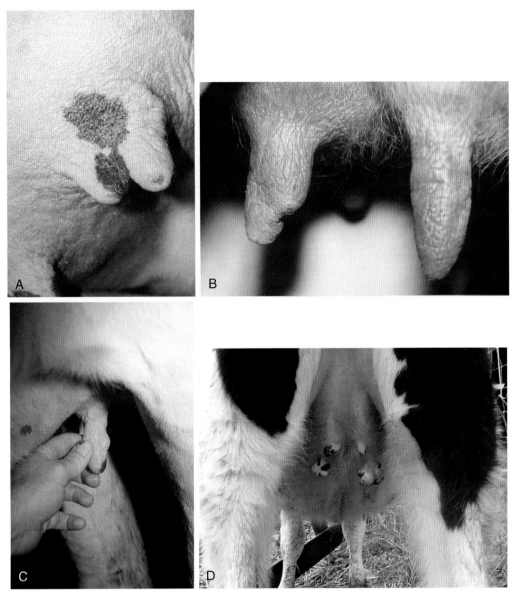

• **Fig. 8.13** **A,** Webbed teats may appear as a distinct teat. **B,** An enlarged proximal portion of teat. **C,** Only as a small tissue mass on a normal-sized teat. **D,** Or as clusters.

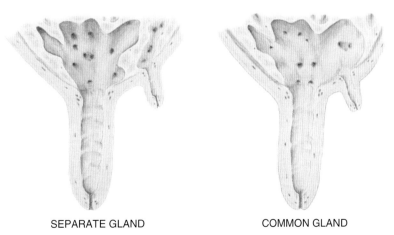

SEPARATE GLAND   COMMON GLAND

• **Fig. 8.14** Conjoined supernumerary teats may communicate with a separate gland or the gland of the major teat. Image courtesy of Dr. Laurie Peek.

teat meets the skin of the udder. A suitable antiseptic is applied to the wound after removal, but sutures generally are not used except when a cosmetic appearance is required immediately. Care must be exercised when removing supernumerary teats, lest a true teat be removed accidentally.

If confusion exists as to which teats are the primary ones, the heifer should be allowed to grow for a few months and then be rechecked. It is important, however, to force owners to check for supernumerary teats when the heifers are young so that surgical removal is easier for both the animal and the veterinarian. Removing supernumerary teats on a 2-year-old heifer that is already springing can be difficult and unpleasant for all involved parties.

Supernumerary teats conjoined to a major teat (webbed teats) need to be repaired surgically rather than just snipped off. The repair should be performed when the teat is large enough to be manipulated easily and then sutured. Many

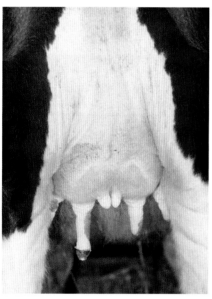

• **Fig. 8.15** Keratin corn on the left hind teat of a heifer. Note two caudal supernumerary teats are also present.

surgeons prefer to operate on animals at approximately 8 months of age. Aseptic technique is essential because infection of the future mammary gland may be a major risk. After an 8- to 12-hour fast, the heifer is sedated with xylazine (4-5 mg/100 lb body weight IV), tied in dorsal recumbency, and the hair is clipped from the udder near the extra teat. After routine preparation, a fenestrated drape is placed, and the supernumerary teat is excised by scalpel or scissors. This excision is nearly flush with the skin of the main teat but should leave enough skin to close the wound (Fig. 8.16). After excision, the mucosa of the rudimentary teat should be closed with 3-0 or 4-0 fine synthetic absorbable suture (e.g., Monocryl; Ethicon, Johnson & Johnson, Somerville, NJ). The skin and stroma are sutured as a single layer using interrupted vertical mattress sutures or alternatively closed with individual layers. Many suture materials are suitable for stroma and skin closure, but absorbable sutures such as 3-0 or 4-0 Vicryl (Ethicon) or Monocryl are popular because they do not require subsequent removal and associated restraint. Antibiotics such as IM penicillin (22,000 U/kg once daily) should be administered preoperatively and for 2 to 3 days postoperatively.

When surgery is done at this early age, it does not matter whether the ancillary teat has a separate gland. If, however, surgery is delayed until after the first parturition, surgical repairs may become considerably more complicated because of the need to connect separate gland cisterns to the major teat (see *Farm Animal Surgery,* Fubini and Ducharme, 2nd edition).

Keratin corns or keratomas may be surgically dissected from the teat ends, but simpler means of therapy exist. A light teat bandage held on the teat by adhesive tape may be used to moisten the keratinized material, and the keratinized material may be gently separated from the teat itself after several days of soaking. Saline, lanolin and aloe mixtures, and ichthammol ointment have all been used successfully to soften keratin corns and allow subsequent removal.

Successful removal of tumors associated with the teat has been described. Future production was not destroyed in

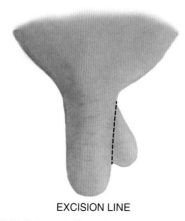
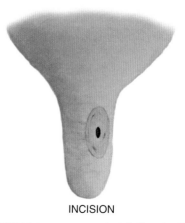

EXCISION LINE   INCISION

• **Fig. 8.16** Schematic illustration of excision line for conjoined supernumerary teat (*left*) and outline of a resultant incision (*right*). The *inner circle* in the incision represents mucosa, and the *outer circle* indicates skin. Image courtesy of Dr. Laurie Peek.

these animals; nonetheless, a guarded prognosis is justified in such cases.

Teat-End Injuries

Etiology

Teat ends are the most common site of mammary injury in dairy cattle and such injuries are the most common reason for owners to seek veterinary consultation regarding the teats of dairy cattle. Teat-end injuries may affect the sphincter muscle, the streak canal, or both. Injuries to the teat end are most often caused by the digit or medial dewclaw of the ipsilateral limb of the affected cow or by injury from neighboring cows stepping on the teat. Teat-end injuries are more common in cows with pendulous udders or in older individuals whose support laminae have lost some degree of integrity. Acute injuries cause inflammation, hemorrhage, and edema within the distal teat stroma and sphincter muscle. Subsequent soft tissue swelling in the teat end mechanically interferes with proper milk release from the streak canal. In addition, the streak canal epithelium and keratin may be disrupted, crushed, lacerated, partially inverted into the teat cistern, or partially everted from the teat end. Occasionally, distal membranous obstruction occurs as a result of teat injuries followed by local fibrosis (Fig. 8.17). Obvious laceration of the distal teat skin may be present concurrently but frequently is not. When present, lacerations also tend to be at the teat end. Degloving injuries to the teat end are also occasionally encountered subsequent to claw or limb trauma when the teat becomes trapped against solid flooring. Repeated or chronic teat-end injury leads to fibrosis of the affected tissues, granulation tissue at the site of any mucosal or streak canal injury, and continued problems with milkout. Subclinical teat-end injury has been associated with defective milking machine functions such as increased vacuum pressures or overmilking.

In addition to traumatic injuries, teat-end ulceration is a common problem that may involve individual cows or be endemic in certain herds. Crater-like ulcers filled with dried exudate and scabs make milkout very difficult and predispose to mastitis. Many causes, including irritation from teat dips, excessive vacuum pressure, and mechanical abrasions, have been suggested, but the exact cause of the lesion often is difficult to ascertain.

Signs

Painful soft tissue swelling of the distal teat is the cardinal sign of acute teat-end injury. The skin may be hyperemic or bruised (Fig. 8.18). The cow resents any handling or manipulation of the teat end and objects to being milked. A combination of mechanical interference with milkout and pain-induced reluctance to let down milk predisposes to incomplete milkout from affected quarters. Mastitis is the feared and frequent sequela to incomplete milkout in cows with teat-end injuries. The cow is further predisposed to mastitis if the physical defense mechanism of the streak canal is compromised.

Chronic teat-end lesions often include a history of acute injury followed by continued difficulty in milking. Palpation of the teat end allows detection of fibrosis in the sphincter muscle or granulation tissue dorsal to the streak canal and sphincter muscle at the ventral-most portion of the teat cistern. Pain is not as apparent with chronic teat-end injuries as in acute cases.

Treatment

Treatment of acute teat-end injuries should address both the injury and any management factors that might lead to further injury, such as overcrowding, lack of bedding, and milking machine problems.

Treatment considerations must be acceptable and logical to the milkers because they are responsible for any ongoing therapies. Milkers also are subject to the consequences of the cow's pain caused by manipulation of the acutely

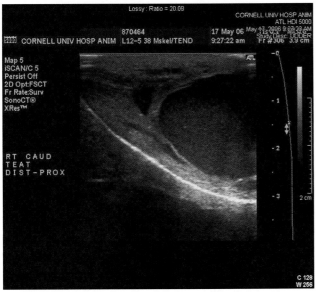

• **Fig. 8.17** Sonogram of the distal aspect of the teat made with a linear 12.5 MHz probe (distal is to the left). A focal occlusion at the distal aspect of the teat cistern is identified as a 3-mm band of tissue. The rosette of Furstenberg and the streak canal (thin hyperechoic line at the tip of the teat) are normal. Courtesy of Dr. Amy Yeager, Cornell University.

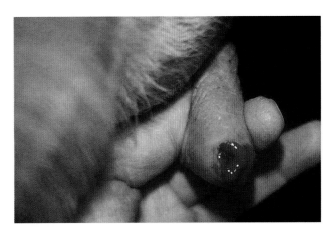

• **Fig. 8.18** Acute teat-end injury showing diffuse swelling and a blood clot extruding from the streak canal.

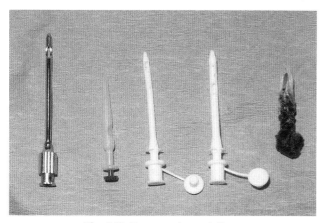

• **Fig. 8.19** Teat cannulas and dilators.

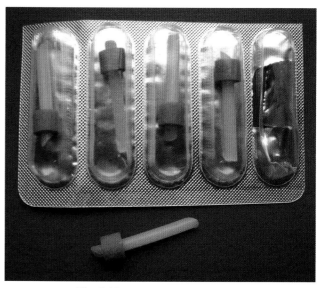

• **Fig. 8.20** NIT natural wax teat inserts.

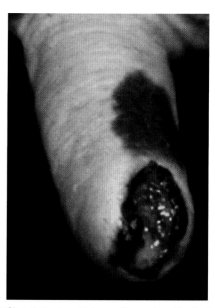

• **Fig. 8.21** Chronic teat-end injury with an ulcerative bed of granulation tissue ringed by crusted edges. This type of wound repeatedly produces a crusty scab that interferes with effective milkout and is an extremely common sequela to acute teat-end injuries.

injured teat. Unless one has milked cows, it may not be apparent exactly how difficult it is to remain patient when being kicked at by cattle that object to having their injured teats handled. Client compliance necessitates empathy for the patient, as well as the people responsible for milking the cow. Advice regarding patient restraint, minimizing pain, and preventing mastitis must be included in any treatment regimen.

The best treatments for acute teat-end injury include symptomatic antiinflammatory therapy and reducing further trauma to the teat end. Each injury must be assessed individually. If milkout is simply reduced but not prevented, milkers sometimes use dilators of various types between milkings to stretch the sphincter muscles, thus allowing machine milkout. If milkout is difficult, or prevented, it is best to avoid further machine milking and to use a teat cannula to effect milking twice daily while the other quarters are being machine milked. If cannulas are used, the milker must exert extreme care to avoid exogenous inoculation of the teat cistern with microbes. Therefore the teat end must be cleaned gently, and alcohol must be applied before introducing the sterile cannula. Usually a disposable 1-in plastic cannula is used for this purpose. After complete milkout, the teat end is dipped as usual and a repeat dip performed in 10 minutes. Alternatively, we recommend indwelling SIMPL silicone or NIT (natural teat insert) wax implants that seal the teat between milkings. In addition, several types of plastic or metal cannulas (Fig. 8.19) are available commercially which may be capped between milkings. In addition to facilitating milkout, these indwelling cannulas act as dilators that may reduce the possibility of streak canal adhesions or fibrosis. Teat dilators impregnated with dyes are not favored because they seem to induce chemical damage to the streak canal. However, many owners use such dilators anyway. Wax and silicone teat inserts may retain patency with less risk of iatrogenic mastitis. The wax insert is recommended for initial use, but it disintegrates after several days. Insertion of silicone teat inserts after the wax (NIT) has disintegrated is recommended. The NIT and silicone teat inserts have comparable efficacy and antibacterial properties. Both inserts are readily available in the United States. Alternatively, milk

can be drained from the gland, intramammary antibiotics infused, and a wax teat insert (Fig. 8.20) placed in the teat followed by icing and bandaging the teat with no further milkout for 2 to 3 days.

Nursing care is helpful but unfortunately is often not readily available on modern dairy farms. Soaking the injured teat with concentrated Epsom salts in a cup of warm water for 5 minutes twice daily helps reduce edema and inflammation. It is most important to avoid further trauma to the teat end and to minimize the risk of developing mastitis. Therefore avoidance of machine milking is indicated for at least several days whenever possible.

Problems associated with teat-end lesions include crusts, necrosis, chronic ulceration (Fig. 8.21), and mastitis. All result in continued pain to the patient and mechanical interference with milkout as a result of scab or exudate buildup. Gentle soaking in warm dilute Betadine solution (Purdue Pharma, Cranbury, NJ) followed by removal of crusts or exudate aids complete milkout. Teat injury predisposes the cow to mastitis, particularly infections with gram-positive organisms.

Gradual return to normal milking is hoped for in 3 to 7 days after acute teat-end injury. Subacute or chronic injuries that continue to interfere with milkout may necessitate surgical intervention. Surgery should be avoided in acute teat-end injury because any sharp injury to an already damaged sphincter muscle and streak canal only serves to worsen the acute inflammation and hemorrhage, as well as the ensuing fibrosis. If milk flow is still obstructed after edema has resolved, examination should determine the site of the injury and the location of the obstructing fibrosis or granulation tissue. Granulation tissue at the most dorsal aspect of the streak canal or most ventral part of the teat cistern is common. Fibrosis of the sphincter musculature also is very common. Instrument manipulation or sharp surgery on the teat end is then indicated. Wax or silicone inserts should be used to decrease stricture post-instrumentation.

Before surgical intervention, the quarter should be full of milk. Experienced owners will not milk out the affected quarter before the veterinary visit, but if they have forgotten, the cow should be given 20 units of oxytocin IV to fill the quarters. Without adequate milk in the quarter, it is impossible to assess how much the obstruction has been relieved.

For surgical correction of obstructed teat ends, the teat should be washed, cleaned, and disinfected with alcohol (Box 8.1). The cow should be restrained or sedated (or both) before surgery. A teat bistoury or knife, preferably one with a small single cutting edge and blunt tip, should be used. The aim of this procedure is to relieve the stricture in the streak canal through two to four angled cuts made at 90-degree intervals (Fig. 8.22). The cuts are made into the dorsal sphincter muscle but tapered so as not to cut the distal sphincter or teat end. We prefer the use of a Larsen teat blade because it allows for better control of the depth of the cut and facilitates the creation of a tapered incision. These radial incisions release the sphincter and frequently are the only treatments required. Some veterinarians use wax inserts to reduce hemorrhage after this procedure and to diminish subsequent inflammation and swelling that may impede milkout.

A Moore's teat dilator also has been used for relief of sphincter muscle fibrosis. This instrument is inserted into the teat after routine preparation and advanced slowly to stretch the sphincter muscle without sharp surgery.

Masses of granulation tissue in the streak canal can act as an obstruction between the canal and teat cistern. They are generally a result of injury to the rosette of Furstenberg. These masses or growths are generally removed with the aid of a Hug's teat tumor extractor. This instrument can be opened to allow excessive tissue to be grasped and cut off by the sharp edge of the extractor. It is a commonly used teat instrument, but care should be taken not to excise healthy mucosa when removing granulation or fibrous tissue from the streak canal. The collateral mucosal damage associated

---

• BOX 8.1 Preparation for Teat Surgery or Treatment

Infusion of Quarter or Placement of Cannula

Wash and completely clean teat and base of udder with mild soap or disinfectant.
Dry.
Alcohol swab teat end carefully.
Treat or cannulate with sterile devices.
Alcohol swab teat end carefully.
Apply teat dip used by owner.

Surgical Manipulation Through the Teat Canal

Restrain or sedate the cow.
Wash and completely clean teat and base of udder with soap or disinfectant.
Dry or alcohol swab until dry.
Ring block base of teat if prolonged manipulation anticipated.
Alcohol swab teat end carefully.
Perform procedure with sterile, cold-sterilized or disinfected instruments.
Alcohol swab and teat dip (unless the owner is to strip quarter frequently).

Surgical Thelotomy or Repair of Full-Thickness Lacerations and Fistulae

Decide on position (standing, tilt table, dorsal recumbency), means of restraint, and required sedation.
Aseptic technique, including clipping hair on udder, surgical preparation, ring block of base of teat, and fenestrated drapes are indicated.
Use sterile instruments.
Administer preoperative and postoperative antibiotics.

---

with the blind use of the teat tumor extractor frequently results in recurrence of the stenosis. To precisely remove diseased tissue and leave adjacent healthy tissue undisturbed, thelotomy with sharp incision is indicated (see teat-cistern obstructions). Minimally invasive fiberoptic theloscopy in combination with electrosurgery is preferable, but the equipment is expensive, although it leads to improved long-term outcomes. The equipment is available from the Karl Storz Company (Charlton, MA).

Occasional instances of prolapsed streak canal mucosa are observed after crushing teat-end injuries. This tissue should be cut off flush with the teat end and then gently probed with a teat cannula to replace any everted tissue back into position within the streak canal.

Most veterinarians initially are too cautious and conservative when treating teat-end fibrosis. Experience is necessary to know "how much to cut" to allow not only short-term results but also to avoid the need for subsequent reoperation because of recurrence of the problem. However, if in doubt, it is best to be conservative because the procedure always can be repeated. Most experienced veterinarians not only want to see a reduced resistance to hand milkout but also a slight dripping of milk immediately postoperatively. This dripping usually subsides as sphincter tone improves after resolution of dilatation associated with surgical instrumentation.

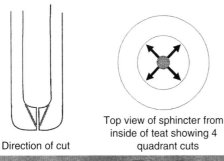

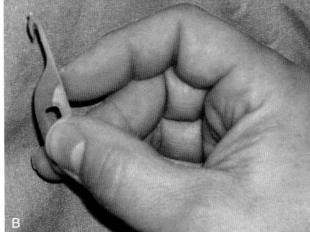

• **Fig. 8.22** **A,** Schematic illustration of teat knife incisions required to relieve sphincter muscle fibrosis. **B,** Preferred teat bistoury for radial cut for treatment of streak canal fibrosis. Note that the cutting edge is in the acute angle and thus allows control of the depth of the incision. In addition, if the operator flexes his or her wrist while pulling distally, only the proximal half of the streak canal will be incised.

Repeated self-induced teat-end trauma to a specific teat dictates evaluation for known causes. Foot-induced trauma may be detected by smearing dye on the medial dewclaw and observing the teats for dye transmission onto the teat. In such cases, removal of the medial dewclaw may help prevent injury in the future. Cows with pendulous udders that sustain repeated teat-end injuries usually have to be culled.

Teat-end necrosis or ulceration is difficult to manage because buildup of scab material in the crater-like ulcer recurrently interferes with milking. Gentle soaking and mechanical removal of the scabs are necessary for milkout. A mild teat dip with glycerin or lanolin for softening is indicated in these patients. Some require surgical manipulation if continued irritation or overmilking damages the sphincter muscle or dorsal streak canal. When teat-end necrosis is observed in more than one cow in a herd, the milking machinery and procedures should be examined carefully to rule out excessive vacuum pressure. The possibility of physical or chemical irritants in teat dip or bedding should also be investigated in such cases (Fig. 8.23).

Acquired Teat-Cistern Obstructions
Etiology
Teat-cistern lesions resulting in obstructed milk flow may be focal or diffuse. Most teat-cistern obstructions result from proliferative granulation tissue, mucosal injury, or fibrosis,

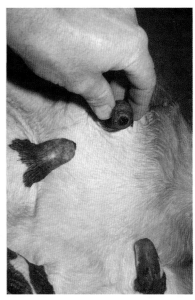

• **Fig. 8.23** Chronic proliferative teat-end lesions caused by excessive vacuum pressure or overmilking. Such lesions are hyperkeratotic or proliferative and circular, and tend to be present in more than one quarter in each affected cow. The problem usually appears in multiple cows within the herd.

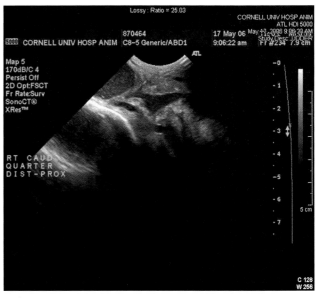

• **Fig. 8.24** Sonogram of the junction of the teat and gland cistern made with a convex 8.5 MHz probe (distal is to the left). At this location, the lumen abruptly narrows from 2 cm to 3 mm because the wall of the teat is thick and irregular. Also, a 3-mm thick band of tissue occludes the lumen of the teat cistern. Courtesy of Dr. Amy Yeager, Cornell University.

all secondary to previous teat trauma. Occasional cases have no history of previous acute injury. Both focal and diffuse lesions in the cistern cause an increasing degree of restriction to flow that interferes with effective milk delivery to the streak canal during machine milking. With ultrasound examination, obstruction at the junction of the gland and teat cistern can be identified (Figs. 8.24 and 8.25). This type of obstruction leads to slow refill of the teat cistern such that the affected gland cannot be milked by machine. However, it can be milked by teat cannula or siphon. In addition

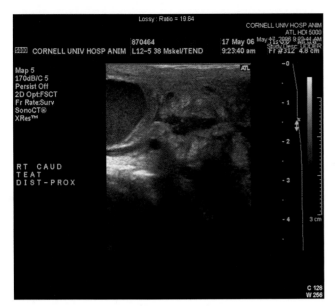

• **Fig. 8.25** Sonogram of the junction of the teat and gland cistern made with a linear 12.5 MHz probe (distal is to the left). The high-resolution image demonstrates the 7-mm-thick, irregular, hyperechoic scar tissue in the wall of the very narrow region of the cistern. Also, a 3-mm-thick band of tissue occludes the teat cistern. Courtesy of Dr. Amy Yeager, Cornell University.

to fixed lesions, floating objects known as "milk stones" or "floaters" may cause problems in milkout because they are pulled into the teat and mechanically interfere with milking by obstructing the proximal aspect of the streak canal. These floaters may be completely free or may be attached to the mucosa by a pedunculated stalk. Mucosal detachments are also sometimes encountered secondary to external teat trauma. The detached mucosa folds onto the opposite teat wall, creating a valve effect as milking progresses. Submucosal hemorrhage or edema from previous trauma is thought to cause the detached mucosa; however, the problem may not become apparent until resolution of the submucosal fluid allows the detached mucosa to become mobile within the cistern.

"Pencil" obstructions are usually caused by adhesions secondary to mural and mucosal trauma that may ultimately obliterate either part of, or the entire, teat cistern. The lesions may be mucosal adhesions or, more often, granulation tissue bridging areas of mucosal tissue that adheres itself to the opposite wall of the lumen. Pencil obstructions may follow diffuse teat injury that causes the entire teat to be swollen, with severe stromal edema and hemorrhage. Palpation of pencil obstructions reveals a longitudinal (vertical) firm mass that appears to obstruct the teat cistern. The most severe lesions will also involve fibrosis of the gland cistern (Fig. 8.26).

Signs

Depending on the individual lesion, teat-cistern obstructions cause partial, intermittent, or complete interference with milk flow during hand and machine milking. Focal lesions tend to cause partial or intermittent milk flow disturbance because of the valve effect they create. Similarly,

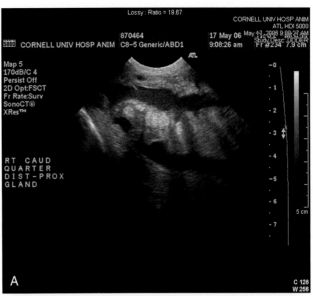

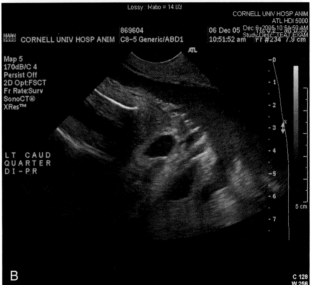

• **Fig. 8.26** A, Sonogram of the distal aspect of the gland cistern made with a convex 9.5 MHz probe (distal is to the left). The gland cistern is diffusely narrow (1 cm in diameter) because the wall is thick as a result of soft tissue swelling (fibrous tissue or edema). The gland cistern is the hypoechoic lumen located in the near field; the anechoic lumen in the far field is a normal vein. B, For comparison, sonogram of the distal aspect of a normal gland cistern made with a convex 9.5 MHz probe (distal is to the left). Teat (0.7 cm in diameter) and gland (2.5 cm in diameter) cisterns are normal. Courtesy of Dr. Amy Yeager, Cornell University.

floaters may lead to intermittent cessation of milk flow. If the floater is completely free, it will only cause obstruction after sufficient milkout allows the floater to enter the teat cistern from the gland cistern. Floaters occur primarily in recently fresh cows from the release of sterile fibrous or granulomatous masses and concretions that had resided in mammary ductules. However, floaters or milk stones occasionally may develop in cows further advanced into lactation. Palpation of the teat and hand milking to determine the degree of obstruction are necessary for diagnosis. These conditions usually are not painful to the patient unless they have been caused by recent trauma.

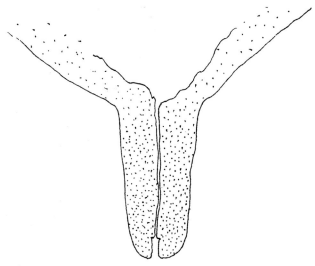

• **Fig. 8.27** Schematic illustration of acute, diffuse teat swelling. Notice that the stroma is diffusely infiltrated, and sharp instrument manipulation of the teat lumen therefore is contraindicated.

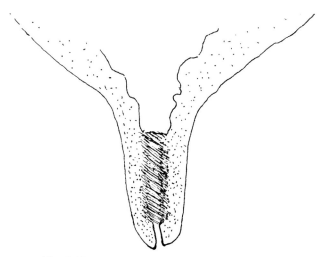

• **Fig. 8.28** Schematic illustration of a pencil obstruction.

Focal detachment of mucosa after injury leads to intermittent or gradual obstruction as milking progresses. Palpation of the detached mucosa can be appreciated best during hand milking when the mucosa is felt to "slip" between the fingers and thumb as milk is expressed from the teat. This sensation is similar to that felt while slipping fetal membranes for pregnancy diagnosis.

Diffuse teat swelling from recent injury may collapse the teat cistern such that the teat feels turgid and swollen, and is painful to the cow (Fig. 8.27). No distinct mass can be felt in the teat cistern, and passage of a 2- to 3-in stainless steel teat cannula allows milk to be obtained from the gland cistern.

Pencil obstructions are palpated as firm longitudinal masses in the teat cistern. They may fill part of, or the entire, teat cistern (Fig. 8.28). Sometimes the lesion extends into the gland cistern. Milk flow is severely altered, and passage of a teat cannula may be met with resistance as the cannula grates against granulation or fibrous tissue. Passage of

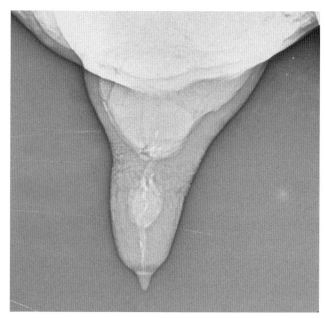

• **Fig. 8.29** Positive contrast study showing a distinct obstructive lesion within the teat cistern. Courtesy of Dr. Norm G. Ducharme.

the teat cannula has a similar feel to passing an insemination pipette through a cervix. Pencil obstructions may occur after known trauma, overly aggressive surgical approaches to focal obstruction, or after injury or infection during the dry period.

Diagnosis

In the past, the diagnosis was reached by history, palpation, and probing with teat cannulas. Current methods for evaluating teat obstructions include ultrasonography, radiographs, xeroradiographs, and contrast radiographic studies. Radiographic contrast studies can be obtained by injecting 10 mL of an iodine-based radiopaque material into the teat and gland cistern and then radiographing the teat and ventral gland cistern (Fig. 8.29). In our experience, ultrasound examination is the most practical diagnostic aid for evaluation of patency of the teats and gland cistern (see Video Clips 8.1 and 8.2). It is best performed before milking because the absence of milk in the teat cistern will cause an apposition of the mucosal lining, giving the false appearance of stenosis (see Video Clips 8.3 to 8.5). The ultrasound examination can be facilitated by placing a water-filled cup over the teat and examining through the wall of the cup. Teat and gland cistern obstruction can be readily identified because the normal luminal appearance is compromised. One has to be careful not to cause deformation of the teat and gland cistern with pressure from the probe; therefore the teat should be examined with minimal pressure. A complete examination is performed by utilizing both transverse and longitudinal imaging.

Treatment

Each cow with teat-cistern obstruction must be evaluated individually for treatment options. Conservative therapies such as drying the quarter off or continued milking with a teat cannula are possibilities for any cisternal obstruction that prevents machine milking. However, the loss of production associated with drying off such quarters and the likelihood that the obstruction will still be present in the next lactation may not make drying off an attractive option to the owner. Continued milking with a cannula may be an alternative to maintain productivity and allow further time for healing in acute or subacute cisternal obstructions. The negative side of continued cannula use is the risk of mastitis. Cows with focal or diffuse cisternal obstructions that are near the end of lactation should be dried off to rest the injured area and then examined after 4 weeks to evaluate whether the lesion is better, worse, or unchanged.

Treatment for focal cisternal obstruction may be provided by either open or closed teat surgery. If closed surgery is chosen, the veterinarian must be careful that instrument manipulations do not worsen the condition through excessive damage to the teat mucosa adjacent to the lesion. Overly aggressive instrumentation with teat knives or Hug's tumor extractors can destroy healthy mucosa and result in more granulation tissue, further fibrosis, and membranous adhesions. Well-demarcated fibrous cisternal teat obstructions are the best candidates for closed surgical removal using a tumor extractor or bistoury. Acute or subacute focal cisternal obstructions should not be approached by closed teat manipulation. Surgery (performed via thelotomy or when possible theloscopy) has the following major advantages; it allows a view of the lesion; more exacting dissection of the lesion is possible; and mucosal defects can be closed or oversewn with healthy mucosa. Open thelotomy is performed as follows: The cow is sedated and placed in dorsal (preferable) or lateral recumbency. Local anesthetic is applied at the base of the teat (ring block). After aseptic preparation of the teat, a metal cannula is inserted through the streak canal into the teat cistern. Using a #15 or #10 Parker-Kerr blade, a skin incision is made on the side of the teat opposite the lesion (in show cows, the incision is placed medially). The incision is started proximally on the teat cistern but distal to the base of the teat because one wants to avoid the highly vascular annular venous plexus. The incision then is extended distally but stops proximal to the streak canal. It is *critical* that the incision does not extend into the streak canal or proximally into the annular venous plexus at the base of the teat. The incision is extended into the teat cistern, and the obstruction is addressed. The detached mucosa is reattached by suturing to the adjacent mucosa, the granulation tissue is removed and the adjacent mucosa sutured to cover the defect, or the granulation tissue is removed and an implant placed to prevent recurrence of granulation tissue. Closure is obtained by reapposing the mucosa of the teat cistern using a simple continuous pattern (penetrating the mucosa) using 4-0 absorbable monofilament suture. If only a larger-size suture is available, the submucosa is reapposed using a continuous Cushing pattern (it is important with a suture larger than 4-0 that the mucosa is not penetrated). The stromal tissue is reapposed using a 0-0 absorbable suture, again

using a simple continuous pattern. The skin is closed with a monofilament suture using a simple interrupted pattern.

With thelotomy as described, although the risk is small, there is a potential for teat fistula formation if wound repair fails. In addition, a lack of confidence and experience in open-teat surgery may discourage the practitioner. Both open and closed surgery techniques also predispose to infection of the quarter.

Currently, open thelotomy performed by an experienced surgeon offers the best chance for correction of focal cisternal obstructions and prevention of recurrence. This is because open thelotomy permits surgical resolution of the mucosal defect after removal of focal lesions, including those that cannot be fully bridged with mucosa.

Theloscopy is most helpful for teat cistern lesions. The procedure is best performed with the cow restrained in lateral or dorsal recumbency. After local anesthesia is applied at the base of the teat and extra anesthetic has been injected through the streak canal into the teat cistern, a Penrose drain is applied at the most proximal aspect of the teat cistern. A 4-mm arthroscope is inserted through a stab incision in the lateral wall and the teat examined under CO_2 insufflation (further details can be found in the section by Dr. Steiner in *Farm Animal Surgery*, 2nd edition, Fubini and Ducharme).

Floaters can be removed by slowly and patiently dilating the streak canal and sphincter muscle with a small pair of mosquito or straight forceps. Usually this takes 5 to 8 minutes. Before dilating the streak canal, the quarter is hand milked until the floater enters the teat cistern and can be held there. After the sphincter muscle stretches sufficiently to allow entrance of the forceps, the floater may be grasped and removed through the streak canal. Many times, the floater can be "milked out" without any manipulations inside the teat cistern after the sphincter muscle has been stretched adequately. The veterinarian may open the jaws of the hemostat to stretch the streak canal while exerting firm milking pressure to the dorsal teat cistern to cause a jet of milk to eject the floater. Alternatively, if the floater is in the streak canal, it can be forced out by slowly rolling two smooth syringe cases down the teat. Regardless of the technique used, after removal, the teat should be iced for 20 minutes at least three times on the day of the procedure and appropriate antiinflammatory therapy administered depending on the degree of suspected trauma. After removal, the quarter should be treated prophylactically with antibiotics or watched carefully for signs of mastitis. The streak canal and sphincter typically return to normal function 24 to 48 hours after being dilated.

Mucosal detachments or tears that impede milkout are best treated by drying the quarter off or by open thelotomy. Closed-teat instrumentation may increase mucosal injury in the cistern or lead to granulation tissue in areas of mucosal detachment. Open surgery allows the mucosa to be repaired and "tacked down" to the underlying stroma in areas of detachment. If an open approach is used, after the teat incision is performed, the tissue underneath the mucosa is debrided, and the mucosa is then brought back into its original site. Detached mucosa is then sutured to the adjacent secured mucosa using 4-0 monofilament absorbable suture using a simple continuous pattern.

Diffuse swelling of the teat associated with recent injury should be managed medically. Severe edema, hemorrhage, and inflammation within the stromal tissues cause the cistern to be swollen shut. There may or may not be associated mucosal injury. Surgery or instrument manipulation is contraindicated, lest the mucosa be further damaged. Epsom salt soaks and lanolin or aloe ointments to protect the teat should be used immediately. If a stainless steel teat cannula passes easily through the teat cistern to the gland cistern, it can be used to allow twice-daily milkout. If a cannula cannot be passed easily, the quarter should be dried off or consideration given to eventual open surgery and implant placement.

Diffuse pencil obstruction of the cistern is best treated by open surgery and implantation of silicone or polyethylene tubes unless the owner elects to dry off the quarter. Closed manipulation or surgery with sharp instruments is contraindicated and will only worsen existing damage. Much has been learned about diffuse teat-cistern obstructions because open-teat surgery has been more widely used. The ability to see the gross pathology and obstruction within the cistern has been a great education and has encouraged veterinarians to devise new surgical techniques. Although the prognosis for diffuse teat-cistern obstructions (pencil obstructions) remains guarded, many successes have been recorded thanks to specific surgical intervention either with or without implants. An implant technique initially reported by Donawick has been modified by Ducharme. This technique uses thelotomy to identify gross pathology, permit surgical removal of the obstructing tissue in the teat cistern (with or without application of a mucosal graft), and implantation of a Silastic tube into the teat cistern before surgical closure of the wound. Sterile Silastic silicone medical tubing with an inside diameter of 7 mm and an outer diameter of 10 mm is measured during thelotomy and placed into the teat cistern. The distal end of the tube abuts against the distal end of the teat cistern, and the proximal end of the tube is fenestrated and lies flush with the junction of the gland cistern (Fig. 8.30). Two to three polypropylene nonabsorbable 2-0 sutures are placed parallel to the long axis of the teat to secure the tubing to the teat stroma. It is important to anchor the tubing well and yet to take care not to distort or malposition the tubing while placing the anchoring sutures. This is done by placing the securing sutures with a teat cannula placed through the streak canal into the tubing, serving as a rigid implant and thus maintaining proper alignment. After standard closure of the teat and removal of the cannula, machine milking is instituted. If this is unsuccessful, the cow may temporarily require a teat cannula for milking or flushing with sterile saline to free blood clots from the implant. Occasional cows require the use of wide-bore milk liners to effect milkout because of the increased thickness or diameter of the teat.

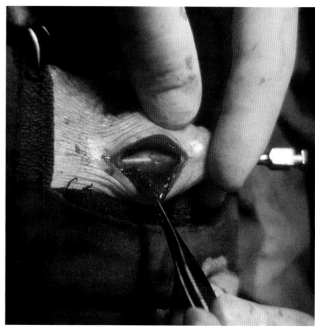

• **Fig. 8.30** Sterile Silastic silicone tubing implant being placed in a teat having a pencil obstruction. Courtesy of Dr. Norm G. Ducharme.

The tubing is left in place permanently unless it loosens or breaks away from the teat cistern. Complications may include an increased incidence of mastitis, lower long-term milking success, and abnormal milking times compared with teats undergoing thelotomy without implants. However, despite the risks of complication, this technique currently is the best hope for preservation of teat function in cattle with diffuse cisternal obstructions. Before the introduction of these techniques, most diffuse cisternal obstructions resulted in permanent drying off or in a hopeless prognosis for the affected quarter. With careful case selection, 50% or more of diffuse cisternal obstructions may be helped by implants and allow completion of the lactation. Implant techniques are unlikely to help cows with combined diffuse teat-cistern obstructions and gland cistern obstruction or fibrosis. In addition, and importantly, implant techniques are contraindicated if mastitis has already complicated the teat injury.

Fistulas

Etiology

Teat fistulas may be congenital or acquired secondary to full-thickness teat injuries that enter the teat cistern. Congenital teat fistulas are a smaller variant of webbed or Siamese teats and often are not detected until lactation begins (Fig. 8.31). Congenital teat fistulas may communicate with the teat cistern of the major teat but usually represent outflow from a separate gland.

Acquired teat fistulas may occur after accidental full-thickness wounds, lacerations, or surgical thelotomy and always communicate with the teat cistern of the major gland. Ineffectual closure or healing leading to breakdown of the mucosal layer is thought to cause most fistulas in surgically repaired teat injuries.

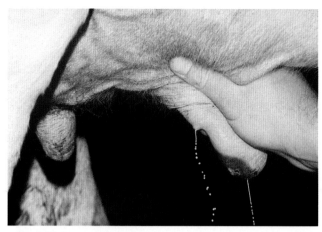

• **Fig. 8.31** Congenital teat fistula that was not apparent until lactation started. Milking causes milk to escape from both the fistula and the streak canal.

Leakage of milk from fistulas predisposes the gland to infection. Even when the fistula represents a separate gland, infection is undesirable because the major quarter may be exposed to contagious organisms by leakage of mastitic milk from the fistula. In addition, leakage of milk from acquired fistulas is likely to unbalance the udder and be unsightly for show cattle. Depending on the location of the fistula on the teat, machine milking may or may not provide effective milkout.

Signs

Congenital fistulas usually are not observed in calves but become apparent in bred heifers or after freshening when milk is noticed to leak from the wall of the teat. A small raised area of skin may be present around the fistula, but this skin usually is less prominent than that observed in a webbed teat. Acquired teat fistulas have a history of teat injury or surgery penetrating into the teat cistern followed by leakage of milk from the scar or incision. Acquired teat fistulas have obvious scar tissue around the fistula and often are larger in diameter than congenital fistulas.

Diagnosis

The diagnosis is obvious based on clinical signs. Ultrasound examination allows determination of the direction and extent of the fistula, the presence of associated damage, and whether one or two glands are present. If ultrasonography is not available, dye injected into the fistula followed by milkout of the major teat or contrast radiography may be indicated to determine whether one or two glands are present. New methylene blue (10–30 mL) may be used for dye injection into the fistula. Milking of the major teat then allows differentiation of fistulas (or webbed teats) that have their own accessory gland (no dye in milk) or have a common gland with the major teat (dye in milk).

Treatment

Surgical repair of fistulas is identical to repair of webbed or Siamese teats. When webbed teats are repaired in calves,

determining the presence of an accessory gland is impractical and unnecessary because complete closure will ensure eventual pressure atrophy of the accessory gland. Congenital fistulas that attach to accessory glands rather than to the gland of the major teat but are not detected until the onset of lactation may be managed in two ways:

1. Surgical repair (see Fig. 8.16) as performed in calves and a nonmilking gland. This approach relies on pressure atrophy of the accessory gland for resolution. This technique is best performed during the dry period to allow 4 full weeks of healing before the next lactation. This technique may also result in some unbalancing of the udder as the accessory gland atrophies. This may make the affected quarter somewhat slack.

2. Surgical repair through thelotomy. The common wall between the two glands is removed, and the mucosa of each gland is sutured over the defect, again using 4-0 absorbable suture. This allows a communication to be established between the teat cistern of the major teat and the cistern of the fistula. This technique is only recommended if the fistula is discovered after calving and initiation of lactation. The advantages of this technique are preservation of milk production from the accessory gland (which may be almost as large as the "major" gland in some cattle) and the cosmetic appearance of the quarter. The disadvantages are that greater technical skills are required to establish communication between the cisterns and to suture mucosa to preserve the communication. In addition, if the common wall mucosal suturing fails, there is a chance of obstructive granulation tissue forming.

The technique for repair of fistulas is well accepted and involves a fusiform incision around the fistula, debridement of necrotic or fibrous tissue (in acquired fistulas), dissection of the mucosal layer, exacting closure of the mucosal defect, and routine teat closure as described under closure of a thelotomy. Teat cannulas are used as guides to allow accurate incision and dissection of the fistula (Fig. 8.32). Acquired fistulas with severe cicatricial fibrosis are more challenging because tissue compliance and healing are negatively influenced. This is especially problematic in fistulas that are very distal in the teat cistern near the teat sphincter. The size of the fusiform incision should be sufficient to allow removal of the fistula and associated fibrous tissue but not so large as to interfere with ease of closure. Previous dogma suggested that the best time for repair of teat fistulas was during the dry period. This allowed several weeks for tissue repair without concern of endogenous milk pressure or exogenous milking pressure being applied to the incision. More recent reports seem unconcerned about this advantage; if repair is done during lactation, the most important feature is to use small suture (4-0) to close the mucosa in a simple continuous pattern as described later. It may still be preferable to perform closure during the dry period after the udder is completely slack and the cow still has 3 to 4 weeks to go before freshening.

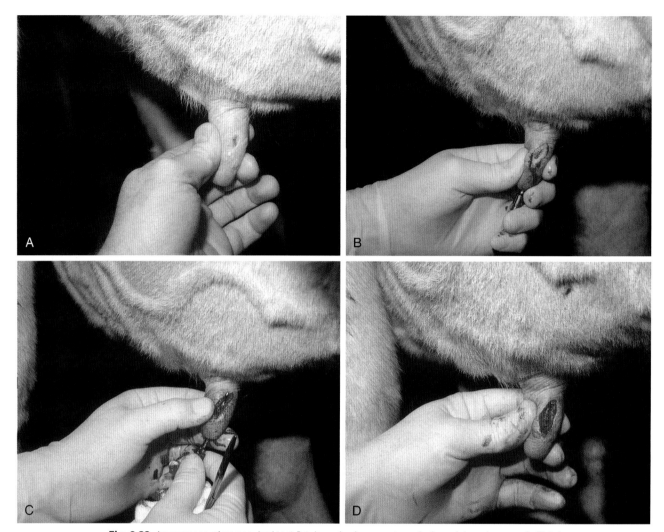

• **Fig. 8.32** Appearance of an acquired teat fistula and subsequent surgical repair in a dry cow. **A,** Fistula surrounded by fibrotic cicatricial tissue. **B,** Fusiform skin incision. **C,** Teat cannula protruding from mucosal defect after en bloc resection of an elliptical skin piece and the fistula tract. **D,** Mucosal closure with continuous absorbable suture.

Fine 4-0 absorbable suture material (3-0 if performed during the dry period) placed in a simple continuous pattern is preferred for mucosal closure. Surgeon preference dictates selection of suture material and pattern for stromal and skin closure. Generally, 3-0 polyglactin 910 or other absorbable material such as Monocryl is used for the stroma in an interrupted fashion, and interrupted 2-0 or 3-0 nonabsorbable sutures such as polypropylene are used in the skin. Some surgeons close the stroma and skin in one layer with interrupted 2-0 or 3-0 nonabsorbable sutures in a vertical mattress fashion. Sutures are placed closer together than in other areas of skin closure in the hope of achieving a more uniform closure pressure. Although not successful in our hands, some surgeons have used tissue adhesives for fistula closure and full-thickness teat lacerations. Skin staples or Michel wound clips also have been used, mainly for skin repair. If fistulas are repaired during lactation, it may be wise to use indwelling teat cannulas that are left open to prevent endogenous pressure on the incision until healing is complete; however, the use of these should be balanced by legitimate concerns for introducing intramammary pathogens. If inserted, indwelling milk tubes should be changed daily, or alternatively, silicone (SIMPL) or wax (NIT) inserts may be used. Wax inserts deteriorate after several days and can be replaced by silicone inserts. Both insert types are commercially available in the United States. The inserts have been shown to improve surgical results in lactating cattle.

Lacerations

Etiology

Trauma from the patient's hind foot or medial dewclaw, trauma by a neighboring cow, or lacerations from barbed wire or other sharp objects may cause teat lacerations. Lacerations may involve skin only, skin and stroma, or enter the teat cistern after mucosal laceration. All lacerations are problematic because of mechanical interference with teat cup placement, milkout, and pain to the patient. Associated

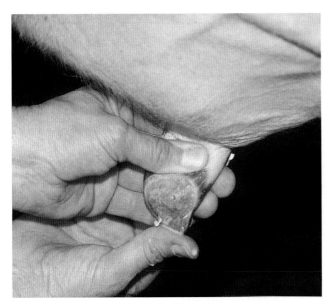

• **Fig. 8.33** Degloving injury.

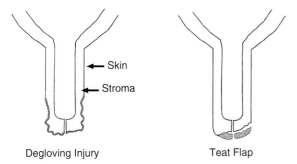

• **Fig. 8.34** Schematic illustration of degloving and teat flap lacerations.

mucosal damage, avulsion, or detachment may lead to focal or diffuse cisternal obstruction. Full-thickness lacerations are considered emergencies and require repair of all layers to avoid mastitis or fistula formation.

Degloving injuries peel away a circumferential section of skin on the distal teat (Fig. 8.33). Teat flaps are created by incomplete removal of skin on the teat. Although flaps of skin may be created by any horizontal laceration of the teat, the term *teat flap* usually is reserved for a lesion that extends through skin, stroma, and a portion of the sphincter muscle (Fig. 8.34). The streak canal is often transected, but a portion of the streak canal and sphincter remains proximal to the laceration and suffices for sphincter tone, barring future injury.

Lacerations may be vertical, horizontal, or circumferential. The depth of laceration and duration of time since injury are important determinants when surgical repair is being considered. The more acute the injury, the more likely surgery will be successful, and the less likely infection has already occurred within the wound and/or quarter.

Signs

These are obvious in most cases of teat laceration. The injured teat is swollen and bleeding, and the cow resents any handling of it. Regardless of depth, teat lacerations may cause sufficient swelling to interfere mechanically with teat

cup placement, cause pain during milking, lead to incomplete milkout, and predispose to mastitis. Full-thickness lacerations may be obvious because of milk leakage but sometimes are plugged with fibrin and blood clots that mask the extent of the lesion. Teat flaps often appear to have milk leaking out of the teat cistern (Fig. 8.35, *A*). In fact, the distal flap of tissue is so swollen as to suggest laceration above the sphincter. Fortunately, close examination of the wound often reveals functional streak canal and sphincter muscle above (dorsal to) the swollen flap.

Diagnosis

The clinical signs followed by careful cleansing of the wound to allow detailed evaluation of depth suffice for diagnosis. The cow may need to be restrained or sedated to allow cleansing and inspection of the wound.

Treatment

Owners neglect many superficial teat lacerations but tend to call veterinarians when the lacerations enter the cistern or cause mechanical interference with milking. Similar to lacerations anywhere on the body, teat lacerations are best approached as soon after injury as possible. Repair of teat lacerations involving only skin and stroma may be performed with sutures, wound clips, or cyanoacrylate products. Before repair (see Box 8.1), careful cleansing of the wound is essential, and gentle debridement with a #15 scalpel blade is helpful. In general, vertical lacerations heal better than horizontal or circumferential ones. Flaps that transect the streak canal should be clipped off with scissors because repair of the transected streak canal is impossible (Fig. 8.35, *B* and *C*).

Full-thickness lacerations that enter the cistern are sutured similarly to the repair of teat fistulas described previously. All principles are identical to repair of a surgical wound into the cistern, but in the words of Dr. Bruce Hull, professor of large animal surgery at the Ohio State University, "The wound is made with a manure-laden foot rather than a sterile scalpel." This statement helps explain the frustration and failures that frequently follow full-thickness repairs. Small details make large differences. Careful debridement, aseptic technique, carefully placed sutures, and precise closure of the mucosal layer are all important (see closure of fistula or thelotomy). Use of indwelling cannulas after surgery helps decrease internal pressure on the wound. The cannula should be left open to drain continually for several days. Systemic antibiotics are used for 3 to 5 days, and the quarter is infused with antibiotics after repair.

Blind Quarters and Membranous Obstructions
Etiology

Blind quarters appear to be laden with milk at freshening but are nonpatent. Congenital or acquired lesions that impair milk flow from the gland cistern cause blind quarters. Complete teat-cistern obstruction may be congenital, acquired before first lactation, or acquired as a diffuse cisternal or pencil obstruction during the dry period.

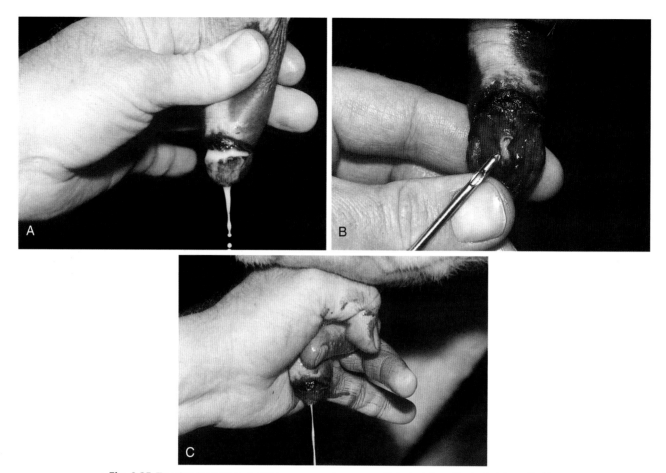

• **Fig. 8.35** Teat flap laceration. **A,** Milking appears to cause milk to leak from the teat cistern. **B,** Eversion of the lacerated flap, however, confirms the presence of remaining streak canal and sphincter muscle proximal to the flap. **C,** Removal of the flap restores teat function.

Degeneration of the gland cistern and connecting ducts is the most common lesion found in freshening heifers that have either small amounts or no milk from a quarter that appears to be of normal size. The condition is thought to be caused by intramammary infection (IMI) or blunt trauma during calfhood. Such infections can be initiated through aggressive cross-sucking by incompletely weaned heifers. At the time the blind quarter is identified, however, mastitis is usually not present in the affected quarter.

Signs

Anticipated quantities of milk cannot usually be obtained from the affected quarter. The teat usually feels flabby and meaty rather than turgid, as expected with normal milk filling. Palpation of the teat may suggest diffuse obstruction in cases in which congenital or acquired cisternal obstruction is present, and palpable fibrosis may extend dorsally toward the gland cistern.

Diagnosis

Ultrasonography is the most accurate technique to fully evaluate the extent and location of the obstruction. However, if there is no milk in the teat cistern, the ultrasound will merely show a collapsed teat cistern, which appears consistent with complete fibrosis of the cistern. The readers are cautioned against this misinterpretation. Careful probing of the teat cistern and gland cistern with a 3- or 4-in (7.5–10.0 cm) sterile teat cannula is recommended to verify integrity of the streak canal and geometry (size and distensibility) of the distal end of the teat cistern where no milk is present. Internal manipulation with a blunt teat cannula also allows detection of membranous or fibrous obstructions at the base of the gland cistern. This technique also allows assessment of any teat-cistern obstruction and may permit milk to be obtained for examination. If the lesion extends proximally so that no gland cistern is detected during ultrasonography, treatment is not possible at that time. It is important to establish the presence and productivity of the glandular tissue before any heroic attempts at surgical fenestration, lest the latter be completely futile.

Treatment

Treatment of fibrous or membranous obstructions at the base of the gland cistern is not likely to be successful. Fenestration of single membranes at the junction of the teat and gland cisterns has been successful rarely, but most surgical interventions are unsuccessful. Treatment of teat obstruction is as described in diffuse teat-cisternal obstruction.

Temporary or permanent teat implants offer the best success rates for heifers and cows that have normal glands and gland cisterns. Success rates of 50% or more are likely for this type of teat obstruction when implants are used.

Stenosis or atresia of the teat end is treated by slow dilation of the streak canal when the canal can be seen or by sharp puncture of the apparent dimple at the teat end when a streak canal cannot be identified. Usually a sharp 14-gauge needle is directed into the teat lumen at the apparent dimple that correlates with where the streak canal should have been. After needle puncture, the stenosis can be opened further with a bistoury.

Leaking Teats

Etiology and Signs

Many cows leak milk just before normal milking times because of intramammary pressure; this is considered normal or physiologic. Cows with high peak milk flow, short teats and teat canal protrusion are also predisposed to leaking just prior to milking. However, constant leaking of milk and that which occurs at times other than milking or that affects show potential are considered abnormal.

Generally, milk leaking is more common in previously injured teats. Presumably, the injury has disturbed normal sphincter tone or integrity of the teat end by fibrosis or loss of tissue such that leaking now occurs.

Diagnosis

Only the history and physical inspection of the teat are required for diagnosis. The teat may be probed to assess the streak canal diameter but seldom is this necessary.

Treatment

Injecting about a drop of Lugol's iodine solution with a tuberculin syringe at four equidistant spots in the sphincter muscles has been reported to correct leaking in approximately 50% of cases. Alternatively, ophthalmic 1% sodium hyaluronate can be used.

Skin Lesions of the Teat and Udder

Viral Causes

Bovine Papillomavirus

Etiology. Bovine papillomaviruses (BPVs) may induce papillomas (BPV6) or fibropapillomas (BPV1 and BPV5). Although these subtypes represent the classic etiologic description of teat and udder "warts" in cattle, other strains (BPV 7, 8, 9, and 10, as well as putative BPV types BAPV4 and BAPV9) have been recently found on the teats and udders of dairy cattle. The most common lesion in dairy cattle is the flat "rice-grain" fibropapilloma caused by BPV5. Frond-shaped warts, which have more epithelial projections on the skin of the teat or udder, are usually caused by types BPV1 (teats) or BPV6 (udder). The frond-shaped types are most problematic when they occur on teat ends. Warts are contagious and spread primarily by milking machines and milkers' hands that carry the virus, which then infects the skin in areas of abrasion. There is increasing evidence that

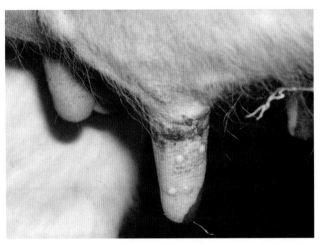

• **Fig. 8.36** Flat "rice-grain" fibropapillomas on the skin of a teat. The abrasion on the proximal teat skin is unrelated.

BPV DNA can be found even in normal, healthy bovine skin using more sensitive modern, molecular techniques. Viral and host-specific factors that dictate when and to what extent individual cattle develop papillomas are still uncertain. Exactly how BPV2 is involved in the carcinogenesis of bladder wall tumors for example is similarly unknown.

Signs. Flat or rice-grain fibropapillomas generally are multiple, may involve one or several teats, and tend to spread through a herd (Fig. 8.36). Young cows are most commonly affected, and in many individuals, the tumors regress spontaneously over several months. Fibropapillomas do not cause problems unless the teat end is involved. Florid warts that appear as classical papillomas or fibropapillomas with epithelial projections may be more clinically significant. These warts may be large enough to cause some mechanical interference with teat cup placement, and larger growths may become torn, causing pain to the cow and bleeding. Warts at the teat end sometimes interfere with effective milkout and always predispose to mastitis because of environmental contaminants. Herds experiencing endemic problems with this type of wart can be extremely challenging because the means to stop spread are limited. Teat warts are extremely common in dairy cattle.

Diagnosis. If signs are not pathognomonic, excisional biopsy is confirmatory. Some specialized laboratories are able to identify subtypes of BPV through molecular techniques.

Treatment and Prevention. Usually no treatment is required for flat, rice-grain (BPV5) lesions unless they interfere with milkout at the teat end. Snipping off frondlike BPV1 and BPV6 warts is commonly necessary, especially when the lesions are near the teat end. Whenever large numbers of cattle are affected, freezing of the warts by application of a steel rod chilled to liquid nitrogen temperature will be curative. Salicylic acid (10%) and fig tree latex applied every 5 days have also been shown to be effective.

Virucidal teat dips may be indicated when faced with an endemic herd problem as a result of BPV. Chlorhexidine is one example, and Udder-Gold is also thought to have antiviral properties. Milking affected cows last makes good sense but is difficult in free-stall barns. Minimizing trauma

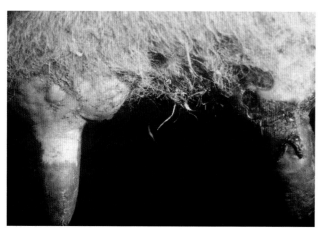

• **Fig. 8.37** Herpes mammillitis. Vesicles are present on the skin of the teat–gland junction at left, and ulcers and crusts are present on the teat and gland to the right.

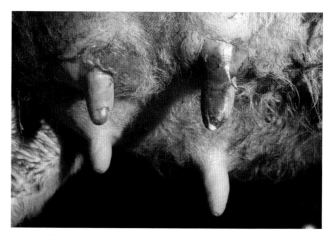

• **Fig. 8.38** Severe herpes mammillitis. A large ulcer is present on the skin above the right hind teat, and the right front teat is sloughing.

to the skin of teats also may decrease the incidence. This is accomplished primarily by improving bedding, good milking technique, and the use of a nonirritating teat dip. Commercial and autogenous vaccines have been used, but efficacy studies are not reported in the literature.

Although most skin warts in cattle are thought to disappear spontaneously by 3 to 6 months, this is not always the case with teat warts, which may persist for years.

The use of common utensils during udder washing and drying should be avoided; udders should be washed and dried with individual paper towels before milking.

Herpes Mammillitis

Etiology. Bovine herpes virus 2 (BHV2) causes skin lesions of both the teat and udder. The disease is known as herpes mammillitis and has its highest incidence in naive first-calf heifers joining herds in which the virus persists in recovered older cattle. Introduction of BHV2 into a naive herd through replacement stock may also cause lesions in cows of any age. Outbreaks usually begin in the autumn and continue sporadically through the winter. The incidence varies but is often higher in a naive herd than in the more typical situation of immune adult cattle but susceptible first-calf heifers. Annual reoccurrence is possible on endemic farms. The exact means of spread is unknown because rather deep inoculation of the virus into the skin of the teat wall is required for experimental reproduction of the disease. Several authors suggest an insect mode of transmission, but this theory does not coincide with the peak seasonal (fall and winter) incidence. Until further work denies the possibility, milking equipment and personnel should be suspected in the transmission of BHV2.

Signs. The types and appearance of early lesions vary but may include vesicles, edematous plaques, and serum crusts. Initially, vesicles form on the skin of the teat and udder, and the skin appears edematous. However, the vesicles quickly rupture, such that they may not be observed. Within 1 to 2 days, erythema, serum oozing, crusting, and ulceration of the skin predominate (Fig. 8.37). Lesions range widely in size from a few millimeters to several inches in diameter and

vary in number in infected cattle. After several days, dense crusts and dark-colored scabs cover the ulcerations and persist for 10 to 14 days until healing begins. Sometimes the entire teat becomes necrotic (Fig. 8.38). Regardless of the size of individual lesions, the affected individual resents handling of the teats and udder, does not milk out well, and frequently develops mastitis. This is especially true for first-calf heifers, who tend to develop the infection shortly after freshening when they have not yet fully acclimated to being milked anyway. The lesions are the most severe skin lesions of the teat and udder seen in dairy cattle. Multiple teat and udder skin lesions, especially in first-calf heifers, with a seasonal incidence beginning in the autumn, should alert the veterinarian to the diagnosis of herpes mammillitis. Up to 50% of affected heifers may subsequently be lost or sold for salvage because of mastitis. Calves that nurse affected cows may develop oral lesions. Concurrent, severe udder edema can make the clinical presentation of BHV2 mammillitis catastrophic in first-calf heifers.

Diagnosis. Clinical signs, history, and diagnostic laboratory tests help confirm the diagnosis. If vesicles are observed in very early cases, fluid should be aspirated into a syringe and submitted for viral culture or PCR. Other useful tests include biopsy of early skin lesions or the edges of ulcers to look for intranuclear inclusions that help differentiate the disease from pseudocowpox (intracytoplasmic inclusions). Some laboratories may offer serology because infection does confer detectable serum antibodies. Natural infection is thought to impart resistance for at least 2 years.

Treatment. There is no effective treatment for BHV2 mammillitis. Supportive measures include careful milking to minimize mastitis, application of softening creams to the teat lesions, use of iodophor teat dips to inactivate the virus, and milking affected animals last. Individual paper towels should be used for washing and drying udders during milking. Live vaccines prepared from the vesicular fluid of early lesions from herdmates injected away from the udder probably may work well but are difficult to obtain and administer. There is no evidence to corroborate the use of either killed or modified live BHV1 vaccines to confer protection against herpes mammillitis. Dietary measures to control udder edema in

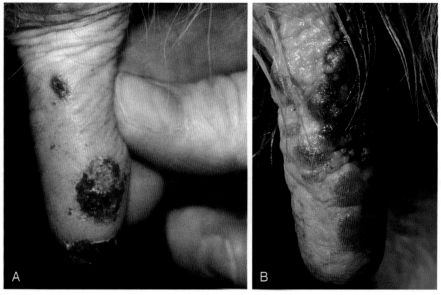

• **Fig. 8.39 A,** Pseudocowpox lesions covered by thick scabs. **B,** Earlier lesion of pseudocowpox with papules.

first-calf heifers during the winter months in endemic herds make intuitive sense and can lessen lesion severity.

Recently, BHV test–negative teat lesions that appeared very similar to BHV2 mammillitis were described in dairy cows in England. *Treponema* phylogroups were identified in the lesions. Further work is necessary to confirm the role of these organisms in what was called "ischemic teat necrosis."

Pseudocowpox

Etiology. The etiologic cause of pseudocowpox lesions on the teats of cattle is a member of the genus *Parapoxvirus* within the family Poxviridae. The pseudocowpox virus is very similar to the papular stomatitis virus and the virus that causes contagious ecthyma (orf) in sheep and goats. Pseudocowpox causes painful papules, vesicles, and denuded circular raised areas that heal under a thick scab. This feature helps to differentiate pseudocowpox from the cowpox or vaccinia viruses, which are orthopoxviruses (and may be the same virus) that tend to cause ulcerative lesions. Cowpox or vaccinia are extremely rare and currently may not be present in the United States. When cowpox or vaccinia is present, cows usually have become infected from a milker recently vaccinated against smallpox with the vaccinia virus. By comparison, pseudocowpox is common in dairy cattle.

Signs. Lesions occur on the teats and ventral udder. Individual lesions consist of multiple white papules that erupt and then are covered by a thick scab. The lesions may be 1.0 to 2.5 cm in diameter and circular or horseshoe shaped (Fig. 8.39). After the lesion heals under the scab, it becomes proliferative and raised rather than ulcerated (Fig. 8.40). Lesions usually heal within 2 to 3 weeks but may become chronic for unknown reasons. Lesions are painful in early but not in the advanced stages. Pseudocowpox virus is spread by milking equipment and milkers' hands. New infections slowly appear in the herd over several weeks, then may disappear for a time, and then recur. Some outbreaks

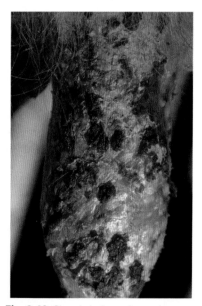

• **Fig. 8.40** Chronic lesions of pseudocowpox.

do not seem to end for months. Milker's nodules may be reported on the hands or other skin areas of milkers working with the herd. The major complication for infected cows is mastitis, but the incidence of mastitis and severity of lesions with pseudocowpox are much less than with herpes mammillitis. Calves sucking affected cows may develop oral lesions indistinguishable from papular stomatitis.

Diagnosis. Because of the public health significance of pseudocowpox and the similarity to cowpox, vaccinia, and exotic diseases, it is best to make a definitive diagnosis through viral isolation or PCR from tissue or vesicular fluid. Alternatively, electron microscopy should be performed on vesicular fluid. Standard histopathology of a biopsy specimen may show intracytoplasmic inclusions, but this will not identify the exact poxvirus. Cattle should be examined for other mucosal disease lesions if illness accompanies the teat lesions because pseudocowpox is *not* associated with systemic illness. There have been several outbreaks of teat lesions resembling pseudocowpox in cattle for which a definitive diagnosis could not be reached.

Treatment. There is no specific treatment for pseudocowpox. Efforts to reduce teat abrasions and to milk affected cows last may or may not be possible. It is not known which teat dips, if any, may control the virus, but those likely to be virucidal (chlorhexidine and chlorous acid–chlorine dioxide) could be tried. Milkers should be instructed to wear gloves to prevent infection and to avoid contact with scabs because the virus is extremely hardy and resistant to environmental destruction. Individual paper towels should be used for washing and drying udders.

Vesicular Stomatitis

Etiology. The rhabdovirus that causes vesicular stomatitis (VSV) has been identified in cattle in some southwestern United States in recent years. For historical reasons VSV in the United States has been divided into distinct Indiana and New Jersey strains. Antigenic forms of both of these strains have been isolated from clinical cases during epidemics in the southwestern United States in the late 1990s and early 2000s. Although the exact means of transmission is unknown, insect vectors are suspected because of the typical spring and summer incidence of disease. Transmission of the Indiana strain of VSV has been confirmed experimentally using the biting midge *Culicoides sonorensis*. The virus has also been isolated from several other insect species, including blackflies and sand flies. VSV is infectious for horses and swine, as well as cattle, and has caused an influenza-like disease in people. Clinical signs are very similar to those of foot-and-mouth disease; therefore regulatory agencies should be notified whenever the disease is suspected so that appropriate samples to confirm the diagnosis and rule out exotic transboundary diseases may be obtained.

Signs. In dairy cattle, the disease may either be sporadic or epizootic. Serologic studies during recent North American outbreaks suggest that the majority of infections in cattle are subclinical. Oral lesions consisting of vesicles and sloughing tissue coincide with vesicles on the teats. Occasional cows show lesions on the coronary bands and interdigital areas. Mastitis secondary to contaminated teat lesions and refusal to let down milk due to pain is common. Milking equipment and practices may spread the disease. Fever may be present but is transient and can be overlooked. Salivation, anorexia, and lip smacking are also often observed.

Diagnosis. When signs consistent with VSV are present in cattle, state and federal regulatory agencies should be notified to assist in appropriate sample submission and quarantine procedures. Appropriate samples to submit include the epithelium of surface vesicles, vesicular fluid, swabs of lesions, and serum. Virus isolation, antigen-capture enzyme-linked immunosorbent assay, and polymerase chain reaction tests for viral RNA are the tests that confirm the diagnosis. Exclusion of other exotic vesicular diseases is

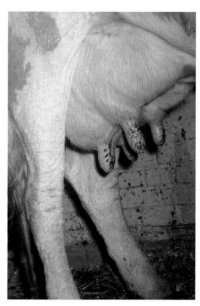

• **Fig. 8.41** Teat lesions and dermatitis of the legs in an adult cow. The cause was unproven, although the cow was polymerase chain reaction positive in blood for bluetongue virus.

important but is typically performed under the guidance of the administering regulatory officials.

Treatment. Treatment is supportive and is usually dictated by the appropriate regulatory officers. People working with the animals or diagnostic material should be warned concerning the zoonotic potential of the disease.

Other Viral Infections

Although rare or not present in the United States, the viruses of foot-and-mouth disease and rinderpest may cause herd epidemics of teat lesions. If there is reasonable doubt about the diagnosis, consultation with regulatory veterinary services should be considered.

Bovine viral diarrhea virus occasionally causes teat lesions that are characterized by hyperkeratosis, fissuring, and erosive dermatitis.

Some herds have endemic or even epidemic disease affecting the teats, udder, or legs for which no etiology can be proven (Fig. 8.41). Although bluetongue and epizootic hemorrhagic disease rarely cause clinical disease in cattle, some skin and teat lesions may occur as an immune response to these viruses. MCF can cause vasculitis in any tissue, and some cattle with MCF have multiple raised papules on the skin of the udder but seldom on the teats. *Mycoplasma wenyonii* infection has been associated with pyrexia, swollen painful teats, edema of the hindlimbs and rarely anemia in cows. The diagnosis can be confirmed by whole blood PCR (see Chapter 16).

Bacterial Causes

Staphylococci (Udder Impetigo)

Multiple small pustules and papules on the udder sometimes involve the dorsal aspect of the teat or the entire circumference of the teat in herds with udder impetigo. This disease has been discussed under causes of udder dermatitis. The diagnosis is confirmed by culture of the organism and ruling out other causes. Chlorhexidine and Udder-Gold may be helpful dips in these herds, and udders may need to be clipped and cleaned gently with antiseptics. Filthy environments or bedding should be identified and corrected.

Chemical and Physical Causes

Etiology

Irritating dips or udder washes may produce teat dermatitis during cold weather and low relative humidity. Teat dips that lack glycerin or emollients may contribute to the problem. Teat dips that have been frozen and then thawed may separate into dermatopathic components. Chemicals such as fly sprays, lime or limestone in bedding, and sanitizers for milking machines are other potential chemical teat irritants.

Causes of physical teat injury include sunburn, frostbite, direct trauma, periparturient edema, and insect bites. Sunburn and photosensitivity may be severe in lightly pigmented cattle and in cows with udder edema or pendulous udders. Similarly, frostbite tends to be more likely in cattle with severe periparturient edema, especially first-calf heifers. Compromised circulation of blood as a result of severe edema predisposes to frostbite of the teats when temperatures reach 0.0°F (-17.78°C) or lower. Wind chill also may contribute to frostbite. Obviously, this problem is usually limited to free-stall cows or cows housed outdoors. Trauma has been discussed (under the section on teat injury and obstructions). Photosensitization is rare but certainly can affect nonpigmented skin on the teats and udder. Primary and secondary causes of photosensitization must be considered in dairy cattle, and porphyria is a genetic disease that may lead to photosensitization. In today's management systems, it is possible that some animals may never have enough exposure to sunlight to show signs of photosensitization. Photosensitization of the skin of the teats and udder subsequent to induction of calving by corticosteroids has also been reported. The frequent use of automatic milking machines has caused an increase in circular muscular hypertrophy of the teat sphincter muscle as a clinical entity.

Signs

Signs that are associated with physical and chemical teat injuries include erythema, blistering or chapping, and pain. Again, pain leads to a vicious cycle of resentment that is manifested by kicking off equipment and milkers, incomplete milkout, leaking milk, and finally an increased incidence of environmental mastitis. Sunburn appears just as in humans, with generalized redness to areas of nonpigmented skin and blisters or vesicles in severe cases. Skin cracks may appear after 2 to 3 days because of necrosis resulting from ultraviolet irradiation. Frostbite initially appears as extremely pale, cold swelling of one or more teats. As the skin begins to slough, the teat becomes more swollen, erythematous or blue, and painful; the skin becomes leathery and dry. In severely frostbitten teats, the entire teat becomes leathery and black and eventually sloughs. Small patches of frostbite-damaged skin slough, leaving an ulcerated surface. Signs of frostbite must be differentiated from those of herpes

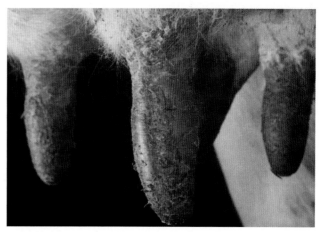

• **Fig. 8.42** Photosensitization of the nonpigmented skin of the teats and udder.

mammillitis because dark sloughing scabs on the teats and udder may be present in both diseases.

Bites from the stable fly (*Stomoxys calcitrans*) can contribute to teat injuries and increase the incidence of staphylococcal mastitis, particularly in heifers. Therefore a high incidence of staphylococcal mastitis in calving first-calf heifers should raise concern about fly control.

Photosensitization may lead to erythema, necrosis, and sloughing of exposed nonpigmented skin (Fig. 8.42). Generally, the lesions are more severe on the lateral aspect of the teats and udder. Absence of lesions on pigmented skin aids in the diagnosis of photosensitization. Sloughing frequently occurs in other areas besides the skin of the teats and the udder. Cattle with congenital porphyria may have discolored dentine giving rise to the colloquial name "pink tooth" as well as urine that fluoresces under ultraviolet light. Cattle with secondary photosensitization caused by hepatic disease may be jaundiced. Cattle that have eaten photosensitizing plants but are free of liver disease appear healthy except for the skin necrosis.

Treatment

Treatment is different for each condition. The use of chemical irritants should be discontinued. Assess all teat dips for their ingredients and discard any freeze-damaged products or dips that do not contain skin protectants. Treatment of affected cattle is symptomatic and includes lanolin or aloe ointments and protection of irritated tissues from sunlight.

Frostbite may be treated by tepid water soaks to restore circulation slowly and soften the skin. Unfortunately, the damage has usually already been done by the time a diagnosis is made in cases of frostbite. Therefore, putting the cow in a warm area and protecting any injured skin with lanolin creams constitute the best treatment for the majority of affected cattle. Leathery skin should be allowed to separate naturally unless infection develops subcutaneously or the leathery, darkened skin interferes with machine milking.

Excessive fly bites or retrospective suspicion of fly bites suggested by endemic mastitis in freshening heifers should be approached through fly control using pyrethrin-based insecticides, baited fly traps, and fly paper. Seldom is fly control as much a problem as environmental or management factors that allow a buildup of mud and manure.

Photosensitization must be treated by removal of affected animals from exposure to sunlight and determination of the cause of photosensitization. Primary photosensitization is best treated by avoidance of the causative chemical or toxin coupled with avoidance of sunlight. Secondary photosensitization caused by liver pathology from toxins or individual disease requires consideration, and porphyria should be considered and ruled out.

Mastitis

To simplify an extremely complex topic, mastitis has historically been broken down into contagious organisms that colonize the mammary gland and that can be spread by milking machines and milkers, and into environmental pathogens that do not normally infect the mammary gland but can do so when the cow's environment, the teats and udder (or injuries thereof), or the milking machine is contaminated with these organisms and they gain access to the teat cistern. Although the distinction between contagious and environmental pathogens is still a useful learning tool, the distinction is not always clear; for example, *Streptococcus uberis* displays both "contagious" and "environmental" properties.

Common contagious organisms include *Streptococcus agalactiae, Streptococcus dysgalactiae, Staphylococcus aureus,* and *Mycoplasma* spp. Environmental organisms include *Escherichia coli, Klebsiella pneumoniae, Enterobacter aerogenes, Serratia* spp., *Proteus* spp., *Pseudomonas* spp., and other gram-negatives, coagulase-negative staphylococci (CNS), environmental streptococci, yeast or fungi, *Prototheca, T. pyogenes,* and *Corynebacterium bovis.*

From a therapeutic perspective (see Tables 8.1, 8.2 and 8.3), it is also helpful to consider where the highest concentration of an infectious organism may be located because this is helpful in determining the likelihood of successful treatment with intramammary therapy, the duration of therapy needed, and whether or not systemic antibiotics may be indicated:

1. Milk and lining epithelial cells (*S. agalactiae*, coagulase-negative *Staphylococcus* spp., and *S. dysgalactiae*)
2. Deep tissue of the gland (*S. aureus, S. uberis,* and *T. pyogenes*)
3. Simultaneous infection of the udder and other body organs (coliforms)

Contagious organisms are spread by milking procedures, contaminated equipment, and the hands of milkers. *S. agalactiae* is the classic example of this group of bacteria because it is highly contagious and an obligate inhabitant of the mammary gland. Although it does not invade the glandular tissue to cause fibrosis and abscesses as does *S. aureus, S. agalactiae* colonizes epithelial surfaces and results in subclinical or intermittent clinical signs of mastitis. *S. dysgalactiae* is not as contagious as *S. agalactiae* but is similar in the means by which it spreads within a herd. *S. aureus* is probably the worst of

the contagious bacterial organisms because it causes chronic, deep infections of glandular tissue and is extremely difficult to cure. Most contagious organisms cause new intramammary infections (IMIs) within the first 2 months of lactation and many are capable of causing subclinical mastitis that results in decreased production. Estimates of financial losses as a result of subclinical mastitis are frequently quoted or estimated in lay and veterinary publications. Although exact financial figures are subject to debate, anyone connected with the dairy industry realizes that there is significant economic loss associated with chronic, subclinical mastitis. These losses include unrealized production, costs of medication and discarded milk, and imposed milk-quality penalties based on high somatic cell counts (SCCs) or bacterial plate counts. It is estimated that every doubling of SCC over 50,000 cells/mL results in a loss of approximately 0.5 kg/milk/day. Proper hygiene during udder preparation and milking, post-milking dipping of teats, segregation or culling of infected cows, appropriate treatment of clinical cases, regular milking machine maintenance, and dry cow therapy are key points in the control of contagious bacterial mastitis.

Mycoplasma mastitis may be impossible to cure unless self-cure occurs. Therefore the aforementioned procedural efforts to reduce new infections become even more important, and segregation or culling of infected cows is essential.

Environmental organisms can best be discouraged by clean bedding, clean housing, avoidance of wet environments (including mud and filthy manure packs), proper udder preparation, only milking dry udders, fly control, decreasing teat-end injuries, and implementation of proper milking procedures. Teat dipping and dry cow therapy have less impact on new IMI with the environmental bacteria, but teat sealants are moderately effective.

CNS possess traits of both environmental and contagious pathogens. Although they are not normal inhabitants of the mammary gland, they commonly colonize the skin of the teat, the teat end, teat injuries, and the hands of milkers. Therefore they can be mechanically spread and present major risks for cows with teat-end injuries. They also have been shown to infect teat ends after fly bites and may be a major cause of heifer mastitis. It is uncertain how gram-positive organisms gain entrance into the udder of prepartum heifers in all cases. They are presumed to enter via the teat end and are generally the same strains as those found on the skin of a heifer's udder or in mastitic milk from adult lactating cows. The incidence of prepartum infections in some herds may exceed 30%. A single intramammary infusion with an appropriate antibiotic, such as pirlimycin, 10 to 14 days before freshening can reduce the infection rate.

Environmental organisms that invade the mammary gland result in clinical mastitis that may be peracute or acute. Some of these organisms are also capable of establishing chronic infection of the gland. Environmental organisms first must be present in the cow's environment and then be given an opportunity to invade and overcome the normal defense mechanisms of the teat and udder to establish infection.

The dry period is considered an important time for new IMIs with environmental pathogens such as *S. uberis* and *E. coli*. In many cows, multiple organisms (e.g., *S. uberis, E. coli,* or coagulase-positive staphylococci) may be cultured from the same gland during the dry period, suggesting a synergy between them. This differs from *Corynebacterium* infections, which often exist as the only isolate. The proportion of quarters from which positive cultures involving major bacterial pathogens may be obtained increases from 3.8% at the end of lactation to 15.6% just before calving. If dry cow therapy and the use of teat sealants are not incorporated, this increase in mammary infection during the dry period may be as high as 20%.

Streptococcus agalactiae

Etiology

S. agalactiae is an obligate pathogen of the bovine mammary gland and is spread in a contagious manner during milking. It commonly causes very high SCCs and is shed in large numbers into the milk, causing high bacterial counts in the bulk tank milk as well. Over the past 40 years, the herd prevalence of *S. agalactiae* has greatly decreased with the routine use of dry cow therapy and improved sanitary milking procedures, which include wearing gloves, use of effective postmilking teat dips, and single-use towels to clean and dry teats. When present, the reemergence of this and other contagious pathogens is likely due to their reintroduction via new herd additions or due to a low level of infected animals in the herd with a break in milking procedure protocol. Reports of spread within robotically milked herds have also been reported.

Signs and Diagnosis

S. agalactiae can cause clinical mastitis; however, the majority of infections are subclinical in nature. Although herds with *S. agalactiae* can maintain a low level of clinical mastitis (2%–4%), a much higher percentage of the herd may be subclinically infected (>50% has been reported). Clinical signs associated with *S. agalactiae* infection are transient, frequently comprising abnormal milk with or without inflammation or swelling of the quarter. Systemic signs, such as fever, inappetence, and depression, are uncommon with this organism but may occur at the time of initial infection. Cows with subclinical infections exhibit reduced milk production and very high SCCs (in the millions per mL) which may be detected with routine SCC testing or a California Mastitis Test (CMT). Because of its contagious nature, it is common for cows to be infected in more than one quarter.

The diagnosis is based on aerobic culture. *S. agalactiae* is a gram-positive coccus that appears in chains on Gram stain and can be confirmed in most laboratories by a positive Christie-Atkins-Munch-Petersen (CAMP) reaction. A positive CAMP reaction is the result of the "lytic phenomenon," which is a characteristic of the Lancefield group B streptococci. This reaction occurs when *S. agalactiae* is aerobically cultured on blood agar containing β-hemolysin

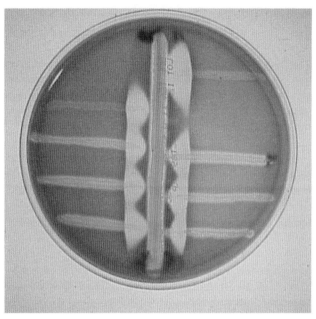

• **Fig. 8.43** Positive Christie-Atkins-Munch-Petersen (CAMP) reactions from *Streptococcus agalactiae* (horizontal streaks) cultured perpendicular to a β-hemolytic strain of *Staphylococcus aureus* (vertical streak). "Arrowhead" hemolysis of red blood cells in the media is interpreted as a positive reaction.

from *S. aureus* or co-cultured with a β-hemolytic strain of *S. aureus*. The presence of *S. agalactiae* will be revealed by enhanced hemolysis of red blood cells in the agar. The blood agar under the *S. agalactiae* that is within 5 to 6 mm of the *S. aureus* will be lysed, creating a "half-moon" or "arrowhead" appearance. This positive CAMP test result differentiates *S. agalactiae* from most other hemolytic streptococci, although a small percentage of other streptococci such as *S. uberis* can produce a similar CAMP reaction. In addition, a few strains of *S. agalactiae* are negative on a CAMP test, and in either situation, if there is a question based on other morphologic features, advanced diagnostic testing should be performed to confirm the result (Fig. 8.43).

Treatment

The goal for every herd should be to be *S. agalactiae* free. After *S. agalactiae* has been truly eliminated from a herd, the only way it is likely to be reintroduced is from a new infected animal entering the herd. Generally, cows with *S. agalactiae* infections respond well to intramammary therapy with a response rate of 85% to 95% when treated with appropriate products. β-lactam antibiotics, especially penicillin and amoxicillin, work well for lactating therapy. Because *S. agalactiae* responds well to treatment and there is a lack of environmental sources for the organism, it is possible to eradicate this type of infection from a herd. It is important to use an approved product that will achieve a high enough concentration of antibiotic to be effective. In vitro testing has not given any indication of antibiotic resistance. When treating infected individuals, all four quarters should be treated because of the potential risk of spreading the infection between quarters. All known infected cows should be treated at the same time rather than piecemeal. When left untreated, cows have a self-cure rate of 25% or less.

Several strategies have been used successfully to eliminate *S. agalactiae* from a herd. Systematic sampling of every cow in the herd to identify all infected individuals is recommended so that cost-effective treatment and management strategies can be developed. If infection prevalence is low, the most cost-effective strategy may be to cull the infected individuals from the herd.

If culling is not an option, known infected animals should be segregated from the uninfected portion of the herd and milked last during treatment and until a negative culture result has been obtained. The whole herd should be sampled, infected animals treated and this process repeated every 3 weeks until no more animals are found with the infection. Animals that are still infected after two rounds of treatment should be milked last until they can be culled. These animals are likely chronically infected and may not respond to therapy despite repeated attempts; thus, they can serve as a potential reservoir of infection.

Another option is "blitz therapy," in which every cow in the herd is treated with antibiotics. This may be a viable option in smaller herds in which the infection rate is very high. If elimination of *S. agalactiae* is a herd goal, culturing all lactating cows within the herd about 3 weeks after treatment is necessary to identify the individuals that did not respond to initial therapy. Bulk tank milk samples should also be cultured regularly (weekly) to ensure that the infection is not reemerging. It is recommended that new additions to the herd, including purchased animals as well as recently calved dry cows and heifers, be milked last until their milk can be sampled and shown to be free of *S. agalactiae*. All cows should be treated with an approved dry cow therapy at dry-off to reduce the risk of a subclinical infection being carried through the dry period.

Infected animals that are treated successfully should show a bacteriologic cure when recultured. In addition, milk quality and value should increase because of lower SCC and bacteria count. Milk production of previously infected individuals should measurably increase. Because of the high cure rate and consistent improvement in milk quality, *S. agalactiae* is considered economically beneficial to treat and eradicate from the herd.

Prevention and Control

Spread within a herd can be mitigated with appropriate hygiene during milking, including use of pre- and postdip disinfectants, wearing gloves, wiping with individual towels, and establishing standardized milking procedures. A high-quality pre- and postmilking teat dip should be used on every cow, and the entire teat should be covered with dip. All milkers should wear gloves while milking and should change or clean, sanitize, and dry their gloved hands often during milking. Individual towels should be used to prevent contamination between cows when drying teats before milking. The use of a common cloth or udder wash bucket can facilitate the spread of the infection because these

organisms can survive on towels immersed in disinfectant for several hours. Milkers should be trained in the milking protocol specific to the farm, and the information should be refreshed often. Using such practices alone can decrease the new infection rate by 75%. Management should monitor milking procedures several times each year (monthly to quarterly depending on management) to quickly identify deviations from the established milking protocol.

Problem cows (high-SCC individuals, those with recurrent clinical signs, and those with abnormal milk) should be milked last, and the units should be cleaned before they are used on another cow. After a herd is free of *S. agalactiae* infection, new IMIs with this pathogen can be prevented through biosecurity measures. Regular bulk tank sampling is a good tool for screening the herd for all contagious pathogens, although false-negative results are possible, especially in very large herds.

Streptococcus dysgalactiae
Etiology

S. dysgalactiae is a pathogen that exhibits both contagious and environmental characteristics, requiring management of both the milking parlor and the cow's environment to control the spread of infection. This pathogen does not typically reach the same infection level in herds compared to other contagious organisms such as *S. agalactiae*; however, this may be because it is more likely to result in clinical signs, prompting treatment. Although one strain may predominate on any single farm, more than one strain can often be found, illustrating the potential for both cow-to-cow transmission and environmental sources of infection. *S. dysgalactiae* can be found in the milk from infected cows, manure, bedding, and other sources of organic matter on the farm, making animals of any lactation or stage of lactation at risk for infection, although those late in the dry period and early lactation are at the highest risk. Good transition cow management, with a focus on energy balance and minimizing stress, may decrease the risk of infection during the fresh period. The organism has been isolated from common cattle flies, which can be responsible for spreading bacteria to the teat skin, so fly control may be helpful in the summer months. Different strains may contain genes for different virulence factors, implying that only a small number of virulent organisms may be required to establish a new IMI after gaining access to the mammary gland. The duration of infection is relatively short; it is believed that many unidentified subclinical infections are eliminated by the cow's immune system. About 20% of infections can become chronic.

Signs and Diagnosis

S. dysgalactiae is more likely to cause clinical signs of mastitis than *S. agalactiae*. Signs are typically limited to the mammary gland and include abnormal milk with clots or flakes with or without palpable inflammation and swelling of the quarter. Definitive diagnosis is based on culture. Bovine strains of *S. dysgalactiae* are gram-positive cocci that are nonhemolytic or α-hemolytic. *S. dysgalactiae* is classified as Lancefield group C.

Treatment and Prevention

S. dysgalactiae infection responds well to approved intramammary antibiotics in the β-lactam family. Few strains when tested in vitro show resistance to antibiotics, although several studies have found resistance to pirlimycin. Multidrug resistance is uncommon compared with *S. uberis.*

Prevention and control require that the cow's environment be kept clean and dry and that milking procedures include teat disinfection and other practices to prevent the spread of infection from cow to cow. Milking equipment should be maintained properly, and teats should be dried well before unit attachment to help avoid liner slips, which may push bacteria into an uninfected quarter. The use of gloves and individual towels to remove teat dip during milking will help reduce the contagious spread. Inorganic bedding such as sand reduces the growth of these bacteria in the environment; however, recycled sand may sometimes serve as a reservoir for new infections.

Streptococcus uberis

Etiology

S. uberis is a gram-positive coccus and considered an environmental pathogen. In some regions of the world, *S. uberis* is considered to be the predominant and most economically important environmental mastitis pathogen. An increasing prevalence of *S. uberis* has been reported throughout the world and it is reported to cause 14% to 26% of clinical mastitis in the United States, Canada, the United Kingdom, and the Netherlands. As a cause of mastitis the organism does not appear to be restricted to farms with confinement housing because it is one of the most significant pathogens in New Zealand and Australia, where cows are pasture based. One explanation for the increase in prevalence of this pathogen is that the improved management and control of contagious pathogens has left a niche that has been filled in part by *S. uberis.* Although *S. uberis* has been considered the most common species of environmental streptococci, research has indicated that other *Streptococcus* species have the potential to be misidentified as *S. uberis,* which may lead to some overestimates regarding the frequency of this infection.

Similar to other environmental pathogens, the potential reservoirs for the organism include all aspects of the cow's environment, encompassing manure, bedding, soil, and the animal herself, including the vulva, lips, nares, and teat skin. *S. uberis* proliferates well outside of the host, implying that the environment serves as the major reservoir, and it appears that proliferation is highest in straw and hay compared with sawdust or shavings as bedding sources. Levels found on heavily used pastures can reach similar numbers to other types of bedding within confinement housing. Because of this, infection can occur either between or during milkings if there is insufficient disinfection of the teat skin during preparation. New IMIs can occur during lactation, in dry cows, and in preparturient heifers.

Recent research in New Zealand and investigations of *S. uberis* outbreaks in the United States have identified the potential development of dominant strains of *S. uberis* in some herds. When a dominant strain is present in a herd, infection appears to spread in a more contagious manner, most likely during milking. Strain typing has supported this theory when the same strain of *S. uberis* is found in more than one quarter. Effective infection control methods are likely to be different in herds with one or more dominant strains. Additional control strategies may include the identification and segregation of known infected cows that are milked as a segregated group. The presence of a dominant strain of *S. uberis* can usually only be identified through molecular methods.

Signs and Diagnosis

S. uberis can cause clinical and subclinical mastitis in both lactating and non-lactating (multiparous dry and nulliparous prefresh) animals. Some studies have shown that the majority of *S. uberis* infections result in clinical mastitis, which can then evolve into a chronic subclinical state. Others have identified large populations of animals in herds with subclinical infections but no history of clinical disease. Clinical signs of infection range from mild illness purely associated with abnormal milk containing clots and flakes to severe disease with fever, anorexia, and decreased ruminations. Those with subclinical mastitis often experience chronic infection with a lengthy duration and very high SCCs, and potentially serve as an additional reservoir for infection within the herd and cause higher bulk tank SCCs.

Definitive diagnosis of these gram-positive, β-hemolytic, esculin-positive cocci is made via microbiologic methods. *S. uberis* infections are generally caused by only one strain, supporting the hypothesis that more virulent strains outcompete others that may have been present at the time of initial infection. As a result, aseptically collected samples frequently grow a pure culture. The increasing use of advanced molecular techniques in diagnostic laboratories has highlighted potential flaws in traditional microbiologic methods for identification of *S. uberis.* Research comparing these standard methods with newer molecular techniques has identified the potential for other pathogens to be misidentified as *S. uberis,* most commonly *Streptococcus parauberis,* although *Lactococcus, Enterococcus,* and *Aerococcus* spp. can all be misidentified as *S. uberis.* Use of sorbitol fermentation as a confirmatory test appears to increase the sensitivity and specificity of *S. uberis* identification by differentiating it from *Lactococcus* spp.

Treatment and Prevention

Infection with *S. uberis* appears to respond well to intramammary β-lactam antibiotics with increasing rates of resolution associated with extended duration of therapy with ceftiofur (8 days). Some studies that have seen poorer responses to treatment have identified that differences in strains may explain poor cure rates. Some strains can show a variety of results to antibiograms, so not all cases may respond to therapy as expected. Other pathogens erroneously identified as *S. uberis* may also impact the response to therapy on different farms because these other pathogens are more likely to be resistant to antibiotic therapy. Farms that are seeing poor cure rates in cows with *S. uberis* should discuss the value of molecular diagnostics to confirm the precision of pathogen identification and reliability of antibiotic sensitivity testing.

Some strains of *S. uberis* appear to have different virulence factors, allowing them to outcompete other strains. Some show resistance to phagocytosis by neutrophils; this may be overrepresented in strains with a hyaluronic acid capsule. The capsule may prevent binding of antibodies and complement to the surface of the bacteria, reducing recognition by the immune system. Other strains excel in adherence and invasion of mammary epithelia and macrophages.

Production of different host bacteriocins (small, antimicrobial peptides) can result in the death of closely related species and strains of bacteria. Because 15% to 18% of the genome can differ among *S. uberis* strains, there is significant variation in the virulence and susceptibility to treatment within a population of bacteria. Vaccines for *S. uberis* mastitis have been developed, but poor efficacy against these heterogeneous strain populations makes them less valuable to the industry.

The effectiveness of *S. uberis* infection control depends on the prevalence within the herd of clinical versus subclinical infections. Because of the known environmental component, cow hygiene and stall cleanliness are essential to reduce new IMIs. Cleaning stalls several times a day, frequent manure removal from cow traffic areas, adding fresh bedding when necessary, and avoiding overcrowding are all essential management tools to reducing the risk of infection. Appropriate udder preparation that provides clean dry teats at milking time should substantially reduce new infection risk during milking. For herds with a larger population of subclinically infected cows, identification and management of that population may be economically beneficial to reduce the risk of contagious spread via the milking machine. Management options may include treatment, dry-off, or culling.

"Other" *Streptococcus* spp.
Etiology

This category includes any gram-positive, catalase-negative cocci that cannot be more accurately identified by the diagnostic laboratory. Differentiation of this group is based on the diagnostic tools available and microbiologic tests performed. Organisms may be from the genera *Streptococcus*, *Enterococcus*, *Lactococcus*, or *Aerococcus*. Because of their diversity, clinical signs and response to therapy can vary significantly, and generalizations are difficult to make. However, they are generally considered environmental organisms and can be found in manure, bedding, on the animal's skin, and occasionally within the mammary gland itself. At this time, little is known about specific management practices that may predispose a dairy to this group of mastitis pathogens.

Signs and Diagnosis

As with *S. uberis*, these other gram-positive cocci frequently result in clinical signs of infection, causing abnormal milk and swollen quarters. Cows may also exhibit systemic signs of infection, becoming acutely ill with a fever and inappetence. High SCCs can be found in infected animals. There is less known about the potential for chronic, subclinical infection with these organisms and the area warrants further study, although recent research has documented outbreaks of subclinical *Lactococcus* spp. mastitis on dairy farms in both New York and Minnesota.

Treatment

Treatment of this group is approached similarly to that of *S. uberis* with the recommendation of extended therapy. Interpretation of antibiograms is difficult because break points for susceptibility and resistance are not well established for these organisms for all of the available intramammary antibiotics. Case studies on farms with larger numbers of animals experiencing IMIs with *Lactococcus* spp. indicate an increased risk for chronic infection. There is no useful current literature assessing the in vivo response to any of the commercially available products in the United States and additional clinical research is warranted.

Staphylococcus aureus
Etiology

After it has become established within a herd, *S. aureus* is difficult, if not impossible, to eliminate. Chronic infections, resistance to antibiotics, and difficulty in diagnosis typify the organism. *S. aureus* is not an obligate organism of the mammary gland but may colonize unhealthy skin on the teat or udder, vagina, tonsils, and other areas of the body. However, the major source of mastitic infection is secretions from infected quarters spread by the hands of milkers and milking equipment.

Calves can acquire infection with *S. aureus* from cross-sucking after the feeding of mastitic milk. Heifers 3 months of age and older may also acquire *S. aureus* infections by fly-bite irritation of the teat end and vector transmission of the organism by flies. Therefore insects and a dirty environment may contribute to a high incidence of *S. aureus* mastitis in freshening heifers and will severely damage milk production.

Subclinical infections are the rule, but acute mastitis or recurrent flareups are more common with *S. aureus* than the contagious streptococci. Typically, infection with *S. aureus* is chronic, and self-cures are rare. In addition to decreased productivity, infected glands suffer permanent parenchymal damage with fibrosis and microabscess formation.

Single cultures before antibiotic therapy are considered to have a satisfactory sensitivity for most bacterial causes of mastitis *except S. aureus* infections, for which the sensitivity may be less than 75%! Therefore misleading negative cultures may erroneously suggest clinical cure after antibiotic therapy, and subsequent clinical relapses may be incorrectly attributed to a new infection. Such regrowth explains clinical experience with relapses after apparent cures. Furthermore,

S. aureus commonly acquires resistance to antibiotics. Incomplete killing of the bacterium by penicillin and cephalosporin drugs may give rise to L-forms, which regrow after cessation of antibiotic therapy. L-forms are cell wall–deficient variants that may not grow on standard culture media. Phagocytes do not provide effective defenses against L-forms. Freezing and thawing of milk samples may allow improved culture detection as intracellular organisms are released from phagocytes. Collectively, these observations make antibiotic therapy of *S. aureus* mastitis very challenging.

Signs

Signs in subclinical infections may be mild and nonspecific and include abnormal milk (e.g., clots, flakes, or watery secretion) observed on the strip plate and a positive CMT result. Acute or peracute mastitis is not unusual with *S. aureus*, however. Clinically infected glands have intermittent acute attacks usually noticed by the owner. During acute flareups or an initial infection, the affected cow may be febrile, have a swollen, painful, warm quarter, and show a slightly reduced appetite. Secretion tends to be creamy or purulent with alternating serum-like secretion interspersed with clots, flakes, or creamier contents. The character of the secretion is in no way pathognomonic for any specific intramammary organism, and it should be emphasized that the ability to predict the causative organism of mastitis based on appearance of the milk has been shown to be poor in several field studies.

Peracute *S. aureus* illness occurs most commonly in recently fresh cows or in cows with an initial infection. Peracute signs involve systemic illness characterized by high fever (105.0° to 107.0°F [40.56° to 41.67°C]); depression; inappetence; and a hard, swollen, painfully inflamed quarter. Affected cows may become lame because of inflammation and pain in the affected gland. Gangrenous mastitis is the worst example of peracute *S. aureus* mastitis. Gangrenous cases occur most frequently in postpartum cows. Although other organisms including anaerobes are capable of causing gangrenous mastitis, *S. aureus* is the most frequent cause of gangrenous mastitis in dairy cattle. Signs of systemic toxemia worsen when gangrene develops, and the greatly swollen, firm quarter changes color from pink to red to purple to blue within a few hours. Affected cattle have tachycardia, gradually diminishing fever, profound toxemia, marked depression, and inappetence. The quarter progresses from a red and hot quarter (Fig. 8.44) to a purplish color, becomes cold, and may develop intrafascicular emphysema. A line of demarcation between healthy and gangrenous skin usually is apparent on the skin of the udder (Fig. 8.45, *A* and *B*). Later the skin becomes necrotic and sloughs (Fig. 8.45, *B* and *C*). The secretion is typically serosanguineous, indicating the presence of vascular disturbance. The dermonecrotic and vasoconstrictive α toxin of *S. aureus* is thought responsible for the tremendous tissue damage associated with gangrenous infection. Other toxins and a leukocidin may contribute as well. Compromised defense mechanisms in the recently fresh cow are thought to contribute to such overwhelming infection and toxemia.

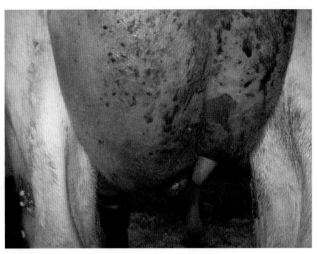

• **Fig. 8.44** Red and White Holstein cow with gangrenous *Staphylococcus aureus* mastitis. Despite removing the left teat, cellulitis spread throughout the left and right rear glands, necessitating an incision into, and drainage of, each quarter.

Heifers freshening with chronic *S. aureus* mastitis acquired as calves usually have ricelike clots or pus in the secretion from the infected quarter or quarters. The quarters are firm, edematous, and warm, but because of periparturient edema, they may be difficult to identify as infected by observation or palpation alone.

Chronic *S. aureus* mastitis commonly results in palpable fibrosis of the mammary gland. Although many cows are suspected of having chronic *S. aureus* infections based on abnormal milk or acute flareups, others remain subclinical and escape detection. Careful palpation of the mammary glands can be a helpful diagnostic tool and can reveal the obvious permanent damage to productivity. Chronic subclinical infections remain a major reservoir of *S. aureus* and represent a substantial risk to uninfected herdmates.

Diagnosis

Strip plate evidence of creamy or puslike secretion from forestrippings and a history of recurrent bouts of mastitis may suggest *S. aureus* mastitis, but definitive diagnosis requires culture of these coagulase-positive organisms. Approximately 75% of *S. aureus* infections are identified by single quarter samples. The sensitivity of cultural isolation can be increased to 94% and 98% by sampling two or three times, respectively.

Increases in bulk tank SCC and standard plate counts (SPCs) are not sensitive indicators of a *S. aureus* herd problem. Up to 50% of the cows in a herd may be infected by *S. aureus* before bulk tank SCC or SPCs become alarmingly elevated. This is in distinct contrast to *S. agalactiae* herd infections, in which even a few heavily shedding infected cows may dramatically increase the bulk tank SCC and SPCs. Therefore SCCs and CMT results are not as reliable as individual quarter cultures in the diagnosis of *S. aureus* mastitis. However, cows with linear SCC scores above 4.5 are undoubtedly the best candidates for individual quarter samples to detect contagious mastitis organisms such as *S. aureus*.

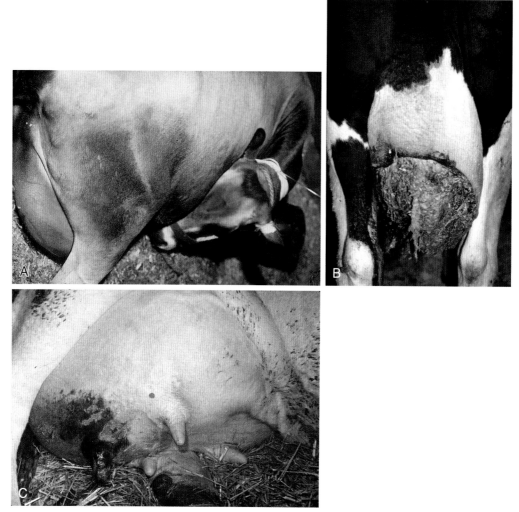

• **Fig. 8.45** **A,** Gangrenous mastitis of the right hindquarter caused by *Staphylococcus aureus* in a Jersey cow; notice the distinct discoloration of part of the gland. **B,** Sharp line of demarcation between healthy and necrotic tissue in a cow that had survived the acute stages of gangrenous mastitis. **C,** Gangrenous mastitis of the right hindquarter caused by *S. aureus* in a recently fresh cow.

Treatment and Prevention

Treatment of *S. aureus* mastitis includes both lactation therapy for acute mastitis flareups and dry cow therapy. Acute flareups require treatment during lactation to reduce the shedding of large numbers of bacteria and somatic cells into bulk tank milk. Unfortunately, the true cure rate with lactation therapy is probably less than 40%. Reasons for the low cure rate during lactation include incorrect drug selection, using a reduced dosage or compromised length of treatment, resistant strains of the organism, decreased activity of the drug because of the environment in the mammary gland (pH, biofilm production by staphylococci, inflammatory debris, high SCC), and inability of the drug to reach the organism (intracellular location of *S. aureus*, existence of abscesses and fibrotic lesions containing organisms). The inability of a drug to reach the organism is partially related to duration of infection; bacteriologic cure rates for newly acquired infections (<2 weeks) may be as high as 70%. Younger cows (<48 months) have also been shown to have higher cure rates (81%) than cows older than 96 months

of age (55% cure rate). Early lactation infections are more commonly cured than infection in other stages of lactation, and cows with only one quarter infected are twice as likely to be cured than cows with multiple quarter infections. Cure rates are higher for front quarters compared with hindquarters and decrease with increasing SCC as well as duration of infection. The most significant treatment factor affecting cure is treatment duration, but economics often mitigate against protracted antimicrobial use.

Gangrenous cases should be treated with systemic antibiotics (ceftiofur or tetracycline), fluids, and flunixin meglumine. If the teat is purple, it should be removed with an emasculator or emasculatome to allow drainage of the necrotic quarter. If the gland is necrotic but the teat is not, then an incision into the gland to allow drainage should be performed.

There may be an advantage to combined systemic and local therapy that is continued for up to 5 days when treating clinical, nongangrenous *S. aureus* mastitis. Penicillin has been used systemically in several studies with success, but results suggest that antibiotic selection based on culture and sensitivity results may have the best chance of cure when using a combination of systemic and local therapy. Penicillin resistance is the best-documented antimicrobial resistance demonstrated by *S. aureus*, but the prevalence of penicillin-resistant strains from bovine mastitis cases appears to have decreased in recent years in the United States. Similarly, combination therapy using ceftiofur and pirlimycin has resulted in greater cure rates than either drug given alone just intramammary or systemically. Local therapy alone is highly unsuccessful in effecting clinical cure but may yield clinical improvement or remission that masquerades as a cure to the owner. Extra-label use of intramammary products (e.g., three tubes per treatment) may provide higher cure rates but will result in prolonged withdrawal times. The success of therapy is related to not only choosing the right antibiotic but also to the duration and extent of the mastitis and the immune status of the cow.

Culture and susceptibility testing of *S. aureus* infected quarters is always indicated, and antibiotics selected for local treatment should be used at least four times at 12-hour intervals or for longer if necessary. Cloxacillin and approved cephalosporins are most commonly used for local treatment of flareups during lactation. Pirlimycin is also frequently used in cattle with gram-positive mastitis. Milkers should handle the teats of infected cows carefully to minimize spread of infection. Infected cows to be treated should be milked last or at least have mandatory backflushing or dipping of teat cups and milking machine claws into disinfectants performed. Iodine sanitizers may be used for disinfection of milking machines when diluted to a final iodine concentration of 200 parts per million (ppm); the shell and claws are dipped before and after milking an infected cow. Teat dip may be used before and after milking. Because the infected cow's milk is not going into the tank, the extra iodine in milk caused by these procedures is not a problem. This same technique can be used prophylactically for fresh cows or heifers that are thought to be at high risk for mastitis based on concurrent diseases, uterine discharges, and the like.

Dry cow therapy for *S. aureus* is reported to be much more successful at curing infection than lactation therapy. Wide-ranging estimates of cure percentages exist, and some authorities believe that 80% to 85% of *S. aureus* quarters may be cured by dry cow therapy with benzathine cloxacillin or other antibiotics. Higher percentage estimates of success seem hard to believe given the long list of potential reasons for failure mentioned in the discussion of lactation therapy. Less dilution of the drug, longer duration of the drug within the udder, and fewer opportunities for the bacteria to form biofilms and L-forms during the dry period may account for the greater success rate of dry cow therapy. Concerns remain however as to what determined "cure" in these studies. A negative posttreatment culture may or may not indicate success because of the existence of L-forms, intermittent shedding, or low but persistent numbers of intracellular organisms. Given the apparent success of dry cow therapy as treatment for *S. aureus*, all quarters in infected herds should

be treated at dry-off and a teat seal applied. Selection of the appropriate dry cow formulation should be made after assessment of antibiotic sensitivity of the predominant *S. aureus* strains in that herd. Dry cow therapy is also helpful in reducing new IMI during the early part of the dry period by both *S. aureus* and *S. agalactiae*. Thus dry cow therapy helps both reduce existing IMI and decreases the incidence of new IMI. Dry cow therapy has also been used for heifers before calving when high incidences of *S. aureus* exist in freshening heifers on a particular farm.

Autogenous and commercial bacterins have also been advocated and used for chronic *S. aureus* mastitis in problem herds. Commercial bacterins may or may not contain the same strain of *S. aureus* that exists on the farm in question. Furthermore, more than one strain may be present on a given farm experiencing *S. aureus* mastitis. Autogenous bacterins may be somewhat helpful in decreasing new infections, but they do not clear existing infections. Systemic immunization during the dry period may be more effective than during lactation and mainly induces IgG1 immunoglobulin, helps neutralize toxins, and may improve opsonization. Local immunization (of mammary lymph nodes) may be more dangerous as regards delayed hypersensitivity reactions but would be expected to generate more IgA and IgM and to improve cell-mediated defenses. Recent work also suggests that immunized heifers are significantly less likely to develop *S. aureus* mastitis. Bacterins may be incorporated into the control scheme for *S. aureus* problem herds but should never be substituted for improved milking management. It is hoped that improved vaccines for prevention of *S. aureus* mastitis will be available in the future.

Dry-off of affected quarters and culling are the last components of treatment and control of *S. aureus* mastitis. Valuable brood cows that cannot be cured and cannot be culled can be dried off permanently or have the affected quarters killed. Culling of problem cows that are chronically infected may be necessary for the sake of milk quality control and reducing the risk of new IMIs. Veterinarians and producers need to be aware of the inverse relationship between duration of infection and the likelihood of cure when selecting individual cows for treatment in endemic or high-prevalence herds, lest unrealistic expectations regarding cure rates be established.

The future may hold significant hope for treatment of *S. aureus* mastitis without antibiotic therapy. Interest in non-antimicrobial treatment of *S. aureus* mastitis has in part been fueled by the limited efficacy of traditional treatments combined with the growth of the organic dairy business. Bacteriocins that are natural bactericidal proteins are being produced by molecular techniques and marketed for treatment of streptococcal and *S. aureus* mastitis and for use in teat dips. Lysostaphin, originally isolated from *Staphylococcus simulans*, has been reproduced by recombinant techniques and used in clinical trials. Nisin, another bacterial peptide originally isolated from *Lactococcus lactis*, has been reproduced by similar techniques and may be marketed soon. Immunomodulating cytokines, including various interleukins, have also shown promise (experimentally) as non-antibiotic modes of therapy for *S. aureus*. Combination cytokine and antibiotic therapy may improve the bactericidal efficacy of certain antibiotics. Other immunomodulators such as β-1,3 glucan have either unproven efficacy or have shown no benefit in small clinical trials. It is possible in the future that transgenic cows may be developed, expressing antibacterial endopeptidase in the mammary gland, which enhances resistance to mastitis.

Calves should never be fed unpasteurized mastitic milk, and heifers should be raised in clean, dry environments where fly control can be maintained to reduce the incidence of *S. aureus* teat canal colonization and subsequent infection of developing glands.

Coagulase-Negative Staphylococci

Etiology

Coagulase-negative staphylococci are normal flora of the skin of the teat and external orifice of the streak canal. Strictly speaking they are neither categorized as strict contagious nor environmental pathogens but rather as opportunists. It is important to note that the term CNS refers to a group of bacterial species, each of which may behave differently in the udder. Although there have been up to 48 species identified, recent research has shown that only a few species usually account for the majority of IMIs. Mastitis due to CNS organisms usually results in subclinical mastitis, elevated SCC from infected glands, but minimal to no effect on milk production.

Current research has identified *Staphylococcus chromogenes, Staphylococcus epidermidis, Staphylococcus haemolyticus, Staphylococcus simulans,* and *Staphylococcus xylosus* as the most common species. However, within the CNS group the majority of IMIs are associated with *S. chromogenes*, followed by *S. simulans*, suggesting that these species may be better host-adapted. *S. haemolyticus* can be an opportunistic pathogen causing IMI, but it can also occupy a variety of habitats. Little is known about the epidemiology of *S. xylosus*, and *S. epidermidis* is considered a human-adapted species; most cases of IMI associated with this organism appear to arise from human sources.

Factors that contribute to teat skin irritation or teat end injury increase the numbers of CNS at these locations. Bulk milk may be heavily contaminated with CNS if milking procedures are inadequate, hygiene is poor, teat skin is irritated, or postmilking teat dips are not used. These organisms are commonly cultured from the milk of prepartum and first-calf heifers. Older cows may also be infected but at a lower prevalence, supporting the efficacy of both dry cow and lactation therapy in resolving subclinical CNS udder infections.

The individually increased SCC seen with CNS tends not to cause as dramatic an effect on bulk tank numbers as seen in contagious *S. agalactiae* outbreaks. In fact, up to 50% of the herd may be infected with CNS before the bulk tank SCC causes great concern. Mastitis caused by CNS is reported to be common, with some sources claiming that it is the most common IMI in many herds. Infections most commonly occur during early and late lactation or in the dry period if dry cow therapy is not used. Calves 3 to 9 months of age can develop staphylococcal mastitis from contamination by mastitic milk or by contaminated flies that feed on injured teat ends.

Signs

Other than a positive CMT result and elevated SCC, no clinical signs exist that specifically identify coagulase-negative *Staphylococcus* spp. Heifers freshening with mastitis should be suspected to have a CNS infection.

Diagnosis

Culture of individual quarters from all cows is essential for the identification, treatment, and prevention of new IMI infections. Development of new molecular techniques, including gene sequencing and fingerprinting, is allowing further analysis of the epidemiology of CNS infections, but currently not all methods have been validated in ruminants.

It is important to note that CNS are commonly found on the skin and may easily contaminate milk samples, leading to false positives. Careful aseptic technique must therefore be followed to minimize the risk of contamination, and multiple positive cultures from the same quarter may be necessary to confirm the diagnosis. Individual cow SCC (or linear score) as well as bulk tank SCC may assist the initial diagnosis but are not sufficient for detection, monitoring treatment response, or as a sole means of control.

Treatment and Control

Improved milking hygiene, correction of milking machine problems to minimize teat end damage, postmilking teat dipping with iodine teat dips, and dry cow therapy are very effective in the control of CNS. Obvious causes of teat skin irritation should be eliminated. Wet milking or poor udder preparation are notorious problems that can lead to high numbers of CNS in bulk tank milk and an increased incidence of mastitis resulting from these organisms. Antibiotic therapy may be used if the cow is sufficiently early in lactation that treatment costs are outweighed by production losses if left untreated. Dry cow therapy is also indicated in herds with a high percentage of IMIs due to CNS. Antibiotic therapy should be based on sensitivity reports, with antibiotics having efficacy against β-lactamase–positive organisms preferred. Iodine teat dips have been reported to be superior to other chemicals, and backflushing milking machine claws will reduce spread of these organisms. Calves should not be fed mastitic milk, especially if kept in common calf pens. Heifers should be kept in clean, dry environments, and fly control should be emphasized to decrease staphylococcal infection before calving. If there is a herd problem with CNS in heifers at freshening, treatment with a cephalosporin or pirlimycin 1 to 2 weeks before freshening may be indicated (but this is more than a little challenging practically!).

Mycoplasma Mastitis

Etiology

Mycoplasma mastitis is a contagious and costly disease of dairy cattle that significantly impacts animal health and milk production. *Mycoplasma bovis* is the most common cause of mastitis associated with *Mycoplasma* spp., but up to 11 other species have been isolated from milk in various parts of the United States. Historically, *Mycoplasma californicum* has been a common isolate in California. In a recent study in New York of the 845 *Mycoplasma* isolates investigated, 627 were *M. bovis* from 68 farms (78% incidence), 22 *Mycoplasma alkalescens* from 15 farms (17% incidence), 119 *Acholeplasma laidlawii* from 10 farms (11% incidence), 15 *Mycoplasma bovigenitalium* from 9 farms (10% incidence), 16 *Mycoplasma canadense* from 9 farms (10% incidence), 35 *Mycoplasma californicum* from 3 farms (3% incidence), 3 *Mycoplasma arginini* from 2 farms (2% incidence), 3 *Mycoplasma bovirhinis* from 1 farm (1% incidence), 4 *Acholeplasma oculi* from 1 farm (<1% incidence), and 1 *Acholeplasma pleciae* from 1 farm (<1% incidence).

Mycoplasma spp. cause herd endemics of acute mastitis that subsequently evolve into chronic infections. After acute attacks, cattle may show chronic mastitis or intermittent acute flareups or may have subclinical infection requiring culture confirmation. Mastitis may occur in only one quarter but frequently appears in two or more quarters in each affected cow. Much of the current evidence suggests that herd outbreaks occur via horizontal transmission, most likely from asymptomatic carriers. The possibility of internal transmission to the udder from other internal organs within an asymptomatic cow also challenges the view that *Mycoplasma* is purely contagious from cow to cow and spread in an identical fashion to other contagious causes of mastitis, such as *S. aureus* and *S. agalactiae*, which are predominantly spread during milking. *M. bovis* may be found on mucous membranes and secretions from the respiratory and urogenital tracts.

Infection may be introduced by a purchased animal from an infected herd or may appear spontaneously after mechanical transmission of organisms by contaminated workers or equipment. Isolates, to include *M. bovis*, *Mycoplasma dispar*, *Mycoplasma bovirhinis*, *Mycoplasma bovigenitalium*, *Mycoplasma canadense*, *Mycoplasma alkalescens*, and *M. californicum* have been isolated from single herds. *Mycoplasma* populations usually are highest in calves and heifers, but within non-mammary tissues. These *Mycoplasma* species have been implicated in causing mastitis as well as other reproductive and respiratory diseases in dairy cattle, although not all species have been comprehensively studied. Although *M. bovis* is considered the most prevalent, contagious, and clinically important *Mycoplasma* species and has been well researched, very little has been reported about the distribution and role of other species or *Acholeplasma* spp. in mastitis.

Clinical signs of *Mycoplasma* infection, including respiratory disease, otitis interna and otitis media, arthritis, and reproductive problems, may or may not be obvious or reported in problem herds, but *Mycoplasma* spp. can often be cultured from the respiratory or reproductive tracts in young cattle and adults on affected farms. Therefore, although purchase of infected cattle represents a risk for the introduction of *Mycoplasma* mastitis, perhaps the greater risk is chance contamination, transmission, and spread of the organisms from infected nasal, urogenital, or joint secretions to the udder, most likely from animals without evidence of clinical disease. After infection of one or more lactating cows, the disease may then spread as a contagious mastitis. Fresh cows appear to be at greater risk than cows in midlactation. The management of sick and fresh cows also potentially contributes to the spread of this organism. Fresh cows should not be housed in the same pens, or milked with the same equipment, as sick cows or cows with mastitis. The feeding of waste milk from infected cows to calves is another source of *Mycoplasma* transmission throughout the herd. Cold, wet seasons also may increase the incidence of infection because the organisms may persist longer in the environment.

Signs

Acute mastitis in one or more quarters is the typical history. The affected quarters are warm, swollen, and firm. Secretions are variable in appearance. Early secretions may be watery and have flakes with "sandy material," but this is not observed frequently enough to be diagnostically useful. The secretion may evolve over several days to a tannish serous-like material, containing clots, flakes, or pus. Although acute *Mycoplasma* mastitis is associated with fever (103.0° to 105.5°F [39.44° to 40.83°C]), affected cows may not appear outwardly ill. Some acutely infected cows may be slightly off feed, perhaps coincident with fever. Milk production decreases dramatically in those with acute *Mycoplasma* mastitis but may not be obviously reduced in subclinical cases. Acute mastitis involving multiple quarters and swollen, painful joints occurring in several cows within a short period should alert the veterinarian to the increased possibility of *Mycoplasma* mastitis. Unfortunately, the signs are less suggestive in chronic *Mycoplasma* mastitis, for which subclinical infections predominate. Intermittent acute flareups will be present but may not be as dramatic as the signs of acute *Mycoplasma*, especially when the organism is first introduced into a herd. Generally, by the time a diagnosis of *Mycoplasma* mastitis is confirmed, at least 10% of the herd is already infected. Arthritis, lameness, reproductive problems, calf pneumonia, otitis interna or otitis media, and adult cow respiratory disease may be other owner complaints when procuring a history in herds with *Mycoplasma* mastitis. These other diseases may or may not be associated solely with *Mycoplasma* spp. Frequently the existence of multiple health problems more likely indicates management deficiencies and overcrowding of cattle. Increased incidence of *Mycoplasma* respiratory disease and arthritis has been confirmed in several herds that were monitored for several years because of *Mycoplasma* mastitis. The fact that occasional outbreaks of *Mycoplasma* spp. mastitis occur in the absence of new purchases and herd additions reinforces the view that some cattle can remain asymptomatic carriers for extended periods. The introduction of bred heifers, reared off farm or purchased commercially, appears to be a particularly common antecedent event to acute herd outbreaks of *Mycoplasma* mastitis.

Diagnosis

Definitive diagnosis of *Mycoplasma* mastitis requires isolation from milk. Most *Mycoplasma* organisms will not grow on culture media that is routinely used to identify other bacterial pathogens. Therefore *Mycoplasma* mastitis should be suspected when obvious mastitis is present, bacterial culture yields negative results, and antibiotic treatment has failed to improve the signs. Special media such as Hayflick's medium incubated at 37.0°C and kept in 10% CO_2 are necessary for culture of *Mycoplasma* spp. *Mycoplasma* is shed in great quantities in milk, and consequently culture of bulk tank milk may be used as a sensitive method for early identification of infection in only a few cattle. After growth of *Mycoplasma* spp., speciation is indicated and requires an indirect immunoperoxidase assay or fluorescent antibody (FA) technique performed by a competent laboratory. *Mycoplasma* may be grown after freezing of milk. Identification of one or more specific species may assist an epidemiologic investigation for predisposing factors that contributed to the development of a *Mycoplasma* mastitis problem. In addition, one saprophytic organism, *Acholeplasma laidlawii*, is commonly isolated from tank milk both on its own and also in association with other *Mycoplasma* spp. Alternative molecular methods that can rapidly confirm a bacteriologic diagnosis of *Mycoplasma* as well as further speciate the isolate are of value to a mastitis laboratory. New molecular diagnostic methods (polymerase chain reaction [PCR]) allow much faster (1–2 days) and accurate differentiation of *Mycoplasma* to the genus or species level. A number of research groups have also developed various PCR-based strategies to discriminate between *Mycoplasma* spp. and *Acholeplasma* spp., speciate bovine Mycoplasmas, or to rapidly identify a species of concern, particularly *M. bovis*.

Treatment

Approved antibiotics in the United States are ineffective against *Mycoplasma* mastitis. Macrolide and tetracycline antibiotics that are used to treat *Mycoplasma* infection in other organ systems have not been successful against *Mycoplasma* mastitis. Fluoroquinolones are legal in Europe for mastitis treatment and would be the preferred treatment. However, it is not legal to use fluoroquinolones in lactating dairy cattle in North America. Because of this lack of therapeutic options, culling of all infected cattle should be considered. Cows that continue to have clinical mastitis and agalactia are easier for an owner to cull than cows that apparently recover and continue to produce milk. Because of the high number of cattle that are affected initially, culling as many as 10% or more of a herd may be required. This is seldom acceptable to an owner. Lag times between

collection of milk samples and positive identification of infected cattle after milk culture allow new infections to occur. Therefore, when more cows become positive based on follow-up cultures, the owner becomes discouraged, having already culled what was perceived to be "all" positive cows based on initial culture. Owner compliance with culling is much more likely if only a few cows are infected initially and the subsequent new infection rate is low because of effective management changes. Segregation of infected and non-infected cattle has been practiced in California and other regions when large numbers of cattle are infected and owners are unwilling or economically unable to cull all infected cattle.

Control

The goal of *Mycoplasma* mastitis control is the identification of infected animals and their isolation and segregation from uninfected herdmates. After *Mycoplasma* infection has been identified in a herd, quarter samples from all cows should be submitted for culture, all cows should be dipped with 1% iodine dips after milking, milking claws and teat cups should be rinsed with 30 to 75 ppm iodine and sanitized or backflushed with the same solution between cows, and all milking procedures should be evaluated carefully. After quarter culture results become available infected cattle should be culled or segregated from their non-infected herdmates. Cultures should be collected from all quarters of the remaining cows monthly, and new positives should be identified and culled. After herd cultures are negative, milk filters should be cultured monthly, and aggressive quarter culturing and culling programs should be reinitiated if *Mycoplasma* is reisolated. Ideally, infected milk should not be fed to calves, but pasteurization has become an attractive option for some larger dairies.

The feeding of waste milk from infected cows to calves is another source of transmission and perpetuation of this disease throughout the herd. Calves fed infected milk may develop pneumonia, joint infections, and head tilts related to ear infections. Milk from infected cows should not be fed to calves. There are differences in the thermal resistance patterns of different *Mycoplasma* spp., so periodic quality-control checks of on-farm pasteurization equipment are critical. Submitting pasteurized milk samples as fed to calves for routine bulk tank testing, to include specific *Mycoplasma* culture, is an important part of the preventive calf health program on larger dairies that pasteurize waste milk.

Infected cows may recover from acute infections and become productive, but others develop chronic mastitis and/or lameness. The frequency with which the long-term carrier status occurs and the shedding patterns of recovered cattle in milk are unknown. Infection with one species of *Mycoplasma* does not confer immunity against other species. In addition, active immunity to a single species is likely to be short lived. One report concerning *M. bovis* showed that cattle that recovered from *Mycoplasma* mastitis were resistant to reinfection in all quarters for 55 days and were resistant in previously infected quarters for up to 180 days, but they became susceptible to reinfection in all quarters by 1 year after initial recovery.

A vaccine for *M. bovis* is commercially available, MpB Guard, both as a licensed product or on a custom basis; however, efficacy is not well established. Further use in field settings will eventually determine its usefulness for control of the infection in cattle. The wide variation in antigenicity between different species and strains of *Mycoplasma* does not bode well for cross-protection against all currently encountered *Mycoplasma* spp. for the prevention of mastitis, arthritis, or respiratory disease.

Trueperella pyogenes (Formerly Arcanobacterium pyogenes, Corynebacterium pyogenes and Actinomyces pyogenes)

Etiology

Classically, *T. pyogenes* causes "dry cow" or "summer" mastitis. Infection is extremely purulent, and abscessation of affected glands is common. Most, but not all, infections occur during the dry period, and the incidence of infection is increased by keeping dry cows in unhygienic environments. Because *T. pyogenes* is a common skin organism of cattle, it is routinely isolated from abscesses and wounds in a variety of tissues. The organism may be spread by flies and fly bites of the teat end during summer months but can occur year round in some operations. Teat injury may predispose to *T. pyogenes* as well as other grampositive infections. Most infections begin after the udder has been dry for 2 weeks or more. Epidemics with up to 25% of the dry cows being affected are possible, and devastating.

T. pyogenes infection of the gland in heifer calves has been reported in England and in warm-weather zones of the United States. Affected calves were at pasture during the summer months and ranged in age from 5 to 22 months. The degree of damage to infected glands based on future productivity was not reported. Fly control reduced further incidence of the disease.

Signs

Swelling of infected quarters is usually acute and results in a very firm or hard, inflamed, painful gland or glands. Fever and inappetence may accompany acute infection. Cattle that are closely observed may have a less severe and gradual inflammation of the infected gland. Therefore "acute" cases may in fact be well advanced when finally recognized and represent fulminant abscessation of a longer standing, subacute, or chronic infection. Cows having truly acute infections are febrile and have firm, inflamed quarters and watery secretion with thick clots or ricelike clumps in the secretion. Cows with subacute or chronic infections do not appear ill systemically but have extremely hard, greatly swollen glands with toothpaste-like or thick malodorous pus as the major secretion. Milking the affected quarter may be difficult because of the viscosity of the secretions. Abscesses may appear in chronic cases and can be located anywhere in the gland. Such abscesses eventually drain percutaneously through the skin of the udder (Fig. 8.46) with the typical discharge and odor associated with

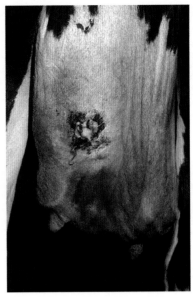

• **Fig. 8.46** *Trueperella pyogenes* mastitis causing a firm, swollen left rear quarter in a dry cow. A draining abscess is apparent.

T. pyogenes. Most chronically infected glands are ruined by the infection. Dry cows with *T. pyogenes* occasionally may abort because of toxemia and fever in acute cases. Occasionally, *T. pyogenes* will be isolated from a recurrent or chronic case of mild clinical mastitis in a cow with a history of coliform mastitis or mastitis caused by some other primary pathogen. The presumed pathogenesis in these cases is vascular damage, tissue infarction, and subsequent colonization of necrotic or compromised mammary tissue from pyogenic foci elsewhere in the body, or via the teat.

Diagnosis

The diagnosis is confirmed by culture of secretions from the quarter.

Treatment

Although the prognosis is guarded, early recognition of *T. pyogenes* mastitis before abscessation offers the best opportunity for resolution. Before intramammary administration of antimicrobials, infected quarters must be milked out completely.

Penicillin should be administered systemically (22,000 U/kg IM twice daily) for a minimum of 1 week. Penicillin should also be infused into the quarter once or twice daily using approved lactational intramammary products. Most cattle that improve require 7 to 14 days of this combined approach to antibiotic therapy. Cattle that do not improve eventually develop draining udder abscesses and cease lactating in the infected quarter or quarters. Gradual softening of an infected quarter is the desired response. Other signs of improvement include reduced size of the gland and a more fluid secretion. Prevention of *T. pyogenes* mastitis revolves around provision of clean, dry environments for non-lactating cows and heifers, frequent observation of dry cows' udders for evidence of overt swelling or asymmetry, fly control, and aseptic administration

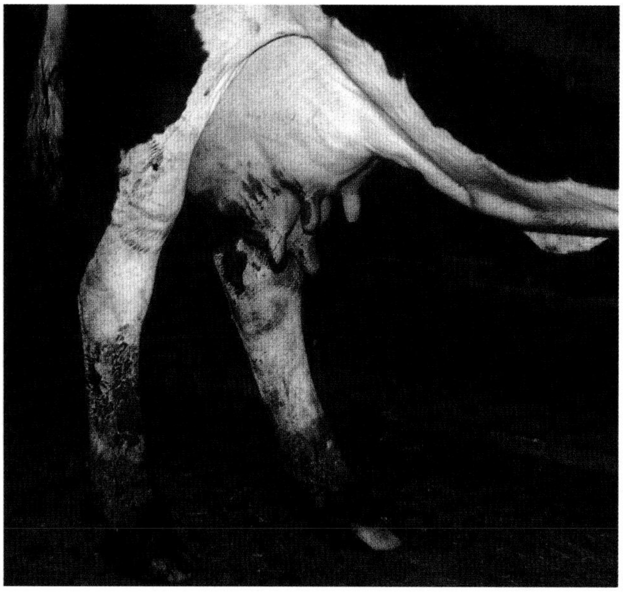

• **Fig. 8.47** *Trueperella pyogenes* mastitis of both rear quarters in a dry cow. Notice that the cow has been kept in a filthy environment as evidenced by dried mud on the udder and rear legs.

of dry cow treatments. Although dry cow preparations certainly discourage *T. pyogenes* infections, careless administration of dry cow products may actually introduce *T. pyogenes* to the teat cistern. Despite being protective with respect to many mastitis pathogens, dry cow formulations will be ineffective in conditions of overwhelming bacterial challenge (Fig. 8.47). Cure rates have been so low historically for *T. pyogenes* mastitis that practitioners have frequently elected to attempt to dry off the affected quarter or chemically sterilize it. In some cases, attempted dry-off or chemical sterilization meets with the identical outcome as the natural progression of the disease, namely, abscessation, and eventual spontaneous drainage from the skin of the affected gland.

Coliform Mastitis

Etiology

The lactose-fermenting gram-negative rods such as *E. coli*, *Klebsiella* spp., and *Enterobacter* spp. are the causative organisms of coliform mastitis. Coliform mastitis is familiar to all bovine veterinarians because of the mortality associated with the infection in dairy cattle and because farmers call on veterinarians to treat coliform mastitis more often than any other type of mastitis. Coliform mastitis also is the subject of heated debate regarding proper therapeutics, drug residues, and drug withdrawal times. *E. coli*, *Klebsiella* spp., and *Enterobacter* spp. will be referred to collectively as coliforms in this discussion unless a specific point needs to be made.

Coliform mastitis is the classic example of an environmental form of mastitis. Management factors that contribute to a buildup of environmental coliforms increase the risks of coliform mastitis. Deep mud in barnyards, for example, greatly increases the likelihood of coliform organisms contaminating the udder. Summer heat and humidity contribute to multiplication and persistence of coliforms in the environment such

that the incidence of coliform mastitis usually is increased during the summer months. However, because of the widespread use of free-stall housing for cattle, the damp barn environment present in free stalls predisposes to coliform mastitis, regardless of seasonality. Contact of the teat end by retained fetal membranes or uterine discharges may also increase the risk of coliform infection.

Sawdust bedding, especially when wet, has been known to harbor high levels of coliform organisms. Epidemics of *Klebsiella* mastitis have been associated with the use of wet sawdust. Within days of being placed as bedding and although still appearing clean, fresh sawdust may harbor 10^7 coliform/g, and it has been shown that even 10^6 coliform/g of bedding increases the risk of coliform mastitis. Kiln-dried sawdust may be better but is harder and more expensive to obtain. Straw bedding would seem to be a better choice than sawdust, and inorganic bedding materials such as sand and crushed limestone will reduce the environmental exposure to coliform bacteria still further. In terms of both cow health and comfort, sand should be viewed as a preferable bedding material for free-stall housing. Any advantage conferred by selection of a specific type of bedding, however, will be negated by a lack of daily maintenance because any bedding material will continue to accumulate coliform bacteria, although some simply do it faster than others. An advantage of sand is that it is pushed out of the free-stall bed by the cows more slowly than sawdust. However, if beds are not picked and scraped free of manure daily, coliform counts will quickly increase. Recycling of sand is becoming an attractive economic option for larger free-stall dairies that use this bedding material. It appears that properly recycled sand does not carry forward high-risk gram-negative bacterial populations, although persistence of environmental streptococci may be an issue. The addition of hydrated lime to bedding has been helpful in many barns but is labor intensive and, if too concentrated, can initiate skin and mucous membrane irritation.

Cows are at greater risk for coliform mastitis in the immediate postpartum period than at other stages of the lactational cycle. Cows in herds with low SCCs experience the highest incidence of clinical mastitis within the first 30 days of lactation. Udder edema, incomplete milkout, hemorrhage into the gland, sprinkling cows with water, and leaking milk between milkings are important contributing factors to coliform mastitis in fresh cows. Leaking of milk allows environmental mastitis pathogens to enter the teat cistern and gland. Concurrent metabolic diseases such as hypocalcemia that cause the cow to remain recumbent also may increase the exposure to environmental coliforms. Other concurrent diseases in the postpartum period, such as hepatic lipidosis or retained placenta, may depress neutrophil function and alter the intramammary defenses. Neutrophils may respond to infection of the gland at a slower rate in recently fresh cows than in those in mid-lactation.

Dry cows exposed to heavy numbers of environmental coliforms may remain inapparently infected until the periparturient period. Indeed, higher rates of new IMIs caused by coliforms occur during the dry period than during lactation. Dry cows are at greatest risk for infection just after drying off and just before calving, when intramammary lactoferrin concentrations are lowest. Coliform mastitis is most frequently seen in herds in which contagious causes of mastitis have been controlled. The reasons for this association are unclear. However, the high rate of contagious IMIs in herds with poor mastitis control probably results in high SCCs in a large proportion of cows, and somewhat paradoxically, high concentrations of intramammary neutrophils have been shown to deter coliform mastitis via the rapid engulfment of coliforms gaining access to the quarter. Milking procedures and teat-end injuries are also important contributing factors to coliform mastitis. In some herds with a low level of contagious mastitis, coliforms are not only the most common cause of clinical mastitis but also may be the most common organism cultured from the milk of subclinical cases. The common presentation of severe, peracute disease allied with the fact that it is a potentially fatal disease heightens producer and veterinarian awareness of this form of mastitis over most others.

Poor udder sanitation before milking is an obvious problem and predisposing factor. Similarly, failure to dry teats and udders before milking or use of contaminated wash water for udder disinfection contributes to outbreaks of coliform mastitis. Mechanical or procedural milking problems such as vacuum fluctuations leading to squawking or drop-off can reverse milk flows at the teat end that inject coliform-contaminated milk droplets into the teat end and streak canal. High bulk tank coliform counts indicate poor udder preparation, too much filth in the environment, or both, but do not necessarily correlate with the incidence of coliform mastitis.

Teat-end injuries caused by abrasive surfaces, skin chafing, excessive milking vacuum, overmilking, trauma, infections, and irritants all predispose to colonization of glandular tissues by coliforms. These injuries also cause pain, which leads to incomplete milkout and a tendency to leak milk between milkings; both of which predispose to coliform infection.

Coliforms multiply rapidly by 16 hours after entering the streak canal and overcoming local resistance mechanisms. The bacteria are normally destroyed by phagocytosis and intracellular killing within phagocytes. However, in the course of bacterial lysis, the release of endotoxin initiates a cascade of inflammatory mediators, which in turn leads to the local and systemic signs of coliform mastitis. The endotoxin-induced mediator cascade is complicated and involves both the cyclooxygenase and lipoxygenase pathways. Inflammatory mediators, including histamine, serotonin, and eicosanoids, are activated or released during the process. Production of prostaglandins such as prostaglandin F2 alpha ($PGF2_\alpha$), prostaglandin E2 (PGE2) and thromboxane B2 has been detected in cows with coliform mastitis. Oxygen free radicals probably are produced during acute coliform infections because studies have shown a reduced severity of coliform mastitis in herds that have adequate vitamin E and selenium levels. Endotoxins cause rumen stasis and ileus and delay calcium absorption from the gut. Hypocalcemia is likely to be a clinical problem in affected individuals because the inappetence also reduces calcium intake in the face of continued calcium drain from lactation.

Hypokalemia can be a major contributing cause to weakness or recumbency in cows with coliform mastitis. This electrolyte disturbance is thought to occur via a combination of decreased potassium consumption, decreased potassium absorption from the gut, and ileus-related metabolic alkalosis. Clinical signs associated with coliform mastitis probably become apparent after bacterial levels have peaked and the inflammatory cascade is maturing.

The efficient bactericidal activities of neutrophils that have been recruited by liberated endotoxin may explain the inability of clinicians to isolate coliforms from some acutely infected quarters. Delaying collection of milk for culture or previous treatment further contributes to negative cultures. Freezing of milk samples may increase the sensitivity of bacteriologic culturing by releasing bacteria that are engulfed in phagocytes that would have been killed normally in vivo. Cattle can spontaneously clear intramammary coliform infection as early as 10 days post-infection; however, some chronic infections do occur. The role of host (cow) factors in deciding whether or not a cow will develop severe systemic illness and potentially die appears to be more important than that of pathogen-specific factors in coliform mastitis. Gram-negative bacterial isolates associated with even fatal disease do not belong to the more virulent strains of *E. coli*, such as enterotoxigenic or enteropathogenic *E. coli*. Undoubtedly, the size of the inoculum plays a role, and therefore the level of environmental contamination on the farm is an important control point, but the metabolic and immunologic status of the transition cow are very important factors in deciding the prevalence and severity of new, coliform IMIs in dairy cattle.

Chronic cases of coliform mastitis once were thought to be rare but are now confirmed in at least 10% of infected quarters. Chronically infected quarters may be nonproductive or may have subclinical mastitis with intermittent flareups that mimic other causes of acute mastitis. Unfortunately, spontaneous cure is difficult for those cows that have become chronically infected. Many cows die as a result of coliform mastitis, not only because of lipopolysaccharide (endotoxin) and its effects but also from bacteremia. Also, somewhat neglected by research, are those cows that have chronic active infection deep within the glandular tissue or infarction within infected mammary tissue (Fig. 8.48). These cows do not recover spontaneously and certainly do not have sterile quarters. Coliform mastitis–associated bacteremia may be present in up to 40% of severely infected cows, sometimes causing concurrent uveitis, arthritis, meningitis, or tenosynovitis.

Clinical Signs

Acute or peracute inflammation of a quarter accompanying systemic signs of illness typifies coliform mastitis in dairy cattle. Affected quarters are warm and swollen. The degree

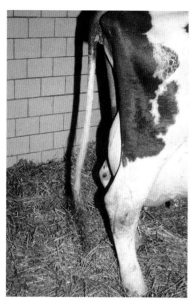

• **Fig. 8.48** A Red and White Holstein cow with chronic coliform mastitis and a "rock hard" right rear quarter. On postmortem examination, the gland had areas of infarction.

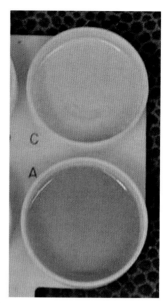

• **Fig. 8.49** Milk secretions from a recently fresh cow with coliform mastitis. Note thick yellow colostrum appearance in C and watery discolored milk in A.

of "firmness" varies, with some cows having only doughy or edematous quarters in contrast to those in whom the affected gland is very firm. Peracute inflammation may cause only subtle swelling of the quarter in some periparturient cows that may be masked by normal periparturient edema. Regardless of the degree of swelling, the secretion in coliform mastitis (acute) is more watery than that in unaffected quarters (Fig. 8.49). The typical secretion is described as "serum-like" or "watery" by most experienced clinicians and is best detected by first stripping normal milk from an unaffected quarter onto a black-colored plate and then milking secretions from the affected quarter onto the normal milk. Watery milk is easily detected under reflected light. Intramammary subcutaneous and intrafascicular emphysema may be detected in some coliform-affected quarters.

In addition to the local signs in the affected quarter, the cow has systemic illness (Fig. 8.50). Owners first notice inappetence and depression as typical early signs. Rectal temperatures ranging between 104.0° and 107.0°F (40.0° and 41.67°C) occur in acute cases of coliform mastitis. Cows with concomitant periparturient hypocalcemia may however be hypothermic rather than febrile. Additional signs from endotoxemia, hypocalcemia, and mediator cascade include inappetence, fever, rumen stasis, tachycardia, tachypnea, diarrhea, weakness, and dehydration. Some affected cows shiver and have their hair stand on end as early nonspecific signs that are associated with fever and endotoxemia. Ophthalmic consequences of the toxemia associated with coliform mastitis may include scleral injection, miosis, hypopyon, and hyphema. Cows may become recumbent from the profound weakness due to the combination of electrolyte disturbance, hypocalcemia, and endotoxemia. Recumbency worsens the prognosis and may interfere with detection of the mastitis. The udders of *all* recumbent cattle, especially those in the early periparturient

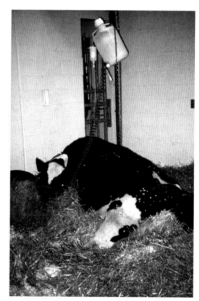

• **Fig. 8.50** Cow with severe toxemia caused by *Klebsiella* mastitis. The individual was recumbent, severely dehydrated, and acidemic.

period, should be examined to exclude the possibility of coliform mastitis.

Systemic complications include musculoskeletal injuries secondary to recumbency, laminitis, metabolic disorders such as hypocalcemia, hypokalemia, shock with lactic acidosis, and multiple organ failure involving the kidneys, liver, and cardiopulmonary systems. Disseminated intravascular coagulation and thrombocytopenia occasionally are observed. Leukopenia and neutropenia are often associated with coliform mastitis and may predispose affected cows to other infectious diseases such as metritis and pneumonia, as well as infection in other quarters of the udder. Some patients that have been treated with high doses of dexamethasone have developed fatal bacterial or fungal septicemia. Overuse of NSAIDs combined with disruption of the rumen microflora may result in abomasal ulceration.

Rarely, cattle with peracute coliform mastitis have developed lactic acid indigestion after ingestion of large meals of high-moisture corn. In these cases, the profound rumen stasis from endotoxemia was thought to have contributed to malfermentation of the grain.

The severity of endotoxic signs varies tremendously in cattle with coliform mastitis. Infections by *Klebsiella* spp. cause the most dramatic and persistent signs of endotoxemia of all the coliform bacteria. Many cattle affected with acute coliform mastitis subsequently confirmed to be due to *Klebsiella* spp. remain anorectic, depressed, and weak for up to 7 days, regardless of the rate of therapeutic response in the udder.

Diagnosis

In both peracute and acute coliform mastitis, the combination of local and systemic signs is a highly reliable indicator of the diagnosis. The most specific signs of coliform mastitis include serum-like secretion, a swollen and hard quarter, tachypnea, tachycardia, fever, weakness, and shivering. Although these signs are not absolute, they probably are even more specific when the cow resides in a herd with an overall low SCC; is living in a wet, damp, or dirty environment; or has recently freshened.

The importance of careful examination of the milk with a black strip plate cannot be overemphasized. Plates should be examined under reflected lighting to detect subtle changes that may occur early during coliform mastitis.

Tests based on increased milk pH are used for the detection of coliform mastitis in Europe, but such tests are less available in the United States. A CBC may also suggest coliform mastitis because the acute infection and endotoxemia frequently result in a degenerative left shift, with leukopenia, neutropenia, and band neutrophils observed.

Definitive diagnosis can be achieved through bacteriologic cultures of milk. Freezing and thawing the samples before inoculation onto media increases the sensitivity of the test but could also kill some sensitive bacteria. Lack of culture sensitivity despite preculture freezing and thawing is probably the result of phagocytosis and destruction of the causative organisms by mammary gland phagocytes before collection.

Treatment

Treatment of coliform mastitis has been controversial because of the administration of extra-label drugs without specific knowledge of antibiotic withdrawal times and the lack of controlled therapeutic trials under rigorous, blinded conditions. Many experimental studies of coliform mastitis emphasize that infection resolves spontaneously as a result of the inflammatory neutrophilic influx into the gland and that most clinical signs simply represent the effects of endotoxin and other mediators of inflammation on the cow. Although these studies suggest that antibiotics may not be a necessary component of treatment, they are counterbalanced by the high mortality rate from coliform mastitis. Clinically, it is impossible to distinguish signs that are associated with persistent infection from those of persistent endotoxemia, and furthermore, continued signs of endotoxemia may imply continued persistence of infection. Even knowing about these studies, the practicing veterinarian may not wish to withhold antibiotic therapy when faced with a greatly distressed or litigious owner whose valuable cow becomes gravely ill with coliform mastitis. Although the majority of experimental studies demonstrate that antibiotic therapy confers no benefit on induced coliform mastitis, there are a smaller number of studies that do show favorable outcomes when severe field cases are treated with antibiotics such as ceftiofur. These findings, taken with the repeated demonstration of true bacteremia in a proportion of cows with naturally occurring coliform mastitis, are strong arguments in favor of systemic antibiotic administration. The pros and cons of antibiotic therapy, albeit controversial, should be understood by bovine practitioners. The pharmacology and likely benefits or risks associated with each antibiotic should be known (see the pharmacology discussion). Currently approved antibiotics for use in lactating cattle in the U.S. are listed in Table 8.1. Antibiotics should be at least considered as therapy for coliform mastitis to ensure complete elimination of the infection and avoidance of chronic infection, and we recommend their use in severe cases.

Studies that report antibiotic susceptibility of gram-negative bacteria causing mastitis have been published; the accumulated data from these studies alongside literature reviews and more recent culture and antibiotic sensitivity results indicate the following:

1. Third-generation cephalosporins and amikacin (which should not be used without strict adherence to prolonged withdrawal guidelines and only in a rare if ever situation when its use is considered important for survival of the cow) work against most coliforms in vitro.
2. Cephalothin works against approximately 60% of isolates in vitro.
3. Ampicillin and tetracycline work against approximately 40% of isolates in vitro.

Inflammation and serum leakage into the gland increase the pH of the milk to nearly physiologic levels (7.2), which inhibits diffusion of some alkaline drugs into the glandular tissue. Inflammation, cellular debris, and decreased ability to diffuse throughout the quarter diminish the effectiveness of all antibiotics, especially intramammary antibiotic infusions. Therefore the pharmacology of each drug considered, regardless of antibiotic sensitivity results in vitro, must be evaluated. By and large, whereas weak acids are better choices for intramammary administration in the treatment of clinical mastitis, the weak bases achieve better tissue levels when given systemically. Macrolide antibiotics and sulfonamides, when given systemically, establish high milk-to-plasma ratios in healthy cattle because these drugs are weak bases. Tetracyclines attain a fair to good milk-to-plasma ratio when given systemically. Penicillin and ampicillin,

TABLE 8.1	Food and Drug Administration–Approved Antibiotics for Intramammary Use in Lactating Dairy Cattle					
Active Ingredient	Drug Type	Milk Withholding Time (hr)	Meat Withholding Time (days)	Product Name	Manufacturer or Marketer	Frequency of Treatments and Number of Treatments
Amoxicillin	Rx	60	12	Amoxi-Mast	Merck Animal Health	q12 hr/3
Ceftiofur hydrochloride	Rx	72	2	Spectramast LC	Zoetis, Inc	q24 hr/2–8
Cephapirin	OTC	96	4	Today	Boehringer Ingelheim Vetmedica, Inc.	q12 hr/2
Cloxacillin	Rx	48	10	Dairy-Clox	Merck Animal Health	q12 hr/3
Hetacillin	Rx	72	10	Hetacin-K	Boehringer Ingelheim Vetmedica, Inc.	q24 hr/3
Penicillin G	OTC	60	3	Hanfords	G.C. Hanford Mfg. Co.	q12 hr/3
Pirlimycin	Rx	36	9*	Pirsue	Zoetis, Inc.	q24 hr/2–8

OTC, Over the counter; *Rx,* prescription.
*Nine-day meat withholding after infusion twice at 24-hour interval; at least a 21-day meat withholding for any therapy extended beyond two infusions.

weak acids, attain limited ratios in the milk of healthy cows after parenteral administration. Systemic ceftiofur and the aminoglycosides have the poorest distribution in the glandular tissue of mastitis patients.

Results of studies examining experimental and natural coliform mastitis treatments are highly confusing. In one field study, no apparent benefit resulted when systemic gentamicin was used in the treatment of coliform mastitis. The reported success in cows treated systemically with gentamicin (to which the organisms were sensitive) was no better than in cows treated systemically with erythromycin, even though the causative organisms were resistant to erythromycin, or in non-treated control animals. All quarters in this study were treated with cephalothin, regardless of the systemic antibiotic chosen. This differs from another study that demonstrated a beneficial effect of ceftiofur treatment in cows with severe coliform mastitis. It is no wonder that most practitioners develop an individual or clinic-based approach to the therapy of coliform mastitis in the field, heavily based on their own experiences. It has become increasingly important that treatment decisions are made within the framework of federally regulated drug approvals and with due diligence with respect to residue avoidance, especially when extra-label drug use is performed.

Many practitioners use oxytetracycline HCl systemically when treating coliform mastitis. Although the likelihood of sensitivity of the organism to oxytetracycline is only moderate, distribution of the drug to the udder should be good, and the drug may provide some antiinflammatory properties within the udder. Nephrotoxic effects may occur in dehydrated cows treated with oxytetracycline! It is impossible to recommend one treatment above all others because of geographic differences in bacterial populations, resistance

patterns of coliform organisms present on each farm, and many other factors. Culture and sensitivity results should be obtained for isolates from each farm to better determine appropriate antibiotic therapy when faced with an acute coliform mastitis case or cluster of cases.

New antibiotics such as florfenicol, a derivative of chloramphenicol that is not associated with aplastic anemia, and the fluoroquinolones such as norfloxacin are drugs that have been shown to have good distribution via systemic and intramammary routes for bovine mastitis. Despite the therapeutic efficacy of the fluoroquinolones against coliforms, the U.S. Food and Drug Administration (FDA) has prohibited the use of those drugs in dairy production animals. Florfenicol is also not approved for lactation-age dairy cows in the United States.

Obviously, the dosage, vehicle, degree of inflammatory debris or plugging of milk ductules, and nature of the secretion may alter patterns of distribution (Fig. 8.51). New formulations will continue to appear on the market after testing, and it is hoped that the pharmacokinetics and efficacy of approved drugs will be further evaluated. Although most farms harbor a multitude of coliforms, culture and antibiotic sensitivity results from previous cases of coliform mastitis should be catalogued for individual farms to provide background data that may be useful in selecting initial therapy for future cases.

Every cow with coliform mastitis should be evaluated individually as to present and future productive and genetic value before a decision to treat with antibiotics is made. Cows of marginal economic or emotional importance may best be culled before initiation of potentially expensive therapy. Prolonged residues in meat and milk as a result of extended use of antibiotics should be avoided

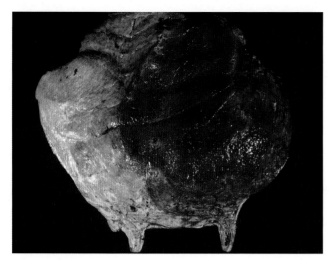

• **Fig. 8.51** Necropsy view of a fatal chronic coliform infection showing a large infarcted zone in the infected gland. Methylene blue was administered intravenously (IV) before euthanasia. It is apparent that neither IV nor local therapy can counteract the walled-off infection in such cases.

unless the cow is deemed valuable enough to remain on the farm and salvage for meat is not an option. If the cow's life is in jeopardy and extra-label drugs or dosages are deemed necessary to save the cow, the owner and practitioner are responsible for ensuring that adequate withdrawal times are observed. Because of fear of residues, antibiotic therapy is often withheld or compromised by lack of intensity, reduction in dosages, or shortened duration of treatment. All of these factors not only limit the potential for successful treatment but also increase the likelihood of chronic infection and resistant organisms. Although many cases of coliform mastitis are life threatening, the destruction of glandular tissue is generally less than what occurs with gram-positive infections, and if the cow survives and quickly clears the infection (with or without antibiotics), return to near maximum production may be possible in the next lactation.

Supportive measures are extremely important for a successful therapeutic outcome in cases of coliform mastitis. Supportive therapy should be administered independent of the decision for or against antibiotic therapy. Frequent milking out of the affected quarter has previously been considered the most valuable nursing procedure. The philosophy behind frequent stripping was that it removed organisms, endotoxins, and mediators of inflammation, as well as neutrophils and macrophages whose products further foster inflammation. Historically, stripping every 1 or 2 hours had been advocated, but that has now been refuted with respect to outcome, and current guidelines call for stripping no more than every 4 to 6 hours, even in peracute cases. Too frequent stripping may actually cause the teat sphincter to remain open, allowing other organisms to gain entrance. Chronic cases may also benefit from stripping up to 4 times a day. Oxytocin (20 units) may be administered systemically to facilitate milk letdown so as to remove accumulated endotoxin from the quarter. Alternatively, one or more calves may be placed in a box stall with the affected cow to nurse the quarters frequently.

Nonsteroidal antiinflammatory drugs should be used in an effort to block the prostaglandin-mediated inflammation associated with endotoxemia. Flunixin meglumine is the most potent of these drugs in common use and may be given IV for two to three treatments. Aspirin, although not approved for use in lactating cattle, has been used at 1.0 grain/kg at 12-hour intervals as an alternative. It is important to realize that the NSAIDs have been shown to be most effective when administered prophylactically. Obviously, however, in clinical practice, their use is never prophylactic because clinical signs only appear after endotoxemia already has occurred. Nevertheless, NSAIDs are most effective when administered early in the course of the disease. NSAIDs should be used cautiously because they are potentially toxic to the gastrointestinal tract and kidneys. Abomasal ulceration is the most frequent gastrointestinal complication of overdosage, prolonged use, or use of these drugs (especially flunixin meglumine) in very dehydrated patients. Renal papillary necrosis and renal infarcts may develop in cattle treated with NSAIDs, and dehydration of the patient increases the risk of renal problems. Therefore IV or oral fluids should be administered to correct existing dehydration whenever NSAIDs are used in critically ill patients.

Corticosteroid use in coliform-affected cattle is controversial. Some clinicians use intramammary corticosteroids such as 10 to 20 mg of dexamethasone as a one-time treatment. Other clinicians administer 10 to 40 mg of dexamethasone systemically. Although corticosteroids may alleviate the inflammatory cascade, they probably increase the risk of chronic infection and deter defense mechanisms. Corticosteroids should never be used as maintenance therapy, and "shock" dosages, such as 100 to 200 mg of dexamethasone, have been suggested by some clinicians but should be considered as being very dangerous to cattle. A low-dose, one-time treatment may be acceptable in nonpregnant dairy cows with coliform mastitis, but high-dose or continued treatment is contraindicated.

Intravenous fluid therapy is indicated whenever dehydration is obvious or when appetite or water consumption is depressed by the disease. Balanced electrolyte solutions such as lactated Ringer's solution are usually the best choice, but severely affected cattle that show signs of shock coincident with acidemia may require replacement bicarbonate therapy as well. Although metabolic alkalosis is the most common acid–base disturbance in off-feed cattle, peracute or acute coliform mastitis is one of the few common illnesses in adults that is often associated with metabolic acidosis. If the patient shows profound weakness, an acid–base and electrolyte panel should be submitted to guide further fluid and electrolyte replacement. Many clinicians use hypertonic saline (1–3 L IV) as therapy for dehydrated, endotoxemic patients, but it is important to remember that there needs to be

TABLE 8.2	Food and Drug Administration–Approved Antibiotics for Injectable Use in Lactating Dairy Cattle in the United States				
Active Ingredient	Drug Type	Milk Withhold Time	Meat Withhold Time (days)	Label Dose and Duration	Precautionary Statements
Ampicillin trihydrate.† (Polyflex)	Rx	48 hr	6	2–5 mg/lb body weight once daily; not to exceed 7 days	The dosage of Polyflex will vary according to the severity of infection and the animal's response. Polyflex is to be given by IM injection.
Ceftiofur crystalline-free acid (EXCEDE)*	Rx	None	13	1.5 mL/100 lb body weight SC at *base of ear*	EXCEDE is to be administered as a SC injection at the base of the ear. *Do not* administer SC in the neck.
Ceftiofur hydrochloride (EXCENEL)*	Rx	None	4	0.5–1.0 mg/lb body weight for 3 to 5 days SC	Treatment should be repeated at 24-hr intervals for a total of 3 consecutive days. Do not inject more than 15 mL per injection site.
Ceftiofur sodium (Naxcel)*	Rx	None	4	0.5–1.0 mg/lb body weight for 3–5 days IM	Treatment should be repeated at 24-hr intervals for a total of 3 consecutive days. May also be used on days 4 and 5 for animals that do not show a satisfactory response (recovery) after the initial 3 treatments.
Oxytetracycline.†	OTC	96 hr	28		Several formulations of oxytetracycline are available for use in lactating dairy cattle. Doses and routes of administration vary. Consult product label for dose, route of administration, duration of treatment, and approval for lactating dairy cattle.
Penicillin G (procaine)†	OTC	48 hr	4–10	3000 units/lb body weight†	The daily treatment schedule should not exceed 5 days in lactating dairy cattle.

IM, Intramuscular; *OTC,* over the counter; *Rx,* prescription; *SC,* subcutaneous.

*The U.S. Food and Drug Administration has restricted extra-label use of these products in lactating dairy cattle relative to dose, duration and mode of administration. Extra-label drug use for therapeutic indication such as mastitis is permitted.

†If higher dosage levels, extended duration, or increased frequency of administration are used for ampicillin, oxytetracycline or penicillin G, extended withdrawal periods are necessary. Consult the Food Animal Residue Avoidance Databank (FARAD; http://www.farad.org) for precautionary statements and withdrawal times.

follow-up administration of large-volume IV or, more practically, oral fluids after the infusion of such hypertonic solutions.

Calcium should be administered to all multiparous cows that develop coliform mastitis because of the likelihood of clinical or subclinical hypocalcemia. In cattle with coliform mastitis that are able to stand, calcium is more safely administered subcutaneously or diluted in 5 to 20 L of IV fluids. Cattle that are recumbent may require careful and slow IV administration.

Antihistamine therapy also is controversial. Many authors comment that no true indication exists for the use of antihistamines, but some experimental studies confirm the presence of increased concentrations of histamines in the milk of cattle with coliform mastitis. These studies have been taken to indicate the potential therapeutic benefits of antihistamine therapy in coliform-infected cattle. Nursing procedures include packing the quarter in ice or snow and application of an udder support. Cows with persistent anorexia may require repeated treatment with IV or oral fluid supplementation, rumen transfaunations and feeding of slurries with alfalfa pellets, rumen bypass fats, and probiotics to reestablish rumen function.

Blanket implementation of a single protocol for treatment of coliform mastitis in dairy cattle seems futile because of varying economic factors, differences among cows with respect to clinical severity, availability of approved drugs, intended future use of the patient, and past experiences of the attending veterinarian. Therapeutic guidelines are offered in Tables 8.1 and 8.2 and Box 8.2. Culture and antibiotic sensitivity testing should be completed in all cases.

TABLE 8.3 Food and Drug Administration–Approved Antibiotics for Intramammary Use in Non-lactating Dairy Cattle

Active Ingredient	Drug Type	Milk Withholding Time	Meat Withholding Time (days)	Product Name	Manufacturer or Marketer
Ceftiofur hydrochloride	Rx	None*	16	Spectramast DC	Zoetis, Inc
Cephapirin	OTC	72 hours	42	Tomorrow	Boehringer Ingelheim Vetmedica, Inc.
Cloxacillin	Rx	None	30	Dry-Clox	Boehringer Ingelheim Vetmedica, Inc.
Cloxacillin	Rx	None*	28	Orbenin-DC	Merck Animal Health
Penicillin G	OTC	72 hours post-calving	14	Hanfords	G.C. Hanford Mfg. Co.
Penicillin G/Novobiocin	OTC	72 hours post-calving	30	Alba Dry Plus	Zoetis, Inc.

OTC, Over the counter; *Rx,* prescription.
*Do not use with in 28 days of calving.

• BOX 8.2 Recommended Guidelines for Therapy for Cattle Having Coliform Mastitis*

Treatment for Coliform Mastitis with Minimal Systemic Signs

1. Strip out quarter q6hrs for first day ± oxytocin before stripping.
2. Administer calcium SC.
3. If antibiotics are to be administered, intramammary therapy after the first and last milkout of the day can be performed.
4. If there is improvement in 24 hours, continue 1 and 3 or administer an approved intramammary antibiotic twice daily for six to eight total treatments. (The decision as to milk out frequently or treat quarters twice daily will be made based on how much secretion is obtained via frequent stripping. If secretion is obtained with each stripping, it is beneficial to continue four times/day strippings and treat with intramammary antibiotics at night. If little or no secretion is obtained because of agalactia, twice-daily treatment after milking-time stripping is indicated.)

Treatment for Coliform Mastitis with Moderate Systemic Signs

1. Strip out quarter q6hrs ± oxytocin before stripping.
2. Administer flunixin 0.3 mg/kg IV three times daily.
3. Administer calcium SC.
4. Assess and correct hydration deficits.
5. Administer intramammary therapy as above.
6. Systemic antibiotics; the systemic drug should be the same drug as used intramammary or one that attains good distribution to the udder after systemic administration.
7. If there is improvement within 24 hours, continue stripping as well as intramammary and systemic antibiotics for at least 3 days.

Treatment for Coliform Mastitis with Severe Systemic Signs and Endotoxemia

1. Strip out quarter after oxytocin injection, repeat, but no more than q6hrs.
2. Administer flunixin 1.0 mg/kg once daily IV.
3. Administer calcium SC if standing or very slowly IV if recumbent.
4. Administer 20 to 40 L of balanced IV fluids, or 2 to 3 L of hypertonic saline followed by at least 10 gallons of oral electrolytes either voluntarily or by orogastric tube, and consider submission of blood acid–base and electrolytes to guide fluid therapy.
5. Administer intramammary antibiotics as discussed previously.
6. Administer systemic antibiotics as discussed previously.
7. Consider ancillary drugs such as antihistamines, intramammary corticosteroids, or dexamethasone 30 mg IM (once only; do not use in late pregnancy).
8. Continue to address fluid needs and consider feeding via stomach tube twice daily.

Treatment for Chronic or Intermittent Coliform Mastitis with Minimal Systemic Signs

1. After completion of culture and antibiotic sensitivity results, treat quarter for at least eight consecutive times after milking or select appropriate dry cow formulation to treat when dry.

IM, Intramuscular; *IV,* intravenous; *SC,* subcutaneous.
*Antibiotic usage should be considered as ancillary to the other suggested treatments.

Prevention

Other than implementation of good milking management and the provision of a hygienic, clean environment, no reliable specific prevention for coliform mastitis currently exists. However, attempts at prevention of the disease or at least a reduction of severity in the clinical endotoxemia through the use of *E. coli* J-5 vaccine is indicated. Currently, the J-5 strain of *E. coli*, which is an R-mutant strain possessing core antigens similar to other coliform organisms, has been shown to be effective in decreasing severe disease due to coliform infections in cattle. Briefly, an *E. coli* J-5 bacterin has been used to immunize dairy cattle and has resulted in a decreased incidence of coliform mastitis in vaccinates versus controls in study herds. Use of J-5 bacterin has also been shown to be of economic benefit in well-managed herds. The vaccine is licensed for administration to dairy cattle at 7 and 8 months of gestation and then a third time around 2 weeks postpartum. Regardless of the efficacy of the J-5 vaccine, bacterins must not be used as an excuse for poor management or dirty conditions. No vaccine can counteract overwhelming environmental contamination or poor milking procedures.

Other Gram-Negative Bacterial Causes
Etiology

Pseudomonas spp. and *Serratia* spp. occasionally cause mastitis in dairy cattle. Infections may be epidemic, sporadic, or endemic within a herd. Epidemics of *Pseudomonas* mastitis have been associated with contaminated wash hoses and water supplies in milking parlors. Water tanks, hoses, and pipeline connectors should be suspected as harboring *Pseudomonas* spp. whenever cases of this type of mastitis are diagnosed. Antibiotics or sublethal concentrations of sanitizers may allow proliferation of *Pseudomonas* spp. or the development of resistant strains phenotypically expressing glycocalyx or slime. Contaminated udder infusion vials, cannulas, or syringes, are other common sources of *Pseudomonas* spp. Filthy environments and lack of udder preparation may predispose to mastitis due to *Pseudomonas* spp. as well.

Although sporadic infection from *Pseudomonas* spp. is possible because of poor management and milking procedures, herd epidemics usually have a point source that is often linked to contaminated water sources used in sanitizing milking systems or contaminated teat dip.

Serratia spp., another opportunistic environmental pathogen, may also survive in chlorhexidine digluconate and quaternary ammonia products. The organism does not survive in recommended concentrations of iodine or chlorhexidine acetate. Contaminated dipper cups, spray bottles, transfer jugs, teat dip drum pumps, infusion devices, and intramammary infusions are all potential sources of *Serratia* infection.

Signs

Pseudomonas spp. cause acute, necrotizing, endotoxic mastitis. The affected quarter remains very hard, swollen, and warm. The secretion is serum-like or blood tinged and often contains clots. After initial infection, the quarter may remain hard and agalactic or may improve somewhat but remains clinically abnormal with clots or pus in the secretion. Chronic mastitis with intermittent clinical flareups or subclinical infection is also possible. Somatic cell values are elevated during herd outbreaks.

Serratia liquefaciens and *Serratia marcescens* cause a chronic subclinical or clinical mastitis that has no unique signs. Secretion tends to be serous with clots. A high SCC and several new IMIs may be the only suggestive finding on an affected farm. Persistent infection is likely after *Serratia* spp. have colonized the mammary gland.

Diagnosis

Both *Pseudomonas* spp. and *Serratia* spp. require culture for confirmation because signs are nonspecific. Environmental samples and samples from milking equipment (e.g., teat dip cups, wash hoses) should be cultured after these organisms have been identified from clinical cases in a herd.

Treatment

Treatment of *Pseudomonas* spp. infection rarely is successful because of tissue necrosis within the gland, the resistance of the bacterium to many antimicrobials, the tendency of the organism to spread septicemically, and the difficulty in penetrating the udder by effective antimicrobials. Chronic infections may appear to improve clinically, but infected cattle usually shed *Pseudomonas* spp. for the remainder of their lives. Treatment of a valuable cow should be based on results of culture and sensitivity tests because of the frequent antibiotic resistance associated with the organism. Sterilization of a *Pseudomonas*-infected quarter is unlikely even with large doses of antimicrobials. When obvious chronic mastitis or agalactia is present, affected cattle should be culled.

Treatment of *Serratia* spp. should also be based on culture and sensitivity results for cows deemed valuable enough to treat. Because mastitis resulting from *Serratia* spp. tends to be chronic, treatment should be intense and continue for several consecutive days to yield the best chance of success. Many cows appear to spontaneously resolve the infection. Cows that remain culture positive after treatment should receive an appropriate intramammary dry treatment medication at dryoff. Therapy and prevention must also address the source of infection in endemic situations. An epidemiologic investigation and cultures from possible fomites should be completed.

Pasteurella spp. or *Mannheimia* spp.

Pasteurella spp. and *Mannheimia* spp. are gram-negative bacteria that are normal inhabitants of the respiratory tract yet capable of occasionally causing acute or chronic mastitis in individual animals. How these pathogens spread to an intramammary location is unknown. Typical clinical signs of mastitis are production of a thick, creamy, yellow secretion with foul odor. Although *Pasteurella* spp. and *Mannheimia* spp, appear susceptible to many antibiotics in vitro, infected animals respond poorly to intramammary or systemic antibiotics. Infected animals may require culling or the infected quarter may need to be sterilized.

Yeast Mastitis
Etiology

Yeast mastitis is most commonly caused by *Candida* spp. This yeast typically infects the mammary gland iatrogenically through contaminated infusion cannulas, syringes, or multidose mammary infusion solutions. Yeast mastitis almost always is secondary to a primary acute bacterial mastitis that required treatment by the owner. Persistent swelling of the gland and abnormal secretion finally force the owner to seek veterinary advice.

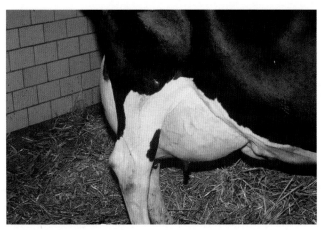

• **Fig. 8.52** Swollen udder on a cow with yeast mastitis in all four glands.

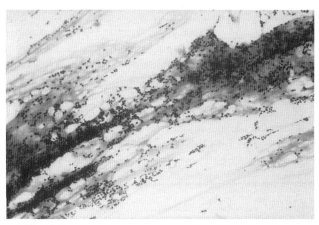

• **Fig. 8.53** Gram stain of milk culture from the cow in Fig. 8.52.

Yeast grows very well in the presence of some antibiotics. Therefore continued use of antibiotics or combinations of antibiotics by the owner in an effort to cure this "resistant" infection only serves to perpetuate the yeast infection. Corticosteroids worsen the condition. Yeasts reside on the mucosal lining and cause inflammation from this location.

Signs

Yeast infections produce a diffusely swollen, dough-like quarter. The affected cow may have fever (103.0° to 106.0°F [39.44° to 41.11°C]) but does not appear severely depressed or endotoxic. Cows with high fever may be depressed and partially anorectic, but the majority of infected animals remain alert and appetent. Invariably, the owner of a cow with yeast mastitis relays a history of chronic mastitis (1–3 weeks' duration) that has not responded to therapy with a variety of intramammary antimicrobials, sometimes mixed with a corticosteroid. The degree of swelling in yeast-infected quarters varies but is often dramatic (Fig. 8.52). Edema and moderate inflammation create the doughy consistency. Because the glandular parenchyma is not infected, the quarter seldom feels "hard." The secretion varies from almost normal milk that is slightly watery to one with clots or flakes. The secretion from an infected gland may change appearance from day to day.

Diagnosis

The chronic history, appearance of the infected gland, and good systemic condition of the affected cow suggest the diagnosis. A stained smear of milk from the quarter or culture provides definitive diagnosis (Fig. 8.53).

Treatment

Spontaneous cure will occur in most cows affected with yeast mastitis if all antibiotic therapy is stopped and the affected quarters are milked out four or more times daily. However, resolution of the infection usually takes 2 to 6 weeks. Despite the likelihood of spontaneous cures, owners need reassurance of success to resist the temptation to try yet another antibiotic over such a lengthy time period. A variety of antifungal or anti-yeast preparations have been used to treat yeast mastitis. Antifungal medications and iodine in ether preparations have been used historically, but most of these treatments are now illegal. It is difficult to scientifically evaluate success of any therapy because of the high rate of spontaneous cure.

Prevention should be addressed whenever yeast mastitis is diagnosed. Although most cases are sporadic, endemic incidence has been observed as a result of contaminated multidose mastitis formulations. Client education is essential whenever iatrogenic problems occur as a result of intramammary therapy.

Other Yeast and Fungal Agents

Aspergillus spp. and other opportunistic fungi can gain access to the udder through the same mechanisms as *Candida*. Severe, potentially fatal mastitis has been documented in association with *Trichophyton beigelii* in the United States. *Nocardia*, a partially acid-fast, zoonotic bacterium, has also been isolated rarely from cattle. Little is known regarding the likelihood of spontaneous cure, treatment, or prognosis with these organisms. Culture is essential for definitive diagnosis. Cows with hard quarters and persistent fever should have the gland killed if it is desirable for the cow to stay in the herd.

Cryptococcus neoformans has been reported to cause mastitis and represents a public health risk if contaminated raw milk is consumed.

Prototheca spp.

Prototheca spp. are algae, assigned to the genus *Prototheca*, family Chlorelaceae. They are ubiquitous in nature, living predominantly in aqueous environments containing decomposing plant material. Within the known *Prototheca* spp., only *P. zopfii* (type 2), *P. wickerhamii*, and *P. blaschkeae* have been associated with disease in humans and animals. In veterinary medicine, *P. zopfii* is reported as the most common cause of *Prototheca* mastitis. Until recently, the genus *Prototheca* was considered a rare pathogen in dairy cattle and only associated with infection in the presence of certain predisposing factors, such as poor environmental conditions and insufficient milking hygiene; however, cases of clinical and chronic mastitis are increasingly recognized, and mastitis caused by *Prototheca* is becoming endemic worldwide. Bovine IMIs are most frequently caused by *P. zopfii* infection, but *P. wickerhamii* infection is occasionally seen. *Prototheca* spp. IMI due to either *P. zopfii* or *P. wickerhamii* appears to be more common in water buffalo herds. Almost all *Prototheca* isolates from bovine milk in Europe and Asia belong to *P. zopfii* genotype 2, suggesting that it is the principal causative agent in *Bos taurus*. However, others have also reported the involvement of *P. blaschkeae* in bovine mastitis cases.

Diagnosis

The diagnosis of *Prototheca* spp. mastitis is typically based on morphologic characteristics on culture media. The use of specialized *Prototheca* isolation media has been shown to improve the chances of positively identifying *Prototheca* in milk samples. Wet mounts and smears stained with Gram or methylene blue will quickly confirm the diagnosis. Molecular methods (PCR) are available to confirm the species and genotype if necessary. When evaluating environmental samples the ability to differentiate type 1 and type 2 *P. zopfii* is helpful because type 1 *P. zopfii* is not considered to be an important mastitis pathogen and the clinical relevance of it being isolated should therefore be downplayed. Strain typing of *Prototheca* is accomplished through PCR technology.

Roesler et al found that because *P. zopfii* infection induces a specific local and systemic antibody response, serologic examination can be used to identify both acutely and chronically infected animals as well as intermittent shedders. They found that 14.8% of infected cows could be identified as *Prototheca* positive by enzyme-linked immunosorbent assay (ELISA) (serum or milk) as many as 6 months before they first tested positive by culture. Presently, there are no commercially available ELISA tests for *Prototheca* spp. in the United States, but it has been suggested that a combination of milk culture and ELISA testing could enhance the identification of infected cows and reduce the time necessary for effective elimination of the infection on farm.

Signs

Clinical signs of *Prototheca* spp. infection range from a merely watery appearance to the milk without glandular changes to palpable swelling, edema, and firmness of the affected quarters. Asymptomatic subclinical infections also exist.

Pathogenesis and Risk Factors

After these organisms have gained access to the mammary gland, *Prototheca* spp. invade both macrophages and glandular udder tissue, creating a chronic granulomatous lesion.

These organisms are ubiquitous in nature, often found in many locations in a dairy farm environment, including water, manure, bedding, forages, and other locations associated with high moisture levels and decaying organic matter. *Prototheca* spp. organisms have been found in the feces of many species of animals, including dairy cattle, cats, rats, and swine. About 20% to 70% of fecal samples from dairy cattle without a history of *Prototheca* mastitis have been found to contain *Prototheca* spp.

Prototheca spp. were originally classified as environmental, opportunistic mastitis pathogens. However, after a critical number of infections has been established in a herd, cow-to-cow transmission during milking becomes the dominant means by which new IMIs occur. The presence of *Prototheca* organisms in the claw and liners after milking an infected cow has been demonstrated, thereby increasing the risk for infection in the next cow to be milked with that unit. In one outbreak in which infected cows were housed in a hospital pen, it was determined that *Prototheca* infection risk increased for any individual cow once she entered the hospital pen. Regardless of what other infection prompted a cow to enter the hospital pen, individuals were emerging from that location with new *Prototheca* infections.

The presence of healthy, subclinically infected cows is common in endemic herds and those experiencing outbreaks of *Prototheca* mastitis. In one study of a large confinement herd in Germany involving 248 infected cows, 74% of the cows identified with *Prototheca* infections had clinical signs of mastitis; 80 cows were identified as infected from a whole-herd survey but without a history of clinical mastitis. A total of 27% of the cows were infected in more than one quarter.

Prototheca mastitis can be especially problematic and endemic on farms located in tropical areas. Increased prevalence of infection is seen during periods of warm weather and heavy rainfall. Farms in northern climes may see an increased number of clinical cases in the summer and fall months. Herds using recycled sand as bedding that is washed with effluent from a lagoon have been shown to be at greater risk for outbreaks of *Prototheca* mastitis.

In a recent study in Ontario, Canada, the final logistic regression model for herd-level risk factors included use of intramammary injections of a non-intramammary drug; the number of different injectable antibiotic products being used; and the use of any dry cow teat sealant (external or internal). Cow-level risk factors included being in the second or greater lactation. Unsanitary or repeated intramammary infusions, antibiotic treatment, and off-label use of injectable drugs in the udder might therefore promote *Prototheca* udder infection. Risk factors identified by other researchers also included increasing parity and a history of clinical mastitis.

Treatment

There are no known effective or approved therapies for *Prototheca* mastitis. Because most infections become chronic with periodic shedding of infective organisms, recommended management includes segregation and culling of culture-positive animals.

Prevention and Control

One strategy for control includes stopping lactation in the infected quarter by infusion of an iodine solution. In one published study, cessation of lactation was successful by this means, but viable *Prototheca* organisms were still isolated from all treated quarters sampled 5 to 10 days after treatment.

SCC numbers in milk are greatly increased in animals with acute *Prototheca* spp. infections compared with chronically infected cows. The SCC of milk from chronically infected but still culture negative animals is not significantly increased. Data recently analyzed from an endemically infected herd showed that 24% of *Prototheca*-infected cows (culture positive) had linear scores below 4.0, but the remaining 76% of infected cows had a mean linear score of 5.3 (range, 4.0–9.6) at the time of diagnosis. The existence of a large portion of unidentified healthy, subclinically infected shedders in a herd complicates any herd plan to control and eliminate *Prototheca* mastitis.

Most *Prototheca* spp. infections are chronic and unresponsive to therapy. Segregation and culling of known infected cows is recommended. Herd-level infection is maintained by outwardly healthy, subclinically infected shedders. Whole-herd sampling is necessary to identify subclinically infected animals and better control cow-to-cow transmission. Because infected animals are periodic shedders, several herd samplings may be necessary to reduce infection risk to an acceptable level. Environmental sampling may be helpful in identifying the initial source of infection.

Corynebacterium bovis

Considered a minor mastitis pathogen, *Corynebacterium bovis* may be cultured from individual quarters and composite milk samples when milking procedures are poor. The organism has been shown to colonize teat skin and the streak or teat canal and may spread from animal to animal during milking. True infections of the mammary gland are rare, but SCCs can be slightly elevated. Isolation of *C. bovis* from milk cultures typically indicates poor teat dipping procedures or products. Effective teat dipping, coupled with dry cow therapy, should correct the problem.

Gram-Positive Bacillus spp.

Many gram-positive *Bacillus* spp. may be found in soil, water, dust, air, manure, wounds, and abscesses. Most species are considered commensal and nonpathogenic. *Bacillus* spp. are often contaminants in bulk tank and individual animal milk samples because of poor aseptic sampling technique. True IMIs often result from improper treatment technique, contaminated treatment materials, and improper teat end sanitation before intramammary treatment. Although mastitis caused by these organisms is infrequent, herd outbreaks have occurred, and some cases have been fatal.

Bacillus cereus

Although rare, *Bacillus cereus* has been linked to severe, gangrenous, toxic mastitis (see also Chapter 7). When introduced to the mammary gland, this environmental pathogen causes acute hemorrhagic necrosis of the mammary gland, toxemia, and death. As a contaminant of the bulk tank, sporulation of *B. cereus* during pasteurization can lead to decreased shelf life and spoilage of dairy products.

Clostridium perfringens Type A

Clostridium perfringens type A is a rare cause of gangrenous mastitis in first-calf heifers. Affected heifers are acutely ill from septicemia, and the udder is discolored and has a crepitant feel because of gas production by the organism. It should be noted that gas in the udder is not pathognomonic for *C. perfringens* because other causes of gangrenous mastitis, including *S. aureus*, *Pseudomonas aeruginosa*, *Corynebacterium* spp., *B. cereus*, and *T. pyogenes*, can be associated with palpable gas in the udder. Additionally, some cows with coliform mastitis also have palpable gas in the udder; it is unclear if this is a superinfection with anaerobic bacteria or if it occurs from unusually frequent stripping action allowing air to enter the udder.

Diagnosis

First-calf heifers with acute gangrenous mastitis and large amounts of crepitus in the udder are likely candidates for the diagnosis. Gram stain of the milk will reveal large numbers of large gram-positive rods. Anaerobic cultures will confirm the diagnosis.

Treatment

The treatment of *Clostridium perfringens* mastitis is three pronged; administration of high levels of penicillin, both systemically and intramammary; treatment for exotoxemia and shock (fluids, flunixin); and drainage of necrotic tissue via teat removal or incision through necrotic skin and into the udder. With aggressive early treatment, the prognosis for survival is good, but future production from the affected quarter is unlikely. (See Tables 8.1 and 8.2 for available drugs and dosages.)

Causes of Mastitis Requiring Public Health Concern (Table 8.4)

Detection and Monitoring for Udder Health

Comprehensive mastitis surveillance requires a combination of cowside and laboratory tests. Although not all herds require all available tests, the veterinarian should be familiar with those tests that supplement physical examination of the udder and that may detect subclinical mastitis.

Cowside Tests

Strip Plate or Cup

A black-colored strip plate is invaluable in detecting abnormal secretions in forestrippings. Although flakes and clots may be palpable or obvious on other surfaces, subtle serum-like or watery milk can best be detected by mixing with milk

TABLE 8.4 Causes of Mastitis That Require Public Health Concern

Organism	Means of Infection of Udder	Signs	Diagnosis	Treatment and Control
Salmonella Dublin	Environmental contamination by feces of carrier cows most likely leading to septicemic spread to udder. Steroids may cause acute clinical flareup	Usually subclinical and chronic (≥6 mo). Increased somatic cell count may be present	ELISA (PrioCHECK, Thermo Fisher Scientific/Life Technologies, Grand Island, NY) performed multiple times over an 8-month period on serum or milk to detect antibodies in carrier cows. Culture/PCR of milk and feces	No specific treatment will likely cure carrier status. Detection and culling of carriers should be performed to avoid milk contamination. Prohibit drinking of raw milk
Listeria monocytogenes	Septicemic spread to udder usually occurs following fecal-oral contamination from environment	Neurologic signs. Abortions	Only diagnostic signs appear in neurologic form ("circling" disease). Culture (requires cold enrichment), PCR may be available	Prohibit drinking raw milk. Pasteurization of milk regardless of intended use
Brucella abortus	Septicemic spread to udder	Abortions	Serology. Culture	Prohibit drinking raw milk. Regulatory intervention
Staphylococcus spp.–producing enterotoxin	Contagious or environmental mastitis pathogen	Subclinical ± acute mastitis flareups. Elevated SCC	Culture. Culture of bulk tank raw milk	Inadequate refrigeration or prolonged storage should be avoided. Pasteurization essential. Do not drink raw milk
Nocardia asteroides	Contaminated intramammary multiple-dose vials, syringes, or cannulas	Acute mastitis in recently fresh cows with fever and hard quarters	Culture	Treatment seldom successful
	Environmental contamination by infected secretions	Mild or subclinical mastitis in cows further into lactation. These cows then may develop acute, severe mastitis after their next freshening or may remain chronically infected with subclinical or intermittent acute flareups. Fibrosis of the gland is progressive in most infected cattle, and some cows develop pyogranulomatous reactions in infected quarters. This may lead to fistulas or draining abscesses		Identification and culling of infected cows. Do not drink raw milk
Cryptococcus neoformans (rare)	Contaminated intramammary products	Acute mastitis and mammary lymph node enlargement. Thick gray-white secretion	Culture. Stained smears. Udder biopsy	Cull affected cows. Do not drink raw milk

ELISA, Enzyme-linked immunosorbent assay; *SCC,* somatic cell count; *PCR,* polymerase chain reaction

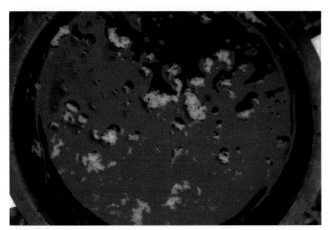

• **Fig. 8.54** Milk clots on a strip plate from a cow with mastitis. Almost any etiologic agent could cause a similar appearance to the milk. It is difficult to predict the causative agent merely from the appearance of the milk!

TABLE 8.5	Relationship of Linear Scores to Actual Somatic Cell Counts	
CMT Score	**Approximate Somatic Cell Count**
Negative	0-200,000
Trace	150,000-500,000
+1	400,000-1 million
+2	800,000-5 million
+3	>5 million
Linear Score	**Somatic Cell Count Midpoint**
0	12,500
1	25,000
2	50,000
3	100,000
4	200,000
5	400,000
6	800,000
7	1.6 million
8	3.2 million
9	6.4 million

from other quarters on a black background with surface illumination (Fig. 8.54). Large milking parlors may have black floor tiles placed strategically under the cow's udder to evaluate forestrippings for the presence of gross mastitis. The problem with this technique is that forestripped milk hitting the floor will spray or spatter, making it difficult to pool the milk as one can do by gently stripping into a strip plate. In addition, this spraying of milk may spread contagious organisms.

California Mastitis Test

The CMT qualitatively estimates the amount of DNA in milk secretions. This is useful because the concentrations of DNA and white blood cells (WBCs) in milk are directly correlated. The CMT reagent lyses the cells and gels the DNA. The degree of gel formation can be used to estimate the numbers of WBCs in the milk sample. The test is subjectively read as negative, trace, +1, +2, and +3; these scores equate well with somatic cell levels as listed in Table 8.5. The CMT is most helpful in detecting subclinical mastitis and, although accurate, serves little purpose in acute clinical mastitis.

A CMT will tend to have a high score in recently fresh cows and in cows at the end of lactation just before dry-off; in both cases it should not be over-interpreted as indicative of subclinical mastitis. A CMT is also elevated in secretions from cows whose milk production has decreased precipitously because of illness. For example, cows in peak lactation that become acutely ill as a result of traumatic reticuloperitonitis may have milk production plummet acutely. Although these cows do not have mastitis based on normal udder palpation and strip plate evaluation, the CMT result will be positive. The high CMT scores represent a failure of fluid milk production to dilute the somatic cells.

Because results of the CMT are interpreted subjectively, discrepancies may arise among evaluators, and estimates of how SCC correlates with CMT score vary greatly. Therefore the values listed in Table 8.5 are composites of several reported values for CMT scores versus SCC. Ample evidence demonstrates that loss of production correlates directly with

CMT scores. This factor may be useful when convincing owners to use mastitis detection aids. For example, production losses from quarters with CMT trace values may be 5% or more, and losses from quarters having CMT +3 values may be 25% to 50%. For herds that do not perform individual SCC on a monthly basis with a testing laboratory, the use of the CMT test can be extremely valuable in identifying cows with subclinically infected quarters that are contributing high numbers of somatic cells to the bulk tank. This information can even be entered into a spreadsheet to track individual cows and to calculate approximations for infection risk at the herd level.

pH Indicator Papers

These test strips, which are widely used in Europe, detect the more alkaline pH of milk in quarters with mastitis. Whereas normal milk has a pH of approximately 6.5 to 6.7, mastitic milk often approaches the plasma pH of 7.4.

Palpation of the Udder

Perhaps becoming a lost art, udder palpation once formed the heart of mastitis-control programs. Careful udder palpation is particularly helpful for detection of fibrosis caused by chronic subclinical contagious *S. aureus* infection. Palpation also is useful for differentiation of mastitis-related high CMT results from false-positive high CMT scores as a result of acute dry-off or systemic illness (see previous section on CMT). The palpation of a swollen gland coupled with serum-like appearance to mastitic milk are findings that suggest the cow will need to be treated for several days. Palpation also is valuable after resolution of acute clinical mastitis to detect glandular changes that may be associated with infarction, abscessation, or chronic infection.

Somatic Cell Counts

The SCC has become the most widely used indicator of mastitic infection for individual cows and within herds. Monitoring of somatic cell numbers has been simplified by automated cell counters that allow large numbers of milk samples to be evaluated quickly. Monitoring individual quarters or composite samples from all four quarters provides specific information that is helpful in making treatment and culling decisions. Monitoring bulk tank samples for SCC gives the owner and veterinarian a frequent reminder of the overall effectiveness of mastitis control in the herd.

Mastitis increases the relative proportion of neutrophils in mammary secretions to 95%. Other cell types in mastitic milk include mononuclear and sloughed alveolar epithelial cells. Economic losses are caused by reduced productivity that begins whenever the SCC reaches 50,000 cells/mL and increases with each doubling of the SCC from 50,000 up to 400,000 cells/mL. Above 400,000 cells/mL of milk, production losses continue to increase but not as dramatically as below this level. A bulk tank sample showing an SCC of 500,000 cells/mL or greater typically indicates a higher than 50% infection rate.

As regards bulk tank SCC, just a few cows with acute *S. agalactiae* mastitis may markedly elevate the total tank SCC because large numbers of neutrophils tend to be produced in acute *S. agalactiae* infection. Perhaps more dangerous is the fact that contagious *S. aureus* may be present in 50% or more of the herd before the bulk tank SCC reaches the alarm level of 500,000 cells/mL. SCCs, as discussed under CMT, tend to be higher for individual cows during the first 2 weeks and last 2 weeks of lactation and lower during peak lactation. A decrease in daily milk production of 20 lb, for example, increases the SCC because of nonspecific concentration of cells. Somatic cells tend to be higher in afternoon milkings, which undoubtedly occurs because of the shorter milking interval and lesser fluid milk dilution of sloughed epithelial cells. Therefore increased frequency of milking (three or four times/day) may slightly elevate SCC from individual cows but may benefit the herd because with increased milking frequency there is less time for new IMIs to develop. Therefore the tendency for slightly increased SCC caused by shorter milking intervals may be offset by a lesser incidence of mastitis in well-managed dairies. Other factors such as season, age of cows, and relative numbers of cows at various stages of lactation may influence SCC from bulk tanks or individual animals. Debate continues concerning the effect, if any, of aging on the SCC. Some experts state that SCC increases with age, but others argue that this just reflects increased probability of infection or the consequences of previous infection in older cattle. There is also debate about what cut-off level should be used to determine if a cow is infected, but many in the industry use a level of 200,000 cells/mL.

Because of the variation in SCC as a result of multiple factors, the linear score method was devised and is used by many dairy herd improvement (DHI) cooperatives and mastitis control services. The relationship between linear scores and SCCs is listed in Table 8.5. Whereas a linear score less than 4 indicates less than a 10% probability of infection, a linear score greater than 5 indicates a greater than 90% probability of infection with causes of contagious mastitis. Correlation between SCC and linear score is not as good for environmental pathogens, however. Linear score values can be averaged and are reported as current, average, and last year's on DHI records. When examined concurrently with culture results, linear score values are very helpful to decision making for treatment of infection, dry cow therapy, and culling. Heifers may lose an average of 200 lb of production with each linear score value of 3 or more during their first lactation. Multiparous cows may lose an average of 400 lb of production per lactation with each increase in linear score starting at 3. Goals for herds include linear scores of less than 4, and concern is amplified by any linear score of greater than 5. SCCs from all individual cows are more valuable than only bulk tank SCCs because a treated cow's milk does not enter the tank. Because of this, a high incidence of clinical mastitis could exist despite a normal bulk tank SCC. Combining the tank SCC with bacterial plate counts and cultures from the bulk tank may add more information, in particular this may reveal milking and storage problems, but information from individual cows may be essential when mastitis problems exist.

Goals for bulk tank samples include a SCC of less than 300,000 cells/mL, and ideally this figure should be no more than 200,000 cells/mL in well-managed dairies. Many herds that practice good milking techniques and hygiene, alongside effective control of contagious mastitis problems, have bulk tank SCCs of less than 100,000 cells/mL, and this level should be sought by all dairies striving for excellent milk quality. Milk with low SCCs yields cheese with superior flavor and in greater quantity. The National Conference of Interstate Milk Shipments lowered the allowable bulk tank SCC standard in the Grade "A" Pasteurized Milk Ordinance to 750,000 cells/mL from the previous level of 1 million cells/mL several years ago. Dairies are monitored by at least four bulk tank SCC tests every 6 months. If the SCC exceeds limits in three of five samples, the producer's permit for grade A milk will be suspended. In some states, sanctions will be imposed if two of the four samples have SCCs greater than 750,000 cells/mL. Individual states may further restrict SCC limits, and the trend for the future will almost certainly be a continued reduction in allowable SCC limits. Some milk cooperatives are lowering their unofficial limit to 400,000 cells/mL because of recent restrictions on milk exports to the European markets.

Electrical Conductivity

More recently, the technology to determine the electrical conductivity of milk in order to detect both clinical and subclinical mastitis has become available. These devices can be placed either in the milkline for automatic detection or else be handheld. The basic premise is that conductivity is increased in mastitic milk because of an increase in Na^+ and Cl^- concentration and a decrease in lactose and K^+ levels. The recorded conductivity value is then either compared with an established threshold value or used in combination with the data from the cow's other quarters or historical averages to determine the likelihood that an individual has mastitis. Although this detection method is being used on some dairies, the accuracy and usefulness of this diagnostic test are still being investigated.

Culturing

Bulk tank cultures may be used as an indication of specific contagious mastitis organisms such as *S. agalactiae* and *Mycoplasma* spp. or as an indicator of milking hygiene. Filthy environments, poor udder preparation, milking wet udders, and other procedural problems during milking may increase the numbers of coliforms and other environmental bacterial numbers on plate counts. Other causes of increased bacterial numbers in bulk tank samples include inadequate cooling of milk as a result of mixing or refrigeration problems and poorly sanitized equipment or pipelines.

Many different culture methods have been recommended for bulk tank milk, but probably the most important are the standard plate count (SPC), laboratory pasteurized count (LPC), *Mycoplasma* culture, coliform count, and cultures for other contagious forms of mastitis. The milk should be agitated before collecting the sample, and it should be collected by a sterile dipper into the tank rather than from the outlet valve, which might have a high concentration of environmental bacteria and yield false positive results.

Public health concerns may dictate special culture procedures for zoonotic pathogens. Bulk tank milk can be contaminated by organisms that pose a human health threat such as *Salmonella* spp. or *Listeria monocytogenes*. These organisms may be concurrently causing other bovine health problems in the herd (see Table 8.4).

Bulk tank cultures may identify high numbers of specific contagious organisms (*S. agalactiae*) and indicate a herd problem that requires individual cow cultures. *Mycoplasma* spp. and *S. aureus* may be shed intermittently in milk by a small percentage of the herd and may be detectable only after repeated cultures.

Except for cases of *S. agalactiae* and possibly mastitis due to other *Streptococcus* spp., SPCs are general indicators of milking and management problems. The SPCs do not reflect cases of coliform mastitis because the affected milk would most likely be discarded or affected animals would be agalactic because of the more serious systemic effects of the condition. Therefore high bulk tank milk coliform counts usually reflect a combination of poor hygiene, bad milking technique, refrigeration failures, or unsanitary milking equipment rather than clinical cases of coliform mastitis. Coliform counts should be well below 50 CFU/mL. Excellent SPCs should record fewer than 1000 CFU/mL milk, but counts greater than 100,000 CFU/mL cause milk to

be rejected by processing plants. Plate counts should be less than 5000 CFU/mL in well-managed herds, and counts of 10,000 CFU/mL or more warrant a complete evaluation of milking procedures and mammary health in the herd.

The LPC, which measures heat-resistant bacterial numbers in postpasteurized milk, is run by the processing dairy and may give helpful information to the farm. Bacteria that survive pasteurization are environmental contaminants from udder skin or from contaminated milking equipment, including pipelines. Biofilms on the surfaces of milking equipment make excellent incubators for pasteurization-resistant bacteria. LPCs of greater than 200 CFU/mL are most often caused by equipment cleaning problems. The preliminary incubation count (PIC), performed by holding the tank milk at 55°F for 18 hours before culturing, gives an indication of on-farm sanitation. If the PIC is three times the SPC, and the SCC is less than 250,000 CFU/mL, it would indicate a problem with milking and storage sanitation.

Individual cow (composite) or quarter samples provide the most in-depth means of monitoring herd mastitis status and provide the only clear-cut method to monitor new IMIs. Debate exists as to whether milk samples for culture should be collected before or after machine milking. Currently, the New York State Quality Milk Production Service recommends postmilking samples because fewer contaminants occur. The teats should be clean and dry. Alcohol swabs should be used to wipe the teat end carefully before and after sampling. Collection tubes should be sterile and held horizontally with the cap downward to minimize contamination by the teat end or material falling off the udder. After collection, milk should be stored at 4.0° to 5.0°C for a maximum of 24 hours until cultures are instituted. If samples need to be stored longer, freezing is recommended.

On-farm cultures of mastitis cases may be accomplished using various culture methods such as the Minnesota Easy Culture System II and the Petrifilm culture system. These on-farm culture systems and other laboratory-based programs are being successfully used by some farms to allow true pathogen-based treatment programs. This means that for mild and moderate clinical mastitis on these farms, intramammary antimicrobials are delayed for 1 day until the results of the culture are determined. At that point, the decision to treat or not treat along with the intramammary antimicrobial choice is based on the culture results.

Well-managed herds free of contagious organisms with excellent bulk tank and individual cow SCC monitoring may not need to culture as often, or as many cows, to stay abreast of current pathogens and new IMIs. Whenever contagious organisms are identified or high SCCs persist, every cow should be cultured to establish the causative organism(s), and the potential for successful lactation or dry cow therapy should be factored into all cull decisions.

Veterinarians should encourage clients to enlist the services of mastitis control experts to aid in interpreting results and institute programs to improve udder health in every herd.

Prevention and Control of Mastitis

Milking Hygiene

Milking hygiene includes the pre- and postmilking routines as well as the cleanliness of the equipment used to milk the cows. Premilking procedures may consist of predipping, dry wiping, forestripping, and cleaning or drying of the teats and teat ends. At the start of each milking or for any procedure that requires handling of the teats, all persons involved should put on latex or nitrile gloves to reduce the risk of transferring mastitis-causing organisms from one cow to the next via the milkers' hands. Gloved hands should be cleaned and disinfected when they become contaminated with milk or other organic matter. Gloves should be disinfected with a solution consisting of 50 ppm of iodine or other disinfecting solution. Torn gloves should be removed and replaced.

Premilking hygiene may include disinfecting the teats when permitted. The teats should be disinfected with an approved premilking teat dip to reduce the environmental pathogen load on the teat. Milkers should be instructed to refrain from wetting the udder during the premilking process as water with mastitis-causing organisms will flow from the udder skin down the teat into the teat cup, thus increasing the risk of an infection and increasing the bacterial count of the milk. Iodine, chlorhexidine, or chlorine dioxide as a predip is recommended. Predip should remain in contact with the teat for 30 seconds to allow for proper disinfection. Applying teat dip with a dipper cup is recommended over spraying of the teats because the sprayed dip does not always lead to uniform teat dip coverage. With proper application of teat dip, the environmental load of bacteria on the teat should be reduced significantly. Predips can be applied as a liquid or as foam; neither method has been proven to be superior to the other. An individual-use paper or cloth towel should be used to clean the barrel of the teat and the teat end. The process of cleaning the teat should focus on the teat end. Data have shown that the use of disinfectant and an individual towel removes the highest concentration of bacteria from the teats compared with cleaning the teats without a disinfectant or with a towel alone. Do not use a common towel or wash solution to clean the teats of multiple cows because this increases the risk of transferring mastitis-causing organisms such as *S. aureus* and *S. agalactiae* from cow to cow. In arid areas, it is common for cows to be sprayed with water in a wash pen. In those situations where wash pens are in use, it is important that at least 15 minutes elapse between wetting of the cow and the cow entering the parlor to allow for the excess water on the udder to dry.

Forestripping is a vital component of the premilking routine because it allows milkers to identify abnormal milk, and it also acts as a form of stimulation, leading to the release of oxytocin. Cows that have a mammary gland infection may have inflammation, swelling, redness, or a hot quarter, any of which may be identified by an astute and attentive milker during forestripping. The process of forestripping may take place before or after predipping; the timing does not appear to influence milk quality.

The use of postdips after removal of the milking unit is designed to prevent new infections caused by contagious organisms. Postdips usually contain a higher disinfectant concentration as well as emollients that are designed to keep the teats from drying and cracking. The higher disinfectant concentration is also important in controlling new environmental infections, noting that the teat end may remain open for 1 hour or more after milking. Postdip should be applied to the entire teat with a droplet forming at the teat end. Organic matter on the teat and especially the teat end rapidly inactivates teat dips, thus the importance of higher concentration postdips. Disinfecting classes of teat dips include, but are not limited to, iodine, chlorhexidine, chlorine dioxide, hydrogen peroxide, sodium hypochlorite, and quaternary ammonia. Iodine teat dips are still the most popular class of postdip with a 1% iodine concentration being common. Iodine teat dips maintain their disinfecting properties because they are created as an iodophor. Iodophors contain iodine and complexing agents in a state of equilibrium; this prevents I_2 molecules from bonding with one another. The unbound I_2 molecules are considered free iodine and disinfect the teat skin when released from the complexing agent.

Barrier dips add an additional latex or acrylic layer of protection to the teat. Barrier dips are designed to protect the teats from infection for an extended period of time compared with conventional dips. Barriers remain wetter for a longer period of time when cows return to their housing area after milking; thus, it is important that cows stay standing for close to 1 hour if barrier dips are used. Light bedding materials such as manure solids may quickly adhere to barrier dips if cows return to the housing area and promptly lie down. Barrier dips require significant physical scrubbing of the teat to remove the barrier during the premilking process.

Storage, proper mixing, and "use by" dates are all important components to keep in mind when working with teat disinfectants. More and more teat dips are mixed on farms today, and it is important to make sure that the water source is not contaminated when this is performed. The majority of teat dips manufactured today are mixed with water from a municipality; thus, contamination of the dip from water is of less concern than when well water is used. Teat disinfectants should be stored in areas that prevent freezing because the process of freezing will cause the components of the teat dip to separate. The complexing agents of a teat dip and/or the high concentration of the active ingredient in the dip may cause severe teat irritation when freezing has occurred. All teat disinfectants have "use by" dates that should be abided by because when these dates are exceeded, the disinfecting efficacy of the dip is greatly reduced.

Backflushing of the milking unit (claw and teat cups) is another form of disinfection that may reduce the spread of mastitis-causing organisms from cow to cow via the milking unit. Backflushing the milking unit with 30 to 50 ppm of iodine will reduce but not eliminate mastitis-causing organisms. The use of iodine or sodium hypochlorite as a backflush will lead to ocular irritation of the liner necessitating a shorter interval between liner changes. The cost of mechanical backflushing equipment may be prohibitive; however, manual backflush is always an option. Manual backflush is the process of taking a water hose that is treated with iodine and inserting the hose nozzle into the liner and flooding the liner and claw. This process expels milk residue from the other three liners while disinfecting the claw and liners. This process should be used after milking cows with a high SCC or when a cow with clinical mastitis is identified in the parlor.

Teat dip selection should be based on the mastitis-causing pathogens known to be present in the herd and the teat skin condition at the time. Any "diagnosed" inadequacy in premilking routine may also influence which teat dip is used. The National Mastitis Council (NMC) produces a set of protocols to follow to prove the efficacy of a teat dip and also maintains a bibliography of dips that have been tested under scientific guidelines. Therefore it is recommended that teats dips chosen for use on farm are selected from the NMC bibliography. Dairy operations that have a high incidence of contagious mastitis should focus on postdip selection, and operations with environmental mastitis issues should focus on predips.

Milking Procedures and Equipment

Recent investigations on the influence of milking procedures on milk harvest efficiency and udder health have demonstrated the importance of adequate stimulation of milk letdown and time spacing of milking procedures (prep-lag time). Studies have shown that premilking stimulation provided by forestripping, washing, and wiping of teats and the time interval required to take full advantage of oxytocin release and milk letdown are critical with respect to peak milk flows and shorter unit on time. Milk is stored as two distinct fractions in the udder. Cisternal milk is stored in the gland and teat cisterns. It accounts for only approximately 20% of stored milk but is immediately harvestable. Alveolar milk accounts for the remaining 80% of milk in the udder and requires the action of oxytocin to be harvestable in a timely manner.

Ten to 20 seconds of vigorous teat stimulation is required to stimulate the release of oxytocin from the pituitary gland. The time period from the initiation of stimulation to milk letdown is referred to as the prep-lag time. Optimal prep-lag time can be influenced by a number of factors, including parity, stage of lactation, presence of a calf, and negative stimuli that may startle or induce a flight reaction in the cow. Forestripping three squirts of milk from each teat provides the best opportunity to visually evaluate milk from each quarter and provides the necessary stimulation to induce milk letdown. It is believed that a period of 60 to 90 seconds is the optimal prep-lag time. Adequate prep-lag time can be achieved by organizing other premilking procedures, including predipping, cleaning, and drying of teats.

The dynamics of milk flow are important and can influence the development of teat-end hyperkeratosis, which is a recognized risk for new infections when these lesions become severe. Characteristics of optimal milk flow from a properly prepared cow include a rapid increase to peak flow and maintenance of a relatively uniform peak flow until milk-out is complete. The initial increase in the milk flow rate and peak flow are strongly influenced by the level of teat stimulation and prep-lag time. The decline phase of milk flow is largely an individual cow characteristic and appears not to be influenced by milking procedures.

The milk flow rate can be assessed simply by observing the flow of milk from the cow into the claw of the milking unit. The first milk to be harvested immediately after the milking unit is attached will be the cisternal milk. If adequate stimulation and prep-lag times have been provided, milk flow will be uninterrupted until all alveolar milk is harvested from the cow. If stimulation of letdown is inadequate, or prep-lag time is short, milk flow into the claw will decrease substantially or cease for a period after cisternal milk is harvested (often 1 minute or more), and letdown of alveolar milk then occurs. A more precise means of measuring milk flow from individual cows is via the use of a LactoCorder (WMB AG, Balgach, Switzerland). The milk flow graphs in Figs. 8.55 and 8.56 were generated with the LactoCorder. These graphs can provide a valuable diagnostic tool and teaching aid for milker training.

A basic understanding of the milking machine and equipment is essential when evaluating mastitis or milk quality problems on a dairy. The following information is condensed and summarized from three basic references pertaining to milking machines. Although slight differences exist, the major principles and techniques are very similar. Poorly functioning or poorly maintained milking equipment may contribute to the spread of both contagious and environmental pathogens, cause short- and long-term damage to teat ends, and create teat-end impacts secondary to large irregular vacuum fluctuations such as those that occur with liner slips. Poorly cleaned equipment may contribute to high bulk tank bacterial counts and increased postpasteurization counts.

Schematic illustrations of the open (milk) and closed (massage) phases of the two-chamber teat cup are illustrated in Fig. 8.57. The inside of the liner and teat end are under constant vacuum supplied from the short milk tube of the claw. During the open (milk) phase, the liner maintains its normal shape because vacuum is also applied between the outside of the liner and the shell in the space known as the pulsation chamber. This leads to a dilating force on the teat end, which opens the streak canal and allows milk to flow. During the closed (massage) phase, the pulsator allows atmospheric air to rush into the pulsation chamber, and the liner collapses around the teat end. This force massages the fluids that have accumulated in the teat end during the open (milk) phase back toward the base of the udder. If pulsation did not occur, application of a constant vacuum on the teat end would produce edema and blood engorgement of the teat walls and teat end. As milking progresses and the gland cistern empties, there is a gradual reduction in the slight positive pressure of the gland cistern and teat cistern. This reduces milk flow, which in turn leads to an increase in

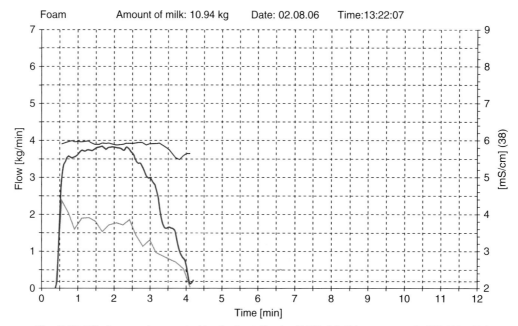

• **Fig. 8.55** Milk flow graph generated by the LactoCorder (WMP AG, Wegenstrasse 6, CH-9436, Balgach, Switzerland. http://www.lactocorder.ch). This graph demonstrates a desirable milk flow curve (Blue line). Peak milk flow is achieved within 15 to 30 seconds and is sustained uninterrupted. Milk is completely harvested in less than 4 minutes. Foam percentage (Brown line); Temperature (Red line).

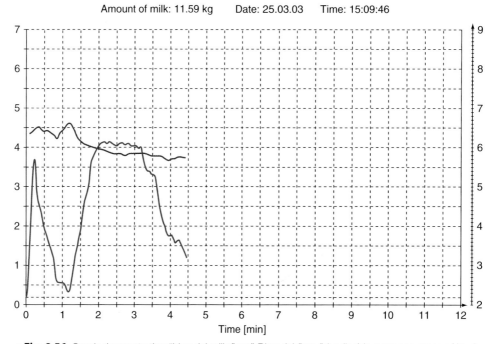

• **Fig. 8.56** Graph demonstrating "bimodal milk flow." Bimodal flow (blue line) is a consequence of inadequate stimulation of milk letdown, inadequate prep-lag time, or a combination of both issues. Bimodal milk flow results in inefficient milk harvesting by extending machine-on time. The extended machine-on time results in overmilking and excessive trauma to teat ends, which may increase teat-end hyperkeratosis and the risk for new mastitis infections.

teat-end vacuum and many times a rise in the vacuum in the mouthpiece chamber of the liner. At this point in milking, depending on the specific design of the liner, weight of the shell and claw, vacuum level, and individual characteristics of the teat, the liner may move up on the teat and lead to an obstruction of milk flow from the gland cistern into the teat cistern. When the teat is subjected to vacuum under conditions of low or no milk flow for prolonged periods of time, teat damage can occur. This is because the massage phase is less effective at reducing the congestion at this point,

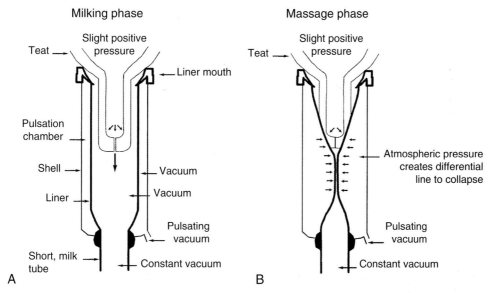

Milking phase

Massage phase

• Fig. 8.57 Schematic illustration of the milking (**A**) and massage (**B**) phases of a two-chamber teat cup milking machine.

and the force applied to the teat is greater because of the higher vacuum. Reducing the time spent in low milk flow (<1 kg/min [2.2 lb/min]) and therefore mitigating the negative effects on the teat during this period has been a major area of focus on many modern dairies. An excellent milking routine as outlined in the previous section combined with appropriate vacuum levels and automatic take-off settings can dramatically reduce the risk of damage to individual teats. Modern liners are designed with a narrower bore to help maintain a snug fit along the entire length of the teat and lessen the chances of liner slips, air leaks, and riding too high on the teat. These latter problems may occur more commonly with wide-bore liners. Proper unit alignment so that an even weight is placed on all four teats is also critical to promote even milk-out of all four quarters.

There are well-established parameters for the design and testing of milking equipment in the United States by the American Society of Agricultural Engineers (ASAE) and the NMC, and worldwide by the International Organization for Standardization (ISO). Dynamic testing during milking is the most critical component because it relates directly to the interaction of the milking equipment with the teat. Determining the average claw vacuum at peak flow for a 5- to 20-second interval on at least 10 cows gives a value that is used to determine what the system vacuum should be. This critical distinction—that the claw vacuum drives the system vacuum rather than the other way around—is a point that the veterinarian needs to be crystal clear on and reinforce when troubleshooting mastitis problems on farm. Testing the pulsator parameters with the unit on the cow and milk flowing is also recommended, at the very least, for comparative purposes with the static or dry pulsator tests (done with teat plugs and vacuum to the liner but no milk in the unit). A third dynamic test is to record the milkline vacuum over a period of time to determine if there are excessive fluctuations; if present this indicates that further diagnostic testing

is warranted. Veterinarians should encourage producers to have the milking equipment service provider perform regularly scheduled maintenance on the system and do a complete system evaluation at least once a year.

Average claw vacuums at peak flow for a 5- to 20-second interval are typically recommended to be in the range of 9.5 to 12.5 inches of Hg (32–42 kPa). The pulsation rate is normally from 55 to 62 pulsations per minute (ppm) with many farms set at 60 ppm. Pulsation ratios are listed as ratios of open (milk phase) to closed (massage phase) and can vary from 50:50 to 70:30. It is important to note that the same ratio in two different milking systems can have very different b phases (open or milk) and d phases (closed or massage); therefore, it is important to use the values from those pulsator tests specifically performed on a particular farm to determine if there is an issue. ASAE recommendations state that proportionately the b phase should be greater than 30% whilst the d phase should not be less than 15% nor less than 150 msec in duration. The more common recommendations in the U.S. dairy industry, though, are that the b phase should be greater than 45% and the d phase not less than 20%. The duration of the d phase (closed or massage) is always a compromise with too short potentially leading to not enough massage and too long potentially leading to a compressive force being placed on the teat end for an excessive period of time.

It is recommended that the milking equipment manufacturer be consulted as to the proper vacuum and pulsation settings for a given combination of claw, shell, and liner. It is further recommended that the liners should be replaced according to the manufacturer's recommendations. Worn-out liners do not function properly in terms of milking characteristics, thereby increasing the risk of mastitis. They are also difficult to clean and disinfect effectively when worn, which can increase the risk of contagious mastitis transfer and decrease milk quality because of bacterial contamination.

Excessive machine stripping (pulling down on the unit or placing an additional weight on the unit) at the end of milking should be avoided because it contributes to liner slips and large irregular vacuum fluctuations, which can both increase the risk of mastitis. At the end of milking, the vacuum should be shut off to the milking unit and then a slight time delay instituted to allow the vacuum to decay before the liners are removed from the teats.

When troubleshooting a mastitis problem, it is important to remember that there are currently thought to be three primary ways by which milking equipment is directly related to mastitis; (1) liners can facilitate the spread of contagious and environmental mastitis organisms by transferring them from cow to cow; (2) milking machines can cause teat damage if they are not properly set up and maintained; and (3) large, irregular vacuum fluctuations primarily caused by liner slips and units being kicked off can lead to teat end injury leading to a higher rate of new IMIs. In some cases, it will be necessary to consult mastitis control professionals as well as milking equipment manufacturers or their dealerships to determine if an issue exists with the milking equipment.

Teat Sealants

The use of teat sealants (e.g., bismuth subnitrite) as a component of dry cow therapy or as an "organic" alternative to intramammary infusion of antibiotics at the beginning of the dry period has become more commonplace. There is currently evidence to support a combination of teat sealant and intramammary antibiotic infusion at dry-off, particularly in cattle that have experienced late lactation mastitis during the previous lactation. Furthermore, teat sealant usage on its own at dry-off has been shown to reduce the prevalence of new IMIs in the subsequent lactation compared with non–dry-treated, unsealed controls. This offers considerable promise for producers who elect not to use antibiotic therapy at dry-off for reasons of residue avoidance.

Natural Resistance Mechanisms of the Udder

Physical Mechanisms

The streak canal (teat canal) provides the most important physical deterrent to the entry of pathogens. Keratin in the streak canal not only serves as a physical barrier that tends to block and trap bacteria but also inhibits pathogens through a chemical defense system composed of antimicrobial lipids and proteins. Bacteria attached to keratin in the teat canal may be sealed in this location by tight closure of the sphincter muscle or extruded during milking as keratin desquamates. Thinning of the keratin layer predisposes to mastitis, as does any relative dysfunction in the tight muscle tone of the teat sphincter. Because milking opens the teat canal for up to 2 hours, management procedures such as feeding cows after milking to keep them standing may lessen the chances of environmental mastitis.

Fear of excessive dilatation of the streak canal during dry cow treatment has led to research concerning the advantages of partial insertion of the dry cow infusion cannula. This technique may significantly decrease the number of new IMIs during the dry period.

As discussed in the section on staphylococcal mastitis, dirty environments, fly bites, and nursing by a group of poorly weaned calves fed mastitic milk may all play roles in teat-end colonization by staphylococci. Infection of the teat canal may lead to overt staphylococcal mastitis before or at the onset of lactation.

The udder is most susceptible to new IMIs during the early dry period before the teat canal has formed a thick keratin plug and is most resistant to new infections during the middle of the dry period.

Cellular Mechanisms

Macrophages and neutrophils along with sloughed alveolar epithelial cells constitute the majority of somatic cells in milk. Lymphocytes constitute a small fraction of these cells as well. Macrophages may be the most populous in noninflamed glands, but neutrophils predominate ($\geq$90%) in inflamed glands. After infection, neutrophils home toward the distal teat end and may migrate through the parenchyma rather than the cistern of the gland. Neutrophils work in conjunction with the keratinized teat canal defense mechanism to trap and kill bacteria before they can infect glandular tissue. Because neutrophils have a relative functional impairment in milk compared with blood, large numbers of neutrophils are necessary for an effective response to bacterial infection. This impairment of neutrophils in milk is thought to be because of a lack of opsonins, lack of an energy source, and interference with phagocytosis by casein and fat. Experimental attempts to stimulate neutrophil numbers in the mammary gland, and consequently the teat end, have used indwelling intramammary devices of various types. Plastic and polyethylene coils, either smooth or braided, and chains of small glass beads are some of the types of intramammary devices that have been used. The goal has been to produce enough neutrophils or somatic cells to prevent bacterial colonization in the milk. This is an offshoot of the research that demonstrates a reduced coliform incidence in herds or cows with high SCC because of subclinical mastitis. Controversy continues regarding the usefulness and success of these devices in preventing new IMIs, but one large field study in Israel using abraded devices showed decreased clinical mastitis and increased milk yield. Other studies have shown less dramatic results and a slightly negative production response. Research with intramammary devices will likely be ongoing. Although a high SCC is probable with such devices, the neutrophils tend to be near the teat end, and forestripping may remove a large proportion of them.

Mammary cellular defense mechanisms are altered at different stages of lactation. The SCC increases dramatically in noninfected quarters during the dry period and decreases dramatically in the peripartum period because of dilution. Macrophages predominate followed by lymphocytes and then neutrophils in noninfected dry quarters. Lymphocyte numbers and IgA concentrations may be increased in dry cow secretions and colostrum compared to normal milk.

Secretory Antibodies

Systemically derived IgG is the major antibody class in milk; IgA and IgM are in lower concentrations and are locally synthesized and transferred through the mammary epithelium. Immunoglobulins are selectively transported to the udder in the 3 weeks before freshening to concentrate in colostrum. Despite the high concentration of colostral antibodies at this time, the udder still remains susceptible to infection. As regards defense of the udder versus pathogens, antibodies primarily act non-specifically to aid opsonization of bacteria. Subclinical mastitis with a variety of typical udder pathogens does not seem to generate a sufficient immune response to eliminate most infections. Attempts at systemic and local immunization have been attempted for *S. aureus* for many years, and the results have been variable (see section on staphylococcal mastitis).

Elegant basic research and field trials support the use of the J-5 *E. coli* vaccine, a molecularly engineered vaccine that stimulates protection against lipopolysaccharide to ameliorate some of the pathophysiologic events associated with coliform mastitis. In well-managed herds that have a minimal incidence of contagious pathogens, coliform mastitis may be the predominant cause of acute mastitis. Vaccination of large numbers of dairy cattle in California during controlled studies shows that J5 bacterins significantly reduce the prevalence of coliform mastitis.

Lactoferrin and Other Soluble Factors

Lactoferrin, a whey protein, chelates iron in the presence of bicarbonate and therefore reduces iron availability for some pathogenic bacteria, particularly coliforms and most staphylococci. Conversely, streptococci require very little iron for optimal growth and hence lactoferrin is of less relevance in protecting against this genus of bacteria. Lactoferrin increases markedly in the well-involuted dry cow mammary gland and helps prevent new IMIs associated with coliform organisms during this time. Citrate is low and bicarbonate is high in the involuted gland. As parturition approaches and colostrum is secreted into the udder, lactoferrin levels are reduced, and citrate, which competes with lactoferrin for iron, is increased. Therefore more iron becomes available for bacterial growth during the late dry period, helping to partly explain the temporal susceptibility to new coliform infections at this time.

Lysozyme and lactoperoxidase are other soluble components of the defense mechanisms of the mammary gland. Cattle with low concentrations of lysozyme in milk are more prone to mastitis than cows with normal levels. Lactoperoxidase, an enzyme that is produced by mammary epithelial cells, oxidizes thiocyanate to hypothiocyanite in the presence of H_2O_2. This oxidation reaction liberates free radicals that induce bactericidal cell membrane damage.

Mammary Gland Therapy-General Comments

Mastitis is considered the most costly infectious disease of dairy cattle in the United States and throughout much of the world. It is the most common reason for administration of antimicrobials to dairy cattle. Dairy farmers spend millions of dollars on mastitis treatments annually. The financial impact of mastitis, particularly clinical cases, varies greatly depending on the infecting pathogen and the severity of the infection. Clinical mastitis in the first 30 days in milk (DIM) is estimated to cost approximately $400 per case.

Milk antibiotic residues became a prominent consumer issue in the 1990s, resulting in a significant change in the approach of many veterinarians to mastitis therapy. Before this time, the dominant approach to clinical mastitis therapy included treatment of the majority of clinical cases with intramammary antibiotics. This approach contributed to an increase in antibiotic residues in milk and resulted in greatly increased regulatory intervention and screening for antibiotic residues (specifically, the β-lactams) in milk at the milk tanker level. The residue controversy prompted many veterinarians and farmers to markedly limit their use of antibiotics in the treatment of mastitis and rely much more on supportive care. Although this approach resulted in substantially reduced treatment costs, over time, it caused an increase in chronic, subclinical infections at the herd level. The increase in subclinical infections (largely associated with increased environmental streptococcal IMIs) contributed to higher SCCs and reduced milk quality and value. It should be emphasized that efforts to reduce the incidence of residue violations through education and testing at the farm and tanker levels have been very successful. For example, the percentage of residue violations at the tanker level for 2015 was only 0.012%.

Today's consumers are still concerned about the use of antibiotics in food animals, however, the emphasis has switched to the contribution of animal agriculture to the development of antimicrobial resistance (AMR). It is estimated that 50% to 70% of treatments for clinical mastitis are unnecessary and not effective. This has led to the development of a "pathogen-based treatment" concept founded on the medications approved for use in lactating cattle (see Tables 8.1 and 8.2). This concept is focused on treating cases that are most likely to be responsive to antibiotic therapy and managing the remainder by other means. We know that some of the most common mastitis pathogens, chiefly streptococcal and CNS species, most often respond to intramammary treatment with the approved antimicrobial products currently available. Other mastitis organisms, including yeasts, *Prototheca* spp., *Mycoplasma* spp., and *T. pyogenes,* respond poorly, if at all, to intramammary or systemic therapy with antimicrobials. Most gram-negative bacilli respond poorly or not at all to antimicrobial therapy. Mild *E. coli* and *Klebsiella* spp. infections (i.e., those not showing systemic signs of disease) may have bacteriologic cure after intramammary therapy with ceftiofur; however, spontaneous cure of *E. coli* mastitis is also common within days after the initial signs of inflammation, especially in well-vaccinated herds.

Pathogen-Based Therapy

Several trials of pathogen-based treatment protocols have been presented recently. These trials produced similar

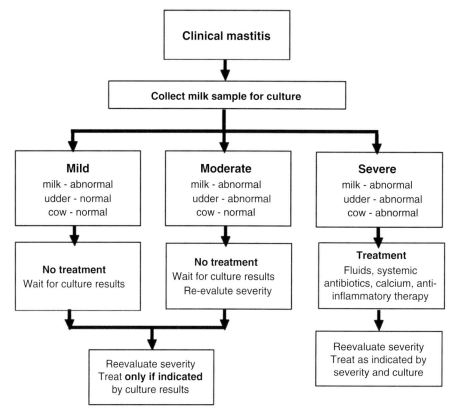

• **Fig. 8.58** Algorithm for pathogen-based mastitis management.

results. A trial in New York run on a 3500-cow herd used a randomized design for cows with a clinical severity score of 1 or 2. Cows with a clinical score of 3 were excluded from the trial. Samples were collected aseptically and submitted to the laboratory on a daily basis, and culture results were available to the farm by direct electronic upload within 24 hours of the samples being received by the laboratory. Cows were assigned to one of two groups. The first received an arbitrary blanket intramammary treatment for 5 days (compliant with the product label). The other group received no treatment for 24 hours until culture results became available. Those who were culture positive for streptococcal, staphylococcal (coagulase negative), or *Enterococcus* spp. received treatment that consisted of two intramammary infusions of sodium cephapirin twelve hours apart. Cows positive for other organisms received no treatment. Any cow with a positive result for *Prototheca, Mycoplasma, S. aureus,* or *S. agalactiae* was culled. A total of 489 clinical events were enrolled; 247 cows were assigned to the pathogen-based therapy group, and 242 cows were assigned to the blanket therapy group. A total of 164 cows in the pathogen-based group (33.5%) received no treatment, and 83 (17%) received cephapirin treatment. A total of 113 (13%) cows were not enrolled in the trial because they were classified as severity score 3 (severe clinical signs). No statistically significant differences were observed between the two groups with respect to days to clinical cure and next test day milk production. Risk for culling before 30 days after enrollment was the same for both groups, as was the risk for culling 60

days after enrollment. Days out of the bulk tank were significantly higher for the blanket therapy group (8.9 days) than for the pathogen-based therapy group (6.9 days). The cost analysis, including the cost of sample submission and laboratory fees, showed a substantial benefit to the pathogen-based treatment group of $32,287 per 1000 cows. In this herd trial, there would have been a 60% reduction in the treatment of the mild and moderate clinical cases of mastitis and a substantial reduction of antibiotic use if the pathogen-based treatment approach became the herd protocol.

There are some specific resources necessary for implementing a pathogen-based treatment protocol as described in (Fig. 8.58) on farm. The most critical requirement is the availability of a timely microbial diagnosis for the people responsible for making and implementing treatment decisions. A microbial mastitis diagnosis can be conducted at the farm by well-trained personnel. On-farm diagnostics can take a variety of forms, including a simple growth/no-growth, gram-positive/gram-negative identification, or more complex diagnostic systems that are capable of identifying treatable and non-treatable genera of pathogens. The Lago et al. trials for pathogen-based antimicrobial therapy utilized on-farm culture methods for decision making. Any on-farm diagnostic system or a practice-based mastitis diagnostic protocol should always include some sort of additional third-party laboratory confirmation or quality assurance program.

Establishing a mastitis or milk quality diagnostic service represents an opportunity for veterinary practitioners to expand services to their clients and become more involved in monitoring animal health issues and managing drug use on the farm. Veterinary practices in intensive dairy production areas have established daily courier pickup of milk samples, which can greatly simplify sample submission and the timeliness of the diagnostic process.

Easy and timely access to a reference or diagnostic laboratory is available to some practices and farms. The technology exists today to provide accurate and rapid communication of test results to the farm and veterinary practitioner, often through on-farm herd management software. In most situations, a preliminary culture result and pathogen identification can be made within 24 hours after the receipt of the sample at the laboratory. Twenty-four-hour aerobic culture results could be followed up with a 48-hour reading to note any change in test interpretation.

The other prerequisite for a pathogen-based treatment approach is a qualitative but simple system that assesses the clinical severity of the infection or inflammatory response. The following simple but effective classification system provides three categories of severity:

Mild: Signs of mastitis are limited to an abnormal appearance to the milk.
Moderate: Signs in the affected cow include abnormal appearance of milk and a painful or visibly swollen quarter(s). No other signs of systemic illness are present.
Severe: Signs include abnormal appearance of milk; a painful or visibly swollen quarter; and systemic signs of severe inflammation, which may include a fever above 103.5°F (39°C), anorexia, reduced rumen motility, and dehydration.

There may be some concern that delaying therapy until milk culture results are available for animals with mild to moderate signs of clinical mastitis will permit progression to more severe disease. However, many field observations, as well as the published clinical trials from those farms that have adopted this approach to therapy, do not support this concern. However, it is recommended that animals yet untreated be observed closely and reevaluated daily.

Severe clinical cases only represent about 10% to 15% of all mastitis cases. Animals with mastitis classified as severe need immediate therapy, which should consist of IV (hypertonic saline, 4 mL/kg) followed by oral fluids, antiinflammatory medication, and perhaps a systemic antibiotic (see Table 8.2). The primary purpose of systemic antibiotics is to lessen the likelihood of bacterial septicemia, although some antibiotic classes do also cross from the bloodstream into the udder. Antiinflammatory medication should reduce the inflammatory response by mitigating the cytokine cascade, which in turn should reduce the likelihood of bacterial septicemia and multiorgan failure.

A protocol for pathogen-based therapy can be relatively simple; however, implementation is greatly enhanced when training is provided to those responsible for detection and treatment. Fig. 8.58 graphically depicts the decision-making method.

The decision-making process in pathogen-based therapy starts when a clinical case is detected, usually in the course of milking. The cow and affected quarter are identified and the individual diverted to the hospital pen. A milk sample can be taken by the milker at the time of detection or as the cow enters the hospital pen for further evaluation; at this point the cow is assigned a severity score. The milk sample is submitted for culture according to the farm protocol. If classified as severe, therapy is started as soon as possible. If classified as mild or moderate, case management is delayed until the culture result is available. Those with a culture result of streptococcal (including *Lactococcus* spp.) or staphylococcal species (non *S. aureus*) are treated according to the farm protocol developed in concert with the veterinarian of record. Animals with a positive culture for *Mycoplasma* spp., *Prototheca* spp., and *S. aureus* should be culled. Those with other culture results, including no-growth or no detectable organisms, should not be treated with intramammary antibiotics, and cases are managed by other means, which may include culling, dry-off, "killing" the quarter, or discarding milk until the clinical signs are resolved.

The pathogens prevalent in a herd will change over time. Changes may be seasonal or associated with changes in herd management or the introduction of new animals to the herd. Routine monitoring and review of clinical cases alongside consistent pathogen speciation can ultimately contribute greatly to the udder health of the herd and present greater opportunities to intervene sooner and alter treatment protocols and case management. Fig. 8.59 demonstrates a systematic means of monitoring clinical mastitis within individual cows in the herd over time. Use of this algorithm does require that managers record individual clinical cases in a systematic fashion and maintain good records such as those provided by on-farm herd management software or dairy health improvement association (DHIA) records. The mastitis control team can establish herd-specific goals for clinical cases. An ideal goal for clinical mastitis in a herd is less than 2% of the lactating herd on a monthly basis. Evaluators can distinguish between new clinical cases or repeated cases in individual cows. In many herds, 50% of cows that have an initial clinical case of mastitis will have a repeat clinical case in the same lactation. A 30% repeat case rate is considered an acceptable level. An incidence rate of 15 new cases per 100 cows per lactation is achievable in good herds and whenever this number is exceeded further investigation is warranted. Studies suggest that at least in the United States, the average incidence for all herds is closer to 30% of all cows per lactation. Following the process in an organized manner allows the investigator to identify infection risk for both the lactating and dry periods.

Monitoring and Managing Subclinical Mastitis

Milk from subclinically infected cows is the leading cause of elevated bulk tank somatic cell counts (BMSCCs). Milk quality standards are regulated at the federal level through the Pasteurized Milk Ordinance enforced by the FDA. The

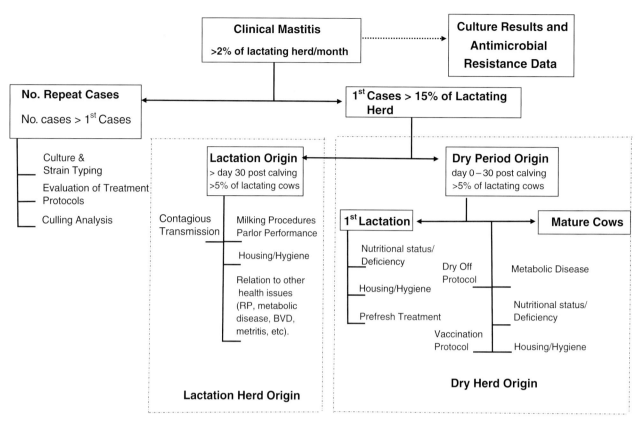

• **Fig. 8.59** Algorithm for clinical mastitis analysis.

U.S. BMSCC regulatory standard for grade A milk remains at 750,000 cells/mL. However, since January 2012, most milk processors have complied with the European standard of a geometric mean BMSCC of 400,000 cells/mL for all producers whose milk is eligible for export. Many milk processors also provide financial incentives to producers to achieve and maintain very low BMSCC (<200,000 cells/mL). Improved milk quality has value. As a result, the identification and management of cows with subclinical mastitis has become more important for maintaining a higher level of milk quality as measured by SCC.

Treatment of subclinical infections takes place at the cow level; however, the management of milk quality takes place at the herd level. A pathogen-based approach to therapy also works well for cows identified as being subclinically infected; however, identification of cows eligible for treatment is somewhat more complicated. Test day data from herds enrolled in DHI programs provide the most reliable data for identification of these individuals. Regular use of other diagnostic methods, including routine use of CMT scores, can also be used but requires additional time and labor.

Fig. 8.60 illustrates the process of managing individual cows' SCC to maintain herd-level SCC at an acceptable level. Most herds will have a small percentage of lactating cows that are contributing the greatest proportion of the BMSCC above any herd goal. Treatment of all subclinically infected cows is not recommended, and there are criteria that should be used to identify cows eligible for treatment. Treatment of cows with a new infection identified by a recent herd test is not recommended because a majority of these animals are likely to self-cure by the next monthly test. Therapy and management should focus on animals with two consecutive high linear scores (>4.0). All quarters from selected animals are evaluated with the CMT, and results are recorded. Milk from CMT-positive quarters is aseptically sampled and submitted to the laboratory. Intramammary treatment is limited to quarters infected with gram-positive pathogens (streptococci and CNS species and, in some herds, first or second lactation animals with new *S. aureus* infections). Milk from animals with no-growth or other pathogens is managed by other means, including no intervention, segregation, dry-off, or "killing" of the quarter. Cows with more than five consecutive test periods with elevated cell counts are less likely to respond to therapy, as are cows greater than third parity. Cure rates of cows with more than one infected quarter will also be significantly lower. Chronic coliform infections are very unlikely to respond to intramammary (IMM) therapy.

Dry Cow Therapy

Dry cow therapy is an important component of mastitis management (see Table 8.3). It has been a popular mastitis control method since recommendations first began in the 1960s and became widely adopted in the 1970s. The primary goal of dry cow therapy is to cure those infections that exist at dry-off. A secondary goal is to prevent new

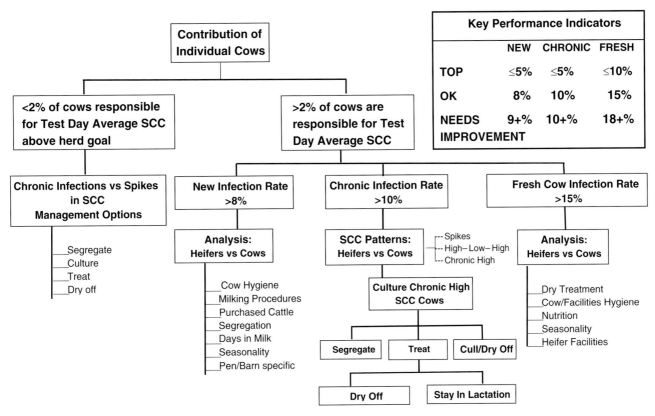

• **Fig. 8.60** Algorithm for analysis of high somatic cell count (SCC) investigations.

infections during the dry period extending into early lactation. Blanket dry cow therapy; treatment of all cows and quarters after the last milking, provides the most significant protection against new IMIs as opposed to selective treatment of cows and quarters. However, blanket therapy creates a selective pressure on pathogen populations, which can contribute to the development of antimicrobial resistance.

Blanket treatment, however, currently accounts for a significant proportion of antimicrobial use in the dairy industry, and this approach to infection control is being questioned because of its potential contribution to antimicrobial resistance (AMR). Many dairy-producing nations have been reevaluating the concept of blanket dry cow therapy in an effort to reduce antimicrobial use and the development of AMR by zoonotic pathogens to medically important drugs. Some nations have restricted dry cow therapy to only those cows with confirmed or suggested infections based on culture or elevated SCC. It is very likely in the future that efforts to reduce antimicrobial use on dairy farms both in North America and worldwide will result in greater and greater adoption of selective dry cow therapy.

Efficacy trials of various antimicrobials used for both blanket and selective dry cow therapy have shown varying results. Such variable outcomes may relate to different trials examining treatment outcomes for differing farm-specific pathogens such as *S. aureus, Klebsiella, Prototheca* spp., and other gram-negative organisms. Furthermore, studies have varied as to their definition of cure, and the

inevitable differences in other aspects of study design have contributed to the conflicting results. Broadly speaking, however, the choice of specific dry cow antibiotic does not appear to be an important variable, with no single product being demonstrated to be superior to another. The target for dry-off cure rates at the herd level should be 80% or higher. If selective dry cow therapy is chosen then this will limit the secondary goal of preventing new infections during the dry period. However, widespread adoption of internal teat sealants has improved prevention of new infections, independent of intramammary dry cow antibiotics.

Specific criteria for culling and selective therapy should be established on a farm-by-farm basis. Appropriate criteria include udder health history during the current lactation (including SCC), recent and repeated clinical mastitis episodes, and the specific pathogen(s) identified. Penicillin-resistant *S. aureus* presents a particular problem in some herds. Research has shown that animals in herds infected with penicillin-resistant *S. aureus* have a substantially lower cure rate than herds in which the majority of *S. aureus* isolates are penicillin sensitive. The lower cure rate for penicillin-resistant *S. aureus* also extends to other non-penicillin antibiotics. Culling these animals is likely a better option for effective control of *S. aureus* and milk quality at the herd level. Parity will also be an important factor in decision making as older cows (≥4th lactation) are less likely to respond to antimicrobial therapy. Additional factors affecting udder health influence the success or failure of selective dry cow therapy such as dry cow housing and management, predominant mastitis pathogens on the farm, teat condition, and nutrition and feeding management.

It is likely that blanket dry cow therapy will remain the preferred approach for most dairies until farms and veterinarians consistently have better diagnostic tests and data management methods at their disposal to allow for pathogen-based treatment methods at dry-off. Selective dry cow therapy could then be used in those herds with a low prevalence of infection at dry-off combined with a low risk of new infection during the dry period.

Obtaining effective levels of antibiotics in milk by either systemic or intramammary routes is difficult. The following discussion highlights the major points regarding antibiotic therapy for mastitis. Systemically administered antibiotics must reach the udder and be able to effect inhibitory concentrations in milk and, for many pathogens, the udder parenchyma. Appropriate systemic antibiotics must be used at effective dosages and frequency and for sufficient duration to successfully eliminate bacteria. Unfortunately, compromises often are made by veterinarians because of drug costs and expense of discarded milk, as well as fear of contaminating food products with antimicrobial residues. Intramammary antibiotics must diffuse well into the gland and must work in the presence of milk and inflammatory debris. Clinical and bacteriologic cures are not always coincident. This is especially true with organisms such as *S. aureus* where intracellular bacteria or L-forms produced subsequent to β-lactam antibiotic therapy may not grow in standard media yet may remain alive and active within mammary tissue.

The effectiveness of blood-to-milk transfer of systemic drugs depends on three factors:
1. Lipid solubility: More lipid solubility equates with better passage across biologic membranes.
2. Degree of ionization: Poorly ionized drugs enter milk better.
3. Degree of protein binding: Less protein bound equates to better transfer into milk.

In addition, the concentration gradient, which serves as a driving force for drug secretion into various tissues, is a function of a drug's total dose, frequency of administration, and rate of absorption from the administration site. The higher the dose or frequency of administration, the greater the concentration gradient pushing the drug to different areas of the body. Without question, failure to establish effective concentration gradients may be one of the most routine pitfalls in dairy cattle treated with systemic antimicrobials. As is well known to clinicians, on-farm antibiotic dosages, frequency of administration, and duration of treatment are often less than optimal in order to satisfy regulatory agencies with respect to residue avoidance.

Milk has a pH of about 6.5 versus a plasma pH of 7.4. Therefore after systemic administration, weak bases such as erythromycin and other macrolides diffuse into milk at higher concentrations than in plasma. However, when mastitis develops, the pH of milk increases and may approximate that of plasma. The higher pH reduces the concentration of erythromycin for example that diffuses into the gland.

Conversely, penicillin, amoxicillin, and ampicillin are weak acids that normally do not diffuse into the milk very well after systemic administration. Serum levels of penicillin after systemic administration may be 37 times higher than milk levels in healthy quarters but may only be 15 times higher than those in mastitic milk because of the higher pH of mastitic milk. Ampicillin may achieve serum levels eight times greater than in normal milk and six times greater than in mastitic milk. In one pharmacokinetic study ceftiofur levels in mastitic milk were demonstrated to be approximately 0.28 µg/mL compared with 1.0 µg/mL in the serum, an approximately 4-fold difference. Tetracycline, which is amphoteric, tends to be distributed equally into healthy and mastitic quarters. Although higher doses of relatively nontoxic drugs may be used to improve concentrations of certain drugs in mastitic milk, it is extremely important to adhere to regulatory requirements regarding legal drug use – for example, off-label use of third generation cephalosporins such as ceftiofur in the United States is currently prohibited.

Partitioning and ionization of alkaline drugs in fluid with pH less than their pKa or greater than the pKa in the case of acidic drugs lead to ion trapping and enhancement of antimicrobial efficacy within the udder. The site of injection into the cow may affect drug absorption and distribution as well. Sick or dehydrated cattle will not absorb non-IV administered drugs at normal rates and have prolonged tissue and milk levels because of reduced drug circulation, metabolism, and elimination.

In acute or peracute mastitis with severe edema and swelling, stripping out may not only be therapeutic but may also greatly enhance the passage of systemically administered antibiotics such as gentamicin, ticarcillin, and polymyxin B. This could be especially important because many drugs, especially the aminoglycoside antibiotics, tend to be poorly distributed to the udder. However, it is important to remember that increasing the frequency of stripping, beyond every 4-6 hours, has not been shown to confer a beneficial effect for cattle suffering from coliform mastitis.

Regarding systemic antibiotics, the previous examples of distribution represent useful information rather than specific recommendations. Because regulations controlling antibiotic usage in dairy cattle are changing constantly, some of these drugs may or may not be available for label or extralabel use in the future. In all instances, it is the veterinarian's responsibility to know what can be legally used and to know appropriate withdrawal times for saleable milk and meat.

Intramammary (local) therapy is governed by pharmacologic principles affecting distribution that should be considered. As with systemically administered drugs, intramammary antibiotics may diffuse back into plasma depending on the pKa of the drug, the pH of the milk, the degree of inflammation in the gland, and other factors. Oils added to mastitis preparations reduce the rate of distribution and inhibit drug diffusion out of the udder. Mixing of drugs with an oil vehicle is particularly effective in dry cow preparations in which aluminum monostearate or benzathine is used to delay systemic absorption of the antibiotic from the udder.

The effect of inflammatory debris on the activity of an antibiotic is a concern when intramammary treatment is chosen. Increased dosages of antibiotics may be necessary and helpful to some cows, especially those with large udders. A double or triple dose of a commercially approved mastitis treatment may be advantageous as an initial treatment for mastitis in cows with large udders but would prolong milk withdrawal times. Antibiotics in milk may also affect neutrophil function; whilst most drugs have a negative effect, enrofloxacin actually enhances neutrophil activity. Unfortunately, the latter cannot legally be administered by the intramammary route in lactating cattle in the United States.

A limited number of products are approved for lactation and dry cow therapy - these are likely to change over time. The appropriate selection and effective use of intramammary products requires extensive background information regarding the mastitis status of each herd. Periodic reevaluation of treatment strategies is aided by complete culture surveys and thorough mastitis control programs. As with systemically administered drugs, intramammary antibiotics are differentially distributed in the udder. Intramammary erythromycin, macrolides (except spectinomycin), pirlimycin, ampicillin, hetacillin, amoxicillin, novobiocin, rifampin, and fluoroquinolones have good distribution. Intramammary penicillin G, cloxacillin, cephapirin, ceftiofur, and oxytetracycline have intermediate distribution, and the aminoglycosides and polymyxin B have poor distribution. In all cases, drug distribution may be further influenced by the pH of mastitic milk (being more alkaline, and therefore closer to the pH of plasma than normal milk).

Clinical improvement after initial treatment should dictate continuation rather than discontinuation of therapy. The fact that bacteriologic cure rates are frequently lower than "clinical" cure (the cow and quarter improve, but bacteria still can be cultured intermittently from the gland, and the quarter may suffer flareups) is partly because of premature cessation of treatment. It should also be noted that there is some evidence that cure rates with drugs with in vitro sensitivity to the mastitic agent are no different than cure rates when a drug having in vitro resistance is used. This may indicate a large number of "self-cures," inflammation from the drug or vehicle providing a secondary beneficial effect, or sensitivity in vivo despite in vitro resistance.

Veterinarians are responsible for all drugs used in food-producing animals when a valid doctor–client–patient relationship exists. Although legislative and regulatory guidelines are available for approved and extra-label usage of drugs, the ultimate decision rests with the veterinarian. Recently, the American Veterinary Medical Association has supported a 10-Point Quality Assurance Program to help maintain the safety of milk and meat. Practicing veterinarians must remain informed on approved drugs and extra-label drug restrictions. Many milk residue antibiotic detection screening tests are available. Newer tests have greatly increased the sensitivity of detection of drug residues. Testing to detect infinitesimally low levels of antibiotics is illogical to rational people but not to zealots who look for reasons to condemn farming and the consumption of dairy and beef products.

Perhaps more worrying is the fact that many of the newer tests used to detect antibiotics in milk may yield false-positive results. Plasma or serum leaking into inflamed quarters because of coliform mastitis (particularly if untreated) seems to be commonly responsible for a false-positive antibiotic residue test result. Therefore cows with mastitis that have not been treated with intramammary antibiotics could show a false-positive test result, necessitating milk discard and causing significant economic losses. An inherent problem with the use of tests such as the Penzyme Milk Test, Delvo-SP, and Snap β-lactam assays is that they are intended, and have been validated, for use with comingled milk from tankers before processing for food. In field situations, these same tests are often used with milk from individual cows, and recent studies have shown that although they may demonstrate high sensitivity and specificity, they have only modest positive predictive values when assaying milk from mastitic cows that have undergone antibiotic treatment.

Stray Voltage

Stray voltage consisting of as little as a 10V potential difference has been suggested as a cause of milk letdown failure and mastitis. The relationship between mastitis and stray voltage is thought to result from cow discomfort, poor letdown because of apprehension, and incomplete milkout. Decreased production can be explained by both incomplete milkout and a decreased appetite or water consumption associated with the stray voltage. Cows apparently react to recurrent flow or amperage, although voltage may be the measured assessment.

Experimental attempts to create stray voltage and then monitor productivity and appetite have yielded varying results. When there is stray voltage, cows can be subjected to voltage potential differences between electrified water cups or milking machines and their milking platform. There are numerous causes of stray voltage, including short circuiting of electrical wiring through the milking machines, induction currents in ground through power lines, and direct voltage leaks from distant high-intensity electrical sources. Cows that are subjected to stray voltage may be reluctant to enter milking areas, may kick at milking units, or may show decreased appetite and water consumption. The economic importance of stray voltage in individual cases is controversial, however, because at least one study has not detected lowered production in dairy cattle exposed to low levels of stray voltage, but others have shown significant improvements in productivity after correction of stray voltage in the dairy barn. For example, a study that exposed cows to 1.8 V for prolonged periods found no detrimental effects on the cows.

Given the controversy concerning the economic effects of stray voltage, obvious management deficiencies contributing to mastitis or other bottlenecks of productivity should not be overlooked on problem farms. Unless the cow's behavior suggests stray voltage problems, low-level stray voltage may not be as important as other management components when mastitis problems exist in a herd.

Milk Allergy

Milk allergy is the result of an immediate autoallergic reaction in cattle that are sensitized to their own casein. Milk allergy occurs most commonly within hours of dry-off. Although observed in all major dairy breeds, the condition has the highest incidence in Jersey and Guernsey cattle. Retention of milk for any reason can also stimulate this immediate hypersensitivity. The mediator release results in variable degrees of urticaria and dyspnea. The condition may be life threatening when dyspnea caused by pulmonary or laryngeal edema develops. The condition is characterized by urticarial swellings of the eyelids, lips, vulva, and skin. Other instigating causes of milk allergy include delayed milking or "bagging" a cow for a show, sale, or photography session. The physiologic mechanisms that initiate the attack are unknown because these same cows that developed allergic disease after several hours of dry-off seem to tolerate routine 12-hour milking intervals without problems. A cow may have only one episode or may develop repeated episodes so that drying-off is impossible. A genetic basis for milk allergy is suspected.

Treatment includes immediate milkout, NSAIDs, antihistamines, and epinephrine if necessary for fulminant anaphylaxis. Corticosteroids may only be used in nonpregnant cows; pregnant animals being dried off routinely should not be treated with corticosteroids.

Teat Amputation or Mastectomy

Teat amputation is indicated when the teat canal presents a barrier to effective drainage of a severely infected mammary gland that threatens the cow's life. A decision is based on the potential value of the affected cow and is only considered when it is acceptable for the future productivity of the affected gland to be lost. Typically, severe toxic or necrotizing mastitis has caused thick clots or toothpaste-like secretions that cannot be milked out of the teat in an efficient manner. Gangrenous mastitis and clostridial mastitis are two other possible indications for teat amputation. Badly mangled teats that have sustained repeated trauma with secondary mastitis sometimes are amputated to allow salvage of the cow. It is not recommended that teats be amputated when a contagious mastitis pathogen is known to be present and there is not life-threatening illness. A teat that is leaking milk containing a known contagious mastitis organism can contribute significantly to that pathogen's load in the environment, thus increasing the risk of infectious spread to other cows.

After anesthesia of the teat, amputation is performed by first clamping a Burdizzo at its base. The proximal udder should not be damaged because of the large venous plexus present in that location. After clamping with the Burdizzo, the teat is excised with heavy serrated scissors below the emasculatome. Anesthesia of the teat is unnecessary if it is gangrenous. It is recommended that the excision be performed before releasing the emasculatome. If the teat and quarter are gangrenous, anesthesia and Burdizzo clamping before excision are not necessary.

There are also reports from field veterinarians of applying a tight elastrator band near the base of the teat to affect amputation. This may control milk leakage from the remaining stump better than teat excision but would not be the method of choice in life-threatening illness when more rapid drainage is desired.

Pain management may be indicated when teat amputation is performed. One product for the veterinarian to consider is meloxicam given orally at a dose of 50 mg per 100 lb. The prescribing veterinarian needs to provide a meat and milk withholding time for this product.

Mastectomy has been performed in some cows with chronic mammary gland disease (see description earlier in this chapter). This procedure must be performed by an experienced surgeon due to the considerable anatomic and hemostatic challenges.

Cessation of Lactation in a Single Quarter

A quarter that continues to produce grossly abnormal milk, has frequent clinical flareups that require treatment, or has chronic active necrotizing inflammation may be a candidate for cessation of the lactation process in that quarter. The two main options would be to stop milking this quarter or attempt chemical destruction of the lactiferous tissue. Simply not applying a milking machine to a quarter to cause cessation of lactation has worked successfully in some situations, especially for chronically infected quarters. The veterinarian should recommend that the quarter and cow be monitored closely for signs that the cow is becoming systemically ill. These cows should be appropriately marked and a notation made in the cow's record for future reference so that milkers do not inadvertently attach a milking unit.

Chemical destruction or "killing" of a quarter obviously requires the teat to be fully functional to hold in whatever chemical is used. Therefore amputation of the teat cannot be performed at the same time as chemical destruction. Chemical destruction of a quarter tends to be used for chronic problems that are not life threatening to the patient but require treatment, make the cow slightly ill, or could be spread to other cows. Glands chronically infected with *T. pyogenes* or *S. aureus* probably constitute the majority of cases that undergo chemical destruction. Teat amputation, on the other hand, is indicated in situations of acute or chronic life-threatening inflammation of the gland. Chemical destruction should not be considered in peracute or acute mastitis because it tends to worsen toxemia and illness associated with the primary problem. Chemical destruction has been performed with a variety of preparations over the years, all of which have met with variable success. All are infused into the quarter in sufficient volume to penetrate the entire gland; thus, a sizeable volume of chemical or chemical plus diluent may be necessary. The solution is left in the udder and, if possible, never milked out. All solutions cause inflammatory swelling, edema, and discomfort within 24 to 48 hours. However, unless the patient acts ill (inappetence, fever), the solution should not be milked out. If the cow acts ill, the quarter may be stripped out at 24 to 48 hours after instillation of the chemical. Successful chemical destruction of a gland will be indicated by progressive atrophy of the gland after the initial acute inflammatory reaction has subsided.

Intramammary administration of any of the listed compounds below does not conform to the existing FDA regulations regarding approved drug use in food-producing animals. The systemic absorption of these compounds is unknown, and several of the chemicals are proven carcinogens. For chemicals that are noncarcinogenic, valid voluntary waiting periods are still unknown; consequently, the use of any drying-off agent to a food-producing animal cannot be recommended.

Chemicals that have been used and have some published data include:

1. 120 mL of 5% povidone-iodine solution after milkout has been used to stop lactation in chronically infected *S. aureus* quarters. In one study, this was a preferable method to chlorhexidine infusion.
2. Chlorhexidine, 60 mL: There is no transference of chlorhexidine into nontreated quarters; however, the disinfectant is present in infused quarter samples for as long as 42 days. Chlorhexidine is not very effective in killing the gland and may require multiple infusions to be effective. On rare occasions, systemic adverse effects (neurologic signs) may be seen.

Use of other compounds has been reported, but most are considered illegal drug treatments, and there is no useful, published literature about their efficacy. These compounds include:

1. 100 mL of 10% formalin diluted to 500 mL with sterile saline and 30 mL of lidocaine: Infusion of as much as the quarter will hold by gravity flow has been suggested.
2. 50 to 100 cc of 3% silver nitrate solution.
3. 20 mL of 5% $CuSO_4$.
4. Acriflavine 1 g/500 mL in sterile water: Administration of 250 mL by gravity infusion.

The practicing veterinarian may obtain withdrawal information in individual farm situations from the Food Animal Residue Avoidance Databank at http://www.farad.org.

Abnormal Milk Flavor

Although not a "disease," a rancid flavor to milk can have a serious impact on consumers. Milk with a rancid flavor is soapy or bitter. Lipase activity that forms free fatty acids from milk fat continues to occur until milk is pasteurized. Intact protein membranes normally encapsulate milk fat molecules and protect the fat from enzyme activity. Conditions that interfere with or destroy protein membranes accelerate milk fat breakdown and should be avoided. S. E. Barnard of Pennsylvania State University states that

rancidity may be found in as much as 70% of regular milk bought by consumers. He lists the following potential causes of milk rancidity:

1. Lack of adequate protein in the cows' diet
2. Milking cows greater than 305 days
3. Air leaks in pipeline milkers
4. Foaming or flooding of pipelines and receivers
5. Holding raw milk more than 48 hours after collection
6. Partial or less than every-other-day collection of milk from farms
7. Failure to empty and wash raw milk storage tanks on every processing day
8. Exposure of milk to copper or oxidizing metals
9. Contamination by chlorine sanitizers or acid water
10. Exposure of milk to fluorescent lights
11. Ingestion of onions, *Helenium* (sneezeweed), or *Hymenoxys* spp. by lactating cows
12. Excessive agitation of milk in bulk tank
13. Low dietary vitamin E; feeding high levels of vegetable fats, soybeans, and cottonseed meals
14. High iron or copper content in the drinking water
15. Diets that have strong odors, such as butyrous feed stuffs
16. Diets that are low in green forage or that depress milk fat

Rancidity of milk fats may cause more than 50% of the objectionable flavors detected in retail milk. Rancidity is produced by hydrolysis of the fatty acids from the glycerol backbone of the triglyceride. The release of the fatty acids produces a "goat acid" or rancid taste to the consumer. Rancidity can be detected using the acid degree value (ADV) test, in which the short-chain fatty acids are measured. The test is recommended for use on individual farm samples rather than in tanker truck or composited creamery samples. The ADV of nonrancid, sweet-tasting milk is less than 0.8. Rancid milk usually has an ADV of 0.8 or greater.

Suggested Readings

Almeida, A., Albuquerque, P., Araujo, R., et al. (2013). Detection and discrimination of common bovine mastitis-causing streptococci. *Vet Microbiol, 164*, 370–377.

Anderson, K. L., & Walker, R. L. (1988). Sources of Prototheca spp in a dairy herd environment. *J Am Vet Med Assoc, 193*, 553–556.

Anderson, K. L., Smith, A. R., Gustafsson, B. K., et al. (1982). Diagnosis and treatment of acute mastitis in a large dairy herd. *J Am Vet Med Assoc, 181*, 690–693.

Arighi, M., Ducharme, N. G., Honey, F. D., et al. (1987). Invasive teat surgery in dairy cattle. Part II. Long-term follow-up and complications. *Can Vet J, 28*, 763–737.

Arruda, A. G., Godden, S., Rapnicki, P., et al. (2013). Randomized noninferiority clinical trial evaluating 3 commercial dry cow mastitis preparations: II. Cow health and performance in early lactation. *J Dairy Sci, 96*, 6390–6399.

Barkema, H. W., Green, M. J., Bradley, A. J., et al. (2009). Invited review: The role of contagious disease in udder health. *J Dairy Sci, 92*, 4717–4729.

Barkema, H. W., Schukken, Y. H., & Zadoks, R. N. (2006). Invited review: the role of cow, pathogen, and treatment regimen in the therapeutic success of bovine Staphylococcus aureus mastitis. *J Dairy Sci, 89*, 1877–1895.

Bayoumi, F. A., Farver, T. B., Bushnell, B., et al. (1988). Enzootic mycoplasmal mastitis in a large dairy during an eight-year period. *J Am Vet Med Assoc, 192*, 905–909.

Berry, E. A., Johnston, W. T., & Hillerton, J. E. (2003). Prophylactic effects of two selective dry cow strategies accounting for interdependence of quarter. *J Dairy Sci, 86*, 3812–3919.

Bleul, U. T., Schwantag, S. C., Bachofner, C., et al. (2005). Milk flow and udder health in cows after treatment of covered teat injuries via theloresectoscopy: 52 cases (2000-2002). *J Am Vet Med Assoc, 226*, 1119–1123.

Bloomquist, C., & Davidson, J. N. (1982). Zearalenone toxicosis in prepubertal dairy heifers. *J Am Vet Med Assoc, 180*, 164–165.

Bowman, G. L., Hueston, W. D., Boner, G. J., et al. (1986). Serratia liquefaciens mastitis in a dairy herd. *J Am Vet Med Assoc, 189*, 913–915.

Bozzo, G., Bonerba, E., Di Pinto, A., et al. (2014). Occurrence of Prototheca spp. in cow milk samples. *New Microbiol, 37*, 459–464.

Brka, M., Reinsch, N., & Kalm, E. (2002). Frequency and heritability of supernumerary teats in German Simmental and German Brown Swiss cows. *J Dairy Sci, 85*, 1881–1886.

Burvenich, C., Van Merris, V., Mehrzad, J., et al. (2003). Severity of E. coli mastitis is mainly determined by cow factors. *Vet Res, 34*, 521–564.

Bushnell, R. B. (1984). The importance of hygienic procedures in controlling mastitis. *Vet Clin North Am Large Anim Pract, 6*, 361–370.

Bushnell, R. B. (1984). Mycoplasma mastitis. *Vet Clin North Am Large Anim Pract, 6*, 301–312.

Butler, J. A., Sickles, S. A., Johanns, C. J., et al. (2000). Pasteurization of discard Mycoplasma mastitis milk used to feed calves: thermal effects on various Mycoplasma. *J Dairy Sci, 83*, 2285–2288.

Cha, E., Bar, D., Hertl, J. A., et al. (2011). The cost and management of different types of clinical mastitis in dairy cows estimated by dynamic programming. *J Dairy Sci, 94*, 4476–4487.

Chester, S. T., & Moseley, W. M. (2004). Extended ceftiofur therapy for treatment of experimentally-induced Streptococcus uberis mastitis in lactating dairy cattle. *J Dairy Sci, 87*, 3322–3329.

Clegg, S. R., Carter, S. D., Stewart, J. R., et al. (2016). Bovine ischaemic teat necrosis: a further potential role for digital dermatitis treponemes. *Vet Rec, 16*, 71–75.

Constable, P. D., & Morin, D. E. (2003). Treatment of clinical mastitis using antimicrobial susceptibility profiles for treatment decisions. *Vet Clin North Am Food Anim Pract, 19*, 139–155.

Couture, Y., & Mulon, P. Y. (2005). Procedures and surgeries of the teat. *Vet Clin North Am Food Anim Pract, 21*, 173–204.

Cullor, J. S. (1991). The Escherichia coli J5 vaccine: investigating a new tool to combat coliform mastitis. *Vet Med August*, 836–844.

Deluyker, H. A., VanOye, S. N., & Boucher, J. F. (2005). Factors affecting cure and somatic cell count after pirlimycin treatment of subclinical mastitis in lactating cows. *J Dairy Sci, 88*, 604–614.

Denamiel, G., Llorente, P., Carabella, M., et al. (2005). Anti-microbial susceptibility of Streptococcus spp. isolated from bovine mastitis in Argentina. *J Vet Med B Infect Dis Vet Public Health, 52*, 125–128.

Detilleux, J., Kastelic, J. P., & Barkema, H. W. (2015). Mediation analysis to estimate direct and indirect milk losses due to clinical mastitis in dairy cattle. *Prev Vet Med, 118*, 449–456.

Ducharme, N. G., Horney, F. D., Baird, J. D., et al. (1987). Invasive teat surgery in dairy cattle. Part I. Surgical procedures and classification of lesions. *Can Vet J, 28*, 757–762.

Edmondson, P. (2010). Blitz therapy and Streptococcus agalactiae. *Vet Rec, 166*, 342.

Erskine, R. J., Tyler, J. W., Riddell, M. G., Jr., et al. (1991). Theory, use, and realities of efficacy and food safety of antimicrobial treatment of acute coliform mastitis. *J Am Vet Med Assoc, 198*, 980–984.

Erskine, R. J., Eberhart, R. J., Hutchinson, L. J., et al. (1988). Incidence and types of clinical mastitis in dairy herds with high and low somatic cell counts. *J Am Vet Med Assoc, 192*, 761–765.

Erskine, R. J., Bartlett, P. C., VanLente, J. L., et al. (2002). Efficacy of systemic ceftiofur as a therapy for severe clinical mastitis in dairy cattle. *J Dairy Sci, 85*, 2571–2575.

Erskine, R. J., Bartlett, P. C., Johnson, G. L., 2nd., et al. (1996). Intramuscular administration of ceftiofur sodium versus intramammary infusion of penicillin/novobiocin for treatment of Streptococcus agalactiae mastitis in dairy cows. *J Am Vet Med Assoc, 205*, 258–260.

Erskine, R. J., Wilson, R. C., Tyler, J. W., et al. (1995). Ceftiofur distribution in serum and milk from clinically normal cows and cows with experimental Escherichia coli-induced mastitis. *Am J Vet Res, 56*, 481–485.

Erskine, R. J., Unflat, J. G., Eberhart, R. J., et al. (1987). Pseudomonas mastitis: difficulties in detection and elimination from contaminated wash-water systems. *J Am Vet Med Assoc, 191*, 811–815.

Erskine, R. J., Wagner, S., & DeGraves, F. J. (2003). Mastitis therapy and pharmacology. *Vet Clin North Am Food Anim Pract, 19*, 109–138.

Foret, C. J., Corbellini, C., Young, S., et al. (2005). Efficacy of two iodine teat dips based on reduction of naturally occurring new intramammary infections. *J Dairy Sci, 88*, 426–432.

Fox, L. K. (2012). Mycoplasma mastitis: causes, transmission, and control. *Vet Clin North Am Food Anim Pract, 28*, 225–237.

Fox, L. K., Kirk, J. H., & Britten, A. (2005). Mycoplasma mastitis: a review of transmission and control. *J Vet Med B Infect Dis Vet Public Health, 52*, 153–160.

Galton, D. M., Petersson, L. G., & Erb, H. N. (1986). Milk iodine residues in herds practicing iodophor premilking teat disinfection. *J Dairy Sci, 69*, 267–271.

Galton, D. M., Peterson, L. G., & Merrill, W. G. (1988). Evaluation of udder preparations on intramammary infections. *J Dairy Sci, 71*, 1417–1421.

Gibbons-Burgener, S., Kaneene, J. B., Lloyd, J. W., et al. (2001). Reliability of three bulk tank antimicrobial residue detection assays used to test individual milk samples from cows with mild clinical mastitis. *Am J Vet Res, 62*, 1716–1720.

Gioia, G., Werner, B., Nydam, D. V., et al. (2016). Validation of a Mycoplasma molecular diagnostic test and distribution of Mycoplasma species in bovine milk among New York dairy farms. *J Dairy Sci, 99*, 4668–4677.

Godden, S., Rapnicki, P., Stewart, S., et al. (2003). Effectiveness of an internal teat seal in the prevention of new intramammary infections during the dry and early-lactation periods in dairy cows when used with a dry cow intramammary antibiotic. *J Dairy Sci, 86*, 3899–3911.

Goff, J. P. (2006). Major advances in our understanding of nutritional influences on bovine health. *J Dairy Sci, 89*, 1292–1301.

González, R. N., Sears, P. M., Merrill, R. A., et al. (1992). Mastitis due to Mycoplasma in the state of New York during the period 1972–1990. *Cornell Vet, 82*, 29–40.

González, R. N., Cullor, J. S., Jasper, D. E., et al. (1989). Prevention of clinical coliform mastitis in dairy cows by a mutant Escherichia coli vaccine. *Can J Vet Res, 53*, 301–305.

Green, M. J., Green, L. E., Bradley, A. J., et al. (2005). Prevalence and associations between bacterial isolates from dry mammary glands of dairy cows. *Vet Rec, 156*, 71–77.

Grohn, Y. T., Gonzalez, R. N., Wilson, D. J., et al. (2005). Effect of pathogen-specific clinical mastitis on herd life in two New York State dairy herds. *Prev Vet Med, 71*, 105–125.

Gunderlach, Y., Kalscheuer, E., Hamman, H., et al. (2011). Risk factors associated with bacteriological cure, new infection, and incidence of clinical mastitis after dry cow therapy with three different antibiotics. *J Vet Sci, 12*, 227–233.

Hallberg, J. W., Wachowski, M., Moseley, W. M., et al. (2006). Efficacy of intramammary infusion of ceftiofur hydrochloride at drying off for treatment and prevention of bovine mastitis during the nonlactating period. *Vet Ther, 7*, 35–42.

Hemmatzadeh, F., Fatemi, A., & Amini, F. (2003). Therapeutic effects of fig tree latex on bovine papillomatosis. *J Vet Med B Infect Dis Vet Public Health, 50*, 473–476.

Hill, A. W., Shears, A. L., & Hibbitt, K. G. (1979). The pathogenesis of experimental Escherichia coli mastitis in newly calved dairy cows. *Res Vet Sci, 26*, 97–101.

Hillerton, J. E., & Berry, E. A. (2003). The management and treatment of environmental streptococcal mastitis. *Vet Clin North Am Food Anim Pract, 19*, 157–169.

Hillerton, J. E., & Kliem, K. E. (2002). Effective treatment of Streptococcus uberis clinical mastitis to minimize the use of antibiotics. *J Dairy Sci, 85*, 1009–1014.

Hillerton, J. E., Bramley, A. J., Staker, R. T., et al. (1995). Patterns of intramammary infection and clinical mastitis over a 5 year period in a closely monitored herd applying mastitic control measures. *J Dairy Res, 62*, 39–50.

Hoe, F. G., & Ruegg, P. L. (2005). Relationship between antimicrobial susceptibility of clinical mastitis pathogens and treatment outcome in cows. *J Am Vet Med Assoc, 227*, 1461–1468.

Hoeben, D., Burvenich, C., & Heyneman, R. (1997). Influence of antimicrobial agents on bactericidal activity of bovine milk polymorphonuclear leukocytes. *Vet Immunol Immunopathol, 56*, 271–282.

Hogan, J., & Smith, K. L. (2003). Coliform mastitis. *Vet Res, 34*, 507–519.

Hortet, P., & Seegers, H. (1998). Calculated milk production loss associated with elevated somatic cell counts in dairy cows: review and critical discussion. *Vet Res, 29*, 497–510.

Janett, F., Stauber, N., Schraner, E., et al. (2000). Bovine herpes mammillitis: clinical symptoms and serologic course. *Schweiz Arch Tierheilkd, 142*, 375–380.

Jarp, J., Bugge, H. P., & Larsen, S. (1989). Clinical trial of three therapeutic regimens for bovine mastitis. *Vet Rec, 124*, 630–634.

Johnson, A. P., Godden, S. M., Royster, E., et al. (2016). Randomized noninferiority study evaluating the efficacy of 2 commercial dry cow mastitis formulations. *J Dairy Sci, 99*, 593–607.

Jones, G. F., & Ward, G. E. (1990). Evaluation of systemic administration of gentamicin for treatment of coliform mastitis in cows. *J Am Vet Med Assoc, 197*, 731–735.

Jones, T. O. (2004). Correct use of intramammary treatments at drying off. *Vet Rec, 154*, 799.

Kang, J. H., Jin, J. H., & Kondo, F. (2005). False-positive outcome and drug residue in milk samples over withdrawal times. *J Dairy Sci, 88*, 908–913.

Keefe, G. (2012). Update on control of Staphylococcus aureus and Streptococcus agalactiae for management of mastitis. *Vet Clin North Am Food Anim Pract, 28*, 203–216.

Keefe, G. P. (1997). Streptococcus agalactiae mastitis: a review. *Can Vet J, 38*, 429–437.

Kessels, J. A., Cha, E., Johnson, S. K., et al. (2016). Economic comparison of common treatment protocols and J5 vaccination for clinical mastitis in dairy herds using optimized culling decisions. *J Dairy Sci, 99*, 3838–3847.

Klaas, I. C., Enevoldsen, C., Ersbøll, A. K., et al. (2005). Cow-related risk factors for milk leakage. *J Dairy Sci, 88*(1):128–36.

Knight, A. P. (2004). *Plants affecting the mammary gland. A guide to plant poisoning in North America.* Ithaca, NY: Teton NewMedia, IVIS.

Kristula, M. A., Rogers, W., Hogan, J. S., et al. (2005). Comparison of bacteria populations in clean and recycled sand used for bedding in dairy facilities. *J Dairy Sci, 88*, 4317–4325.

Lago, A., Godden, S. M., Bey, R., et al. (2011). The selective treatment of clinical mastitis based on on-farm culture results: Effects on lactation performance, including clinical mastitis recurrence, somatic cell count, milk production and cow survival. *J Dairy Sci, 94*, 4457–4467.

Lago, A., Godden, S. M., Bey, R., et al. (2011). The selective treatment of clinical mastitis based on on-farm culture results: effects on antibiotic use, milk withholding time and short term clinical and bacteriological outcomes. *J Dairy Sci, 94*, 4441–4456.

LeBlanc, S. J., Lissemore, K. D., Kelton, D. F., et al. (2006). Major advances in disease prevention in dairy cattle. *J Dairy Sci, 89*, 1267–1271.

Leininger, D. J., Roberson, J. R., Elvinger, F., et al. (2003). Evaluation of frequent milkout for treatment of cows with experimentally induced Escherichia coli mastitis. *J Am Vet Med Assoc, 222*, 63–66.

Leitner, G., Pinchasov, Y., Morag, E., et al. (2013). Immunotherapy of mastitis. *Vet Immunol Immunopathol, 153*, 209–216.

Letchworth, G. J., & Carmichael, L. E. (1984). Local tissue temperature: a critical factor in the pathogenesis of bovid herpesvirus 2. *Infect Immun, 43*, 1072–1079.

Lindeman, C. J., Portis, E., Johansen, L., et al. (2013). Susceptibility to antimicrobial agents among bovine mastitis pathogens isolated from North American dairy cattle, 2002-2010. *J Vet Diagn Invest, 25*, 581–591.

Lundberg, A., Nyman, A., Unnerstad, H., et al. (2014). Prevalence of bacterial genotypes and outcome of bovine clinical mastitis due to Streptococcus dysgalactiae and Streptococcus uberis. *Acta Vet Scand, 56*, 80–92.

Mahommod, Y. S., Mweu, M. M., Nielsen, S. S., et al. (2014). Effect of carryover and presampling procedures on the results of real-time PCR used for diagnosis of bovine intramammary infections with Streptococcus agalactiae at routine milk recordings. *Prev Vet Med, 113*, 512–521.

Makovec, J. A., & Ruegg, P. L. (2003). Characteristics of milk samples submitted for microbiological examination in Wisconsin from 1994 to 2001. *J Dairy Sci, 86*, 3466–3472.

McDermott, M. P., Erb, H. N., & Natzke, R. P. (1982). Predictability by somatic cell counts related to prevalence of intramammary infection within herds. *J Dairy Sci, 65*, 1535–1539.

McDonald, J. S., & Anderson, A. J. (1981). Experimental intramammary infection of the dairy cow with Escherichia coli during the nonlactating period. *Am J Vet Res, 42*, 229–331.

McDougall, S. (1998). Efficacy of two antibiotic treatments in curing clinical and subclinical mastitis in lactating dairy cows. *N Z Vet J, 46*, 226–232.

McDougall, S. (2003). Intramammary treatment of clinical mastitis of dairy cows with a combination of lincomycin and neomycin, or penicillin and dihydrostreptomycin. *N Z Vet J, 51*, 111–116.

McLennan, M. W., Kelly, W. R., & O'Boyle, D. (1997). Pseudomonas mastitis in a dairy herd. *Aust Vet J, 75*, 790–792.

Middleton, J. R., Timms, L. L., Bader, G. R., et al. (2005). Effect of prepartum intra-mammary treatment with pirlimycin hydrochloride on prevalence of early first-lactation mastitis in dairy heifers. *J Am Vet Med Assoc, 227*, 1969–1974.

Middleton, J. R., Hebert, V. R., Fox, L. K., et al. (2003). Elimination kinetics of chlorhexidine in milk following intramammary infusion to stop lactation in mastitic mammary gland quarters of cows. *J Am Vet Med Assoc, 222*, 1746–1749.

Millar, M., Foster, A., Bradshaw, J., et al. (2017). Embolic pneumonia in adult dairy cattle associated with udder cleft dermatitis. *Vet Rec, 180*(8):205–206.

Milne, M. H., Biggs, A. M., Barrett, D. C., et al. (2005). Treatment of persistent intramammary infections with Streptococcus uberis in dairy cows. *Vet Rec, 157*, 245–250.

Minst, K., Märtlbauer, E., Miller, T., et al. (2012). Short communication: Streptococcus species isolated from mastitis milk samples in Germany and their resistance to antimicrobial agents. *J Dairy Sci, 95*, 6957–6962.

Morin, D. E., Shanks, R. D., & McCoy, G. C. (1998). Comparison of antibiotic administration in conjunction with supportive measures versus supportive measures alone for treatment of dairy cows with clinical mastitis. *J Am Vet Med Assoc, 213*, 676–684.

Nickerson, S. C. (1985). Immune mechanisms of the bovine udder: an overview. *J Am Vet Med Assoc, 187*, 41–45.

Nickerson, S. C., & Owens, W. E. (1993). Staphylococcus aureus mastitis: reasons for treatment failures and therapeutic approaches for control. *Agri-Practice, 14*, 18–23.

Nickerson, S. C. (1987). Resistance mechanisms of the bovine udder: new implications for mastitis control at the teat end. *J Am Vet Med Assoc, 191*, 1484–1488.

Nickerson, S. C., & Pankey, J. W. (1983). Cytologic observations of the bovine teat end. *Am J Vet Res, 44*, 1433–1441.

Nielsen, P. K., Petersen, M. B., Nielsen, L. R., et al. (2015). Latent class analysis of bulk tank milk PCR and ELISA testing for herd level diagnosis of Mycoplasma bovis. *Prev Vet Med, 121*, 338–342.

Nydam, D., Virkler, P. D., Capel, M., et al. (2016). *Pathogen based treatment decisions for clinical mastitis.* Syracuse, NY: Proceedings NMC Regional Meeting.

O'Brien R. T. (2017). Over bagging in dairy show cows: an ethical crisis. *J Am Vet Med Assoc, 251*, 271–272.

Ogawa, T., Tomita, Y., Okada, M., et al. (2004). Broad-spectrum detection of papillomaviruses in bovine teat papillomas and healthy teat skin. *J Gen Virol, 85*, 2191–2197.

Oliver, S. P., Gillespie, B. E., Ivey, S. J., et al. (2004). Influence of prepartum pirlimycin hydrochloride or penicillin-novobiocin therapy on mastitis in heifers during early lactation. *J Dairy Sci, 87*, 1727–1731.

Oliver, S. P., & Matthews, K. R. (1994). Analytical review of new teat dip efficacy claims. *Bov Pract, 26*, 79–83.

Oliver, S. P., Almeida, R. A., Gillespie, B. E., et al: Efficacy of extended ceftiofur intramammary therapy for treatment of subclinical mastitis in lactating dairy cows, *J Dairy Sci* 87:2393–2400.

Oliver, S. P., Almeida, R. A., Gillespie, B. E., et al. (2003). Efficacy of extended pirlimycin therapy for treatment of experimentally induced Streptococcus uberis intramammary infections in lactating dairy cows. *Vet Ther, 4*, 299–308.

Owens, W. E., Watts, J. L., Boddie, R. L., et al. (1988). Antibiotic treatment of mastitis: comparison of intramammary and intramammary plus intramuscular therapies. *J Dairy Sci, 71*, 3143–3147.

Owens, W. E. (1988). Evaluation of antibiotics for induction of L-forms from Staphylococcus aureus strains isolated from bovine mastitis. *J Clin Microbiol, 26*, 2187–2190.

Owens, W. E., Ray, C. H., Watts, J. L., et al. (1997). Comparison of success of antibiotic therapy during lactation and results of antimicrobial susceptibility tests for bovine mastitis. *J Dairy Sci, 80*, 313–317.

Parkinson, T. J., Vermunt, J. J., & Merrall, M. (2000). Comparative efficacy of three dry-cow antibiotic formulations in spring-calving New Zealand dairy cows. *N Z Vet J, 48*, 129–135.

Persson, W. K., Bengtsson, M., & Nyman, A. K. (2014). Prevalence and risk factors for udder cleft dermatitis in dairy cattle. *J Dairy Sci, 97*, 310–318.

Phuektes, P., Mansell, P. D., Dyson, R. D., et al. (2001). Molecular epidemiology of Streptococcus uberis isolates from dairy cows with mastitis. *J Clin Microbiol, 39*, 1460–1466.

Pieper, L., Godkin, A., Roesler, U., et al. (2012). Herd characteristics and cow-level factors associated with Prototheca mastitis on dairy farms in Ontario, Canada. *J Dairy Sci, 95*, 5635–5644.

Pinzón-Sánchez, C., & Ruegg, P. L. (2011). Risk factors associated with short-term post-treatment outcomes of clinical mastitis. *J Dairy Sci, 94*, 3397–3410.

Pol, M., & Ruegg, P. L. (2007). Relationship between antimicrobial drug usage and antimicrobial susceptibility of gram-positive mastitis pathogens. *J Dairy Sci, 90*, 262–273.

Polk, C. (2001). Cows, ground surface potentials and earth resistance. *Bioelectromagnetics, 22*, 7–18.

Povey, R. C., & Osborne, A. (1969). Mammary gland neoplasia in the cow. *Pathol Vet, 6*, 502–512.

Power, E. (2003). Gangrenous mastitis in dairy herds. *Vet Rec, 153*, 791–792.

Pryor, S. M., Cursons, R. T., Williamson, J. H., et al. (2009). Experimentally induced intramammary infection with multiple strains of Streptococcus uberis. *J Dairy Sci, 92*, 5467–5475.

Punyapornwithaya, V., Fox, L. K., Hancock, D. D., et al. (2012). Time to clearance of Mycoplasma mastitis: the effect of management factors including milking time hygiene and preferential culling. *Can Vet J, 53*, 1119–1122.

Querengasser, J., Geishauser, K., Querengasser, K., et al. (2002). Comparative evaluation of SIMPL silicone implants and NIT natural teat inserts to keep the teat canal patent after surgery. *J Dairy Sci, 85*, 1732–1737.

Reed, D. E., Langpap, M. S., & Anson, M. S. (1977). Characterization of herpesviruses isolated from lactating dairy cows with mammary pustular dermatitis. *Am J Vet Res, 38*, 1631–1634.

Ricchi, M., De Cicco, C., Buzzini, P., et al. (2013). First outbreak of bovine mastitis caused by Prototheca blaschkeae. *Vet Microbiol, 162*, 997–999.

Roberson, J. R., Warnick, L. D., & Moore, G. (2004). Mild to moderate clinical mastitis: efficacy of intramammary amoxicillin, frequent milk-out, a combined intramammary amoxicillin, and frequent milk-out treatment versus no treatment. *J Dairy Sci, 87*, 583–592.

Robert, A., Seegers, H., & Bareille, N. (2006). Incidence of intramammary infections during the dry period without or with antibiotic treatment in dairy cows—a quantitative analysis of published data. *Vet Res, 37*, 25–48.

Rollin, E., Dhuyvetter, K. C., & Overton, M. W. (2015). The cost of clinical mastitis in the first 30 days of lactation: An economic modeling tool. *Prev Vet Med, 122*(3), 257–264.

Ruegg, P. L., Oliveira, L., Jin, W., et al. (2015). Phenotypic antimicrobial susceptibility and occurrence of selected resistance genes in gram-positive mastitis pathogens isolated from Wisconsin dairy cows. *J Dairy Sci, 98*, 4521–4534.

Ruegg, P. L. (2003). Investigation of mastitis problems on farms. *Vet Clin North Am Food Anim Pract, 19*, 47–74.

Sargeant, J. M., Scott, H. M., Leslie, K. E., et al. (1998). Clinical mastitis in dairy cattle in Ontario: frequency of occurrence and bacteriological isolates. *Can Vet J, 39*, 33–38.

Scherenzeel, C. G. M., Uijl, I. E. M., van Schaik, G., et al. (2011). Evaluation of the use of dry cow antibiotics in low somatic cell count cows. *J Dairy Sci, 97*, 3606–3614.

Schukken, Y. H., Bennett, G. J., & Zurakowski, M. J. (2011). Randomized clinical trial to evaluate the efficacy of a 5 day ceftiofur hydrochloride intramammary treatment on non-severe Gram negative clinical mastitis. *J Dairy Sci, 94*, 6203–6215.

Sears, P. M., González, R. N., Wilson, D. J., et al. (1993). Procedures for mastitis diagnosis and control. *Vet Clin North Am Food Anim Pract, 9*, 445–468.

Sears, P. M., Smith, B. S., English, P. B., et al. (1990). Shedding pattern of Staphylococcus aureus from bovine intramammary infections. *J Dairy Sci, 73*, 2785–2789.

Sears, P. M., Fettinger, M., & Marsh-Salin, J. (1987). Isolation of L-form variants after antibiotic treatment in Staphylococcus aureus bovine mastitis. *J Am Vet Med Assoc, 191*, 681–684.

Serieys, F., Raquet, Y., Goby, L., et al. (2005). Comparative efficacy of local and systemic antibiotic treatment in lactating cows with clinical mastitis. *J Dairy Sci, 88*, 93–99.

Shim, E. H., Shanks, R. D., Morin, D. E., et al. (2004). Milk loss and treatment costs associated with two treatment protocols for clinical mastitis in dairy cows. *J Dairy Sci, 87*, 2702–2708.

Smith, G. W., Lyman, R. L., & Anderson, K. L. (2006). Efficacy of vaccination and antimicrobial treatment to eliminate chronic intramammary Staphylococcus aureus infections in dairy cattle. *J Am Vet Med Assoc, 228*, 422–425.

Smith, G. W., Gehring, R., Craigmill, A. L., et al. (2005). Extralabel intramammary use of drugs in dairy cattle. *J Am Vet Med Assoc, 226*, 1994–1996.

Smolenski, G. A., Broadhurst, M. K., Stelwagen, K., et al. (2014). Host defence related responses in bovine milk during an experimentally induced Streptococcus uberis infection. *Proteome Sci, 12*, 19–32.

Sol, J., Sampimon, O. C., Snoep, J. J., et al. (1997). Factors associated with bacteriological cure during lactation after therapy for subclinical mastitis caused by Staphylococcus aureus. *J Dairy Sci, 80*, 2803–2808.

Steiner, A. (2017). Teat surgery. In S. L. Fubini, & N. G. Ducharme (Eds.), *Farm Animal Surgery* (2nd ed.) (pp. 485–496). St. Louis: Elsevier.

Taponen, S., Simojoki, H., Haveri, M., et al. (2006). Clinical characteristics and persistence of bovine mastitis caused by different species of coagulase-negative staphylococci identified with API or AFLP. *Vet Microbiol, 115*, 199–207.

Thornsberry, C., Marler, J. K., Watts, J. L., et al. (1993). Activity of pirlimycin against pathogens from cows with mastitis and recommendations for disk diffusion tests. *Antimicrob Agents Chemother, 37*, 1122–1126.

Tovar, C., Pearce, D., Zaragoza, J., et al. (2016). *Effect of the selective treatment of Gram-positive clinical mastitis cases versus blanket therapy.* Glendale, AZ: Proceedings NMC Annual Meeting.

Tozato, C. C., Lunardi, M., Alfieri, A. F., et al. (2013). Teat papillomatosis associated with bovine papillomavirus types 6, 7, 9, and 10 in dairy cattle from Brazil. *Braz J Microbiol, 44*, 905–909.

Tyler, J. W., Wilson, R. C., & Dowling, P. (1992). Treatment of subclinical mastitis. *Vet Clin North Am Food Anim Pract, 8*, 17–28.

Verbeke, J., Piepers, S., Supré, K., et al. (2014). Pathogen-specific incidence rate of clinical mastitis in Flemish dairy herds, severity, and association with herd hygiene. *J Dairy Sci, 97*, 6926–6934.

Waage, S., Mork, T., Roros, A., et al. (1999). Bacteria associated with clinical mastitis in dairy heifers. *J Dairy Sci, 82*, 712–719.

Waage, S., Odegaard, S. A., Lund, A., et al. (2001). Case-control study of risk factors for clinical mastitis in postpartum dairy heifers. *J Dairy Sci, 84*, 392–399.

Warnick, L. D., Nydam, D., Maciel, A., et al. (2002). Udder cleft dermatitis and sarcoptic mange in a dairy herd. *J Am Vet Med Assoc, 221*, 273–276.

Wedlock, D. N., Buddle, B. M., Williamson, J., et al. (2014). Dairy cows produce cytokine and cytotoxic T cell responses following vaccination with an antigenic fraction from Streptococcus uberis. *Vet Immunol Immunopathol, 160*, 51–60.

Wenz, J. R., Garry, F. B., Lombard, J. E., et al. (2005). Short communication: efficacy of parenteral ceftiofur for treatment of systemically mild clinical mastitis in dairy cattle. *J Dairy Sci, 88*, 3496–3499.

Wenz, J., Garry, F. B., & Barrington, G. M. (2006). Comparison of disease severity scoring systems for dairy cattle with acute coliform mastitis. *J Am Vet Med Assoc, 229*, 259–262.

Wenz, J., Barrington, G. M., Garry, F. B., et al. (2001). Bacteremia associated with naturally occurring acute coliform mastitis in dairy cows. *J Am Vet Med Assoc, 219*, 976–981.

Werner, B., Moroni, P., Gioia, G., et al. (2014). Short communication: genotypic and phenotypic identification of environmental streptococci and association of Lactococcus lactis ssp. lactis with intramammary infections among different dairy farms. *J Dairy Sci, 97*, 6964–6969.

Wilson, D. J., Gonzalez, R. N., Case, K. L., et al. (1999). Comparison of seven antibiotic treatments with no treatment for bacteriological efficacy against bovine mastitis pathogens. *J Dairy Sci, 82*, 1664–1670.

Wilson, D. J., Kirk, J. H., Walker, R. D., et al. (1990). Serratia marcescens mastitis in a dairy herd. *J Am Vet Med Assoc, 196*, 1102–1105.

Woolford, M. W., Williamson, J. H., Day, A. M., et al. (1998). The prophylactic effect of a teat sealer on bovine mastitis during the dry period and the following lactation. *N Z Vet J, 46*, 12–19.

Wraight, M. D. (2003). A comparative efficacy trial between cefuroxime and cloxacillin as intramammary treatments for clinical mastitis in lactating cows on commercial dairy farms. *N Z Vet J, 51*, 26–32.

Wraight, M. D. (2005). A comparative field trial of cephalonium and cloxacillin for dry cow therapy for mastitis in Australian dairy cows. *Aust Vet J, 83*, 103–104.

Yamagata, M., Goodger, W. J., Weaver, L., et al. (1987). The economic benefit of treating subclinical Streptococcus agalactiae mastitis in lactating cows. *J Am Vet Med Assoc, 191*, 1556–1561.

Younis, A., Krifucks, O., Fleminger, G., et al. (2005). Staphylococcus aureus leucocidin, a virulence factor in bovine mastitis. *J Dairy Res, 72*, 188–194.

Zadoks, R. N., Middleton, J. R., McDougall, S., et al. (2011). Molecular epidemiology of mastitis pathogens of dairy cattle and comparative relevance to humans. *J Mammary Gland Biol Neoplasia, 16*, 357–372.

Zadoks, R. N., Allore, H. G., Barkema, H. W., et al. (2001). Cow and quarter level risk factors for Streptococcus uberis and Staphylococcus aureus mastitis. *J Dairy Sci, 84*, 2649–2663.

Zdanowicz, M., Shelford, J. A., Tucker, C. B., et al. (2004). Bacterial populations on teat ends of dairy cows housed in free stalls and bedded with either sand or sawdust. *J Dairy Sci, 87*, 1694–1701.

Ziv, G. (1992). Treatment of peracute and acute mastitis. *Vet Clin North Am Food Anim Pract, 8*, 1–15.

9

Reproductive Diseases

ROBERT O. GILBERT

Efficient reproduction is critical for the economic success of any dairy unit. Reproductive disorders increase risk of culling and compromise welfare of dairy cows. Their treatment often involves use of antimicrobials with concomitant human health and environmental concerns. Therefore recognition, prevention, and efficient and efficacious treatment of reproductive disorders, based on the best available scientific information, are important for dairy producers and veterinary practitioners. Additionally, newer technologies that promise to enhance reproduction and genetic progress are emerging and are briefly reviewed here.

Congenital Conditions

Freemartinism

Development of the reproductive tract is compromised in about 95% of female calves born co-twin to a male. Affected calves are called "freemartins." (The origin of the term is not known.) In twin pregnancy, the chorions of both conceptuses fuse, establishing a shared circulation. Early development of the male gonad leads to production of anti-Müllerian hormone, which not only drives regression of the paramesonephric ducts (origin of the female tubular genitalia) of the male fetus but also those of his female co-twin. Later production of androgens by the male gonads contributes further to masculinization. Note that some freemartins may be born as apparent singletons after the in utero death of their male co-twin. At birth, the vulva and vestibulum of affected heifers are essentially normal; they develop from the urogenital sinus rather than the paramesonephric ducts. The clitoris may be prominent, and there is sometimes a prominent tuft of hair on the ventral vulvar commissure. Vaginal development cranial to the vestibulovaginal junction is rudimentary, as are the cervix and uterus. There are often vesicular glands (male accessory sex organs) at the level of the cervix, which may be palpated in older animals. The gonads are variable but are often ovotestes. The male twin is essentially unaffected, although there are some reports of reduced testicular size and fertility. Affected females can be recognized at birth by failure of vaginal development cranial to the vestibulovaginal junction (the area of the vestigial hymen), confirmed by gentle probing with a gloved finger, a small speculum, or an appropriately sized test tube. The diagnosis can be confirmed by karyotyping (both calves will be chimeric with XX/XY chromosomes). If the male calf is available, a blood smear may reveal "drumsticks" in some cells—small projections from nuclei, most easily seen on neutrophils, that indicate presence of two X chromosomes, proving that chimerism exists. This confirms, indirectly, the diagnosis of freemartinism in the female twin.

Segmental Aplasia of the Paramesonephric Ducts

Failure to develop may affect any part of the paramesonephric duct derivatives—the uterine tubes, uterine horns and body, cervix, or vagina. Partial or complete failure of the uterine tubes to develop completely may be difficult to diagnose unless hydrosalpinx (fluid accumulation cranial to an obstruction) develops. In the uterus, the lesion may involve a whole uterine horn or just a few millimeters of the structure. One consequence is that uterine gland secretions may accumulate proximal to a segmental lesion, resulting in a fluid-filled structure that can become secondarily infected to form an abscess. Failure of one whole uterine horn to develop (uterus unicornis) may be diagnosed as an incidental finding in cows that have had one or more successful pregnancies. Of course, conception depends on ovulation occurring from the ovary adjacent to the intact uterine horn. However, because luteolysis in cows depends on the action of prostaglandins secreted by one uterine horn having a luteolytic effect on the ipsilateral ovary, ovulation on the side of the undeveloped horn may result in a corpus luteum that persists for up to 3 months. This is a problem in herds that are bred on observed estrus without use of ovulation synchronizing drugs. This condition may be managed by checking the side of dominant follicle development and inseminating only when it occurs ipsilateral to the intact uterine horn or by prophylactic surgical removal of the ovary on the side of the aplastic uterine horn.

Failure of Fusion of the Paramesonephric Ducts

Fusion of the caudal portion of the paramesonephric ducts forms the uterine body, cervix, and (cranial) vagina. Complete failure of fusion results in uterus didelphys, a condition in which the uterine body, cervical canal, and cranial vagina are all duplicated. Pregnancy and normal birth have been reported in affected cows. More often, the duplication is partial, with a single uterine body and completely or partially duplicated cervical canal. There may be a caudal (vaginal) cervical os that ends blindly without connecting to the uterine body, adjacent to a second cervix and cervical canal that are complete. Partial or complete duplication of the cervix is often an incidental finding.

Paraovarian Cysts

Cystic remnants of the mesonephric duct system can sometimes be found in the mesosalpinx, where they may vary in size from a few mm to 20 mm or more. Large cysts can be mistaken for ovaries or ovarian structures during palpation but are generally of no functional significance. Cystic remnants of the mesonephric duct may also be found in the broad ligament of the uterus, where they are also of no consequence, or under the mucosa of the caudal vagina in a ventrolateral position, where they are known as Gartner's duct cysts. Although they may be quite prominent, they do not cause complications unless secondarily infected.

Congenital Vulvar Conditions

An abnormally small vulva as a cause of dystocia has been reported in Holstein and Jersey cows. In some cases, the vulva lips remain partially fused to each other. The more cranial tract is usually normal. In Jerseys, the condition has been seen among closely related individuals, suggesting a genetic basis.

Puberty and Breeding

Heifer rearing accounts for about 15% to 20% of the total cost of milk production. It is therefore important to feed and manage replacement heifers to achieve target body size and weight because milk yield is influenced by frame size, body weight, and age at calving. For Holstein heifers, the optimal age range at first calving (considering milk yield, reproductive performance, and herd life) seems to be 21 to 24 months.

Complications of Pregnancy

Embryonic Death

Fertilization rates in cows are generally high (≈90%), but the number of pregnancies diagnosed at 28 days or later after ovulation is much lower. The causes of early embryonic losses (those occurring before time of pregnancy diagnosis) are generally unknown and hence commonly remain undiagnosed but include endometritis, heat stress, nutritional deficits, failure of pregnancy recognition mechanisms, infectious agents, and teratogens. The prevalence of genetic causes of early wastage in cows is not known.

In high-producing dairy cows, substantial embryonic loss occurs even after pregnancy diagnosis, especially when diagnosis is early, as when ultrasonography is used, with as many as 15% of pregnancies diagnosed at 28 days after insemination lost by 60 days. Losses are greater in cows bred when already pregnant, cows with endometritis, and in cows with high milk somatic cell counts. Cows previously suffering from periparturient diseases such as dystocia, metritis or endometritis, or mastitis have increased risk of late embryonic death, as do cows with prolonged postpartum anovulation. Heifers are less likely to suffer embryonic loss than lactating cows.

Abortion

Sporadic losses occurring after 60 days of pregnancy are categorized as abortion. It is a frustrating but important fact to remember that diagnostic investigation of abortion in dairy cattle is commonly unrewarding. Establishing realistic expectations for anxious clients is important in the face of individual or groups of abortion cases. The emphasis historically has always been on the diagnostic identification of infectious causes, but even when fresh fetal and placental tissue are available along with blood or milk from the dam, an infectious etiology may only be identified in about 65% of cases. See Chapter 18 for diagnostic sample submission.

Hydrops

Etiology

Uterine dropsy or hydrops is a sporadic condition usually occurring during the last trimester of pregnancy. Hydrops of the amnion (hydramnios) is usually accompanied by fetal anomalies that may contribute to fluid accumulation. Hydramnios accounts for only approximately 10% of the cases of hydrops. Hydrops of the allantois (hydrallantois) is the more common condition and is usually accompanied by abnormal placentation characterized by adventitious placentation (multiple areas of adhesion between the endometrium and allantochorion, appearing as miniature or diffuse placentomes). It is not clear whether this contributes to the pathogenesis of the condition or is a consequence of a common inciting cause. Hydrallantois tends to cause rapid (days to weeks) abdominal distention that results in a rounded abdominal appearance as the patient is viewed from the rear, but hydramnios usually results in a slowly progressive enlargement with eventual pear-shaped appearance. Twinning or multiple fetuses are more likely associated with hydrallantois. Pregnancies that are the result of modern in vitro reproductive technologies such as those producing cloned or transgenic fetuses are more commonly beset by abnormal placentation and subsequently represent a greater risk for hydrops. The incidence of hydrops and calf respiratory or cardiopulmonary, hepatic, and umbilical problems associated with cloning appears to have decreased from the alarmingly high numbers seen in the early 2000s.

It is possible for nutritional deficiencies to cause hydrallantois. Fetal hydrops may occur because of accumulation of cerebrospinal fluid (hydrocephalus) or from ascites or anasarca (usually in Ayrshire calves). Fetal hydrops is also seen at a higher prevalence in fetuses established using in vitro techniques. These calves, if delivered alive, can survive, but should not be used for breeding.

Signs

The major outward sign of hydrops is progressive abdominal distention during the last trimester that worsens to such a degree as to decrease appetite and cause difficulty in moving or rising (Fig. 9.1). Although abnormal fetuses causing hydramnios rarely can cause abdominal distention as early as midpregnancy, this is much less common than hydrops that appears during the last 4 to 6 weeks of pregnancy. Weakness results both from reduced feed consumption and from the increased weight of uterine fluids. Secondary ketosis and other metabolic conditions are possible complications as a result of decreased feed intake and fetal nutritional needs, especially if twins are present in cows with hydrallantois. Rectal examination may help to differentiate hydramnios and hydrallantois. In hydramnios, the fetus and placentomes are palpable, but the uterine horns are more difficult to palpate. In hydrallantois, the distended uterine horns appear to fill the abdomen, but palpation of the fetus and placentomes may not be possible because the uterus is stretched tightly by the increased fluid content. Rectal or transabdominal ultrasound examination is helpful in making a diagnosis. Unless the conditions are diagnosed promptly, musculoskeletal complications in the dam such as exertional myopathy, hip injuries, hip luxations, and femoral fractures can occur because of struggling to rise or slipping brought on by the tremendous abdominal weight. (As much as 200 L of additional fluid may accumulate in the case of hydrallantois.) Rupture of the prepubic tendon and ventral hernias also may occur. Because hydrallantois tends to cause more rapid fluid accumulation, musculoskeletal injuries appear to be more common with this condition than in the slowly enlarging hydramnios patients.

If cattle with hydrops calve or abort spontaneously, the thick, viscous amniotic fluid present in hydramnios also can help differentiate this condition from the watery, transudative, excessive fluid discharged from cattle with hydrallantois.

Cattle with hydrops have normal temperatures but will show progressive tachycardia, anxiety, reduced appetite, and dehydration associated with severe abdominal distention. Fetal hydrops may cause dystocia.

Treatment

Treatment decisions must be tempered by the potential immediate and delayed complications anticipated. The prognosis usually is worse for hydrallantois because abnormal maternal placentation may be expected to cause severe and intractable problems with retained placenta and metritis, making future fertility extremely unlikely. If neglected or allowed to "run their course," most cattle with hydrallantois will progress to recumbency, cardiovascular collapse, and overwhelming myopathy. Hydramnios may have fewer severe immediate complications with retained placenta and metritis. In both conditions survival of the fetus is unlikely. Perhaps the most important consideration is the overall systemic state of the dam. Most hydrops cattle are in a negative energy balance, are 4 to 6 weeks from parturition, have slack udders, and may or may not come into lactation—at least to anticipated, productive lactation levels. Therefore salvage should be considered unless the cow is particularly valuable or is within 2 weeks of term. Cattle that are recumbent and unable to rise or that already have severe musculoskeletal injuries should be euthanized.

When treatment is elected, several options exist. Induction of parturition is preferable if the uterus has not already been stretched beyond physiologic limits, which is unfortunately usually the case. If cesarean section is elected, uterine fluid should be released over a period of 30 minutes to 2 hours, via a Foley catheter or small-bore stomach tube, while intravenous (IV) fluids are administered rapidly. This is also advisable if vaginal delivery is to be attempted following pharmacologic induction once the cervix is sufficiently dilated (Fig. 9.2). Hypertonic saline (1–2 L) administered

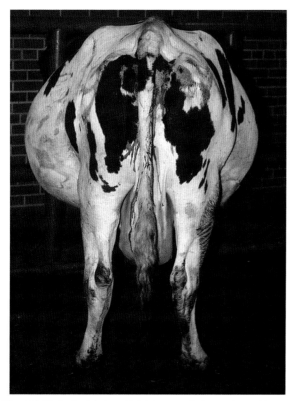

• **Fig. 9.1** Hydrallantois in a Holstein cow that was 8 months pregnant.

IV is practical and can quickly expand intravascular volume. This prevents the rapid onset of shock, which may result from venous fluid shifting into the splanchnic pool during abdominal decompression. Although some authors have not found hydrops patients to be markedly dehydrated, our experience differs and supports the comments of Roberts that such patients usually are dehydrated. Dehydration further increases the risk of compartmental pressure changes, subsequent splanchnic pooling, and shock for hydrops patients treated by cesarean section.

If induction of parturition is elected, it can be achieved by injection of 20 mg of dexamethasone followed in 24 hours by 25 mg of prostaglandin $F_{2\alpha}$ ($PGF_{2\alpha}$). Most cattle treated with this combination calve within 36 to 48 hours and should be monitored closely. Intravenous fluids including hypertonic saline are administered to cattle showing any degree of dehydration or inappetence. Supportive glucose or calcium may be indicated when ketosis or hypocalcemia is present. Treated cows are kept in well-bedded box stalls with good footing and are monitored closely because they may require assistance in calving. Periodic assessment of cervical dilation and fetal position after induction is prudent. Milking is started as soon as the fetus is delivered, even when little milk is present in the udder. Most fetuses or calves delivered are abnormal, small, or nonviable. If the calf is more valuable than the cow, close to term, and ultrasound examination indicates a viable fetus, treatment of the cow with dexamethasone for 3 days at high doses (50 mg) might help accelerate fetal lung maturation such that cesarean section 24 hours later would provide the best chance of obtaining a live calf. In the case of an apparently viable calf, colostrum should be provided from another cow because the patient seldom has normal colostrum. Prognosis is better for those cows near term. Metritis and retained fetal membranes (RFM) should be anticipated in cows with hydrallantois and prophylactic antibiotic therapy instituted. Clinicians should anticipate that the cow will have an unusually large, atonic uterus after calving and will experience highly protracted and challenging involution.

Because of the common complications of intractable retention of fetal membranes and associated metritis and infertility, alongside the poor prognosis for survival of the fetus, culling of the cow with hydrallantois may represent the most economical option. Survival and subsequent fertility are much more likely in cows with hydrops amnios, but they should not be bred again to the same sire.

Rupture of the Prepubic Tendon and Ventral Hernia

Etiology

Rupture of the prepubic tendon and ventral abdominal hernias usually occur during the last month of pregnancy. Contributing causes include the weight of a gravid uterus and periparturient edema of the ventrum. Further predisposition occurs in cattle with twin or multiple pregnancies and those with hydrops. Although more common in multiparous cattle with a pendulous abdomen, the condition may occur in primiparous cattle. Injuries from direct trauma (especially from animals with horns), being cast or trapped on inanimate objects, or slipping on treacherous footing may be contributing or initiating factors. Factors that increase the uterine mass remain the major cause in cattle. Rarely, spontaneous rupture of the body wall in the flank area with hematoma formation and obvious swelling occurs at parturition.

Clinical Signs and Diagnosis

Rupture of the prepubic tendon causes a bilateral and complete loss of fore udder definition and the fore udder points ventrally in continuum with the pendulous, ventrally directed abdominal wall (Fig. 9.3). The patient assumes a sawhorse stance because of exquisite pain in the abdomen and is reluctant to lie down (Fig. 9.4). When the cow does lie down, she tries to assume lateral recumbency to avoid putting pressure on the ventrum. Abdominal distention usually is obvious. Overt or atypical extensive abdominal distention may be observed before rupture of the tendon, and cows may have the rupture preceded by both extreme abdominal distention and a large plaque of ventral edema.

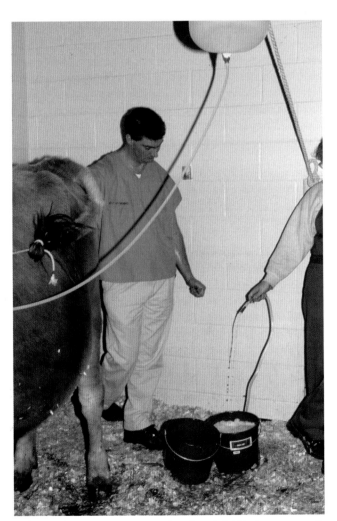

• **Fig. 9.2** Slow drainage of excessive allantoic fluid in Jersey cow with hydrallantois. Note concurrent administration of intravenous fluids.

These characteristics have been referred to as "impending rupture of the prepubic tendon" and are a grave sign.

Cattle with ventral hernias have the same predisposing causes as for rupture of the prepubic tendon but may have unilateral abdominal sagging coupled with an abnormal relationship of the fore udder to the affected side of the abdomen. Ventral hernias have been reported to be more common on the right side in cattle but can occur on either side.

Cattle with either condition become acutely painful at the moment that an "impending" situation becomes a hernia. Tachycardia, tachypnea, an anxious expression, reluctance to move or lie down, and a sawhorse stance are typical findings. Prepubic tendon rupture usually results in more overt pain than ventral hernia.

Rectal examination may help to differentiate the conditions. When true rupture of the prepubic tendon has occurred, the cranial brim of the pelvis may be tipped slightly upward, and the hand may be cupped under the brim because of loss of the prepubic tendon. In ventral hernias, the hernia may or may not be palpable, but the intact prepubic tendon can be palpated in the caudal abdomen as it attaches to the pelvic brim.

Cattle with either condition may require assistance in calving because pain and an inability to generate normal abdominal press may lead to dystocia. In addition, twins or hydrops may be present and increase the chances of dystocia. Cows with rupture of the prepubic tendon should be

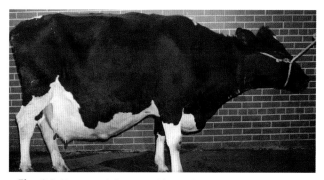

• **Fig. 9.3** Rupture of the prepubic tendon in a 6-year-old Holstein cow.

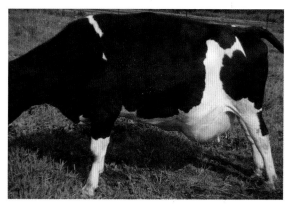

• **Fig. 9.4** Rupture of the prepubic tendon in a first-calf heifer that was confirmed to have twins. The heifer has a sawhorse stance and would not lie down because of severe abdominal pain.

salvaged or euthanized because they are in extreme pain. Cows with ventral hernias that do not appear to be in severe pain may be kept for the current lactation but should not be bred back. Cattle thought to be showing signs of "impending rupture" or those suspected to have hydrops should be induced to calve immediately or undergo elective cesarean section in an effort to prevent herniation or rupture of the prepubic tendon. Cattle with either condition that are recumbent and unable to stand or those already having secondary musculoskeletal complications should be euthanized.

When parturition is induced in these cases, it should always be attended. Inserting a nasotracheal or orotracheal tube helps limit the extent and degree to which the dam can abdominal press to prevent further exacerbation of the abdominal wall rupture, while the calf may still be delivered by traction.

Rupture of the prepubic tendon and ventral hernias are specifically diagnosed based on clinical signs alone but should be differentiated from large hematomas or abscesses cranial or dorsal to the udder, severe preparturient ventral edema, and inflammatory ventral edema or edema secondary to thrombosis of the mammary vein. The anatomic relationship of the udder to the ventral abdomen usually suffices to differentiate these conditions. Ultrasound examination will help in making a more definitive diagnosis. Anemia would be present with large udder hematomas, and fever might be present with abscesses. Ultrasonography could be very useful whenever the diagnosis is in doubt to definitively identify whether or not a continuous abdominal wall is still present. Impending rupture may be identified and monitored ultrasonographically by edematous separation of the muscular layers. Experience is necessary to distinguish intramuscular edema and fiber separation from the rather more common but frequently extensive subcutaneous edema that is common and more benign in modern, high-producing, periparturient cows and heifers.

Uterine Torsion

Etiology

Uterine torsion is well known as a cause of dystocia in dairy cattle. Although the exact cause of torsion seldom is discovered in an individual case, prolonged confinement, sudden falls or slipping, a pendulous abdomen, strong fetal movements, and poor uterine muscle tone may predispose. Unicornual pregnancy (in which the conceptus fails to occupy both uterine horns) and especially unicornual twin pregnancy may cause instability of the uterus and predispose to torsion. Torsion is less common in *Bos indicus* breeds, in which the uterine broad ligament is attached over a greater length of the uterine horns than in *Bos taurus* cows. Many parturient torsions occur during the latter part of the first stage of labor or early in the second stage. Partial torsions of between 45 and 180 degrees may be maintained in this position for weeks or months during late gestation but do not result in signs unless further rotation occurs that interferes with fetal or uterine blood supply.

Although most cases of uterine torsion occur during the first stage of labor, uterine torsion can also result in clinical signs during the second or third trimester well before term. Such cattle have torsions greater than 180 degrees, and colic signs similar to intestinal obstruction may occur. Roberts states that uterine torsions in the cow have been observed as early as 70 days of gestation.

Clinical Signs and Diagnosis

Although an uncommon cause of colic, uterine torsion should be considered in the differential diagnosis of any cow more than 4 months pregnant and showing colic. The early signs shown by these cows are similar to those observed in the more common term uterine torsions and include restlessness, treading, anxiety, tachycardia, reduced appetite, and swishing of the tail. The cow may be reluctant to lie down or may get up and down frequently. As the condition progresses, complete anorexia, progressive tachycardia, and true colic with kicking at the abdomen may appear. Because the condition is seldom suspected in cattle in midgestation, a further delay in diagnosis may occur if the signs are interpreted as intestinal in origin and treated symptomatically. Rectal examination allows definitive diagnosis. Most symptomatic midpregnancy torsions are greater than 180 degrees. The right broad ligament will be pulled downward under the torsed organ while the left broad ligament is pulled over the top of the reproductive tract in the case of a clockwise or right torsion. The opposite arrangement occurs in counterclockwise or left torsions. The viability of the calf should be determined by palpation or ultrasound examination. Counterclockwise torsions are slightly more common because the uterus rolls toward and over the more commonly nongravid left horn.

Treatment

Unlike treatment methods available for term uterine torsions (e.g., manual detorsion, mechanical detorsion, "plank in the flank" [Fig. 9.5], and rolling), mid-trimester uterine torsions are best managed by manual correction during laparotomy.

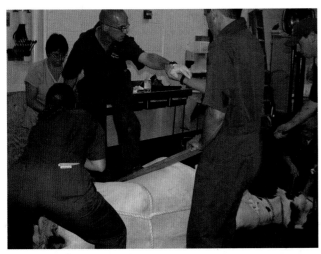

• **Fig. 9.5** Adult cow, cast and positioned in right lateral recumbency for correction of a clockwise uterine torsion via the "plank in the flank" technique.

Attempts to roll the cow or use the plank-in-the-flank technique are usually unsuccessful because of lack of fetal mass and tend to further damage the already compromised uterus while risking hemorrhage or further transudative or exudative peritoneal effusion. When rolling was attempted in some early cases, the technique failed, and subsequent laparotomy revealed severe serosanguineous peritoneal effusion and some frank hemorrhage. When diagnosed early and corrected by laparotomy, cattle with midpregnancy uterine torsions have a better chance of delivering a live calf. Fetal death and eventual abortion are likely after correction in neglected cases, severe torsions, or those with obvious vascular compromise. Prolonged cases can have uterine necrosis and die from septic shock. Intraoperative assessment of the peritoneal cavity, uterine status, and fetal viability should be used to dictate supportive therapy such as fluids, systemic antimicrobials, and antiinflammatory drugs.

Anovulation and Acquired Ovarian Disorders

Ovarian cysts and other forms of anovulation are functional disturbances of the ovary. In the United States, approximately 23% of postpartum cows fail to ovulate by the end of the postpartum voluntary waiting period (60–65 days). These cows have lower pregnancy rates than ovulatory cows and are at higher risk of embryonic loss. Conversely, cows ovulating early in the postpartum period have improved reproductive performance. Importantly, the time to first postpartum ovulation and the risk of anovulation persisting up to or beyond 60 days in milk are much more highly heritable than most reproductive traits ($\approx$17%–23%), providing a potential selection tool for enhanced fertility.

The major contributor to anovulation is negative energy balance in early lactation. Body condition score at calving and at the onset of the breeding period and especially body condition loss over this period are predictive of anovulation, as is the presence of any disease condition during the postpartum period. There is little direct effect of milk yield on anovulation.

Ovarian follicular cysts may be regarded as a special form of anovulation. In this case, follicles develop up to and beyond the normal ovulatory size (usually 15–18 mm). These follicles produce physiological amounts of estradiol but fail to induce a preovulatory luteinizing hormone (LH) surge even though pituitary LH concentrations are normal. Treatment with gonadotropin-releasing hormone (GnRH) may evoke a physiological LH surge, resulting in ovulation or luteinization of another mature follicle (not ovulation of the cystic follicle). Treatment with progesterone may restore the hypothalamic ability to induce an ovulatory surge of LH by appropriate GnRH release. Therefore GnRH, LH analogues (e.g., human chorionic gonadotropin), or progesterone are all potentially suitable treatments for cows with ovarian follicular cysts.

Oophoritis (ovaritis) is a rare lesion in cows. Occasionally, ovarian abscesses may be encountered. They are often large and rounded with a smooth surface and may be mistaken for tumors. Ovarian abscesses may arise by chance as a consequence of bacteremia or may be a consequence of transvaginal oocyte recovery, with contamination accompanying ovarian puncture. Viral oophoritis and transient infertility may follow infection with bovine viral diarrhea virus, or with infectious bovine rhinotracheitis (IBR) virus. *Mycoplasma* spp. have also been associated with oophoritis.

Granulosa cell tumors are the commonest form of bovine ovarian neoplasia. These tumors are common in surveys of slaughtered animals but are less commonly diagnosed in live animals, perhaps being mistaken for nonresponsive ovarian cysts. Granulosa cell tumors may occur at any age and in pregnant and nonpregnant cows. They may attain a very large size but seldom metastasize. Clinical signs vary from anestrus to frequent estrus depending on the profile of hormones produced by the neoplastic cells.

Ovarian fibromas have also been reported in cows. They are generally benign. Lymphosarcoma may invade the ovaries but within the female reproductive tract this neoplasm is more likely to involve the uterus. Other ovarian tumors are rare in cows.

Acquired Disorders of the Uterine Tubes

Lesions of the uterine tubes are common in slaughterhouse surveys but are difficult to diagnose clinically. These may take the form of adhesions between the uterine tube or mesosalpinx and the ovary, or tubal occlusion resulting in hydrosalpinx. Ovariobursal adhesions may vary from thin strands of fibrous tissue, often originating from the site of an ovarian corpus albicans, to multiple, dense adhesions completely encasing the ovary in the ovarian bursa. Some of these adhesions appear to result from spontaneous hemorrhage from ovulation sites. Others may follow damage to ovarian structures during palpation or be the result of local or generalized peritonitis. There is evidence that uterine exudate may flow through the uterine tubes in a retrograde manner and mediate ovarian bursitis and peritubal adhesions, either spontaneously or as a consequence of lavage as a form of treatment for puerperal metritis.

Very small, delicate adhesions between the ovary and mesosalpinx are probably inconsequential for fertility, but more severe adhesions, especially those involving the fimbriae, effectively render the involved utero-ovarian unit nonfunctional, with bilateral involvement resulting in complete infertility.

Although the uterine tubes are not palpable per rectum, being very delicate and small in diameter, it is possible to insert two to four fingers into the ovarian bursa. To do so, gently grasp the ovary and pull it upward, so that the ovarian ligament is ventral. Then run the fingers ventral to the ovary in a ventrolateral direction. The confines of the ovarian bursa can readily be discerned, and this procedure allows diagnosis of ovariobursal adhesions. When the operator's fingers are in the ovarian bursa, the uterine tube will run along the tips of the fingers (although it cannot be identified if normal). Running the thumb along the fingertips

allows appreciation of focal or extensive distention of the tube. Any such distention implies blockage with subsequent loss of function of that tube.

Although diagnostic tests for tubal patency have been described (depending on retrograde flow of dye through the tubes with rapid absorption via the peritoneum or transport of starch granules through the tubes to be identified by staining of cervical mucus with iodine), they are laborious and not completely reliable. Attempted recovery of embryos after superovulation probably provides the best diagnostic test of tubal patency and function.

Acquired Uterine Disorders

Uterine Rupture

Etiology

Uterine rupture is an unfortunate but rare consequence of dystocia in cattle. The condition is extremely rare after unassisted delivery, and most cases occur after forced traction, uterine torsions, fetotomy, or delivery of emphysematous fetuses. Prolonged dystocia, emphysematous fetuses, and failure to lubricate sufficiently during extraction can increase the resistance and "drag" between the fetus and maternal reproductive tract and predispose to rupture of the uterus. Pressure of the uterus against the pelvic brim can also cause tissue necrosis and spontaneous uterine rupture.

Clinical Signs

When a veterinarian is present for the dystocia, manual examination of the cervix and uterus through the vagina should be performed after delivery of the calf. Full-thickness uterine tears (and a second calf if present) usually can be diagnosed at this time unless the injury occurs in the uterine horns distal to the reach of the veterinarian.

When the condition is undetected initially, clinical signs usually appear within 1 to 5 days postpartum. Depression, inappetence, fever, tachycardia, rumen stasis, and abdominal guarding because of peritonitis appear as the major signs. Some cattle progress rapidly to a condition of septic shock because of massive peritoneal contamination. This is especially common when prolonged dystocia, RFM, or a dead or emphysematous fetus allows bacterial inoculation of the uterus that quickly spreads to the abdomen at, or shortly after, parturition. The fetal membranes may enter the abdominal cavity through the uterine tear and cause severe, potentially fatal peritonitis. Cattle with large uterine tears and tenesmus associated with dystocia may prolapse intestine through the reproductive tract and have these organs appear at the vulva. Spontaneous rupture caused by unattended dystocia occasionally has resulted in the calf or fetus being extrauterine, at least in part, within the abdomen.

Signs of overt peritonitis greatly worsen the prognosis because fibrinous adhesions spread quickly through the abdomen and lessen the chances for uterine repair. When the condition is suspected, a manual vaginal examination after careful preparation of the perineum and vulva is indicated.

If the cow is less than 48 hours post partum, a hand may enter the uterus easily, but rapid cervical involution makes this difficult after 48 hours. A speculum may be helpful, but manual palpation of the tear remains the best means of diagnosis. Most spontaneous tears are dorsal and just cranial to the cervix. When uterine rupture is detected immediately after delivery, options should be discussed with the owner. Salvage is the best option for cows of average value. Conservative treatment may be attempted when the uterine tear is dorsal and small (a few inches). Broad-spectrum systemic antibiotics and repeated administration of oxytocin (5 IU every 6 hours) have been used for conservative therapy. The success of conservative therapy is often poor because of the primary problems of dystocia allowing heavy bacterial contamination of the uterus and abdomen. Cows that experience small dorsal uterine tears after manipulation or delivery of a live calf and in which fetal membranes do not contaminate the abdomen have the best prognosis. Uterine tears are a potential complication of uterine torsion, and cattle that have undergone correction of a torsion without laparotomy should be evaluated and monitored for signs of peritonitis. This would be particularly true of cattle in which repeated and unsuccessful attempts at correction have been made using the "plank in the flank" technique.

When the cow is judged to be extremely valuable, direct aggressive therapy, including repair of the uterine tear, may be necessary.

Treatment

Specific therapy includes surgical correction of the laceration, intensive antibiotic therapy to treat or prevent peritonitis, and supportive measures that may vary in each case. Surgical repair has been accomplished through the birth canal, but obviously this is difficult, is often done blindly, and is frequently unsuccessful. Epidural anesthesia and special extra-long surgical instruments facilitate this technique, but it remains, at best, difficult. This technique is possible only when the condition is recognized immediately and the cervix is open enough to allow two-handed manipulation.

Surgical repair after laparotomy is a better choice but also has inherent difficulties because the site of the tear often is dorsal and close to the cervix; consequently, it is difficult to reach and to suture effectively from a flank approach after uterine involution has commenced. Incisions for this type of repair need to be made as far caudal in the paralumbar fossa as possible to facilitate visualization and repair of the rupture. It may be helpful to have an assistant direct the reproductive tract toward the operator by placing an arm through the birth canal. Flank laparotomy also is necessary for those rare cases having the fetus or fetal membranes free in the abdomen.

We have attempted repair of uterine tears in dairy cattle after medical prolapse of the uterus by inversion through the caudal birth canal. This technique is only possible during the first 24 hours after parturition because it requires near complete cervical dilation. It requires pharmacologic relaxation of the organ to allow manual prolapse. A slow IV infusion of 10 mL of 1:1000 epinephrine is administered by an assistant while the veterinarian holds the uterus after passing a gloved arm through the cervix. As uterine relaxation occurs, the uterus is retracted through the vagina, and a surgical repair of the uterine tear is completed. The uterus then is returned to normal position similar to replacing a spontaneous uterine prolapse. Despite the epinephrine-induced relaxation of the organ, retraction still may be difficult. In addition, the cardiovascular consequences of IV epinephrine constitute a risk to the patient but may be the lesser of two evils when contrasted with the disadvantages and challenges of other repair methods.

Antibiotics are indicated preoperatively and for at least 2 weeks postoperatively if repair has been successful. Intraperitoneal lavage with saline and antibiotics or very dilute povidone-iodine (tea-color Betadine) is indicated and facilitated when the uterine tear is repaired through a flank approach. Further supportive therapy such as IV fluids, or short-acting corticosteroids for cattle showing early signs of shock, may be indicated. Prognosis is poor to guarded for cattle with uterine rupture in which any significant degree of abdominal contamination has occurred, especially in the event of a dead or emphysematous fetus.

Uterine Prolapse

Etiology

Prolapse of the uterus occurs immediately (within 24 hours and usually within 6 hours) after parturition. In dairy cattle, the condition is not thought to be inherited and seldom recurs in subsequent parturitions. The fundamental pathogenesis depends on uterine flaccidity, which can be predisposed to by dystocia and hypocalcemia. Primiparous cows can be affected, but multiparous cows are at greater risk. Prolapse of the uterus also is fostered by confinement, lack of exercise, and gravitational effects when cattle are allowed to calve with their hindquarters lower than their forequarters, as happens when confined cows calve into the drop of conventional (tie stall) barns. The incidence of the condition is about 2 per 1000 births.

Clinical Signs and Diagnosis

The clinical signs are dramatic and suffice for definitive diagnosis (Fig. 9.6). Conspicuous placentomes on the exposed endometrium make the prolapsed uterus impossible to confuse with any other organ. The cow may appear healthy otherwise; this is often the case in primiparous cattle. Multiparous cows with uterine prolapse often show varying degrees of hypocalcemia such as weakness, depression, subnormal temperature, anxiety, struggling or prostration, and coma. Tenesmus is common to most cases. Signs of shock should be differentiated from those of hypocalcemia because a small percentage of prolapse patients may develop hypovolemic shock secondary to blood loss (internal or external), laceration of the prolapsed organ, or intestinal incarceration within the prolapsed organ. Extreme pallor, a high heart rate, and prostration are grave signs in such cattle. Rarely, the cow

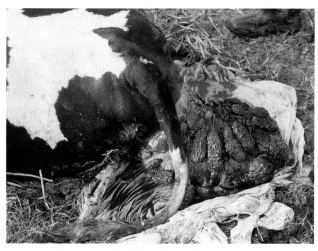

• **Fig. 9.6** Uterine prolapse.

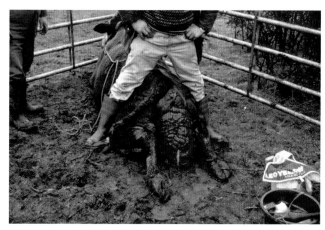

• **Fig. 9.7** Adult cow positioned in sternal recumbency for replacement of uterine prolapse. (Courtesy of Dr. Nigel Cook.)

is found dead, especially when an unobserved calving has occurred. The prolapsed uterus often is heavily contaminated with bedding, feces, dirt, and placenta. Some bleeding is common from exposure injuries to the placentomes or endometrium. If the affected cow is able to stand and walk, the massive organ hangs down toward the hocks and can be stretched, traumatized, or lacerated as it flops back and forth against the rear quarters. More dangerously, the uterine and ovarian blood vessels may be stretched or snapped, with fatal consequences. In an individual that is still standing, the lower the organ hangs, the greater the apprehension the veterinarian should have that catastrophic hemorrhage has already occurred.

Treatment

Uterine prolapse is one of the true emergencies in bovine practice, and rapid owner recognition followed by prompt veterinary treatment greatly improve the prognosis. When notified of the condition, the veterinarian should instruct the owner to keep the cow quiet and to cleanse the exposed organ and keep it moist. Warm water containing dilute (1%) iodine and a clean towel or sheet work well for this purpose. If possible, the owner also may be instructed to elevate the organ to the level of the ischium or higher to relieve vascular compromise and subsequent edema, as well as lessen the chance of injury. When the veterinarian arrives at the scene, overall assessment of the situation is in order before proceeding with specific treatment. The cow's position, overall physical status and the environment should be assessed. Specifically:

1. Can the cow's position be altered easily given the available help and environment to provide a mechanical advantage for replacement?
2. Is the cow hypocalcemic? Would correction of the hypocalcemia be beneficial immediately, or can it wait until after replacement of the organ? Would the cow be more likely to stand if treated with calcium? Some practitioners prefer replacement with the animal standing; others do not. Calcium treatment increases uterine tone and makes it substantially more difficult to replace; deferment until

after uterine replacement is preferred if the cow can withstand the delay.
3. Is the cow in shock? If so, the owner should be made aware of the poor prognosis.
4. Is footing adequate to allow the cow to stand, or should moving the cow to better footing be considered?

This overall assessment and a very quick history and cursory physical examination can be completed within minutes and may improve the end results greatly.

Specific treatment is subject to great individual variation as regards when to administer calcium, whether to perform the replacement with the patient recumbent or standing, when to give certain drugs, and aftercare. The basic premises are, however, agreed on by most practitioners:

1. An epidural anesthetic is administered to relieve tenesmus during replacement.
2. The cow is positioned to the veterinarian's advantage. The cow already may be able to stand, or the veterinarian may choose to treat the cow for hypocalcemia and allow her a few minutes so that she may stand for the procedure. If the cow remains recumbent but struggles persistently, light sedation may be considered to facilitate positioning of the animal to the veterinarian's advantage. Recumbent cows on a flat surface that have the hind legs pulled behind them so they are in sternal recumbency with the hind legs pulled caudally so the animal lies on the cranial stifle areas are easier to correct (Fig. 9.7), but this position may predispose to coxofemoral injury if the cow struggles to get up. Positioning the cow in this way tips the pelvis forward and allows a mechanical and gravitational advantage. If the cow is in an uneven posture, it also may be possible simply to angle her front end downhill to give significant mechanical advantage. In difficult situations when labor is unavailable or the environment is not conducive to gaining a mechanical or gravitational advantage, hip slings can be used to elevate the cow's rear quarters to hasten replacement. In some cases, it may be possible to hoist the hindquarters of the cow using farm equipment such as a skid steer. Although this does facilitate replacement of the uterus, care must

be taken to support the uterus as the cow's hindquarters are raised. Excessive tension on the prolapsed uterus may result in rupture of the uterine artery, already compromised by stretching within the prolapsed organ.

3. The uterus should be elevated to at least the level of the ischium to relieve vascular compromise and edema. One or two assistants can do this by suspending the organ in a towel, sheet, or prolapse tray when the cow is standing. In recumbent cows, the assistant can sit on the cow's sacral region facing backward and elevate the organ by holding it in his or her lap or suspended by a towel or sheet.

4. The uterine surface should be gently and thoroughly cleaned of debris and dirt and the placenta removed carefully. Usually the edematous placentomes allow easy separation of cotyledons from caruncles. Dilute antiseptics can be added to the water used for this purpose and the organ protected from further contamination. During this cleansing, gentle pressure and kneading of the organ are helpful to start restoration of uterine tone and relieve edema.

5. Systemic injection of oxytocin or ergonovine before replacement is controversial. The author prefers to postpone administration until after replacement of the uterus.

6. After the cow is positioned and the organ cleansed, replacement begins by slowly kneading and pushing the organ starting at the cervical end nearest the vulva. Lubrication with mild soaps and water or obstetric lubricants is essential to safely facilitate these manipulations. Glycerol, if available, makes a useful lubricant because it is also hygroscopic and reduces uterine edema. The veterinarian must be careful not to push fingers through the friable endometrium or uterine wall; cupped hands work best. If iatrogenic uterine tears occur, they should be sutured with an inverting pattern. Candid discussion with the client regarding salvage should be undertaken when significant abdominal contamination is deemed to have occurred through uterine tears acquired after prolapse. Individual caruncles must be eased through the vulva, and rest periods during extreme tenesmus may be necessary. A slow, gradual replacement usually ensues until only a portion of the gravid horn remains exposed. At this time, the tip of the horn is identified, and hand and arm pressure is exerted to evert the horn and uterus completely back into the abdomen. When everted, the organ should be rocked gently and shaken to ensure complete eversion of the horns and minimize the chances of reprolapse. Some practitioners also use a bottle as an "arm extension" to aid in complete eversion of the horns. It is very important to completely evert both gravid and nongravid horns to prevent tenesmus from causing reprolapse after the epidural wears off. It is common to need to repeat epidural anesthesia during the replacement of a challenging prolapse.

7. Oxytocin or ergonovine and calcium are administered systemically after replacement and the organ palpated further to assess the response (i.e., increased tone). Systemic antibiotics such as penicillin or ceftiofur should be used for 3 to 4 days to counteract the anticipated metritis. The cow should not be allowed to lie with her hind end "downhill" or in a gutter.

In cows, prolapse of the previously gravid horn is the rule. The nongravid uterine horn is contained within the prolapsus, in its normal configuration. It is sometimes possible to find the open base of the nonprolapsed horn. If so, the effort to replace the uterus may be commenced at this site. It is often easier to replace the nonprolapsed horn and uterine body in this way, leaving a smaller mass of tissue to replace without the contained nongravid horn, to complete the process. When it is possible, replacing the uterus in this way is easier than the traditional method of starting at the vulva and slowly replacing the whole organ.

Retention sutures placed in the vulva after replacement of uterine prolapses are not indicated, yet commonly done. They are ineffective for prevention of reprolapse and may rarely mask the condition by allowing the uterus to become trapped in the vagina. Because the common predisposition for uterine prolapse is uterine atony, complete restoration of the uterus to its normal position and treatment to enhance uterine tone are sufficient to prevent recurrence of the condition.

Prognosis

The prognosis for uncomplicated uterine prolapse is good, and most cows that respond promptly will breed back after routine monitoring and treatment of their metritis. The fatality rate is approximately 10% to 20%. Most surviving cows have satisfactory fertility although calving to conception interval may be moderately ($\approx$10–20 days) prolonged. Furthermore, dairy cows that have had prolapses do not have a higher incidence of the problem at future calvings.

Of cows that do not do well, some die as a result of intestinal incarceration in the prolapse or bleed out, some develop severe peritonitis or perimetritis from uterine tears, and some do irreparable damage to the prolapsed organ. The owner should be made aware that the cow could die at any time during or after replacement when shock is obvious. Reprolapse is an extremely bad sign, and cows that repeatedly prolapse after initial correction seldom do well. It is wise to reexamine all prolapse patients 3 days after repair to assess the overall systemic state and make specific recommendations regarding metritis or uterine injury. Decisions on further antibiotic and other therapy can be discussed with the owner at this time. Uterine amputation is a heroic, and rarely successful, salvage procedure for cattle with repeated prolapse (Figs. 9.8 and 9.9). The risk of fatal hemorrhage is very high.

Retained Fetal Membranes
Etiology

Retained fetal membranes or retained placenta is a very common condition in dairy cattle, with an incidence typically ranging from 5% to 15%. Fetal membranes should

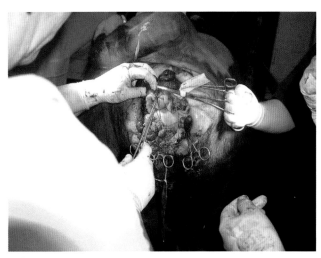

• **Fig. 9.8** Intraoperative appearance of standing surgery for uterine amputation. (Courtesy of Dr. Liz Santschi.)

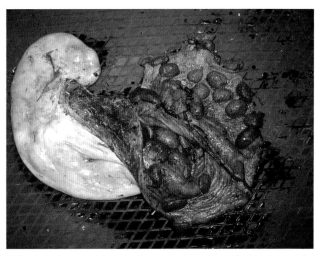

• **Fig. 9.9** Amputated uterus from surgery in Fig. 9.8. (Courtesy of Dr. Liz Santschi.)

be expelled in less than 8 hours after normal parturition; therefore retention for longer than 8 to 12 hours is considered abnormal, although retention for more than 24 hours is the most common definition of the condition. Abortion or premature birth for any reason frequently results in RFM. Hydrops, uterine torsion, twinning, and dystocia result in increased incidence of RFM compared with normal parturitions. Heat stress and periparturient hypocalcemia also predispose to the condition. Cows induced to calve by pharmacologic means such as exogenous corticosteroid administration are at increased risk. Nutritional causes such as overconditioning of dry cows and carotene and selenium deficiencies also have been incriminated. Low levels of vitamin A as occur in hyperkeratosis and polybrominated biphenyl toxicity are associated with RFM, metritis, and abortion. In selenium-deficient areas, cattle that have low selenium values may have an increased incidence of RFM, metritis, and cystic ovaries. Vitamin E, which has been shown to enhance neutrophil function, also may be involved. Cattle fed stored feeds from areas that are

selenium deficient should be monitored for selenium status and supplemented routinely. Selenium and vitamin E could be related to RFM either as a result of pure deficiency or altered neutrophil function.

Cattle that have RFM after parturition may be at greater risk of the condition in subsequent years, and a genetic component of the pathogenesis is likely. Cows with RFM have a higher incidence of metabolic diseases, mastitis, metritis, and abortion in the subsequent pregnancy. Therefore, despite the fact that many cows with RFM remain asymptomatic as regards immediate uterine health, associated diseases are a definite risk. Decreased resistance to uterine and other infections in cattle with RFM is partially explained by proven neutrophil dysfunction associated with the condition in periparturient cows. In addition to impaired neutrophil function, cattle with RFM frequently exhibit severe neutropenia. Although septic metritis or chronic endometritis does not occur in most cattle with RFM, the urge to treat RFM is based primarily on the inability to predict which cows will develop clinically significant sequelae.

Recent evidence strengthens the hypothesis that RFM is mediated by impaired neutrophil function beginning in the late dry period. Reduced neutrophil migration toward tissue extracts of placentomes can be detected as long as 2 weeks before calving in cows that go on to develop RFM. Other neutrophil functions, such as oxidative burst (a component of neutrophil bacterial killing action), are also impaired in these cows. Impaired neutrophil function has also been recorded in hypocalcemic cows. Indeed, many of the etiologic factors associated with RFM have also been correlated with impairment of neutrophil function, including vitamin and mineral deficiencies, heat stress, or exogenous corticosteroid administration. The poor neutrophil function in affected cows extends into the postpartum period and probably mediates most of the complications usually associated with RFM. Increasing evidence for the critical role that transition cow management plays in the pathogenesis of early postparturient diseases such as RFM and metritis links factors such as overcrowding, pen changes or movement, feed availability and type, to health determinants such as neutrophil function in the physiologic response to infectious diseases. The role of dystocia, prolonged unassisted labor, and induced parturition have long been recognized, but when the incidence of RFM on a farm in either heifers or cows increases in the absence of these conditions, practitioners are advised to consider late gestation and transition cow management factors.

Clinical Signs and Diagnosis

Clinical signs are obvious when the fetal membranes protrude from the vulva or hang ventral from the vulva to the escutcheon, rear udder, or hocks (Fig. 9.10). The condition is less apparent when the membranes are retained within the uterus or only project into the cervix or vagina and require a vaginal examination to be detected. Other clinical signs are completely dependent on evolution of associated diseases. Metritis is the most common secondary complication, and

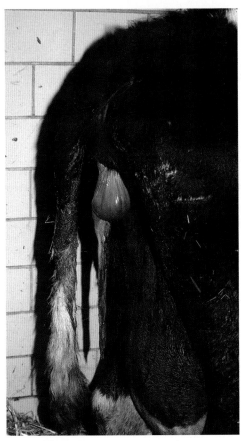

• **Fig. 9.10** Retained fetal membranes.

clinical signs of metritis or endometritis in association with RFM are identical to those discussed in later sections of this chapter. As previously mentioned, mastitis, metabolic diseases, ascending urinary tract infections, and displaced abomasa may be associated with RFM complicated by metritis or, in the case of infectious disease, because of less than optimal neutrophil function.

Tenesmus may appear in some cattle because of constant tension and irritation of the caudal reproductive tract by the protruding membranes. Eventually, a fetid odor emanates from the RFM, especially when metritis develops, and this may be the initial prompt for producers to seek veterinary attention or instigate treatment themselves. Untreated, most RFMs separate and fall away 3 to 12 days after calving.

Treatment

In general, it seems preferable not to treat uncomplicated cases of RFM but to treat when signs of illness (metritis) are detected. Cows with RFM that had dystocia, twinning, induced parturition, obesity, or hepatic lipidosis should be considered at high risk for metritis and probably justify prophylactic therapy. It is likely that the greatest benefits will accrue when measures are taken to improve management of cows in late gestation rather than focus attention purely on individual animals actually with RFM. If treatment is given, systemic administration of ceftiofur currently represents the most appropriate balance of antimicrobial efficacy and drug residue avoidance. Administration of hormones

such as oxytocin, $PGF_{2\alpha}$ or estrogens has been shown to be ineffective. Physical removal of the membranes has no beneficial effect and may be harmful. Gross contamination of the udder and escutcheon can be limited by tying the membranes into a clean plastic bag (e.g., a rectal examination sleeve) or by cutting the membranes off above the hocks. Although many practitioners prefer not to trim the protruding membranes in the belief that the weight of the dependent membranes speeds detachment, there is no supporting evidence for this view. Indeed, even fetal membranes left intact at cesarean surgery in a predominantly intrauterine location are usually expelled spontaneously within a few days.

Acute Puerperal Metritis

Etiology

Postparturient metritis is common in dairy cattle (occurring after 10%–25% of calvings). Septic metritis (acute puerperal or postpartum metritis, toxic metritis) refers to a severe puerperal uterine infection of the endometrium and deeper layers that results in systemic signs of toxemia. Puerperal metritis usually occurs from 1 to 10 days postpartum. "Metritis" is sometimes used as a general term for postpartum uterine infections of the endometrium, or endometrium and deeper layers, that may or may not cause systemic signs but may have implications for future reproductive performance. Infectious causes of reproductive failure such as brucellosis, leptospirosis, trichomoniasis, and campylobacteriosis may also cause varying degrees of metritis, but this discussion will be limited to conventional postpartum metritis.

Bacterial contamination of the uterus after parturition is extremely common during the first 2 weeks postpartum. As many as 93% of dairy cattle may have some bacterial contamination during this early postpartum period, but most infections appear to clear spontaneously because the infection rate decreases to 9% by days 46 to 60. Dystocia, RFM, twins, unhygienic calving facilities, hepatic lipidosis, negative energy balance, uterine atony, and iatrogenic vaginal contamination increase the occurrence of metritis. Heifers are more likely to develop metritis than multiparous cows.

Early (days 1-3) uterine infection with *Escherichia coli* appears to be a common factor in pathogenesis. Specific strains of *E. coli*, with specific virulence factors, appear to be involved. This infection paves the way on days 3-7 for gram-negative anaerobes, particularly *Fusobacterium necrophorum*, *Bacteroides* spp. and *Prevotella melaninogenica*, which are the most abundant pathogens in the uterus at the time of diagnosis of metritis, as revealed by metagenomic analysis of the uterine microbiome in healthy and diseased cows. *Trueperella pyogenes* is a pathogen in more chronic infections of the reproductive tract and when purulent exudate is noted.

Fertility is depressed in cows with metritis, but the consequences of postpartum metritis are not limited to reproductive matters, and many bovine practitioners believe that clinically significant metritis is *the* most common primary predisposing cause to displacement of the abomasum for cows in many herds. Affected cows are also predisposed to mastitis and clinical or subclinical endometritis.

Normal postpartum uterine discharges tend to be mixtures of mucus and blood, with more mucus representing the better finding. Blood associated with normal uterine involution will often color uterine discharges red or orange or give the appearance of tomato soup. The consistency and "anaerobic" odor of postpartum uterine discharges are important clues to the presence and severity of metritis in dairy cattle. Highly mucoid discharges in the early postpartum period (<10 days) usually indicate healthy uterine involution and minimal, if any, pathologic inflammation.

Although normal cattle have the greatest amount of lochia (several liters) within the first 48 hours postpartum, the amount subsequently discharged from the vulva varies from less than 100 mL (primipara) to 1 L or more (multipara), and some may be absorbed via the uterus. Lochia consists of mucus, sloughing maternal placental tissue, and blood. Discharge of lochia begins immediately postpartum and continues through day 10. Around day 9 or 10 postpartum, the yellow-brown to red discharge may show increasing amounts of pink, brown, or red blood coinciding with sloughing of the maternal caruncles and their stalks, which leaves a denuded vascular surface. Such bloodstained mucoid discharge may be apparent as late as day 15 to 18. Cows with excellent postpartum health generally have their first postpartum ovulation around day 15, the second around day 32 or 33, and subsequent ones at regular 21-day cycles. Most first postpartum ovulations do not result in observable behavioral signs of estrus.

On rectal palpation, early postpartum uteri have good muscular tone and may have palpable longitudinal ridges associated with muscular contraction. Multiparous cows usually have a uterus that is too large to retract manually or to palpate fully before days 10 to 14. Some primiparous cows may have sufficient involution to allow full definition of the uterus per rectum by days 10 to 14. Rectal palpation may not, however, be the best means to detect abnormalities in uterine involution during the first 14 days after parturition, and veterinarians should not hesitate to perform clean vaginal examinations and a vaginal speculum examination as adjuncts. The onset of estrus causes a remarkable difference in the size of the organ in most cattle, and slightly cloudy or clear mucus may be massaged from the uterus and cervix at this time. Most palpably detectable uterine involution is completed by 25 to 30 days postpartum, although the uterine horns still may feel thicker or more doughy than normal until days 35 to 40. The process of involution is completed more quickly in primiparous cattle than older cattle, in cattle free of metritis, cattle without RFM, cattle without metabolic disease, and cattle that have not had dystocia. Normally during a vaginal examination at 2 days postpartum, a hand cannot be passed through the cervix, and by day 4, only two fingers can be passed into the cervix. Cervical involution may be delayed by dystocia, cervical trauma, or RFM.

Perimetritis is the most severe manifestation of metritis in cattle. Infection progresses through the entire uterine wall to cause serosal inflammation, exudation, and fibrinous adhesions. Almost invariably, this condition is a consequence of dystocia because physical compromise and trauma to the uterus and caudal reproductive tract promote dissemination of bacteria from the uterine lumen and endometrium to the deeper layers. Vascular compromise as occurs in severe uterine torsions and subsequent manipulations to deliver the calf also predispose to perimetritis. True perimetritis results in peritonitis because this condition is not limited to retroperitoneal tissues. Extensive peritoneal exudates, fibrin deposition and adhesions to other viscera, and localization of septic exudates are common in perimetritis patients.

Clinical Signs and Diagnosis

Cattle with septic or toxic metritis become ill within the first 10 days—usually the first 7 days—postpartum. Signs of toxemia such as fever (103.0° to 106.5°F [39.5° to 41.39°C]), tachycardia, inappetence, decreased production, rumen stasis, depression, dehydration, and diarrhea are common. Note that fever may be absent in some cows with acute puerperal metritis. Extremely severe infection may cause recumbency secondary to toxemia, weakness, and metabolic disorders, and death may ensue. A fetid watery uterine discharge may be obvious at the vulva, may stain the tail, or may require a vaginal examination to be detected. Such uterine discharges vary in color from brown to amber to gray or red but always are fluid, low in mucus content, and purulent, and they have an extremely fetid odor that permeates one's clothes, hair, and arm even when guarded by an obstetric sleeve. Because these patients are very early postpartum, uterine infection and resultant appetite and gastrointestinal (GI) consequences predispose to metabolic diseases such as hypocalcemia and ketosis. The general term *toxemia* is used because (depending on the exact mix of causative organisms) absorbed endotoxins, exotoxins, and other mediators may be involved in the pathophysiology of the systemic signs.

Rectal examination usually reveals a flaccid or atonic uterus with fluid distention. Physometra also may be present and cause the gas-fluid–filled uterine horn to be confused with other viscera such as a distended cecum. Although attempts to retract the uterus should not be forced, gentle massage of the uterine body, cervix, and anterior vagina quickly causes fetid uterine discharges to be expelled from the vulva. Evidence of pain upon rectal palpation of the uterus is common and can be recognized by the cow arching her back during, and immediately after, palpation. A vaginal examination after cleaning of the perineal area is useful because this procedure allows differentiation of necrotic vaginitis or cervicitis and also allows detection of RFM and other pathology. However, the presence of caudal reproductive tract disease and toxic metritis are not mutually exclusive; severe dystocia or over-aggressive fetal extraction being possibly to blame when both are present concurrently in some cases. Transabdominal ultrasound examination can be useful in determining size of the uterus, thickness of the wall, and the presence of fetal membranes or intrauterine gas. Cattle with septic metritis are at increased risk of abomasal displacement as a result of toxemia-induced GI stasis and secondary metabolic conditions. A complete physical examination should be completed to rule out concurrent abomasal displacement and other conditions such as septic mastitis.

Clinical signs usually suffice for definitive diagnosis of septic metritis. Ancillary data support an overwhelming infection as evidenced by a degenerative left shift in the leukogram and elevated fibrinogen and other acute phase proteins. Acute recruitment of neutrophils to the uterus out of the bloodstream depletes the patient's available cellular defenses against other infections, especially mastitis. A mild metabolic alkalosis is anticipated in cattle with GI stasis. Differential diagnosis includes consideration of septic mastitis, peritonitis of any source, and acute pyelonephritis.

Perimetritis and peritonitis are manifestations of the severest forms of metritis and usually occur only after dystocia and compromise of the uterine wall. Ancillary data may be helpful when perimetritis and peritonitis must be differentiated from retroperitoneal inflammation caused by vaginal perforations or extensive pelvic hematoma formation or inflammation secondary to dystocia. Abdominal paracentesis will indicate peritonitis based on increased protein and white blood cell counts in perimetritis patients but may be normal or have only moderately increased protein in retroperitoneal conditions. Transabdominal ultrasound examination can be useful to assess the degree of peritonitis and serosal fibrin accumulation. A complete blood count usually shows a degenerative left shift when perimetritis is peracute or acute. Neutrophilia is possible in subacute or chronic cases. Serum albumin tends to be decreased because of extensive protein loss into the uterus and peritoneal cavity in severe perimetritis cases (Fig. 9.11). Vaginal examination may be indicated to rule out purely vaginal conditions and should be performed very gently after epidural anesthesia to avoid "malignant tenesmus," which is a constant straining initiated and then perpetuated by persistent movement of air into the rectum.

The prognosis is guarded for septic metritis and extremely poor for perimetritis; many cows with this condition die within 1 to 7 days after diagnosis. If the cow's value allows intensive treatment, systemic broad-spectrum antibiotics should be started immediately. Intravenous fluid therapy is necessary because the extensive peritonitis usually results in complete anorexia. Penicillin, oxytetracycline, ampicillin and ceftiofur are the most common antibiotics used for systemic therapy for either condition. Local or intrauterine therapy is contraindicated in most cases of perimetritis because extensive compromise of the uterine wall increases the risk of perforation or leakage! Prostaglandins may be used to encourage evacuation of the uterus but probably are of limited value because the uterus quickly adheres to adjacent visceral and parietal peritoneum. Epidural anesthesia may be necessary if tenesmus exists. Nonsteroidal antiinflammatory drugs (NSAIDs) may be helpful during the first few days of treatment to counteract endotoxemia and provide a degree of

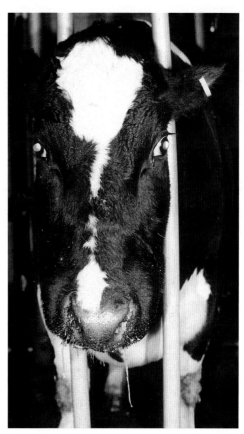

• **Fig. 9.11** Severe facial edema caused by hypoproteinemia secondary to perimetritis.

analgesia, although their use in postpartum cows is generally discouraged because they impair beneficial inflammatory processes that are a component of uterine involution. The dosage and duration of therapy with these drugs must also be limited to minimize the potential for abomasal or renal toxicity.

Cattle that survive perimetritis show slow but continual improvement as evidenced by a gradual return to normal temperature and normal heart rate alongside the return of appetite. Long-term (3–4 weeks) antibiotic therapy is indicated, and attempts to palpate the reproductive tract should be minimal during this 3 to 4 week period so as not to disturb adhesions. Surviving cows will always have extensive adhesions of the reproductive tract in the caudal abdomen and pelvis following perimetritis. It is best to allow complete sexual rest; prostaglandins should be administered at 14-day intervals to encourage uterine evacuation, although this may be hampered by uterine adhesions. The cow should be assessed by rectal palpation once monthly. Despite the initial presence of extensive adhesions, surviving cattle eventually may resolve many of these over a 5- to 6-month period and conceive. Frequently, these cows only "work on one side"—meaning that one uterine horn, uterine tube, or ovary (or all of these) continue to be confined by adhesions. Therefore such cows may conceive only when an ovulation occurs on the healthy or non-adhered ovary. Careful evaluation of the caudal reproductive tract and the presence of mature fibrous adhesions within the pelvic canal are critical before a decision as to breeding the cow back is made. Some cattle with persistent adhesions may be able to conceive and carry a pregnancy to term but should undergo elective cesarean section rather than attempting a natural or assisted vaginal delivery. Individual cattle of high genetic merit that survive may be considered candidates for in vitro fertilization (IVF) procedures or conventional embryo transfer as a means of maximizing their reproductive potential.

Cattle that do not improve after initial intensive therapy may either die as a result of diffuse peritonitis within the first few days after parturition or else linger as chronic peritonitis patients with persistent low-grade fever, partial anorexia, abdominal distention, hypoproteinemia resulting from albumin and globulin loss into the uterus or peritoneal space, and wasting.

Clinical Endometritis or Purulent Vaginal Exudate

The term "purulent vaginal exudate" is now preferred over the previously used "clinical endometritis" because many cows with visible vaginal exudate do not have demonstrable inflammation of the endometrium. Although definitive confirmation is not yet available, it is assumed that the source of the exudate in these cases is most commonly a primary cervicitis. As many as 15% to 30% of cows in North American dairy herds are affected per lactation. Risk factors include dystocia, RFM, and puerperal metritis.

The presence of purulent vaginal exudate may be confirmed by appreciation of externally visible material; by vaginoscopy; by "sweeping" the cranial vagina with a sterile, gloved hand and examining vaginal content; or by use of a dedicated instrument, the "Metricheck" (Simcro Inc., Lawrence, KS, 66047). Depending purely on visible exudate or palpation findings will result in missing as many as 40% of cases of purulent vaginal exudate.

Multiple studies have confirmed that purulent vaginal exudate diagnosed after 4 weeks postpartum has a detrimental effect on reproduction as measured by pregnancy to first postpartum artificial insemination (AI) rate, time to conception, percentage of cows remaining open after 150 or 300 days, and the risk of culling for reproductive failure. Purulent vaginal exudate also increases the risk of subsequent pregnancy failure. It is difficult, or impossible, to distinguish a pathological mucopurulent discharge from normal inflammation associated with postpartum uterine remodeling before 3 weeks postpartum.

There are few effective treatment options for purulent vaginal exudate. In many countries, but not in the United States, a formulation of cephapirin specially fabricated for intrauterine administration is available and has been shown convincingly to improve reproductive performance when administered to affected cows after 4 weeks postpartum. There is currently no evidence in favor of intrauterine infusions other than cephapirin, and they should be avoided. Although $PGF_{2\alpha}$ is often used for treating purulent vaginal discharge, there is no convincing evidence of its efficacy, although it may have beneficial effects on reproduction independent of endometritis.

Subclinical Endometritis or Cytologic Endometritis

Subclinical endometritis can be defined as endometrial inflammation of the uterus, usually determined by cytology, in the absence of purulent material in the vagina. It is only of significance at or after the stage at which normal involution should be complete (i.e., after about 4 weeks postpartum). In animals without signs of clinical endometritis, subclinical disease can be diagnosed by measuring the proportion of neutrophils present in a sample collected by flushing the uterine lumen with a low volume (20 mL) of sterile saline solution or using a cytobrush. Although investigation of subclinical endometritis is at an early stage, the presence of greater than 5% neutrophils after about 40 days postpartum constitutes a level of inflammation related to significantly impaired reproductive performance in affected cows. Alarmingly, several studies in different parts of the United States have indicated that as many as 50% of cows meet this definition.

Use of endometrial cytology in individual cows is not economically feasible, and attention should be devoted to preventing this disease, which has been associated with depressed dry matter intake beginning 2 weeks before parturition, negative energy balance, and impaired immune function.

Treatment with intrauterine infusion of cephapirin has been associated with improved conception to first service and fewer days open, although this would not currently be legal in the United States. Although routine $PGF_{2\alpha}$ treatment is often associated with improved reproductive performance, this effect does not seem to be mediated by resolution of endometritis, and no effect of such treatment on the prevalence or consequence of endometritis has been demonstrated.

Intrauterine Therapy

Intrauterine antibiotics have fallen largely into disfavor despite having been used for decades in the treatment of metritis in cattle. Intrauterine antibiotics also are often absorbed from the uterus to establish blood and milk levels that cause concern for milk residues and discard, resulting in significant economic losses. Absorption is more likely from healthy uteri, at the time of estrus, and after uterine involution. Certain antibiotics may interfere with phagocytic cell function, may be made inactive by β-lactamase–producing bacteria, may irritate the endometrium, or may not work well in the relative anaerobic state thought to exist in the uterus. Large amounts of uterine fluid may simply overwhelm or inactivate small doses of locally administered antibiotics. Cephapirin, a first-generation cephalosporin, is available in some countries in a formulation designed specifically for intrauterine administration (Metricure, Merck Animal Health). It is not available in the United States. In several trials, it has been found to be beneficial for treatment of clinical and subclinical endometritis. Its use in acute puerperal metritis has not been reported.

Systemic Antibiotics

Systemic antibiotics have become the standard treatment for metritis in dairy cattle over the past decade. The use of systemic antibiotics is justified and often required for metritis that causes systemic illness. However, systemic therapy is definitely overused in cattle with postparturient metritis or RFM that do not have a fever or who are not systemically ill. This overuse results in significant economic loss for owners because of antibiotic costs and loss of income resulting from discarded milk, although ceftiofur can be used without having to do the latter. Veterinarians inexperienced with other treatment options do not discriminate or differentiate metritis based on severity, duration, or association with systemic signs and may be too quick to suggest systemic antibiotic therapy. The same situation can arise when the decision to treat is made by laypeople, as is frequently the case on many modern dairies.

Systemic antibiotics are indicated when metritis causes systemic illness early postpartum. Procaine penicillin (22,000 U/kg once daily) would likely maintain effective concentration in the uterus and be an appropriate treatment for *Fusobacterium* and other anaerobic bacteria often associated with the fetid smell so easily noted in cows with septic metritis. Ceftiofur may be more effective against coliforms and has been found to have lower mean inhibitory concentration (MIC) against *T. pyogenes* and anaerobic bacteria cultured from the uterus compared to oxytetracycline. Ceftiofur derivatives have been shown to reach concentrations in both uterine tissue and uterine fluid of healthy postpartum cows that exceed the MICs for *E. coli, F. necrophorum, Bacteroides* spp., and *T. pyogenes*. Twice-daily penicillin therapy may maintain uterine fluid and tissue levels above the MIC for the anaerobic uterine pathogens and can be administered instead of, or in addition to, ceftiofur. Oxytetracycline dosed at 11 mg/kg twice daily may only establish uterine tissue concentrations of 5 µg/kg—a level thought to be less than that required to kill *T. pyogenes*. Ampicillin provides an effective alternative and is cheaper than ceftiofur but like penicillin and oxytetracycline requires milk withholding.

Hormonal Therapy

Historically, estrogenic compounds have been administered systemically to cows with metritis or endometritis, usually in subacute to chronic cases. Double-blind, prospective clinical trials have established convincingly that estradiol treatment of postpartum cows has no merit for improving health, survival, or later reproductive success, and its use is contraindicated.

The use of $PGF_{2\alpha}$ or other prostaglandin analogues for treatment of metritis and endometritis is not supported by experimental data. Even though $PGF_{2\alpha}$ use (often routine) has been associated with improved reproduction in many cases, the mechanism of such improvement does not lie in resolution of endometrial infection or inflammation. Similarly, oxytocin treatment in the early postpartum period is not associated with accelerated release of fetal membranes,

clinical recovery from metritis, or improved reproductive performance.

Summary Comments About Treatment of Cattle with Acute Puerperal (Septic) Metritis

Acute puerperal metritis requires therapy for systemic manifestations and control of local infection in the uterus. Systemic antibiotics should be administered once or twice daily. Oxytetracycline (13.2–15.4 mg/kg) administered IV once or twice daily (renal injury from the tetracycline must be considered at the higher dosage or in dehydrated cows), procaine penicillin G (22,000 U/kg) given intramuscularly (IM) once or twice daily, ceftiofur (2.2 mg/kg) once daily, ampicillin (11.0 to 22.0 mg/kg) once or twice daily, and sulfadimethoxine with or without oxytetracycline have all been used for systemic treatment. Some antibiotic resistance has been reported for all major uterine pathogens against these antibiotics. Most practitioners now use ceftiofur. Supportive treatment includes parenteral dextrose, calcium, and oral or IV fluids. Although NSAID treatment is no longer routinely recommended at calving or as treatment for RFMs because of an association with increased risk of metritis and poorer reproductive performance, they are frequently used as supportive treatment for cattle with septic puerperal metritis and life threatening systemic illness. Associated or secondary hypocalcemia and ketosis are common problems. Cows that are completely off feed benefit from IV fluids, but those with functional rumen activity can be economically rehydrated and provided with an energy substrate with fluids and alfalfa meal administered through a stomach tube.

Intrauterine treatment is generally not recommended. Uterine lavage carries a significant risk of uterine rupture and risk of retrograde flow of uterine exudate through the uterine tubes into the ovarian bursa and peritoneal cavity. Physical disturbance of the uterus may also increase the risk of uterine rupture or worsening bacteremia. If drainage is attempted in sick cows with septic metritis with the hope of removing the toxic fluid it must be done with great caution and only if the cow is already being treated with systemic antibiotics. Dr. Robert Hillman, to whom this book is dedicated, has performed this procedure on hundreds of clinically ill cows with septic metritis. His technique has been to infuse by gravity a liter of non-irritating lavage fluid through a clean, soft stomach tube which has been placed gently through the cervix and then immediately the fluid is drained from the uterus by lowering the end of the tube to the ground allowing a siphon effect to occur. This can be repeated until the color of the retrieved fluid is similar to that of the fluid administered. This is performed only after proper cleaning of the vulva and distal vagina with a non-irritating soap or disinfectant scrub solution. An epidural may be required if any discomfort or straining is expected, or observed, from the procedure.

Summary Comments About Treatment of Cows with Clinical and Subclinical Endometritis

Intrauterine infusion of cephapirin in a formulation designed specifically for this purpose (Metricure) has consistently been beneficial. It is not, however, permitted in the United States currently. No other intrauterine infusion can be supported by the available evidence. Systemic administration of antibiotics has not been tested as a treatment for endometritis. Although $PGF_{2\alpha}$ and its analogues have been beneficial to dairy cow reproduction, they do not appear to exercise this effect by reducing the prevalence or severity of endometritis.

Uterine Abscesses and Adhesions

Etiology

Uterine abscesses and adhesions may originate from spontaneous compromise of the uterine wall during calving, small uterine perforations, or extension of endometrial infection through the uterine wall or uterine tube. Such causes result in focal or diffuse inflammation and infection. A major iatrogenic cause is pipette injuries to the uterine body. Attempts to infuse cows less than 14 days postpartum are the usual cause of pipette injuries to the dorsal uterine body just proximal to the interior os of the cervix. Partial- or full-thickness uterine tears created in this way allow seeding with bacteria that result in abscesses or adhesions, especially when postpartum endometritis has existed. Pipette injuries can also occur during conventional reproductive procedures involving the uterus, such as insemination or embryo transfer manipulations.

Clinical Signs and Diagnosis

There are usually no systemic signs, and the conditions are not recognized until subsequent routine rectal palpation is performed for reproductive purposes. A history of dystocia, endometritis, retained placenta, and treatment for these conditions is typical but not invariable. On palpation, uterine wall abscesses are firm, round or oval masses intimately attached to the uterine body or horn. Abscesses vary in size from 2 to 30 cm or more and may have a network of fibrinous or fibrous adhesions associated with their juncture at the uterus. Such masses require differentiation from tumors, hematomas, and cysts. Differentiation may be difficult by palpation alone, but ultrasonography or aspiration may provide definitive diagnosis. In some cattle with uterine wall abscesses, intermittent or persistent purulent discharge from the vulva is noticed by the owner. These abscesses have a communicating tract into the uterine lumen. Other affected cattle have no evidence of purulent discharge. Blood work seldom is helpful because the leukogram and hemogram usually are normal, and serum globulin is elevated only when the uterine wall abscess is large and of chronic duration. *T. pyogenes* is the usual isolate identified in these abscesses.

Uterine adhesions generally are found as sporadic problems in cattle without systemic signs but with possible historical evidence of parturient or immediate postparturient uterine problems. A history of cesarean section is an obvious predisposing factor. A network of adhesions may involve part of or the entire reproductive tract, and it usually is impossible to fully retract the uterus as adhesions hold the organ in the cranial pelvis, at the pelvic brim, or along the caudal prepubic tendon region. Some adhesions may be friable, thin, or fibrinous and can be broken down

manually. However, it is best to leave these undisturbed so as not to tear the uterine tubes or horns. Cattle with extensive adhesions may have residual endometritis because the dependent arrangement of the uterus interferes with effective evacuation of luminal contents. The patient may or may not have been noticed in estrus depending on the magnitude of ovarian involvement and health of the uterine endometrium. Rectal palpation often suffices for diagnosis but can be significantly and helpfully augmented by transrectal ultrasonography.

Treatment

Conservative therapy for uterine abscesses consists of systemic antibiotics. Penicillin (22,000 U/kg once daily) for 2 to 4 weeks or ceftiofur (Excenel RTU EZ® 2.2 mg/kg once daily) for 5 days are common treatments. Ceftiofur treatment may be repeated but in the United States must always conform strictly to the product license label in terms of dose, route of administration, and duration of use. Twenty percent sodium iodide administered IV at 30 g/450 kg once followed by 1 oz of organic iodide orally, once daily, until signs of iodism appear, can be an additive treatment but milk from the cow cannot be used for human consumption. Conservative therapy is not very successful, however. Valuable cattle with uterine abscesses usually require surgical drainage or amputation of the affected horn through a caudal flank or inguinal incision. When the uterine body is involved, surgical drainage coupled with the aforementioned medical therapy usually is attempted. Cattle with uterine wall abscesses confined to one horn may be candidates for removal of the affected horn, abscess, and ipsilateral ovary. Such surgery is often difficult because of problems gaining adequate exposure to the abscess and the fact that coexisting adhesions may further limit delivery of the mass into a flank incision. Rarely, a uterine abscess will drain into the uterine lumen and resolve spontaneously. Subsequent endometritis can be managed by systemic antibiotic therapy.

Uterine adhesions are best managed conservatively and with protracted rest. Many of these cows can conceive eventually if given sufficient time for natural resolution of the adhesions. Usually 4 to 6 months of reproductive rest is necessary, so the cow must be deemed valuable enough to allow a prolonged lactation. Cattle with uterine and reproductive tract adhesions should be palpated gently once or twice monthly by the same examiner to monitor progress. Those with associated endometritis can have intermittent injections of prostaglandin ($PGF_{2\alpha}$ or analogues) to encourage evacuation of purulent material, especially if palpation confirms the presence of a functional corpus luteum. Attempts at intrauterine therapy are contraindicated because further damage may result. Systemic antibiotics and iodide can be administered as outlined previously for treatment of uterine abscesses but seem less important than time. Interestingly, the slow and steady stretching of the pregnant uterus and passage of time frequently cause the majority of the adhesions to resolve by the time of next calving. Some cows are left as "one-sided" breeders because severe inflammation and adhesions permanently destroy function of one ovary, one uterine tube, or one horn. The extent and location of adhesions may also impact the ability of the cow to deliver a calf vaginally or the accessibility of the uterus to the conventional left-sided approach for cesarean section. These potential issues should be evaluated and discussed with the owner during late gestation. Breedings in these animals can be adjusted for ovulation from the functional ovary by prostaglandin therapy after palpation, or the ovary on the affected side can be removed via colpotomy or celiotomy. Cattle with bilateral ovarian or uterine tube involvement and those with persistent endometritis have a poor prognosis.

Pyometra

Etiology

Pyometra is defined as intrauterine accumulation of pus accompanied by a persistent corpus luteum. Apparent failure of the endometrial luteolytic factor or endogenous prostaglandin to cause luteolysis makes cows with pyometra fail to cycle. Pyometra usually occurs when a cow ovulates early postpartum in the presence of persistent uterine infection. (Uterine infection usually delays the first postpartum ovulation, fortunately most cows ovulating early postpartum have a healthy uterus and high fertility.) Functional closure of the cervix prevents uterine drainage and allows accumulation of exudate. Pyometra also may occur after conception and embryonic death associated with infection. *T. pyogenes* is the usual organism isolated, but it may not initiate the condition. When it is a plausible differential, trichomoniasis always should be considered, especially if more than one case occurs on the premises or in a bull-bred herd.

Clinical Signs and Diagnosis

Clinical signs are limited to failure to show estrus, palpable or ultrasonographic evidence of persistence of a corpus luteum, and fluid accumulation in the uterus (Fig. 9.12). Many cases have intermittent or frequent mucopurulent discharge from the reproductive tract that has been noticed by the owner. Pyometra must be differentiated from pregnancy. Absence of a fetus, fetal membranes, and placentomes confirms nonpregnancy. The amount of fluid in pyometra cases varies from several ounces to several gallons. The ultrasound appearance of pyometra is quite distinct from pregnancy.

Treatment

Currently, $PGF_{2\alpha}$, cloprostenol, and other analogues are the most satisfactory treatment. Most pyometra cases can be successfully evacuated by one or more injections of prostaglandin drugs. Treatments may be repeated at 14-day intervals. $PGF_{2\alpha}$ (35 mg) or 500 µg of cloprostenol have given excellent results. This treatment also works well for many cases of mummified fetus, although in some cows even repeat injections are not successful. On occasion, fetal mummification or maceration is refractory to exogenous hormonal attempts at abortion. The remaining fetal tissues in such circumstances may be removed by hysterotomy via a caudal flank or inguinal incision, but this may be technically challenging (Fig. 9.13).

In general, the prognosis in cases of pyometra is good for health and fertility. However, the duration of pyometra is

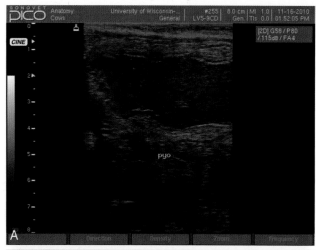

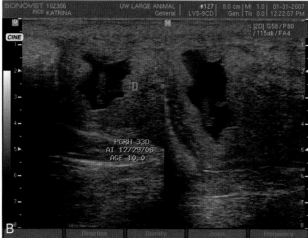

• **Fig. 9.12** **A,** Transrectal ultrasound image of pyometra demonstrating characteristic appearance of echogenic uterine fluid. **B,** Normal transrectal ultrasound appearance of a 33-day pregnancy for comparison with *A*. (Courtesy of Dr. Harry Momont.)

inversely related to subsequent fertility. Cattle with pyometra for longer than 2 months and those with large amounts of pus have lesser chances of subsequent fertility.

Uterine Tumors

Etiology

The most common neoplasm to affect the uterus of dairy cattle is lymphosarcoma. Adenocarcinomas, leiomyomas, fibromyomas, fibromas, and others are rarely reported.

Clinical Signs and Diagnosis

Cattle with lymphosarcoma of the uterus usually have detectable tumors of lymph nodes or other target organs in addition to lesions in the reproductive tract. Because of routine rectal palpation for reproductive examination, the uterine masses may be discovered either before the cow shows systemic signs or at the onset of illness associated with multifocal lymphosarcoma (see the section on lymphosarcoma in Chapter 16). Lymphosarcoma can appear in several forms in the reproductive tract such that focal, multifocal, or diffuse neoplastic infiltration is possible. The uterus is the most common portion of the reproductive

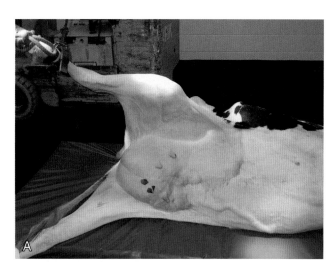

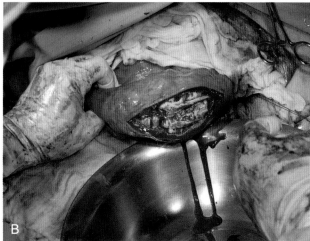

• **Fig. 9.13 A,** Cow positioned for inguinal approach for removal of macerated fetal remnants by hysterotomy. **B,** Bony fetal remnants being removed at surgery. (Courtesy of Dr. Mike Pritchard.)

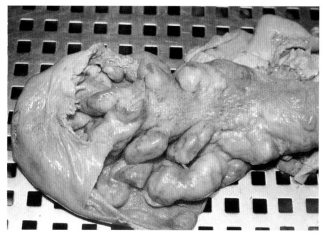

• **Fig. 9.14** Lymphosarcoma of the uterus.

tract to be affected, but the ovaries, uterine tubes, cervix, and caudal reproductive tract can also be involved. The typical uterine form of lymphosarcoma consists of multiple firm umbilicated masses in the uterine wall that feel similar to residual maternal caruncles (Fig. 9.14). Diffuse, firm thickening of the uterine horns, body, or both may be found in other cows. Occasionally, only a single smooth- or rough-surfaced uterine wall mass is palpated. A complete physical examination will usually allow identification of other lymphosarcoma tumors in affected cattle. In the United States, cattle greater than 2 years of age with lymphosarcoma will be bovine leukosis virus positive in the great majority of cases.

Cattle with uterine tumors other than lymphosarcoma usually are asymptomatic, and the tumors are identified as incidental findings during prebreeding examinations. Some affected cattle are examined because of repeat breeding or failure to conceive. Pulmonary metastases and subsequent respiratory signs have been described in association with uterine adenocarcinomas and may become clinically evident long before the primary tumor. Adenocarcinomas tend to be hard, rough surfaced, and involve one uterine

horn. Leiomyomas are firm and rounded and have distinct borders. Other tumors vary in gross appearance, shape, and consistency. Depending on the tumor type, metastases may or may not constitute a risk. Rectal ultrasonography and biopsy transvaginally or via laparotomy are helpful ancillary procedures.

Treatment

Cattle with lymphosarcoma of the uterus usually will be dead in less than 6 months as a result of multicentric disease. Pregnant cattle with lymphosarcoma of the uterus usually deliver small or nonviable calves if several weeks or months remain until term. Pregnant cattle that are less than 6 months' pregnant at the time of diagnosis seldom produce viable calves, and if a live calf is born, it will likely have been vertically infected with the bovine leukemia virus. Therefore treatment for this tumor is usually not indicated.

Unilateral horn neoplasia resulting from other tumors may be treatable by partial hysterectomy if the condition is detected early and the cow is deemed valuable enough to warrant surgical approach through a caudal flank incision by an experienced surgeon.

Acquired Cervical Disorders

Cervical lacerations may occur at calving and frequently remain undiagnosed. Small lacerations may predispose to cervicitis, which impairs fertility. Cervicitis, as distinct from endometritis, appears to be an independent and significant condition affecting as many as 20% of dairy cows. Indeed, an enlarged cervix or delayed return of the cervix to normal size has long been associated with infertility and has been regarded as a sign, or comorbidity, of "endometritis." Cervicitis may or may not be accompanied by grossly visible reproductive tract exudate. No effective treatment has been described, but the condition may resolve with time (Fig. 9.15). Cicatricial fibrosis of the cervix may complicate insemination and future cervical dilation at parturition. It is, however, true to say that the bovine cervix is remarkably "forgiving" when it comes to functional recovery postinjury.

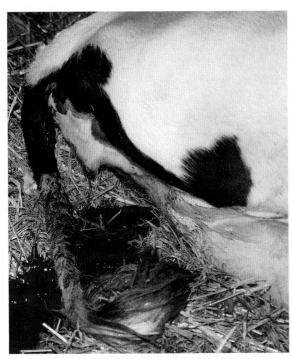

• **Fig. 9.15** Hemorrhage from the cervix that recurred at each of the first three postpartum heats after dystocia. The exact site of the origin in the cervix could not be seen, and the condition resolved.

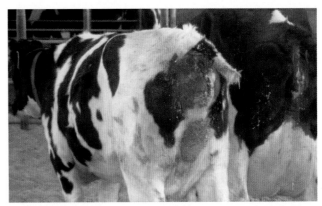

• **Fig. 9.16** First-calf heifer with extensive cellulitis and crepitant edema in the perineal region associated with necrotic vulvovaginitis after forced fetal extraction. Multiple cases were observed on the farm over a 1-month period.

Prolapse of a cervical fold is seen in parous cows. In this condition, one or more cervical folds protrude caudally through the external os of the cervix. Prolapse of a cervical fold does not seem to interfere with fertility.

Leiomyomas are the most common cervical tumor of cows. Fibromas are sometimes seen. Adenocarcinomas are extremely rare. The benign cervical tumors are usually only important as space-occupying lesions that may impede cervical function.

Acquired Vulvo-Vestibulo-Vaginal Disorders

Lacerations and contusions of the vagina and vulva are common parturient injuries. Sequelae include distortion secondary to scar tissue formation, which may impair normal vulvar closure, with chronic pneumovagina or infection of the cranial tract. Tears should be carefully inspected immediately after parturition and repaired if necessary to maintain vulvar function. Vaginal, perivaginal, vulvar, and perivulvar contusions are important for two main reasons. Large hematomas may form and become abscesses after secondary infection. These abscesses may be carefully drained, either into the vagina or via the ischiorectal fossa. Postparturient contusions also provide a hospitable locus for reactivation of clostridial spores with potentially fatal myositis or tetanus. Sporadic infection with other anaerobic or tissue necrotizing organisms may also occur (Fig. 9.16). Aggressive antibiotic therapy is justified in cows with severe contusion of the caudal reproductive tract sustained at calving.

Less obvious, but possibly more consequential, is subtle damage to the vestibulovaginal junction that may occur during parturition when traction is applied before dilation of the caudal tract is complete. This is often the case when less valuable dams are carrying potentially valuable offspring, but it may occur in any assisted delivery. Premature interference with parturition can be an unintended consequence of greater maternity pen vigilance and misguided human attempts to provide obstetric assistance. On farms where involvement of nonveterinarians in the calving pen is the usual first-line approach to calving assistance, it is critical that staff are educated in not only proper hygiene and technique but also about the perils of forced extraction before adequate cervical and vaginal dilation. Financial programs for maternity pen employees that reward purely according to the number of live calves delivered would represent a particularly risky scenario. The consequences of such interference may be appreciated by problems such as an increase in RFM and metritis early in the postpartum period but also by increases in caudal reproductive tract abnormalities later in lactation such as perivaginal adhesions and urovagina. Distortion of the vestibulovaginal junction may result in ongoing urovagina by altering the position and orientation of the urethral orifice such that some urine splashes on the roof of the vestibular vault and is reflected cranially into the vagina. There it causes chemical endocervicitis and may potentially lead to endometritis. Urovagina causes infertility and may be difficult to diagnose. It can be managed surgically by urethral extension or by creating a dam by placing a circumferential purse-string suture into the hymenal fold to prevent cranial flow of urine. The latter surgical technique is simple and effective. A specialized surgical instrument (modified Deschamps needle) can greatly facilitate the placement of such sutures, especially in large, multiparous older cows (Fig. 9.17). The suture should be pulled tight enough to allow only enough space for insemination. The procedure will need to be repeated after the subsequent calving.

In addition to physical conditions that result in vaginitis, specific infectious diseases can cause vaginitis.

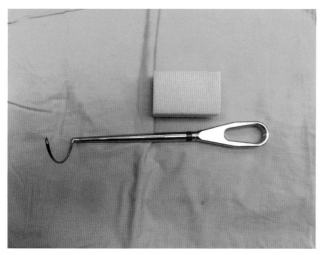

• **Fig. 9.17** Modified Deschamps suture device used to place purse-string suture for correction of urovagina. (Courtesy of Dr. Mike Livesey.)

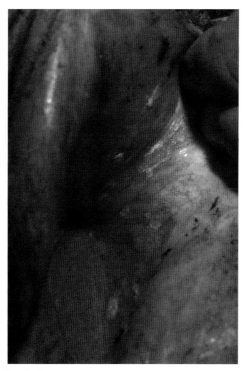

• **Fig. 9.18** Vulvar plaques caused by bovine herpesvirus.

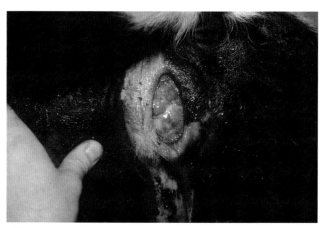

• **Fig. 9.19** Large vaginal fibropapilloma protruding from the vulva of a bred Holstein heifer.

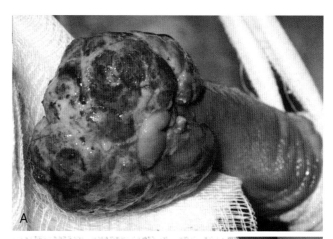

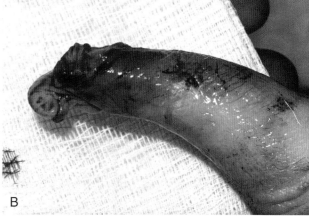

• **Fig. 9.20** **A,** Fibropapilloma on the penis of a 2-year-old Holstein bull. **B,** The same tumor as shown in A following debulking and before cryosurgical treatment of the base of the mass.

Causative organisms include *Mycoplasma* spp., *Ureaplasma* spp., *Histophilus somni,* IBR virus (Fig. 9.18), and others. Such organisms can cause endemic or epidemic vaginitis in dairy cattle and will be discussed separately. More recently, an outbreak of vulvovaginitis caused by *Porphyromonas levii* has been reported.

Fibropapillomas are occasionally observed in the vulva or vagina of young cattle and heifers (Fig. 9.19). These tumors are caused by a bovine papillomavirus and are also common on the penises of young bulls (Fig. 9.20 and 10.15). Venereal transmission is possible when natural service is practiced. Fibropapillomas of the vulva and vagina are probably more common than we realize because only large warts that protrude from the vulva or bleed cause detectable signs. These tumors are benign and usually regress spontaneously but may require treatment when large enough to protrude through the vulva because they then result in bleeding and tenesmus.

In adult cattle, many tumor types are possible. Squamous cell carcinoma (SCC) of the vulva (Fig. 9.21) in older cattle with a lightly pigmented perineum can be an aggressive

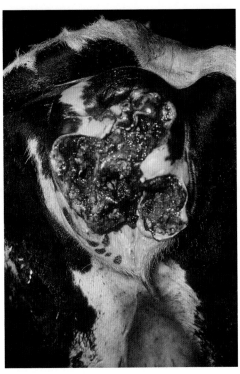

• **Fig. 9.21** Squamous cell carcinoma on the vulva of a 12-year-old Holstein cow.

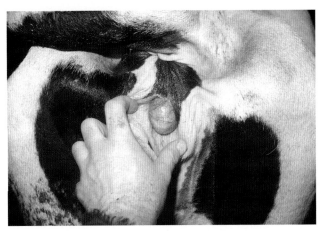

• **Fig. 9.22** Cystic Bartholin gland in a mature Holstein cow.

tumor that spreads by both local infiltration and metastasizes unless diagnosed early. Lymphosarcoma can involve the vagina, especially when diffuse neoplasia of the reproductive tract occurs.

Unexplained bleeding from the vulva, vaginal discharge, tenesmus, or an obvious mass protruding from the vulva may signal a vaginal or vulvar tumor. Vaginal examination by speculum determines the extent of the lesion and allows surgical or excisional biopsy. Fibropapillomas may be left untreated unless they disturb the heifer or are large enough to protrude from the vulva.

Squamous cell carcinoma causes raised or ulcerative (or both) pink cobblestone-like tissue proliferation on the vulva. The tumor is more common in cows with nonpigmented vulvas and more frequent in geographic areas where cows receive a great deal of exposure to sunlight. The lesion may be singular or multifocal and causes progressive erosion of the affected tissue. Neglected cases have a characteristic necrotic odor, purulent or crusted discharge and may invade deeper structures or metastasize to regional lymph nodes and other visceral locations. Sometimes precursor plaquelike lesions or warty epitheliomas precede carcinomas similar to the progression of lesions observed in ocular SCC.

Other tumors are extremely rare, and biopsy is indicated to identify the tumor type and offer treatment or prognostic information. Although lymphosarcoma can involve the caudal reproductive tract, tumor masses in other target organs are more likely to be responsible for clinical signs, and therefore lymphosarcoma in this region usually is an incidental finding.

Treatment

Removal of large fibropapillomas and those that protrude from the vulva or that are located on the penis may be necessary. Surgical debulking or removal should be followed by cryosurgical destruction of the tumor base to prevent recurrence. Vaginal fibropapillomas occasionally have a very thick and vascular base that bleeds profusely if the tumor is simply excised. Hemostasis may be difficult in such cases, and the surgeon should anticipate this problem. Bulls with penile warts may spread the problem to many heifers. The efficacy of wart vaccines as preventive medicine for such fibropapillomas is debatable, and wart vaccines are not an effective form of treatment.

Treatment of SCC of the vulva is most successful when the condition is diagnosed early. Affected areas should be treated with cryosurgery, radiofrequency hyperthermia, or other means. Radiofrequency hyperthermia is best used for small, superficial lesions. Cryosurgical destruction of early vulvar SCC is often successful. Serial injections of Bacillus Calmette–Guérin are usually avoided as a treatment option in dairy cattle despite their potential efficacy because these injections could sensitize the cow to tuberculin and cause a false-positive result on a tuberculin test. Intralesional chemotherapy with cisplatin and 5-fluorouracil or topical imiquimod as used in horses may become useful in the future, but as yet, sufficient experimental data are lacking and the legality of their use is uncertain. Advanced cases that have invaded the pelvic region or regional lymph nodes usually are hopeless.

Cystic Bartholin Glands

Cystic Bartholin (or vestibular) glands occasionally are noticed by owners when an affected cow lies down and the pink or red cystic structure protrudes through the vulvar cleft (Fig. 9.22). It may be confused with a mild vaginal prolapse. One gland exists on each lateral vestibular wall, and cyst formation is thought to be the consequence of obstruction or atresia of the emptying duct. Most are unilateral, and the condition is sporadic, perhaps seen once a year in bovine practice. Some cattle with lesser degrees of the condition may escape detection because the cystic structure does not protrude from the vulva. Usually the condition goes unobserved until the cyst is greater than 5 cm in diameter. The cyst is soft, smooth, and fluid filled. Chronic exposure damage may change the appearance and predispose to contamination of the caudal reproductive tract as the cyst repeatedly prolapses and then returns to the vaginal region.

Treatment merely involves scalpel incision of the cyst, which will usually drain a thick, slightly cloudy, mucoid fluid. Occasionally, the condition coexists with cystic ovaries, but the two generally are considered unrelated. It simply may be that increased laxity of the caudal reproductive tract associated with cystic ovaries allows the cyst to protrude more easily.

Infectious Causes of Vaginitis

Infectious Bovine Rhinotracheitis and Infectious Pustular Vulvovaginitis

Bovine herpesvirus I type 2 causes infectious pustular vulvovaginitis (IPV). This form of IBR manifests as typical plaques (see Fig. 9.18), erosions, ulcers, and inflammation of the vaginal and vulvar mucous membranes. Swelling and discharge are apparent at the vulva, and affected animals may be uncomfortable. Although not as common as the respiratory or conjunctival forms of IBR, IPV is observed occasionally. The condition may be spread by coitus from infected bulls with lesions on the prepuce or penis and through use of infected semen. As with other forms of IBR, a septicemic spread of the virus does occur despite localization of signs to the caudal reproductive tract. Therefore systemic signs of fever, depression, and inappetence may accompany the genital lesions. Lactating cattle or those under stress for other reasons are more likely to show systemic signs than heifers. The condition may appear as the only sign of IBR in a group or may appear in conjunction with the respiratory form. Abortion is a possible sequela as a result of septicemia and is more common when severe systemic signs appear. Abortions are not as common with IPV as with the other forms of IBR but always are a risk when the disease occurs. Abortions may occur at any stage of pregnancy but are more common in cattle in the last half of gestation.

Diagnosis

Clinical signs in acute cases are pathognomonic and include white plaques, erosions, and ulcers of the vulvar and vaginal mucous membranes. Historically, diagnosis has been confirmed by smears subjected to fluorescent antibody (FA) testing or viral cultures. Currently, however, the diagnostic emphasis for IBR and IPV lies with viral nucleic acid identification using polymerase chain reaction (PCR) assays performed upon appropriate samples. If lesions are older than 7 to 10 days, virus may no longer be present in the lesions, and serologic (paired) testing is indicated. It has been reported, however, that a neutralizing antibody response may occur very slowly after IPV in females or similar lesions in bulls (infectious balanoposthitis). Therefore FA, PCR, and virus isolation procedures may be indicated even after the acute phase if serology does not yield definitive information. Abortions may occur during the recuperative period or be delayed for weeks after clinical signs of IPV and other forms of IBR. Therefore cattle that subsequently abort are usually seropositive and may not show an increase in titer with paired samples. Latent recrudescence of the virus is always possible once an animal has been infected.

Treatment and Prevention

No specific treatment exists. Prevention includes using semen from IBR-negative bulls and ensuring adequate immunization against IBR in all cattle (see IBR in Chapter 4). Young stock should be vaccinated after maternal antibodies subside; good primary immunity is established by two vaccinations at 2- to 4-week intervals when killed or inactivated products are used. Thereafter, cattle should be boostered against IBR every 6 to 12 months for life.

Granular Vulvitis Complex

A condition of controversial significance and uncertain etiology, granular vulvitis is diagnosed when signs of vaginitis, including a cloudy or mucopurulent discharge, appear chronically or intermittently; infertility or repeat services recur as an epidemic or endemic problem; and typical vulvar lesions that are comprised of raised nodules, granules, or lymphoid follicles are found on the vulvar mucous membrane, especially near the clitoris. It is not known whether these lesions are specific, semispecific, or simply represent nonspecific lymphoid hyperplasia tissue responses to any of the potential opportunistic or pathogenic organisms inhabiting the caudal reproductive tract. Lesions are more common in heifers and younger cows but can be seen at any age. Mild lesions also can be observed in normal cows with no known reproductive problems. Moderate to severe lesions occurring with a high prevalence in a herd experiencing reproductive problems and vaginal or vulvar discharges should be considered abnormal and suggestive of contagious infection.

Many causes have been suggested for the condition, but currently *Mycoplasma* spp., *Ureaplasma diversum*, and *Histophilus somni* have received the most attention and will be discussed here. That these organisms may be isolated from the caudal reproductive tracts of both healthy and diseased cattle further frustrates a clear-cut definition for the disease.

Ureaplasma diversum

U. diversum has been associated with granular vulvitis and caudal reproductive tract infection. The organism resides primarily in the vagina and vulva but can gain entrance to the uterus during insemination. Although *U. diversum* usually does not cause chronic endometritis, experimental inoculation of the organism into the uterus of susceptible cows produces endometritis and salpingitis. Experimental infection of pregnant cows has resulted in abortion. Natural infections of the uterus are thought to be cleared relatively quickly but may create an unhealthy environment for implantation or cause the death of early embryos if present at the time of insemination. Early embryonic deaths also have been observed in field outbreaks of this disease. Experimental infection of the vulva causes red or tan, granular vulvitis lesions and may in severe cases produce heavy purulent discharge, swelling of the vulva, and pus-filled white nodules several millimeters in diameter on the vulvar mucous membranes. These lesions may be confused with those seen with IBR-IPV. However, IPV tends to be erosive or ulcerative.

Bulls commonly have *U. diversum* as a commensal (or pathogen) in their urethra or prepuce and can spread the organism to cows through natural service or via fresh or frozen semen. Although *U. diversum* has been shown to establish infection in the vesicular glands of bulls when inoculated there experimentally, infection of accessory sex glands in bulls is thought to occur less often than urethral contamination of semen.

Field infection with *U. diversum* may be sporadic and tends to go undiagnosed unless an endemic or epidemic condition involving multiple cows within a herd appears. Cloudy or mucopurulent discharges on the vulva, tail, and perineum signal the condition. Many of the affected cows will not have been observed to have endometritis during the early postpartum period and may have had "clean" early postpartum reproductive examinations. Discharge may be found in cows at any stage of lactation but is most common in cows due to be bred and cows that have been bred but returned to service. Some cows may not show obvious discharge until a few days after breeding.

Examination of affected cattle usually reveals typical lesions of granular vulvitis or atypical, more purulent, focal vulvar lesions. Repeat services at regular or irregular (suggestive of early embryonic death) intervals and early abortions frequently accompany clinical signs of vulvar discharges in these infected herds. Sporadic cases in herds not considered to be having reproductive problems usually are dismissed as cases of chronic endometritis or chronic vaginitis. Crowding, dirty environments, and other stressors may contribute to herd infections, and selenium deficiency has been identified as a coexisting problem in a few dairy herds investigated. It is not known how the organism spreads in non-natural service herds. Overcrowding and spread by tails has been theorized, as has "sniffing" by cows during heat activity that might spread the organism via respiratory secretions. Dogs licking discharges from infected cattle and transmitting the pathogen to other cows also has been theorized but seems unlikely on most farms. After *U. diversum* establishes infection, it persists for a prolonged period and apparently fails to cause any effective immune response.

Positive diagnosis requires isolation of *U. diversum* from multiple cows that have had signs of disease. Ideally, these signs include discharges, granular vulvitis lesions, and reproductive failure. A single isolate is less than conclusive because the organism has often been found as an apparent commensal in the reproductive tract of both cows and bulls. Treatment and control measures are as follows:

1. Improve management to minimize overcrowding, clean dirty facilities, and improve sanitation.

2. Avoid natural service if it is currently practiced in the herd. Most AI stud services add antibiotics to semen to control both *Mycoplasma* spp. and *Ureaplasma* spp. in processed semen.
3. Inseminate cows using "double-sheathing" techniques to avoid contamination of the uterus with vaginal organisms.
4. Consider use of systemic antibiotics in specific animals.
5. Assess the herd for concurrent diseases and nutritional status. Assess selenium levels in feed and blood when the disease occurs in unsupplemented herds that reside in selenium-deficient areas.

Mycoplasma spp.

Although *Mycoplasma* spp. are linked less specifically to granular vulvitis than *U. diversum,* they have been isolated from cows with the condition, and *Mycoplasma* spp. can infect the reproductive tract to cause infertility. Similar to *U. diversum, Mycoplasma* spp. also can be isolated from the caudal reproductive tract of healthy cattle without overt reproductive disorders. Therefore cause-and-effect relationships, data on experimental infections, and significance of individual isolates often are questioned.

Mycoplasma bovigenitalium can be cultured from the vagina or cervix of many cattle. Some of these cows may have histories of reproductive failure or granular vulvitis lesions. Uterine infection appears much less commonly than caudal reproductive tract infection, and some strains of *M. bovigenitalium* may be more pathogenic than others. One study found that heifers bred to an infected bull developed purulent infections and had biopsy-confirmed evidence of endometritis. *M. bovigenitalium* (at least some strains) definitely can infect the prepuce, urethra, and vesicular glands of bulls. Because of this, antibiotic mixtures of gentamicin, tylosin, and lincocin-spectinomycin commonly are added to collected semen to be used in AI. Natural service use of infected bulls would likely constitute a major risk.

Mycoplasma bovis does not appear to infect the reproductive tract of cows or bulls very commonly, but when experimental infections have been produced, severe uterine, uterine tube, and vaginal pathology can occur.

Based on current understanding, *M. bovigenitalium* appears to be a more common isolate from the caudal reproductive tract of cows. This organism tends to remain in the caudal reproductive tract but, similar to *U. diversum,* could be introduced to the uterus by insemination and cause transient endometritis, interfere with implantation, or result in early embryonic death. It should be considered a pathogen only when signs of granular vulvitis, discharge, and reproductive failure in multiple cattle are found in conjunction with identification of the organism by culture or PCR. Control measures are similar to those for *U. diversum* but also include antibiotic additives to semen for bulls in AI use. In addition, systemic treatment of infected cattle with tetracycline appears effective.

Histophilus somni

H. somni can be isolated with great regularity from the cervicovaginal area of cows with and without signs of reproductive tract infection. Similar to *Mycoplasma* spp. and *U. diversum*, the significance of an isolate may be difficult to determine. This gram-negative pleomorphic coccobacillus is discussed further in Chapters 4 and 13. It is capable of causing infection in several organ systems of cattle. Neurologic disease, including thrombotic meningoencephalitis in growing cattle, meningitis in adult dairy cattle, polyarthritis, pneumonia, myocarditis, upper respiratory tract infections, septicemia, and reproductive conditions, have all been attributed to the organism. Although microbiologists disagree regarding the existence of strain differences among isolates as regards organ tropism and pathogenicity, field outbreaks suggest that strain variation is real. Some strains may cause neurologic disease but not reproductive disease and vice versa. The pathophysiology and route of infection sometimes are difficult to determine, but the respiratory tract appears the most likely entry point. Septicemia is thought to follow infection regardless of entry site. Because of the frequent isolation of *H. somni* from the reproductive tract, some have theorized that this may be a site of entry. Isolation of the organism from the reproductive tract of healthy, fertile cattle raises questions as to the pathogenicity of the organism, but perhaps again this reflects strain differences.

Klavano worked with field outbreaks of infertility associated with *H. somni* isolates and was then able to reproduce clinical disease experimentally, confirming that the *H. somni* from the original patients was capable of causing vaginitis with acute mucopurulent discharge and persistent isolation of the organism for almost 2 months. Therefore vaginitis certainly is a possible consequence of *H. somni* infection.

Uterine infections also have been attributed to *H. somni*. Such infections may represent ascending postpartum infection from the caudal reproductive tract or be the result of septicemia. Abortion and early embryonic death also have been attributed to *H. somni* both in field studies and in some experimental infections.

In addition to the frequent isolation of *H. somni* from the caudal reproductive tract of cows, the organism is often isolated from the sheath and semen of bulls. Infection of the reproductive tract or accessory glands is possible, but the organism frequently is isolated from bulls with neither macroscopic nor histologic lesions. Infected bulls can have reduced semen quality and certainly could transmit the disease through natural breeding or semen. Semen usually is treated with antibiotics to minimize this possibility, as discussed already.

A diagnosis of *H. somni* infertility should be based on isolation of the organism from several animals, aborted fetuses, or other samples. Treatment recommendations or indications are nebulous, but it appears that systemic treatment with tetracycline is preferable to local intrauterine or intravaginal therapy.

Control is best attempted by immunization using *H. somni* bacterins even though proof of vaccine efficacy in preventing or controlling reproductive infections is sparse. Animals should be vaccinated twice within 2 to 4 weeks or according to manufacturer's recommendations and then given booster shots annually or semiannually depending on perceived risk and farm history. Little is known regarding immunity to the organism, but vaccines generally are considered helpful regardless of the organ system infected. Vaccines may be improved significantly in the future if distinct strains of *H. somni* are identified and strains having specific organ tropism confirmed. Some manufacturers currently attempt to address this issue by formulating bacterins from clinical isolates obtained from specific organ systems.

Vaginal Prolapse

Etiology

In dairy cattle, vaginal prolapse occurs primarily in dry cows that are overconditioned or that have had anatomic injuries at previous parturitions that resulted in excessive pelvic or perineal laxity. Increasing estrogenic influence during late gestation further contributes to laxity of the caudal reproductive tract. The condition is observed when the cow is lying down and especially if the cow lies with her rear parts lower than the foreparts, as occurs in confined cattle that lie over, or in, a gutter. Apparently, the abdominal contents help push the cervix and vagina caudally. Laxity, deformity of the vulvar lips, and obesity predispose to vaginal prolapse as well.

When vaginal prolapse is observed in cows that are not in advanced gestation or as a cluster of cases that occurs over a short period of time, excessive estrogen levels should be suspected. Cystic ovaries and highly estrogenic feeds may be responsible for some cases. Zearalenone, a mycotoxin, can cause vaginal prolapse in addition to other problems such as swollen vulva, cystic ovaries, and premature udder development when moldy corn or other feed containing the mycotoxin is fed. Rarely, a cow that suffered severe dystocia with marked physical stretching and perhaps damage to pelvic innervation may develop recurrent or persistent vaginal prolapse that does not respond to simple corrective measures. This specific form of vaginal prolapse has the most devastating impact on productivity and future fertility.

Clinical Signs and Diagnosis

The diagnosis is obvious based on clinical signs of a round pink or reddened mucosal prolapse that protrudes from the vulva (Fig. 9.23). Usually the ventral vagina protrudes because the prolapse invariably begins with the ventral floor of the caudal vagina rolling over the vestibulovaginal junction, and the cervix and lateral vaginal walls only appear in more severe cases. In many dry cows, the condition is benign, only appears when the cow lies down, and the prolapsed tissue returns to its normal position when the cow rises. If the cow is close to term and the condition is mild, it may be neglected. Cattle that are weeks or months from term usually require treatment, lest a vicious cycle of vaginal prolapse, vaginal irritation and exposure damage, vaginitis, and tenesmus develops. Such cows suffer vaginal irritation simply from drying of the mucosa and abrasions created by their own tails. Exposure damage may result in edema, inflammation, superficial necrosis, or the formation

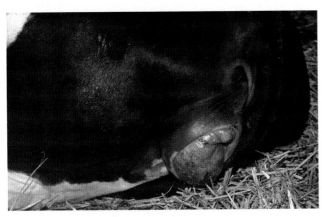

• **Fig. 9.23** Vaginal prolapse in a dry cow.

of diphtheritic membranes as the vaginal mucosa continues to be exposed during recumbency. Eventually, persistent tenesmus and vaginitis make the cow uncomfortable and disturb appetite. In severe cases that expose the cervix and a large part of the vagina, cervicitis and abortion are possible. Hematoma of the vagina, cystic vestibular glands, and tumors may be mistaken for vaginal prolapse.

Cattle that are not pregnant should be examined for the presence of ovarian cysts. Mycotoxins such as zearalenone should be considered, especially when more than one animal in the herd or group of heifers has signs of vaginal prolapse. Cattle that develop persistent or recurrent vaginal prolapse after dystocia usually have had a "big calf," and physical examination will detect extreme laxity of the perineum, vulva, pelvic ligaments, and ischial region. These cattle may also have partial loss of innervation to the caudal reproductive region, perineum, and bladder. Vaginal prolapse is also encountered in cows repeatedly superovulated for embryo recovery because of the chronically high estrogen level to which they are exposed.

Treatment

Mild vaginal prolapse in dry cows that are near term may not require any therapy. These cows may be helped by removal from confinement and placement in a well-bedded box stall, clean maternity area, or pasture where their rear quarters are less likely to be dependent or over a gutter.

Pregnant cows with mild to moderate vaginal prolapse that have weeks or months until term can be treated by the aforementioned management changes or may be helped by aluminum or rope trusses that are held in place by rope surcingles around the neck and chest. Pessaries have also been used in the past but are seldom used today.

More severe vaginal prolapses require surgical intervention. Procedures that simply close the vulvar lips are ineffective at preventing prolapse and do not contain it effectively. Buhner's method consists of a buried suture that constricts the vestibule region. In this method, incisions are made below the lower commissure of the vulvar lips and above the dorsal (close to the anus but not in the anal sphincter) commissure. A Görlach ("Buhner's") needle, which is a 12-in-long needle with the eye in the point, is passed through

from ventral to dorsal, and the procedure is repeated on the opposite side of the vulva. This "purse-string" suture then is tied tightly. The well-placed suture will migrate cranially and come to lie close to the vestibulovaginal junction, the area where the prolapse begins. Correctly performed, this suture prevents recurrence. The suture should be tightened to a point where two fingers can enter the vagina. The suture should then be knotted, leaving long ends that will ease removal when calving is imminent. When postpartum cattle are treated, the sutures may be left in place until fibrosis occurs in the vestibular caudal vagina, thereby reducing the chances of recurrence.

Minchev's method achieves permanent pexy of the vagina by passing heavy suture from the cranial vagina through the gluteal region, where the suture is anchored by buttons or other devices. Abscessation and damage to sciatic nerve branches have developed occasionally after this technique; it is thus not recommended. Similarly, radical techniques such as cervopexy rarely are indicated in dairy cattle. Reefing procedures that resect large areas of affected vaginal mucosa could be considered only for extremely severe cases when the cow's value justifies the surgery.

Early intervention is perhaps the best means of ensuring successful management of vaginal prolapse in dairy cattle and preventing the vicious cycle of events that result in vaginal injury and tenesmus. Simple techniques work most effectively when used before severe vaginal exposure damage, edema, necrosis, and diphtheritic membrane formation have resulted.

All of the aforementioned surgical techniques require epidural anesthesia, careful cleansing of the exposed area of vagina, replacement of the organ, and then surgical repair. Rarely, the bladder is also prolapsed within the tissue, preventing easy replacement of the vagina; aspiration of urine through the prolapsus will decrease its size and allow replacement. Antibiotics and other supportive measures are seldom necessary except in neglected cases. Cows having severe exposure damage and vaginitis that result in tenesmus may require repeated epidural anesthesia for a day or longer until vaginal irritation subsides.

There is an inherited predisposition to vaginal prolapse and owners should be made aware of this. It is advisable to exclude affected animals and their offspring from breeding programs. Cows with vaginal prolapse attributable to repeated superovulation for embryo recovery can be exempt from this judgment.

Infectious Causes of Infertility

Campylobacteriosis (Vibriosis)

Campylobacter fetus subsp. *venerealis* is the cause of campylobacteriosis, formerly called vibriosis in cattle. Although the disease rarely, if ever, occurs in dairy herds using only AI with semen from commercial production, it still is common in beef cattle and could be introduced to dairy cows or dairy heifers if infected bulls or heifers are purchased. *C. fetus* subsp. *venerealis* is an obligate parasite of the reproductive tract of cattle, particularly the prepuce of older bulls. After infection of the vagina, the organism quickly establishes an endometritis that persists for weeks to months. Salpingitis also may occur. The major consequences of the disease are early embryonic death, fetal death, and infertility. Immunity slowly develops after infection, and most cows subsequently conceive after two or more repeat services even when the organism continues to persist in the caudal reproductive tract. Young bulls (2 years old or younger) are difficult to infect but can act as mechanical carriers of the infection from infected to susceptible heifers and cows during natural service. Older bulls (>5 years) more commonly are found to be chronically infected, harbor the organism in their prepuce, and contaminate semen with the organism.

Endometritis associated with *C. fetus* subsp. *venerealis* usually is subclinical and seldom causes detectable evidence of infection on rectal examination. Purulent discharge is unusual. Immunoglobulins of the IgG type eventually are produced and found in the uterus in recovered animals, and IgA antibodies are found in the vagina. Infertility in infected cows may be apparent as repeat services at regular or irregular intervals. Irregular intervals are associated with embryonic death. Abortion can also occur, and although most observed abortions occur at 4 to 7 months' gestation, truly speaking a greater incidence probably occurs at less than 4 months but remains undetected or is only suspected following a return to heat.

Diagnosis of the disease requires culture of the organism from vaginal mucus or reproductive discharges of infected cows and heifers, aborted fetuses (lung and stomach contents), or sheath aspirates from bulls. Material can be collected with sterile insemination pipettes passed through an insemination straw or speculum for cranial vaginal mucus or via sheath samples in males. Diagnostic laboratories should be contacted before sample collection to determine appropriate handling, transport media, and temperature for shipment and samples should reach the laboratory within 6 hours of collection. Antibodies may be detected in vaginal mucus by an agglutination test, but this test has low sensitivity and may be more useful if multiple individuals from a herd are tested. Cultures are more likely to be diagnostic but the organism is fastidious, requiring selective media and microaerophilic conditions. *C. fetus* subsp. *venerealis* must be differentiated from *C. fetus* subsp *fetus*, an inhabitant of the intestinal tract which is usually non-pathogenic but may cause occasional abortions. The conventional means of differentiation is that *C. fetus* subsp. *venerealis* is sensitive to 1% glycine whereas *C. fetus* subsp. *fetus* is not. Unfortunately, this test is not completely reliable. Molecular (PCR) methods of detection and differentiation of *Campylobacter* spp. have been developed but are also susceptible to subspecies misidentification.

Control of the disease includes using only commercial antibiotic-treated semen from AI companies and avoiding natural service. Vaccination also is effective as both a control and treatment method because it evokes IgG production that results in elimination of infection from the uterus of cows and sheath of bulls. Vaccination should be performed according to manufacturer's instructions and repeated yearly. If natural service is continued, it must be emphasized that noninfected vaccinated bulls may transmit the disease mechanically even though they themselves are immune.

Trichomoniasis

Etiology

Tritrichomonas foetus, a flagellate protozoan, is the cause of trichomoniasis, a venereal disease of bull-bred cattle. Although herds using semen from commercial AI stud services as the exclusive source of semen are not at risk, herds that use custom collected and frozen semen or natural service are at risk. The disease is much more prevalent in beef cattle but deserves mention to remind us that dairy cattle are susceptible.

Trichomoniasis is spread by carrier and infected bulls. Older bulls are more likely to be infected chronically because *T. foetus* establishes infection on the epithelium and in the epithelial crypts of the prepuce and glans. These crypts become deeper and more numerous as bulls age, thereby causing greater risk for older bulls.

Infected bulls have no outward signs of infection and may shed large numbers of *T. foetus* when mated to only a few cows. Heavy breeding, as occurs during seasonal breeding in beef animals, tends to dilute or reduce the number of organisms shed during coitus, thereby somewhat reducing infectivity. Infected bulls kept on dairy farms and bred year round would likely be more infective at all breedings. Even noninfected bulls and bulls that develop immunity or resistance (rare) to *T. foetus* may act as mechanical carriers of infection between infected and noninfected females.

Cows infected with *T. foetus* usually clear the infection spontaneously within 3 to 4 months. The mechanisms of immunity involved in this self-limiting infection are unclear, but few cows remain persistently infected or become carriers. Cattle that have been infected, resolve the infection, conceive, and calve but who are subsequently reinfected seem to clear the new infection more rapidly, which suggests some immune responsiveness. Infected cows suffer from infertility thought to be the result of early embryonic death. Such embryonic death is related to uterine and oviductal inflammation. Infected cows either become repeat breeders or return to estrus at irregular intervals, suggesting early embryonic death. Most infected cattle resolve the infection spontaneously within 3 to 4 months and then are able to conceive and maintain a normal pregnancy. A small percentage of infected cows develop pyometra or suffer abortion. The occurrence of multiple cases of pyometra in a bull-bred herd should be considered as a major indicator of trichomoniasis. Abortions usually occur before the fifth month of gestation, and those that occur before 90 days seldom are observed. When abortion is observed, the fetus is autolyzed and may be macerated.

After inoculation of the organism into the reproductive tract of susceptible cows, infection is established in the vagina, cervix, endometrium, and tubules. Some cattle show postcoital discharge several days after breeding, and mild vulvovaginitis and cervicitis are also possible. However, most cows have little observable discharge. The vaginal infection usually resolves within 1 to 2 months because of vaginal antibody production, but the uterine infection lingers for 3 to 4 months, after which time immunity or resistance is established.

Clinical Signs and Diagnosis

Clinical signs other than infertility may be minimal. Therefore a careful history and examination of breeding records may be required before the disease is suspected. Postcoital discharges, pyometra, and abortion are helpful signs but are far less common than simple return to service at either regular or irregular intervals.

The diagnosis requires identification and isolation of *T. foetus*. It is recommended that bulls be sampled by preputial scrapings and aspirates. These are collected using a dry pipette inserted into the preputial fornix, simultaneously scraping while aspirating any available smegma. Because the organism lives in the mucosal crypts, the procedure must be done vigorously. The pipette also may be introduced through a dry straw, and preparation of the prepuce should include clipping preputial hair. Several specialized devices for preputial sample collection are commercially available. Cows and heifers may be sampled by collection of cranial vaginal mucus but are not as likely to yield organisms from this technique unless infected recently. Pyometra cases may yield the organism if fluid is aspirated directly from the uterus, and the abomasal fluid of aborted fetuses also is worth sampling. Sampling of bulls is considered the prime means of both diagnosis and surveillance in infected herds.

Field samples may be transferred to sterile physiologic saline solution or lactated Ringer's solution and quickly transported to a qualified diagnostic laboratory for identification. Preferably, the collected samples should be inoculated immediately into appropriate isolation media. Diamond's medium is time tested for isolation of *T. foetus*. Inoculation of samples into screw-top culture tubes containing Diamond's medium or In-Pouch TF medium chambers (Biomed Diagnostics, Santa Clara, CA) in the field is advisable to reduce loss of viable organisms in traditional transport diluents. In-Pouch TF medium may allow more rapid detection of *T. foetus* and superior detection of infection when smaller inocula are collected.

Although the morphology and motility of *T. foetus* are characteristic, there are other species of trichomonads that may complicate and confuse diagnosis. Use of PCR methods may provide more specific confirmation of the diagnosis. While PCR may offer higher sensitivity and specificity than culture alone, diagnostic accuracy is improved by serial testing and by combining culture and PCR test results.

Treatment and Control

Elimination of infected and carrier animals coupled with prevention of reintroduction of the disease are the hallmark features of a control program. In dairy herds, this can be simplified by stopping all natural breeding; getting rid of all bulls; and using only reputable, commercially prepared semen. If bull breeding must still be practised, only virgin bulls should be introduced, they should be tested, and regularly replaced. Treatment, in jurisdictions where it is permitted, currently consists of three injections of 15 to 30 g (deeply IM) of ipronidazole at 24-hour intervals. Because this imidazole ring compound (ipronidazole) may be inactivated by the normal preputial flora that includes micrococcal organisms, systemic antibiotics should be administered for several days before starting ipronidazole. One injection of long-acting tetracycline or daily injections of penicillin for 2 to 3 days have been used for this purpose. Ipronidazole is very acidic and irritating to tissue, so injection site abscesses are common. Other imidazoles including metronidazole and dimetridazole also have been used but have disadvantages (IV use for metronidazole and the unpalatability and GI tract dysfunction associated with dimetridazole) compared with ipronidazole. Practitioners should familiarize themselves with the legality of administering antibiotics belonging to the azole family in their respective geographic region before use. **For example, use of the substituted azoles (metronidazole, dimetridazole, and ipronidazole) in food-producing animals is currently forbidden by the Food and Drug Administration in the United States.**

Infected cows may be segregated, allowed several months of sexual rest, or repeatedly cycled with prostaglandin or analogues to hasten elimination of the infection from the reproductive tract. There are currently very few vaccines available worldwide against *T. foetus*; the one product that is available in the United States is a whole-cell product with no efficacy claim regarding protection in bulls. The best treatment is to eliminate natural service and use only commercially prepared semen by AI.

Neosporosis

Neospora caninum has been identified as a major cause of abortion in cattle worldwide. Domestic dogs are the primary host and shed oocysts in their feces that are infectious to cattle. Abortions may occur between 3 and 9 months, with the majority occurring at 4 to 6 months' gestation. After transplacental infection, the central nervous system of the fetus is the major target area, and protozoal encephalomyelitis ensues. In addition to abortions, calves may be born weak or with obvious neurologic deficits. Some cattle that have aborted once because of *Neospora* spp. infection may subsequently deliver calves with neurologic lesions and concurrent paresis as a result of congenital *Neospora* infection. On-farm studies of precolostral antibody levels in calves on endemic premises suggest that the risk of endogenous vertical transmission by a chronically infected dam may be as high as 95%, but the vast majority of congenitally infected calves are clinically normal.

Vertical transmission is the primary mode of transmission after the infection has been introduced into a herd. Experimental confirmation of vertical transmission in cattle is well documented. Nonsuppurative myocarditis has also been reported in fetuses or calves with congenital focal necrotizing encephalomyelitis. *Neospora* parasites have been isolated from aborted fetuses. In addition, other workers have found protozoan abortion in one herd of cattle that was concurrently infected with *Hammondia pardalis* thought to be related to a large feral cat population.

In most affected herds, protozoal abortion has seemed to be associated with close confinement of cattle. Abortions may be sporadic, endemic, or epidemic, and the prevalence varies greatly. Clinical signs are limited to abortion and the birth of calves with neurologic signs secondary to congenital infections of the central nervous system. Infected cows are asymptomatic. The diagnosis is based on immunohistochemical staining of fetal or calf tissues and an enzyme-linked immunosorbent assay (ELISA) test on serum. The current immunohistochemical procedure performed on tissue samples is an immunoperoxidase test using antisera against *N. caninum* or the bovine *Neospora* (BPA1) isolate in paraffin-embedded sections. All tissues should be examined, but the fetal brain and heart are most likely to show lesions. The ELISA test currently is recommended for screening of cattle and precolostral calves showing signs or considered at risk of congenital infections. Serology may be a helpful screening procedure to detect the presence of the *Neospora*-like organism in a herd or suspect calf. If all tested animals are negative, the disease is not likely to exist on that farm, and immunohistochemical staining may not be indicated. A milk ELISA test may be useful to assess herd status. Diagnostic laboratories studying aborted fetuses will need to use immunohistochemical stains to detect the organism in fetal tissues. Practitioners should inquire regarding the availability of these tests before sending samples to specific laboratories. A vaccine has recently become available in many parts of the world. Although reportedly efficacious in reducing incidence of abortion, it does not eliminate it.

Epizootic Bovine Abortion
Etiology

Epizootic bovine abortion is a disease of uncertain etiology that occurs in the foothill regions of the Sierra Nevada Mountains, including parts of Nevada, Oregon, California, and northern New Mexico. Although the specific etiologic agent is unknown, the disease occurs only in areas harboring *Ornithodoros coriaceus,* so the disease is thought to be tickborne. Cattle and deer are the primary hosts of this tick. *Chlamydia* was long considered to be the cause, but this assumption appears to be erroneous. Spirochetes and more recently a novel delta protobacterium have also been incriminated in the etiopathogenesis of the disease.

Abortions occur 3 months or more after tick exposure and tend to be correlated with seasonal implementation of grazing. Resistance to the disease appears to develop and is important for prevention and control. Susceptible cows and heifers moved to tick-infested areas for the first time are at greatest risk. Abortion generally occurs during the last trimester of pregnancy. After initial exposure, cattle develop

resistance, and therefore cattle sometimes are moved to tick-infested areas several months before first breeding in an effort to allow protective immunity to develop. The duration of immunity is unknown but appears adequate for one or two seasons.

Clinical Signs and Diagnosis

Infected cattle show no signs other than abortion or delivery of weak calves, and diagnosis requires laboratory confirmation of compatible histopathology in aborted fetuses or calves. Gross lesions include lymphadenopathy, splenomegaly, and hepatomegaly. Ascites is present in some fetuses. Histopathology identifies lymphohistiocytic infiltration of many tissues. This infiltration suggests chronic inflammatory disease that may have a proliferative component. Lymphoreticular tissues and other organs may be involved, and thymic lesions are extensive. The disease can be experimentally reproduced in susceptible animals by inoculation of thymic tissue from aborted fetuses.

Control measures other than avoiding endemic areas or preimmunizing cattle by exposure to tick-infested areas several months before breeding await further elucidation of the specific etiology.

Prolonged Gestation
Etiology

Prolonged gestation in dairy cattle most commonly results from fetal anomalies and requires differentiation from fetal loss or fetal mummification because in both scenarios affected cattle fail to show signs of impending parturition at their due date. Abnormalities in the fetal pituitary-adrenal axis are the usual cause of prolonged gestation and although adrenal abnormalities can be responsible, the primary lesion in prolonged gestation cases usually involves the fetal pituitary gland. The condition is reported in Holsteins and Ayrshires, and I have observed it in Brown Swiss cattle; it is thought to represent a recessive trait. Dams with this form of prolonged gestation appear normal but do not show signs of udder edema or pelvic laxity at the predicted calving date. Gestation may be prolonged 1 to 3 months or more. Palpation of the cow reveals a large fetus; errors in breeding dates or records must be ruled out before confirming the condition. Fetuses with pituitary or adrenal insufficiency may be normally formed, are very large (up to 150 to 250 lb in Holsteins and Brown Swiss), and usually require delivery via cesarean section (Fig. 9.24). Spontaneous parturition seldom occurs in true prolonged gestation unless the fetus dies in utero. If induction of parturition is elected, dystocia should be anticipated. If the fetus is born alive, it will be nonviable and most calves with this condition die shortly before, during, or within 48 hours of birth.

Prolonged gestation may also occur in calves produced by cloning, IVF, or sometimes embryo transfer as part of the "large offspring" syndrome. The possibility of prolonged gestation in such calves is sufficiently high enough that induction protocols frequently form part of the reproductive management discussion. This form of large offspring

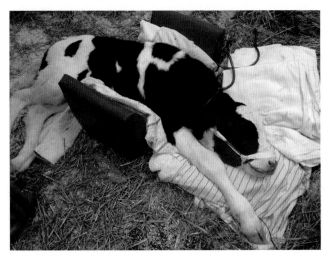

• **Fig. 9.24** An 11-month gestation bull calf delivered alive by C-section and euthanized on day 2. The calf weighed 88 kg and had a normal pituitary gland but abnormal adrenal glands on necropsy examination.

is mediated by altered genetic imprinting mediated by the in vitro procedures. Although anasarca, umbilical hemorrhage of abnormally large umbilical vessels, and respiratory distress are common in these calves, some cases do survive.

Another form of prolonged gestation occurs with fetal anomalies involving the skull and brain. Affected calves are miniature rather than giant and may have a cyclopeanlike head deformity with accompanying adenohypophyseal hypoplasia or pituitary abnormalities. A recessive trait is suspected as the cause of this condition in Guernseys, Ayrshires, and Swedish Red and White cattle. Roberts also has observed another anomaly of the skull and brain that includes cerebral hernia as a cause of prolonged gestation. Adrenal, hypophyseal, and pituitary anomalies are also likely with this form, and calves are large, often requiring cesarean section.

The prognosis should always be guarded for dams experiencing prolonged gestation and a frank conversation undertaken with the owner following diagnosis because:
1. They usually are not prepared to produce milk.
2. They usually experience dystocia or require cesarean section.
3. Inheritance is suspected as the cause; except in the case of cloned or IVF calves.

Reproductive Monitoring of Dairy Cattle

Although this section cannot, and will not try to, address the broad subject of reproductive management in dairy cattle fully, a brief synopsis, review, and summary will follow. Bovine practitioners should consult standard theriogenology and reproductive textbooks for more in-depth reading.

Reproductive programs have been, and will continue to be, devised and revised based on herd management styles, owner preferences, veterinary preferences, available labor, and pharmacologic manipulations. Veterinarians tend to be products of their education and experience when it comes to recommending or devising reproductive monitoring

programs for their clients. It is idealistic yet unrealistic for veterinarians to assume that clients will always accept a set protocol. In fact, veterinarians will suffer less damage to their egos and gain better client compliance when a reproductive monitoring program evolves from collective bargaining between client and doctor. Such negotiation minimizes client reservations, allows consideration of time-tested successful components on each farm, and allows the veterinarian to suggest and implement new or corrective measures to address unsuccessful components. Above all, the program should be tailored to the individual farm. Monthly herd checks may be acceptable for cow herds of 40 but obviously are unacceptable for herds with a population of 400 or more. Decisions as to which open cows should be monitored also will vary. Some herds have all postpartum cows evaluated, but others check only those 30 days or more postpartum and those with known postpartum problems. Ideally, all cows not observed in heat by 30 to 40 days should be examined; however, the intensity and effort put into estrus detection is extremely herd variable, and many larger herds now prefer to arbitrarily schedule reproductive examinations for all cows beyond a certain number of days in milk before first breeding. Regardless of the program chosen, it is imperative that a program exists that allows a regular, timely, and interactive relationship between veterinarian and client that forces both to concentrate on the herd's reproductive performance.

Postpartum cows should be evaluated regularly by routine rectal examinations to monitor involution and to allow detection of postpartum abnormalities such as endometritis, cervicitis, vaginitis, and cystic ovarian disease. In some herds, all postpartum cattle are included on the check list; in others, only those fresh 2 weeks or more are palpated. Rectal palpation of recently fresh cows (<14 days) is limited in value because uterine retraction is not always possible. However, evaluation of the uterine tone, degree of muscular contraction, and palpation of obvious abnormalities may still be helpful. In addition, repeated pressure directed downward and backward on the cervix and anterior vagina allows the examiner to propel discharges to the vulva and thereby evaluate reproductive tract discharges that might be missed otherwise. Vaginal and speculum examinations are indicated for cows less than 14 days postpartum suspected to have endometritis, RFM, necrotic vaginitis, or other caudal reproductive tract pathology.

Estrus Cycle

Cattle undergoing normal involution usually ovulate for the first time 13 to 15 days after calving. This ovulation usually does not result in detectable signs of heat but will be associated with a palpable follicle, increased uterine tone, and increased amounts of mucus discharge. The mucus discharge may be mixed with purulent material or bloody lochia or may appear fairly clear. The second ovulation follows another shorter than 21-day cycle and generally occurs 30 to 35 days after parturition. This ovulation is more likely to result in observable signs of heat than the first ovulation but still may go undetected in approximately 50% of cows. After this second ovulation, dairy cows usually assume a regular estrus interval of 20 to 23 days. A small percentage of cows will have cycles that are regular but shorter or longer by a few days compared to the average 20- to 21-day cycle.

Veterinarians monitoring reproductive programs try to determine whether cows are cycling normally and to anticipate heat dates (based on rectal palpation findings). An accurate history, including observed heats, reproductive tract discharges, treatments for postpartum conditions, and notes recorded at the time of earlier examinations, is essential when palpating cows during prebreeding examinations. Uterine tone, the cervix, the oviducts, reproductive tract discharges, and ovarian structures constitute the major palpable entities during routine rectal palpation of the nonpregnant cow.

Follicular development during the estrus cycle in cattle is characterized by two or three waves of follicular growth that produce 5 to 10 follicles on each ovary. Of these follicles, one usually becomes dominant and larger than the others within 1 to 2 days of the start of the wave, and the others undergo atresia. In cattle that have two follicular waves during their cycle, one may start on the day of the previous ovulation, and the second wave starts around day 10 of the cycle. The dominant follicle from the first wave enlarges for 5 to 6 days, becomes stationary for 5 to 6 more days, and then regresses. The dominant follicle from the second (or third) wave is the eventual ovulatory follicle. It follows that a palpable follicle may be present from about day 4 or 5 until ovulation because regression of the first wave–dominant follicle overlaps with the production of the second wave–dominant follicle. Ovulatory follicles usually are 12 to 18 mm in diameter. Nonovulatory dominant follicles reach a similar size. Therefore the presence of a follicle should not be interpreted mistakenly always to mean a cow is near heat. Some research suggests that many cows have three waves of follicular activity, and some may even have four. Cows that have three follicular waves have the waves start at about days 0, 9, and 16 of the cycle. Cows with three wave cycles tend to have longer luteal phases and correspondingly longer cycles of 22 to 24 days.

The dominant follicle of the last wave is the ovulatory follicle. Luteolysis is associated with increased concentrations of $PGF_{2\alpha}$ in the uterine endometrium that eventually reach the corpus luteum following transport into the uteroovarian veins and then into the ovarian artery. Regression of the corpus luteum causes reduced progesterone levels and triggers a large secretion of LH from the anterior pituitary gland after hypothalamic release of GnRH. At the same time that LH is peaking, estradiol levels are increasing and result in estrus behavior. The dominant follicle is being acted on by both LH and follicle-stimulating hormone (FSH) as follicular maturation occurs in the preovulatory period. Whereas LH acts on theca interna cells and increases androgen synthesis, which eventually has effects on granulosa cells, FSH enhances estradiol production.

The preovulatory LH peak is associated with complex and poorly understood effects on the follicle, but the result is follicular rupture, ovulation, and corpus luteum production. The estradiol peak associated with follicular maturation is thought to be responsible for the physical and behavioral signs of heat or estrus. Increased uterine tone, clear mucus discharge, hyperemia of the reproductive tract, and a palpable follicle 12 to 18 mm in diameter occur as the cow approaches "standing heat." Cows in heat should have a palpably small or barely detectable, regressing corpus luteum.

Estrus and Heat Detection

Estrus is usually regarded as lasting 10 to 18 hours, but there is evidence that estrus in modern high-yielding dairy cows is much shorter, probably about 8 hours. Ovulation generally occurs about 12 hours after estrus ends or 24 to 30 hours after the onset of estrus. Heat detection has been the traditional heart of all reproductive programs and cannot be overemphasized. The observed duration of heat may be less than 10 hours and can be split in some cows such that physiologic duration of heat may be longer than that which is apparent based solely on observation. Despite urging by lay publications, the availability of heat detection techniques and aids, and veterinary encouragement, many farms continue to do a poor job of heat detection. A study from the 1970s revealed that at that time approximately 50% of estrus periods went undetected on the average dairy farm in the United States; current biology and management of high-yielding cows mean that far fewer estrus periods are detected now. Owners who insist that cows do not show heats are reluctant to accept rectal palpation findings that suggest normal cyclic activity in their cows. Veterinarians who have grown up or worked on dairy farms know all too well the reasons for poor heat detection. When the labor force is spread too thin, assigned to field or mechanical chores, or fails to turn out confined cows, heat detection will be compromised. Some dairy farm workers and owners simply are poor observers, are impatient, or only check cows for a 5- to 10-minute period each day. Veterinarians must understand owner limitations but must not reinforce bad habits by agreeing that all cows have had "silent heats." Owners should be encouraged to observe cows several times daily. Bonuses may be paid to workers who detect heats, and this may encourage workers to observe the cattle more closely. Owners who refuse to turn cows out or only do so once a day for a short time are at an automatic disadvantage. Free-stall housing is not limited by turnout time but can suffer heat detection problems for other reasons. Because estrus occurs over a limited period of 12 to 18 hours, cows showing estrus at night frequently go undetected. Owners should check tails and perineums for clear mucus discharges that suggest proximity to, or recent, estrus; metestrus bleeding can be detected in the same manner. Cows suspected to be in or near heat because of previous heat charting, prostaglandin treatment, or rectal palpation findings should be observed closely and perhaps have a rectal examination performed by the person responsible for insemination. Increased uterine tone or clear mucus discharge can be detected by this examination. Behavioral or physical signs of standing for other cows to mount, decreased milk production, increased activity, frequent mounting of other cows, roughed-up topline, or foot stains along the flank region from allowing other cows to mount are things to look for in cows showing heat. Mechanical aids include heat detector strips attached to the tail head, progesterone levels, pedometers, teaser bulls of various types, instruments to measure the electrical resistance of vaginal mucus (lower resistance or increased conductivity occurs during estrus because of increased chloride levels), an organized highly visible heat expectation chart, and easily observed means of animal identification. When video monitoring of cattle to detect heat is compared with observed visual detection of heats, the pattern of heat detection is brought into perspective. For the first three postpartum heats, approximately 20%, 44%, and 64% were observed by visual observation, but the video camera recorded approximately 50%, 94%, and 100%.

Not all blame for failure to detect estrus accrues to labor, however. High-producing cows consume more dry matter to sustain the high yield. High dry matter intake, in turn, stimulates increased liver blood flow and liver size, both of which result in increased metabolism of steroid hormones. These cows have lower circulating concentrations of progesterone and estrogens, which undoubtedly contributes to reduced intensity of estrus expression and potentially to poorer pregnancy recognition and higher rates of pregnancy failure.

Time of Insemination

After heat is detected, the next problem is deciding when to breed the cow. Ovulation generally occurs 24 to 30 hours after the onset of estrus or 12 hours after the end of estrus. Much debate exists regarding the appropriate time for insemination. Some farms breed in the afternoon for morning-observed heats and breed the following morning for afternoon-observed heats. Others breed once daily. If breeding is in the afternoon, cows in heat that morning are bred, and cows in heat that afternoon are bred the next day. Although recommendations vary greatly, it appears clear that conception rate is improved if insemination occurs before ovulation, and insemination probably should be performed within 12 to 20 hours after the onset of heat.

A small percentage of pregnant cows will show heat despite being pregnant. Although this is more commonly observed in the early months of pregnancy, some cows show heats at regular intervals throughout pregnancy.

After ovulation, a corpus luteum forms from the theca and granulosa cells of the follicle under the influence of the LH surge and begins to secrete progesterone. The postovulatory ovary and uterus usually have characteristic, palpable changes that are present for the first few days of the cycle. The early corpus hemorrhagicum is friable, crepitant, or spongy and generally smaller than the mature corpus luteum. In addition, the uterus feels edematous and thickened, has progressively decreasing tone, and may be flaccid. These changes occur more quickly in some cows than others, and persisting uterine tonus accompanying a small corpus luteum can cause confusion between a preheat and postheat palpation, especially in the 48 hours before or after heat. Usually other determinants such as a dominant preovulatory follicle; a small, firm, regressing corpus luteum; a clear mucus discharge; or metestrus bleeding will assist in accurate determination of the cycle stage, but this may not always be easy. Metestrus bleeding may occur 1 to 3 days after heat, especially in younger animals and usually signals that a heat occurred 2 days previously. Although suggestive that ovulation has successfully occurred, this bleeding has nothing to do with conception or lack thereof, despite lay opinions to the contrary.

Rectal palpation after recent ovulation may reveal uterine edema and reducing tone for up to 7 days, after which time a mature corpus luteum is palpable and "normal" midcycle tone returns to the uterus. Increased uterine tone develops as the next heat approaches and is more obvious in young cows than in older ones. As mentioned previously, it is common and expected to palpate dominant follicles throughout the estrous cycle of cattle. Therefore palpation of uterine tone and corpus luteum size, consistency, shape, and other factors must be evaluated jointly when predicting stage of cycle and anticipated time of heat. It always is useful to attempt to "back-rake" cervical and vaginal discharges forcefully per rectum during routine evaluations, especially in older cows in whom uterine tone can be misleading because the appearance of clear mucus discharge may signal an impending heat, and cloudy or purulent discharge may allow diagnosis of inflammatory conditions.

Reproductive Goals and Programs

Each farm must have an established set of goals for reproductive performance. Criteria to be considered include heat detection efficiency (or AI submission efficiency), average days to first service, average days open, services per conception, and the duration of the voluntary waiting period. Each farm likely has strengths, weaknesses, and different goals.

"Pregnancy rate" is a parameter calculated by many electronic record systems. It calculates the number of cows becoming pregnant in each 21-day period (estrous cycle length) as a proportion of all cows eligible to be bred (taking into consideration the voluntary waiting period and pregnancy diagnosis status). This calculation reflects upon estrus detection (or AI submission) as well as the number of inseminated cows becoming pregnant. In modern herds, a pregnancy rate above 20% can be considered satisfactory and above 25% good.

With more herds depending heavily on synchronization of ovulation as a substantial component of their reproductive management, some simple guidelines are helpful in assessing success of programs.

Target parameters to aim for could be:
- No cows beyond 100 days in milk (DIM) at first insemination

- More than 40% of cows pregnant to first insemination
- No more than 42 days between inseminations
- High fertility at second and subsequent inseminations (e.g., >35%).

These parameters are useful because they take into account the difficulty frequently experienced in getting cows pregnant after failure to become pregnant to the first insemination, something that requires effective detection of estrus as well as successful insemination.

Ovsynch is an ovulation synchronization protocol that allows timed insemination of cattle without the need for heat detection. It has become a very popular approach to reproductive management in recent years, especially on larger free-stall dairies. This technique involves administration of GnRH at random stages of the estrous cycle followed by $PGF_{2\alpha}$ 7 days later. Forty-eight hours after the $PGF_{2\alpha}$, a second shot of GnRH is administered, and the cow is inseminated 16 to 20 hours later. Fertility in Ovsynch programs is increased when cows receive the first injection during the early to midluteal phase. Therefore fertility is further improved when cows on the Ovsynch program are presynchronized by administering $PGF_{2\alpha}$ one or two times before initiating Ovsynch. The second (or only) presynchronizing prostaglandin injection is administered 12 days before Ovsynch is begun. Presynchronization may also involve the use of back-to-back Ovsynch protocols, so-called "Double Ovsynch," which aims to ensure all cows begin the second Ovsynch protocol at the optimal stage of the cycle and ovulate to the first GnRH injection of the second Ovsynch. A problem recently identified in Ovsynch programs is the failure of complete luteolysis at the prebreeding prostaglandin injection. Some practitioners counteract this problem by including two prostaglandin injections on the same day. (This has been found to be superior to simply increasing the prostaglandin dose.)

One advantage of Ovsynch is that previously anovulatory cows can become pregnant using this protocol, although a lower proportion do so compared with previously cycling cows. Fertility in previously anovulatory cows can be improved by use of Double Ovsynch or by incorporating a source of progesterone into the protocol, such as CIDR-Synch, in which Ovsynch is modified by introducing an intravaginal progesterone-releasing device coincident with the first GnRH injection of Ovsynch. Previously anovulatory cows remain at increased risk of pregnancy loss after initial pregnancy diagnosis even if they do become pregnant to these protocols. Attention should therefore be focused on management of body condition score to ensure cows calve in optimal body condition (score, 3.5 to 3.75 of 5) and lose as little condition as possible in early lactation.

Nutritional Causes of Infertility

Poor nutrition and poor body condition have significant and negative influences on fertility. Field observations and many scientific references implicate poor body condition and inadequate energy balance as causes of reduced fertility.

Cows that calve in poor condition because of deficiencies in dry cow management are more likely to have prolonged anestrus postpartum. In addition, those cows with the greatest decline in body condition postpartum have more problems reproductively. Negative energy balance in early lactation may depress luteal function, lower progesterone levels, and lower fertility. Therefore regardless of specific pathophysiology, cows that freshen in less than desirable body condition or those that lose more condition than desirable during the first 5 to 8 weeks of lactation are likely to have reduced fertility. Although it is expected that early lactation is a time of negative energy balance because of peak production preceding peak dry matter intake, cows that suffer the most severe losses will be likely to have altered fertility and metabolic diseases that could further compromise reproductive performance. Cows with severe energy imbalances do not cycle, or cycle but fail to show heat. Repeat services are common even in such cows that do show heat.

Cattle with extreme energy imbalances have a reduced tendency to cycle normally, have reduced conception rates, and may suffer early fetal losses. These cows should not be bred until they are in a positive energy balance. Negative energy balance increases hypothalamic sensitivity to estradiol, resulting in negative feedback by GnRH and gonadotrophins. Dominant follicles in affected animals regress before they reach ovulatory size or produce estradiol. (This mimics the endocrinology of prepubertal heifers.)

Dietary protein is another nutritional factor that affects fertility. Inadequate protein significantly lowers conception rates, and too much protein with resultant increases in urea nitrogen levels may do the same. Excessive urea or ammonia levels resulting from excessive dietary protein may affect spermatozoa or early embryos, but the exact mechanism of infertility is unknown. Discrepancies in the results of various studies on excessive protein levels in the diet of dairy cows may be explained somewhat by the variations in protein sources. Experimental studies and field work support the theory that excessive rumen-degradable protein is harmful to reproduction. Experimentally, diets that result in serum urea nitrogen levels greater than 20 mg/dL have been associated with infertility. This work is supported by field observations that confirm a high incidence of repeat breedings, early embryonic death, and cystic ovarian disease in herds feeding excessive rumen-degradable protein. It has been recommended that 35% of dietary protein be present as rumen bypass protein and that excessive protein may not only be harmful to reproduction but also expensive. In addition, certain protein supplements derived from cotton sources may contain excessive gossypol, which has negative implications for both reproductive performance and cow health.

In selenium-deficient areas, low selenium levels in dairy cattle can have a significant negative effect on reproduction. In addition to an increased incidence of RFM, selenium-deficient herds have a higher incidence of endometritis, cystic ovarian disease, failure to show estrus, and embryonic death. Supplementation with selenium to correct blood-selenium deficiencies results in dramatic improvement in the herd reproductive status within 60 days. Selenium supplementation is best performed by adding the mineral to the ration at approved rates rather than administering selenium in slow-release boluses or by injection. Herds confirmed as selenium deficient should have periodic assessment of selenium status provided by analysis of blood samples from cows in various stages of lactation and from heifers. Practitioners in selenium-deficient areas that have identified selenium-deficient herds and observed response after dietary supplementation remain perplexed by the logic behind recent regulatory efforts that limit selenium supplementation to livestock. The supposition that dairy cattle in selenium-deficient areas somehow release excessive selenium into the environment seems unlikely to say the least.

Heat Stress and Infertility

High ambient temperature and humidity can create heat stress in dairy cattle, especially when management deficiencies in ventilation or cooling exacerbate the problem. Cows experiencing heat stress may secrete higher levels of progesterone to a degree that interferes with the LH surge of estrus. Alteration in the steroidogenic function of ovarian tissue and the resultant negative implications for folliculogenesis are likely primary physiologic forces behind the diminished reproductive performance observed during periods of severe heat stress in dairy cattle. Anestrus and reduced evidence of estrus behavior may be observed. Thyroxine and triiodothyronine levels decrease to effect lower heat production to help the cow accommodate, but these same reductions lower feed intake. Reduced feed intake can contribute to decreased production and energy imbalances. The combined effects of high temperature and humidity result in heat stress. Conception rates plummet in cows under severe heat stress, and some farms discontinue breeding during periods of high temperature and humidity because of frustration with poor heat detection and poor conception. Heat stress has been associated with increased numbers of abnormal embryos and unfertilized ova. Conception failure, early embryonic death, and even abortion can be observed in herds suffering heat stress. Late gestation cows may calve early with resultant RFM and have metabolic problems that are amplified by decreased feed intake. Cows tend to be inactive, do not want to move about to feed bunks or demonstrate estrus activity, and tend to congregate in areas of better ventilation or around water troughs. Severe heat stress causes some cows to show open-mouth breathing, and all cows to show tachypnea. Heat stroke is a possible sequela.

Management must anticipate the possibility of heat stress caused by weather extremes during warm months and ensure adequate ventilation by proper barn construction that includes escape of hot humid air through the roof, increased use of powerful fans, water misters, open or screened sides, and other measures to ameliorate cow comfort and performance during hot weather. Decreased dry-matter intake and electrolyte losses through panting, sweating, and salivation may contribute to a decrease in rumen pH. Supplemental buffers such as bicarbonate and additional potassium may aid appetite and increase rumen pH value. Cattle that have not fully shed out winter hair coats should be clipped to help avoid heat stress.

Cold Stress

Cold stress during periods of inclement weather is largely a problem for free stall–housed dairy cattle that must increase energy intake to maintain body heat. In this instance, thyroid hormones may increase to enhance dry-matter intake. However, regardless of exact pathophysiology, reproductive performance is diminished. Cows are reluctant to interact, tend to lose weight, may suffer production losses as more energy is directed toward body heat, and do not like to move about on icy floors and hard irregular surfaces created by frozen manure. Roughened hair coats and losses in body condition are observed in many animals in cold-stressed herds. Heat detection and conception suffer. A more energy-dense ration may need to be formulated when herds suffer from cold stress–induced fertility problems, metabolic problems, or production losses.

Slippery Surfaces

Slippery surfaces may exist in free-stall barns without grooved floors, on frozen icy surfaces of free stalls during cold extremes, in poorly cleaned free stalls, muddy areas, and frozen barnyards. Cattle that fall on slippery surfaces are reluctant to stand for, or mount, other cows and therefore show reduced estrus activity or shortened evidence of behavioral estrus.

Lameness and Other Stresses

One of the most common causes of sporadic individual infertility and an occasional cause of reduced herd fertility in dairy cattle is lameness. Lame cows do not want to stand, move about, or interact with other cows. The obvious consequences are less time spent eating, less movement to bunks, subsequent weight and production losses, and failure to show heat. Extreme lameness with weight loss causes a negative energy balance and can cause anestrus. Special consideration for lame cows must be made. Treatment and alleviation of the pain associated with lameness must be the foremost considerations, and the cow should be placed in a well-bedded box stall or bedded pack with good footing. If this is not possible, the cow is likely to suffer other musculoskeletal injuries, be battered by herdmates, and develop secondary conditions in addition to having infertility. Lame cows in negative energy balance are unlikely to conceive, and breeding is best attempted after correction of the lameness and following evidence that positive energy balance has been restored. Even when lame cows are in estrus, they do not interact for fear of injury or pain and therefore are reluctant to stand to be mounted. Herd epidemics of lameness caused by laminitis, foot rot, hairy heel warts, or interdigital fibropapillomas can have a drastic effect on herd fertility for all of the previous reasons.

Nonspecific stress associated with infectious, metabolic, musculoskeletal, environmental, and nutritional conditions also can have a negative impact on fertility. It is impossible to quantify or scientifically explain "stress," but veterinarians recognize the importance of this poorly defined condition. Most explanations theorize that cortisol levels are increased. Studies wherein heifers were given exogenous adrenocorticotropic hormone during proestrus resulted in delayed LH surges, delayed onset of estrus, and shortened behavioral estrus. Progesterone and cortisol levels both may be elevated in cattle under stress. Progesterone alone may prevent estrus, or other hormonal interactions may contribute to the problem. In any event, estrus may be shortened or nonexistent, and fertility suffers. Recognition and treatment of conditions that cause cow stress are essential to restoration of fertility in affected cattle.

Semen Quality and Delivery

Many dairy farms own their own semen tanks to store commercial semen from a variety of bull stud services regardless of whether insemination is performed by professional representatives of AI studs or a farm employee. Errors in semen handling can have profound effects on conception rates and frequently are overlooked as a cause of reduced fertility. A well-maintained semen tank is critical to preservation of quality semen. The temperature must remain at −196.0°C in liquid nitrogen tanks and even brief periods of exposure to ambient temperatures can be disastrous. Temperatures above −120.0°C can lead to recrystallization that allows water molecules to leave ice crystals, which attach to other crystals, creating some that are large enough to damage cellular structures within spermatozoa. Straws of semen are much more subject to damaging thermal variations than the older semen ampules because of volume differentials. Recrystallization damage may be cumulative. Tanks must be monitored closely, and a repeated need to add liquid nitrogen to a tank may signal a vacuum leak that eventually could cause severe problems. If vacuum is lost completely, all liquid nitrogen may be gone within 24 hours.

American Breeders Service has produced a monitoring device composed of ampules with color detectors that can signal inappropriate temperature increases in semen tanks. These devices are available from Minitube of America (Madison, WI).

Expertise of the inseminator is another concern, especially when a recently trained or neophyte farm employee assumes the role of inseminator. The uterine body is the best site for semen deposition, and personnel involved in insemination must be trained properly to deliver semen to this location. There is a great deal of variation in the skill of individual inseminators, and profound conception rate decreases associated with a new inseminator warrant investigation of technique. Surprisingly, conception rates often decline steadily over time even for experienced inseminators. In such instances retraining, with emphasis on proper technique, semen handling, and hygiene often result in a return to previous, acceptable conception levels.

Pregnancy Diagnosis

Accurate and safe diagnosis of early pregnancy in dairy cattle is a required skill for bovine practitioners. Economics dictate that cows be checked for pregnancy as early as possible so that open cows not observed in heat after breeding be identified promptly. Practitioners must be confident and comfortable with whatever limit of detection is established for each herd. Most practitioners choose to diagnose pregnancy any time after 35 days, but some only feel confident at 40 days or more. Heifers and young cows can be diagnosed as early as 30 days by conventional rectal palpation in most instances. It is now recognized that even healthy dairy cows experience a considerable degree of spontaneous pregnancy failure in the period after initial pregnancy diagnosis. This can reach 15% between 30 and 60 days of pregnancy. It is therefore important to confirm pregnancy at 60 to 70 days after insemination to avoid complacency and failure to reinseminate cows deemed to be pregnant but that have subsequently lost the pregnancy. It is also prudent to confirm pregnancy at the stage of drying off at the end of lactation.

Four cardinal signs may confirm pregnancy during transrectal palpation. These are detection ("slipping") of the fetal membranes (chorioallantois), palpation of the amniotic vesicle, palpation of the fetus itself, and identification of placentomes. Uterine asymmetry and fluid content and an ipsilateral corpus luteum are suggestive, but not confirmatory, findings. Transrectal ultrasonography is useful for confirmation of pregnancy as early as 20 to 28 days after insemination. This technique allows detection of fetal heart rate and evaluation of fetal fluids, which may indicate early fetal distress and death. Determination of fetal sex is possible by ultrasonography at 55 to 75 days of pregnancy.

Slipping of fetal membranes is best performed between days 35 and 90. Membrane slip must be performed gently to avoid injury to the fetus or membranes. This technique is most helpful when differentiating pregnancy from other causes of uterine fluid accumulation, such as pyometra and mucometra. It also is helpful when diagnosing pregnancy in bull-bred herds or herds that do not practice prebreeding examinations that would tend to rule out previous uterine pathology.

The diagnosis of pregnancy by palpation of the amniotic vesicle can be used for pregnancy diagnosis as early as 30 days but must be performed very gently to avoid embryonic injury, which may result in fetal death or atresia coli. As with membrane slipping, palpation of the amniotic vesicle is also valuable when prebreeding examinations have not been performed to rule out pathologic fluid distention of the uterus.

Abnormal pregnancies are usually characterized by lesser amounts of fluid in the gravid horn than would be expected based on experience and normal variation for cows bred a specific number of days. When pregnancy determinations are made before 40 to 45 days, less fluid than normal usually equates to embryonic death that has not yet resulted in expulsion or absorption of the uterine contents. Any cow suspected to have an abnormal pregnancy based on decreased amounts of fluid in the gravid horn should be rechecked in 1 to 2 weeks unless she returns to estrus before this. Some of these cows also will have decreased uterine tone or edematous-feeling gravid horns that further raise suspicion that embryonic death already has occurred. Because some biologic variation exists in the volume of fluid present at any specific day, however, discretion is called for, and a recheck in 1 to 2 weeks is a safer alternative than immediate $PGF_{2\alpha}$ treatment. Experimental induction of embryonic or fetal death has demonstrated that expulsion or resorption of dead embryos and fetal fluids, as well as return to estrus, can be delayed well beyond the time of death.

It is not rare for pregnant cattle to demonstrate behavioral evidence of estrus at regular intervals. This is most common during the first half of pregnancy, but some cows show behavioral signs of heat at regular intervals throughout a normal pregnancy. Many cows have palpable increased uterine tone when palpated on days 21, 42, and 63 after breeding despite having a normal pregnancy; therefore some evidence of a tendency for cyclicity during pregnancy seems likely based on clinical observations.

Cows diagnosed pregnant that subsequently develop purulent or bloody discharges or that have behavioral signs of estrus should be rechecked by rectal palpation; they are also excellent candidates for ancillary examination using ultrasonography. Ultrasound examination for pregnancy is being routinely used by many bovine practitioners today, which enables diagnosis of pregnancy as early as 20 days and allows earlier detection of open cows in need of rebreeding. Ultrasonography is also being used to identify twin pregnancies, which is a major problem in the dairy industry. Some experienced practitioners will then facilitate early ultrasonographic twin reduction, such is the reluctance of some producers to allow both fetuses to proceed to term. Transrectal ultrasonography has numerous applications for bovine reproduction and could be used in problem breeders, cattle suspected to have abnormal pregnancies, and cattle suspected to have uterine fluid accumulations that require differentiation from pregnancy. Use of ultrasonography, uterine cultures, and uterine biopsies should be practiced more when individually valuable cattle have fertility problems. Ultrasonography is also used in select circumstances for fetal sexing, typically between the eighth and tenth weeks of gestation. Determination of fetal sex may be of greater economic benefit to the beef rather than dairy industries, although clients may believe that pregnant, genetically superior dairy cattle may economically justify the expense of fetal sexing before contract sale of a calf. Semen sorting into sex-specific spermatozoa may also become a common service offered by the commercial AI industry in the near future, allowing clients to choose the likely sex of the fetus at the time of breeding.

Disorders of the Reproductive Tract in Dairy Bulls can be found in Chapter 10

Assisted Reproductive Technologies

Artificial Insemination and Sexed Semen

Artificial insemination is well established in the dairy industry. A major recent development has been the commercialization of sexed semen. Flow cytometric sperm separation provides greater than 85% certainty for offspring of the desired sex. The process is time consuming and labor intensive. Therefore the product is expensive, and the number of sperm packaged per insemination dose is a mere 10% of that of conventional frozen semen. As a result, fertility is lower. Very disappointing results are usually obtained if sex-sorted semen is used in mature, lactating cows, and even worse results may be expected in superstimulated embryo donors. Sex-sorted semen is best reserved for use in heifers, whose fertility is high, and for in vitro embryo production, in which appropriate sperm–oocyte relationships can be ensured. The proportion of heifers pregnant per insemination with sex-sorted semen can be expected to be 15 to 20 percentage points lower than results with conventional semen on the same farm.

In farms with excellent reproductive management and results, it is generally economical to use sex-sorted semen for the first two inseminations of heifers. After that conventional semen should be used. Farms with average reproductive performance should use sex-sorted semen for just the first insemination of virgin heifers. Farms with poorer reproductive performance can usually find more cost-effective means to make progress than using sex-sorted semen.

Embryo Transfer

The feasibility of embryo transfer was demonstrated in 1890 in rabbits, but application to cattle breeding came much later, with the first calf born in 1951. In the 1960s and 1970s, nonsurgical methods were introduced for recovery and transfer of uterine-stage embryos, and cryopreservation of embryos followed soon after. Better understanding of follicular dynamics in cattle (1980s) permitted refinement of ovarian superstimulation programs.

In its simplest form, embryo transfer depends on induction of multiple ovulations by providing sufficient exogenous FSH to rescue subordinate follicles in a follicular cohort from atresia. Multiple follicles become functionally dominant and ovulate. The donor cow is then inseminated and fertilized embryos recovered from the uterus at 6 or 7 days after estrus. (In cattle, the zygote completes tubal transit in about 4 days.) These embryos are identified under a stereoscopic microscope, evaluated based on stage of development and morphology, and transferred to synchronous recipients.

At first, embryo transfer was simply used to multiply offspring from genetically valuable females. In dairy cattle, systematic use of ovarian superstimulation and embryo transfer in multiple ovulation and embryo transfer (MOET) herds also allowed generation of large full-sib or half-sib cohorts from young donors, permitting genetic evaluation of sisters rather than daughters of potential AI sires, thus generating reliable breeding values in much less time. This formed the basis of more rapid genetic progress and shorter generation intervals. Mastery of embryo transfer techniques is also important for establishing pregnancies in recipients using embryos created by in vitro embryo production methods or by cloning (somatic cell nuclear transfer).

There is some risk of disease transmission involving embryos, but health standards and embryo-handling procedures have been developed to allow safe commerce in embryos, domestically and internationally. Indeed, embryos can be transported internationally with less risk of disease or injury than transport of mature animals, and much more cheaply. Additionally, resulting calves are born to (recipient) dams with native immunity appropriate for their location and prosper more readily than adult animals translocated to a new environment. There is, however, an obvious imperative to ensure that recipient females are screened for, and clear of, vertically transmissible infectious diseases both at the time of transfer and throughout pregnancy. Biosecurity programs for recipient herds become just as important as the status of the genetically superior donor animals for all forms of assisted reproduction.

Embryo transfer has also been used to increase reproductive performance in some circumstances. For example, high-producing mature cows tend to have lower pregnancy rates when inseminated than when receiving donated embryos, suggesting that their own oocyte quality is reduced. This is especially marked during periods of heat stress, when use of donated embryos can reduce the detrimental impact of heat stress on normal fertility.

In vitro techniques can also be applied to oocytes recovered as part of a terminal procedure from donors with catastrophic injury or acute terminal illness. The number of viable oocytes may be increased if there is time for superstimulation, although ethical concerns must be addressed before undertaking exogenous hormone administration because of the added time delay. In the event of illness being the causative reason rather than catastrophic injury, there will most likely be a negative impact on oocyte viability and subsequent pregnancy numbers. Fever and conditions that give rise to severe systemic inflammation, as well as neoplasia (especially multicentric lymphosarcoma), appear to be associated with very poor results when terminal oocyte harvest is attempted.

Genomic Prediction of Breeding Value

Recent progress in bovine genomics has permitted evaluation of the breeding value of animals by identifying genetic markers. Large databases allow imputation of genetic sequences in DNA in between specific markers (single nucleotide polymorphisms [SNPs]), meaning that reliable breeding value estimates can be obtained even when relatively few (from a few thousand to almost 1 million) markers are identified in each individual. Current estimates are approximately as reliable as conventional bull breeding values calculated from about 40 daughters; they have the added advantage of being immediately available and inexpensive. Holstein Association USA offers genomic testing commercially. The least expensive option uses a custom-designed chip that queries 9000 SNPs for a current price (April, 2017) of $46. This provides an estimated predicted transmitting ability (PTA) for milk yield with a reliability of some 72%. (For comparison, pedigree analysis provides about 40% reliability.) In addition, for no additional charge, the following is included: parentage verification, PTA for health and other production traits, carrier status for certain known autosomal recessive traits such as bovine leukocyte adhesion deficiency, deficiency of uridine monophosphate synthase, complex vertebral malformation and citrullinemia, and genetic information on casein subtypes that are important in milk processing. It is also possible to detect Y chromosome–specific sequences for diagnosis of freemartinism and known haplotypes shown to be associated with infertility caused by embryonic or fetal death (HH1, HH2, and HH3). For additional charges, testing is available for other genetic conditions using the same samples. Existence of reliable breeding values when animals are only weeks old has revolutionized selection of dairy bulls and heifers.

Far fewer bulls than before now enter artificial breeding organizations, and they do so with far greater likelihood of being genetically superior sires. This considerably reduces the costs of bull maintenance and shortens the generation interval, allowing even more rapid genetic progress. On the heifer side, genetically superior heifers can be selected as donors for oocyte recovery and in vitro embryo production, beginning even before conventional breeding age and providing superior replacement heifers for the next generation. Average or below average heifers can be used as recipients of in vitro–produced embryos or can be sold.

In Vitro Embryo Production

The first calf produced after IVF was born in 1981, using an ovulated oocyte. Since then, methods have been refined for oocyte recovery, oocyte maturation (resumption of meiosis and development to the metaphase II stage, accompanied by cytoplasmic maturation), IVF (requiring sperm selection and capacitation), and embryo culture. Oocytes may be obtained from selected donors by transvaginal oocyte recovery or OPU ("ovum pickup"). For this procedure, the donor is restrained in stocks, and epidural analgesia is provided. An ultrasound with a needle guide is advanced to the cranial vagina. The needle guide allows the operator to predict the path of the needle when it is advanced. By transrectal manipulation of each ovary in turn, visible follicles can be aligned with the needle path, the needle advanced, and follicular contents aspirated, typically using a vacuum pump that provides a constant and controlled negative pressure. Too little negative pressure results in lower recovery of oocytes, and too much strips off the surrounding cumulus oophorus cells, without which normal oocyte maturation is impaired.

Oocytes may be recovered from donors twice weekly without any ovarian stimulation or every 2 weeks with superstimulation. The overall number of oocytes recovered in a 2-week cycle is roughly comparable by the two methods, but superstimulation requires only one recovery attempt, rather than four, and has been shown to be associated with a higher proportion of oocytes developing to transferable embryos. On average, about 14 oocytes can be expected every 2 weeks, of which about 5 may develop to blastocyst stage, resulting in two live calves born under optimal conditions. Recipient animals need to be synchronized in advance, before knowledge of embryo development is available, which increases the cost of the overall procedure. (Heifers prepared as recipients but not used, or not becoming pregnant, may result in an older average age at first calving in herds using this technology.) Successful application of in vitro embryo production requires good animal health and excellent animal management, as well as skilled operators (for oocyte recovery and embryo transfer) and laboratory support. Oocytes may be obtained by transvaginal aspiration from immature heifers and from pregnant animals, further increasing the utility of this technology. Some bulls produce semen that functions better than others in in vitro embryo production systems for as yet unidentified reasons. IVF-produced embryos may be frozen (usually by vitrification) but result in lower pregnancy proportions than frozen-thawed embryos produced in vivo. Techniques for cryopreservation of bovine oocytes are under development but still not commercially available.

Cloning

Cloning by somatic cell nuclear transfer resulted in the birth of the sheep "Dolly" in 1996, with the first calf born the following year. This technique requires a mature oocyte, from which the nuclear DNA (metaphase II plate and first polar body) has been removed, which is fused with the nucleus of a somatic cell from the donor animal. The resulting embryo contains the nuclear DNA of the donor but the mitochondrial DNA of the oocyte donor. In cattle, the oocytes used are usually matured in vitro. The removal of the nuclear material is accomplished by micromanipulation under microscopic control. It may be facilitated with fluorescent DNA dyes. The enucleated oocyte is called a cytoplast. The donor DNA may come from embryonic or fetal cells or from adult epithelial cells or fibroblasts. (This cell is referred to as the karyoplast.) The cytoplast and karyoplast are fused with an electrical pulse and the oocyte activated with a calcium ionophore. For optimal programming, the donor cell needs to be at the G0 or G1 stages of the cell cycle. Recently, a simplified method for producing cloned embryos has been described. It is referred to as "handmade cloning" and does not require micromanipulators. Instead, the procedures are performed by hand under

a conventional dissection (stereo) microscope. Two (half) oocytes are fused with a selected karyoplast.

The success rate for producing cloned offspring is still very low. Blastocyst production is usually less than 10% and less than 10% of those result in live offspring, although the initial pregnancy rate may be much higher. Several reasons have been advanced for the disappointing performance of cloned embryos. Chief among these is improper epigenetic reprogramming. This results in abnormal placental development, among other anomalies. Cloned embryos are subject to high rates of embryonic loss and abortion. There are frequently aberrant placentas, with few, but very large, placentomes. Recipients carrying cloned calves are at higher risk of hydrallantois. Gestation may be prolonged. Frequently, the normal sequence of events that identify visible first-stage and especially second-stage labor are incomplete, protracted, or absent in recipients carrying cloned embryos. At birth, cloned calves may have enlarged umbilical vessels (Fig. 9.25) and pulmonary hypertension. Cloned calves are often very large (Fig. 9.26); they may be lethargic and lack normal reflexes, including the suckling reflex. They may experience transient diabetes. These phenotypic abnormalities,

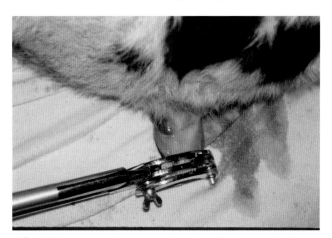

• **Fig. 9.25** Large umbilical vessels in a cloned Holstein heifer. Hemostasis was achieved with an emasculatome.

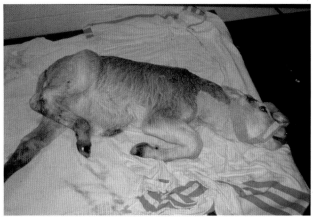

• **Fig. 9.26** Phenotypically abnormal newborn cloned Brown-Swiss calf. Note the distended abdomen.

taken with the tendency for prolonged gestation and the inherent risk of dystocia and increased neonatal morbidity as a consequence, lead to discussions regarding elective cesarean section or induction of parturition. Similar conversations are frequently undertaken regarding the management of parturition in IVF recipients, although the prevalence and severity of problems in this population appears to be less than for cloned or transgenic fetuses. There are no evidence-based studies that identify an ideal induction protocol or optimal timing for elective cesarean section for fetuses produced by either technique, but it is uncommon for dams to be allowed to go to term. Strongly held opinions regarding breed differences and the best approach to management or parturition are often held by people with experience. These empiric experiences currently offer the largest dataset rather than the scientific literature. As a consequence, veterinarians are advised to consider such neonates as being at high risk for a number of common (failure of passive transfer, dystocia trauma, perinatal asphyxia or hypoxia) and less common (umbilical hemorrhage or abnormalities, abnormal GI function, musculoskeletal weakness) health issues. Nevertheless, cloned calves that survive the neonatal period are usually clinically normal after that and appear to pass none of these abnormalities to their own offspring.

The availability of cloning procedures opens the door for bovine transgenesis because a transgenic nucleus may be used for a karyoplast, and these are readily produced.

Suggested Readings

Abbitt, B., Ball, L., Kitto, G. P., et al. (1978). Effect of three methods of palpation for pregnancy diagnosis per rectum on embryonic and fetal attrition in cows. *J Am Vet Med Assoc, 173*, 973–977.

Akagi, S., Geshi, M., & Nagai, T. (2013). Recent progress in bovine somatic cell nuclear transfer. *Anim Sci J, 84*, 191–199.

Allrich, R. D. (1993). Estrous behavior and detection in cattle. *Vet Clin North Am Food Anim Pract, 9*, 249–262.

Almeira, S., & Lopez-Gatius, F. (2013). Bovine neosporosis: clinical and practical aspects. *Res Vet Sci, 95*, 303–309.

Anderson, M., Barr, B., Rowe, J., et al. (2012). Neosporosis in dairy cattle. *Jpn J Vet Res, 60*(Suppl), S51–S54.

Anderson, M. L., Blanchard, P. C., Barr, B. C., et al. (1991). Neospora-like protozoan infection as a major cause of abortion in California dairy cattle. *J Am Vet Med Assoc, 198*, 241–244.

Antony, A., & Williamson, N. B. (2001). Recent advances in understanding the epidemiology of Neospora caninum in cattle. *N Z Vet J, 49*, 42–47.

Ball, H. J., & McCaughey, W. J. (1979). Distribution of mycoplasmas within the urogenital tract of the cow. *Vet Rec, 104*, 482–483.

Ball, L., Dargatz, D. A., Cheney, J. M., et al. (1987). Control of venereal disease in infected herds. *Vet Clin North Am Food Anim Pract, 3*, 561–574.

Barr, B. C., & Anderson, M. L. (1993). Infectious diseases causing bovine abortion and fetal loss. *Vet Clin North Am Food Anim Pract, 9*, 343–388.

Barr, B. C., Conrad, P. A., Breitmeyer, R., et al. (1993). Congenital Neospora infection in calves born from cows that had previously aborted Neospora-infected fetuses: four cases 1990–1992. *J Am Vet Med Assoc, 202*, 113–117.

Barth, A. D. (1993). Factors affecting fertility with artificial insemination. *Vet Clin North Am Food Anim Pract, 9*, 275–290.

Bisinotto, R. S., Ribeiro, E. S., & Santos, J. E. (2014). Synchronization of ovulation for management of reproduction in dairy cows. *Animal, 8*(Suppl. 1), 151–159.

BonDurant, R. H. (1985). Diagnosis, treatment, and control of bovine trichomoniasis. *Compend Contin Educ Pract Vet, 7*, S179–S184.

Borchardt, K. A., Norman, B. B., Thomas, M. W., et al. (1992). Evaluation of a new culture method for diagnosing Trichomonas foetus infection. *Vet Med, February*, 104–112.

Bretzlaff, K. N., Ott, R. S., Kortiz, G. D., et al. (1983). Distribution of oxytetracycline in genital tract tissues of postpartum cows given the drug by intravenous and intrauterine routes. *Am J Vet Res, 44*, 764–769.

Brisville, A. C., Fecteau, G., Boysen, S., et al. (2013). Neonatal morbidity and mortality of 31 calves derived from somatic cloning. *J Vet Intern Med, 5*, 1218–1227.

Brown, M. P., Colahan, P. T., & Hawkins, D. M. (1978). Urethral extension for treatment of urine pooling in mares. *J Am Vet Med Assoc, 173*, 1005–1007.

Butler, W. R., & Smith, R. D. (1989). Interrelationships between energy balance and postpartum reproductive function in dairy cattle. *J Dairy Sci, 72*, 767–783.

Carvalho, P. D., Guenther, J. N., Fuenzalida, M. J., et al. (2014). Presynchronization using a modified Ovsynch protocol or a single gonadotrophin releasing hormone injection 7 d before an Ovsynch-56 protocol for submission of lactating dairy cows to first timed artificial insemination. *J Dairy Sci, 97*, 6305–6315.

Carvalho, P. D., Souza, A. H., Amundson, M. C., et al. (2014). Relationship between fertility and postpartum changes in body condition and body weight in lactating cows. *J Dairy Sci, 97*, 3666–3683.

Chenault, J. R., McAllister, J. F., Chester, S. T., Jr., et al. (2004). Efficacy of ceftiofur hydrochloride sterile suspension administered parenterally for the treatment of acute postpartum metritis in dairy cows. *J Am Vet Med Assoc, 224*, 1634–1639.

Curtis, C. R., Erb, H. N., Sniffen, C. J., et al. (1985). Path analysis of dry period nutrition, postpartum metabolic and reproductive disorders, and mastitis in Holstein cows. *J Dairy Sci, 68*, 2347–2360.

Dargatz, D. A., Mortimer, R. G., & Cheney, J. M. (1985). Bovine trichomoniasis. *Bov Clin, Fall*, 3–5.

Dinsmore, R. P., White, M. E., & English, P. B. (1990). An evaluation of simultaneous GnRH and cloprostenol treatment of dairy cattle with cystic ovaries. *Can Vet J, 31*, 280–284.

Dinsmore, R. P., Stevens, R. D., Catall, M. D., et al. (1994). Oxytetracycline residues in milk following intrauterine infusion of dairy cows. *Bov Prac, 26*, 186–187.

Dirandeh, E., Roodbari, A. R., & Colazo, M. G. (2015). Double-Ovsynch compared with presynch with or without GnRH improves fertility in heat stressed lactating dairy cows. *Theriogenology, 83*, 438–443.

Doig, P. A., Ruhnke, H. L., & Palmer, N. C. (1980). Experimental bovine genital ureaplasmosis: I. granular vulvitis following vulvar inoculation. *Can J Comp Med, 44*, 252–258.

Doig, P. A., Ruhnke, H. L., & Palmer, N. C. (1980). Experimental bovine genital ureaplasmosis: II. granular vulvitis, endometritis, and salpingitis following uterine inoculation. *Can J Comp Med, 44*, 259–266.

Dubey, J. P., Lindsay, D. S., Anderson, M. L., et al. (1992). Induced transplacental transmission of Neospora caninum in cattle. *J Am Vet Med Assoc, 201*, 709–713.

Dubey, J. P., & Schares, G. (2011). Neosporosis in animals – the last five years. *Vet Parasitol, 180*, 90–108.

Elad, D., Friedgut, O., Alpert, N., et al. (2004). Bovine necrotic vulvovaginitis associated with *Porphyromonas levii*. *Emerg Infect Dis, 10*, 505–507.

Ellington, J. E., & Schlafer, D. H. (1993). Uterine tube disease in cattle. *J Am Vet Med Assoc, 202*, 450–454.

Elliott, L., McMahon, K. J., Gier, H. T., et al. (1968). Uterus of the cow after parturition: bacterial content. *Am J Vet Res, 29*, 77–81.

Elmore, R. G. (1992). Focus on bovine reproductive disorders: managing cases of placental hydrops. *Vet Med, January*, 73–77.

Erb, H. N. (1984). High milk production as a cause of cystic ovaries in dairy cows: evidence to the contrary. *Compend Contin Educ Pract Vet, 6*, S215–S216.

Erb, H. N., Martin, S. W., Ison, N., et al. (1981). Interrelationships between production and reproductive diseases in Holstein cows. Path analysis. *J Dairy Sci, 64*, 282–289.

Erb, R. E., Hinze, P. E., Gildow, E. M., et al. (1958). Retained fetal membranes: the effect of prolificacy of dairy cattle. *J Am Vet Med Assoc, 133*, 489.

Ferguson, J. (1986). The effects of protein level and type on reproduction in the dairy cow. In *Proceedings: Annual Meeting Society of Theriogenologists* (pp. 164–185).

Forro, A., Tsousis, G., Beindorff, N., et al. (2015). Factors affecting the success of resynchronization protocols with or without progesterone supplementation in dairy cows. *J Vet Sci, 16*, 121–126.

Fortune, J. E., & Quirk, S. M. (1988). Regulation of steroidogenesis in bovine preovulatory follicles. *J Anim Sci, 66*, 1–4.

Frazer, G. S. (2005). A rational basis for therapy in the sick postpartum cow. *Vet Clin North Am Food Anim Pract, 21*, 523–568.

Garverick, H. A., & Smith, M. F. (1993). Female reproductive physiology and endocrinology of cattle. *Vet Clin North Am Food Anim Pract, 9*, 223–247.

Gearhart, M. A., Curtis, C. R., Erb, H. N., et al. (1990). Relationship of changes in condition score to cow health in Holsteins. *J Dairy Sci, 73*, 3132–3140.

Gilbert, R. O., Grohn, Y. T., Guard, C. L., et al. (1993). Impaired postpartum neutrophil function in cows which retain fetal membranes. *Res Vet Sci, 55*, 15–19.

Gilbert, R. O., & Oettle, E. E. (1990). An outbreak of granulomatous vulvitis in feedlot heifers. *J S Afr Vet Assoc, 61*, 41–43.

Gilbert, R. O., Shin, S. T., Guard, C. L., et al. (2005). Prevalence of endometritis and its effects on reproductive performance of dairy cows. *Theriogenology, 64*, 1879–1888.

Gilbert, R. O., & Schwark, W. S. (1992). Pharmacologic considerations in the management of peripartum conditions in the cow. *Vet Clin North Am Food Anim Pract, 8*, 29–56.

Gilbert, R. O., Wilson, D. G., Levine, S. A., et al. (1989). Surgical management of urovagina and associated infertility in a cow. *J Am Vet Med Assoc, 194*, 931–932.

Ginther, O. J., Kastelic, J. P., & Knopf, L. (1989). Composition and characteristics of follicular waves during the bovine estrous cycle. *Anim Reprod Sci, 20*, 187–200.

Gonzalez-Carmona, L. C., Sanchez-Ladino, M. J., Castaneda-Salazar, R., et al. (2012). Determination of Trichomonas foetus in uterine lavages from cows with reproductive problems. *Rev Bras Parasitol Vet, 21*, 201–205.

Gonzalez-Martin, J. V., Astiz, S., Elvira, L., et al. (2008). New surgical technique to correct urovagina improves the fertility of dairy cows. *Theriogenology, 69*, 360–365.

Gröhn, Y. T., Erb, H. N., McCulloch, C. E., et al. (1990). Epidemiology of reproductive disorders in dairy cattle, associations among host characteristics, disease, and production. *Prev Vet Med, 8*, 25–40.

Grooms, D. L. (2004). Reproductive consequences of infection with bovine viral diarrhea virus. *Vet Clin North Am Food Anim Pract, 20*, 5–19.

Grummer, R. R., Wiltbank, M. C., Fricke, P. M., et al. (2010). Management of dry and transition cows to improve energy balance and reproduction. *J Reprod Dev, 56*, S22–28.

Guitian, J., Thurmond, M. C., & Hietala, S. K. (1999). Infertility and abortion among first-lactation dairy cows seropositive or seronegative for Leptospira interrogans serovar hardjo. *J Am Vet Med Assoc, 215*, 515–518.

Gustafsson, B. K. (1984). Therapeutic strategies involving antimicrobial treatment of the uterus in large animals. *J Am Vet Med Assoc, 185*, 1194–1198.

Habel, R. E. (1957). Prevention of vaginal prolapse in the cow. *J Am Vet Med Assoc, 130*, 344.

Haddad, J. P., Dohoo, I. R., & Van Leewen, J. A. (2005). A review of Neopsora caninum in dairy and beef cattle—a Canadian perspective. *Can Vet J, 46*, 2302–2343.

Hall, C. A., Reichel, M. P., & Ellis, J. T. (2005). Neospora abortions in dairy cattle: diagnosis, mode of transmission and control. *Vet Parasitol, 128*, 231–241.

Hammon, D. S., Evjen, I. M., Dhiman, T. R., et al. (2006). Neutrophil function and energy status in Holstein cows with uterine health disorders. *Vet Immunol Immunopathol, 15*(113), 21–29.

Hjerpe, C. A. (1990). Bovine vaccines and herd vaccination programs. *Vet Clin North Am Food Anim Pract, 6*, 171–260.

Hoeben, D., Mijten, P., & de Kruif, A. (1997). Factors influencing complications during caesarean section on the standing cow. *Vet Q, 19*, 88–92.

Kassam, A., BonDurant, R. H., Basu, S., et al. (1987). Clinical and endocrine responses to embryonic and fetal death induced by manual rupture of the amniotic vesicle during early pregnancy in cows. *J Am Vet Med Assoc, 191*, 417–420.

Kastelic, J. P. (1994). Understanding ovarian follicular development in cattle. *Vet Med, January*, 61–71.

Kastelic, J. P., Knopf, L., & Ginther, O. J. (1990). Effect of day of prostaglandin F-2-alpha treatment on selection and development of the ovulatory follicle in heifers. *Anim Reprod Sci, 23*, 169–180.

Kennedy, P. C. (1990). Epizootic bovine abortion. In C. A. Kirkbride (Ed.), *Laboratory diagnosis of livestock abortion* (3rd ed.). Ames, IA: Iowa State University Press.

Kesler, D. J., & Garverick, H. A. (1982). Ovarian cysts in dairy cattle: a review. *J Anim Sci, 55*, 1147–1159.

Kimura, K., Goff, J. P., Kehrli, M. E., Jr., et al. (2002). Decreased neutrophil function as a cause of retained placenta in dairy cattle. *J Dairy Sci, 85*, 544–550.

King, G. J., Hurnik, J. F., & Robertson, H. A. (1976). Ovarian function and estrus in dairy cows during early lactation. *J Anim Sci, 42*, 688–692.

Kirkbride, C. A. (1987). Mycoplasma, Ureaplasma and Acholeplasma infections of bovine genitalia. *Vet Clin North Am Food Anim Pract, 3*, 575–591.

Klavano, G. G. (1980). Observations of Haemophilus somnus infection as an agent producing reproductive diseases: infertility and abortion. In *Proceedings: Annual Meeting Society of Theriogenologists* (pp. 139–149).

Konigsson, K., Gustafsson, H., Gunnarsson, A., et al. (2001). Clinical and bacteriological aspects of the use of oxytetracycline and flunixin in primiparous cows with induced retained placenta and postpartal endometritis. *Reprod Domest Anim, 36*, 247–256.

LaFaunce, N. A., & McEntee, K. (1982). Experimental Mycoplasma bovis seminal vesiculitis in the bull. *Cornell Vet*, *72*, 150–167.

LeBlanc, S. J., Duffield, T. F., Leslie, K. E., et al. (2002). The effect of treatment of clinical endometritis on reproductive performance in dairy cows. *J Dairy Sci*, *85*, 2237–2249.

Lee, C. N., Maurice, E., Ax, R. L., et al. (1983). Efficacy of gonadotropin-releasing hormone administered at the time of artificial insemination of heifers and postpartum and repeat breeder dairy cows. *Am J Vet Res*, *44*, 2160–2166.

Lein, D. H. (1986). The current role of Ureaplasma, Mycoplasma, and Haemophilus somnus in bovine reproductive disorders. In *Proceedings: 11th Technical Conference on Artificial Insemination and Reproduction* (pp. 27–32).

Lindell, J. O., Kindahl, H., Jansson, L., et al. (1982). Postpartum release of prostaglandin $F_{2\alpha}$ and uterine involution in the cow. *Theriogenology*, *17*, 237–245.

Lucy, M. C. (2001). Reproductive loss in high-producing dairy cattle: where will it end? *J Dairy Sci*, *84*, 1277–1293.

Magdub, A., Johnson, H. D., & Belyea, R. L. (1982). Effect of environmental heat and dietary fiber on thyroid physiology of lactating cows. *J Dairy Sci*, *65*, 2323–2331.

Maiorka, P. C., Favaron, P. O., Mess, A. M., et al. (2015). Vascular alterations underlie developmental problems manifested in cloned cattle before or after birth. *PLoS One*, *10*, 137–141.

McArt, J. A., Caixeta, L. S., Machado, V. S., et al. (2010). Ovsynch versus Ultrasynch: reproductive efficacy of a dairy cattle synchronization protocol incorporating corpus luteum function. *J Dairy Sci*, *93*, 2525–2532.

Miller, H. V., Kimsey, P. B., Kendrick, J. W., et al. (1980). Endometritis of dairy cattle: diagnosis, treatment and fertility. *Bov Pract*, *15*, 13–23.

Miller, R. B., Lein, D. H., McEntee, K. E., et al. (1983). Haemophilus somnus infection of the reproductive tract of cattle: a review. *J Am Vet Med Assoc*, *182*, 1390–1391.

Morrow, D. A. (1986). *Current therapy in theriogenology* (2nd ed.). Philadelphia: WB Saunders.

Murray, R. D., Allison, J. D., & Gard, R. P. (1990). Bovine endometritis: comparative efficacy of alfaprostol and intrauterine therapies, and other factors influencing clinical success. *Vet Rec*, *127*, 86–90.

Newman, K. D., & Anderson, D. E. (2005). Cesarean section in cows. *Vet Clin North Am Food Anim Pract*, *21*, 73–100.

Nightingale, C. R., Sellers, M. D., & Ballou, M. A. (2015). Elevated haptoglobin concentrations following parturition are associated with elevated leucocyte responses and decreased subsequent reproductive efficiency in multiparous Holstein dairy cows. *Vet Immunol Immunopathol*, *164*, 16–23.

Olson, J. D., Ball, L., & Mortimer, R. G. (1985). Therapy of postpartum uterine infections. *Bov Pract*, *17*, 85–88.

Parish, S. M., Maag-Miller, L., Besser, T. E., et al. (1987). Myelitis associated with protozoal infection in newborn calves. *J Am Vet Med Assoc*, *191*, 1599–1600.

Peter, A. T., & Bosu, W. T. K. (1988). Relationship of uterine infections and folliculogenesis in dairy cows during early puerperium. *Theriogenology*, *30*, 1045–1052.

Prado, T. M., Schumacher, J., Hayden, S. S., et al. (2007). Evaluation of a modified surgical technique to correct urine pooling in cows. *Theriogenology*, *67*, 1512–1517.

Pursley, J. R., Mee, M. O., & Wiltbank, M. C. (1995). Synchronization of ovulation in dairy cows using PGF2 and GnRH. *Theriogenology*, *44*, 915–923.

Randel, R. D. (1990). Nutrition and postpartum rebreeding in cattle. *J Anim Sci*, *68*, 853–862.

Refsal, K. R., Jarrin-Maldonado, J. H., & Nachreiner, R. F. (1987). Endocrine profiles in cows with ovarian cysts experimentally induced by treatment with exogenous estradiol or adrenocorticotropic hormone. *Theriogenology*, *28*, 871–889.

Reichel, M. P., Moore, D. P., Hemphill, A., et al. (2015). A live vaccine against Neospora caninum abortions in cattle. *Vaccine*, *33*, 1299–1301.

Rhoads, M. L., Rhoads, R. P., Gilbert, R. O., et al. (2006). Detrimental effects of high plasma urea nitrogen levels on viability of embryos from lactating dairy cows. *Anim Reprod Sci*, *91*, 1–10.

Risco, C. A., Donovan, G. A., & Hernandez, J. (1999). Clinical mastitis associated with abortion in dairy cows. *J Dairy Sci*, *82*, 1684–1689.

Risco, C. A., & Hernandez, J. (2003). Comparison of ceftiofur hydrochloride and estradiol cypionate for metritis prevention and reproductive performance in dairy cows affected with retained fetal membranes. *Theriogenology*, *60*, 47–58.

Risco, C. A., & Reynolds, J. P. (1988). Uterine prolapse in dairy cattle. *Compend Contin Educ Pract Vet*, *10*, 1135–1143.

Roberts, S. J. (1986). *Veterinary obstetrics and genital diseases (theriogenology)* (3rd ed.). Woodstock, VT: published by the author.

Ruegg, P. L., Marteniuk, J. V., & Kaneene, J. B. (1988). Reproductive difficulties in cattle with antibody titers to Haemophilus-somnus. *J Am Vet Med Assoc*, *193*, 941–942.

Souza, A. H., Ayres, H., Ferreira, R. M., et al. (2008). A new presynchronization system (Double-Ovsynch) increases fertility at first postpartum timed AI in lactating dairy cows. *Theriogenology*, *70*, 208–215.

St. Jean, G., Hull, B. L., Robertson, J. T., et al. (1988). Urethral extension for correction of urovagina in cattle: a review of 14 cases. *Vet Surg*, *17*, 258–262.

Saint-Jean, G., Rings, D. M., Hoffsis, G. F., et al. (1988). Adenocarcinoma of the uterus with pulmonary metastasis in two cows. *Compend Contin Educ Pract Vet*, *10*, 864–867.

Samuelson, J. D., & Winter, A. J. (1966). Bovine vibriosis: the nature of the carrier state in the bull. *J Infect Dis*, *16*, 581–592.

Schonfelder, A., & Sobiraj, A. (2005). Etiology of torsio uteri in bovines: a review [article in German]. *Schweiz Arch Tierheilkd*, *147*, 397–402.

Scott, H. M., Schouten, M. J., Gaiser, J. C., et al. (2005). Effect of intrauterine administration of ceftiofur on fertility and risk of culling in postparturient cows with retained fetal membranes, twins, or both. *J Am Vet Med Assoc*, *226*, 2044–2052.

Sheldon, I. M., Bushnell, M., Montgomery, J., et al. (2004). Minimum inhibitory concentrations of some antimicrobial drugs against bacteria causing uterine infections in cattle. *Vet Rec*, *155*, 383–387.

Sheldon, I. M., Lewis, G. S., LeBlanc, S., et al. (2006). Defining postpartum uterine disease in cattle. *Theriogenology*, *65*, 1516–1530.

Sirois, J., & Fortune, J. E. (1988). Ovarian follicular dynamics during the estrous cycle in heifers monitored by real-time ultrasonography. *Biol Reprod*, *39*, 308–317.

Sprecher, D. J., Nebel, R. J., & Whittier, W. D. (1988). Predictive value of palpation per rectum vs milk and serum progesterone levels for the diagnosis of bovine follicular and luteal cysts. *Theriogenology*, *30*, 701–710.

Sprecher, D. J., Strelow, L. W., & Nebel, R. L. (1990). The response of cows with cystic ovarian degeneration to luteotropic or luteolytic therapy as assigned by latex agglutination milk progesterone assay. *Theriogenology*, *34*, 1149–1158.

Stoebel, D. P., & Moberg, G. P. (1982). Effect of adrenocorticotropin and cortisol on luteinizing hormone surge and estrous behavior of cows. *J Dairy Sci*, *65*, 1016–1024.

Théon, A. P., Pascoe, J. R., Carlson, G. P., et al. (1993). Intratumoral chemotherapy with cisplatin in oily emulsion in horses. *J Am Vet Med Assoc*, *202*, 261–267.

Thurmond, M. C., & Picanso, J. P. (1993). Fetal loss associated with palpation per rectum to diagnose pregnancy in cows. *J Am Vet Med Assoc, 203*, 432–435.

Trimberger, G. W. (1948). Breeding efficiency in dairy cattle from artificial insemination at various intervals before and after ovulation. Nebraska Agricultural Experimental Station Research Bulletin, *153*.

Vaillancourt, D., Bierschwal, C. J., Ogwu, D., et al. (1979). Correlation between pregnancy diagnosis by membrane slip and embryonic mortality. *J Am Vet Med Assoc, 175*, 466–468.

Villa-Godoy, A., Hughes, T. L., Emery, R. S., et al. (1988). Association between energy balance and luteal function in lactating dairy cows. *J Dairy Sci, 71*, 1063–1072.

Weaver, L. D. (1987). Effects of nutrition on reproduction in dairy cows. *Vet Clin North Am Food Anim Pract, 3*, 513–532.

Wehrend, A., Reinle, T., Herfen, K., et al. (2002). Fetotomy in cattle with special reference to postoperative complications—an evaluation of 131 cases [article in German]. *Dtsch Tierarztl Wochenschr, 109*, 56–61.

Weiss, B., Hogan, J., & Smith, L. (1994). Vitamin E and selenium: key nutrients for health. *Hoard's Dairyman, April, 10*, 288–289.

West, J. W., Mullinix, B. G., & Sandifer, T. G. (1991). Changing dietary electrolyte balance for dairy cows in cool and hot environments. *J Dairy Sci, 74*, 1662–1674.

White, M. E., & Erb, H. (1980). Treatment of ovarian cysts in dairy cattle—a decision analysis. *Cornell Vet, 70*, 247–257.

Wiltbank, M. C., Gumen, A., & Sartori, R. (2002). Physiological classification of anovulatory conditions in cattle. *Theriogenology, 57*, 21–52.

Wolfe, D. F., & Baird, A. N. (1993). Female urogenital surgery in cattle. *Vet Clin North Am Food Anim Pract, 9*, 369–388.

Yao, C. (2013). Diagnosis of Tritrichomonas foetus-infected bulls, an ultimate approach to eradicate bovine trichomoniasis in US cattle. *J Med Microbiol, 62*, 1–9.

Younquist, R. S., & Braun, W. F., Jr. (1993). Abnormalities of the tubular genital organs. *Vet Clin North Am Food Anim Pract, 9*, 309–322.

10

Diseases Specific to or Common in Dairy Bulls

DONALD R. MONKE, JUSTIN L. TANK, ANTHONY E. GOOD, AND
ELIZABETH A. LAHMERS

Management Considerations of Dairy Bulls

Many dairy bulls are raised in an artificial insemination center (AIC) for semen collection in order to widely distribute quality genetics to the dairy industry. Although veterinarians are less likely to encounter diseases common to dairy bulls at a routine dairy herd visit, they may be called to consult on or examine a bull within an AIC. This chapter addresses common management and special health problems of dairy bulls resident in an AIC.

The management and treatment of dairy bulls includes a number of unique characteristics compared with the much larger population of dairy heifers and cows. One important difference is the restraint required to conduct a thorough physical examination, to perform diagnostic tests, and to administer treatments. A docile bull may be restrained in a physical manner by simply walking it into a restraint chute; however, sedatives may be needed for some bulls to assist in the restraint. If adult bulls are regularly handled at a work site, a large and sturdy restraint chute system is essential. There may also be circumstances in which restraint is conducted with sedatives while the bull is partly restrained with a halter tied to a fence or with the head of a bull restrained in a specially adapted self-catch head lock. After the bull is adequately restrained so that it can be approached safely, the conduct of a physical examination should be as described in Chapter 1 and diagnostic tests and treatments administered as explained in Chapter 2.

Because bulls are acquired by commercial AICs with the intent to produce high-quality semen for domestic and international markets, it is vital to the financial success of the AIC that the bulls are repeatedly tested free of specific infectious diseases and are housed in a manner so as to retain their biosecurity status. Although this aspect of bull management is not directly concerned with clinical disease, it is an integral component of veterinary work at an AIC. Health problems associated with dairy bulls retained by an owner for natural service will not be specifically considered herein.

Dairy bulls resident in an AIC have a unique position in the dairy industry. Almost every dairy bull resident in an AIC has a potentially high value ascribed to it by either a conventional progeny testing program or by genomic evaluation criteria. However, a meaningful financial value is only achieved when the bull regularly has good-quality semen collected that can be sold domestically or internationally without constraints of positive diagnostic health test results. Therefore, veterinarians working for an AIC must practice and provide counsel about preventive medicine management programs (biosecurity), offer a "well-animal" medical program that keeps the bull functioning at a high level, and provide care of sick or injured animals when required.

Dairy bulls are most likely to require veterinary assistance at four stages of their lives:

1. As calves on a dairy farm being evaluated for transport and entry to the admittance unit of an AIC
2. As calves recently procured and admitted to the isolation unit of an AIC
3. As yearling bulls during initial semen collection
4. As older bulls and adults when on a regular semen collection schedule

Keeping Healthy Bulls Healthy

From the strategic management perspective of an AIC, a dairy bull is either being raised or maintained so it can have semen collected or is on a regular semen collection schedule. In either situation, the bull must be in good health so that a satisfactory quantity and quality of semen can be collected. Good health begins with a balanced nutrition program. It is not the intent of this chapter to provide nutritional guidelines, but when corn silage is included in the ration, it is preferable to feed bulls a total mixed ration (TMR) compared with multiple feedings of individual feed ingredients. It is the authors' experience that feeding a TMR of corn silage, grass hay, and pellets (formulated to complement the forages) markedly reduces the occurrence of displaced abomasum, especially in yearling dairy bulls. Abomasal displacement has not been a problem for bulls fed free-choice hay along with either grain or pellets.

It is important that dairy bulls not be fed a dairy cow ration. There are concerns that the high levels of calcium fed to dairy cows may, in older bulls, contribute to excessive bone deposition along the thoracolumbar vertebrae, leading to ankylosing spondylosis and associated neurologic problems such as deficits in conscious proprioception of the hind limbs and feet. Other problems may include thyroid hyperplasia and calcification of specific soft tissues. Rations for bulls should be formulated to have a calcium:phosphorus ratio of 1.5:1, although a higher ratio of 1.8:1 may be more practical to achieve. Although non-nutritional factors may also play a role in development of ankylosing spondylosis, it remains important to feed the bulls a non–dairy cow ration.

Regardless of the nutrition program, it is important to regularly evaluate body condition score (BCS) of bulls to monitor each animal's response to its ration, so that the quantity of feed can be increased or decreased as needed. (Refer to the Appendix for Body Condition Scoring at the end of Chapter 15 on metabolic diseases.) The frequency of conducting a BCS may be variable, but a quarterly evaluation represents a good data set for comparative purposes. If a bull is in good health, one should feed it so the variance in BCS is less than 0.5 between scoring intervals, based on a 5-point BCS scale. It is important to remember that adult bulls should be fed a maintenance ration so they do not gain excessive weight. Bulls that are overconditioned relative to their body frame may exhibit reduced libido and be reluctant to mount the teaser animal. Overconditioning also causes adipose tissue deposition around the neck of the scrotum, which may decrease semen quality by negatively affecting the testicles' thermoregulatory mechanism.

Adequate shelter that protects bulls from severe weather conditions is also a necessity. In cold climates, shelter from high winds and precipitation when the ambient temperature is less than 0°F is needed to prevent frostbite of the scrotum. If such protection is not provided, the blood flow to the scrotal epithelium can be markedly reduced. This results in tissue anoxia and resultant frostbite (Fig. 10.1). Because the bull will draw its testicles upward toward the abdomen in cold weather, the first clinical sign may be blood from the injured scrotum on the medial aspect of the bull's hocks. Severe cases of scrotal frostbite may cause adhesions within the distal scrotum. Resolution of the frostbite lesion is slow, but after several months, the ventral scrotal scab will eventually slough, and a permanent scar may be all that remains of the injury.

High ambient temperatures, especially when associated with high humidity, may also be associated with a decline in semen quantity and quality. The thermoregulatory process of the scrotum causes the testicles to descend ventrally within the scrotum. The result on seminal quality is bull dependent; some dairy bulls tolerate high ambient temperatures, but others do not. If the production of high-volume and satisfactory quality spermatozoa is important for a specific bull, it should be housed in an air-conditioned room with good ventilation and air exchange to reduce the accumulation of ammonia in the stall.

Hematology and Serum Chemistry of Dairy Bulls

In a typical production agriculture setting, it may be uncommon to evaluate cattle using clinical pathology tests because the cost of the testing may not be economically warranted. However, the potential high value of genetically proven and genomically tested dairy bulls may provide the impetus to conduct diagnostic testing, especially in difficult or protracted cases. When hematologic and serum chemistry tests are conducted at a veterinary diagnostic laboratory, a report is generated that may show which diagnostic parameters are outside of normal reference ranges. The normal reference ranges used by many diagnostic laboratories are based on data for cows. Tables 1.2 and 1.3 in this textbook are examples of such reference ranges for cattle. Extrapolating recommended reference ranges from cows to bulls can be acceptable for many variables, but there are a few specific instances in which an erroneous conclusion may be reached unless one recognizes that the normal reference values for bulls can be different. Furthermore, there are age-related differences for selected parameters.

For example, when evaluating the hemogram of a bull, it may be helpful to know that the reference range for leukocytes is significantly lower in adult bulls ($3.3–8.0 \times 10^3/\mu L$) compared with yearling bulls ($7.6–16.4 \times 10^3/\mu L$). But because the normal reference range for leukocytes in cows ($4.9–12.0 \times 10^3/\mu L$) overlaps the normal leukocyte ranges

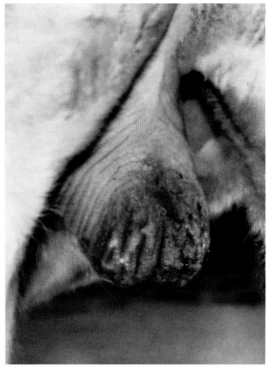

• **Fig. 10.1** Adult Holstein bull with acute scrotal frostbite.

TABLE 10.1	Total Neutrophils and Lymphocytes in Bulls: Normal Reference Ranges (x10³/µL)		
Variable	Yearling Bulls	Adult Bulls	
Segmented neutrophils	1.7-9.0	1.9-5.9	
Lymphocytes	3.1-9.2	0.5-2.4	

TABLE 10.3	Albumin and Globulin: Normal Reference Ranges (g/dL)		
Variable	Yearling Bulls	Adult Bulls	
Albumin	3.0-3.6	3.0-3.7	
Globulin	2.6-3.8	3.8-5.3	

TABLE 10.2	Creatinine: Normal Reference Ranges (mg/dL)		
Variable	Yearling Bulls	Adult Bulls	Cows
Creatinine	1.0-1.6	1.9-3.0	0.4-1.0

TABLE 10.4	Normal Complete Blood Count Values for Dairy Bulls	
Variable	6–18 Months	>48 Months
Erythrocytes		
RBC (x10⁶/µL)	6.3–9.0	5.9–8.9
Hemoglobin (g/dL)	8.7–13.1	10.5–16.2
Hematocrit (%)	23–34	28–43
MCV (fl)	33–41	44–54
MCHC (g/dL)	36–41	36–39
Leukocytes		
WBC count (x10³/µL)	7.6–16.4	3.3–8.0
Band neutrophils (x10³/µL)	0–0.5	0–0.2
Segmented neutrophils (x10³/µL)	1.7–9.0	1.9–5.9
Lymphocytes (x10³/µL)	3.1–9.2	0.5–2.4
Monocytes (x10³/µL)	0–1.1	0–0.6
Eosinophils (x10³/µL)	0–3.9	0–0.9
Basophils (x10³/µL)	0–0.3	0–0.1

MCHC, Mean corpuscular hemoglobin concentration; *MCV*, mean corpuscular volume; *RBC*, red blood cell; *WBC*, white blood cell.
Reproduced with permission from Monke DR, Kociba GJ, DeJarnette MS, et al: Reference values for selected hematologic and biochemical variables in Holstein bulls of various ages, *Am J Vet Res* 59:1386-1391, 1998.

for both age groups of bulls, interpretation of the total leukocyte value is probably not affected. However, when the differential leukocyte values are evaluated, the difference in age and gender becomes important.

The absolute number of both segmented neutrophils and lymphocytes is lower in adult bulls compared with yearlings. However, the normal number of lymphocytes more markedly declines as bulls get older (Table 10.1). The neutrophil:lymphocyte (N:L) ratio in yearling bulls is 0.85, which is not different from adult cows using the reference range for adult cows published in Schalm's 1957 laboratory report, which many laboratories still use. An updated reference range (N:L ratio) in adult BLV negative cows of 1.2:1 has been reported by Dr. Jeanne George, a classmate of Dr. Rebhun. The N:L ratio in adult bulls is 2.5:1, which is considerably higher than any of the abovementioned adult cow reference ranges. This is an important distinction for adult bulls. The comparative neutrophil and lymphocyte values in both yearling and adult bulls are presented in Table 10.1.

Clinical disease of the urogenital system in bulls is almost exclusively of the genital tract. However, when a serum chemistry test is conducted from a bull for any reason, especially on an adult bull, the report will inevitably show that the bull's creatinine value is above normal if reference intervals for cows are used (Table 10.2). This could cause concern to the inexperienced clinician, particularly if some medication is being administered that has nephrotoxicity as a possible adverse reaction. It is important in such a case that it be recognized that creatinine concentrations increase with age in bulls and a "high" value may simply be correlated with protein metabolism associated with a bull's large muscle mass.

Evaluation of blood protein variables (i.e., albumin and immunoglobulins) is important in the detection of chronic inflammatory and infectious disease in bulls and for monitoring recovery. A bull infected with a chronic infectious disease may not exhibit clinical signs of disease for many months. But if hyperglobulinemia accompanied by a lower than normal albumin:globulin (A:G) ratio is determined from a serum chemistry test conducted on a bull that is not eating, has an unthrifty hair coat, or has a low body

condition score, then further investigation of a probable chronic infectious condition is warranted. A common and notorious example of this is chronic bronchopneumonia.

Albumin levels are not different between yearling and adult bulls, but the normal reference range for globulin is much higher in adult bulls. The comparative values are illustrated in Table 10.3. The normal A:G ratio in a yearling bull is about 1.0, but the normal A:G ratio in an adult bull is 0.78. If an A:G ratio is less than 0.6 or the globulin concentration is greater than 5.0 g/dL, then a diagnosis of chronic inflammation and possible infection is warranted in an adult bull.

Recommended reference ranges for hematologic and serum biochemistry variables for yearling dairy bulls (6–18 months) and adult bulls (>48 months) are provided in Tables 10.4 and 10.5.

TABLE 10.5	Normal Serum Biochemistry and Plasma Protein Values for Dairy Bulls	
Variable	6–18 Months	>48 Months
Alkaline phosphatase (IU/L)	110–310	30–80
Aspartase transaminase (AST) (IU/L)	50–120	50–190
Bilirubin: total (mg/dL)	0–0.2	0.1–0.3
Blood urea nitrogen (BUN) (mg/dL)	8–15	13–24
Calcium (mg/dL)	9.3–10.5	8.0–9.7
Chloride (mEq/L)	92–103	87–102
Creatine kinase (CK) (IU/L)	100–340	70–470
Creatinine (mg/dL)	1.0–1.6	1.9–3.0
ɣ–Glutamyl transferase (GGT) (IU/L)	11–35	23–47
Glucose (mg/dL)	45–90	45–80
Magnesium (mg/dL)	1.5–2.3	1.6–2.2
Phosphorus (mg/dL)	7.0–9.6	5.0–8.1
Potassium (mEq/L)	3.8–6.3	4.1–6.0
Protein: plasma (g/dL)	6.1–7.3	7.3–8.5
Protein: serum (g/dL)	5.9–7.1	7.1–8.6
Albumin (g/dL)	3.0–3.6	3.0–3.7
Globulin (g/dL)	2.6–3.8	3.8–5.3
Albumin:globulin (A:G) ratio	0.8–1.3	0.6–0.9
Sodium (mEq/L)	133–142	127–143
Triiodothyronine (T_3) (ng/dL)	90–290	60–225
Thyroxine (T_4) (µg/dL)	4.0–8.0	3.2–6.8

Reproduced with permission from Monke DR, Kociba GJ, DeJarnette MS, et al: Reference values for selected hematologic and biochemical variables in Holstein bulls of various ages, *Am J Vet Res* 59:1386-1391, 1998.

Injuries to Bulls Residing in Group Housing

It has been common practice in the AI industry since the 1970s to house young bulls in small groups of 3 to 15 bulls per pen. Group-housed bulls are typically not on semen collection and are waiting results of the traditional progeny test sire summary. Group housing has been considered favorable because of lower cost of construction per animal unit and efficiency of labor. The primary concern for housing bulls in groups pertains to the possibility of injury. It has been perceived that the risk of injury to bulls in communal housing would increase as they reached adult size at 3 to 5 years of age. Accordingly, group housing has gradually been restricted to bulls less than 3 years old. Although injuries occur infrequently in bulls housed in groups, there are five clinical problems that deserve special mention: slipped

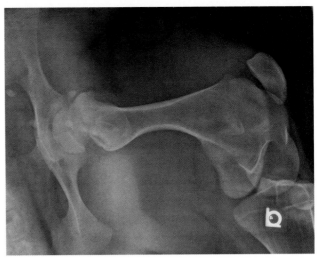

• **Fig. 10.2** Radiograph of a slipped capital physis in the left hindlimb of an acutely lame 7-month-old Holstein bull.

capital femoral epiphysis (SCFE), spiral fracture of the humerus with accompanying radial nerve paralysis, brachial plexus injury, soft tissue stifle injuries, and testicular trauma resulting in tunic rupture and scrotal hematoma.

The advent of genomic evaluation of young sires and a lesser reliance on traditional progeny test programs has provided an impetus to house bulls in individual stalls. The frequency of traumatic injury in bulls housed in groups is therefore anticipated to decline.

Slipped Capital Femoral Epiphysis

Clinical Signs

A bull in group housing with acute onset of non–weight-bearing hind limb lameness should have SCFE included in the differential diagnosis. Because closure of the femoral capital epiphysis is considered to be complete by 3.5 years of age, cases of SCFE may only occur in bulls younger than this. Physical examination reveals signs of pain and crepitus over the greater trochanter when the limb is manipulated. If the case is not observed when acute, muscle atrophy will be present in the affected limb. Most bulls prefer to be recumbent and are reluctant to stand and walk. When they do stand, the affected limb is rotated externally. Confirmation of a diagnosis of SCFE compared with coxofemoral luxation can only be achieved with radiography (Fig. 10.2).

Treatment and Prognosis

If surgery is an option, then it should be approached by open reduction with internal fixation using intramedullary pins across the fracture. When surgery has been conducted on bulls weighing less than about 500 kg, about half of the cases had a successful outcome. Larger bulls had an unfavorable prognosis. This is a serious fracture, and if a conservative, stall-rest approach is the only treatment option because of economic concerns or inability to transport to a facility where surgery can be conducted, then it is suggested that the bull be humanely euthanized.

Spiral Fracture of the Humerus

Clinical Signs

When a bull housed in a group is observed to be acutely lame on a front limb, cannot advance the front limb, and drags the toe of the hoof on the ground, the diagnosis of a spiral fracture of the humerus with resulting radial nerve paralysis should be considered (Fig. 10.3).

Manipulation of the affected limb is painful. When the condition is chronic, the affected limb will have generalized muscle atrophy. Radiographs provide confirmation and more detailed evaluation of the extent and severity of the fracture (Figs. 10.4 and 10.5).

Treatment and Prognosis

Treatment consists primarily of stall rest, although nonsteroidal antiinflammatory drugs (NSAIDs) and hydrotherapy are appropriate during the acute stage of treatment. The bull's stall should be well-bedded so it can lie comfortably and reduce injury to the dorsum of the hoof of the affected limb.

Many bulls that are 1 to 2 years old at the time of the injury recover well enough to get around in their stalls, maintain an average BCS, and after several months of rest can be walked a short distance to a collection arena. Because the injury does not involve a hind limb, young bulls with this problem can mount and successfully produce viable semen after the stress associated with the injury has dissipated. The prognosis declines as the bull gets older because of the gradually progressive weight and stress applied to the contralateral front limb. If the bull is considered a valuable animal, it is advised to collect and inventory semen while the bull is able to mount because the duration of this ability may be limited to several months.

Brachial Plexus Injury

Etiology

Brachial plexus injury most often occurs when a bull, typically in group housing, mounts another bull and its front

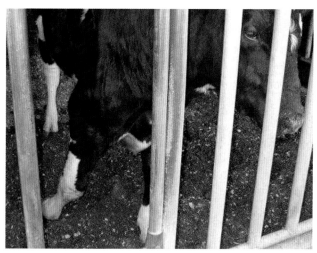

• **Fig. 10.3** Yearling Holstein bull with a spiral fracture of its humerus and radial nerve paralysis. Notice the posture of the right front limb with the dorsum of the toe touching the ground.

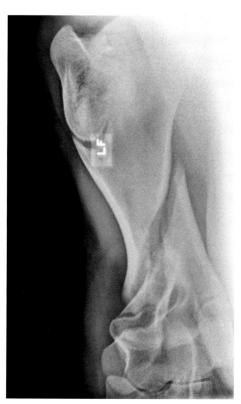

• **Fig. 10.4** Radiograph (AP view) of a spiral fracture of the humerus from an acutely lame 2-year-old Holstein bull.

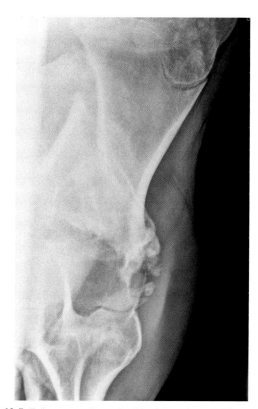

• **Fig. 10.5** Follow-up radiograph of the injury shown in Fig. 10.4 subsequent to 2 months of stall rest and conservative treatment. At the time the image was obtained the bull was sound at the walk.

limb drags across the other bull's back. This action of mild abduction combined with full extension can be an awkward enough posture to cause stretching and damage to the nerves within the brachial plexus. Occasionally, damage or tearing of the suprascapular nerve occurs. This problem is observed more frequently than spiral fracture of the humerus.

Clinical Signs

An affected bull presents as three-legged lame similar to a humeral fracture, but the limb is not painful nor is crepitus felt when the affected limb is manipulated during examination. The bull cannot extend its forelimb to step forward. When the condition becomes chronic, the animal tends to accommodate by "flipping" the limb forward during use. If the suprascapular nerve is irreversibly damaged, the supraspinatus and infraspinatus muscles atrophy, and the spine of the scapula is easily observed ("sweeney"). Similar to a fracture of the humerus, the contralateral limb has to compensate and tends to break down over time.

Treatment and Prognosis

Treatment includes antiinflammatory medication and stall rest. Daily improvement may be observed if permanent nerve damage has not occurred. Most bulls do not permanently damage the suprascapular and subscapular nerves emanating from the brachial plexus. After 1 or 2 weeks of stall rest and therapy, many bulls return to normal.

Stifle Injury

Clinical Signs

Stifle injuries caused by mounting activity can be a cause of hind limb lameness in bulls in both group housing or in semen production situations. When the injury is observed in the acute phase, the bull will be mild to moderately "toe-touching lame" with visible abduction of the affected limb distal to the injured stifle joint (Fig. 10.6). Before the clinician concludes the bull has an injured stifle, the hooves

of the affected limb should always be examined to rule out more common issues associated with the hoof such as a sole ulcer, an abscess extending from the white line, or a toe abscess. Upon examination of the stifle, joint effusion will be present along with pain on manipulation. Increased joint laxity may be noted depending on the severity of the damage to the stifle joint. If the stifle injury is chronic in origin, muscle atrophy of the quadriceps may be present. For more details concerning examination of the stifle, refer to Chapter 12.

Treatment and Prognosis

A juvenile bull diagnosed with a stifle injury should be removed from group housing and medically managed with an antiinflammatory regimen. With stall rest and pain management, the prognosis for return to production is fair to good.

Scrotal Hematoma

Etiology

Injury to the testicles and scrotum of a bull residing in group housing is speculated to be caused by a bull accidentally stepping on the exposed scrotum of a recumbent bull or from a bull's scrotum being head-butted or kicked by another bull.

Clinical Signs

The injury is typically unilateral, and the scrotum is markedly distended (Fig. 10.7). Regardless of the cause, a traumatic

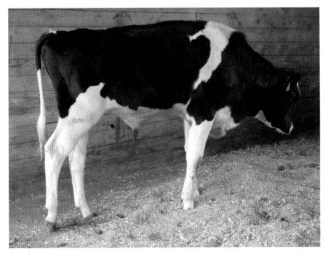

• **Fig. 10.6** Yearling Holstein bull with an injured right stifle. Note how the bull touches its toe to the ground when standing and the moderate swelling of the stifle joint.

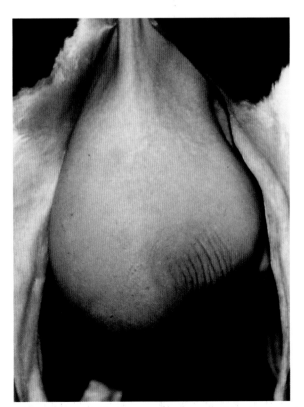

• **Fig. 10.7** Unilateral enlargement of the left side of the scrotum subsequent to a traumatic injury resulting in a scrotal hematoma.

insult to the scrotum can cause rupture of the testicular tunics (Fig. 10.8), resulting in extensive hemorrhage and a large scrotal hematoma. In the acute phase, it may cause the bull to have a minor gait abnormality because of pain and discomfort even at a walk.

Treatment and Prognosis

Although hydrotherapy may provide some benefit, treatment is typically conservative with the bull residing in an individual stall. Over an interval of several months, the clot is resorbed followed by fibrosis, but this is typically accompanied by complete degeneration of the affected testicle. Most bulls are still able to have satisfactory semen collected after the affected testicle has degenerated and the inflammatory response has subsided, but the quantity of spermatozoa is diminished for obvious reasons. Hemicastration of the affected testicle has been performed by Dr. Hillman to speed return to service.

Problems Observed During a Breeding Soundness Examination

The breeding soundness examination (BSE) of a bull is an important management tool that helps determine the breeding potential of male cattle. Most BSEs in veterinary practice are conducted on beef bulls because of the extensive use of artificial insemination in the dairy industry. However, practitioners may be called to evaluate a dairy bull at an AIC that has reproductive problems. The four items that should be covered in a BSE include general examination, external reproductive examination, internal reproductive examination, and semen evaluation. In an AIC, semen evaluation is thoroughly performed by the quality control laboratory and is not discussed in this chapter. It is important to remember that a BSE cannot directly determine a bull's libido or mating ability without observing the mating process. Several management items and problems of young dairy bulls that may be encountered when conducting a BSE are presented here.

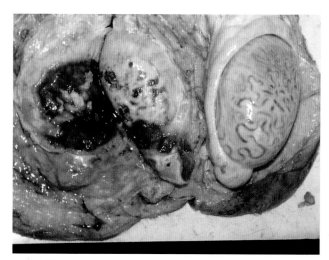

• **Fig. 10.8** Rupture of the left testicular tunic and area of scrotal hematoma subsequent to a traumatic injury.

External Reproductive Examination

The external exam focuses on reproductive structures visible and palpable outside the bull. External tissues to be examined include the scrotum, testes, epididymides, prepuce, and penis. Each genital structure has its own characteristics that should be evaluated for potential abnormalities (Table 10.6). Most important, the scrotum should be palpated to determine testicular and epididymal tone and measured to determine scrotal circumference (SC).

The Value of Scrotal Circumference Measurements

The SC provides useful information about the potential ability for a bull to produce sperm. Because testicular growth as measured by SC is about 2 cm/month from 5 to 10 months of age and approximately 1 cm/month through 15 months of age, a meaningful table for evaluating SC of yearling dairy bulls must provide an average SC for each month of age through 18 months. This is provided in Table 10.7. Without such a table, a 6- or 7-month old dairy bull with a normal SC might be considered to have testicular hypoplasia if its SC was evaluated based on an average SC for a 6- to 12-month-old bull. It is important to note that the normal SC for Jersey bulls aged 5 to 18 months is about 1.5 cm less than the normal measurements provided for Holstein bulls.

TABLE 10.6	External Genitalia to Evaluate During a Breeding Soundness Examination	
External Structure	**Characteristics Examined**	**Potential Abnormalities**
Scrotum	Circumference, shape, epithelial health	Excessive adipose tissue, adhesions, hernia, frostbite
Testicles	Size, tone, symmetry, position, mobility	Hypoplasia, degeneration, orchitis, calcification, incomplete descent, cryptorchid, adhesions
Epididymis	Size, tone	Epididymitis, sperm granuloma, hypoplasia, aplasia, detachment
Prepuce	Length, degree of eversion, epithelial health	Lacerations, adhesions, abscesses, frostbite
Penis	Erection, protrusion, epithelial health	Persistent frenulum, fibropapilloma, hematoma (fractured penis), adhesions, deviation, avulsion, insensitivity

Reproduced with permission from Ayars WH: Applied reproductive strategies in beef cattle. *Proceedings, Breeding Soundness Exam: Beef Bulls*, St. Joseph, Missouri, 2006, pp 265-268.

Incomplete Testicular Descent

Retention of a testicle in the neck of the scrotum (Fig. 10.9) is commonly referred to as incomplete testicular descent. Retention of a testicle in the inguinal canal or abdomen is considered cryptorchidism. This distinction may be only an issue of semantics, but the cases observed by the authors have reliably fallen into the category of incomplete descent of the testicle. From evaluation of 13,460 bulls by the authors over a 36-year interval, incomplete testicular descent was diagnosed in 25 bulls (0.19%). This is similar to the incidence of cryptorchidism reported from a study of 10,940 BSEs of 0.13%. Affected bulls typically have one normally descended testicle with the other only partially descended into the neck of the scrotum. The incompletely descended testicle does not develop normally (Fig. 10.10). The prognosis is that the bull will only have one functional testicle. This is considered a congenital anomaly. Heritability has been considered, but there have been insufficient cases to establish a mode of inheritance.

Pathology of the Epididymis

The epididymis is a single, long convoluted tubule, and it is divided into three anatomical parts: the caput (head), corpus (body), and cauda (tail). Testicular fluid is resorbed, and spermatozoa continue to mature during their 2-week transit through the epididymis from the testis to the cauda segment. The cauda epididymidis is the segment most easily palpated at the distal portion of the scrotum and contains the mature sperm before ejaculation. The normal diameter of the cauda epididymidis of a yearling bull is about 1.5 cm. Pathology of the epididymis is associated with changes in the palpable size of the cauda or nonpatency of the duct caused by congenital malformation or acquired injury.

From 1979 through 2014 (36 years), the veterinarians at Select Sires have empirically assessed the size of the cauda

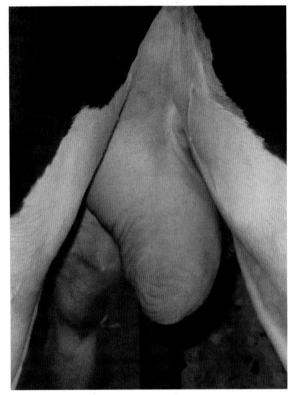

• **Fig. 10.9** Incomplete testicular descent in a 9-month-old Holstein bull. Note the marked asymmetry of the scrotum.

TABLE 10.7	Average Scrotal Circumference Measures for Holstein Bulls Aged 5 to 18 Months		
Age		**Scrotal Circumference (cm)**	
Month	**Days**	**Mean**	**SD**
5	153–182	18.9	1.6
6	182–213	21.9	2.5
7	214–243	24.3	2.4
8	244–274	26.6	2.4
9	275–304	28.6	2.3
10	305–335	30.5	2.1
11	336–365	31.7	2.2
12	366–396	32.7	2.0
13	397–426	33.7	2.0
14	427–457	34.7	2.1
15	458–487	35.2	2.4
16	488–518	35.9	2.3
17	519–548	36.1	2.2
18	549–579	36.4	2.1

SD, Standard deviation.
Reproduced with permission from Hueston WD, Monke DR, Milburn RJ: Scrotal circumference measurements on young Holstein bulls, *J Am Vet Med Assoc* 192:766-768, 1998.

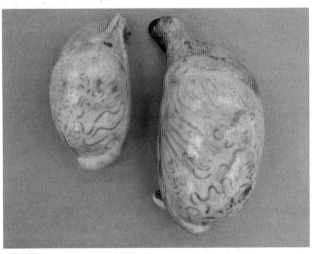

• **Fig. 10.10** Testicles surgically excised from the Holstein bull in Fig. 10.9. The left testicle is markedly underdeveloped.

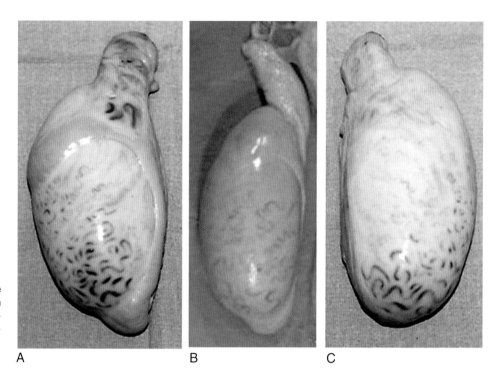

• **Fig. 10.11** Comparative size of the cauda epididymidis in yearling Holstein bulls: **A**, A normal size cauda epididymidis **B**, A hypoplastic cauda epididymidis; **C**, An aplastic cauda epididymidis.

A   B   C

epididymidis on every bull entering the herd and thereafter at 6- or 12-month intervals. The cauda receives a score of either N for normal or a hypoplasia score of H1, H2, H3, H4, or H5, meaning the cauda is considered smaller than normal in 20% increments. The letters A for aplastic and L for larger than normal are also assigned at each examination. From evaluations on 13,460 yearling bulls during the 36-year interval, 16 (0.12%) were found to have unilateral segmental aplasia of the cauda epididymidis (Fig. 10.11). Of these 16 bulls, 8 had left and 8 had right segmental aplasia. These bulls were culled because even though both testicles were present, spermatozoa would be gleaned from only one testicle. From this same population, 391 young bulls (2.9%) were detected to have significant unilateral or bilateral hypoplasia of the cauda early in their life (see Fig. 10.11); however, from this group with marked hypoplasia, only 32 were eventually culled (0.24%) by 18 months of age because of low sperm production associated with a hypoplastic cauda epididymidis. The majority had acceptable sperm production numbers, and the cauda did not remain markedly hypoplastic.

An enlarged, usually fibrotic, cauda epididymidis (Figs. 10.12 and 10.13) occurs less frequently than aplasia and hypoplasia, with an incidence of 11 cases (0.08%) during the same interval of time and from the same population of bulls. An enlarged cauda epididymidis may not be apparent on observation of the scrotum (Fig. 10.14), but it is readily palpated.

Occlusion of the epididymis is typically associated with a congenital, blind-ended efferent ductule. As spermatogenesis progresses and the young bull reaches puberty, a spermatocele will develop in the region of the caput epididymidis if one or more efferent ductules are blind ended. In this situation, the sperm accumulate in the blind-ended tubule. When the tubular epithelium degenerates, spermatozoa extravasate into epididymal stroma,

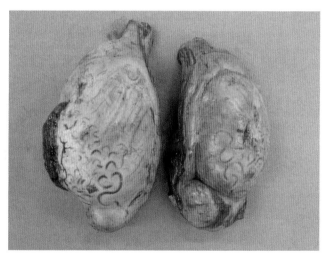

• **Fig. 10.12** Unilateral cauda epididymitis in a yearling Holstein bull. The right cauda is markedly enlarged.

causing an inflammatory response. A sperm granuloma develops, which is palpated as a fibrotic enlargement on the dorsal pole of the testis about 2.5 to 4 cm in width. This is a very unusual problem in yearling dairy bulls as evidenced by the fact that only five bulls have been culled (0.04%) for this problem within our AIC during the 36-year period.

Penile Fibropapillomatosis

Etiology

Penile fibropapillomas are caused by the bovine papillomaviruses and manifest as multinodular warts on the glans penis of young bulls (Fig. 10.15 and Figs. 9.20 A&B). Penile warts are thought to originate from viral infection of abrasions of the preputial and penile epithelium as a result of mounting and mating behaviors. The significance of

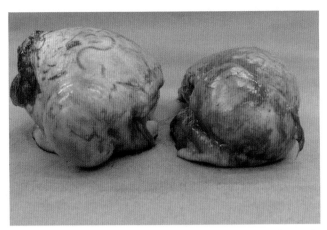

• **Fig. 10.13** Unilateral cauda epididymitis, viewed from the distal pole of the testis. From this perspective one can more fully appreciate the extent of the epididymitis, but also the difference in size of the testicles; the right testicle is in a degenerative phase, evidenced by its smaller diameter compared to the left testicle.

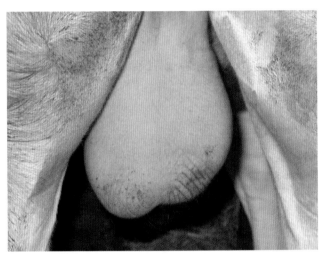

• **Fig. 10.14** Scrotum of the yearling bull from which the testicles and epididymides from Figs. 10.12 and 10.13 were taken. Note the asymmetry of the scrotum. This photo illustrates that one must palpate the scrotum to recognize the reason for the asymmetry.

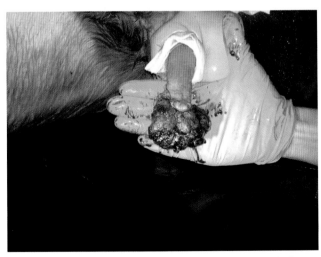

• **Fig. 10.15** Penile fibropapilloma in a yearling Holstein bull.

penile fibropapillomas in an AIC is found in the potential for extensive trauma to the penis during collection, blood contamination of a semen sample from trauma to the mass, and reluctance to exteriorize the penis and mount for collection because of discomfort from a penile wart.

Clinical Signs

Observation of an abnormal mass on the penis, blood coming from the preputial orifice, or a bull with phimosis or paraphimosis may be signs that a penile fibropapilloma is present. Penile warts can range in size but are typically attached to the penile epithelium by a stalk of tissue, creating a pedunculated mass. Even when masses appear to be large and encompassing the penis, further examination often reveals a single tissue stalk of origin. However, diffuse attachment of a penile fibropapilloma does occur and makes surgical correction more difficult.

Treatment

Although some penile warts regress without intervention, surgical removal is indicated if the mass is adversely affecting the semen collection process. Surgical correction can be performed by properly restraining the bull, exteriorizing the penis, and providing local anesthesia around the base of the mass. Ligation of the stalk of the mass is important because penile warts have a very rich vascular supply. Absorbable suture, size 0 or 1, can be used for ligation prior to excision of the mass. Excision can be performed with a surgical blade, but electrocautery or laser techniques can also be used also be used as could debulking and cryotherapy. Care should be taken to avoid accidental trauma to the urethra during excision. Experience has shown that the use of an immunostimulant such as Immunoboost, 1 cc administered intravenously (IV) at the time of surgical correction, helps reduce the recurrence of penile warts. Bulls should be sexually rested for 2 to 4 weeks after surgical correction.

Prognosis

The prognosis for bulls to return to normal collection after routine surgical correction is good. Commercial or autogenous vaccines can be administered with the intent to reduce recurrence, but their efficacy is variable and not well documented.

Persistent Penile Frenulum

Etiology

Persistent penile frenulum is an infrequently observed condition in pubescent bulls in which a congenital band of tissue located between the glans penis and the prepuce does not break down as the bull reaches maturity (Fig. 10.16). This condition may cause the penis to deviate ventrally during mating activity and adversely affect the bull's ability to serve an artificial vagina (AV) or breed a heifer. The condition can easily be treated. A persistent frenulum may have a heritable component, which should be considered in the herd setting.

Clinical Signs

Clinically, a persistent frenulum can be observed during a young bull's first collection and is commonly observed as an

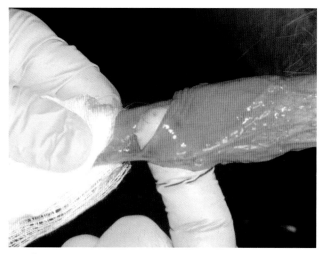

• **Fig. 10.16** Persistent penile frenulum in a yearling Holstein bull.

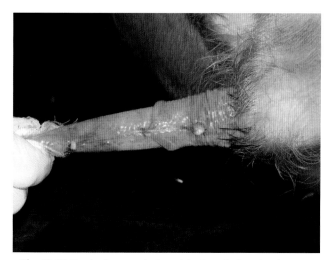

• **Fig. 10.17** Surgically corrected persistent penile frenulum in a yearling Holstein bull.

abnormally shaped glans penis. Some cases have a ventral deviation during erection.

Treatment

A persistent frenulum may break down after repeated erections, but if the tissue remains persistent, surgical correction can be performed. It is important to properly restrain the bull, clean the preputial region and penis, and provide local anesthesia before commencing surgical repair. The penis can be manually extended and held by an assistant. Transfixing ligatures are placed on the proximal and distal aspects of the frenulum using size 0 or 1 absorbable suture and then a cut is made between the sutures (Fig. 10.17). Electrocautery and laser procedures have also been described for repair of a persistent frenulum. Care should be taken to avoid damage to the urethra during correction.

The surgical procedure is routine when the size of the frenulum is distinct and small. In such cases, the bull should be given 1 to 2 weeks of sexual rest to allow for healing. However, if the persistent tissue is extensive and attached at multiple locations along the ventral aspect of the penis,

TABLE 10.8	Internal Genitalia to Evaluate During a Breeding Soundness Examination		
Internal Structure	Characteristics Examined	Potential Abnormalities
Prostate	Size, tone	Abnormalities are rare
Seminal vesicles	Size, symmetry, tone	Seminal vesiculitis
Ampullae	Size, tone	Abnormalities are rare
Inguinal rings	Length, degree of eversion, epithelial health	Hernia, cryptorchid

Reproduced with permission from Ayars WH: Applied reproductive strategies in beef cattle. *Proceedings, Breeding Soundness Exam: Beef Bulls*, St. Joseph, Missouri, 2006, pp 265-268.

the surgery becomes more involved, and time for recovery should be extended.

Internal Reproductive Examination

The internal reproductive examination focuses on genitalia that must be assessed by rectal palpation. These tissues include the prostate gland, seminal vesicles, ampullae, and inguinal rings. Problems associated with these tissues are reviewed in Table 10.8.

Vesiculitis, Seminal Vesiculitis, and Vesicular Adenitis

Etiology

Seminal vesiculitis is an inflammation of one or both vesicular glands located within the pelvic canal of a bull that may also include an infectious component. Bulls of all ages can be affected with vesiculitis, but the problem is most commonly observed in yearling bulls starting on collection or being evaluated as part of a BSE. From evaluations on 13,460 yearling bulls during a 36-year interval, 60 bulls (0.45%) were culled from the genetic testing program because of vesiculitis.

The purulent material that accompanies most cases of vesiculitis can contaminate the ejaculate and is a cause for semen to be discarded from bulls collected at an AIC. Vesiculitis diagnosed in an adult bull is usually chronic and subsequent to vesiculitis as a yearling bull for which treatment may have been administered but only a transient improvement or temporary resolution was achieved.

Vesiculitis has traditionally been considered to be caused by either bacterial or mycoplasmal infection. The most commonly identified microbial agents have been *Trueperella pyogenes, Pseudomonas aeruginosa, Streptococcus* spp., *Staphylococcus* spp., *Proteus* spp., *Escherichia coli, Mycoplasma bovis,* and *Mycoplasma bovigenitalium.* The pathogenic mechanism

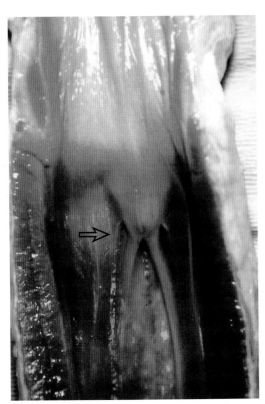

• **Fig. 10.18** Normal excretory ducts on the colliculus seminalis. Vesicular fluid from the vesicles enters the proximal urethra at this site. Note opening to right of arrow.

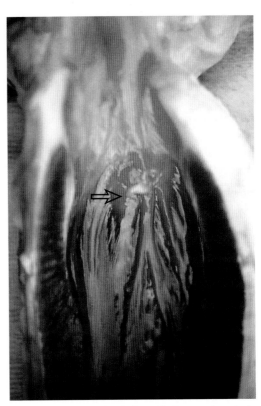

• **Fig. 10.19** Malformation of both the vesicular excretory ducts on the colliculus seminalis. Note absence of excretory duct opening to right of arrow - compare with Fig. 10.18.

by which infection of the vesicular glands occurs is most likely hematogenous and secondary to a systemic or umbilical infection. An ascending route of infection seems unlikely unless the bull has urethritis or penile trauma. A descending route of infection via the ductus deferens and originating from an epididymis or testicle is possible but not as likely. When conventional bacterial species are involved, embolic spread from the lungs, liver, or sinuses or a chronic soft tissue abscess are all potential sources, but with mycoplasmal infection, the possibility of hematogenous spread after inhalation through the respiratory tract or ingestion via the gastrointestinal tract is more likely.

Because many cases of vesiculitis are refractory to antimicrobial treatment, an intriguing possible explanation lies with a congenital malformation of the excretory ducts of the vesicles at the colliculus seminalis on the dorsum of the proximal urethra (Fig. 10.18). In one study, 40% of the dairy bulls with vesiculitis had a congenital malformation at this location (Fig. 10.19).

An abnormal excretory duct orifice is postulated to permit the reflux of semen or urine from the pelvic urethra to pass retrograde up the duct and into the vesicle. When the lining of the excretory tubule or duct degenerates, the semen would enter the parenchyma of the vesicle and be recognized as a foreign body. An inflammatory response would follow.

Clinical Signs

In an AIC setting, the first suggestion that a bull may have vesiculitis is when the laboratory technicians report

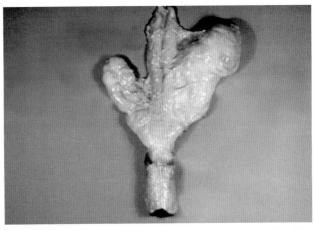

• **Fig. 10.20** Notice the marked asymmetry of the vesicles. The right vesicle was abscessed.

a seminal sample contaminated with purulent material. Most dairy bulls do not have an internal genital examination conducted before the first collection of semen. When palpated, the bull may be found to have one or both vesicles enlarged and possibly fibrotic. When unilateral vesiculitis occurs, there is typically asymmetry in the size of the vesicles (Fig. 10.20). It is very unusual for a bull with vesiculitis to have clinical discomfort, and it is also unusual for a bull to show evidence of pain on rectal palpation of the vesicles. Although vesiculitis may be the primary reason for purulent contamination of semen, other possibilities such as epididymitis, orchitis, and posthitis must be ruled out.

Treatment

Because of the traditional consideration that vesiculitis has an infectious etiology, most bulls are treated with a prolonged-release antibiotic approved for cattle. Because inflammation is also a component of vesiculitis, additional benefit may be achieved when antiinflammatory medication is administered concurrent with the antimicrobial therapy. Because one cannot know from palpation if a bull has a congenital defect at the colliculus seminalis, predisposing the animal to vesiculitis, response to antimicrobial therapy may be useful prognostically; treatment failure may be taken to suggest a congenital defect with a resultant worsening of prognosis. There are reports suggesting that intraglandular injections of antibiotics may provide a positive benefit. For cases that have not responded to antibiotics, surgical excision of the affected vesicle has long been considered the only alternative. The response to surgery is best described as marginally successful for yearling bulls but not successful for adults with chronic infection.

Prognosis

Review of the literature provides conflicting evidence regarding prognosis subsequent to antimicrobial therapy. Some studies report that young bulls may spontaneously recover from vesiculitis, and others report that antibiotics can provide a positive therapeutic result. Other studies report a guarded prognosis or that treatment is often unsuccessful, and the best "treatment" is to cull the bull. Mindful of these conflicting results, when one is attempting to give a prognosis, it is advisable to consider the purpose of the bull and the future reproductive demands on him. If only several hundred to several thousand straws of semen are needed by the owner of a bull, an intensive therapy of antibiotics and antiinflammatory medication *may* occasionally provide a transient improvement adequate to reduce the purulent contamination so that the semen can be collected over the course of 1 or 2 months. If it is a natural service bull, the semen will not be available for regular evaluation, and one may never know the response to therapy other than indirectly via the pregnancy rate in mated females. But these scenarios do not apply to most dairy bulls in an AIC with the intent of producing semen of satisfactory quality several days a week for many years. For this type of dairy bull, a transient improvement is not satisfactory. Because a full resolution of vesiculitis from medical therapy is uncommon, most diseased bulls are eventually found to be unsatisfactory for semen production and are culled in favor of collecting a dairy bull that is not affected with vesiculitis. Whether a bull fails to respond to antimicrobial therapy because of insufficient penetration of the antibiotics into the tissue or if the bull indeed has a congenital malformation of an excretory duct, the end result of lack of response to therapy is the same, and the bull is culled.

Problems Associated with the Collection of Semen in Adult Bulls

As discussed earlier in this chapter, a dairy bull is only profitable when it can mount and have semen of satisfactory

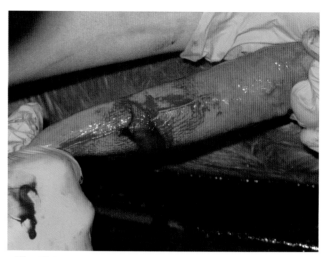

• **Fig. 10.21** Penile epithelial avulsion approximately 6 cm in length. Notice the ventral penile raphe used as a landmark for surgical correction.

quality collected on a regular basis. The typical AIC has rubber mat flooring or clay and sand in collection arenas to provide good footing for the bulls during use. Stalls have mats with bedding and are regularly cleaned to keep dry, or a bedding pack is maintained if the bulls reside in an open-front barn. Livestock technicians are trained to handle bulls in a safe, calm, and consistent manner to minimize negative behavioral factors. The animals the bulls mount, which are usually steers, should be docile, structurally sound, and similarly sized to the bull. These are all important factors in keeping bulls healthy and behaviorally and reproductively sound.

Dairy bulls are about 5 years old when they return to collection after receipt of the progeny test data. This situation is changing to some extent with genomic evaluations because some high-value bulls may remain on collection through 2 or 3 years of age rather than spending 3.5 years waiting for progeny data with no semen collected. Even with excellent management and handling, however, problems do arise. An injury to the penis that may be specific to dairy bulls residing in an AIC is avulsion of the penile integument. Because of the size of a mature dairy bull, variability in conformation, and the repetitive motion of the semen collection process, traumatic musculoskeletal injuries and degenerative joint disease also occur. The most common locations for osteoarthritis in an adult bull involve the vertebral column and major joints of the hind limb. These problems are discussed in greater detail in the following sections.

Penile Epithelial Avulsion

Etiology

A penile epithelial avulsion (PEA) is a tearing or separation of the outermost layer of the penis and commonly occurs at the fornix of the penile and preputial integument (Fig. 10.21). The fornix is the primary location for an avulsion injury because it is the region on the penis where very elastic, flexible mucosa from the preputial integument meets the inelastic, rigid mucosa of the penile integument. PEAs most commonly occur in bulls that return to collection after having several years of sexual inactivity, but they can occur in bulls of any age. The significance of PEAs can be found in the economic potential that is lost because of the bull requiring sexual rest for at least 6 to 8 weeks after injury.

Although the specific etiology remains undetermined, many factors may contribute to the occurrence of a PEA. Both bull and collection process factors appear important. The most common bull factors that may predispose to or increase the severity of PEAs include the inelasticity of the mucosal tissue at the fornix and the intensity of libido and force of thrust of the bull after a period of sexual inactivity. Some collection process factors that may increase the likelihood of PEA include inadequate lubrication of the AV, excessively rough texture of AV liners, insufficiency of water within the AV, and improper AV application. Two important features of AV application are the angle of application onto the penis and the pressure applied by the collector when the bull serves the AV.

Clinical Signs

The most obvious indications that a PEA has occurred are blood within the AV or blood observed at the preputial orifice. Often, an experienced collector will be aware that a problem occurred during collection, and a veterinarian should be contacted immediately because of the likelihood of penile trauma. After a short period of time, an enlargement within the prepuce may be observed as a result of blood and inflammation emanating from the avulsed area.

Visualization of the penis is the most appropriate way to assess the presence and severity of a PEA. Visualization can be achieved by encouraging protrusion of the penis by mounting the bull on a teaser animal or by electroejaculation. Alternatively, a bull can be placed in the lateral recumbent position on a tilt table (commonly used for hoof trimming), and the penis can be exteriorized manually. Before manual extension of the penis for evaluation, parenteral administration of a sedative that relaxes the retractor penis muscles (acepromazine 0.02–0.03 mg/kg IV) is helpful.

Typically, PEAs originate on the ventral aspect of the penis because of the inelasticity of the tissue along the ventral penile raphe. Severe avulsions can radiate dorsally in a spiral pattern around the circumference of the penis as a result of the collagen fiber arrangement of the penile integument. Most lesions range from approximately 3 to 10 cm in length.

Treatment

After examination of the penis to determine the severity of an avulsion, the clinician must determine if the injury can be repaired using suture or should be left to heal by secondary intention. Small lesions (<2 cm) often heal successfully without intervention. Large lesions (>2 cm) typically require placement of sutures to allow for appropriate tissue healing and to avoid large regions of granulation tissue that can lead to abscessation or penile adhesions. The interval

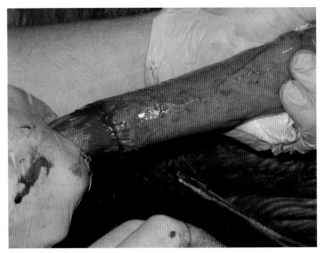

• **Fig. 10.22** Surgically corrected penile epithelial avulsion.

of time from the injury to evaluation plays the biggest role when determining how an avulsion should be repaired. Ideally, PEAs should be repaired within 24 hours of occurrence to allow for the best healing response and to avoid extensive wound contamination. Avulsions that are addressed longer than 24 hours after occurrence can be treated as open wounds by providing a preputial infusion of nonirritating antiseptic solution for several days to ward off contamination. It may be warranted to begin systemic broad-spectrum antibiotics as well.

To repair a PEA, the bull must be physically and chemically restrained to ensure safety to the veterinarian, assisting personnel, and the bull. The authors prefer the use of a tilt table and sedation as previously described. Hair surrounding the preputial orifice is clipped, the ventral abdomen is cleansed using a common surgical scrub, and the area is rinsed to allow for a generally clean working environment. The penis is manually exteriorized by straightening the sigmoid flexure and gradually pulling the preputial skin over the penis until the penile tip is protruding from the preputial orifice. The penile tip can be gently grasped by an assistant using dry 4 × 4 gauze pads to allow for sufficient grip, and the penis should then be fully exteriorized for evaluation of the lesion. Local anesthetic can be injected circumferentially at the most proximal end of the exteriorized penis (carefully avoiding large vessels) to reduce sensation during repair. The avulsed area may require cleansing before suturing can commence. Absorbable suture size 0 or 1 should be used in a simple continuous or simple interrupted pattern to obtain appropriate tissue apposition using the ventral penile raphe as a landmark (Fig. 10.22). After surgical correction, triple antibiotic ointment can be applied to the sutured area and the penis gently released back into the prepuce.

Regardless if repaired by suture or allowed to heal by secondary intention, the most important factor for treatment is sexual rest. Appropriate healing will take at least 6 to 8 weeks and thereafter should be followed by a gradual return to collection. It is critical to be patient when considering a return to collection because premature collection risks reinjuring the penis and may lead to more economic loss because of time off collection.

Prognosis

When treated in a timely manner and allowed appropriate time for healing, the prognosis for a bull's return to normal collection frequency is good. Although repair of the penis should be performed as indicated, it is critical to evaluate the collection process in an effort to prevent PEAs from occurring. It is important to assess the collection technique to ensure proper AV application onto the penis as well as the AV preparation to ensure the appropriate use of lubrication and liners.

Pain Management of Nonspecific Osteoarthritis and Degenerative Joint Disease

Pain relief is an important animal welfare concern in the livestock industry, but the lack of approved analgesic drugs provides a significant challenge to bovine veterinarians. Consequently, the use of any drugs for pain relief in bulls represents an extralabel drug use (ELDU). The Animal Medicinal Drug Use Clarification Act (AMDUCA) of 1994 allows veterinarians ELDU as long as certain conditions are met. Please refer to AMDUCA concerning the criteria for ELDU in food animals in the United States.

Although there are several specific musculoskeletal and neurologic diseases of adult bulls, many bulls have nonspecific osteoarthritis problems for which pain management is important to permit the bull to continue to have semen harvested. NSAIDs are applicable in the treatment of both acute injuries and chronic osteoarthritis because they provide analgesic and antiinflammatory benefits. Commonly used NSAIDs include flunixin meglumine, meloxicam, and aspirin. Flunixin meglumine is provided at a dose of 1.1 to 2.2 mg/kg IV every 24 hours for no more than 3 consecutive days and delivers the most immediate analgesic and antiinflammatory response. Aspirin is provided at a dose of approximately 100 mg/kg orally (PO) every 24 hours and is typically used for mild osteoarthritic cases. Meloxicam is a convenient and effective drug for providing analgesia in geriatric and injured bulls because of its oral administration, longer lasting analgesia, lower cost and higher cyclooxygenase 2:cyclooxygenase 1(COX2:COX1) ratio than both flunixin and aspirin. Therapy with meloxicam is initiated with a single loading dose of 1 mg/kg PO and then continued with a maintenance dose of 0.5 mg/kg PO every other day. More recently, gabapentin, a γ-aminobutyric acid analogue, has been shown to act synergistically with NSAIDs in the management of chronic pain of inflammatory or neuropathic origin.

When an NSAID regimen has been initiated on a bull, prolonged treatment is generally warranted because of the chronic and progressive nature of degenerative joint disease and osteoarthritis. It should be noted that bulls undergoing protracted NSAID treatment regimens are at an increased risk for the development of abomasal ulcers and should be closely monitored for gastrointestinal disturbances. Melena or a decrease in packed cell volume and plasma protein after initiating NSAID therapy could indicate abomasal bleeding, necessitating changes in pain management. Adjunct, nontraditional treatments such as acupuncture and chiropractic manipulation have become increasingly popular for chronic back and osteoarthritic conditions in individually valuable cattle, including bulls. The scientific evaluation of these is lacking, but the combination of anecdotal success, personal experience, and the limitations and side effects of long-term NSAID administration all contribute to their increasing use.

Spastic Syndrome or "Crampiness"

Spastic syndrome is a disease observed occasionally in mature dairy bulls; it is rarely if ever observed in beef bulls. The problem is typically first observed when the bull is 4 or 5 years old, but the onset can be as early as 3 years of age. The disease is characterized by intermittent spasms of skeletal muscle groups, especially when the bull first rises from a recumbent position and adapts to a weight-bearing posture. A spastic syndrome episode may last from 15 to 60 seconds when the bull is standing and then the affected muscle groups relax. Another episode may occur within several minutes, or there may be longer intervals between episodes depending on the severity of the condition. Spasms do not occur when the bull is recumbent.

In early cases, the spasticity may involve only one hind limb. When the bull rises, it will lift the hoof of the affected limb from the ground and shake it in a backward direction. It may also do this when standing or walking. If the bull is being led, the handler may need to pause to let the bull complete a spastic episode. For some bulls, the spasticity does not progress beyond this stage. In other bulls, however, the disease progresses anteriorly to eventually involve the trunk of the body as well as the hind limbs. Bulls will stand with their hind limbs "stretched out" for 30 to 60 seconds during the spasm and then relax (Fig. 10.23). In the most

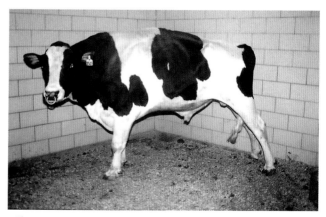

• **Fig. 10.23** Adult Holstein bull with typical signs of spastic syndrome.

advanced cases, the spasms will progress into the neck, causing the bull to lift its head and twist it slightly to one side during the spasm (Fig. 10.24).

Some bulls seem to have an exacerbation of the spasticity when they have a painful hoof problem, such as an abscess or sole ulcer. This can be an acute and focal stressor, and it suggests that a painful stimulus may worsen the spasticity. An extension of this reasoning infers that nonspecific arthritis lesions may also worsen the spasticity condition.

Treatment of spastic syndrome is directed toward reducing painful stimuli by conducting hoof trims to keep the hooves in good health and providing antiinflammatory medication. Muscle relaxant medications have also been used but the benefit from them may be difficult to assess. Bulls with varying levels of spasticity can have semen collected on a regular basis, particularly when they are well managed with antiinflammatory medication.

Posterior Spinal Paresis

Clinical Signs

Posterior spinal paresis (PSP) is a chronic disease of adult to aging bulls; the onset is typically after 6 years of age. It is clinically observed as a progressive hind limb ataxia. Early in the progression of the disease, bulls may have an uncoordinated gait evidenced by weaving from side to side when walking, crossing their limbs excessively when turning a corner, or having inconsistent stride lengths. Some bulls may have reluctance to mount a steer, but many do not show reluctance in the early phase. As the disease progresses, the uncoordinated gait will worsen, and conscious proprioceptive (CP) deficits of one or both hind limbs will be observed (Fig. 10.25). The CP deficits are most remarkable when a bull has good libido, mounts and serves the AV well, and then stumbles or falls on dismount because it does not "know" where its hind feet are positioned.

In many earlier texts or articles, PSP is referred to as posterior spinal paralysis. However, after working with many dairy bulls for almost 4 decades, there has never been a bull affected with PSP that was actually paralyzed. Every bull had reduced muscular strength, hind limb weakness and ataxia, or some CP deficits that were better described by paresis than paralysis.

Similar neurologic signs or deficits in younger bulls are more likely associated with acute problems such as a fracture of a vertebra or a congenital vertebral abnormality such as hemi- or wedged vertebrae.

Etiology

A definitive etiology for PSP has not been determined even though it has been observed and studied for many years. There is an association with vertebral osteophytosis or more specifically with ankylosing spondylitis (Figs. 10.26 and 10.27). Most bulls with PSP that are evaluated postmortem have

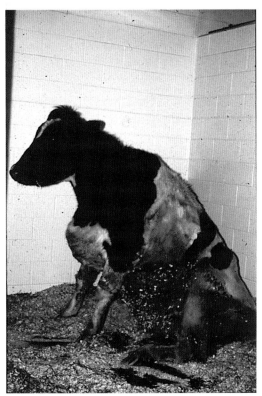

• **Fig. 10.25** Dog-sitting posture of a mature Holstein bull with severe PSP due to ankylosing spondylitis. The bull could stand with assistance but demonstrated severe and dangerous proprioceptive deficits.

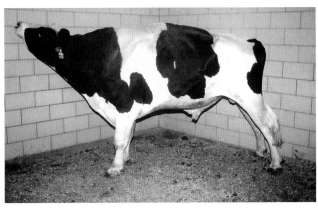

• **Fig. 10.24** Adult Holstein bull with advanced spastic syndrome.

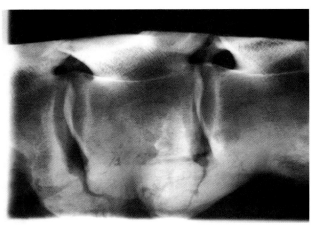

• **Fig. 10.26** Lateral radiographs of lumbar spine from bull in Fig. 10.25 obtained post mortem. Note the severe ankylosing spondylitis.

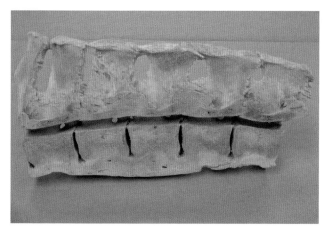

• **Fig. 10.27** T12 to L3 vertebrae recovered from a 9-year-old Holstein bull with clinical signs of posterior spinal paresis. Note the extensive ankylosing spondylitis below the vertebral bodies.

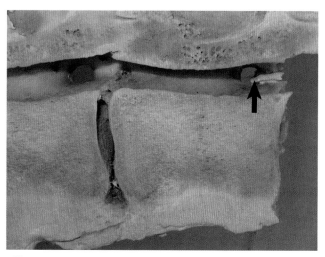

• **Fig. 10.28** Vertebrae L2 and primarily L3. Note the bony spicule near the intervertebral foramen of L3 (arrow). This contrasts markedly with the unimpeded foramen cranial to it.

ankylosing spondylitis, but certainly not every bull with ankylosing spondylitis develops PSP.

Several decades ago, it was common for genetically superior dairy bulls to have been raised on dairy farms and be admitted to an AIC for semen collection when 5 years old. When these bulls developed PSP later in life and were found to have ankylosing spondylitis, it was considered that a diet too high in calcium during their residence on the dairy was the probable cause of the problems observed. Feeding excessive calcium was found to have contributed to thyroid hyperplasia and calcification of selected soft tissues, and it would seemingly contribute toward development of ankylosing spondylitis. However, we have since discovered that when dietary calcium was reduced in the diet of bulls, the incidence of vertebral osteophytosis and ankylosing spondylitis did not decline, suggesting that this initial explanation was too simplistic.

Other studies have evaluated nondietary associations. An attractive concept was that vertebral osteophytosis and ankylosing spondylitis were an "occupational hazard" for a dairy bull, possibly being related to the mechanics of repeated collection. However, studies have determined that it is not associated with ejaculatory thrust when servicing an AV nor associated with frequency of semen collection. The type of housing has been evaluated, and it was determined that the frequency or severity of vertebral osteophytosis was not different whether the bull resided in group housing for an interval of time or always resided in an individual stall. Another study noted an association of the major histocompatibility complex with development of ankylosing spondylitis and hind limb ataxia in older bulls. Some authors have suggested that it is part of the normal aging process in bulls.

It is clear that PSP is a multifactorial condition, and it seems probable that the development of clinical signs of PSP is associated with the extent of the ankylosing spondylitis and whether or not osteophytes or excessive bony deposition along the vertebrae impinge on the intervertebral foramina (Fig. 10.28) and in turn the spinal nerve roots, causing a localized radiculoneuropathy.

Treatment

Treatment for PSP is typically management based. Supportive therapy includes adequate bedding that is changed frequently so the bull can be comfortable and dry. If possible, the bull should reside in a stall not too far from the collection arena to reduce the distance it has to walk. Frequency of semen collection may need to be reduced from 2 or 3 days a week to 1 or 2 days a week and for some bulls, a reduction from two ejaculates per day to one. As PSP advances, collection of semen by mounting may need to be discontinued altogether in favor of careful electroejaculation or collection of semen by ampullae massage. Antiinflammatory medications may be indicated because most adult or aging bulls will concurrently have some osteoarthritis.

Prognosis

Because of the chronic nature of the onset of PSP, each case is managed on its own merits to extend the functional longevity of the bull as best as possible. The problem will not be resolved nor reversed; the bull should be humanely managed until semen quality declines or it is unable to rise from a recumbent position. The interval of this management may vary from several months to 2 years.

Suggested Readings

Almquist, J. O., & Thomson, R. G. (1973). Relation of sexual behavior and ejaculation frequency to severity of vertebral body osteophytes in dairy and beef bulls. *J Am Vet Med Assoc, 163*, 163–168.

Anderson, D. E. (2008). Surgery of the prepuce and penis. *Vet Clin North Am (Food Anim Pract), 24*, 245–251.

Ashdown, R. R. (1962). Persistence of the penile frenulum in young bulls. *Vet Rec, 74*, 1464–1468.

Ashdown, R. R., Ricketts, S. W., & Wardley, R. C. (1968). The fibrous architecture of the integumentary coverings of the bovine penis. *J Anat, 103*, 567–572.

Ayars, W. H. (2006). Applied Reproductive Strategies in Beef Cattle. *Proceedings - Breeding Soundness Exam: Beef Bulls*, 265–268.

Blom, E. (1979). Studies on seminal vesiculitis in the bull. I. Semen examination methods and post mortem findings. *Nord Vet Med*, *31*, 193–205.

Blom, E. (1979). Studies on seminal vesiculitis in the bull. II. Malformation of the pelvic genital organs as a possible factor in the pathogenesis of seminal vesiculitis. *Nord Vet Med*, *31*, 241–250.

Carroll, E. J., Ball, L., & Scott, J. A. (1963). Breeding soundness in bulls – A summary of 10,940 examinations. *J Am Vet Med Assoc*, *142*, 1105–1111.

Coetzee, J. F. (2013). A review of analgesic compounds used in food animals in the United States. *Vet Clin North Am (Food Anim Pract)*, *29*(1), 11–28.

Coulter, G. H., & Foote, R. H. (1979). Bovine testicular measurements as indicators of reproductive performance and their relationship to productive traits in cattle: a review. *Theriogenology*, *11*, 297–311.

Hall, W. C., Nielsen, S. W., & McEntee, K. (1976). Tumours of the prostate and penis. *Bull World Health Organ*, *53*(2-3), 247–256.

Hueston, W. D., Monke, D. R., & Milburn, R. J. (1988). Scrotal circumference measurements on young Holstein bulls. *J Am Vet Med Assoc*, *192*, 766–768.

Hull, B. L., Koenig, G. J., & Monke, D. R. (1990). Treatment of slipped capital femoral epiphysis in cattle: 11 cases (1974-1988). *J Am Vet Med Assoc*, *197*, 1509–1512.

Hull, B. L., Monke, D. R., & Rohde, R. (1992). A new technique for seminal vesiculectomy. *Proceedings 14th Natl Assoc Anim Breeders Tech Conf on AI and Repro*, 100–103.

Kennedy, S. P., Spitzer, J. C., Hopkins, F. M., et al. (2002). Breeding soundness evaluations of 3648 yearling beef bulls using the 1993 Society for Theriogenology guidelines. *Theriogenology*, *58*(5), 947–961.

Larson, L. L., Parker, W. G., & Braun, R. K. (1978). Limb diseases in bulls: Their recognition, prevention and treatment. *Proceedings 7th Natl Assoc Anim Breeders Tech Conf on AI and Repro*, 41–44.

McEntee, K. (1990). *Reproductive pathology of domestic animals*. San Diego, CA: Academic Press, Inc.

McEntee, K., Hall, C. E., & Dunn, H. O. (1980). The relationship of calcium intake to the development of vertebral osteophytosis and ultimobranchial tumors in bulls. *Proceedings 8th Natl Assoc Anim Breeders Tech Conf on AI and Repro*, 44–47.

Monke, D. R. (1980). Avulsion of the bovine penile epithelium at the fornix: incidence, treatment, and prevention. *Proceedings 8th Natl Assoc Anim Breeders Tech Conf on AI and Repro*, 48–55.

Monke, D. R. (1987). Examination of the bovine scrotum, testicles, and epididymides – Part II. *Compend Contin Educ Pract Vet*, *9*, F277–F283.

Monke, D. R. (2003). Bull management: Artificial insemination centres. In H. Roginski, J. W. Fuquay, & P. F. Fox (Eds.), *Encyclopedia of Dairy Sciences* (pp. 198–209). Amsterdam: Elsevier Science Ltd.

Monke, D. R., Kociba, G. J., DeJarnette, M. S., et al. (1998). Reference values for selected hematologic and biochemical variables in Holstein bulls of various ages. *Am J Vet Res*, *59*, 1386–1391.

Park, C. A., Hines, H. C., Monke, D. R., et al. (1993). Association between the bovine major histocompatibility complex and chronic posterior spinal paresis – a form of ankylosing spondylitis – in Holstein bulls. *Animal Genetics*, *24*, 53–58.

Parker, W. G. (1990). The effect of environment on spondylosis in bulls. *Proceedings 13th Natl Assoc Anim Breeders Tech Conf on AI and Repro*, 80–83.

Parker, W. G., Braun, R. K., Bean, B., et al. (1987). Avulsion of the bovine prepuce from its attachment to the penile integument during semen collection with an artificial vagina. *Theriogenology*, *28*, 237.

Pentecost, R., & Niehaus, A. (2014). Stifle disorders: cranial cruciate ligament, meniscus, upward fixation of the patella. *Vet Clin North Am (Food Anim Pract)*, *30*(1), 265–281.

Radostits, O. M., Leslie, K. E., & Fetrow, J. (1994). *Herd Health Food Animal Production Medicine* (2nd ed.).

Rovay, H., Barth, A. D., Chirino-Trejo, M., et al. (2008). Update on treatment of vesiculitis in bulls. *Theriogenology*, *70*, 495–503.

Schefers, J. M., & Weigel, K. A. (2012). Genomic selection in dairy cattle: Integration of DNA testing into breeding programs. *Animal Frontiers*, *2*, 4–9.

Senger, P. L. (2003). *Pathways to Pregnancy and Parturition: Male Reproductive System* (2nd ed.). Pullman: Current Conceptions, Inc. (revised).

U.S. Food and Drug Administration: Animal Medicinal Drug Use Clarification Act (AMDUCA) of 1994 (website): www.fda.gov/RegulatoryInformation/. Legislation/FederalFoodDrugandCosmeticActFDCAct/SignificantAmendmentstotheFDCAct/AnimalMedicinalDrugUseClarificationActAMDUCAof1994/default.htm. Accessed May 19, 2015.

Weisbrode, S. E., Monke, D. R., Dodaro, S. T., et al. (1982). Osteochondrosis, degenerative joint disease, and vertebral osteophytosis in middle-aged bulls. *J Am Vet Med Assoc*, *181*, 700–705.

Wheat, J. D. (1961). Cryptorchidism in Hereford cattle. *J Heredity*, *52*, 244–246.

Wolfe, D. F., & Moll, H. D. (1999). *Large Animal Urogenital Surgery* (2nd ed.). Baltimore: Williams & Wilkins.

Youngquist, R. S., & Threlfall, W. R. (2007). *Current Therapy in Large Animal Theriogenology* (2nd ed.). St. Louis: Saunders Elsevier.

11

Urinary Tract Diseases

THOMAS J. DIVERS

Abnormal Urinary Constituents and Conditions

Urinary tract diseases are less common in dairy cattle than disorders of the gastrointestinal (GI) tract, respiratory tract, musculoskeletal system, and mammary glands. Geographic differences in the incidence of specific diseases also may affect the relative frequency of urinary tract disease in cattle. For these reasons and because signs of renal disease may be subtle, the urinary tract often is overlooked as a cause of illness. Urinalysis, serum chemistry, and evaluation of urine for abnormal constituents may be necessary to confirm urinary tract disease. Additionally, ultrasonographic examination of the kidneys or cystoscopic examination may be warranted in some cases. Transabdominal ultrasound examination of both kidneys can be achieved easily in adult dairy cows and calves through the paralumbar fossae with a 2.5 to 5 MHz probe, and excellent images of the left kidney, ureter, and bladder can also often be obtained during rectal examination using a conventional 5 or 10 MHz reproductive probe. Most practitioners use the gross appearance of urine, evaluation of abnormal urine constituents based on reagent test strips, and signs found on physical examination as indicators of urinary tract disease. Fortunately, urine is easily obtained routinely during completion of physical examination for evaluation of urinary ketones, and this provides a sample for other routine screening processes such as pH, occult blood, urine specific gravity, leukocytes, and bilirubin when indicated. Although midstream samples are usually sufficient for cultures, on rare occasion, it may be necessary to collect a catheterized sample. Catheterization is somewhat difficult in adult cows compared with horses because of the urethral diverticulum, and the technique is shown in Fig. 11.1. Vague illnesses that originate from the urinary system may require more ancillary data in the form of complete urinalysis, serum electrolytes and chemistry, and complete blood counts (CBCs) for diagnosis. Abnormal urinary constituents identified by multiple reagent strips often give direction as to other ancillary tests to be performed.

The following discussion of abnormal urinary constituents will give examples of diseases to be considered in a differential diagnosis.

Proteinuria

Because positive values for proteinuria obtained using multiple reagent test strips are relative rather than absolute, a urinalysis including a sulfosalicylic acid test (SSA) or urine protein/creatinine ratio evaluation of protein are indicated before attributing much significance to positive reagent strip results. For example, highly alkaline urine in ruminants may cause a false-positive protein reaction on reagent test strips (tetrabromophenol blue). An even more specific test is to perform simultaneous protein and creatinine measurements followed by calculation of the urinary protein to urine creatinine ratio (UP:UC). Unfortunately, normal UP:UC values in cattle are not published. In most species, ratios greater than 2 are associated with significant glomerular protein leakage, but in cattle, we have had some acute tubular necrosis cases with a UP:UC ratio of greater than 3, suggesting that this test alone should not be used to distinguish between primary glomerular and tubular diseases (e.g., amyloidosis and tubular necrosis).

Proteinuria may be normal in ruminants younger than 2 days of age that have ingested adequate or large amounts of colostrum. This physiologic phenomenon should correct quickly after this time, and the urine should then be negative or trace for protein. Any insult to the renal glomeruli or tubules could lead to mild or moderate proteinuria. For example, renal infarcts secondary to severe dehydration and reduced renal perfusion could cause mild proteinuria, and glomerulonephritis, tubular nephrosis, amyloidosis, pyelonephritis, and other severe renal diseases lead to more significant proteinuria with eventual hypoalbuminemia. In cattle with glomerulonephritis or amyloidosis, low serum protein and nephrotic syndrome would be expected. Nonspecific inflammation or irritation of the postrenal urinary tract as found in cystitis, urolithiasis, trauma, or neoplasia also may result in proteinuria. Finally, false-positive proteinuria may occur from admixture of urine with vaginal discharges,

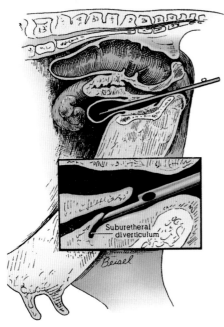

• **Fig. 11.1** Drawing of the urinary system of a cow and proper urinary catheterization technique. The urethral diverticulum makes catheterization difficult as shown in insert.

preputial discharges, uterine discharges, or fecal material and is therefore particularly common in free-catch samples obtained from normal, healthy postparturient cattle.

Glycosuria

In cattle, exogenous sources of glucose such as intravenous (IV) glucose solutions, exogenous corticosteroids, and stress-induced glycosuria account for most positive reactions on multiple reagent test strips. False-positive reactions also may result from other reducing agents present in the urine, such as penicillin, tetracycline, some other antibiotics, and aspirin. Therefore except for use in monitoring parenteral nutrition or aggressive and persistent IV dextrose infusion, this constituent seldom is helpful in dairy cattle.

Ketonuria

Ketone segments contained in multiple test reagent strips (Multistix; Bayer, Elkhart, IN) are specific for diacetic (acetoacetic) acid and do not react with acetone in urine. The urine strip test is approximately 78% sensitive and 98% specific for ketosis (clinical or subclinical) when the lower detection level of 5 μmol/L is used as a positive test result. A Ketostix (Bayer) that measures acetone and aceto-acetate has a high sensitivity and specificity for diagnosing ketosis if interpreted within 5 to 10 seconds. A complete physical examination, anamnesis, and additional serum chemistry testing (possibly including β-hydroxybutyrate [BHBA] quantitation) may be indicated to further evaluate an individual. A BHBA level of 1.2 mmol/L (12.5 mg/dL) or greater is considered indicative of ketosis. The color intensity of conventional reagent strips cannot be used to accurately separate primary from secondary ketosis because

urine specific gravity may influence the color intensity of the ketone reading.

pH

Routine testing of urine can provide a good indication of normal feed intake, especially that of potassium intake. As a general rule, when the pH is above 8, the potassium intake and likely forage intake are high. This does not apply to late pregnant cattle who are on high-ionic diets for prevention of milk fever; these cows should have urine pH of 7 or slightly less. For optimal control of subclinical hypocalcemia, the average urine pH of preparturient Holstein cows should be between 6.2 and 6.8. In Jersey cows, the average urine pH of the close-up (1–3 week) cows has to be reduced to between 5.8 and 6.3 for effective control of hypocalcemia. If the average urine pH is between 5.0 and 5.5, excessive anions have induced an uncompensated metabolic acidosis, and the cows will suffer a decline in dry matter intake. In high-production lactating cows, a urine pH of 7 or less in several cows could suggest a problem with subclinical rumen acidosis.

Hematuria

Whereas gross hematuria is apparent by inspection, occult or microscopic hematuria is detected by a positive reaction on the orthotoluidine test strip of multiple reagent test strips. *This orthotoluidine reagent cannot differentiate among hematuria, hemoglobinuria, or myoglobinuria, and all three must be considered unless urine color, precipitation of red blood cells (RBCs), or complete urinalysis indicates the exact component.*

Microscopic hematuria could originate in the kidney (e.g., infarct, tubular nephrosis, pyelonephritis, or other causes), ureter (e.g., calculi, tumor, or pyelonephritis), bladder (e.g., cystitis, calculi), or urethra, or falsely through blood contamination of urine in the vagina. Gross hematuria usually is associated with pyelonephritis, urinary calculi, urolithiasis, or cystitis in dairy cattle in the United States. In calves, it is important to consider urachal remnant infection as a cause of microscopic hematuria, the index of suspicion and the need for ultrasound examination being heightened if pyuria is also present.

Cattle affected with malignant catarrhal fever (MCF) often have hematuria caused by renal vasculitis or hemorrhage from the bladder due to hemorrhagic cystitis.

Hemoglobinuria

Gross hemoglobinuria may be apparent as reddish or sometimes brown urine (Fig. 11.2) when marked intravascular hemolysis (plasma should be discolored pink or even yellow or icteric if there is a prolonged or severe hemolysis) has occurred and subsequently exceeded the renal threshold for hemoglobin. Such conditions as water intoxication in calves, hypotonic IV fluid administration, onion and rye grass toxicity, bacillary hemoglobinuria caused by *Clostridium hemolyticum*, leptospirosis in calves, babesiosis, theileriosis and postparturient hemoglobinuria may cause obvious hemoglobinuria during acute hemolysis. Early or late stages of

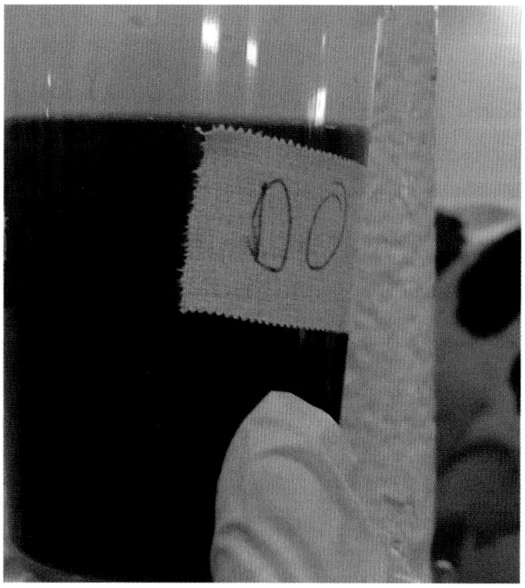

• **Fig. 11.2** Dark-colored urine from a Holstein cow with hemolytic anemia caused by *Theileria buffeli*. The color of this urine is similar to that observed with myoglobinuria.

these diseases may only yield occult hemoglobinuria causing a positive reaction on the blood (orthotoluidine) component of multiple reagent strips. Many plant and heavy metal toxicities also cause hemoglobinuria. Methemoglobinuria is another, very unusual, but sporadic explanation for a reddish-brown tinge to the urine. Severe, oxidative RBC injury may occur with nitrate or chlorate toxicity and both methemoglobinuria and hemoglobinuria may be responsible for the brown discoloration of the urine. Although rare, cattle urine of normal color that is occult blood negative may turn red after a few minutes on bedding or the ground. In these cases, a urine pigment associated with an ingested substance in feeds (e.g., rapeseed meal) causes the urine to turn red following just a short exposure to air.

Myoglobinuria

Gross evidence of myoglobinuria in the form of brown or brownish-red urine may be apparent in severe myopathies such as exertional myopathy in downer cows, coffee weed poisoning, and diffuse nutritional myopathy involving the heavy muscle groups in selenium deficiency (white muscle disease). Frequently, however, occult myoglobinuria is detected in such cases as a positive reaction in the orthotoluidine component in multiple reagent test strips alongside a positive protein reaction. A positive orthotoluidine test result but absence of RBCs in the urine, no reddish discoloration to the plasma, and elevations in serum muscle enzymes heavily suggest myoglobinuria.

Bilirubin and Urobilinogen

Urinary bilirubin may be increased in rare cases of obstructive jaundice in cattle, such as biliary stones, cholangiohepatitis, abscess, or neoplasia. Urobilinogen evaluation has not been of any diagnostic value in cattle.

Specific Gravity

Assessment of urine specific gravity is an essential test when renal pathology is suspected or if serum chemistry confirms azotemia. Isosthenuria (USpG of 1.006-1.014) in dehydrated or azotemic cattle is indicative of renal dysfunction because normal renal function should concentrate urine in a dehydrated patient. Unilateral renal ischemia or disease usually does not result in isosthenuric specific gravity of urine. With acute renal failure, the specific gravity is not always in the isosthenuric range, but it is no higher than 1.022, even in the face of dehydration. Healthy lactating dairy cows and milk-fed calves normally have low urine specific gravity (1.004–1.015), and when the specific gravity is greater than 1.025, dehydration should be considered.

White Blood Cells

Microscopic evidence of white blood cells (WBCs) merely provides evidence of urinary tract inflammation or degeneration. The most common causes include renal inflammation or degeneration, ureteral infection or obstruction, and cystitis. Contamination of free-catch samples by normal lochia or abnormal uterine or vaginal discharges is common in postpartum cows. The finding of 1 to 5 WBCs per high-power field should be considered normal in urine samples obtained from cattle. Tubular degeneration caused by nephrosis or nephritis must be differentiated from lower urinary tract infection (UTI) or inflammation as either may have an increased number of leukocytes in the urine. Gross pyuria is observed most commonly in pyelonephritis or cystitis in cattle. Urine samples demonstrated to have gross or microscopic pyuria should be submitted for bacterial culture; ideally, such samples should be obtained with aseptic preparation and bladder catheterization. In calves, pyuria and cystitis are commonly associated with umbilical remnant infection.

Casts

Hyaline casts usually are composed of protein and are most common in severe nephrosis. Granular casts usually originate from damaged tubular epithelium.

Fractional Excretion of Urinary Electrolytes

Urine fractional excretion (FE) of electrolytes is determined by simultaneous measurement of the electrolyte in question in serum and urine along with serum and urine creatinine. Percentage clearance (FE) is determined by:

$$\text{FE of X} = \frac{(Xur \, / \, Xsr)}{(CRur \, / \, CRsr)} \times 100$$

Xur = concentration of substance X in the urine
Xsr = concentration of substance X in the serum
$CRur$ = concentration of creatinine in the urine
$CRsr$ = concentration of creatinine in the serum

The FE of sodium can be used to help evaluate tubular function as long as diet, age, and the rather wide normal range are considered. Both urine sodium and salivary sodium can be used to help diagnose salt deficiency because both are under the influence of aldosterone. Low magnesium in the urine, cerebrospinal fluid, or aqueous humor can help confirm magnesium deficiency in an animal that has died of presumed hypomagnesemia. Measurement of magnesium in the urine and FE can also help confirm a chronic intracellular deficiency of magnesium, even when the serum magnesium level is normal.

There is moderate variation in urinary FE of sodium in normal dairy cattle according to diet, stage of lactation, and gestational status, but FE sodium values in dairy cattle rarely exceed 1%, although normal cows, especially in peak lactation, may occasionally have higher levels of up to 3%. Neonatal calves typically have urinary fractional sodium excretion values less than 1%. Breeding-age heifers have an average FE of sodium of 1.97%. Sodium concentration in the urine of healthy cattle is often approximately 25% less than serum concentration, but this is highly variable. Normal FE of chloride is slightly higher than sodium FE, and chloride concentration in the urine is therefore often slightly greater than the serum value. FE of potassium is greatly influenced by diet and can range from 15% to >100% in adult cows, with milk-fed calves being at the low end of that range. FE of phosphorus and calcium can be greatly influenced by early lactation and presumed increases in parathormone (PTH) or PTH sensitivity. Urine magnesium concentration has little rapid hormonal regulation and is mostly determined by diet, intestinal absorption of magnesium (potassium inhibits absorption), and urine volume. Cattle with hypomagnesemia are expected to have low serum magnesium (<0.8 mg/dL) and a FE of magnesium of less than 4%. Because age, stage of lactation, and diet can cause such marked changes in FE values, FE testing may not be very useful in routine practice and could easily result in misinterpretation of renal tubular dysfunction.

Renal Diseases

Embolic Nephritis

This condition occurs in septicemic calves and cows (Fig. 11.3) or occasionally in endocarditis patients with left-sided valvular disease. Cattle with severe dehydration resulting from GI obstruction or diarrhea also frequently develop renal infarcts. Fever, other signs of septicemia, and specific-organ dysfunction (e.g., mastitis, joint infections) also may be present. Urine multiple reagent test strips may be positive for blood and protein, and microscopic examination of the urine reveals increased numbers of WBCs, RBCs, and bacteria in some cases. Finding these abnormal constituents in urine from dehydrated patients should arouse suspicion of renal failure and alert the clinician to the need for rehydration and avoidance of nephrotoxic drugs. Nephritis is seldom the most significant component of disease in these animals but is another sign of septicemia. Therapy must be directed against the primary disease.

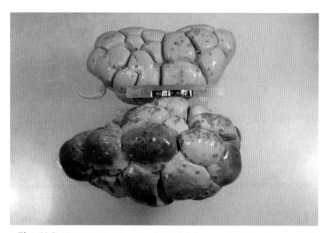

• **Fig. 11.3** Kidneys of a 5-year-old Holstein cow that died from septic metritis. Numerous large infarcts consistent with embolic nephritis can be seen.

Acute Kidney Injury

A common but often undetected problem, acute kidney injury (AKI), occurs in many septic, hypotensive, or dehydrated cattle. AKI is likely a result of decreased renal perfusion with subsequent reduced glomerular filtration in dehydrated patients, or more commonly, altered hemodynamics within the kidney caused by inflammatory mediators, vasopressors or vasodilators, and tubular epithelial dysfunction. Histologic lesions may not be pronounced, confirming that AKI should be viewed as dysfunction more than disease. Mild to moderate tubular epithelial loss into the lumen can be seen in some cases, as evidenced by granular, tubular casts on urinalysis. The loss of tubular epithelial cells may cause variable degrees of nephron obstruction or proximal tubular dysfunction causing decreased absorption of sodium and chloride and increased concentrations of these electrolytes downstream at the macula densa. This results in vasoconstriction of the glomerular afferent arteriole and a decrease in the glomerular filtration rate (GFR) of the affected nephron. Renal dysfunction that occurs with sepsis should not be viewed as a uniform nephron dysfunction; instead, there may be relatively nonfunctional nephrons mixed with normal or even "hyperfunctional" nephrons. Renal failure is more common when sepsis and dehydration are concurrent. Another possible cause of ischemic renal failure is severe ruminal distention.

An increase in serum creatinine of 0.3 mg/dL or more above baseline or expected normal value should arouse suspicion of renal failure or at least prerenal azotemia and alert the clinician to the need for rehydration and avoidance of nephrotoxic drugs such as tetracycline or flunixin. If renal failure is present, urine concentration is 1.022 or less; therefore evaluation of specific gravity is imperative to rule out renal failure. This is especially true when serum chemistry indicates azotemia in dehydrated patients. Prerenal azotemia is properly diagnosed only when a dehydrated, azotemic cow possesses the ability to concentrate urine or when the cow is receiving IV fluid therapy and has hyposthenuria (specific gravity usually <1.006), indicating the ability to dilute urine. A proportionately higher blood urea nitrogen (BUN) concentration compared to the creatinine level might also suggest prerenal azotemia but in ruminants this is not very sensitive for prerenal azotemia. Further laboratory tests that help distinguish between prerenal and true renal azotemia could be used, including FE of electrolytes, particularly sodium. GFRs can be determined using the iodine (Iodixanol) elimination rate in cattle; the GFRs for adult dairy cattle and calves are approximately 2.8 and 2.3 mL/kg/min, respectively. Precise determination of GFR (approximate normal =2.3 mL/kg/min) is rarely required in bovine practice, as knowledge of serum creatinine, BUN, urine specific gravity, packed cell volume, and plasma protein concentration along with a thorough clinical examination will allow accurate assessment of renal function and both prerenal and renal azotemia. As in other species, renal prostaglandin levels are cytoprotective to the kidney during reduced perfusion. Therefore prostaglandin inhibitors such as nonsteroidal anti-inflammatory drugs (NSAIDs) should be used in reduced dosages or not at all in severely dehydrated cattle, lest further ischemic damage with increased infarction or papillary necrosis occurs. If sepsis is present, the benefits of the NSAID would likely outweigh the negative effects on the kidneys, such as might be the case in individuals with severe gram-negative mastitis or severe metritis.

Treatment of AKI should be directed toward the primary disease, and the patient should be rehydrated with IV fluids to improve renal perfusion and urine production and to correct existing prerenal azotemia. If the affected cow or calf develops polyuria within a few hours after fluid therapy is begun, this is a good prognostic sign but does not guarantee an improvement in GFR and functional recovery. Unfortunately, the increase in urine production may be the result of increased flow from a small number of relatively healthy nephrons that only represent a relatively small proportion of the total nephron mass. Ideally, blood pressure and central venous pressure should be monitored during fluid therapy, although the methodology in cattle is challenging and readings can be inaccurate and sometimes misleading. Clinically, if the affected animal becomes euvolemic and perfusion pressure (palpable pulse of ear, face, tail, or elsewhere) normalizes yet the patient is not producing sufficient urine, then administration of vasoactive drugs (norepinephrine, dopamine, vasopressin) should be done in "hopes of" changing intrarenal hemodynamics with improvement of GFR and urine production. These vasoactive drugs may also be considered based upon more precise blood pressure monitoring and evidence of volume expansion, insufficient urine production, and increasing blood pressure. Nephrotoxic drugs such as aminoglycosides, oxytetracycline, and NSAIDs should be avoided if possible.

Toxic Nephrosis

Damage to the renal tubules by organic and plant toxins, drugs, and occasionally ischemia-associated pathophysiologic events can cause severe tubular degeneration, inflammation, and in some instances, interstitial nephritis. Usually both kidneys are affected equally, and microscopic evidence of extensive tubular necrosis with granular casts can be seen.

Etiology

Antibiotics such as aminoglycosides, tetracycline, and sulfa drugs are known to be nephrotoxic. Although rarely used in cattle currently because of limitations on extralabel drug use and a very prolonged withdrawal time for meat, aminoglycosides have been well documented as causing renal tubular damage in cattle and other species. However, because of its frequency of use in practice, oxytetracycline is likely the most common drug-induced cause of acute renal failure in cattle. Renal failure is most common in cattle that receive abnormally large doses of the drug or when recommended doses are used in dehydrated cattle. Propylene glycol and polyvinylpyrrolidone vehicles are used in many oxytetracycline hydrochloride preparations, and these vehicles may also cause hemodynamically mediated reduced renal perfusion, thereby accentuating any basic nephrotoxicity of the antibiotic itself. Sulfa preparations possess the ability to damage kidney tubules and precipitate within them. Most antibiotic-associated nephrotoxicity occurs as a result of administration of the antibiotic to dehydrated patients.

Overuse of calcium salts has also, on rare occasions, caused renal tubular nephrosis, as well as large vessel and dystrophic myocardial calcification. In some instances, recumbent cattle, especially Jersey cattle, have received inordinate amounts of calcium solutions as therapy for hypocalcemia.

Nephrosis also may result from physiologic progression of minor renal ischemia associated with septic conditions, GI diseases, and other problems that reduce renal perfusion and GFR. Early manifestations of renal ischemia include renal infarcts and papillary necrosis. These conditions are much more common in dehydrated cattle than most veterinarians realize but are relatively benign if the cow's primary disease is treated and dehydration corrected. When severe renal ischemia occurs, widespread reduction in renal perfusion results in further organic necrosis of tubulointerstitial renal tissue. Acute renal failure is possible in this instance and would be suggested by azotemia and isosthenuria.

Reduced renal perfusion also is a possible result of overuse of NSAIDs in cattle. Drugs such as flunixin meglumine are potent inhibitors of prostaglandin synthesis within many tissues, including the kidney. Renal prostaglandins are "cytoprotective" because they help maintain renal perfusion through small vessels during times of hypotension or dehydration. Loss of this protective effect occurs when NSAIDs have reduced the production of renal prostaglandins, making the kidneys more susceptible to ischemic damage. Although renal papillary necrosis is frequently associated with the use of NSAIDs, minor (infarction) or major (tubular nephrosis) disease also may occur. Again, the use of NSAIDs in dehydrated patients increases the risk of nephrotoxicity. The risk of toxicity can be further exacerbated by hypoalbuminemia, such as occurs with acute GI diseases, because more of the NSAID being administered will be non–protein bound and therefore pharmacologically active. Therefore reduction of the dosage or total avoidance of these drugs, unless concomitant fluid therapy restores renal perfusion, should be practiced when devising therapy for a dehydrated patient.

Other nephrotoxins include the heavy metals (i.e., lead, mercury, and arsenic) and plant toxicities, such as oxalates, *Lythrum hyssopifolia* (Australia), *Narthecium ossifragum* (Europe), oak (Fig. 11.4), and pigweed that occur in some parts of the United States. Toxicities may involve several animals within a group, thus raising an index of suspicion regarding a toxic etiology. Oak poisoning is the most common plant causing renal failure in cattle in the United States, although it is much more common in beef cattle because of their increased exposure risk compared with adult dairy cattle who are seldom pastured under current management systems. Oak poisoning most commonly affects dairy heifers at pasture, with acorns being ingested in the fall and oak buds or leaves in the spring. Feed deprivation may increase the toxicity of the plant, possibly because of decreased production of proline-rich salivary proteins which can inactivate the primary toxin, gallotannin. In addition to causing renal failure, oak poisoning can also be associated with enteritis and hepatopathy.

Myoglobinuria, often compounded by hypotension, can cause AKI in recumbent, hypotensive cattle with severe myopathy, or in otherwise healthy pastured cattle that develop coffee weed (*Cassia occidentalis*) toxicity. In one large retrospective study on arsenic toxicity, 100% of the cattle were azotemic and had hematuria.

Clinical Signs

Cattle affected with toxic nephrosis usually have nonspecific signs with both septic/hypotensive and nephrotoxic AKI, including depression, anorexia that varies from mild to absolute, dehydration, and potentially, recumbency. Cattle with AKI often have more blatant lesions in other body systems, such as septic mastitis, septic metritis, abomasal disorders, diarrhea, pneumonia, and so forth (Fig. 11.5). Therefore coexisting or primary diseases may mask specific signs of nephrosis. Polyuria may be present in some, but certainly not all, cattle with nephrosis. When present, this sign is helpful because an obviously dehydrated animal with normal renal function would not be observed to void grossly dilute urine frequently. Rectal palpation may suggest enlargement of the left kidney; perirenal edema is common with oak toxicity but can occur with any severe nephrosis and is a poor prognostic finding. Ultrasound examination for AKI is often unremarkable except for toxic nephrosis cases with renal enlargement and perirenal edema.

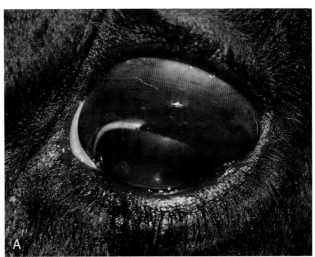

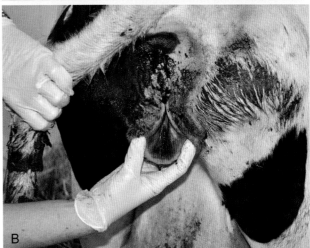

• **Fig. 11.5** A 5-year-old Holstein cow with acute renal failure and disseminated intravascular coagulation (scleral [A] and vaginal [B] hemorrhages) associated with *Klebsiella* spp. mastitis and septicemia. The cow survived with intensive treatments.

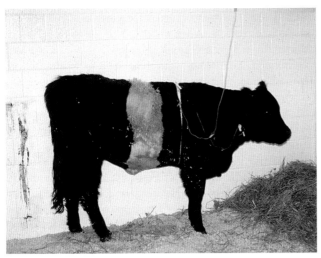

• **Fig. 11.4** An adult Galloway cow with acute renal failure after ingestion of acorns in the fall of the year. The cow had a serum creatinine value of 21 mg/dL but recovered with fluid therapy; the serum creatinine value 3 months later was 1.6 mg/dL.

In nephrosis associated with ingestion of heavy metals, neurologic signs (lead, arsenic) or GI signs (lead, arsenic, and mercury) may be present, raising suspicion of intoxication. In plant toxicities, an absence of historical evidence of previous antibiotic or NSAID use, as well as the absence of obvious infectious diseases, may lead to suspicion of plant poisoning. In many such plant toxicities, however, the diagnosis must be assisted by clinical pathology and necropsy. Uremic encephalopathy is a rare but documented clinical syndrome associated with high blood ammonia and Alzheimer type II cells in the brain on necropsy. Although all the cows with this condition that we have treated have died, we did successfully treat one sheep, implying that recovery may be possible.

Clinical Pathology and Diagnosis

The diagnosis is linked primarily to clinical pathology data and history of AKI. Renal failure will be documented by a urine specific gravity in the isosthenuric range (1.006-1.014 in most cases but always ≤1.022) despite obvious dehydration. RBCs, WBCs, granular casts, and proteinuria usually are confirmed by urinalysis in acute nephrosis. Azotemia is present and characterized by elevations of serum urea nitrogen and creatinine. Specific causes may be suggested by the history (i.e., previous use of aminoglycosides or NSAIDs) or merely suspected (severe dehydration in a patient with salmonellosis). Serum chemistry often confirms hypochloremia, which may be more severe than that seen with intestinal obstruction. The author (TJD) reported on one cow with renal failure and a serum chloride level of only 50 mEq/L but no evidence of mechanical intestinal obstruction. Hypokalemia, hyponatremia, hypocalcemia, hyperphosphatemia, and hypermagnesemia are also common serum chemistry abnormalities (Table 11.1). Plasma fibrinogen is high in many cattle with AKI.

Renal biopsy is the most definitive means of diagnosing the disease process and can be accomplished blindly by percutaneous biopsy of the left kidney, which is pushed during rectal examination into the right paralumbar fossa, or alternatively, and more preferably, either kidney can be biopsied from the right with ultrasound guidance. A Tru-Cut biopsy needle (Baxter Health Care, Deerfield, IL) is used for this procedure. Evaluation of a coagulation panel may be indicated before biopsy because some renal diseases of cattle have been associated with a bleeding diathesis.

Ultrasound study of the kidney may be a helpful ancillary procedure if available.

Treatment

Therapy must attempt to reestablish renal function and to correct primary disorders that may have contributed to nephrosis. Previous use of nephrotoxic drugs should be discontinued and other potentially nephrotoxic drugs avoided in the therapy.

Aggressive fluid therapy to ensure adequate renal perfusion and accomplish diuresis is the primary therapeutic goal. IV fluids that are balanced to address associated electrolyte or acid–base abnormalities must be tailored to the individual patient. Because hypochloremia, hypokalemia, and hyponatremia usually are present, physiologic sodium chloride with supplemental KCl added at 20 to 40 mEq/L is frequently used. Unless the patient is anuric, large volumes of IV fluids are required to address existing dehydration, allow for anticipated fluid losses, and establish diuresis. If an adult patient is anuric or oliguric after an initial 20 to 40 L of IV fluids, 250 to 500 mg of furosemide may be administered IV one or more times at 15- to 30-minute intervals in an effort to initiate diuresis. An alternative is to initially treat with 2 L of hypertonic saline to more rapidly and practically improve cardiac output, renal perfusion, and urine production. If this is successful, then follow-up therapy with physiologic sodium chloride with additional potassium could be instituted. If continual polyionic IV fluid administration is not a possibility, then hypertonic saline treatment could be followed by repeated ororumen tubing with large volumes of electrolytes in water in adults.

Failure to produce urine in the face of hypertonic saline or high-volume fluid therapy alongside diuretic administration should be taken as a negative prognostic sign. Repeated bladder evaluation by rectal palpation or ultrasonography to confirm urine production and accumulation may be a useful monitoring technique, especially in severely dehydrated acute renal disease patients in whom outward confirmation of adequate urine production may take several hours. Patients that are severely hypoproteinemic, produce inadequate urine despite large-volume fluid administration, or show evidence of dependent edema, may need additional monitoring of central venous pressure. A 500-kg cow that is azotemic, isosthenuric, and 10% dehydrated requires 50 L of fluids simply to counteract her existing dehydration. Therefore she may require a total of 80 to 100 L during the first 24 hours of therapy to establish adequate diuresis.

Judicious IV calcium or subcutaneous calcium borogluconate should be used in patients that are hypocalcemic, but if the cow is severely hyperphosphatemic, calcium administration should be used only if clinical signs of hypocalcemia are evident. A low percentage of dextrose may be added to the IV fluids by adding 1 L of 50% dextrose to each 20 L of normal saline/KCl, if desired.

Although adult cows with renal failure resulting from nephrosis seldom become hyperkalemic, calves that have acute diarrhea, azotemia and metabolic acidosis may be hyperkalemic. Therefore initial fluid therapy should be formulated based on the individual patient's measured acid–base and electrolyte status. Acidotic, hyperkalemic calves should receive IV saline, dextrose (half-strength physiologic saline solution [PSS] mixed equally with 2.5% dextrose) and supplemental $NaHCO_3$. Salmonellosis patients (either calves or cows) with secondary tubular nephrosis may be acidotic and require bicarbonate therapy if simple volume expansion by balanced crystalloid administration does not correct the acidosis.

Anuria that is unresponsive to fluid diuresis and furosemide therapy may necessitate dopamine (3–5 µg/kg/min) and/or dobutamine (2–5 µg/kg/min) in 5% dextrose (or both dopamine and dobutamine) if all other therapy fails.

TABLE 11.1   Blood Chemical and Urinalysis Data from 22 Cases of Bovine Renal Disorders

Cow #	BUN (mg/dL)	Creatinine (mg/dL)	Chloride (mEq/L)	Sodium (mEq/L)	Potassium (mEq/L)	Calcium (mg/dL)	Phosphorus (mg/dL)	Magnesium (mEq/L)	Glucose (mg/dL)	Fibrinogen (mg/dL)	Urine Specific Gravity	Urine Protein
1	199	21.3	88	123	3.4	6.3	10.4	2.7	69	600	1.014	tr
2	117	5.0	98	137	4.1	9.9	5.2	3.0	121	200	1.017	tr
3	102	4.4	96	131	4.0	6.9	9.9	1.7	57	700	1.008	+
4	144	15.0	94	125	3.6	8.3	4.7	4.0	61	900	1.008	+
5	163	15.5	96	130	2.2	8.9	5.1	2.4	65	700	1.009	++
6	152	16.5	81	127	3.2	9.0	10.3	2.7	125	1900	1.012	+
7	130	4.2	95	120	2.0	6.8	8.6	4.1	618	1500	1.013	+
8	100	12.6	35	113	3.2	7.5	14.0	3.8	600	1200	1.014	++
9	14	2.5	93	129	1.8	8.5	9.0	1.7	81	600	1.009	−
10	100	20.1	74	127	2.8	11.3	11.2	3.1	74	600	1.021	+
11	295	21.0	56	123	1.6	7.5	11.6	4.7	105	600	1.014	+
12	280	29.5	50	122	3.9	6.2	11.7	3.5	97	1900	1.013	++
13	466	33.0	67	111	5.8	5.3	8.4	2.3	139	800	1.012	+
14	104	5.6	56	119	2.1	7.0	10.6	2.8	276	600	1.012	++
15	105	11.8	67	113	7.6	10.6	18.0	6.0	76	1000	1.016	tr
16	137	14.1	75	146	3.4	7.7	9.5	4.8	74	1400	1.029	++++
17	14	2.2	97	142	4.0	ND	ND	ND	ND	1100	1.015	++
18	82	4.4	93	135	3.4	7.9	8.2	2.4	110	1900	1.016	++++
19	42	2.5	97	144	2.4	10.4	7.5	3.2	93	1000	1.019	tr
20	112	5.6	93	132	4.1	9.6	10.1	2.9	67	1150	1.012	++++
21	172	12.9	86	132	2.4	7.6	16.5	3.5	137	1500	1.008	+
22	161	10.5	50	115	2.2	7.3	13.8	4.2	498	1500	1.012	tr
Normal values*	10–20	0.5–2.0	97–111	132–152	3.9–5.8	9.4–12.2	2.3–9.6	1.2–2.6	40–80	100–600	ND	tr

ND, not determined

BUN, blood urea nitrogen; tr, trace.

*From Divers TJ, Crowell WA, Duncan JR, et al. Acute renal disorders in cattle: a retrospective study of 22 cases. J Am Vet Med Assoc 1982;181:694-699.

Although no vasoactive agent, nor any single drug has been statistically proven effective in treating AKI in humans, that does not mean pressor agents might not work in some cattle. Additionally, dopamine may enhance polyuria, which in itself is highly beneficial in the medical management of AKI. Other potential treatments include mannitol, norepinephrine, vasopressin, and aminophylline.

When diuresis has been established, fluid therapy should be adjusted to maintain diuresis and assist renal excretion of wastes. Serum urea nitrogen and creatinine initially should be monitored each day to establish a trend. In most cases the duration of diuretic fluid therapy varies from a few days to 2 weeks. The prognosis is guarded until normal renal function is reestablished. The more prolonged the azotemia, the more likely the patient is to develop chronic renal failure. Initially, the clinician must proceed with therapy in the hope that nephrosis is acute and reversible. The exact degree of renal damage is impossible to assess initially. Response to therapy and to a lesser degree, the results of renal biopsies, afford the best means of prognosis. Cases of toxic tubular nephrosis seem to respond best to diuretic therapy, although 2 to 3 days may be required for the serum creatinine to drop.

If a potential nephrotoxic drug must be used to treat a primary condition, reduced dosage or preferably prolonged interval and pharmacologic monitoring of blood levels, if available, are essential to continued usage. Supportive care with ororumen transfaunation and substrate feeding (e.g., alfalfa meal, in addition to multi-B vitamins by slow IV administration) are recommended.

Pyelonephritis

Infectious nephritis caused by bacterial infection of the kidney is usually an ascending infection from the lower urinary tract. Pyelonephritis is one of the most commonly diagnosed diseases of the kidney in dairy cattle. This may be a true representation or merely supposed because of the relative ease of diagnosis of pyelonephritis as opposed to other conditions that require more ancillary diagnostics or laboratory data for definitive diagnosis.

Etiology

In cattle, bacterial pyelonephritis has been attributed to ascending infection of the urinary tract by *Escherichia coli* or *Corynebacterium renale* (Fig. 11.6). At least three *C. renale* serotypes exist as normal flora of the caudal portion of the reproductive tract of female cattle and the sheath of male cattle. Unlike most other gram-positive organisms, *C. renale* possesses pili that promote attachment to, and colonization of, the urinary tract mucosa. Conditions that result in physical or chemical damage to the mucosa in the lower portion of the urinary tract such as dystocia or puerperal infection, bladder paralysis, or catheterization, may predispose the cow to pyelonephritis as a result of *C. renale* ascending from the urinary bladder to the ureters and kidneys. *C. renale* causes a humoral antibody response when renal infection develops but not when infection is limited to the bladder. Pyelonephritis as

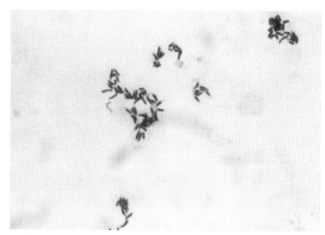

• **Fig. 11.6** Gram stain of the urine from a cow with *Corynebacterium renale* pyelonephritis.

a result of *E. coli* infection has a similar pathogenesis to that caused by *C. renale* in that ascending infection from the lower urinary tract occurs following damage to the caudal portion of the reproductive tract but the disease is not as fulminant. Other studies have found *Trueperella pyogenes*, *Corynebacterium cystitidis*, *Corynebacterium pilosum*, *Staphylococcus* spp., *Streptococcus* spp., *Enterococcus* spp., *Klebsiella* spp. and *Pseudomonas* spp. as potential, yet infrequent, causes of pyelonephritis. In calves, septic nephritis and renal abscessation may occur from umbilical artery infection.

Clinical Signs

Acute primary pyelonephritis causes fever of 103.5° to 105.5°F (39.72° to 40.83°C), anorexia, and a precipitous decrease in milk production. Some cows with acute pyelonephritis have colic manifested by kicking at the abdomen, restlessness, and treading. Signs of colic usually are associated with renal or ureteral inflammation and pain, but urinary obstruction caused by blood clots blocking urine outflow from a kidney (ureter) or bladder (urethra) also may contribute to colic (Fig. 11.7).

Further agitation, such as swishing of the tail, may be observed if the affected cow also has cystitis as a concurrent or precursor lesion to pyelonephritis. Stranguria, polyuria, an arched stance, gross hematuria (see Figs. 11.7 and 11.8), urinary blood clots or fibrin, or pyuria also are observed in some patients with *C. renale* infection. Acute pyelonephritis should be considered as a differential for acute colic in postparturient cattle. Consequently, left kidney and right and left ureteral palpation per rectum should be mandatory components of the physical examination of any sick cow with signs of colic. The ureters may also be palpated per vagina.

Chronic pyelonephritis is associated with weight loss, poor hair coat, anorexia, poor production, diarrhea, polyuria, anemia, stranguria, and gross urinary abnormalities. Lordosis and stretching out may be apparent in some cows affected with chronic pyelonephritis because of renal pain.

Latent or subclinical pyelonephritis may exist in cattle with multiple medical problems, especially during the first few months of lactation. Cattle with concurrent abomasal

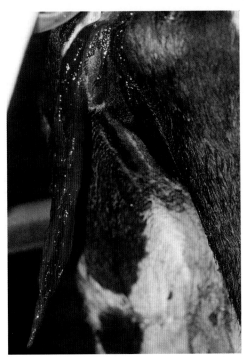

• **Fig. 11.7** Large blood clot protruding from the vulva of a 3-year-old Holstein cow with acute pyelonephritis. The visible clot was part of a larger clot occluding the urethra, causing the animal to show signs of colic.

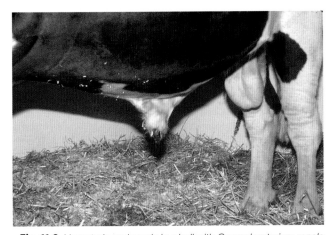

• **Fig. 11.8** Hematuria and pyuria in a bull with *Corynebacterium renale* pyelonephritis.

displacement, metritis, mastitis, or cattle that had dystocia may develop pyelonephritis that is masked by more obvious signs in other systems. Only through screening urine and subsequent urinalysis and ultrasound examination will the condition be confirmed. Specific physical signs of pyelonephritis in these more chronic instances are minimal unless, on rectal palpation, the left kidney is large and painful and has indistinct lobulations, thereby increasing the possibility of pyelonephritis.

Diagnosis

The diagnosis of pyelonephritis is made by combining the clinical signs, rectal palpation findings, vaginal palpation findings, and urinalysis. Fever usually is present in acute pyelonephritis but may be absent in chronic pyelonephritis. Urinalysis abnormalities such as hematuria, pyuria, proteinuria, and bacteriuria may be present in both cystitis and pyelonephritis. However, cystitis does not usually lead to systemic illness, and the ureters would not be enlarged (as one or both are in pyelonephritis) as determined by palpation per vagina or per rectum. Vaginal palpation remains an essential aid to diagnosis because it allows detection of unilateral or bilateral ureteral enlargement that is too subtle to be detected per rectum.

Infection of the left kidney is most common, rectal palpation may therefore reveal enlargement of the left kidney in unilateral left kidney infection or in cases of bilateral disease. Normal lobulations of the kidney may be lost, the kidney may feel "mushy," and there may be a pronounced arterial pulsation. Rectal palpation of the right kidney is rarely possible unless it is greatly enlarged. Ultrasonography is another helpful ancillary aid to diagnosis and may reveal valuable prognostic information (see Video Clips 11.1 and 11.2). Dilatation of the ureter on the affected side is the most common ultrasound finding followed by cystic changes within the kidney.

Other laboratory tests may be performed in valuable cattle or when a definitive diagnosis has not yet been reached. Hypoalbuminemia is present in most pyelonephritis patients and is more severe in chronic pyelonephritis. Proteinuria appears to be very significant in pyelonephritis and occurs in most cases. Serum globulin values may be higher (>5.0 g/dL) if infection has been chronic. Generally, a period of at least 6-14 days of renal infection is necessary to elevate globulin values, and adult cattle tend to have higher globulin levels than calves with chronic infection.

Gross examination of the urine may be diagnostic in acute cases in which fibrin, blood clots, and pus are apparent in voided urine. Some cows with acute pyelonephritis will have severe renal hemorrhage that may obstruct the ureter or urethra, thus leading to intermittent or continuous urinary blockage. On occasion, blood clots may be so substantial as to fill and occlude the bladder and urethra. On a rare occasion, inspissated pus may totally obstruct urine flow on one side leading to hydronephrosis and truly remarkable renal enlargement. Cattle with less obvious urinary abnormalities will have positive blood and protein reactions on reagent test strips, and urinalysis will confirm the presence of RBCs, WBCs, protein, and bacteria. Routine use of multiple test reagent strips to screen urine during the routine physical examination is an excellent means to detect pyelonephritis and other urinary tract diseases.

Urine culture is the most important laboratory aid because it allows identification of the causative organisms and more importantly, permits antimicrobial susceptibility testing. Previous treatment with antibiotics by the owner may interfere with in vitro growth. Therefore, antibiotics should be discontinued for a minimum of 24 to 48 hours before culture of the urine. Urine for culture should be obtained using catheterization or a midstream voided sample to avoid contamination, and a colony count should

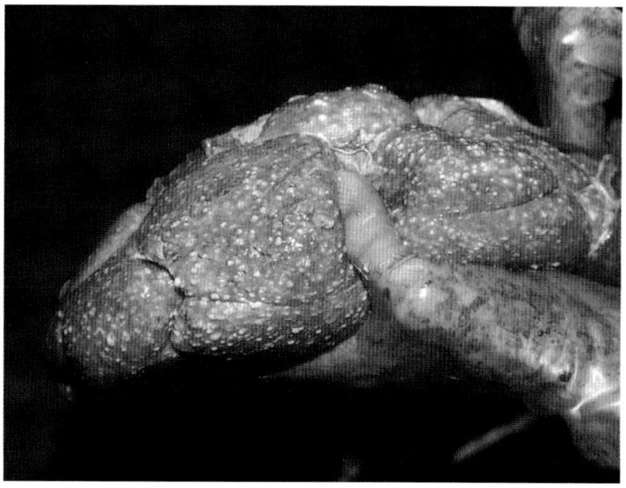

• **Fig. 11.9** Necropsy view of kidney with severe pyelonephritis caused by *Corynebacterium renale* infection in a Holstein cow that died from the disease. Both kidneys appeared similar. (Courtesy of Dr. John M. King.)

be requested. Colony counts of $>10^3$/mL on a catheterized sample or $>10^4$/mL on a midstream voided sample should be viewed as cut-offs for significance and are often necessary to determine the infectious organism(s).

Concurrent azotemia is cause for prognostic concern and may indicate prerenal conditions such as dehydration, bilateral pyelonephritis with subsequent renal failure, or postrenal urinary obstruction.

Postrenal obstruction usually is obvious after the physical and rectal examinations. Prerenal azotemia should be suspected if the animal is very dehydrated but is capable of concentrating urine to a specific gravity greater than 1.022. Prerenal azotemia also should respond to rehydration using oral or IV fluids. Most cattle with pyelonephritis that also are azotemic have bilateral disease and renal failure (Fig. 11.9). These usually are chronic infections and have elevated globulin levels, hypoalbuminemia, and an inability to concentrate urine, and they may have electrolyte abnormalities such as hypochloremia, hyponatremia, hypokalemia, and hypocalcemia. Therefore cattle with bilateral pyelonephritis and azotemia have a guarded prognosis.

Anemia may be suspected based on physical examination or confirmed by a CBC. Anemia may develop from blood loss alone in acute cases or more commonly by blood loss from the urinary tract coupled with reduced erythropoiesis subsequent to renal parenchymal damage and inflammation in chronic cases.

Treatment

The causative organisms, their susceptibility to antimicrobial agents, the existence of bilateral versus unilateral disease, and the presence or absence of azotemia constitute the major data involved in case management and economic decision making. After the organism is identified and antimicrobial susceptibility determined, an antimicrobial agent should be selected that maintains high concentrations in urine, is not nephrotoxic, and is approved for use in cattle. Penicillin, because of its urinary route of excretion, attains

a much higher concentration in urine than in plasma, potentially making the drug effective in vivo against some *E. coli* despite their penicillin resistance in vitro. After a catheterized urine sample has been collected for culture, standard therapy in our clinic consists of penicillin (22,000 U/kg, intramuscularly [IM] every 12 hours), which is given until culture and susceptibility results are available. When *C. renale* is identified, penicillin is continued for 3 weeks because the organism is uniformly susceptible to penicillin. If the disease is severe and peracute, IV penicillin may be administered for the initial treatment. When *E. coli* is identified, penicillin is continued if objective data (e.g., serial urinalyses, temperature) and subjective data (e.g., appetite, attitude) are returning to normal. If no improvement has occurred during the initial 72 to 96 hours of penicillin therapy in patients with *E. coli* pyelonephritis, another antibiotic must be chosen based on antimicrobial susceptibility. Other options include ampicillin, oxytetracycline, or on very rare occasion extralabel use of an aminoglycoside but only if azotemia is absent, the cultured organism is not susceptible to approved drugs, and prolonged withdrawal time is properly discussed, agreed upon, and documented with the owner. If a potentially nephrotoxic antibiotic is needed, the frequency of treatment may be prolonged based on creatinine concentration; for example, if the serum creatinine is 1.8 mg/dL (the reference range in most laboratories for dairy cattle is 1.1–1.5), this value could suggest an approximate 30% decrease in GFR such that the interval of treatment should be extended at least 30%. Recommended antimicrobial therapy for bovine pyelonephritis, as with any UTI, is long term—at least 3 weeks. Short-term antimicrobial therapy is often ineffective or only transiently improves the animal clinically before the condition returns and becomes chronic.

Fluid therapy can be helpful during initial treatment to correct prerenal azotemia, flush debris and bacteria from the urinary tract, and help maintain normal renal blood flow; it is especially important if potentially nephrotoxic antibiotics are being used!

The prognosis for cows with acute pyelonephritis that are treated with long-term antimicrobial therapy is good unless functional or mechanical urogenital abnormalities persist. Cows with severe bilateral pyelonephritis and azotemia have a guarded prognosis. Pyelonephritis secondary to bladder paralysis or rectovaginal fistula after dystocia would have a poorer prognosis because recurrence of UTI would be likely.

The prognosis for chronic pyelonephritis is guarded because abscesses of the kidney or total loss of the normal, functional kidney parenchyma may occur (Fig. 11.10). Cows affected with chronic pyelonephritis also have a greater risk of developing a bilateral infection, leading to azotemia and renal failure. Chronically affected cattle (both calves and adults) also have increased incidence of renal stone formation.

Surgical therapy to remove a massively enlarged and infected kidney occasionally is indicated for treatment of chronic unilateral pyelonephritis (Fig. 11.11). The abnormal kidney usually is palpable per rectum, even if the right kidney is involved. The kidney simply feels like a mass the

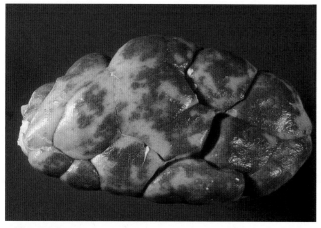

• **Fig. 11.10** Necropsy specimen from a cow with bilateral chronic pyelonephritis showing pale, fibrosed, chronically infected zones of renal cortex. (Courtesy of Dr. John M. King.)

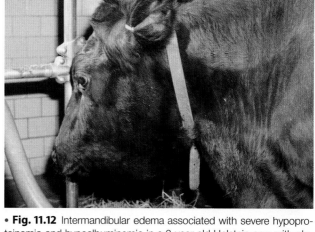

• **Fig. 11.12** Intermandibular edema associated with severe hypoproteinemia and hypoalbuminemia in a 2-year-old Holstein cow with glomerulonephritis of possible genetic origin.

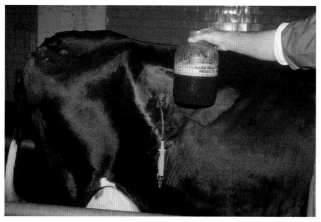

• **Fig. 11.11** Nephrectomy of a right kidney that had ruptured because of chronic pyelonephritis. The red fluid is urine, blood and debris collected from the retroperitoneal space.

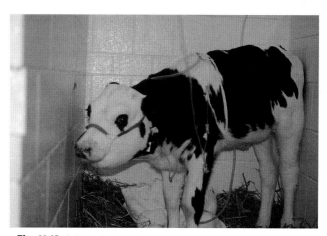

• **Fig. 11.13** A 6-week-old calf with severe edema caused by glomerulonephritis. The calf had marked hypoproteinemia and hypertension.

size of a football and has suffered chronic pyelonephritis, abscessation, and hydronephrosis. This can be further confirmed by ultrasound examination.

Glomerulonephritis

Glomerulonephritis, a rare clinical condition in cattle, causes progressive renal failure and severe proteinuria, hypoalbuminemia, weight loss, and ventral edema.

Etiology

Glomerulonephritis is thought to develop either as a result of antigen–antibody complexes deposited in the glomeruli or specific antibodies produced by the affected animal that attack glomerular basement membranes. In either event, progressive damage to the glomeruli interferes with normal filtration such that protein loss from the kidney occurs and renal failure follows. In cows, glomerulonephritis may be associated with chronic infections in body cavities, the udder, or the uterus and is typically caused by circulating antigen–antibody complexes. Walled-off infections, such

as abscesses that continue to promote antibody production against the somewhat protected antigen, may result in large amounts of antibody, thereby predisposing to glomerulonephritis. One reported case, a 3-year-old Holstein, did not have an apparent predisposing cause.

Dr. Rebhun observed one family of dairy cows in which three full siblings (two heifers and one bull) developed glomerulonephritis and nephrotic syndrome and subsequently died. These animals appeared healthy until 18 to 30 months of age and then developed signs that resulted in death within several months of onset (Fig. 11.12). This familial problem was most likely a genetic disorder with an antibasement membrane antibody responsible for the glomerular lesions. Unfortunately, only one of the three animals was presented for workup and subsequent necropsy.

We have also confirmed renal failure caused by glomerulonephritis in a group of 5- to 8-week-old heifers. The heifers had a rather acute onset of diarrhea and edema caused by the marked proteinuria leading to hypoproteinemia (Figs. 11.13 and 11.14). The heifers

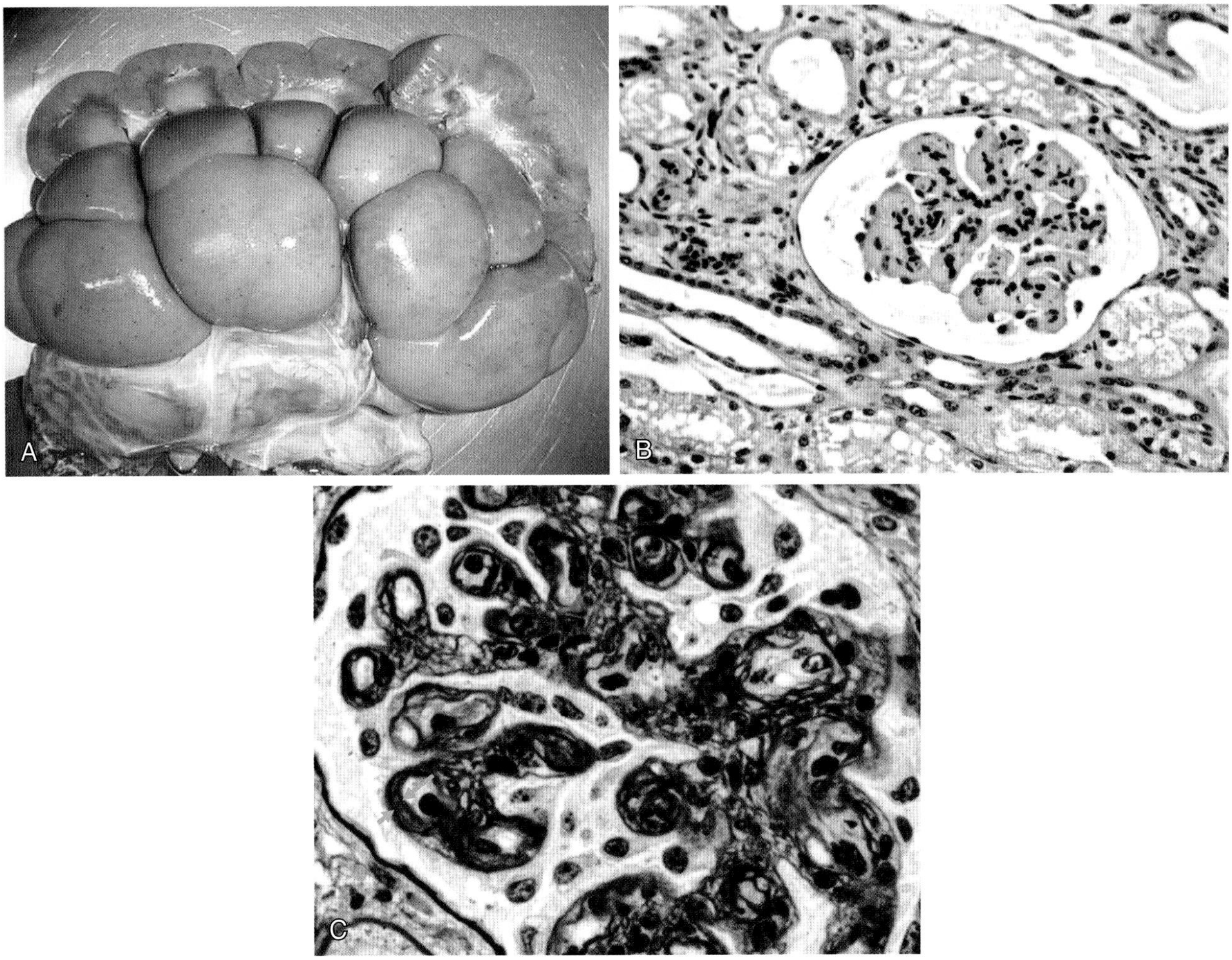

• **Fig. 11.14** **A,** Gross appearance of kidney from the calf in Fig. 11.13. **B,** Microscopic view of the glomeruli from the calf in Fig. 11.13, glomerular loops are expanded by eosinophilic material. **C,** Jone's stain showing increased mesangial cells and marked diffuse thickening of the glomerular basement membrane (green arrows).

were also severely hypertensive. The heifers were from three different farms. The cause of the glomerulonephritis was undetermined, although a common antiserum had been administered to the calves within the first days of life, and resultant antigen–antibody complexes were likely responsible for the glomerulonephritis. This syndrome has been seen sporadically in other areas of the United States.

Clinical Signs

Weight loss, decreased appetite and production, poor hair coat, and ventral edema are typical signs in cattle affected with glomerulonephritis. Some patients have diarrhea. Because these signs are nonspecific and concurrent or chronic infections may be present in affected patients, the possibility of renal disease may easily be overlooked.

Rectal palpation of an enlarged left kidney may be the only specific physical abnormality detected. Proteinuria will be detected by a positive protein reaction on the multiple test reagent strips and can be confirmed by SSA protein or finding a urine protein/urine creatinine ratio greater than 3.

Diagnosis

Because the clinical signs are very similar for glomerulonephritis and amyloidosis, renal biopsy may be essential to differentiate and confirm the diagnosis, although age may be helpful because amyloidosis has not been reported in cows younger than 4 years of age. If the nephrotic syndrome (i.e., ventral edema, hypoalbuminemia, and proteinuria) is present, the condition probably is advanced, and renal failure is present.

Ventral edema, an enlarged left kidney (the right kidney cannot normally be reached) (Fig. 11.15), absence of urinary constituent abnormalities other than proteinuria, and azotemia with isosthenuria should allow a tentative diagnosis of glomerulonephritis or amyloidosis. Renal biopsy will confirm the diagnosis and allows differentiation between these two conditions. Ultrasonography generally is not helpful to the diagnosis but may be useful to guide biopsy. Laboratory data as regards serum urea nitrogen and creatinine and electrolyte levels may show mild abnormalities in early cases or dramatic abnormalities as renal failure progresses. Hypoproteinemia characterized by hypoalbuminemia is present in all cases. Urinary protein to creatinine ratio will generally

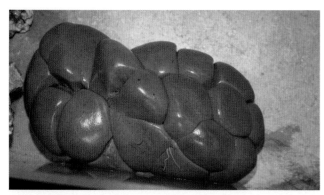

• **Fig. 11.15** Gross specimen of a kidney with glomerulonephritis from a cow that had chronic cellulitis in one hind limb. Both kidneys were enlarged and appeared similar.

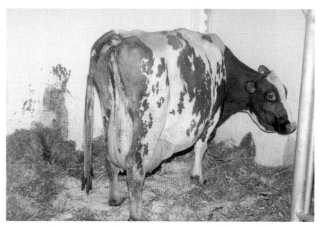

• **Fig. 11.16** An 8-year-old Red and White Holstein cow with amyloidosis causing diarrhea, proteinuria, hypoproteinemia, azotemia, and edema. The kidneys were three or four times the normal size because of the amyloid deposition.

be > 3. Anemia may develop in chronic cases. Diarrhea, although more typical of amyloidosis, may be present in some glomerulonephritis patients if hypoproteinemia is so severe as to lead to edema of the gut wall.

Unfortunately, cattle with glomerulonephritis usually have progressed to renal failure by the time an accurate diagnosis is reached. Therefore attempts at treatment have been limited.

Treatment

Early or acute cases may be treated by supportive care for renal failure and specific therapy directed against any concurrent infections (e.g., mastitis, abscesses), which could be primary to the glomerulonephritis. When renal failure has developed, treatment usually is hopeless. Anecdotally some calves with glomerulonephritis in the absence of renal failure have responded to corticosteroid administration, although long-term follow-up data on fertility and production for these individuals are unavailable.

Amyloidosis

Amyloidosis is an infrequent systemic disease characterized by extracellular deposition of β-sheet amyloid fibrils in the kidney, gut, liver, spleen, and other tissues. Because the kidney appears to be a major site of deposition in cows, proteinuria and a nephrotic syndrome frequently develop in bovine amyloidosis patients. Affected cattle are 4 years of age or older.

Etiology

Both primary and secondary forms of amyloidosis exist. Whereas primary amyloidosis is likely an immune-mediated or metabolic storage disease, secondary amyloidosis (most commonly systemic AA type amyloid) has been associated with chronic infections in various organ systems. The precursor protein of AA is serum amyloid A (SAA), which is synthesized in the acute phase by the liver in response to inflammatory disease. Approximately half of the reported cases in two retrospective case series had evidence of chronic infection that could be interpreted as contributory to the development of amyloidosis. Chronic infection currently is theorized to predispose to both secondary amyloidosis and glomerulonephritis. Inflammatory lesions of hardware disease, chronic pneumonia, mastitis, metritis, pododermatitis, and abscesses have been associated with bovine amyloidosis.

Signs

Weight loss, reduced production, diarrhea, and ventral edema characterize the early signs of amyloidosis in dairy cattle (Fig. 11.16). As the disease progresses, a nephrotic syndrome becomes more obvious with marked ventral edema, hypoalbuminemia, and proteinuria. Appetite may be fair to normal early in the course but tends to decrease as hypoproteinemia worsens and azotemia develops. Rectal palpation may allow detection of an enlarged, firm left kidney with normal lobulations, and test reagent strips confirm marked proteinuria. The retention of normal lobulation helps differentiate other disorders that cause enlarged kidneys, such as lymphosarcoma, hydronephrosis, and pyelonephritis but not glomerulonephritis, in which lobulation is similarly preserved even in advanced cases.

Diarrhea usually is present and may be profuse. Diarrhea is thought to originate from amyloid deposition in the gut. This deposition is not detectable grossly, so it may require microscopic study. Diarrhea probably worsens the hypoalbuminemia because of protein loss from the intestine. Given the relative dearth of clinical signs other than diarrhea, weight loss resulting from Johne's disease or other primary GI conditions need to be considered in the differential diagnosis. Although amyloidosis may be characterized by diarrhea, it should be emphasized that other causes of chronic renal failure or proteinuria also may be associated with diarrhea because of gut and mesenteric edema secondary to hypoalbuminemia.

Diagnosis

The diagnosis of amyloidosis requires renal biopsy or necropsy to differentiate the disease from glomerulonephritis.

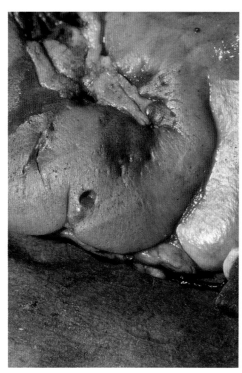

• **Fig. 11.17** Kidney of a cow that died from amyloidosis. Both kidneys were enlarged, tan colored, and firm. Lugol's solution has been poured on the cut surface, and brown dots can be seen in the glomeruli because of the Lugol's staining of the starch component of the amyloid.

Diarrhea, an enlarged left kidney per rectum, weight loss, and other nonspecific signs of chronic illness will also be present. Affected cattle are 4 years of age or older, and this can be a helpful differentiating feature from glomerulonephritis, which often affects younger animals. Other than hypoproteinemia caused by hypoalbuminemia and proteinuria, laboratory tests are not very helpful. The degree of azotemia, electrolyte values, and urine specific gravity vary based on the duration and degree of renal involvement. Terminally, cattle with amyloidosis are azotemic, proteinuric, and isosthenuric.

Hypocalcemia is typical and associated with hypoalbuminemia and calcium-binding principles. At necropsy, affected kidneys are large, pale, and firm.

Kidney biopsy material or gross postmortem tissue may be stained with special reagents to highlight amyloid deposition. Lugol's iodine has been used on gross renal tissue to detect the presence of amyloid (Fig. 11.17). The iodine stains amyloid-infiltrated renal tissue mahogany brown, and further staining with sulfuric acid produces a blue color. Congo red stains highlight amyloid for light microscopy, and electron microscopy identifies a characteristic fibrillar appearance.

Treatment

No practical treatments exist, and the disease is fatal to affected cattle. As a result of the urinary losses of antithrombin III, which is similar in molecular weight to albumin, hypercoagulation may be present, causing an acute clinical demise associated with acute renal vein thrombosis (Fig. 11.18).

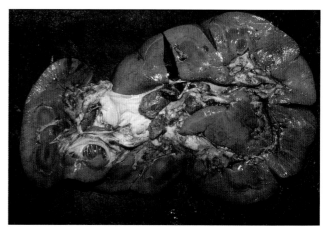

• **Fig. 11.18** A large thrombus in the renal vein of a cow that had renal amyloidosis.

Renal Tubular Acidosis

Renal tubular acidosis (RTA) has only been reported in cattle by Hardefeldt et al from the University of Wisconsin in a beef calf in association with acute renal failure and salmonellosis. Type 1, or distal, RTA most often occurs secondary to systemic inflammatory diseases in other species; failure of one or both of the collecting duct proton pumps (H^+-ATPase and H^+-K^+-ATPase respectively) to excrete H^+ results in an inability to acidify urine to a pH of 5.5 or below; hypokalemia generally accompanies type 1 RTA. Type 2, or proximal, RTA is caused by generalized proximal tubular dysfunction and excessive bicarbonate excretion. Urinary pH may be appropriately acidic because the amount of bicarbonate filtered might not exceed that which can be reabsorbed distally; because of this, type 2 RTA is generally self-limiting. RTA should be considered when there is metabolic acidosis and a normal anion gap (chloride is high). Treatment is to correct the acidosis with oral or IV bicarbonate therapy and to treat renal injury if it is a predisposing cause. The author recently treated an 8-year-old Holstein cow that developed RTA, presumed secondary to oxytetracycline-induced renal failure. After five days of intravenous bicarbonate and crystalloid fluid therapy in addition to 100 grams of bicarbonate administered P.O. twice daily, both the azotemia and severe metabolic acidosis (serum bicarbonate = 12 mEq/L) resolved.

Fanconi Syndrome

Cesbron et al. recently described a heifer with Fanconi syndrome causing growth retardation. Fanconi syndrome is a proximal convoluted renal tubular disorder characterized by impaired proximal reabsorption of glucose, amino acids, phosphate, and bicarbonate leading to increased urinary excretion of these substances. Clinical signs at presentation generally include polyuria, polydipsia, and body weight loss despite a normal appetite. Hypocalcemia, hypophosphatemia, hyponatremia, hypokalemia, and hypochloremia are common serum electrolyte abnormalities.

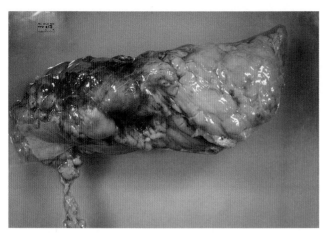

• **Fig. 11.19** Lymphosarcoma involvement of the kidney. The kidney was enlarged, had an abnormal shape, and had lost normal lobulations.

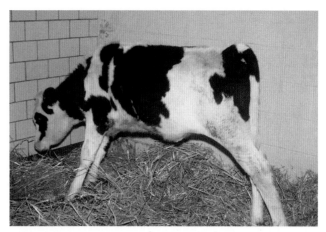

• **Fig. 11.20** A calf demonstrating "colicky" signs (stretching out) because of ureteral obstruction.

Urinalysis findings include glycosuria despite normal blood glucose concentration, proteinuria and phosphaturia, increased urine sodium concentration and aminoaciduria. The syndrome may occur due to either genetic or acquired factors.

Renal Tumors

Although primary renal adenomas, adenocarcinomas, and nephroblastomas are reported in cattle, these tumors are too rare to merit discussion. The neoplasm most commonly encountered involving the bovine kidney is lymphosarcoma (Fig. 11.19). The kidney is one of many organs involved in multicentric lymphosarcoma in cattle. Lymphosarcoma invasion of the left kidney may cause the kidney to develop an unusual shape when palpated per rectum. In most renal lymphosarcoma cases, because of the unilateral nature of the disease, affected cattle do not have renal failure, and clinical signs are attributable to other target organ dysfunction or generalized tumor cachexia.

Disorders of the Ureters

Few specific diseases of the ureters exist. Most conditions affecting the ureters occur by extension from other parts of the urinary tract, either descending from the kidney or ascending from the bladder.

Ureteral inflammation and distention are seen commonly with pyelonephritis, but calculi in the ureter have only been observed rarely in cattle. Either inflammation or calculi in the ureter may result in severe pain that is manifested as colic and requires differentiation from colic of GI origin. Cattle with ureteral calculi may have signs of frequently shifting their weight on their hind limbs, kicking at their abdomen, tail switching, or assuming a sawhorse stance (Fig. 11.20).

When renal or ureteral stones are seen, they are often bilateral, may be associated with chronic infection (Fig. 11.21), and cause intermittent obstruction. Bilateral nephroliths or ureteroliths may also occur without infection and may

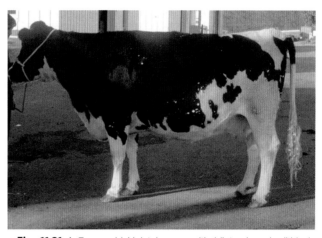

• **Fig. 11.21** A 7-year-old Holstein cow with bilateral nephrolithiasis associated with intermittent obstructive ureterolithiasis. Two episodes of obstruction resulted in severe azotemia which resolved after spontaneous movement of a stone. A third episode of obstruction 1 year after the initial episode resulted in rupture of one kidney, necessitating euthanasia. The histopathological examination of the kidney was diagnostic for chronic pyelonephritis. *Corynebacterium* spp. was cultured from a nephrolith. In this case, it is believed that the chronic pyelonephritis predisposed to calculi formation.

represent calcification of renal papillae in association with NSAID therapy similar to what is described in horses (Fig. 11.22). With bilateral involvement, cattle are generally azotemic and have weight loss and a poor appetite. The diagnosis can be confirmed during rectal palpation of the ureters and by rectal or transabdominal ultrasound examination (Fig. 11.23). Palpation of the ureters is best accomplished per vagina as the ureters cross the pelvic brim. The ureters can be palpated by rolling them gently over the pubis. Transrectal ultrasound examination is also very useful for the evaluation of the left kidney and ureteral abnormalities.

Antibiotic and fluid treatment of cattle with ureteral or renal stones often results in clinical improvement. The ureteral stone may actually move back into the renal pelvis, temporarily relieving the obstruction and granting considerable remission from pain.

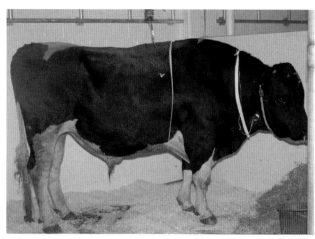

• **Fig. 11.22** Anorexia and azotemia in an adult bull from a bull stud. Calculi were palpated in both ureters, causing bilateral hydronephrosis and renal failure. On necropsy, no evidence of pyelonephritis or infection was found.

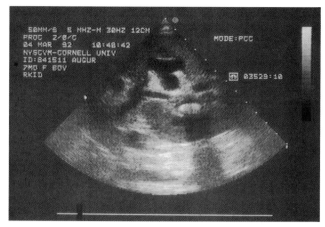

• **Fig. 11.23** Ultrasound of the kidney of the calf in Fig. 11.20 revealing a large nephrolith. *Corynebacterium renale* was cultured from the urine of the calf and was likely the cause for the stones to form.

Congenital ureteral ectopia has been described in a dairy calf. Endoscopy and radiographs were not diagnostic for the case, but it was confirmed during surgery, and the calf recovered after nephrectomy of the affected side.

Lymphosarcoma may invade the ureters in cows with the adult, enzootic form of lymphosarcoma and is the most common tumor of the ureter in our experience.

Disorders of the Bladder

Diseases of the urinary bladder include inflammatory, neurogenic, and neoplastic disorders, as well as formation of cystic calculi.

Cystitis

Etiology

Urinary bladder inflammation and infection occur in adults secondary to bladder paralysis that allows urine stasis, dystocia with ascending contamination from the urethra, or chronic irritation from cystic calculi. Dystocia is a major risk factor for cystitis in dairy cattle because sacral innervation to the bladder may be damaged, thereby decreasing bladder tone, interfering with emptying, and predisposing to infection by either stasis or direct contamination through the urethra.

In calves, cystitis is almost always associated with urachal or other umbilical remnants that act as a nidus of infection or that prevent complete bladder emptying by traction from fibrous adhesions.

Signs

Frequent attempts to urinate small volumes, strangury, tail swishing, treading on the hind limbs, and irritability are common signs of cystitis in cattle (see Video Clip 11.3). Urethritis generally accompanies cystitis and may be responsible for some of these signs. Occasionally, high-strung cows with cystitis may kick at the abdomen, but this sign is not as commonly observed as in pyelonephritis. Scalding of the perineum from urine dribbling is observed in some cattle if

sacral nerve damage has caused relative bladder atony and subsequent urine dribbling. Sandlike particles may be present on the vulvar hair because of excessive crystalluria or uroliths (Fig. 11.24). Umbilical infections in calves frequently produce a mild clinical, or occult, cystitis. Careful observation of calves with urachal or umbilical artery remnant infections may reveal polyuria, but stranguria is not common. Similarly, microscopic urinalysis may reveal pyuria, microscopic hematuria and bacteriuria, but the systemic signs are often mild or attributed to the presence of infection in the umbilical stalk. Pyelonephritis as a consequence of urachal remnant infection and cystitis in calves is extremely rare but may occur.

In adults, rectal palpation may reveal a distended, atonic bladder in cases with sacral nerve damage following dystocia or other neurologic diseases. In primary ascending cystitis without innervation defects, the bladder will be palpated as a firm, thick-walled structure the size of a baseball or softball. Cystic calculi, if present, also can be diagnosed during rectal palpation or during transrectal ultrasonography. Vaginal palpation of the ureters in cases of simple cystitis is normal.

Mature cows with cystitis may void urine with gross evidence of hematuria or pyuria (Fig. 11.25). Multistix (Bayer, Medfield, MA) usually will show positive blood, positive protein, and a variable pH based on the organisms present and the diet. Fever is not common and is one means of differentiating cystitis from acute pyelonephritis. Affected cows do not act ill, but irritation from the infection may cause enough discomfort to affect appetite and thus production.

Diagnosis

The clinical signs, absence of systemic signs, normal ureters, and abnormal urine constituents contribute to the diagnosis. Palpation and ultrasonography of the bladder (per rectum) and kidneys will confirm disease of the bladder and rule out pyelonephritis. Culture and sensitivity of urine for bacteria is helpful to confirm the species responsible for infection and to direct therapy. Bladder endoscopy can be used to determine the severity of mucosal lesions from cystitis (see Video Clip 11.4).

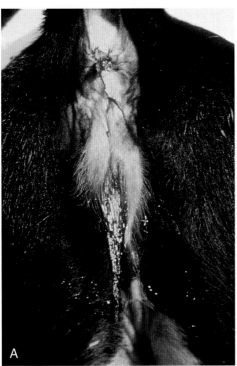
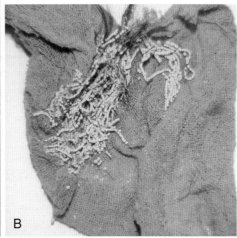

• **Fig. 11.24** **A,** Crystals attached to the vulvar hair of a heifer with chronic *Corynebacterium renale* cystitis. **B,** Sandlike crystals and struvite precipitates removed from the vulvar hair of the heifer.

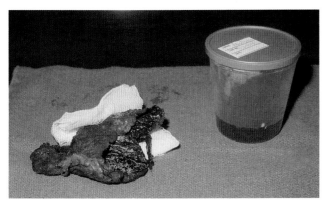

• **Fig. 11.25** Large fibrin cast and urine with hematuria and pyuria from a cow with chronic cystitis. The fibrin cast was removed manually from the urethra where it had lodged.

In calves with cystitis or recurrent cystitis, ultrasonography of the abdomen to detect urachal abscesses or umbilical remnants adherent to the bladder is imperative. On occasion, calves with recurrent cystitis may have resolved the infection within the umbilicus and urachus but have been left with fibrous adhesions between the bladder and abdominal wall, resulting in incomplete voiding and dysuria or pollakiuria. Ultrasonography of the bladder pre and post voiding can be quite informative as to the relative residual volume of urine remaining in the bladder after urination; normally the bladder should be almost impossible to identify in a normal calf immediately following urination (provided the calf was not "interrupted" mid-stream by handling).

Treatment

Bacterial cystitis requires antibiotic therapy based on urine culture and antibiotic susceptibility tests. Therapy should be continued for at least 7 days. Antibiotics that obtain good inhibitory concentrations in urine should be selected when possible. While awaiting urine culture results, penicillin (22,000 U/kg) and ampicillin (11 mg/kg) are both excellent choices for initial therapy. When bladder paresis or atony complicates cystitis, temporary placement of a Foley catheter may improve bladder emptying and decrease inflammatory sediment in the bladder. Bladder paresis decreases the prognosis and predisposes to relapse or reinfection after cessation of antibiotic therapy. Adequate salt and water should be available to encourage water consumption, and in addition to antibiotics a high anionic salt diet may be used to both acidify the urine and promote diuresis.

Bacterial cystitis associated with cystic calculi requires correction of the predisposing risk factors for calculi formation and is discussed in the section on urolithiasis.

Calves with dysuria secondary to umbilical or urachal adhesions and infection require abdominal surgery through a ventral midline approach to free the bladder and resect septic lesions or adhesions (Fig. 11.26).

Bladder Paralysis (Neurogenic Injury, Bladder Atony)

Neurologic injury to the autonomic control of the bladder or direct damage to the bladder musculature can result in bladder atony. The parasympathetic efferent control of the bladder musculature, contraction of which causes bladder

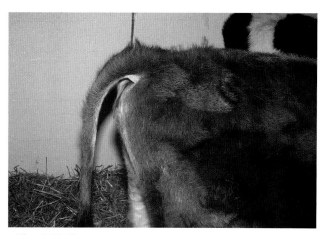

• **Fig. 11.26** Elevated tail head and dysuria in a 6-month-old Brown Swiss heifer with a chronic urachal abscess causing the bladder to be adhered to the ventral body wall. The urinalysis was normal. Surgical removal of the abscess and adhesion as well as part of the bladder alleviated the clinical signs.

emptying, originates with neurons in the sacral spinal cord segments S2 to S4. Afferent information is from pressure receptors in the bladder to the spinal cord and to higher autonomic centers in the brainstem. With injury to the parasympathetic system, bladder distention, dribbling urine, and ease of expression on rectal palpation (lower motor neuron bladder) are expected. The sympathetic innervation of the bladder mainly activates urethral tone and inhibits bladder emptying. Injury to sympathetic innervation may occur in the upper lumbar spinal cord segments, the sympathetic trunk, ganglia of the pelvic plexus, or fibers in the hypogastric and pelvic nerves supplying the bladder and the internal urethral sphincter. Injury in the spinal cord rostral to this area or to micturition centers in the brain may result in upper motor neuron bladder, causing spastic neurogenic bladder paralysis, with spontaneous contractions of detrusor muscles, increased intravesical voiding pressure, and urinary sphincter spasms. The author (TJD) has observed this in an adult cow with rabies. The bladder will be palpably enlarged and tight and difficult to express with applied pressure per rectum. The voluntary control of the external sphincter is mediated by α-motor neurons of the ventral horn in the sacral spinal cord segments (S2–S4), which cause the striated muscle fibers of the sphincter to contract. Cystitis is most likely to occur with a lower motor neuron lesion because of the constant dribbling of urine.

Etiology

Sacral nerve injuries causing bladder dysfunction are most commonly caused by dystocia with intrapelvic injury to the nerves or by crushing injuries to the sacrum and tail head at the vertebral level from riding activity. Occasional cases of direct sacral trauma are observed in modern facilities with poorly designed free-stall dividers or partitions. In either event, the bladder dysfunction seldom is diagnosed until cystitis develops or a large bladder is palpated during routine rectal palpation of the reproductive tract. If suspected in the acute phase after dystocia or crushing tail

head sacral injuries, symptomatic therapy to reduce acute inflammation may be indicated. In some cases, chronic infection and damage to the detrusor muscle of the bladder may cause the paralysis rather than vice versa. Extradural compression of the sacral nerves by lymphosarcoma is another common cause of lower motor neuron bladder paralysis.

Signs and Diagnosis

Dribbling of urine and voiding of small amounts of urine despite obvious and visible efforts at complete urination are the major signs of bladder dysfunction. Urine scalding may be observed in cattle with crushed tail heads from riding injuries. Urine is normal unless secondary cystitis occurs. Cystitis is common after dystocia because of urethral compromise, trauma, and associated vaginitis.

Crystalluria may be seen in cases of chronic cystitis and bladder atony resulting in accumulation of sandy calculi on the vulvar hair ventral to the vulva.

Rectal palpation confirms an enlarged bladder, and although the affected cow cannot empty the bladder when perineally stimulated, it can be expressed during rectal palpation. Lower motor neuron bladder paralysis is more common in cattle than is upper motor neuron dysfunction. Failure to conceive because of urine pooling in the vagina and chemical or bacterial vaginitis is a common reproductive complication to bladder paralysis in cows.

Treatment

In acute cases, placement of an indwelling Foley catheter coupled with prophylactic penicillin therapy may prevent urinary retention and bacterial cystitis. Systemic NSAIDs, dexamethasone (10–20 mg once daily for 3 days), or epidural administration of 5 mg of dexamethasone may be worthwhile to reduce edema and inflammation around the involved sacral nerves in cases related to trauma.

In chronic cases, the same therapy may be attempted but is less likely to be successful; use of antiinflammatory drugs probably is not justified.

When cystitis is present, therapy should be directed against the bacterial pathogen as outlined previously. The prognosis is poor because recurrent cystitis and eventual pyelonephritis are probable.

Hemorrhagic Cystitis Associated With Malignant Catarrhal Fever

Etiology

In addition to the acute severe head and eye form, enteric form, and other milder forms of MCF, acute hemorrhagic cystitis has been observed as a rare manifestation of MCF. The disease is caused by a gamma herpesvirus infection, specifically, ovine herpesvirus type 2 in North America. Instances are sporadic, as are most reports of MCF in dairy cattle. Typically, cattle affected with the hemorrhagic cystitis form have been housed (e.g., fairs) or pastured near sheep at sometime within several months of disease onset. Also see chapter 16.

Signs

Acute onset of high fever (106.0° to 108.0°F [41.11° to 42.22°C]), depression, hematuria, strangury, and frequent attempts at urination constitute the major signs. Affected cattle progress rapidly to severe depression and inappetence, with death occurring in 24 to 72 hours. Other grossly detectable signs of MCF (e.g., oral erosions, lymphadenopathy, and ocular lesions) may not be apparent.

Diagnosis

Necropsy reveals severe hemorrhagic cystitis with a thickened bladder wall and mucosal erosion. A retrospective diagnosis is made based on lesions of vasculitis in all major organs (e.g., kidney, brain, and lymph nodes) and exclusion of other causes of hemorrhagic cystitis. The virus can be identified by polymerase chain reaction using whole blood, and serologic detection of antibodies to the virus can be achieved via competitive enzyme-linked immunosorbent assay.

Prevention

Because the disease is usually fatal, preventing exposure to sheep remains the best management tool for the prevention of MCF in dairy cattle. Although other vectors of the virus have been theorized and are possible, most cases in dairy cattle result from environmental exposure to sheep. Subclinical infection in dairy cattle has been documented in the United States, suggesting that cow-to-cow transmission may also occur, potentially making control for some dairies more challenging.

Enzootic Hematuria

Etiology

Progressive cystitis with tissue metaplasia of the bladder mucosa has been described in cattle allowed to graze bracken fern for extended periods. Sporadic cases also have been observed in cattle with no known exposure to bracken fern or, for that matter, any pasture. Several toxic and carcinogenic factors including ptaquiloside, a glycoside, have been identified in bracken fern plants. Variations in carcinogen concentrations between plants, as well as differences in the amount and duration of toxin ingestion, likely explain geographic distribution of the disease.

There is also a putative role for bovine papillomaviruses (specifically BPV2) combined with bracken fern exposure in the etiopathogenesis of the disease in some parts of the world. Multiple types of urinary tract neoplasia (e.g., transitional cell carcinoma, hemangiocarcinoma) are possible in this syndrome, including both epithelial and mesenchymal origin tumors. Metastases are possible in some cases. Affected animals may also have intestinal carcinomas and bone marrow dysplasia.

Signs

Severe hematuria, strangury, and anemia are found in affected cattle. Absence of fever suggests a noninfectious cause. In most cases, rectal examination allows palpation of multiple masses within the bladder wall; these are also detectable ultrasonographically. Early signs of hematuria may be the result of microscopic lesions in the urinary tract or associated with the pancytopenia typical of chronic bracken fern toxicity.

Diagnosis

The diagnosis is suggested if multiple animals are affected with similar signs after pasturing. In individual cases, necropsy findings of anemia, bladder neoplasia, and hematuria, coupled with exclusion of infectious diseases, allow diagnosis.

Prevention

Removal from the pasture is the best prevention but may not reverse the disease in severely affected cattle. Fortunately, "pasture diseases" such as enzootic hematuria are currently rare in dairy cattle in the United States because of reduced pasture availability and utilization under current management conditions.

Bladder Rupture

Etiology

Bladder rupture is rare in female dairy cattle but has been reported after parturition and in heifers with urachal adhesions or traction adhesions resulting from previous abdominal surgery. Urolithiasis is also uncommon in dairy cattle, thereby decreasing the likelihood of urinary obstruction and secondary bladder rupture. Bladder rupture also has occurred secondary to urethral obstruction by large blood clots in severe cases of acute pyelonephritis in cattle. Although rare in cattle raised for milk production, urolithiasis may occur in dairy calves raised for veal or dairy steers and is discussed later.

Signs

Abdominal distention, depression, inappetence, and a detectable fluid wave during ballottement of the abdomen are typical signs of bladder rupture in cattle. History may reveal previous signs of urinary tract disease (e.g., pollakiuria, tenesmus, and colic), umbilical problems during calfhood, or previous surgery for umbilical or abdominal lesions. Following rupture it will be impossible to palpate the bladder during rectal examination, nor will it be possible to visualize it during transrectal ultrasonography of an adult.

Diagnosis

Failure to palpate the urinary bladder and fluid abdominal distention arouse suspicion of bladder rupture. However, because this problem is rare in dairy cattle, laboratory aids or ancillary diagnostics are essential to diagnosis. Rupture of the intraabdominal portion of a persistent urachus in a neonate may have the identical clinical appearance and laboratory findings of a ruptured bladder. Ultrasound examination of the abdomen will reveal a large amount of anechoic fluid free in the abdomen. Intestinal viscera may be floating up from the fluid. Abdominocentesis should result in copious fluid that may be analyzed for cytology, protein content, and creatinine levels. Comparison of serum creatinine with abdominal fluid creatinine should allow positive diagnosis of urinary bladder rupture because the abdominal fluid creatinine will be much higher (>2 times) than the serum value. Serum electrolytes usually show a mild hyponatremia, hypochloremia, and variable values for potassium. In most species, uroperitoneum results in peripheral hyperkalemia, but reported cases in cattle have not reliably done so.

Confirmation of a ruptured bladder can also be achieved by endoscopic examination of the bladder but this is not available to many practitioners. Laparotomy offers an immediate, and obviously most useful approach to confirmation of bladder rupture if one is considering an attempt at repair.

Treatment

Treatment options include slaughter or surgical repair of a ventral bladder defect. Bladder wall tears in other anatomic locations are not so accessible and hence are rarely amenable to surgical repair. If repair is to be attempted, the patient benefits from preoperative IV fluids (PSS primarily) and slow drainage of urine from the abdomen via a peritoneal drain or Foley catheter (Fig. 11.27). Antibiotics should be used both preoperatively and postoperatively. Because the caudal ventral midline provides the best surgical access to the urinary bladder, adult dairy cows are poor surgical candidates since the udder covers the ideal approach. Repair can also be accomplished by a left or right side flank approach making a caudal, dorsal incision to better allow exteriorization of the bladder. Dorsal tears may sometimes heal without surgery if a Foley catheter with the balloon filled with 45 ml of saline is positioned in the bladder and left in place to allow constant drainage of urine. Antibiotic treatment would also be indicated until the bladder is healed in such cases, as would abdominal drainage. This conservative treatment would likely be successful for many dorsal bladder

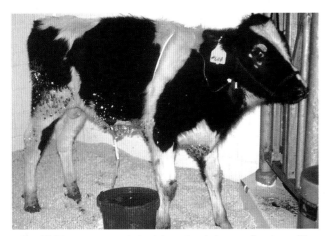

• **Fig. 11.27** Urine being drained from the abdomen of a steer with a ruptured bladder caused by urethral calculi.

tears if the bladder was not chronically distended or diseased prior to its rupture.

Eversion and Prolapse of the Urinary Bladder

Eversion of the bladder through the urethral orifice so that the mucosal surface is exposed has been reported in dairy cattle after severe tenesmus associated with parturition or shortly thereafter. Bladder prolapse, where the serosal surface of the urinary bladder is evident externally, tends to follow a laceration in the floor of the vagina during parturition. A prolapsed bladder usually fills with urine, but an everted bladder obviously cannot contain urine. Both conditions are rare. Bladder eversion or prolapse may grossly mimic vaginal and uterine prolapse but can be differentiated easily after cleansing of the organ and vaginal examination. The bladder may on rare occasions be involved in a vaginal or uterine prolapse and will prevent normal replacement of the vagina until the urine is drained.

The prognosis is guarded for these conditions. Repair of eversion is difficult because of rapid congestion and subsequent edema in the tissue. The female bovine urethra is narrow, making replacement difficult. One case report describes a dorsal urethral incision to aid replacement. Necrosis of the everted bladder may lead to a fatal outcome even if repair has been apparently successful.

Similarly, prolapse of the bladder requires emptying of the bladder, replacement through the lacerated vaginal floor, and repair of the vaginal wound. Peritonitis, bladder necrosis, and adhesions affecting urine outflow are possible complications.

Bladder Neoplasms

Worldwide, bladder neoplasia is seen most commonly in association with enzootic hematuria. Documented tumor types include hemangiomas, hemangiosarcomas, leiomyosarcomas, fibromas, fibrosarcomas, squamous cell carcinomas, transitional cell carcinomas, and papillomas. Experience with enzootic hematuria is limited in the northern United States, where the most common tumor found in the adult bovine bladder is lymphosarcoma. Simply based on the incidence of lymphosarcoma and the potential for this neoplasm to involve any tissue, most neoplastic lesions involving the lower urinary tract (i.e., bladder, urethra, and ureter) prove to be lymphosarcoma. Endoscopy offers the best opportunity for diagnostic biopsy of the bladder (see Video Clip 11.5).

Urolithiasis

Urolithiasis is the most important urinary tract disease in feed lot and range cattle but is seldom a problem in dairy cattle unless dairy veal calves and steers are included. Magnesium ammonium phosphate (struvite) calculi are the most common calculi in confined cattle. The disease is most common in steers, and urethral obstruction mostly occurs at the distal portion of the sigmoid flexure. Struvite calculi are difficult to visualize on radiographs. In modern management systems in the northern United States, few dairy calves, bulls, or cows have problems with urolithiasis, but a basic discussion of the condition is justified because the condition may exist in dairy cattle in other geographic regions. Rarely, Holstein calves may have urethral obstruction from congenital stricture of the urethra.

Etiology

Many causes and contributing factors exist that predispose to urolithiasis in cattle:

1. High-concentrate diets are thought to increase urinary mucoproteins and lead to "solidification" of urine solutes. These diets are a major cause of urolithiasis in feedlot beef animals
2. High-phosphorus diets or improper calcium–phosphorus balance in a ration, again usually associated with a high concentrate diet
3. Pastures containing large amounts of silica or oxalate
4. Vitamin A deficiency and excessive estrogens. Both conditions allow squamous metaplasia of mucosa creating solid nidus formation, narrowing of the urethral lumen, and excessive desquamation of epithelial cells. Estrogens may originate in pastures, feedstuffs, as a mycotoxin (zearalenone) or from estrogenic tissue implants
5. Hypervitaminosis D—perhaps because of increased urinary calcium levels
6. Reduced water intake. Drought or extreme cold with subsequent freezing of water supplies causes severe concentration of urine solutes and encourage calculi formation. During the winter, animals are reluctant to drink normal amounts when water is extremely cold, even though it may not be frozen
7. The mineral composition of the available drinking water, in concert with dietary mineral imbalances, probably contributes more to initiating urolith formation than does the lack of water itself
8. Early castration of male animals contributes to a reduced diameter of the distal urinary tract and is an important contributing feature in beef steers and smaller ruminants
9. Chronic UTIs may predispose to renal, ureteral, or cystic calculi, which may obstruct the urinary tract at their respective sites or move distally into the urethra and cause obstruction at that location

Having reviewed most of the contributing causes of urolithiasis, it becomes obvious that dairy cows, calves, and bulls have few risks compared with beef cattle, sheep, and goats. Sporadic cases may occur in dairy calves or bulls. If endemic problems occur, the veterinarian must investigate all potential causes to rectify the problem as quickly as possible.

Signs

Obstruction of male cattle occurs most commonly at the distal sigmoid region of the urethra. Renal, ureteral, and cystic calculi also are possible, but urethral obstruction is the most common clinical situation. Signs of ureteral obstruction are discussed under the earlier heading "Disorders of the Ureters."

Signs of urethral obstruction include treading, tenesmus, pulsation of the urethra in the escutcheon proximal to the obstruction, colic characterized by kicking at the abdomen, sandy calculi or crystals on the preputial hair, and inappetence. If urine can be passed, it often appears blood tinged. Rectal examination confirms the presence of a greatly distended urinary bladder and pulsating pelvic urethra.

The signs are much different if rupture of the bladder has occurred as a result of prolonged urethral obstruction. Colic is replaced by depression, and tenesmus ceases. Progressive abdominal distention follows. (This is discussed fully under the earlier heading "Bladder Rupture.")

More commonly, rupture of the urethra in males leads to the subcutaneous deposition of urine and appearance of diffuse pitting edema along the sheath and ventral abdomen referred to as "water belly" (Fig. 11.28). This is a severe complication that often results in chemical necrosis and eventual sloughing of the affected tissue.

Diagnosis

The diagnosis is based on clinical signs. Rectal examination or abdominal ultrasonography is imperative to assess an intact bladder. In calves, as in small ruminants, radiography may be helpful to evaluate the number, location, and size of calculi within the urinary tract before surgery.

Treatment

Because of the sigmoid flexure, catheterization usually is impossible in most bulls. Therefore therapy entails urethrostomy or urethrotomy, and this may interfere with future breeding. Complete urethrostomy with penile amputation may be lifesaving but of course renders breeding animals worthless. Postpubic urethrotomy, catheterization, and medical therapy with smooth muscle relaxants and IV fluid therapy with saline solutions could be tried for bulls of valuable genetic base, but the prognosis must be guarded. Aminopromazine (0.2–0.3 mg/kg IV or IM) has been used as a smooth muscle relaxant in feedlot cattle, but a paucity of controlled data exist regarding treatment of intact males and its use in cattle is forbidden in many countries. Aminopromazine should not be confused with acepromazine.

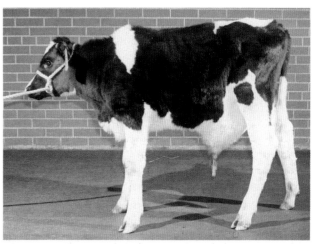

• **Fig. 11.28** "Water belly" or urethral rupture in a Holstein steer with urolithiasis. Sandlike crystals can be seen in chains on the preputial hair.

Where geographic conditions or causes allow single calculus formation, dye studies or ultrasonography to localize the obstruction and specific surgery to remove the calculus would theoretically be possible. It is worth bearing in mind that calculi are rarely single and following removal of one obstructing calculus re-obstruction at the same or another location is quite common.

Prevention

In all instances, correction of the underlying causes or removal from offending pastures or feedstuffs should be used to prevent further cases. The most important measures for struvite calculi (magnesium–ammonium–phosphate) prevention are to increase urinary chloride excretion, decrease urine pH, and provide a calcium:phosphorus ratio of 2:1 in the complete ration. Providing free access to a source of non-frozen water is very important, and adding NaCl to 4% to 5% of the ration will encourage water consumption and reduce precipitation or accumulation of urine solutes. This is especially helpful during extreme cold weather. Ammonium chloride can be used as a urinary acidifying agent (50–80 g/head/day for 240-kg steers). Complete rations with decreased dietary cation–anion difference are also used to prevent struvite calculi; these rations are high in chloride and also result in urinary acidification.

Patent Urachus in Calves

The persistence of a patent urachus in calves is less common than in foals but leads to similar predisposition to septicemia. Clinical signs consist of urine dribbling from the umbilical region or persistent moisture surrounding a small urachal opening at the umbilicus. Unless the urachus closes by 24 hours after birth, intervention is indicated to reduce the likelihood of septicemia. If economics do not permit surgery, prophylactic broad-spectrum antibiotics systemically and cautery of the urachus with silver nitrate, 7% iodine, or Lugol's iodine is indicated. Using a navel dip product with both disinfectant and drying properties would seem to be important in calves.

Umbilical Infections

Etiology

Umbilical infections, hernias, and fetal vascular infections are common problems in calves. Some umbilical lesions (i.e., patent urachus) are evident in the first few days of life, but others, such as small hernias and abscesses, may not become obvious to the owner for 1 to 6 weeks.

The umbilicus does not have a fibrin seal immediately after birth and is a common route (along with the intestinal and respiratory tracts) for bacteria to enter the body; this is especially common in calves with failure of passive transfer of colostral antibodies. Infection in the umbilical region may lead to a multitude of intraabdominal lesions and cellulitis or abscessation external to the body wall. Neonatal infections of the umbilical region result in painful swelling and palpable enlargement of the urachus (most common) or umbilical vessels (the umbilical vein is more commonly infected than the arteries). Septicemia resulting

from bacteria ascending the umbilical vessels or urachus is always a threat. Infection through this route may cause acute septicemia or chronic septicemia with subsequent joint ill, meningitis, uveitis, and so on. In some instances, infection is low grade, and no clinical signs develop until the calf is several months old. Delayed problems often involve infected urachal remnants and bladder dysfunction or recurrent UTI.

Whereas chronic infection of the umbilical vein may cause hepatic abscessation, umbilical artery infection may cause chronic infection involving the urinary bladder and less commonly the kidney. The plethora of pathology possible subsequent to umbilical infection requires that each calf be assessed as to its individual problems (Table 11.2).

Signs and Diagnosis

In acute neonatal umbilical infections, palpation and physical findings may suffice for diagnosis. Affected calves are febrile and have cellulitis in the region of the umbilicus with palpable enlargement of the umbilical vessels.

Signs of septicemia such as septic arthritis, uveitis, meningitis, bronchopneumonia, or peritonitis may be present and would worsen the prognosis.

Subacute infections limited to the umbilicus may have purulent material that drains from the umbilical vessels or urachus after removal of a scab at the exterior umbilicus.

Latent infections of intraabdominal vascular remnants or the urachus are harder to diagnose. Affected calves may be several weeks old before signs of fever and depression occur. Depending on the pathology present, other signs may include signs of peritonitis, septic arthritis, or UTI. The umbilicus may appear normal on external inspection, but deep palpation may detect thickened umbilical remnants intraabdominally.

The diagnosis is greatly aided by ultrasonography to detect the site and extent of infection (see Video Clip 11.6). Ultrasound examination is best performed with a 7.5 to 10 MHz linear probe and the calf in lateral recumbency. The newborn calf differs from the foal in that it has two umbilical veins within the umbilical stalk that merge once within the body wall. Umbilical arteries generally retract rapidly within the abdomen in newborn calves. The width of the external umbilicus should not exceed 2.4 cm at the base and 1.8 cm at the tip. The umbilical vein just inside the body wall should have a diameter of less than 1.7 cm and 1.2 cm, at 1 day and 1 week of age, respectively. The umbilical vein near the liver should be smaller than 0.2 cm by 2 weeks of age. The arteries near the bladder should be smaller than 1.0 cm at 1 week of age and in most calves cannot be visualized after 2 weeks of age. The urachus is not normally identified after the first week unless it is patent or has an infection or an urachal cyst. Thorough ultrasonographic evaluation from the external umbilicus to the bladder is important because some longstanding urachal remnant abscesses can form within a deep segment of the urachus and without any communication to the outside. This is also possible, but less common, with umbilical vein

TABLE 11.2 Treatment of Umbilical Infections*

Physical Findings	Treatment

Neonatal calf, healthy other than palpable cellulitis or vascular thickening with possible fever	1. Remove scab over umbilicus to allow drainage.
	2. Broad-spectrum antibiotic therapy to counteract probable *Trueperella pyogenes* or mixed infection with gram-negative bacteria
	  a. Penicillin 22,000 U/kg once or twice daily
	or
	  b. Ampicillin 11 mg/kg once or twice daily

Neonatal calf with fever, palpable umbilical lesions, and evidence of septicemia	1. Assess adequacy of passive transfer of immunoglobulins.
	2. Remove umbilical scab and culture any discharge.
	3. Consider blood culture if valuable calf.
	4. Intensive broad-spectrum antibiotic therapy for gram-negative organisms.
	  a. Penicillin and amikacin‡, 22,000 U/kg twice daily and 15–20 mg/kg once daily, respectively
	or
	  b. Ceftiofur (Naxcel) 2.2 mg/kg once daily†
	5. Attend localized infections such as septic joints via lavage and so on.
	6. Perform surgical resection of umbilicus after calf is stabilized (1–3 days).

Calf 2 wk or older with fever and evidence of urinary tract infection	1. Urine culture and sensitivity 2. Ultrasonography of extra- and intra abdominal umbilical remnants 3. Surgical resection of umbilicus and urachus or umbilical artery infection 4. Appropriate systemic antibiotics for 7–14 days. *T. pyogenes* and gram-negative organisms are most common.
Calf 2 wk or older with fever and septic arthritis in one or more joints. Umbilicus may appear normal or thickened; vascular remnants may be palpable through the abdominal wall	1. Blood culture and culture of infected joints 2. Resection of umbilicus and infected remnants. This may be complicated by hepatic abscessation or require dissection of multiple adhesions 3. Lavage of infected joints 4. Appropriate systemic antibiotics for 7–21 days. *T. pyogenes* is almost always present but may be complicated by anaerobes or gram-negative organisms.
Apparently healthy calf 1–8 mo of age with umbilical abscess external to body wall	1. Aspirate to confirm the presence of pus. 2. Liberal drainage of abscess followed by daily flushing 3. If concerned about possible intraabdominal lesions, ultrasonography after resolution of external abscess

*Specific therapeutic recommendations must address the pathology present in each patient.
†Ceftiofur (Naxcel) use in the United States must comply with the product license label.
‡Amikacin use in the United States constitutes extralabel drug use – client must be aware of, and agree to comply with, extended withdrawal times in the event that it is used. Use should be limited to valuable calves with clinical and laboratory findings suggestive of life threatening bacteremia.

remnant infections. Attempting to follow or identify such deeper abscesses by scanning from the umbilical region externally may not prove as successful as tracing them from the bladder or liver.

Umbilical abscesses external to the body wall are obvious and are often larger than hernias (Fig. 11.29). They are painful, warm, and irreducible, and they tend to enlarge with time. The diagnosis is based on palpation, ultrasound examination (Fig. 11.30), and aspiration of the lesion. When the patient is placed in lateral recumbency, an enlarged umbilical vein can often be palpated within the abdomen as the examiner gently squeezes the thumb and fingers together while palpating deep to the abdominal wall and rostral to the urachus. This is often resented to a significant degree by the patient.

Treatments

External umbilical abscesses are usually easily treated because they can be drained and the calf treated with penicillin. Treatment with appropriate antibiotics in neonates is often successful early in the disease, but as the structures become inspissated with pus or if there is ascending infection, surgical drainage is generally required. The umbilicus should be examined closely at

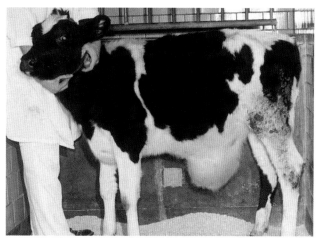

• **Fig. 11.29** Large umbilical abscess in a Holstein heifer.

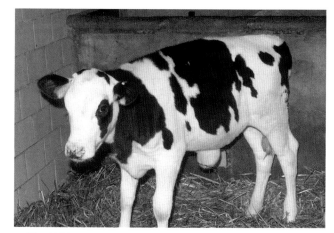

• **Fig. 11.31** Large but reducible umbilical hernia in a Holstein heifer.

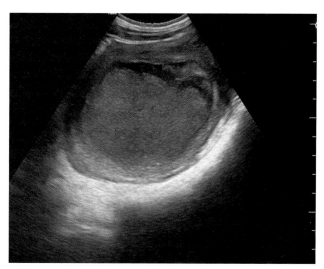

• **Fig. 11.30** Sonogram of a 2-month-old heifer with a 6-cm urachal abscess that is outside of the body wall. Ultrasound examination helps to confirm the safety in simply draining the abscess.

birth and again within the first 5 days of life for swelling, abnormal moisture, and pain. If the umbilici of multiple calves are being palpated, a separate, clean, and gloved-hand examination should be performed for each calf. Table 11.2 gives guidelines for the management of the varying types of umbilical infections in calves. Preventive measures for umbilical infection encompass maternity pen hygiene, decreased residency time of the newborn calf in the maternity pen, adequate colostrum management, and antiseptic umbilical cord care. In a recent randomized controlled trial, Navel Guard (SCG-Solutions Inc., McDonough, GA), 7% iodine tincture and chlorhexidine all had similar efficacy in preventing umbilical infection or health events in calves.

Umbilical Hernias

Etiology and Signs

Uncomplicated umbilical hernias in calves range from 1.0 to 10.0 cm in diameter, are soft and reducible, and are not painful (Fig. 11.31). The omentum and abomasum may be palpated in the hernia. Small hernias (diameter <4.0 cm) often close spontaneously by 3 to 4 months of age. Those that persist require therapy, as do larger hernias. Some hernias are thought to originate secondary to infected umbilical remnants; cordlike remnants of umbilical structures may be palpated in these hernias. Most hernias are of unknown origin. Although inheritance definitely is a possibility, heifer calves usually are not culled because of this problem unless an extremely large hernia exists. Most bull studs will not accept bull calves with hernias (or bulls that have had hernias repaired) for fear of perpetuation of the trait.

Treatment

Manual reduction of small hernias followed by snug taping around the midabdomen with an elastic adhesive tape has been a successful procedure for some practitioners for hernias less than 3 fingerbreadths in diameter. The tape is left in place for several weeks, allowing the abdominal wall to close the defect. In healthy, rapidly growing calves postweaning, the tape may need to be changed at 1- to 2-week intervals to prevent it from becoming too tight. Some owners report successful resolution with repeated manual reduction of small hernias, but these cases may have resolved spontaneously regardless of treatment. In larger hernias or when other therapy fails, surgery is the only option.

Surgery for uncomplicated hernias is performed with the calf sedated with xylazine (≤0.22 mg/kg IV) and regional local anesthesia. The hernia sac is opened and examined for problematic remnants; following this the abdominal wall is closed routinely. Surgical preference dictates the exact suture pattern, but our clinic has been pleased with far–near–near–far suture patterns for large hernias. Dr. Ortved has provided a more detailed description of surgery for umbilical masses in the second edition of Fubini and Ducharme's Farm Animal Surgery Textbook.

Complicated hernias with intraabdominal adhesions or infected umbilical remnants are difficult surgical procedures requiring larger incisions, lengthier general anesthesia,

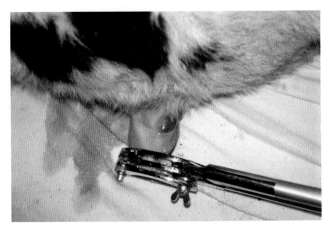

• **Fig. 11.32** Large, edematous umbilicus in a cloned neonate. Emasculation was required to achieve hemostasis.

advanced knowledge of abdominal anatomy, and superior surgical skills. Surgical referral should be considered for these patients.

Umbilical Hemorrhage

Umbilical hemorrhage and hematomas may occur in some calves. These can be especially large and life threating in cloned calves and neonates produced by in vitro fertilization techniques, often requiring double ligation with umbilical tape, emasculation, or the use of some other form of resilient ligation to prevent fatal hemorrhage (Fig. 11.32).

After normal delivery, the umbilicus breaks, and blood vessels contract within the abdomen, leaving a small cord protruding several centimeters from the abdominal wall. The cord should normally shrink over the next 5 to 7 days. If the cord breaks too close to the abdomen or is cut very short, there is increased risk of hemorrhage and infection. All umbilical cords should be dipped with preparations that disinfect and dry the cord.

Suggested Readings

Bertlin, F. R., Baseler, L. J., Wilson, C. R., et al. (2013). Arsenic toxicosis in cattle: meta-analysis of 156 cases. *J Vet Intern Med, 27,* 977–981.

Bertone, A. L., & Smith, D. F. (1984). Ruptured bladder in a yearling heifer. *J Am Vet Med Assoc, 184,* 981–982.

Braun, U., & Nuss, K. (2015). Uroperitoneum in cattle: ultrasonographic findings, diagnosis and treatment. *Acta Vet Scand, 57,* 36–44.

Braun, U., Nuss, K., Wapf, P., et al. (2006). Clinical and ultrasonographic findings in five cows with a ruptured urachal remnant. *Vet Rec, 159,* 780–782.

Braun, U., Nuss, K., Wehbrink, D., et al. (2008). Clinical and ultrasonographic findings, diagnosis and treatment of pyelonephritis in 17 cows. *Vet J, 175,* 240–248.

Carrier, J., Stewart, S., Godden, S., et al. (2004). Evaluation and use of three cowside tests for detection of subclinical ketosis in early postpartum cows. *J Dairy Sci, 87,* 3725–3735.

Cesbron, N., Dorso, L., Royer, A. L., et al. (2017). Aminoaciduria caused by Fanconi Syndrome in a heifer, *J Vet Intern Med, 31*(2), 598–603.

Chandler, K. J., O'Brien, K., Huxley, J. N., et al. (2000). Hydronephrosis and renal failure in two Friesian cows. *Vet Rec, 146,* 646–648.

Defontis, M., Bauer, N., Failing, K., et al. (2013). Automated and visual analysis of commercial urinary dipsticks in dogs, cats and cattle. *Res Vet Sci, 94*(3), 440–445.

Divers, T. J., Reef, V. B., & Roby, K. A. (1989). Nephrolithiasis resulting in intermittent ureteral obstruction in a cow. *Cornell Vet, 79,* 143–149.

Divers, T. J., Crowell, W. A., Duncan, J. R., et al. (1982). Acute renal disorders in cattle: a retrospective study of 22 cases. *J Am Vet Med Assoc, 181,* 694–699.

Divers, T. J. (1992). Assessment of the urinary system. *Vet Clin North Am Food Anim Pract, 8,* 373–382.

Divers, T. J. (1983). Diagnosis and therapy of renal disease in dairy cattle. In *Proceedings: Annual Convention American Association of Bovine Practitioners, 15,* 74–78.

Doce, R. R., Belenguer, A., Toral, P. G., et al. (2013). Effect of the administration of young leaves of Quercus pyrenaica on rumen fermentation in relation to oak tannin toxicosis in cattle. *J Anim Physiol Anim Nutr (Berl), 97*(1), 48–57.

Donecker, J. M., & Bellamy, J. E. (1982). Blood chemical abnormalities in cattle with ruptured bladders and ruptured ureters. *Can Vet J, 23,* 355–357.

Ducharme, N. G., & Stein, E. S., III. (1981). Eversion of the urinary bladder in a cow. *J Am Vet Med Assoc, 179,* 996–998.

Elitok, O. M., Elitok, B., & Unver, O. (2008). Renal amyloidosis in cattle with inflammatory diseases. *J Vet Intern Med, 22,* 450–455.

Fleming, S. A., Hunt, E. L., Brownie, C., et al. (1992). Fractional excretion of electrolytes in lactating dairy cows. *Am J Vet Res, 53,* 222–224.

Flock, M. (2003). Ultrasonic diagnosis of inflammation of the umbilical cord structures, persistent urachus and umbilical hernia in calves [article in German]. *Berl Munch Tierarztl Wochenschr, 116,* 2–11.

Flock, M. (2007). Sonographic application in the diagnosis of pyelonephritis in cattle. *Vet Radiol Ultrasound, 48*(1), 74–77.

Floeck, M. (2009). Ultrasonography of bovine urinary tract disorders. *Vet Clin North Am Food Anim Pract, 25,* 651–667.

Franz, S., Winter, P., & Baumgartner, W. (2004). Cystoscopy in cattle, a valuable additional tool for clinical examination. *Acta Vet Hung, 52,* 423–438.

Hammer, E. J., Divers, T. J., & Tulleners, E. P. (2000). Nephrectomy for treatment of ectopic ureter in a Holstein calf. *Bov Pract, 34,* 101–103.

Hardefeldt, L. Y., Poulsen, K. P., & Darien, B. J. (2011). Secondary renal tubular acidosis in a Hereford calf. *Vet Clin Pathol, 40,* 253–255.

Henniger, T., Schwert, B., Henniger, P., et al. (2013). Renal function tests in milk fed calves—reference values and influence of bovine neonatal pancytopenia (BNP). *Tierarztl Prax Aust G Grosstiere Nutztiere, 41,* 345–352.

Hylton, W. E., & Trent, A. M. (1987). Congenital urethral obstruction, uroperitoneum, and omphalitis in a calf. *J Am Vet Med Assoc, 190*(4), 433–434.

Johnson, R., & Jamison, K. (1984). Amyloidosis in six dairy cows. *J Am Vet Med Assoc, 185,* 1538–1543.

Lefebvre, H. P., Dossin, O., Trumel, C., et al. (2008). Fractional excretion tests: a critical review of methods and applications in domestic animals. *Vet Clin Pathol, 37*(1), 4–20.

Lesser, M., Krüger, S., Nuss, K., et al. (2014). Ultrasonographic findings and treatment of a cow with pyelonephrosis. *Schweiz Arch Tierheilkd, 156*, 336–340.

Roperto, S., Russo, V., Leonardi, L., et al. (2016). Bovine Papillomavirus Type 13 Expression in the Urothelial Bladder Tumours of Cattle. *Transbound Emerg Dis, 63*(6), 628–634.

Mohamed, T., & Oikawa, S. (2008). Efficacy and safety of ultrasound-guided percutaneous biopsy of the right kidney in cattle. *J Vet Med Sci, 70*, 175–179.

Morse, E. V. (1948). *A study of Corynebacterium renale and penicillin therapy in the treatment of specific pyelonephritis of cattle, MS Thesis.* Ithaca, NY: Cornell University.

Mueller, P. O., Hay, W. P., Allen, D., et al. (1999). Removal of an ectopic left kidney through a ventral midline celiotomy in a calf. *J Am Vet Med Assoc, 214*, 532–534.

Müller, K., Kamphues, J., Wolf, P., et al. (2012). Red discolouration of the urine in a dairy cattle herd as a stock problem. *Tierarztl Prax Ausg G Grosstiere Nutziere, 40*, 33–40.

Murakami, T., Inoshima, Y., Kobayashi, Y., et al. (2012). Atypical AA amyloid deposits in bovine AA amyloidosis. *Amyloid, 19*, 15–20.

Murray, G. M., Cert, F. S., & Sharpe, A. E. (2009). Nephrotic syndrome due to glomerulopathy in an Irish dairy cow. *Vet Rec, 164*, 179–180.

Ortved K. (2017). Miscellaneous abnormalities of the calf. In S.L. Fubini & N. D. Ducharme (Eds.), *Farm Animal Surgery* (2nd ed.). St. Louis: Elsevier.

Pérez, V., Doce, R. R., Garcia-Pariente, C., et al. (2011). Oak leaf *(Quercus pyrenaica)* poisoning in cattle. *Res Vet Sci, 91*, 269–277.

Rebhun, W. C., Dill, S. G., Perdrizet, J. A., et al. (1989). Pyelonephritis in cattle: 15 cases (1982-1986). *J Am Vet Med Assoc, 194*, 953–955.

Sharma, R., Bhat, T. K., & Sharma, O. P. (2013). The environmental and human effects of ptaquiloside-induced enzootic bovine hematuria: a tumorous disease of cattle. *Rev Environ Contam Toxicol, 224*, 53–95.

Smith, J. A., Divers, T. J., & Lamp, T. M. (1983). Ruptured urinary bladder in a post-parturient cow. *Cornell Vet, 73*, 3–12.

Sockett, D. C., Knight, A. P., Fettman, M. J., et al. (1986). Metabolic changes due to experimentally induced rupture of the bovine urinary bladder. *Cornell Vet, 76*, 198–212.

Somvanshi, R., Pathania, S., Nagarian, N., et al. (2012). Pathological study of non-neoplastic urinary bladder lesions in cattle and buffaloes: a preliminary report. *Trop Anim Health Prod, 44*, 855–861.

Summers, B. A., & Smith, C. A. (1985). Renal encephalopathy in a cow. *Cornell Vet, 75*, 524–530.

Trent, A. M., & Smith, D. F. (1984). Pollakiuria due to urachal abscesses in two heifers. *J Am Vet Med Assoc, 184*, 984–986.

Tulleners, E. P., Deem, D. A., Donawick, W. J., et al. (1981). Indications for unilateral bovine nephrectomy: a report of four cases. *J Am Vet Med Assoc, 179*, 696–700.

Ulutas, B., & Sahal, M. (2005). Urinary GGT/creatinine ratio and fractional excretion of electrolytes in diarrhoeic calves. *Acta Vet Hung, 53*, 351–359.

Vaala, W. E., Ehnen, S. J., & Divers, T. J. (1987). Acute renal failure associated with administration of excessive amounts of tetracycline in a cow. *J Am Vet Med Assoc, 191*, 1601–1603.

Vogel, S. R., Desrochers, A., Babkine, M., et al. (2011). Unilateral nephrectomy in 10 cattle. *Vet Surg, 40*, 233–239.

Wieland, M., Mann, S., Guard, C. L., et al. (2017). The influence of 3 different navel dips on calf health, growth performance, and umbilical infection assessed by clinical and ultrasonographic examination. *J Dairy Sci, 100*(1), 513–524.

Wiseman, A., Spencer, A., & Petrie, L. (1980). The nephrotic syndrome in a heifer due to glomerulonephritis. *Res Vet Sci, 28*, 325–329.

Yamada, M., Kotani, Y., Nakamura, K., et al. (2006). Immunohistochemical distribution of amyloid deposits in 25 cows diagnosed with systemic AA amyloidosis. *J Vet Med Sci, 68*, 725–729.

Yeruham, I., Elad, D., Avidar, Y., et al. (2006). A herd level analysis of urinary tract infection in dairy cattle. *Vet J, 171*, 172–176.

12

Musculoskeletal Disorders

CHARLES L. GUARD, SIMON F. PEEK, AND GILLES FECTEAU

Digital Lameness—Lesions and Treatments

Throughout this section on therapy of hoof diseases, reference will be made to functional hoof trimming. This refers to the method developed and promoted by the Dutch veterinarian Toussaint Raven and described fully in his excellent book *Cattle Hoof Care and Claw Trimming*. Toes are cut to 75 mm or 3 inches as measured along the dorsal wall from the point near the coronet where the wall becomes hard (this measurement may be increased 3 mm for each 75 kg over 750 kg, or ⅛ inch for every 150 lb over 1600 lb). After this cut, a wedge of sole and wall are removed that is thickest at the toe and tapers toward the heel. The toe thickness is maintained at 5 mm or ¼ inch at the tip where the first cut was made. These dimensions preserve adequate sole thickness (5 mm) at the toe tip to prevent bruising. The heel of the taller claw is trimmed to balance the weight bearing between the two digits. To complete the job, the sole is dished along the axial border of both digits from the heel–sole junction to the point where the axial wall and white line are evident. This is usually between one third and one half the length of the sole.

General principles of therapy for digital diseases are to eliminate the pain first and foremost and then to correct the underlying problem if possible. Hoof horn that is detached from underlying layers of hoof or corium should be removed. Around areas of exposed corium, the wall or sole should be thinned to make the existing hoof capsule more flexible along the border of newly developing cornified epithelium. Bandages do not promote healing but may be used to control hemorrhage or to maintain some antibiotic or antiseptic in contact with a wound. Regardless of original intent, most bandages should be removed in a few days and the lesion left uncovered. Hoof blocks are an essential tool for managing painful conditions, and their use should be routine (Fig. 12.1). Nonsteroidal antiinflammatory drugs (NSAIDs) such as flunixin, ketoprofen (not approved for use in dairy cattle in the United States), or meloxicam (although the latter is not approved and considered extra-label drug use in dairy cattle in the United States

it is increasingly being used as a medication for the relief of musculoskeletal pain) should be considered to reduce the pain of some severe claw horn diseases and after surgery of the digit. Their use is not encouraged enough by most veterinary practitioners.

Basic tools for lame cow therapy include left and right hoof knives and small hoof nippers. Additional tools that are in widespread use are long-handled hoof nippers and electric angle grinders with carbide-toothed chipper wheels. There is a wide variety of restraint devices present on farms, and still some farms have nothing. Practitioners should encourage every client to have a safe and efficient place or device for lameness work because every herd will have lame cows, and most practitioners, at least in the United States, do not travel with a trimming chute to every call. Because most lameness occurs in the rear feet, simple devices for small herds should be made available to make rear limb lifting and examination easy. Examples are illustrated in Fig. 12.2.

Simple Overgrowth

Although not a painful condition itself, overgrowth is considered a predisposing cause of hoof horn problems and is often present in lame cows with painful lesions. The practitioner should trim such hooves to normal conformation when treating lameness. The practitioner should also be aware of the general condition of hoof overgrowth in a herd to advise on the need and frequency of maintenance trimming.

Overwear and Thin Soles

Increasingly in large confinement dairies where cows walk long distances to and from the milking parlor and in some moderate-sized dairies using sand bedding, hooves wear away faster than new hoof is produced (Fig. 12.3). There may be no other hoof diseases, but the lameness caused by subsolar bruising or exposure of the corium at the white line can be very painful. Individual animal treatment is to apply hoof blocks to allow regrowth of the overworn sole.

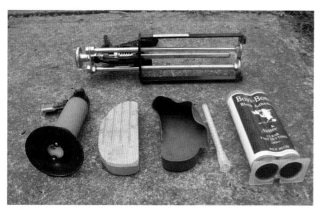

• **Fig. 12.1** Polyurethane hoof block adhesive, two types of blocks, and a heat gun for drying the hoof surface (from right to left).

Some hoof trimmers have suggested placing a layer of hoof block adhesive on the sole to increase its thickness and to reduce wear of the horny tissue. When overwear is present as a herd problem, environmental modification is indicated, which usually means installing rubber in the holding pen and travel lanes to and from the free-stall pens.

White Line Abscess

The most common location for a white line abscess is in the posterior third of the white line of the rear lateral claw. The presence of this lesion may be detected with the response to finger pressure on the bulb of the heel of the affected digit. If the abscess is near the toe tip, it may be necessary to apply pressure with hoof testers to identify the location. In the forelimbs, the most common site is the posterior quarter of the medial claw. Usually white line abscesses are obvious after a thin layer of horn has been removed. There often is dark discoloration of a portion of the white line (Fig. 12.4). Sometimes the white line is fissured with manure packed into the resulting crevice, which must be cleaned before the specific site of the abscess becomes visible. Relieving the pressure within the abscess provides some immediate pain relief. Abscesses near the heel may dissect between layers of sole horn to exit at the heel, resulting in a transverse flap of detached horn. Much less frequently than in horses, abscesses under the wall may erupt at the coronary band. Treatment is to remove the detached horn and trim to allow walking without pressure on the inflamed corium. Large abscesses and those at the toe tip benefit from the use of a hoof block on the healthy digit (Figs. 12.5 and 12.6). Bandaging is discouraged. Most cows recover uneventfully, and reexamination is not necessary. Hoof blocks should be removed in about 4 weeks. Occasionally, white line abscesses will extend into the soft tissue structures of the digital cushion and involve structures posterior to the distal interphalangeal joint. These conditions require surgical intervention, which is described later.

Sole Ulcer

Ulceration of the sole may occur in any digit but is most common in the lateral claws of the rear feet and the medial

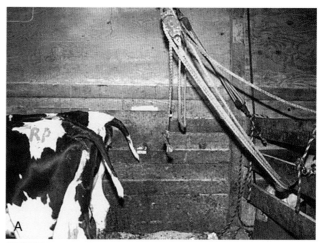

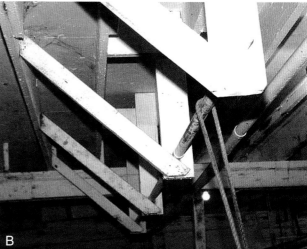

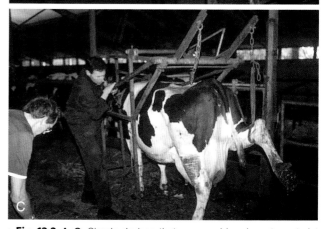

• **Fig. 12.2** A–C, Simple devices that can provide adequate restraint and support for hoof work on rear limbs.

claws of the forelimbs. Symmetrical ulcers can occasionally occur in both rear limbs or both forelimbs. The typical site for ulceration is in the corium that overlies the flexor process of the third phalanx (Figs. 12.7 and 12.8). Ulceration at the toe tip is a less common lesion in housed cattle but the most common lesion in extensive grazing dairies of the Southern Hemisphere. When it occurs in housed cattle, it is thought to be caused by either overtrimming at the toe or from wear that exceeds growth. A third location for ulceration is at the

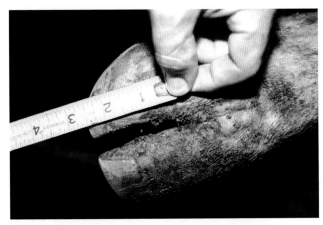

• **Fig. 12.3** Toe length of 2.5 cm in a cow that was part of a herd problem with severe overwear as a result of abrasive sand used as bedding combined with steeply sloped travel lanes. Normal length after trimming is 3 in.

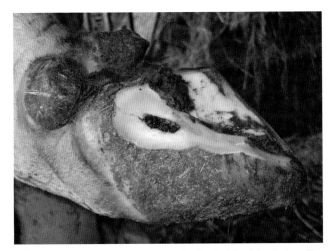

• **Fig. 12.4** White line abscess near the heel of the lateral claw. The heel of this claw was further trimmed to remove weight bearing from this portion of the digit.

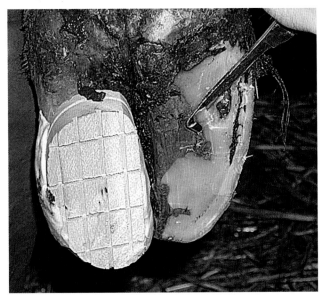

• **Fig. 12.5** White line abscess in the lateral claw.

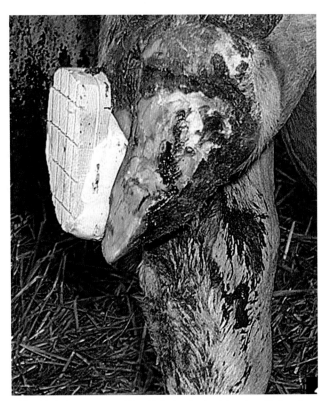

• **Fig. 12.6** Same cow as Fig. 12.5 after further trimming. No bandage was used in the therapy.

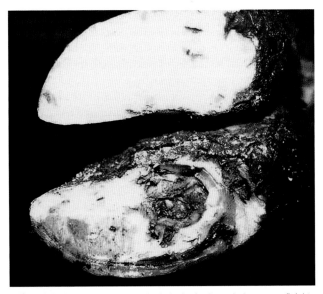

• **Fig. 12.7** Sole ulcer in the typical site in the lateral claw superficial to the flexor tuberosity of the third phalanx.

heel–sole junction. This may occur secondary to severe interdigital dermatitis or, when seen in the medial claw of the rear foot, from unknown causes. The degree of damage to the sole and underlying corium varies from slight hemorrhage visible at trimming to complete absence of a portion of the sole, to extensive necrosis of the underlying corium. The term *complicated sole ulcer* is used for those that have necrosis extending beyond the corium to include other tissues in the hoof.

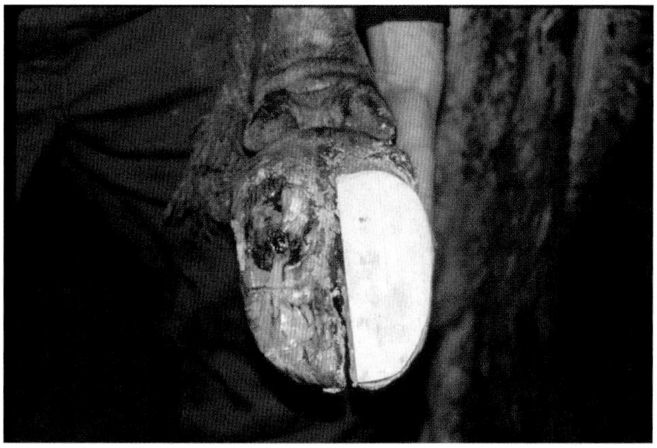

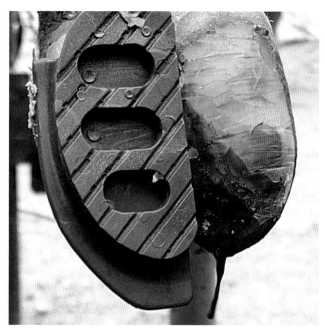

• **Fig. 12.8** Small sole ulcer in right hind lateral claw, trimmed and treated with a wooden block on sound medial claw to facilitate healing.

Treatment for a sole ulcer is to remove weight bearing from the affected portion of the digit. Depending on the location of the lesion and its severity, this may be accomplished by corrective trimming and lowering the heel horn of the affected claw. Most often a hoof block is applied to the healthy claw. If the ulcer is in the typical site or at the heel and there is sufficient heel depth of the healthy toe, a "heelless" trimming method may be used. This method, described by Japanese hoof trimmer H. Manabe, is to remove all wall and sole from the posterior half of the digit to a depth that just preserves a thin layer of sole. When the cow stands, there should be space for a finger between the floor and the remaining portion of the affected area. The use of this technique eliminates the need for a block but is always dependent on the cow having sufficient heel depth on the healthy digit. Bandaging is discouraged. If the corium is intact, the swelling that is usually present throughout the posterior portion of the digit, including protrusion of the coronary corium, will usually subside within a few days.

Reexamination in about 4 weeks is recommended to check the integrity of the hoof block and to trim the sole horn adjacent to the original lesion. Healing time for full-thickness sole ulcers is about 2 months. Reoccurrence in subsequent lactations is likely. Complicated sole ulcers require surgical intervention that is described later.

Toe Ulcer and Toe Necrosis

These conditions result from overwear or overtrimming at the toe tip. The resulting thin sole at this location is more susceptible to deformation from stepping on stones or irregular features in the flooring. If a hematoma results at the toe tip, it may lead to avascular necrosis of the soft tissues at this location (Figs. 12.9 and 12.10). If the lesion is open to the environment, miscellaneous bacteria may invade and produce osteomyelitis or pathologic fracture of the tip of the third phalanx (Fig. 12.11). Conservative therapy with a hoof block and cleaning of the toe tip usually results in a chronic state of infection and mild pain. Our current approach to this problem is to place a hoof block on the sound digit and amputate the distal portion of the affected digit. Either obstetric wire or

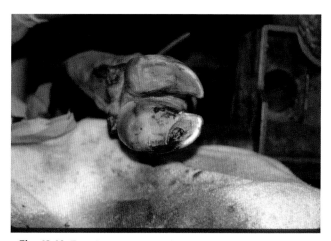

• **Fig. 12.9** Toe ulcer in a heifer from an extensively grazed dairy in Uruguay.

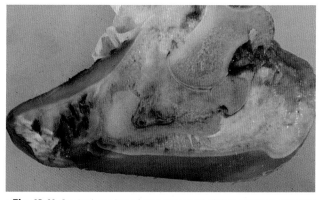

• **Fig. 12.10** Toe ulcer in the lateral hind claw of a 2-year-old show heifer with aggressively trimmed, and very thin, soles during the summer months.

• **Fig. 12.11** Sagittal section of an amputated digit illustrating common changes at the apex of the third phalanx and the remodeling of the associated hoof in chronic toe necrosis.

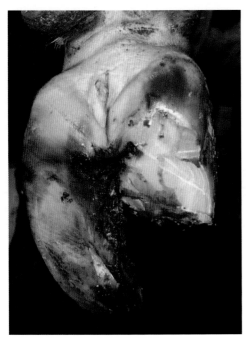

• **Fig. 12.12** Partial toe amputation for toe necrosis. The hoof and all internal structures are resected until only healthy tissue remains.

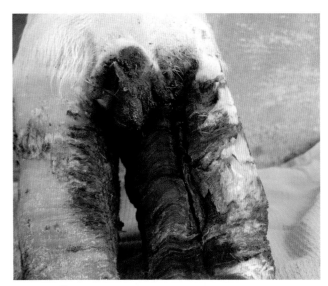

• **Fig. 12.13** Vertical wall crack in a mature dairy cow.

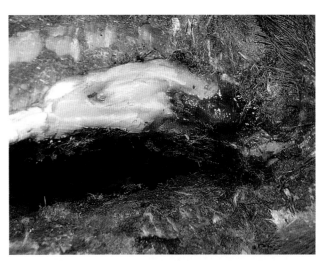

• **Fig. 12.14** Axial wall crack in a yearling dairy heifer.

hoof nippers may be used to remove slices of the affected digit until all tissue exposed appears healthy (Fig. 12.12). A tight bandage is applied over some antibiotic powder to control hemorrhage. The bandage is removed in a few days. There is no need for parenteral antibiotics. Regrowth of functional cornified epithelium will cover the partial amputation in about 1 month. The prognosis is excellent.

Thimbling or Transverse Wall Separation

This condition results from an insult to the coronary corium that results in an interruption in growth and a subsequent break in the continuity of the horn tubules of the hoof wall. It is not apparent until the hoof has grown sufficiently for the break point to be about 5 cm from the coronary band. It is always present in all eight digits but usually noticed because of pain in only one. The distal portion of the hoof capsule separates from the more proximal section along the entire axial, dorsal, and abaxial regions. The sole is normally attached to the younger healthy wall and the older detached wall. Pain occurs when movement of the distal portion relative to the rest of the hoof pinches the corium at the toe tip. The goals of trimming are to minimize weight bearing at the toe tip by shortening as much as possible and thinning the sole at the toe relative to the rest of the hoof. Pain may shift from one limb to another as successive thimbles become more detached from the younger hoof wall. Recovery is complete and without complications as the thimbles wear or are trimmed away.

Vertical Wall Cracks or Sand Cracks

Cracks in the dorsal or lateral hoof wall that extend from the coronary band distally are much more common in

range cattle than in dairy cattle but do occasionally occur (Fig. 12.13). It is important to verify that the crack is the cause of lameness before proceeding. If the crack is causing pain, it should be carefully debrided of foreign material. There may be exposed corium or granulation tissue. Care must be taken to not further extend the hoof wall defect during trimming. Removing granulation tissue may be necessary, followed by controlling hemorrhage and protecting the healing corium from damage during healing. The standard procedure is to stabilize the adjacent portions of the hoof wall with acrylic and to place a block on the sound claw.

Vertical cracks in the axial wall are more common in dairy cattle but are far less frequently seen than ulcers and white line abscesses. The strategy for treatment is similar to that used in range cattle, although acrylic is less often used (Fig. 12.14). The greatest challenge to treatment of axial wall cracks is to visualize and trim affected tissues in the interdigital space. Separated or detached horn should be removed; granulation tissue resected; and a tight bandage with antibiotic powder, usually tetracycline, applied. The tight bandage is to help prevent the formation of new granulation tissue. A hoof block is applied to the healthy digit. Several visits may be required for further trimming and bandage application at about 1-week intervals to achieve complete healing.

Inherited Defects: Corkscrew Claw and Splayed Toes

The appearance of corkscrew claws, although the condition is inherited, does not become evident until the cow reaches 3 or more years of age. Both lateral rear digits, both medial fore digits, or all four may be affected. The entire configuration of the third phalanx, the soft tissues between the claw capsule and bone, and the claw capsule are abnormal. The external appearance is of a hoof that is rotating around an axis perpendicular to the articulation of the third phalanx. The abaxial wall develops a curvature that extends the wall into the normal location of the sole. The axial wall becomes dorsal, and the tip of the toe curls up from the ground (Fig. 12.15). This conformation creates a mild predisposition to lameness, but of more importance is the technique required for routine trimming to prevent exposure of the corium in affected claws. The toe tip should be trimmed slightly longer than normal. Removal of the overgrowth of the abaxial wall can return weight bearing to the sole and wall in a flat plane. Care must be taken near the toe tip because the corium is abnormally close to the exterior, about one fourth of the distance from the toe tip to heel. Thus, the toe tip should be left about 1 cm thick. Exaggerated dishing of the axial margin of the sole may prolong the time until the next trimming is needed.

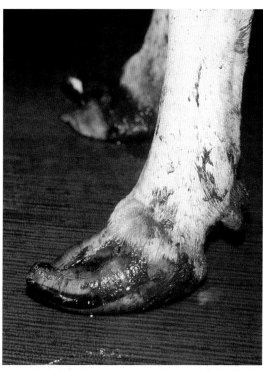

• **Fig. 12.15** Corkscrew claw in a Holstein cow.

Splayed toes is primarily a condition of beef cattle, and predisposes to interdigital fibroma but the condition will not be further considered here.

Traumatic Exungulation

Cows may get a toe caught in a manure grate or floor slot and detach the horny capsule of a claw while extricating themselves. If the corium is not badly damaged and the condition treated as an emergency, regrowth of a new, nearly normal claw capsule can occur. It is important to clean and disinfect the exposed tissues and bandage with a tissue-friendly antiseptic. A hoof block is necessary on the healthy digit, and parenteral antibiotics are recommended for 7 to 10 days. The limitations to recovery seem to depend on the degree of trauma to the soft tissues. If it is apparent that the corium or deeper structures are also significantly damaged, then amputation or slaughter should be chosen.

Fracture of the Third Phalanx

This injury may occur in cattle of any age or size. In a hospital population, it is observed primarily in dairy bulls, but others report that young cattle and young milking cows are predisposed. Excessive dryness of the hoof, leading to reduced cushioning during routine weight bearing, or severe hoof trauma may predispose to third phalanx (P3) fracture. Trauma from a hoof becoming stuck in a floor slot may also result in fracture (Fig. 12.16). The incidence of P3 fractures may be increased when fluorine toxicity exists in a herd. Hoof trauma resulting from blunt injury or falling to the ground after mounting another individual is a suspected cause of some P3 fractures.

Acute severe lameness with no weight bearing in the affected limb is observed. Careful local examination frequently reveals warmth in the affected digit, and flexion of the hoof, hoof tester pressure, and percussion all elicit a painful response from the affected animal. If one digit is affected, the cow will attempt to touch the foot down only on the nonaffected digit, if at all, when forced to walk. Occasional bilateral fractures of the medial P3 in the forelimbs have been

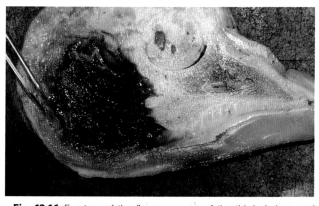

• **Fig. 12.16** Fracture of the flexor process of the third phalanx and hematoma in the heel region.

described wherein affected cattle stand with the forelimbs crossed in an effort to bear all weight on the nonaffected lateral claws. Bilaterally affected cattle may refuse to rise on their front feet and rest on their knees, similar to laminitis patients.

The diagnosis is confirmed by radiographs after elimination of more common causes of lameness through examination and paring of the affected claw. In the absence of obvious hoof lesions in the affected claw, acute laminitis is the most common differential diagnosis when considering a fracture of P3. Radiographs should be taken from at least two views. In addition, lateral radiographs are best obtained by placing the film in the interdigital area such that only the affected digit is evaluated.

Resting the affected digit by use of a standard hoof block applied to the normal claw is the treatment of choice. The affected animal should be placed in a comfortable box stall and the block renewed as necessary during the 4 to 8 weeks required for healing. Based on the size of the animal (e.g., an adult bull compared with a yearling heifer) and individual response to therapy, the exact recuperative time is difficult to predict. Response to therapy is usually good unless underlying nutritional deficiencies or fluorine toxicity exists. In the case of dairy bulls, the animal may require several additional weeks of sexual rest, lest the healing fracture be reinjured during dismounting a cow or an artificial insemination (AI) phantom.

Interdigital Fibroma

Redundant skin in the interdigital space is a hereditary condition associated with lax interdigital ligaments, resulting in a splay-toed conformation. It also occurs in cattle as an acquired problem secondary to chronic interdigital dermatitis. By itself, it is not painful unless the fibroma becomes so large that the cow pinches it between the sole and floor when walking. However, fibromas create a risk for foot rot and are common sites of digital dermatitis in endemically infected herds. For most dairy cattle, fibromas occur secondary to interdigital dermatitis and should not be treated as a specific problem but as a reflection of poor management of hygiene or foot bathing (Fig. 12.17). There exists some pressure from farmers on

veterinarians and hoof trimmers to remove fibromas as part of routine trimming, and this should be discouraged. Rather, the underlying causal factors should be addressed.

If the fibroma is a part of a significant painful process in a cow, then surgical removal is indicated. Anesthesia is discussed in the section on digit surgery. Sharp dissection of the skin around the base of the fibroma follows normal surgical site preparation. It is considered important for prompt healing to remove the interdigital fat and the protruding fibroma. Care must be taken to prevent surgical injury to the distal interphalangeal joint capsule and the cruciate ligaments when removing the fat. Some antibiotic powder may be placed in the wound, but no dressings or packings should be used before bandaging the foot to prevent splaying of the toes. The bandage may be removed in a few days because granulation tissue will fill the defect. Systemic antibiotics are optional.

Foot Rot or Interdigital Phlegmon

Recognition of this acute disease is straightforward. The bacterial causes are *Fusobacterium necrophorum* and *Bacteroides melaninogenicus*, with both required for disease to occur. There may be other important bacterial contributors from the genus *Prevotella*. The cow becomes lame over the course of a day or two with symmetrical swelling above the hoof. Pain may be severe with unwillingness to bear any weight on the affected limb. Rear limbs are more commonly affected. There will be a fissure in the interdigital skin with necrosis of the underlying tissues (Fig. 12.18). Usually this is a dry necrosis with no exudate, but some very virulent strains of *F. necrophorum* may produce tissue liquefaction. The odor of foot rot is strong and characteristic. Corrective claw trimming may be used along with some topical antiseptic to the interdigital space. Bandaging is strongly discouraged so that air may reach the interdigital tissues. Parenteral antibiotics are the most important part of therapy. For almost all cases of foot rot, any one of several types of antibiotics will be effective; hence the specific

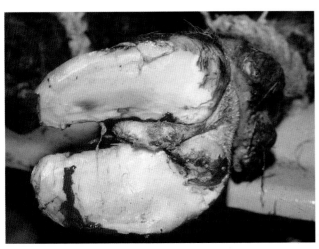

• **Fig. 12.17** Interdigital fibroma in a bull.

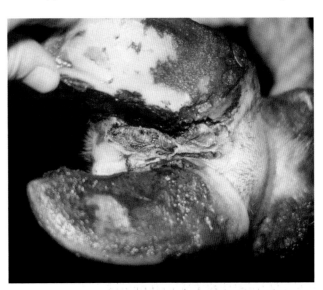

• **Fig. 12.18** Necrosis of interdigital soft tissues in a cow with foot rot.

agent chosen is unimportant. In the United States, as of this writing, ceftiofur is approved for the treatment of foot rot and requires no milk discard. Unfortunately, there are cases of foot rot caused by multiple drug-resistant *F. necrophorum*. Trial and error has determined that these cases respond to treatment with tylosin at label-recommended dosages. Tylosin is only approved for use in non-lactating dairy cattle in the U.S. Recognition of the presence of drug-resistant strains in a herd comes after treatment failure with the usual choice of antibiotic. It is important to verify that the disease problem is foot rot because many cases are diagnosed and treated by farmers or their employees. If the original problem was a sole ulcer, changing antibiotics will not help.

Interdigital Dermatitis, Heel Horn Erosion, and Heel Cracks

Chronic interdigital dermatitis caused by infection with *Dichelobacter nodosus* is very common in cattle that stand in moist environments. The presence of infection may be detected in subclinically affected cattle by nonpainful erosion or ulceration of the interdigital skin (Figs. 12.19 and 12.20). There is usually a moist, white exudate with a characteristic odor distinct from that of foot rot. The infection produces a mild irritation that results in underlying skin hypertrophy and may produce a faster growth rate of the adjacent axial hoof wall. Skin hypertrophy may result in an interdigital fibroma as discussed earlier or excessive horn accumulation along the axial wall. The axial wall may flare toward the interdigital space or cause an abnormally high region in the adjacent sole. Corrective trimming should remove all the excessive horn and open the interdigital space so that it is both more self-cleaning and more accessible to air. If the infection spreads across the heels, it may erode the horny portion of the heel in irregular patterns or create a transverse crack at the heel–sole junction. *D. nodosus* produces proteases that are capable of digesting the keratin of hoof tissues.

Lameness results from interdigital dermatitis when the cracks in the heel combine with hypertrophy of heel bulb skin to change the weight distribution, thereby increasing pressure on the heel. The subsequent tissue discontinuity from sole to heel may also result in pinching of sensitive tissues beneath these cracks. Cows are not usually severely lame but may stand with their heels suspended over the manure gutter or off the rear of a free-stall curb. Usually the problem is symmetrical in both limbs. Rarely, a crack at the heel–sole junction penetrates to expose the corium. Treatment for these heel cracks is to remove the flaps of overlying horn and open the enclosed spaces to air. A hoof block is indicated in the rare case of exposure of the corium. Topical disinfectants such as iodines or copper or zinc solutions are all effective in killing *D. nodosus*.

Digital Dermatitis, Mortellaro, or Heel Wart

This condition goes by a plethora of names including; hairy heel warts; strawberry foot; verrucous dermatitis; digital warts; interdigital papillomatosis; and probably most

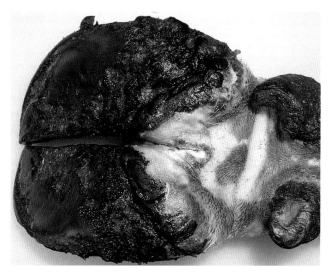

• **Fig. 12.19** Eroded and roughened heels and slight hypertrophy around the interdigital cleft as a result of chronic interdigital dermatitis.

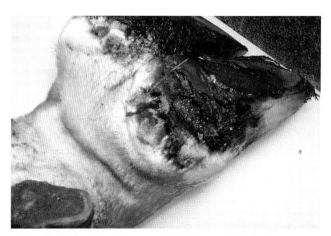

• **Fig. 12.20** Scalloped layers of heel horn typical of heel horn erosion.

correctly, digital dermatitis (or papular digital dermatitis). Since 1994, the disease has progressed to epidemic proportions in most of Europe and spread throughout the United States. One wonders why a disease that was reported originally in 1974 suddenly spread worldwide in dairy cattle in the past few years. Currently, researchers are still trying to define the specific cause(s); several strains of spirochete bacteria from the genus *Treponema* are believed to be responsible for the disease. Histologic specimens of lesions stained with silver demonstrate spirochetes in great numbers throughout the stratum spinosum of the dermis. Various research laboratories are applying genetic tools to characterize these spirochetes and are finding that several strains are usually present within a single lesion. Perhaps different strains or species may be implicated at different depths. Within a farm, the species are consistent but they may vary from farm to farm. There is speculation that some strains or species are capable of initial colonization and that other strains or species can then follow to establish deeper infections. Similar organisms are found in the rumen contents, feces and skin of cattle.

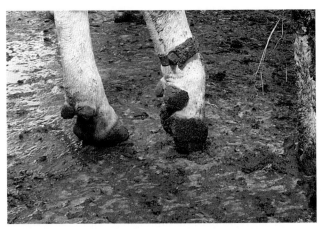

• **Fig. 12.21** Typical posture of a cow with digital dermatitis affecting the plantar surface of the pastern region.

The earliest lesion recognizable as digital dermatitis is a reddened, circumscribed area typically just above the interdigital cleft on the plantar aspect of the pastern; this is the strawberry form of digital dermatitis. The most striking consequence of the condition is the degree of pain expressed by the cow (Fig. 12.21). Hairs at the periphery of the lesion are often erect and matted with exudate to form a rim. As the lesion progresses, focal hypertrophy of the dermis and epidermis leads to raised conical projections appearing similar to wet, gray terrycloth. In even later stages, papilliform projections of blackened keratin may extend 10 to 15 mm from the surface; this represents the hairy wart stage. Typical lesions may be seen affecting any of the limbs, but rear limbs are more commonly involved. The location and extent of affected skin are variable and include interdigital skin, anterior and posterior margins of the interdigital cleft, and distinct lesions that do not touch the coronary band. Many cows have simultaneous infection with *D. nodosus*, leading to significant erosion of the horn of the heels in a hemispherical pattern surrounding the axial space (Fig. 12.22). The hoof may be noticeably misshapen from abnormal wear caused by the altered use of the limb, resulting in short rounded toes and exaggerated heel depth. Interdigital fibromas, regardless of etiology, are commonly infected with digital dermatitis organisms in endemic herds. In our experience, after digital dermatitis has been present in a herd for a year or so, most cases that cause lameness are found in the first-lactation animals even though lesions may be seen on the digits of older cows during routine hoof trimming (Fig. 12.23).

We recommend topical treatment of lame cows with oxytetracycline in the form of 5 to 15 cc of injectable 10% oxytetracycline applied on a cotton dressing with a flimsy wrap. Others use tetracycline powder under some form of bandage with or without a cotton pad. We have examined many of these cows after 2 to 5 days and have been amazed at the regression of the lesion and complete elimination of pain. Because the response is so rapid, we have come to use less and less bandage material so that the cotton will fall off in just a few days. Failure to remove bandages made from highly elastic materials has resulted in deep soft tissue

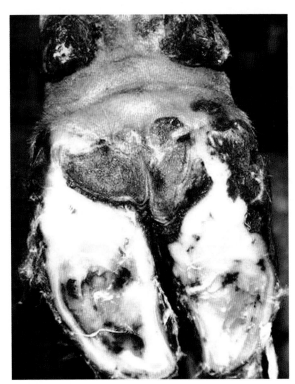

• **Fig. 12.22** Digital dermatitis lesion at the skin–heel horn junction with erosion of heel horn and extension of the digital dermatitis into the solar region.

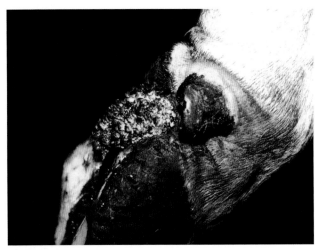

• **Fig. 12.23** Chronic, proliferative lesion caused by digital dermatitis.

fissures or even ischemic necrosis of bandaged digits. Unless the farm has a very reliable method of bandage removal, elastic bandage material is not recommended. A recent report compared a single application of chlortetracycline by spray with the use of salicylic acid under a bandage. Results were significantly better with the salicylic acid.

Unfortunately, reoccurrence in the same cow and even in the same location is common. Research has shown that some treponemes convert from a spirochete to an encysted form that may resist therapeutic efforts. Some cows in an endemic herd never develop lesions. However, all cows in endemic herds will have antibodies to at least two species of treponemes. Autogenous and commercial vaccines have come and gone with none proving efficacious in preventing the development of lesions. An apparently related skin disorder is udder cleft dermatitis on the ventral midline at the attachment of the fore udder. Histologically, this lesion is indistinguishable from digital dermatitis; both conditions are associated with the presence of spirochetes throughout the epidermis. Recent genomic evaluations of gut microbiota have identified the same treponemes in feces and rumen contents as in the skin lesions of digital dermatitis. Furthermore, both sheep and goats have been diagnosed with a similar digital dermatitis that contains the same species of treponemes as implicated in this condition in cattle.

Deep Sepsis of the Digit

Untreated or late-treated foot rot, complicated sole ulcers, white line abscesses that extend into retroarticular structures, and puncture wounds may all result in necrosis or infection of deeper structures important for weight bearing. These problems have in common severe pain that is not relieved by hoof blocks or analgesic medication. Specific diagnosis of the problem may be aided by using a probe to explore fistulous tracts or by inserting a hypodermic needle (14 or 16 gauge) into joints or tendon sheaths but rarely requires radiography (Fig. 12.24). Cows with deep digital sepsis are truly suffering, and a decision should be made at the first recognition of this problem to either euthanize, slaughter, or perform surgery. Too many cases receive no treatment or systemic antibiotics in the hope that the problem will somehow resolve spontaneously (Fig. 12.25). These cows deserve a more humane approach.

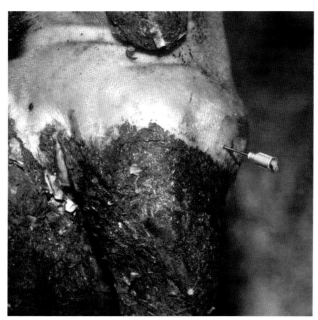

• **Fig. 12.24** Demonstration of pus in the distal interphalangeal joint. The joint capsule enlarges and bulges proximal to the coronary band when the joint is septic.

Surgery of the Digit

Pre-operative anesthesia is most easily performed by intravenous (IV) infiltration of lidocaine distal to a tourniquet on the metatarsus or metacarpus. Lidocaine without epinephrine, 20 to 30 mL, is infused using a butterfly catheter (19 gauge, 15–25 cm in length) (Fig. 12.26). Any accessible vein will result in complete anesthesia of both digits after a few minutes. If no vein can be found, regional perfusion above the intended surgical site is an alternative. The distal limb is scrubbed and disinfected as for any surgery but usually not shaven because the hair is typically very short or absent. Surgical procedures are commonly done in the field and are considered "clean" procedures but not sterile. The goal is to debride necrotic tissues and provide drainage for pus and exudate. If a hoof block is to be used as part of the therapy, it should be attached before the surgery because adhesives require a dry hoof to bond. Injecting the lidocaine followed by applying the block or

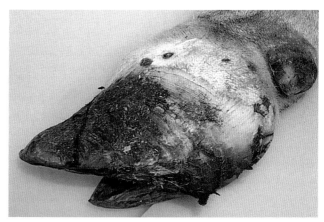

• **Fig. 12.25** Chronic deep sepsis of the digit. Note several fistulous tracts and the upward tilt of the affected digit. Destruction of the deep flexor tendon or its attachment to the third phalanx allows the toe to tip up. This slaughterhouse specimen showed no evidence of attempts at useful therapy.

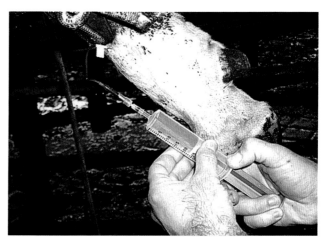

• **Fig. 12.26** Intravenous regional anesthesia with lidocaine injected into the common dorsal digital vein. A butterfly catheter is easier to maintain in the vein than a needle and syringe alone.

scrubbing the area ensures adequate time for diffusion of the anesthetic to all tissues distal to the tourniquet.

Digit Amputation

Amputation of one digit at the proximal interphalangeal joint or just above is a common procedure in cattle practice. After preparation, a skin incision is made in the interdigital space beginning about 2 cm proximal to the interdigital cleft angling upward to a point on the lateral or medial side of the leg even with the distal margin of the accessory digit or dewclaw. All soft tissues can be sharply incised along the line of the skin incision. Obstetric wire is then placed between the digits, and the distal end of the first phalanx is cut (Fig. 12.27). If the cut misses this landmark and a portion of the second phalanx remains proximal to the cut, it should be removed. If the articular surface of the first phalanx is intact, it should be roughened with a knife. Alternatively, the digit may be amputated by sharp dissection to disarticulate the proximal interphalangeal joint (Fig. 12.28). Some practitioners ligate one or two arteries, and others simply use a very tight bandage. The cut surface of the removed portion should be carefully examined for evidence of sepsis or necrosis. If damaged, necrotic tissue extends above the amputation and it is not debrided, the outcome will be poor. After determining that all diseased tissue is removed, the surface of the wound is covered with an antiseptic or antibiotic dressing and a bandage applied to control hemorrhage. The bandage should be removed or changed in about 1 week if there was no need for maintaining drainage of septic regions proximal to the incision. If a tendon resection is performed, the bandage should be removed in 2 or 3 days. Depending on the environment

in which the cow must live after surgery, either no bandage is placed after the first one is removed or a light wrap is used to minimize painful contact with environmental objects. Parenteral antibiotics are usually given for 5 days.

Flexor Tendon Resection

If, after amputation, it is evident that sepsis extends proximally along the deep flexor tendon, it should be resected. A 3-cm incision parallel to the path of the tendon is made over the affected flexor tendon branch beginning just proximal to the accessory digit. There is strong fascia surrounding the sheath of the combined superficial and deep flexor tendons. In fact, the superficial flexor tendon forms a tube around the deep flexor tendon at this level. Sharp dissection oriented along the skin incision through the superficial flexor tendon will reveal the deep flexor tendon. The deep flexor tendon is grasped with a strong instrument such as a dental extractor or exteriorized with the aid of curved hemostats (Fig. 12.29). There may be adhesions of the deep flexor tendon to surrounding structures at the level of the distal transection that require sharp dissection. In some cases, the tendon will simply be pulled to the outside from the proximal incision. The deep flexor tendon is transected at the most proximal exposed part, and surgical drainage tubing is placed through its original course to exit at the distal incision. It may be knotted into a loop or each end affixed by suture. One or two skin sutures are placed in the proximal incision. Systemic antibiotics are routinely given for 5 days. The drainage tubing is removed in 2 weeks.

Retroarticular Abscess

White line abscesses near the heel, penetrating foreign bodies, and deep flexor tendon avulsion or fracture of the flexor process of the P3 all may result in severe lameness with extensive painful swelling of the heel region of a single digit (Fig. 12.30). After anesthesia and standard surgical preparation, an incision is made into the heel bulb. The choices are a vertical incision extending into the sole (after paring away enough sole at the heel so that it is thin enough to make an incision with ordinary

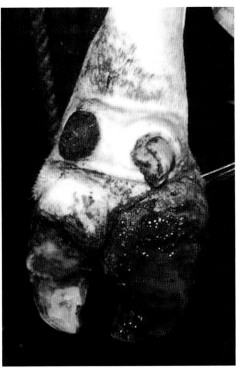

• **Fig. 12.27** Amputation of a digit with a wire saw.

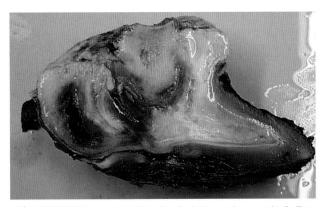

• **Fig. 12.28** Digit amputated by disarticulation and cut sagittally illustrating sepsis of the second phalanx, the third phalanx, the navicular bone, and the deep flexor tendon.

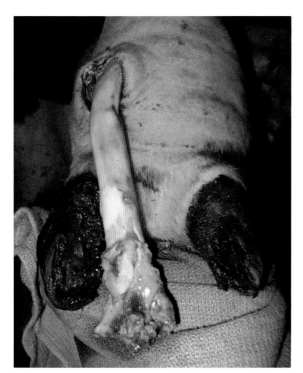

• **Fig. 12.29** Deep flexor tendon with severe inflammation at the distal end resected through an incision above the corresponding accessory digit. A surgical drain was placed in the space left by removal of the tendon and the proximal incision closed with sutures.

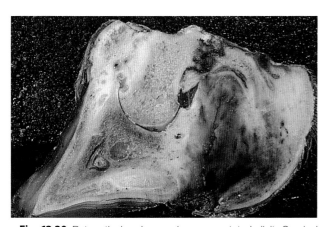

• **Fig. 12.30** Retroarticular abscess in an amputated digit. Surgical debridement and drainage are alternatives to amputation.

surgical instruments) or a transverse incision in the middle portion of the cornified heel. Exploration of the cavity encountered will dictate further steps. If the limits of the abscess or hematoma do not involve the navicular bursa or deep flexor tendon, the prognosis is excellent, and resolution should be prompt. The cavity is flushed with water and a mild disinfectant such as povidone–iodine. A surgical drain is inserted in the wound and affixed with sutures. Antibiotic powder is placed in the cavity, and the incision is closed with a few skin sutures. A hoof block should be placed on the healthy digit. If the condition resulted from mechanical disruption of the deep flexor tendon or an avulsion fracture of P3, there is

risk of involvement of the navicular bone and bursa. If no sepsis is evident, the outcome should still be satisfactory. The cow will probably need the hoof block renewed in 1 month, but no further treatment is necessary.

Septic Distal Interphalangeal Joint

When the distal interphalangeal joint is septic, there is enlargement of the joint space and distention of the joint capsule. This may be observed as painful swelling at the coronary band in the caudal third of the abaxial coronet. It is possible to insert a needle into the joint capsule through the coronary band to verify the nature of the joint contents (see Fig. 12.24). In cases when there is no swelling of the heel or deep flexor tendon, a simple fenestration of the joint may result in a satisfactory cure by allowing ankylosis. Septic distal interphalangeal joints occur most commonly secondary to foot rot or to a complicated sole ulcer. In either case, after distal limb anesthesia and cleaning of the sole, a 7- to 12-mm (⅜–½ inch) drill is used to fenestrate the joint. Beginning in the typical site for a sole ulcer, the drill is directed in a sagittal plane to exit the digit just at the coronary band on the dorsal surface (Fig. 12.31). This will satisfactorily provide drainage of the joint. Surgical tubing or braided nylon rope is passed through the drilled hole and tied around the abaxial side of the hoof (Fig. 12.32). A block is placed on the healthy digit, and systemic antibiotics are given for 5 days. The drain is removed in 2 weeks. Full ankylosis requires several months, but the cow will usually be sound without a block in 1 month.

Extensive Deep Sepsis of the Digit

Amputation is an acceptable therapy for extensive deep sepsis of the digit. However, claw-sparing procedures have been adapted for field use and provide excellent results. We have combined the transverse heel incision (Fig. 12.33) described earlier with drilling through the distal interphalangeal joint, navicular bone resection, and deep flexor tendon resection to resolve some extensive problems with deep sepsis. A hoof block should be applied before beginning surgery. The approach is as for a retroarticular abscess but includes incising deeply just proximal to the navicular bone. This will transect the deep flexor tendon if it is still intact. Through the same skin incision, a more distally directed incision is made to cut the distal attachments of the navicular bone and remove a wedge of tissue. In some cases, the navicular bone and its attachments are so necrotic that it has already disappeared or is easily removed through this incision, allowing visualization of the distal interphalangeal joint (Fig. 12.34). If the collateral ligaments are intact and difficult to incise, use a 5-mm (¼-in) drill to make a hole in the center of the navicular bone. Insert a stout metal rod or screwdriver into this hole to fracture the bone into two pieces. Each piece can then be grasped and twisted to

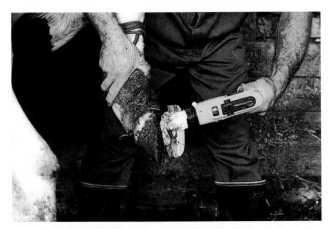

• **Fig. 12.31** Fenestration of the distal interphalangeal joint with a drill to provide drainage and facilitate ankylosis of the joint.

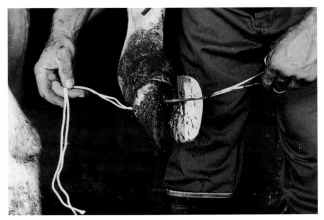

• **Fig. 12.32** Nylon cord placed through the drilled hole to maintain drainage. The cord is removed in 2 weeks.

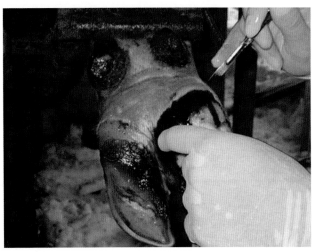

• **Fig. 12.33** Initial incision across the heel bulb for exploration of a digit with deep sepsis.

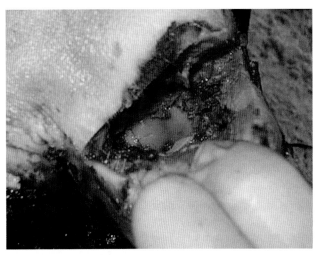

• **Fig. 12.34** Visualization of the distal interphalangeal joint after removal of the navicular bone.

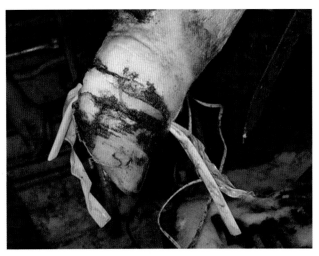

• **Fig. 12.35** Drains placed through the distal interphalangeal joint after drilling through the incision made in Fig. 12.33. Drains are removed in 2 weeks.

rupture any remaining attachments. A useful, inexpensive tool for this procedure is a canine dental extractor. If the flexor tendon is necrotic or septic, it should be resected as described earlier. Use a 7- to 12-mm (⅜- to ½-in) drill to fenestrate the distal interphalangeal joint through the incision. To exit at the coronary band, it is necessary to overextend the distal interphalangeal joint. Surgery tubing should be placed through the joint and secured in a loop around the axial side (Fig. 12.35). If the tendon was resected a drain should be placed there as well. If there was an existing fistula that is not connected to the transverse heel incision, it should also have a surgical drain. After all drains are in place, antibiotic powder is placed in the heel incision, and the incisions are closed with a few skin sutures. Parenteral antibiotics should be given for 5 days, and all drains should be removed in 2 weeks. We do not recommend wiring the toes of the two digits together as is done by others. The intended ankylosis of the distal interphalangeal joint will proceed more quickly if there is no motion in the joint. If the digits are fastened together, every step will cause motion of the joint that underwent surgery. The block may need replacement at 1 month post-operatively.

Functional Anatomy of Cattle Digits: What Goes Wrong That Results in Lameness

Introduction to Biomechanics

The structures of the bovine digit that support her body weight and work in normal locomotion can become diseased in a predictable fashion. The bones, tendons, ligaments, corium, and hooves are all potentially involved when things go wrong. A better understanding of biomechanical relationships within the digits of cattle can help with more rational therapeutics and appropriate preventive maintenance. The things that go wrong with bovine digits from a mechanical perspective are related to the environmental influences of moisture, infection pressure, and standing surfaces. The distance walked and the characteristics of the substrate walked on also contribute in a predictable way. This section describes the interplay between external forces and physiologic and pathologic events in the digits.

What we see as the current condition of the claws on any cow at a particular point in time is the result of continuous growth, continuous wear, and intermittent trimming. The growth rate of hooves is relatively constant but subject to minor modifications. Nutrition can influence hoof growth rate. Hooves do not grow as fast during starvation as during adequate feeding. Because dairy cattle are never intentionally starved, this effect is unimportant. A small variation occurs during the lactation and gestation cycles and with season. Most published reports on the effects of lactation and gestation are difficult to interpret because the cattle described calved seasonally. In a study we conducted at Cornell University on midlactation cows, growth rate was influenced by floor surface within the free-stall pens. Cows grew hoof faster on concrete than on rubber floors. The implication is that hoof growth can respond to environmental conditions by making more hoof when the standing or walking environment is more mechanically abrasive. Typical growth rates are about 6 mm of hoof wall per month with variations caused by environment accounting for less than 10% of the deviation from control rates. Wear rates are much more variable and depend on the abrasiveness of the walking surface and distance walked. Data are not available to compare the wear rates of dry versus wet hooves on the same walking surface but would be interesting and relevant to modern housing systems.

Why do we see more disease in rear feet than fore? Why is there more disease in lateral rear claws than medial? The rear versus fore predilection in dairy cattle has three components. Firstly, the rear limbs of dairy cattle are forced to carry weight in excess of the original design criteria. The wild-type individual that gave us our modern dairy cow never had a large udder, even at calving. As geneticists have selected for more milk production, we do not think they have been able to simultaneously modify the musculoskeletal system to accommodate this extra weight at the rear of the cow. Second, the forelimbs are attached to the body by relatively elastic components compared to the direct bony connections of the rear limbs. Concussive forces created during locomotion must be absorbed by the digital cushion and the flexion of the hock and stifle. Third, rear feet are inevitably more exposed to the bacteria and moisture within manure and urine. The skin near the hooves is more likely to become infected with bacteria as a result of maceration by this moisture, and the hoof capsule is softer because of greater hydration. The lateral versus medial difference is potentially more difficult to explain. Lateral claws grow about 10% faster than medial claws and wear about 8% more in free stall–housed Holsteins. Thus, lateral claws can progressively outgrow medial claws. They are larger even in fetal calves. Larger lateral claws are more heavily loaded than medial claws. This larger load probably results in greater potential for mechanical insult. Cows may adopt a toed-out posture to help equilibrate the weight between the rear claws when overgrowth and some discomfort occur. This toed-out posture, or being "cow hocked," can be used to signal the need to trim an individual cow or by population evaluation to determine when a group or herd needs trimming.

Body weight is supported by the column of digital bones, resulting in the load being approximately evenly divided between the eight digits when normal claws and conformation are present. P3 is the end of this column. The load on P3 is supported by several structures of importance in our concern for lameness. There are laminae in the mural corium that are tightly attached to the lateral and cranial portions of P3 and that interdigitate with laminae in the hoof wall. These have less surface area of mutual contact per unit of supported weight than in the horse. Therefore the laminar region of the bovine digit, although very important, is not as significant as it is in horses for support. There is also support for P3 from ligaments that suspend the caudal portion of the bone and blend with the interdigital cruciate ligaments axially and with the laminar corium abaxially. The tension of the deep flexor tendon on P3, in addition to fixing the bony column in a nearly vertical alignment, pulls the distal tip of P3 ventrally and transfers some weight forward in the claw. Between P3 and the solar corium lies a complex arrangement of fat deposits that cushion and distribute weight transferred to the sole. The fat pad is thickest at the heel and plays a dynamic role in cushioning during walking. The digital cushion has been specifically evaluated for its role in protecting against sole ulcers. Cows that have higher body condition scores have thicker digital cushions and are at a lower risk for sole ulcer. Causation has not been proven, but the association with thinness and lameness has been reported in several observational studies.

The structure of the horny capsule of the claw is different in different regions. Everyone who has trimmed a hoof knows this. The wall horn is the most rigid and hardest. It has the highest density of horn tubules that are arranged in parallel and develop from papillae in the coronary corium. The horn tubules are much less numerous in the sole, and this makes this region more flexible. The horn of the heel has the lowest density of horn tubules, and it is very pliable. The only nontubular horn of the claw is called the cap horn and is produced at the distal ends of the laminae. It serves to cement the sole to the wall and is visually identified as the white line. This cap horn seems particularly vulnerable to the effects of laminitis. It may fail mechanically, allowing the wall and sole to separate, or fall out in segments of the white line, allowing entry of foreign matter.

All of the horny tissue of the claw is able to absorb water. The higher the water content, the softer and more flexible the horn becomes. The most noticeable effect of continuous hydration of the claw is seen in the sole. If the hoof is dry most of the time the horn of the sole flakes away, leaving a concave surface and a relatively thin and consistent thickness of sole. This occurs by slight contraction of the cells of the sole during desiccation and fracture along horizontal planes during walking. Under dry environmental conditions, the moisture within the sole is derived from the corium, and diffuses at a constant rate into the sole, resulting in a constant thickness. In contrast, in free stall–housed cows, where slurry keeps the sole continuously moist, the sole does not flake away, and it must be worn down or trimmed.

When the events commonly known as laminitis occur, a vascular disturbance affects the corium of the laminae and the nonlaminar corium as well. The edema and resulting swelling reduce the ability of normal circulatory dynamics to oxygenate the corium. Some anoxic damage may occur. The mechanical properties of the corium are altered due to edema and anoxia with the consequence being lower tensile strength. As a result, P3 may move within the horny capsule to a greater extent than occurs normally in healthy claws. With the exaggerated movement of P3, two specific lesions may develop. If P3 moves closer to the sole, abnormal pressure may cause further anoxic damage to the solar corium. If mild, this may appear as hemorrhage in the sole at a later trimming. If severe, the solar corium may die, necrose and this results in a sole ulcer. In housed cattle, the ulcer is most common at the caudal portion of P3 in proximity to the flexor tuberosity where the sub-corial fat pad is thin, but in extensively managed cattle, this typically occurs under the distal portion of P3. The abnormal movement of P3 relative to the laminar corium may result in ruptured blood vessels that lead to hemorrhage. If the hemorrhage is very mild, it is later seen as a red line in the sole at the sole–wall junction or white line. If the hemorrhage is more extensive, it can result in a hematoma that later becomes either a sterile abscess or a septic abscess if the white line is separated and permits entry of environmental bacteria. Cattle that must make sharp turns on rough flooring may experience more white line lesions as a result of the lateral forces placed on the wall. During a turn, there may be claw deformation that can pull the wall from the corium or shear the corium if the structural integrity of the tissue is already compromised by edema.

It is important to note that the lesions of the corium that we recognize as, and call, laminitis require weight bearing during the period of primary damage to the corium. No one knows how long episodes of altered permeability and edema last after the chemical messengers from ruminal acidosis.

However, if the cow did not stand during that period, there would be no mechanical damage to the corium. In the vast majority of cases, the lesions within the claw that we call laminitis are the consequence of standing or walking on damaged corium. Standing is perhaps a worse insult to the corium than walking. With each step, there is normal movement of P3 within the horny capsule of the claw. This movement results in periodic perfusion of parts of the corium. When a cow stands without shifting her weight, these periodic changes in blood flow within the corium are probably interrupted. Thus, standing motionless is potentially more damaging to an already insulted corium than walking. As a curious observation, we have seen several down cows that have developed acute laminitis after 2 to 5 days in flotation tanks where they have been standing with the assistance of flotation for extended proportions of each 24-hour period. Whether or not these individuals have also experienced some degree of coincident ruminal acidosis caused by altered feed intake is unknown, but it is interesting to speculate that the forced standing, with very moist corium and potentially altered biomechanics caused by their primary problem, have conspired to cause the laminar separation and pain. Only in the rarest cases do the lesions of laminitis develop while cows are lying down. Thus, the greater emphasis in recent years on cow comfort and maximizing lying opportunities through time management and providing attractive lying surfaces are also potent anti-laminitis efforts.

Claws with abnormal shape, particularly of the ground contact surfaces, are more prone to mechanical insult to the corium. This is most commonly seen when excess horn production occurs at the axial border of the claws near the heel. The horn is probably being produced at an accelerated rate by this portion of the sole in response to stimulation by chronic dermatitis caused by D. nodosus, which is recognized to cause skin hypertrophy at the heels and interdigitally. Unfortunately, this site on the sole where an excess rate of horn production is observed is also that of the common sole ulcer. During weight bearing, the corium deep to the horn buildup will be compressed in a fashion similar to when excessive P3 movement occurs within the claw.

Complications of simpler lesions of the white line may occur when the pressure accumulating within the space between the hoof wall and the mural corium is not released to the exterior. The pressure within an abscess may be great enough to dissect along whatever path presents the least resistance. This may be proximally to the coronary band, axially across the sole, or caudally under the heel. Such abscesses result in greater disruption of the mechanical stability of the claw and necessitate greater horn removal.

Complications of sole ulcer are caused by extension of necrosis to the nearby structures adjacent to the coffin joint. The navicular bursa, deep flexor tendon, and coffin joint are all at risk of sepsis from free entry of bacteria through devitalized tissue. It is unclear whether necrosis of these connective tissue structures must precede invasion by bacteria or whether bacterial infection of a sole ulcer can extend into these other tissues if they are healthy. Penetrating wounds in this region can also have the same pathologic outcome.

Abnormally shaped claws may develop from genetic traits such as corkscrew claw or secondary to chronic or recurrent episodes of laminitis. These laminitic changes may manifest as concavity of the dorsal hoof wall as a result of displacement of the wall from the corium. Weakness of the capsule–corium attachment or corium–P3 attachment in conjunction with mechanical pressure on the hoof at the toe tip can result in turning-up of the toe. Care must be taken in trimming of these claws because Dutch rules will not work unless the dorsal wall is first straightened. The thickening of the white line may be more widely distributed around its entirety, resulting in laterally flared claws. The claw capsule may also seem to twist on its long axis because of laminitis, resulting in an acquired corkscrew claw, although this is distinct from the genetically mediated condition. It is likely that all of these claw shape abnormalities are at least uncomfortable for the cow to walk and stand on. In addition, they predispose to more severe lameness conditions as a result of abnormal loading of the corium. Thus, trimming is of significant value in restoring normal weight bearing to already diseased claws.

Risk Factors for Lameness

Lameness appears to be an increasingly important problem for adult dairy cattle throughout the world. There are both economic and welfare concerns that motivate producers and their advisors to seek answers as to the underlying causes. Specific causes of lameness can be divided into infectious agents that injure either the skin or underlying tissues of the digit with some effect on the horny claw capsule, internal injuries caused by metabolic or circulatory disturbances, and traumatic injuries. Any given cow can have one or more of these causes present to create a painful condition recognized clinically as lameness. The next section discusses what limited literature exists on the environmental risk factors contributing to herd problems of lameness and supplements it with anecdotal information gained in 34 years of examination of individual and herd problems throughout the Americas, Europe, and Australasia.

Environmental Risk Factors for Infectious Causes of Lameness

1. **Foot rot** is caused by specific pathogenic strains of *F. necrophorum* and *B. melaninogenicus* that gain entry through the interdigital skin. These bacteria can persist in wet soil or slurry for very long periods. They are also routinely present in the rumen and colon of cattle, although these are not necessarily pathogenic strains. Intact dry skin is resistant to penetration of both these organisms. Thus, conditions that produce breaks in the interdigital skin such as coarse sand or small stones becoming lodged in the interdigital space by walking through mud may predispose to foot rot. These conditions may prevail in cattle laneways, around water sources, or in riparian zones. Traditional control methods have been to fence cattle away from riparian zones and

mudholes. A different approach for cattle laneways that is in use in the United Kingdom is described by Dr. Roger Blowey from Gloucester. A 40-inch-wide walkway is constructed by excavating to a depth of 12 in. Eight inches of gravel or crushed stone is placed in the trench, covered with geotextile fabric, and the remainder of the excavation is filled with shredded bark. The laneway remains dry on the surface and stands up very well to traffic, and cows move comfortably along.

Foot rot in housed dairy cattle may be predisposed to by maceration of the interdigital skin, which is continuously moist. The severity of foot rot in housed dairy cattle is dependent on manure removal practices, which may influence both the infection pressure and the interdigital skin integrity. Footbathing with antibacterial compounds is a routine procedure to prevent new cases of foot rot.

2. **Interdigital dermatitis** is a chronic superficial infection of the interdigital skin caused by *D. nodosus*. It is very common in housed cattle, with visible lesions often present in the majority of cattle on a single farm, whether housed in free stalls or tie stalls. One reference indicates a lower incidence of lameness as a result of interdigital dermatitis on slatted floors compared to solid floors. Pain and lameness are not often present except in the most obviously infected cattle. Exposure to manure and urine predisposes to infection and influences the clinical severity. Most lameness caused by interdigital dermatitis is secondary either to skin (and possibly hoof sole) hypertrophy or to fissures in the heel horn caused by bacterial elastases that are capable of cleaving the beta-pleated keratin of the hoof. The main environmental risk factors seem to be manure contact with the skin and anaerobic conditions between the manure layer and the skin. Control is as for foot rot.

3. **Digital dermatitis** is an infectious disease of the skin affecting cattle older than about 6 months of age anywhere from the vicinity of the dewclaws distally. The causal organism(s) has not been conclusively identified, but response to therapy with antibacterial drugs and the consistent observation of spirochetes in affected tissues supports a bacterial etiology. Environmental risk factors are the same as for interdigital dermatitis, and the two diseases often occur together with some synergy apparent. Infection with *D. nodosus* may facilitate establishment of the *Treponema* agents of digital dermatitis. Dry conditions, as may occur in dry lots or some pasture conditions, seem to prevent spread of the infection but do not influence the severity in already infected cattle. Control is with footbathing or spraying with the antibiotics oxytetracycline or lincomycin. These, plus some antiseptic solutions including formalin, where permitted, can be used in footbaths for successful control.

Environmental Risk Factors for Claw Horn Diseases

Most concern for the prevention of laminitis has been focused on the nutritional management of cattle to minimize the occurrence of ruminal acidosis. Ruminal acidosis is probably a necessary but not independently sufficient condition for the development of the most commonly observed lesions associated with laminitis, namely, sole and white line hemorrhages, white line abscesses, and sole ulceration. Both environmental conditions and cow behavior appear to modify the final expression of the insult caused to the laminae and corium of the claws by ruminal acidosis. Subacute ruminal acidosis likely occurs in most dairy cattle in North America at some time during lactation. Despite this likely common occurrence, lameness is variable but may be severe in some herds. A great deal of experimental data are available on the ruminal effects of high concentrate diets, yet there are few data on the consequences of dietary manipulations on the claws of cattle. The reports of Manson and Leaver, Livesey and Fleming, and Peterse et al describe the incidence of laminitic lesions in small groups of cattle in experimental herds with dietary treatments that involved either high or low concentrate feeding levels relative to forage. In each study, there were more cases of lameness in the higher concentrate feeding groups. The groups fed low to moderate levels of concentrate were affected with some lesions of laminitis despite attempts to minimize the occurrence of ruminal acidosis.

One of the authors (CLG) participated in a trial of rubber versus concrete flooring in free-stall housing. The experiment was flawed by the cows available to populate the two barns; the groups were not well matched. Nevertheless, there were more lameness events in the cows living on concrete floors versus rubber floors. The consequences of standing on concrete are considered by many to be very important in the development of laminitic lesions. Pressure exerted on specific portions of the claw may contribute to the observed vascular-derived lesions of either hemorrhage or necrosis. Cattle claws are commonly shaped in less than desirable forms. When these misshapen claws are supporting a cow on an unforgiving surface, the localized pressure can contribute greatly to damage of underlying structures. It is these consequences that have led to our suggestion that barn floors be surfaced with something other than concrete and that routine trimming can prevent many of the more severe cases of lameness. It is of interest that the installation of rubber alongside feed alleys, in parlor holding areas, along alleys connecting pens to the milking parlor, and most recently, complete alley covering with rubber mats have been increasing. Thus far, there are no data on the effects of these changes on lameness, but our unquantified observations of cow behavior suggest that we are moving in the right direction.

Lameness incidence (4.75% of 12,010) in bullocks housed on slatted floors in winter in Ireland was twice that of bullocks housed in straw yards (2.43% of 2882). Similarly, a cross-sectional survey of Dutch dairy calves between 2.5 and 12 months of age observed more sole hemorrhages in heifers housed on slatted floors than in straw yards. Calves were examined on 127 farms. The prevalence of sole hemorrhage in straw yards was 5% compared with 45% on slatted floors. A comparison between 11 herds with chronic laminitis problems and 11 control herds was made over a 2 year period by Dr. Christer Bergsten in the vicinity of Skara,

Sweden. There was a correlation between the stall surface material, either concrete or a rubber mat, and the occurrence of hemorrhages. Fewer sole hemorrhages occurred in stalls fitted with rubber mats. The cows were in tie stalls, and bedding use was not found to influence the prevalence of sole hemorrhages, although it was described as minimal for all stall types. The only publication suggesting an effect of environment on laminitis in free-stall housing compared the problem in two herds with the same owner and stall design but managed differently because of the requirements of the manure removal system. The herd with a higher incidence of lameness used less bedding. Both the proportion of animals standing in the alleys and the proportion of animals standing half in the stalls were higher for the herd with more lameness. Increasing the bedding amount in the problem herd resulted in amelioration of the lameness.

Environmental conditions for dairy cattle thus appear to influence the development of laminitis in two main ways. First are environmental conditions that influence feeding behavior. Second are those conditions that predispose to excessive standing time and standing on concrete in particular. Both feeding and lying behavior tend to be synchronized activities within a group of cows. Observations on the behavior of cattle in experimental settings have shown that regardless of feed access, whether 100% can eat at once or 50% at once, most eating will occur in temporal clusters. When feed access is limited, the subordinate cattle will have less time available to eat and will slug feed more often. Second to overcrowding of the feeding space, heat stress probably influences feeding behavior the most adversely with regard to laminitis. Slug feeding is favored by heat stress because the majority of feed consumption takes place when the environment and the body temperature of the cow are comfortable. Heat stress and overcrowding therefore are the major environmental influences on feeding behavior for laminitis, mediating this influence via ruminal acidosis.

Standing time on concrete is heavily influenced by the environmental design of dairy facilities and modified by overcrowding and management activities. Natural synchronization of behavioral activities again leads a group of cattle to mostly lie down at the same time. Overcrowding of free-stall pens prevents some of the subordinate animals from access to a stall. When a stall becomes available, it may signal that the pen is ready to collectively eat or be milked, thus preventing a timid animal from lying down at all. Data from long-term observations of groups of cattle with known dominance structures showed that a very subordinate animal, usually a heifer, might stay in a stall during some group eating times. Reasons for this are speculative, but regardless, the result will be slug feeding by that animal when she does finally leave the stall. Subordinate animals are also more likely to stand entirely in the alley with the head placed in a stall or half in a stall. Interpretation of this behavior is that it provides a reduction in the danger posed by more dominant cattle. Housing first-lactation animals separately from older cows has often resulted in a reduction in the negative effects of these social interactions within the heifer population.

Standing in a free-stall pen is heavily influenced by the design of the free stall itself. Great attention has justifiably been paid during the past 35 years on improving the design of free-stall partitions, beds, and overall dimensions. Cow comfort has been a popular theme in the past decade with most of the emphasis being placed on the stall. This emphasis has in great part been driven by the desire to improve lying time to reduce lameness. The goal of free-stall facility design should be to provide a space for every cow. Cows should enter and exit freely, including lying and rising without interference, and ideally spend about 14 hours per 24 hours lying in the stall. Because mechanical loading of the claws contributes very importantly to the development of the lesions of laminitis, evidence of underutilization of stalls is a cause for alarm. Cows that have had an unpleasant experience in a stall are more reluctant to use a stall the next time it is available. Cows that stand half in and half out of stalls are often increasing the load on the rear digits and are doing so at an unnatural angle. Maintenance of the bedding in stalls is also critical for use and comfort. Hock lesions are a common complaint with many mattress stall designs because of the lack of adequate bedding at the rear of the stall. Plain concrete or hard rubber mat stalls with bedding appear to be the least desirable for overall comfort, utilization, and the development of hock lesions. One notable study made comparison of two free-stall designs using 43 heifers through late pregnancy and early lactation. One stall type was the Dutch comfort with side openings and outfitted with rubber mats. The other was Newton Rigg, which prevented side lunging and had no rubber mat over the concrete base. Lying time was increased, and standing half in stalls was reduced in the Dutch comfort stalls. There were more sole hemorrhages and six cases of acute lameness in the Newton Rigg stalls versus only one lame heifer in the Dutch comfort stalls.

For free stall–housed herds, forced standing time imposed by management activities may contribute to laminitis problems. The milking parlor should be sized to limit the holding period time to 3 hours out of every 24 hours, regardless of milking frequency. Other management activities such as bedding of stalls or veterinary work should be organized to minimize the intrusion on potential lying time.

In many herds in North America, laminitis has a pronounced seasonal occurrence. Late summer through early fall represents the peak in cases of white line abscess and sole ulcers. We believe that there are two primary environmental factors involved in this. First, cows experiencing heat stress will redistribute their meals to eat predominantly in the morning. This slug feeding increases the incidence of ruminal acidosis. Second, and of unknown importance relative to the increase in low rumen pH, is the increase in standing time. Cows stand huddled around waterers. They stand in the stalls, often concentrated where fans move the most air. Sometimes, apparently when stable flies (*Stomoxys calcitrans*) are bothersome, they stand in tight groups at one end of a pen. To avoid fly bites, the goal of a cow is to be in the center of a group where unfortunately the heat stress is likely maximal. Maybe they stand in the stalls because they perceive themselves to be cooler standing than lying down. For whatever constellation of reasons, the slug feeding and excess standing time lead to a large increase in the number of lame cows. Summer ventilation and strategies to cool cows have the possibility to significantly reduce this seasonal lameness problem.

Miscellaneous Environmental Considerations

Floor surfaces may contribute to lameness if they are uneven or have elevated protrusions as with small stones. The softness of moist hooves, as in most free stall–housed cattle, makes them more susceptible to traumatic lesions of the sole. Some floor grooving and some slatted floors have such large voids in the surface that the claws of cows can be injured as they push their claws into the grooves or holes. Small stones on solid floors may come from sand bedding that is not screened to exclude particles larger than about 5 mm or 0.25 inch.

Many herds have experienced excessive lameness when cows have been placed in facilities with new concrete. For the most part, these problems have been caused by excessive wear of the soles, leading to exposure of the corium. Prevention of this problem due to surfaces that are too abrasive at first can be achieved by dragging concrete blocks or scraping with a steel blade after drying and curing but before cattle are introduced to the barn.

Conclusions

Environmental conditions play a significant role in the occurrence of lameness in dairy cattle. Manure and urine in constant contact with the hooves and digital skin may predispose to entry of infectious agents that produce lesions in the skin and hooves, producing lameness. Control is enhanced when hooves and skin are clean and dry. Footbathing with antibacterial solutions in appropriately designed and located baths can reduce the incidence of lameness resulting from infectious causes. Laminitis is predisposed to by ruminal acidosis and augmented by standing on concrete. Design strategies to provide unimpeded access to feed for all members of a group will help minimize slug feeding. Standing time is heavily influenced by facility design. Comfortable stalls and heat stress prevention will greatly minimize the development of lameness resulting from laminitis.

Lameness Above the Digit: Sporadic Diseases

Most upper limb lameness is caused by trauma, although degenerative arthritis does occur occasionally in cattle. The outcome of any case will depend on the severity of the injury, what specific structures are damaged, and the enthusiasm the farm personnel have for nursing disabled or recumbent cows. Many upper limb injuries end in euthanasia or slaughter. It is important to determine a diagnosis and prognosis early for cattle that have no chance of recovery.

Most cattle do not warrant the expense of attempts at surgical correction of major tendon or ligament injuries, which, on the whole, are not very successful anyway. Good hospital pen conditions and management with soft bedding and no competition for food and water are essential. Antiinflammatory medication with steroids such as dexamethasone or NSAIDs such as flunixin, meloxicam, or ketoprofen is an important part of conservative medical therapy.

A second category of upper limb lameness is caused by infection either of muscles, tendons, or joints. Septic arthritis or tendonitis may occur from wounds but more commonly occurs in neonates as a result of failure of adequate colostrum management and poor passive immunity. Arthritis, synovitis and tendonitis caused by *Mycoplasma bovis* appear to be unique conditions that can affect young cattle, typically in the weanling through yearling age group.

Stifle Injuries

Stifle injuries occur most commonly in adult cattle and bulls. Mounting injuries, falls, slipping on poor footing, and exertional activity in downer cows cause most stifle injuries in cattle. Degenerative joint disease also may contribute to stifle injuries in older cows or bulls. Although many specific injuries have been reported for the bovine stifle, only the three most common injuries are discussed in this section.

Cranial Cruciate Ligament Injury

Typical signs of acute stifle lameness characterized by flexion of the stifle and just touching the toe to the ground suggest cranial cruciate ligament rupture. Joint distention may be obvious, and the tibial crest may be more apparent than normal. When weight is forced onto the affected limb or the animal is forced to walk, palpation of the stifle allows detection of an obvious "bone-on-bone" mobility within the joint and an audible "clunking" sound. The degree of pain varies but usually is moderate to severe, and the affected animal is reluctant to bear weight on the limb. Chronically affected cows who tolerate the associated pain may have a severe limp but continue to be profitable members of the herd (Fig. 12.36). A cranial drawer sign may be demonstrated if the animal will bear weight on the affected limb by standing behind the limb with the knees braced against the hock. A pull is exerted on the cranial proximal tibia, which will move back into its normal more caudal position relative to the femur. Although awkward to perform, one can also demonstrate this cranial to caudal instability in the stifle joint as the cow walks and bears weight via palpation from a similar position. In very large animals or animals that will not support weight, this test may not be helpful. Lateral radiographs may support the diagnosis because the femoral condyles appear caudal to the tibial spine, and the cranial joint space seems wider than normal (Fig. 12.37).

Treatment of cranial cruciate ligament injury may be conservative if lameness is only moderate, reflecting subtotal rupture. Conservative therapy consists of box stall rest, good footing, and systemic antiinflammatory therapy. If the

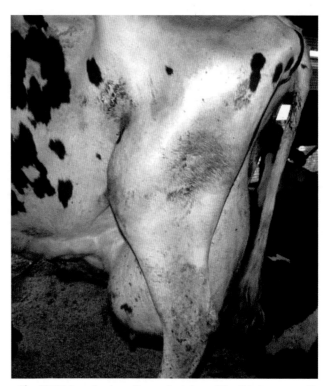

• **Fig. 12.36** Localized swelling and rotation of the tibia in a cow with chronic rupture of the cranial cruciate ligament.

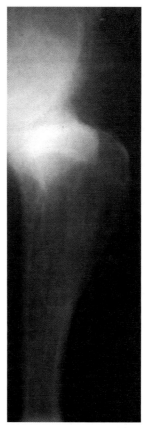

• **Fig. 12.37** Stifle radiograph from cow with a chronic cranial cruciate ligament rupture. The femoral condyles appear caudal to the tibial spine, and the cranial joint space is wider than normal. Degenerative joint changes are present.

affected cow is able to maintain body weight and production, this may suffice. If lameness is severe and obvious pain causes weight loss, poor appetite, and poor production despite conservative measures, slaughter should be considered. The only alternative treatment is referral for surgical procedures that may reduce the abnormal mobility within the joint (see Fubini and Ducharme, *Food Animal Surgery* 2nd edition, 2017). These procedures include attempts at artificial replacement of the cranial cruciate ligament (best) or imbrication procedures to tighten fascia around the joint. These have a low proportion of success in heavy cattle such as adult bulls.

The prognosis is always guarded for cranial cruciate ligament rupture because a cow cannot be managed as an individual in most herds unless the animal is extremely valuable. In addition, the risk of other musculoskeletal injuries increases, especially to the opposite hind limb. We have observed many cattle with cranial cruciate ligament rupture that develop the same lesion or other stifle injuries in the opposite limb within 1 to 2 years of the original injury. This may suggest a predisposition associated with degenerative joint disease or genetics in certain cattle.

Rupture of the Medial Collateral Ligament

Rupture or stretching of the medial collateral ligament results in an abducted limb and weight bearing on the medial claw. The injury is reported to be more common in heifers than adult cattle. Lameness is moderate to severe, and the animal prefers standing with the toe touching the ground and the limb held either forward or behind the normal perpendicular weight-bearing position. Palpation of the medial aspect of the joint usually reveals local sensitivity when digital pressure is placed on the collateral ligament. Radiographs are usually not helpful.

Conservative treatment consisting of box stall rest, good footing, and antiinflammatory medication usually results in improvement within a few weeks. If no improvement is observed, referral for imbrication is the only treatment option. The prognosis is fair for valuable cows that can be individually housed and managed but poor for cattle that must interact with herdmates because continued pain and reinjury are more likely.

Meniscal Injury

Trauma or progressive deterioration secondary to degenerative arthritis may result in meniscal damage or rupture. Nonspecific signs of moderate stifle lameness, including resting the toe on the ground with the stifle flexed and reluctance to bear full weight, are observed. Flexion of the joint may cause pain, but distinct clunking, as in cranial cruciate ligament rupture, is not evident. A palpable click or crepitus is apparent in some acute cases, and joint effusion may also be present. Synovial fluid analysis suggests hemorrhage, trauma, or degenerative joint disease rather than sepsis. Treatment consists of conservative measures as previously described or surgical referral if conservative therapy fails to alleviate the cow's pain. The prognosis is poor because degenerative arthritis either preexists or will likely follow meniscal injury or rupture.

Hip Injuries

The major hip injuries include coxofemoral luxation, fracture of the femoral head or neck, slipped capital femoral epiphysis, pelvic fractures involving the acetabulum, and rupture of the ligament of the head of the femur (round ligament). In heifers and adult animals, these injuries are caused by trauma such as; estrous mounting behavior; falls; slipping on poor footing; splitting the hind limbs by slipping or after obturator nerve paralysis; and struggling secondary to recumbency, myopathies, or neuropathies (Fig. 12.38). When cows struggle to rise on slippery surfaces, especially large cows with hypocalcemia, both hind legs may become splayed in a caudal position. This abnormal hindlimb position creates a high risk for coxofemoral injury. In calves, some of these conditions occur after forced traction during dystocia. Hip lameness resulting from inflammatory or degenerative arthritis (coxitis) also may result in similar signs but is less likely to be as acute as the aforementioned injuries. Septic arthritis of the coxofemoral joint is very rare in neonatal calves and even less common in older cattle. However, mycoplasmal arthritis can be seen in the upper limb joints, including the coxofemoral location in young, maturing animals in whom it is a cause of marked lameness and sometimes a noticeable rounded swelling over the hip (Fig. 12.39).

All of these hip conditions commonly result in severe lameness or recumbency. If the animal can stand, the stifle often will point outward. The animal is reluctant to bear weight, and the limb is advanced with a rolling outward motion and short stride that may cause the toe to drag. The history or posture of the patient may suggest the anatomic location of the problem. This is especially true if the caretaker observed the animal as she slipped and split her hind legs or if the cow tends to lie with the affected limb in forced extension. In newborn calves, a history of forced traction with a posterior presentation to relieve dystocia should arouse suspicion of hip injury or femoral nerve

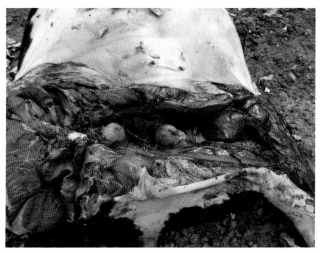

• **Fig. 12.38** Bilateral ventral luxation of the hip joints in a heifer. She was injured by penmates during estrus.

damage. If the affected animal can stand, the symmetry of the greater trochanter and pelvis (tuber ischii and tuber coxae) should be assessed. Craniodorsal luxations are most common, generally are not as painful as caudoventral luxations, and some affected cows may still be able to rise and stand on three legs. In craniodorsal luxation of the hip the affected limb may appear shorter (Fig. 12.40), the greater trochanter may be palpated in a more cranial position than normal (farther away from the tuber ischii), and the limb may be rotated outward. The animal will try to avoid any weight bearing on the limb (Fig. 12.41). In caudoventral luxation, affected cattle are usually recumbent, the greater trochanter may be difficult to palpate, and the femoral head sometimes becomes trapped in the obturator foramen (Fig. 12.42) where it may be palpated per rectum. In either dorsal or ventral luxation, excessive movement of the greater trochanter may be palpated when the limb is manipulated.

In femoral neck fractures, slipped capital epiphysis, round ligament ruptures, and acetabular fractures, crepitus and a grinding sensation will be detected when the limb is manipulated and the greater trochanter is palpated simultaneously.

Regardless of the exact diagnosis, manipulation to flex, extend, rotate, or swing the limb usually causes the animal pain. In recumbent animals, palpation and manipulation are the keys to diagnosis. If the animal is supported

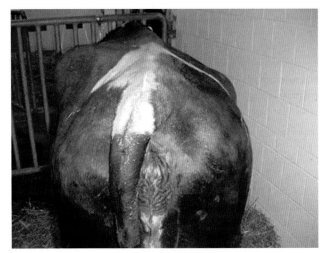

• **Fig. 12.41** An adult cow with right side craniodorsal coxofemoral luxation. Note the swelling over the displaced greater trochanter and the more ventral location of the right tuber coxae, which occurs because of a lack of pelvic support on the affected side.

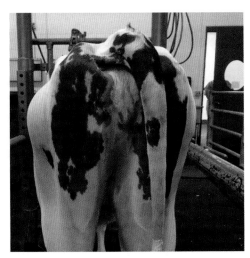

• **Fig. 12.39** A yearling Red and White Holstein heifer with a left coxofemoral joint infection and pronounced swelling over the area. Following joint aspiration and lavage performed standing on two occasions, in addition to systemic antibiotics, the heifer made a complete recovery.

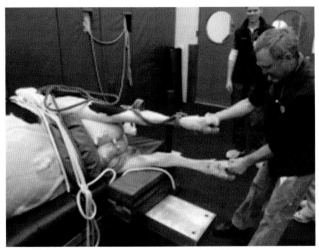

• **Fig. 12.40** A mature Holstein cow with a coxofemoral luxation. It can be noted that the rear limbs do not extend to the same length.

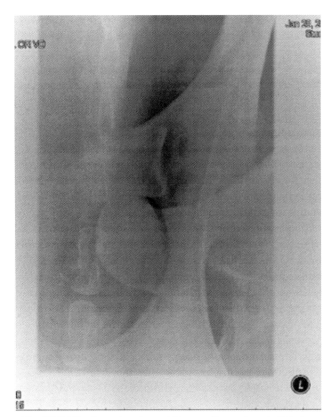

• **Fig. 12.42** Radiographs of an adult cow with caudoventral hip luxation.

by hip slings or other mechanical aids, the leg often is held extended, rotated outward, and is non–weight bearing. Flexion and manipulation of the standing animal (supported) may be done by an assistant while the clinician palpates the hip region externally and then performs a rectal examination to check for acetabular fractures, ventral hip luxation into the obturator foramen, other pelvic fractures, or crepitus in the case of femoral head or neck fractures. We have also used ultrasonography of the hip region to help confirm hip luxation (Fig. 12.43).

Radiographs may be required to confirm acetabular or femoral head fractures. Rupture of the round ligament has been reported in the literature to not be a serious problem. However, we have found that not to be true in all cases because we have managed a few very large and often older cows who have become acutely recumbent, unable to stand and who do not improve with analgesics or flotation tank support that have had rupture of the round ligament with hemorrhage in the immediate area as their only lesion upon euthanasia and necropsy.

The prognosis remains poor for most severe hip injuries and coxofemoral luxations. Therefore if a recumbent cow has obvious signs of hip luxation or a fracture in this area and cannot stand, euthanasia should be at least discussed. Ideally, radiographic visualization of the acetabulum and femoral head and neck should be performed on suspect cases promptly. Closed reduction of coxofemoral dislocation is more successful in our hands when performed promptly (<12 hours) after the inciting injury but is always challenging, not just from the perspective of relocating the femur into the joint, but also in terms of avoiding reoccurrence. For closed reduction of caudoventral luxation, the fact that the femur has moved under the ischium and often into the obturator foramen makes the procedure very challenging because one has to first "lengthen" the limb by pulling the femur while externally rotating it and then either guide it dorsally and internally rotate it back into the joint or hope for spontaneous relocation, often signaled by a gratifyingly palpable and audible "clunk" (see Video Clips 12.1, 12.2, and 12.3). The distance and force required to "pull" the femur out from under the pelvis is typically beyond human strength; hence, pulleys or a calf-jack should be used. From postmortem examinations (Figs. 12.44 and 12.45), it is evident that quite significant hemorrhage can occur into the acetabulum in association

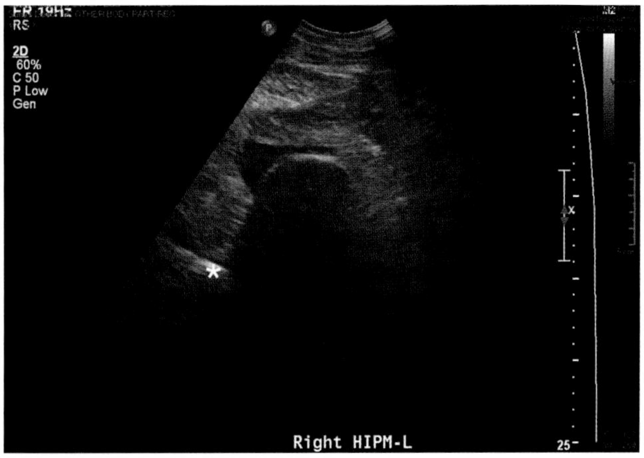

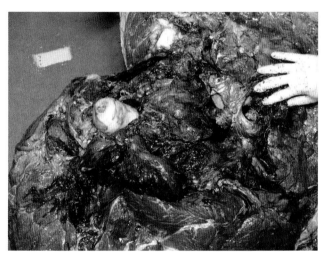

• **Fig. 12.44** Postmortem image of right traumatic coxofemoral luxation in a mature Holstein cow demonstrating substantial hemorrhage in the adjacent thigh musculature and blood clot and hemorrhage within the acetabulum (at the fingertips of the gloved hand).

• **Fig. 12.43** Sonogram of the right hip area of an 850-kg, 8-month pregnant cow that had fallen on the ice 2 days earlier and that had not been able to rise. The sonogram shows obvious displacement of the ball-shaped femoral head from the acetabulum. The acetabulum is not visualized but would be nearly in line with the ilium which can be seen *. The cow was euthanized due to the diagnosis of coxofemoral luxation and size of the cow, recumbency for 2 days and inability to get up on the other limbs even with assistance. On necropsy the cow had a craniodorsal luxation.

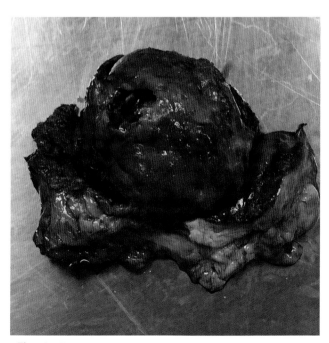

• **Fig. 12.45** Organizing hematoma removed from the acetabulum of the coxofemoral joint during a postmortem examination performed 4 days after luxation. Despite its appearance, this is not an image of the femoral head.

with dislocation, and the longer the clot has to "mature," the more of a physical obstruction it will become to relocation of the femoral head, providing an even greater time impetus to accurate diagnosis and repair. Significant hemorrhage and adjacent thigh muscle damage exacerbate the challenges that accompany any delayed attempts at closed reduction (see Fig. 12.44). At the University of Wisconsin, we routinely heavily sedate or anesthetize adult cattle with physical examination findings consistent with coxofemoral luxation to not only accurately diagnose the problem radiographically but to also facilitate subsequent attempts at closed reduction. Soft tissue swelling, muscle contracture, and pain, all of which worsen with time, make the necessary manipulations all but impossible without the relaxation and relief brought on by at least heavy sedation. For craniodorsal dislocations, the femur is simultaneously pulled down and abducted initially to bring the femoral head lateral to the ilium and to "lengthen" the limb, and then with forthright pressure applied pushing medially over the greater trochanter, the femoral head is pushed back into the acetabulum (personal communication, Drs. Paul Manley and Sheila McGuirk). Again, a gratifying "clunk" will often be palpable and audible by the individual applying the pressure over the femur. The care of adult cattle after relocation of a dislocated hip can be challenging if one wishes to avoid redislocation or catastrophic femoral and pelvic injury. We typically manage such cattle in a sling and with the use of a flotation tank, not permitting the animal to lie down for 10 to 14 days after the injury (Fig. 12.46).

This conservative approach regarding the duration of sling and flotation tank use is hard won from experience of cattle repeating the dislocation as they attempt to rise from a lying position, even if hobbled or assisted to stand by watchful caretakers. Cattle that are not allowed to lie down become exhausted but if supported in a sling will learn to eventually relax and "hang" for periods of time (see Fig. 12.46),

especially if given a little sedation. We have even used this approach successfully when open surgical reduction has been performed and have found that dry cow teat sealant can make an effective waterproof barrier for the skin incision while these individuals are in a flotation tank. As mentioned, we have tried open surgical repair of hip luxation in some valuable, recumbent cows that could not stand before surgery, but unfortunately, very few have recovered. In valuable calves or cows that warrant further diagnostics, radiographs of the pelvis and hip are essential to accurately diagnose, prognose, and offer treatment options, especially if the animal is able to rise and support weight on the three normal limbs, in which case either nonsurgical or surgical replacement are options.

Coxofemoral luxation in calves and adult cows must always carry no more than a fair to guarded prognosis. According to the literature, valuable cows that can rise on the opposite limb may be best treated by open reduction (Fig. 12.47), although this will necessarily only occur for those that are close to a surgical referral facility. The prognosis is better for younger animals and cows that are able to get up and down using the normal opposite hind limb. Recumbent animals that are heavy or have bilateral hip lesions are not good candidates for surgical treatment and have a grave prognosis.

Femoral head and neck fractures, acetabular fractures, rupture of the round ligament, and slipped capital epiphysis carry a guarded to poor prognosis in large heifers or cows. In calves affected unilaterally, surgery may be attempted for repair of some of these conditions, but still with a guarded prognosis in most instances. Reduction with intramedullary pinning has been successful in some calves and young cattle with a slipped capital femoral epiphysis.

Fractures of the wing of the ilium ("knocked-down hip") are relatively common in adult dairy cows and result in an obvious ventral drop of the tuber coxae on the affected side (Fig. 12.48). Initially, there is pain upon palpation of the area and some degree of lameness, but after a few weeks, many animals are nearly sound. If a sequestrum is present

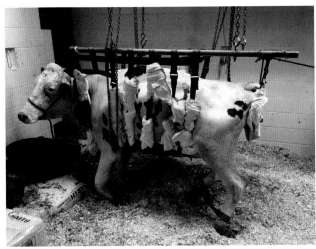

• **Fig. 12.46** Holstein heifer being managed with hobbles, in a sling, and with the use of a flotation tank after closed reduction of coxofemoral luxation. The heifer made a full recovery after 12 days in a sling post-reduction.

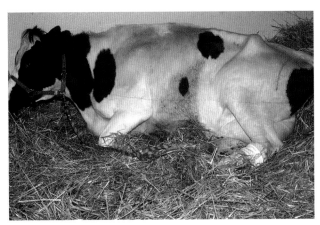

• **Fig. 12.47** A 3-year-old cow that has had surgical repair of a coxofemoral luxation. The halter is loosely tied to the leg that has been repaired to force the cow to lie down on the opposite side. She is housed in a dirt stall with straw bedding.

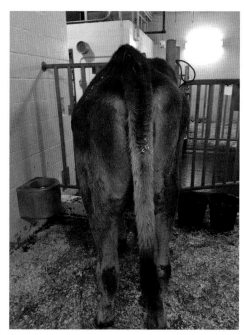

• **Fig. 12.48** An 18-month-old Brown Swiss heifer with a fracture of the left wing of the ilium ("knocked down hip"). The heifer was minimally lame as the fracture had occurred several weeks prior; she was presented to the hospital for decreased appetite which was determined to be a result of a LDA.

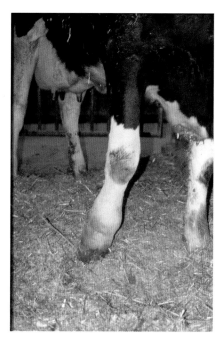

• **Fig. 12.49** Closed fracture of the right distal metacarpus in 2-year-old heifer. Injury was sustained by sudden "flight-or-fright movement" while the forelimb was extended under a stall divider.

or a wound occurs at the time of the initial injury, abscessation of the area may occur. If those are present, surgical intervention may be required to remove the sequestrum and drain the abscess.

Fractures

Although relatively uncommon, fractures require immediate attention and expertise in orthopedics for proper management. The bovine practitioner seldom gets enough experience with fractures to become an "expert" but may handle common fractures, especially those of the lower limbs, on the farm. Economics may preclude the referral of certain cattle or calves for internal or external fixation of fractures, but referral remains the best decision for upper limb fractures involving the tibia, humerus, femur, radius, and ulna. A full discussion of fractures is beyond the scope of this text, and readers are referred to several excellent references concerning bovine fractures such as *Farm Animal Surgery,* 2nd edition, by Fubini and Ducharme.

The diagnosis of a closed fracture is based on non–weight-bearing lameness, limb deviation, and crepitus in the region of the limb deviation. In open or compound fractures, the bone may be grossly visible. Radiographs are required for prognosis in complicated fractures or luxation and are always helpful for decisions regarding initial management and follow-up assessment.

The most common bovine limb fracture in dairy practice involves the metacarpus of young heifers in free-stall housing (Fig. 12.49). Presumably, the forelimb is extended laterally beneath a stall divider during rising, with the divider

as the fulcrum under which the metacarpus fractures. The distal epiphysis is always involved. At the time of examination, there may be minimal displacement of the fracture but severe pain on manipulation. Sedation with xylazine and placement of the patient in lateral recumbency with the affected limb uppermost allow easy alignment of the distal limb and cast application. A fiberglass cast is placed from the hoof to about 10 cm above the distal end of the radius (Fig. 12.50). The cast is removed in 4 to 6 weeks with an excellent prognosis for a normal lifespan.

Fractures of the distal metacarpus or metatarsus are occasionally seen in newborn calves resulting from excessive torque being applied during forced extraction from the uterus. Usually the obstetric chains have been malpositioned in the metacarpal area. These fractures may be associated with vascular compromise to the limb distal to the fracture site because of the "tourniquet effect" of the obstetric chains that caused the fracture or because of sharp bone fragments lacerating vessels supplying the digit. If the tissue distal to the fracture is cold, the prognosis is grave. Calves carry a much better prognosis than adult cattle for fractures in general, and noncontaminated closed fractures have a better prognosis than compound fractures (Fig. 12.51). Standard treatment for metacarpal and metatarsal fractures uses either half-limb or full-limb casts, depending on the anatomic site of the fracture and the size of the animal. A fair to good prognosis is in order for promptly attended noncontaminated fractures of this type.

Fractures above the carpus or tarsus (or involving these joints) require more detailed assessment and planning for successful management. Referral is suggested if the value of the animal warrants this approach. When economics are a concern but the owner wishes some treatment to be

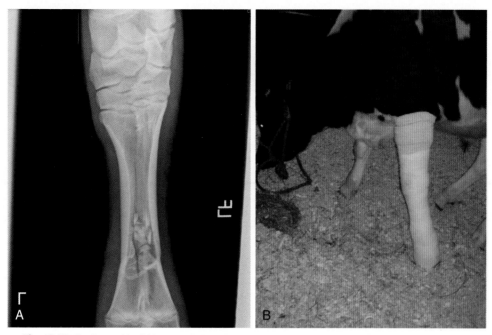

• **Fig. 12.50** Radiographic (**A**) image of closed mid-distal metacarpal fracture in 10-month-old Holstein bull, successfully managed with fiberglass casting to the level of the proximal forearm (**B**). (Courtesy of Dr. Sabrina Brounts.)

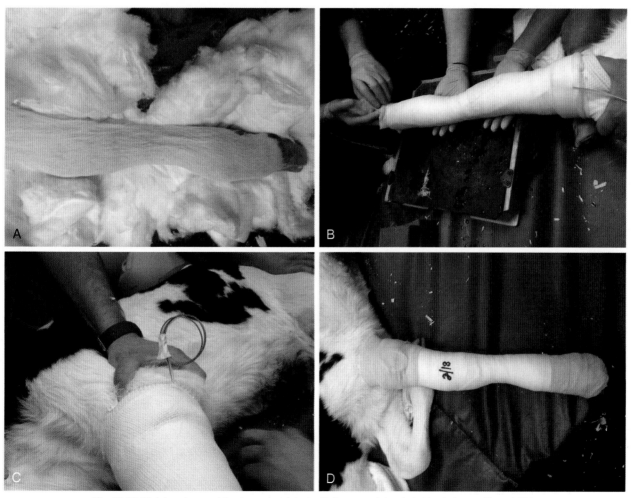

• **Fig. 12.51** Distal metacarpal fracture associated with inappropriate obstetric chain use (**A** and **B**) in a neonatal calf being treated with a fiberglass cast (**C**). Note the wires being incorporated within the cast material (**D**) to facilitate removal at the first cast change. (Courtesy of Dr. Sabrina Brounts.)

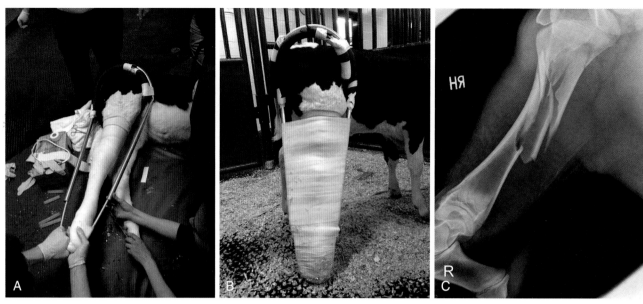

• **Fig. 12.52** Fiberglass limb cast being applied (**A**) and supported with a Schroeder-Thomas splint (**B**) for treatment of a closed tibial fracture in a 3-month-old Holstein calf (**C**). (Courtesy of Dr. Sabrina Brounts.)

attempted, the clinician must use his or her best judgment. Many humeral fractures in calves and heifers have healed with the only treatment being box stall rest. Femoral, tibial, and radius-ulna fractures are not as likely to heal without internal or external fixation. Full-limb casting may suffice for hock and carpal fractures or luxations and for distal radius–ulna fractures. Tibial and femoral fractures are difficult to manage in a field situation and are best managed by modified Thomas splints or internal fixation (Fig. 12.52).

Owners must be made aware of the severity of the problem and informed that referral, hospital-based treatment will likely be very expensive. Therefore, only very valuable or potentially very valuable calves and cows are referred for repair of upper limb fractures. When referring fractures, the practitioner should personally attend to a supportive bandage, splint, or cast, prior to transportation depending on the size of the animal and the bone involved. The support should extend dorsally beyond the joint above the site of the fracture. In this way, transport can be accomplished safely without worsening the injury.

Long bone or vertebral fractures occurring as an epidemic problem in a group of growing animals signals metabolic disease, and nutritional consultation to assess calcium, phosphorus, and vitamin D concentrations in feed is imperative. In modern dairy calf rearing, pathologic fractures and limb deformity associated with rickets caused by hypovitaminosis D have become extremely rare.

Rupture of the Gastrocnemius Muscle or Tendon

The gastrocnemius muscle and tendon in cows are critical structures for normal rising and weight bearing. Rupture of either prevents weight bearing in the affected limb and usually carries a hopeless prognosis. Cattle with hypocalcemia that make repeated efforts to rise or struggle to rise on a

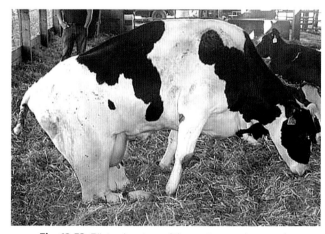

• **Fig. 12.53** Bilateral rupture of the gastrocnemius muscles.

slippery floor are at risk for gastrocnemius rupture. Occasionally, younger animals may be affected if trapped in mud or deep manure or if they have neurologic conditions that cause them to struggle excessively to rise. Tractor front-end loader accidents have also resulted in traumatic gastrocnemius rupture. However, an adult cow with a recent history of hypocalcemia represents the typical patient.

An inability to rise is the typical complaint reported for adult cattle affected with this condition. Usually one limb is affected, but rare cases of bilateral rupture have been observed. The classic appearance of gastrocnemius muscle rupture is described as a "rabbit leg" with the point of the hock resting on the ground such that a 90-degree angle exists between the tibia and metatarsus (Fig. 12.53). Because many heavy cows with gastrocnemius rupture fail to rise even halfway when attempting to get up, the clinician always should stand at the animal's rear to observe the condition when stimulating a recumbent cow to rise. In many cases, the tear occurs within the muscle belly itself and is

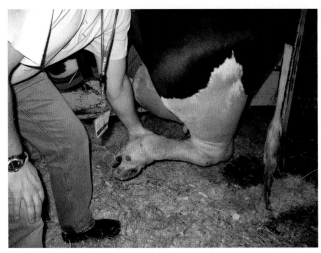

• **Fig. 12.54** Unilateral rupture of gastrocnemius muscle on the left side. Note the significant swelling and hematoma formation on the laterodistal aspect of the musculature.

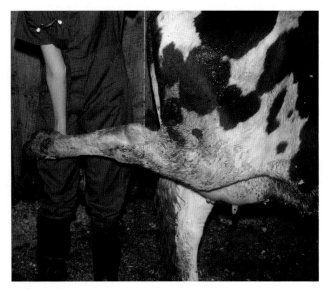

• **Fig. 12.55** Rupture of the fibularis (peroneus) tertius in a recently fresh Holstein cow.

associated with obvious hematoma formation in the distal part of the muscle (Fig. 12.54). The affected gastrocnemius muscle is firm and swollen because of hematoma formation around the rupture site, and the tendon proximal to the hock is relaxed. Less commonly, the gastrocnemius tendon has been ruptured in the area of its origin at the junction of the tendon and muscle belly. These cases can be a bit more challenging diagnostically because less swelling is involved with little to no hematoma formation or muscle swelling. If tendinous rupture is complete, then the animal may be recumbent (predictably so if the injury is bilateral), and it is possible to miss the diagnosis in what will be a down cow. Careful palpation of the gastrocnemius muscles and tendons along their entire length is an important part of the physical examination of a down cow.

Although most cases have complete rupture, partial rupture may occur, resulting in severe lameness in the affected limb; a slightly dropped hock; and a tense, firm swelling in the affected gastrocnemius muscle. The animal can support some weight but prefers to rest the limb in a forward fashion by extending the stifle and flexing the fetlock.

Treatment for adult cattle with complete rupture of the gastrocnemius muscle or tendon is likely hopeless. Calves and younger animals with the problem that can still rise to stand on three legs may be confined to a box stall with good bedding and footing for several months, but the prognosis usually is guarded for these animals as well. Application of a lightweight splint that limits flexion of the tarsal joint while allowing normal extension of the fetlock joint may improve the prognosis.

Rupture of the Fibularis Tertius (Peroneus Tertius)

Rupture of the fibularis tertius muscle, formerly referred to as the peroneus tertius, results in an inability to flex the hock, therefore preventing the normal reciprocal flexion of the hock when the stifle is flexed. Excessive struggling to rise on a

slippery floor with or without concurrent hypocalcemia and slipping backward while trying to rise or mount another cow are the usual causes of rupture of the peroneus tertius.

An extended hock while the stifle flexes results in an inability to advance the limb normally. The toes are dragged, and the dorsum of the pastern or fetlock may sustain abrasion. The gastrocnemius muscle and tendon appear relaxed. As a pathognomonic diagnostic test, the stifle can be flexed with the hock fully extended (Fig. 12.55). A swelling on the craniolateral aspect of the distal tibia and hock joint of the affected limb can sometimes be noticed (Fig. 12.56 A, and B).

Although the prognosis is guarded at best, some affected cattle may recover if placed in a box stall with good footing.

Flexor Tendon Lacerations

The most common cause of laceration to the superficial and deep flexor tendons of the hind limbs is sharp trauma from scraper blades on tractor-mounted manure scrapers in free-stall barns. Alternatively, attendants cleaning stalls with sharp implements may startle a cow that then kicks out and contacts the sharp end of a shovel or other tool. Cattle may also become entangled in a myriad of circumstances and lacerate tendons during their struggle to escape.

Lacerations involving only the superficial flexor tendon allow the limb to bear full weight but will be associated with a slight increase in dorsiflexion of the digit if the superficial flexor is completely transected. In such cases, a thorough inspection of the wound is necessary to rule out partial laceration of the deep flexor, which may progress unless supported more intensively than normal therapy for simple superficial flexor tendon injury. Lacerations that involve both the superficial and deep flexor tendons result in inability to bear weight; the plantar aspect of the fetlock contacts the ground when the animal attempts to bear weight on the affected limb, and the toes point dorsally.

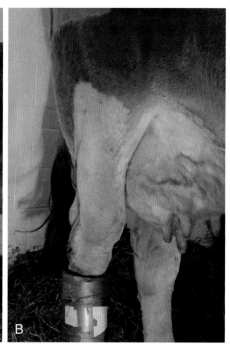

• **Fig. 12.56** A 4-year-old Brown Swiss cow with a right ruptured fibularis (peroneus) tertius (**A**) and swelling over the area of rupture (**B**).

If only the superficial flexor tendon is lacerated, the wound should be cleaned and irrigated and a sterile dressing applied with adequate pressure to prevent exuberant granulation tissue. The wound should be redressed at 3- to 7-day intervals. Antibiotics should be administered for 10 to 14 days.

If the superficial flexor tendon is lacerated and the deep flexor partially lacerated, a splint or cast should be considered because continued stress on the compromised deep flexor tendon could cause a complete rupture. If both the superficial and the deep flexor tendons are lacerated, a splint or cast is required after clipping, cleaning, and irrigation of the wound. For calves and heifers, splints work very well; for adult cattle, however, casts are necessary to withstand the greater weight-bearing stress. Before splinting, the wound is protected by a sterile bandage, and heavy cotton rolls are applied from the ground to the top of the hock. Gauze wrap is used to secure the cotton rolls, and the heel is raised 2.5 to 3.75 cm off the ground with a block or rubber wedge. A piece of polyvinyl chloride (PVC) pipe that has been measured for fit and split lengthwise is then applied to the plantar aspect of the limb from the ground to the top of the hock, and the entire apparatus then is pressure wrapped with strong self-adherent tape. It is important to incorporate the block or wedge pad under the tape to keep the heel raised, thus alleviating tension on the damaged tendons. A waterproof bag or piece of rubber may be applied to the portion of the splint contacting the ground to prolong its life. The animal should be confined to a box stall, and antibiotics should be administered for 1 to 2 weeks. The splint

will need to be changed every few days for the first 1 to 2 weeks and then weekly until 6 to 8 weeks have elapsed. Xylazine is sufficient for sedation and restraint of calves and heifers during this procedure.

For casting, the wound is prepared as with splinting, but only a light sterile dressing is applied followed by a stockinet and the cast. Cast changes are more time consuming than splint changes; therefore adequate restraint under either heavy sedation or anesthesia are necessary during the procedure to prevent reinjury of the healing tendon. Adult cattle may require 6 to 12 weeks in a cast to allow complete healing.

Improper application of the cast or splint and infection of the tendon sheath constitute the major complications. Both casts and splints are in place for extended periods, with only occasional, intermittent veterinary rechecks; therefore it is important to elicit the client's help and educate him or her regarding what to look for to avoid cast or splint complications. The mechanical forces imparted, even by calves, but especially by heavier animals, can result in splints or casts moving from their desired location and skin wounds becoming infected all too frequently from rubbing or loosening. Animals with splints or casts are ungainly and awkward, so one cannot always rely on worsening lameness as a corroborative sign of a complication. Fracture of the limb proximal to the cast has also occurred rarely when the cast application has been improper or patients are housed on slippery floors. In general, the prognosis is fair to good for calves and heifers with flexor tendon lacerations but only fair at best for adult cattle because they have a higher complication rate.

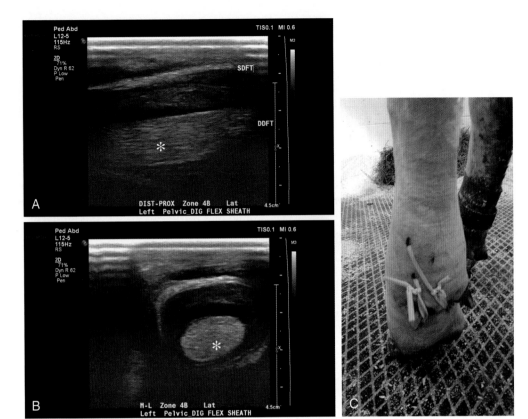

• **Fig. 12.57** Longitudinal **(A)** and cross sectional **(B)** sonographic views of an adult cow with severe lameness due to septic tenosynovitis involving the deep flexor tendon (*) proximal to the left hind fetlock. Excessive mixed echogenicity fluid with fibrin and peritendinous thickening can be seen on both images. The superficial flexor tendon appears compressed possibly due to excessive fluid and inflammation. Surgical drainage of the area was performed **(C)** and both local (regional perfusion) and systemic antibiotics were administered. The lameness improved for a period of 3 months, but the cow was eventually euthanized due to persistent problems in that limb.

Degenerative Arthritis

Degenerative arthritis may be secondary to poor conformation such as extremely straight hind limbs or abducted forelimbs. Previous septic arthritis or osteochondrosis lesions also may contribute to degenerative joint changes. Overnutrition of bulls and genetic factors also have been considered as potential contributors to this condition.

Joint effusion, reduced range of motion in affected joints, a stiff gait, muscle atrophy, and a slow progressive course suggest the diagnosis. Radiographs confirm loss of articular cartilage and osteophyte production within the affected joint or joints. The major joints of the hind limbs are most commonly affected, but occasional cases occur in the shoulder or carpal joints in the forelimbs.

Although no specific treatment is possible, analgesic antiinflammatory treatment with NSAIDs may relieve the animal's pain and allow continued production. In working bulls, these drugs may allow continued semen collection with the use of electroejaculation. Intraarticular corticosteroids may provide transient improvement but contribute to further degeneration of the joint with time. Hyaluronic acid and other intraarticular medications used in horses also may

be beneficial but seldom are used in cattle because of the expense. They may find use in valuable breeding cattle or bulls in AI facilities. Recently, acupuncture and other nontraditional therapies have been used with some success in the treatment of valuable bulls with degenerative arthritis, especially of the vertebral column.

The prognosis is guarded to poor because the condition is progressive. Some animals survive for 1 or more years if kept in comfortable surroundings and treated symptomatically. However, continued deterioration of the joint(s) may eventually cause so much pain that weight loss secondary to musculoskeletal injuries and loss of production are inevitable.

Septic Arthritis

Infectious arthritis is a common problem in dairy calves and a sporadic problem in older animals. A plethora of organisms have been isolated from septic joints in cattle, reflecting the variety of primary endogenous and exogenous sources of infection. Fever and acute lameness are apparent in most cases. The causes, means of diagnosis, and treatment of septic tenosynovitis (Fig. 12.57 A, B, and C) and osteomyelitis are essentially similar to those for septic arthritis and will not be discussed separately. Treatment of septic deep flexor tendon injury is discussed in a prior section of this chapter.

In young calves, septic arthritis typically originates from either umbilical infections or neonatal septicemia. Calves with failure of passive transfer of immunoglobulins are at great risk (Fig. 12.58). Septicemic neonatal calves with septic arthritis or osteomyelitis frequently have other signs of gram-negative sepsis such as enteritis, meningitis, uveitis, or pneumonia. The prognosis for neonatal calves with septic arthritis, especially polyarthritis, secondary to failure of passive transfer of immunoglobulins is often guarded to poor.

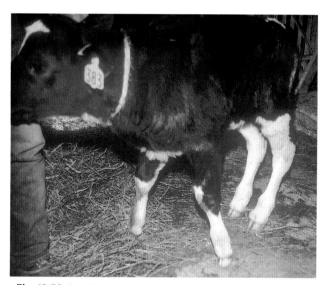

• **Fig. 12.58** A colostrum-deprived calf with septic arthritis and osteomyelitis involving the fetlocks and pastern joints in all limbs.

Calves with umbilical infections may develop septic arthritis in one or more joints due to septicemic spread of a variety of gram-negative and gram-positive organisms. Calves also may develop septic synovitis, osteomyelitis, or arthritis from exogenous abrasions, wounds, and decubital sores that occur secondary to abrasive surfaces. Calves with other medical problems that result in prolonged recumbency are at greater risk. Although *Escherichia coli* may commonly be identified as a cause of septic arthritis or osteomyelitis in neonatal calves, *Salmonella* spp. and *Trueperella pyogenes* are also frequently isolated. The more chronic the infection, the more likely *T. pyogenes* will be involved, in which case the fluid may become so thick that it is difficult to aspirate even with a 14-gauge needle.

Older calves (older than 3 weeks) and heifers may develop septic arthritis subsequent to exogenous wounds, periarticular cellulitis, punctures, or endogenous circulation of pathogens from the intestinal (*Salmonella* spp.) (Fig. 12.59 A, and B) or respiratory tracts (*Histophilus somni* and *Mycoplasma* spp.). *Mycoplasma* arthritis is common in growing calves 3 to 6 months of age, and affected calves frequently have concurrent pneumonia or at least a history of clinically significant respiratory disease. The stifle joint is more commonly affected than with other bacterial causes of septic arthritis.

Uncomplicated trauma to the carpus that results in bruising of the cranial surface may result in a reluctance to flex the carpus when recumbent. If the housing circumstances do not permit extension of the carpus when recumbent, further trauma to other extremities may result. This is not strictly a problem of sepsis, but because of the degree of carpal swelling and pain, the severity of

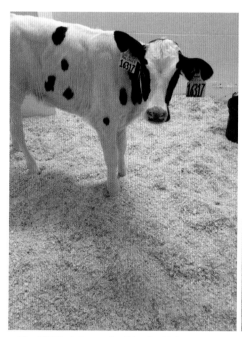
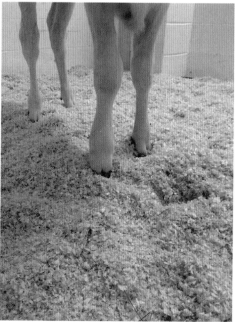

• **Fig. 12.59** A 2-month-old calf with lameness caused by a septic right front fetlock. *Salmonella* Dublin was cultured from the joint, and after flushing and antimicrobial treatment, the calf made an apparent recovery. *Salmonella* organisms were not cultured from her feces.

lameness from nonseptic inflammation may approach that seen with septic arthritis of the same joint. Carpal trauma should be treated with antiinflammatory medication, bandaging when feasible, and appropriate housing. It should be distinguished from sepsis of the carpus, which is less common.

Adult cattle may develop synovitis, arthritis, or osteomyelitis secondary to endogenous diseases such as endocarditis, septic mastitis, pneumonia, lung abscesses, liver abscesses, and chronic foot infections, as well as from exogenous infections secondary to traumatic wounds, decubital sores, and periarticular cellulitis or abscessation. *T. pyogenes* is again the most common organism isolated from septic joints, osteomyelitis lesions, or tenosynovitis in older calves and adult cattle.

Although *Mycoplasma* arthritis was not thought originally to be as common in dairy animals as in beef, the disease probably is underdiagnosed and has been found in many herds in which *Mycoplasma* mastitis exists or in which *Mycoplasma* spp. are also commonly associated with respiratory disease. Isolated cases of polytendonitis or arthritis affecting a single limb in weanling age calves to mature cattle have also been recognized in dairy animals caused by *Mycoplasma bovis*. *Mycoplasma* arthritis may occur concurrently with pneumonia (Fig. 12.60), and the joint fluid typically has a very high protein and neutrophil count, but the neutrophils may be relatively well preserved and non-degenerate.

Signs of septic arthritis include marked lameness with distention of the affected joint capsule; warmth over the joint; and a painful response when the joint is manipulated, flexed, or extended. In young calves experiencing sepsis in multiple joints, especially when present in both carpi,

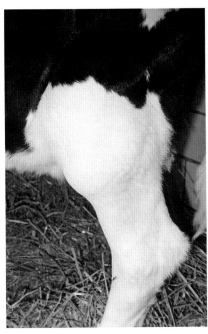

• **Fig. 12.60** Distended left stifle of a 3-month-old calf with *Mycoplasma bovis* arthritis and pneumonia. The tarsi and carpi are the most commonly affected joints in *Mycoplasma* infections.

lameness may not be so obvious as when a single joint is involved. With chronic carpal joint infection, synovial distention may not be as marked as in the tarsus or stifle. Fever usually is present and frequently is low grade (103.0° to 104.0°F [39.4° to 40.0°C]). Cattle may assume an abnormal attitude in recumbency and lie with the affected limb extended or lie in lateral recumbency to extend the affected limb more easily (Fig. 12.61). Calves or cattle with chronic polyarthritis tend to spend excessive time in recumbency and may develop secondary flexor tendon contracture that requires differentiation from primary, congenital flexor tendon contracture (Fig. 12.62).

The definitive diagnosis of septic arthritis or tendonitis is made by examination of fluid aspirates from the affected site. Arthrocentesis after aseptic preparation of the skin over the joint provides synovial fluid for cytology and culture. The diagnosis often is grossly apparent on visual inspection of abnormal synovial fluid, but laboratory analysis is helpful. Cytology of joint aspirates usually reveals a white blood cell (WBC) count greater than 30,000/μL and total solids greater than 3.0 g/dL. Bacteria may be apparent with Gram staining, or culture may be necessary for bacterial identification. In valuable individuals, cytology and culture for aerobic and anaerobic bacteria and *Mycoplasma* spp. are important diagnostic tools. Degenerative neutrophils are apparent in most bacterial arthritis cases but may be missing from acute *Mycoplasma* infections. In chronic septic arthritis, the synovial fluid may be grossly purulent and may require a 14-gauge needle for centesis sampling and lavage. The purulent material that accumulates in chronic mycoplasmal tendonitis and synovitis is always caseous in consistency (Fig. 12.63) and nonodorous in contrast to the characteristic fetid, anaerobic odor associated with *T. pyogenes* infection.

A history and thorough physical examination should be performed to determine the primary cause—umbilical infection, endogenous septicemia, or exogenous infection—and ancillary procedures such as ultrasonography of the umbilical region performed if a primary lesion is suspected in this area. Radiographs of acute joint infection show a widening of the affected joint space because of increased synovial fluid volume, but chronic infections may show a narrowing of the joint space as a result of loss of articular cartilage, erosion of the subchondral bone, bony proliferation, and periostitis. Radiographs are also useful to establish the severity and extent of any osteomyelitis in chronic cases (Fig. 12.64). The subtlety of radiographic lesions in acute cases makes synovial fluid a better diagnostic test, but radiographs are extremely valuable for formulating a prognosis in chronic cases. High-frequency ultrasound examination can be particularly useful for suspect septic tenosynovitis and can help guide aspiration for diagnostic purposes.

Treatment of septic arthritis must address the infected joint or joints, as well as any primary conditions that have predisposed to the condition. Acutely infected joints have a much better prognosis than chronically infected joints that

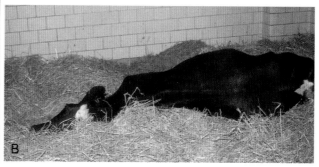

• **Fig. 12.61** A first-calf heifer with a septic left carpus. **A,** Standing. **B,** When recumbent, the heifer assumed lateral recumbency so that the extremely painful joint need not be flexed.

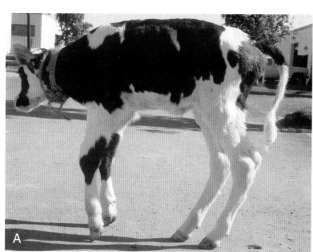

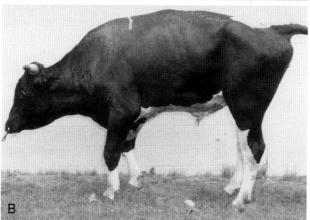

• **Fig. 12.62** Polyarthritis causing a painful stiff gait, an arched stance, and secondary flexor tendon contracture as a result of excessive time spent in recumbency in a calf (**A**) and a Holstein bull (**B**).

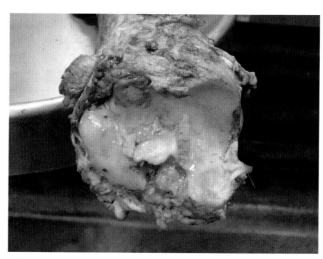

• **Fig. 12.63** Caseous material within the tarsal joint of a 6-month-old Holstein bull with *Mycoplasma bovis*–associated septic arthritis.

contain thick purulent debris. In acute infections, joint lavage is key to successful management. The infected joint should be surgically prepared and lavaged by through-and-through flushing using two 14-gauge needles and buffered lactated Ringer's solution or normal saline (Fig. 12.65); 1 or 2 L per joint suffices. The technique involves arthrocentesis with a 14-gauge sterile needle followed by distention of the joint capsule and subsequent joint puncture by a second 14-gauge needle on the opposite side of the joint. The lavage solution is then pumped through the joint to flush out causative organisms, fibrin, WBCs, and mediators of inflammation. A light sterile dressing is placed over the joint after squeezing as much fluid out of the needles as possible. Systemic antibiotics are more effective than antibiotics injected into the joint or added to the lavage solution and their administration should be initiated as soon as possible. Ideally, antibiotic selection

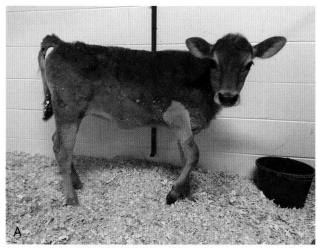

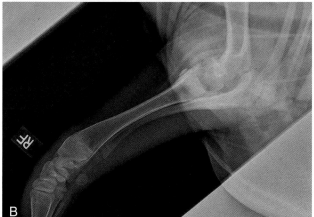

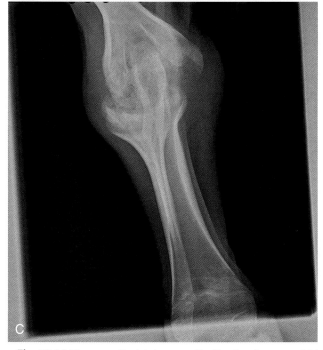

• **Fig. 12.64** Two- month-old Jersey calf with chronic non-weight bearing lameness of right forelimb **(A)**. Lateral **(B)** and anteroposterior **(C)** radiographs demonstrate extensive osteomyelitis and loss of bone in both the proximal radius and distal humerus. Such cases have a grave prognosis.

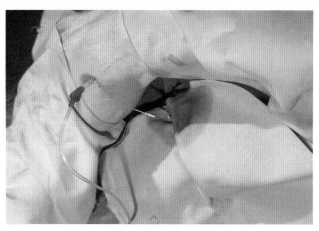

• **Fig. 12.65** Joint lavage in a calf with a septic hock joint.

is based on cytology (Gram stain evaluation) initially and culture results eventually. Alternatively, a broad-spectrum antibiotic such as florfenicol or ceftiofur may be empirically selected without culture results. When *Mycoplasma* is suspected, beta-lactam antibiotics should not be used alone. In adult cattle with septic arthritis or tendonitis, intravenous regional perfusion (IVRP) with antibiotics may be particularly helpful in the treatment. Florfenicol has been administered to young cattle at a dose of 2.2 mg/kg (4–5 mL) via IVRP and resulted in high drug concentrations in both serum and synovial fluid samples collected. Florfenicol (40 mg/kg), tulathromycin (2.5 mg/kg) and gamithromycin (6 mg/kg) have all been shown to establish potentially effective synovial concentrations when given parenterally. A lack of data regarding susceptibility for those bovine pathogens typically associated with chronic synovial infections means that it is hard to predict clinical efficacy with these drugs. However, synovial concentrations of florfenicol when administered parenterally at 40 mg/kg were above the typical mean inhibitory concentration (MIC) for *Fusobacterium necrophorum* and *Bacteroides melanogenicus* but not above the MIC for *Trueperella pyogenes*. Antimicrobial selection should always conform to regulatory requirements with respect to approval for use and withdrawal times.

Joint lavage, with or without antibiotics, is repeated daily (for a minimum of 1–3 days) and then as needed to continue flushing the joint of products of inflammation, organisms, and debris. The degree of lameness and joint distention dictates the need for additional lavage procedures. Most cases require three to seven lavage procedures over a 1- to 2-week course. Appropriate systemic antibiotics are continued for a minimum of 2 weeks, and the animal should be kept in a dry, well-bedded stall.

The following alternative approach to joint lavage has become more popular with surgeons in our clinics, especially in adults: An arthrotomy is performed on the affected joint, the joint is flushed with saline, and surgical drains are placed that permit continuous drainage of joint contents (Fig. 12.66). Repeat flushing of the joint may or may not be performed after the initial procedure. We have had success with septic tarsal joints in adult cattle by simply inserting a

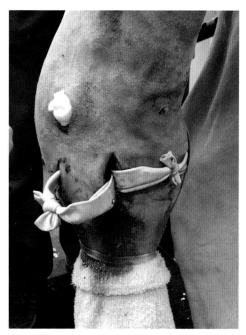

• **Fig. 12.66** Hock arthrotomy image taken from the craniolateral aspect of the right hind limb of a mature Red and White Holstein cow with septic arthritis. (Courtesy of Dr. Russ Freeland.)

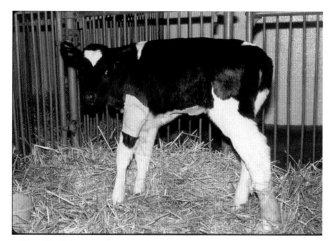

• **Fig. 12.67** A 10-day-old Holstein calf with a septic elbow joint. Although infection of a single joint often has a fair to good prognosis in calves that receive aggressive therapy, this calf did not respond to such therapy. Sepsis of the elbow joint may carry a lower prognosis than infection in other joints.

surgical drain with the use of a Buhner needle after ensuring that the entry and exit points are sufficiently large enough for drainage around the tubing.

Primary predisposing problems must be addressed. Whenever treating septic arthritis in septicemic calves, passive transfer of immunoglobulins and the umbilicus must be evaluated. Blood or plasma transfusions and umbilical resection may be required to prevent further joint seeding. Exogenous wounds and other sites of sepsis must be treated if they are thought to be primary to the septic arthritis.

Chronic septic arthritis carries a guarded prognosis because sterile ankylosis of the joint becomes the only acceptable result. Repeated joint lavage or arthrotomy for drainage of thick purulent joint fluid may be necessary. In calves, chronic infections, usually associated with *T. pyogenes*, require arthrotomy to drain thick pus from the joints. Open lavage of the joint coupled with systemic antibiotics, NSAIDS, and physical therapy to prevent tendon contracture after arthrotomy are all relevant to achieving a good outcome.

Physical therapy may be as simple as manipulation or may necessitate splints or casts for support and immobilization in the most serious cases. Calves are more likely to recover from a single chronic septic joint than an adult animal because calves can more easily support weight on three limbs during the time necessary for treatment and recovery. Treatment of *Mycoplasma* spp. arthritis in cattle is empirical because little documentation of effective resolution of *Mycoplasma* spp. infection in cattle is available. In geographic areas where fluoroquinolones are approved for cattle, they appear to be the first choice. In the United States, newer antibiotics such as florfenicol and macrolides such as tulathromycin are also frequently used as treatment for *Mycoplasma* spp. infection in calves. There are no highly effective, approved antibiotics for this organism available for lactating adult cattle in the United States. Tetracyclines are commonly used in the United States for treatment of mycoplasmal infection in lactating dairy cattle but an increasing number of isolates may be resistant.

The prognosis always should be guarded but is better for acute than chronic cases, better for single joints than multiple ones, better when the primary etiology may be corrected and worse for certain higher limb joints such as the elbow. (see Figs. 12.64 and 12.67).

Osteomyelitis and Bone Sequestra

Both of these conditions usually result in chronic or recurrent purulent drainage from the skin overlying a bony swelling (Fig. 12.68). In some instances, soft tissue swelling precedes drainage of pus and formation of a fistula originating from the necrotic or infected bone. The history may suggest improvement while on antibiotics, but recurrence of the lesion follows cessation of therapy. Affected animals may be slightly to moderately lame and resist palpation of the affected area of bone. Most lesions involve the metatarsus or metacarpus.

The diagnosis is confirmed by radiographs of the area (Fig. 12.69). A bone sequestrum must be differentiated from osteomyelitis because a sequestrum necessitates surgical intervention, but osteomyelitis may require medical therapy or euthanasia, depending on its severity and subsequent effect on the mechanics of the limb. Field removal of a sequestrum is not difficult with the aid of radiographs and a bone-cutting chisel. There is frequently significant cancellous bone surrounding the sequestrum, which must be removed before the sequestrum can be extricated. In addition to radiographs, culture and sensitivity of the purulent discharge should be performed. Although *T. pyogenes* is the most common organism identified, other

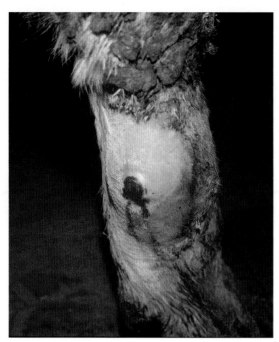

Fig. 12.68 Osteomyelitis in a springing heifer's metacarpal region. Recurrent swelling, lameness, and subsequent drainage had been observed for 3 months.

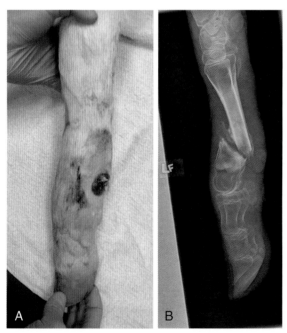

Fig. 12.69 Draining tract (**A**) associated with osteomyelitis and a nonhealing fracture (**B**) of the metacarpus in a 2-month-old Holstein calf. The initially closed fracture was associated with dystocia and managed with a fiberglass cast that remained unchanged for too long, leading to cast sores over the distal cannon region.

organisms requiring broad-spectrum antibiotic therapy occasionally are isolated. Long-term antibiotic therapy (4–6 weeks) is usually required for osteomyelitis. Therefore the animal's value must be sufficient to warrant the costs of therapy.

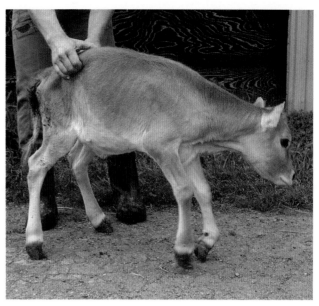

Fig. 12.70 Congenital contracted tendons in a Jersey calf.

Contracted Tendons

Contracted flexor tendons in calves and young cattle are either congenital or acquired. Congenital flexor contracture generally occurs in the forelimbs of calves. If no other congenital defects are present, treatment is indicated for valuable calves. It is important to rule out arthrogryposis as a potential cause. Arthrogrypotic limbs cannot be extended even under heavy sedation or anesthesia, nor can they be corrected by surgical cutting of the flexor tendons. It is a congenital and hopeless condition.

Calves affected by contracture knuckle at the fetlock and may either support weight on the toe or, in severe cases, stand on the dorsum of the fetlock (Fig. 12.70). The carpus also may be slightly flexed in severe cases. When present at birth, the diagnosis is obvious. Acquired flexor tendon contracture occurs when young calves remain recumbent for prolonged periods because of various conditions, including septicemia, white muscle disease resulting in recumbency, polyarthritis, malnutrition, and neurologic diseases. In growing heifers and bulls, recumbency after injury or laminitis predisposes them to forelimb flexor tendon contracture, although polyarthritis and other causes are identified occasionally.

Treatment of flexor tendon contracture requires only physical therapy in the simplest congenital cases. Frequent extension of the digit to gently stretch the tendons and encouraging the calf to stand on the limbs for exercise may be all the treatment required. In severe congenital cases, splints or surgical transection of the superficial, deep, or both flexor tendons followed by application of a cast may be necessary. Splints are elected for individuals that do not appear to respond to physical therapy but are still able to bear weight on the toes (Fig. 12.71). The calf is sedated, and

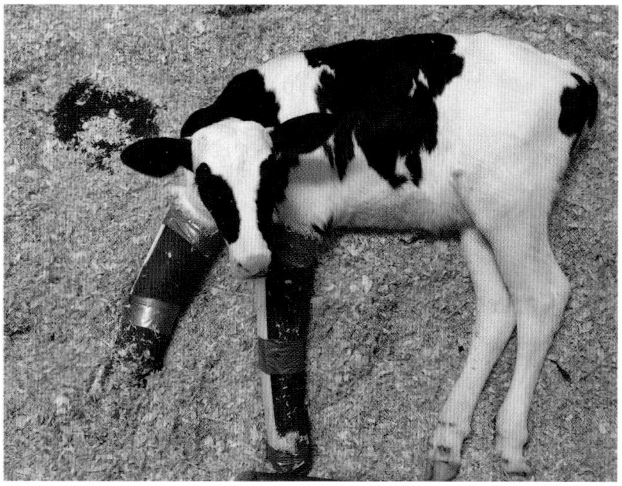

• **Fig. 12.71** Newborn Holstein heifer calf with polyvinyl chloride (PVC) splints applied dorsally and extensive padding as treatment for congenital forelimb contracture that was refractory to physical therapy.

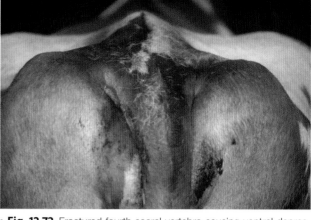

• **Fig. 12.72** Fractured fourth sacral vertebra causing ventral depression of the tail head and diminished ability to move the tail in a Guernsey show cow. The fracture was surgically repaired, and the cow recovered a normal appearance to the tail head and improved function of the tail.

PVC splints are applied over cotton wraps to prevent further knuckling. The splints are changed every week, and the tendons are stretched manually in an effort to gain greater degrees of extension each time the splints are applied. The calf is made, and helped, to stand and exercise several times daily. In valuable calves in which the aforementioned conservative measures fail, surgical referral for tenotomy of the superficial digital flexor or deep digital flexor tendon, or both, may be required. This is best done by surgeons who have experience with equine tendon contracture. Casts are required for several weeks after surgery until the sectioned tendons heal; the prognosis is poor for calves that require tendon section of both the superficial and deep digital flexor tendons. Additionally, in some calves, cutting of the superficial and deep flexor may not resolve the contracture due to contracture of the joint capsule (this will also be true of arthrogrypotic calves). High doses of oxytetracycline, as used in foals for contracted tendons, do not appear to be as effective in cattle, and high-dosage administration is a significant risk for acute renal failure!

In calves or growing animals that develop flexor tendon contracture secondary to other diseases, conservative physical therapy coupled with correction of the underlying condition constitute therapy. The longer that these young animals remain recumbent as a result of their primary disease, the less likely they are to respond to conservative physical therapy for acquired flexor tendon contracture.

Other Musculoskeletal Problems

Ventral Fracture of the Coccyx

"Crushed tail head" is the common term for compression-type fractures or luxations of the sacral and proximal coccygeal vertebrae (Fig. 12.72). This condition is very common in dairy cattle as a result of mounting activity during estrus. Usually, spinal nerves are injured in the process with resulting tail paresis or paralysis in most cases. In intermediate cases, the tail is paralyzed, and the bladder never empties but rather trickles urine into the vagina continuously; however, the cow has normal control of the hind limbs. In more serious cases involving the sacrum, proximal sacral nerves may be damaged, leading to sciatic nerve deficits with bilateral knuckling of the hind limbs.

The diagnosis is made by inspection. The normal alignment of the sacrum and proximal coccygeal vertebrae is disturbed, and abrasions may be apparent over the tail head from mounting activity by other cows. Manipulation of the tail and tail head may be painful to the cow in acute cases. In chronic cases, atrophy of the musculature at the tail head and coccygeal muscles may be apparent. The major long term complication of tail-head injuries that result in tail paralysis is soiling of the perineum and tail with feces and urine. The affected cow is unable to raise her tail to defecate or urinate; subsequently, manure and urine become smeared on the vulva, perineum, and tail. In some instances, this condition promotes vaginal contamination, which may interfere with conception because of ascending reproductive tract infection. Severe sacral fractures also may injure the pudendal nerve with consequential loss of caudal reproductive tract sensation.

Conservative treatment is unlikely to change the clinical signs, but cattle with severe injuries resulting in apparent sciatic nerve damage should be treated with antiinflammatory drugs during the acute period in an effort to reduce edema and inflammation around the sacral nerves. After healing of the luxation or fracture, the pelvic canal may be too small in the dorsoventral plane for normal passage of a calf; if the cow is pregnant, a surgical delivery should be planned.

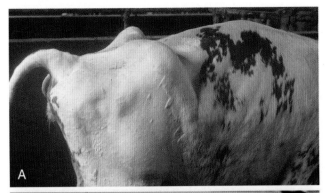

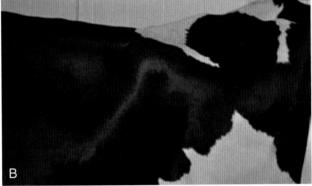

• **Fig. 12.73** Sacroiliac luxation in a mature Ayrshire cow **(A)**. The tuber coxae project dorsally far above the level of the vertebral column. **(B)** Sacroiliac luxation in a 4-year-old Holstein cow. The cow had difficulty rising and was very painful standing for 4 days. She improved after supportive care including use of a flotation tank and was discharged from the hospital with instructions to be housed in a large, deeply bedded box stall until she was fit to be housed with the rest of the herd.

Sacroiliac Luxation

Although rather uncommon, sacroiliac luxation occasionally occurs during the periparturient period, generally 1 week before to 1 week after parturition. The physiologic laxity of ligamentous structures that occurs during the estrogen peak associated with parturition apparently predisposes to sacroiliac luxation or subluxation.

The signs of luxation are apparent by inspection, as the tuber coxae appear raised above the plane of the vertebral column, and they rock back and forth when the cow walks because the hind limbs and pelvis now move independently of the vertebral column (Fig. 12.73 A, B and Video clip 12.4). In subluxation, the tuber coxae may be only slightly raised above the vertebral column or there is small but painful motion between the sacrum and ilium. Some cattle with complete luxation experience severe pain and refuse to move or eat, but others seem to experience less pain, move about with a stiff gait, and continue to eat. If luxation occurs before calving, the cow should be assisted during delivery or may require a cesarean section because of the dorsoventral compression of the pelvic inlet.

The prognosis is guarded to poor in all instances of sacroiliac luxation and favorable for sacroiliac subluxation because scarring of the joint with resultant stabilization will likely

occur in time with the latter. Cattle obviously in extreme pain should be slaughtered. Cattle that continue to eat, give milk, and move about may finish the current lactation. Literature regarding reoccurrence does not exist because of the rarity of the condition. Cattle with complete luxation should not be bred back because dystocia will be inevitable.

The tuber coxae can be traumatically injured without sacroiliac luxation or subluxation; such cattle are often described as having either a dropped hip (see earlier) or a "knocked-down" or "knocked-off" hook bone (Fig. 12.74 A, and B). The most lateral and cranial part of the ilium is typically fractured by a downward force that is insufficient to destabilize the sacroiliac joint but sufficient to fracture the bone. Cattle tend to only be mildly and briefly lame with this condition and often make a full recovery but always look asymmetric as a consequence with the affected hook "dropped" or seemingly absent when viewed from in front or behind. This can be problematic for show cattle, and we have been involved with surgical repair of tuber coxae injury in valuable animals when the cosmetic appearance was important to the intended use of the individual.

Back Injuries

Efforts to rise while accidentally positioned or trapped under stall partitions cause most back injuries in cattle. Cattle in free stalls or tie stalls may become positioned under divider bars if stalls are improperly designed or maintained. Adult cows with lameness or metabolic diseases may also become inadvertently malpositioned. Other causes of back injuries include being ridden by larger cows or falling while being ridden by another cow.

Often cows with injured backs are able but unwilling to stand. Thus, the examination is often conducted on a recumbent cow. An arched stance with the hind limbs placed farther caudal than normal typifies the posture of a cow with a back injury. Inspection of the top line may allow rapid diagnosis if multiple abrasions or hematoma formation is observed (Fig. 12.75). The gait is stiff and shuffling, and the cow may get up and down in a very awkward fashion. The rectal temperature is normal, but heart and respiratory rates may be elevated because of pain. The appetite may be normal or slightly reduced. Palpation of the back and dorsal spinous processes of the cow's vertebrae may elicit a painful response. The history may suggest the diagnosis if back trauma has been observed by the caretaker.

The diagnosis is reached by history, observation, palpation, and the patient's characteristic posture. Other causes of an arched stance, such as localized peritonitis, are ruled out by the physical findings of a normal gastrointestinal tract, normal temperature, and fair to normal appetite. Spastic syndrome may cause the hind limbs to be held caudal to the perpendicular, but spastic cattle tend to lower the loin rather than being arched. In laminitis, cattle may stand with

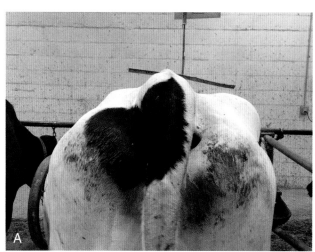
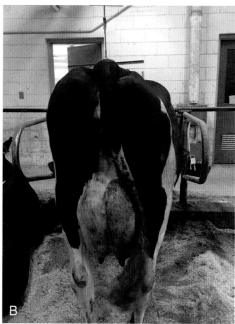

• **Fig. 12.74** "Knocked-down hip" in two mature Holstein cows. Trauma to tuber coxae can cause remarkable asymmetry to the hook bones (left **A**, right **B**) when viewed from behind. When the sacroiliac joint is unaffected, as was the case for both cows in these images, the individual can recover soundness quickly.

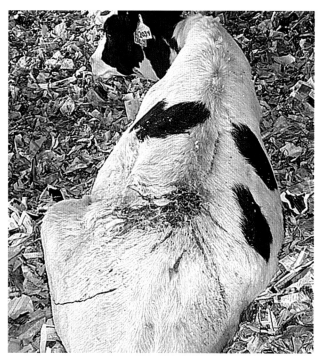

• **Fig. 12.75** Back injury in a cow that became entrapped in a stall. She was unwilling to rise for several days but did recover.

the hind limbs under the body but will show sensitivity to hoof testers and warmth in the claws.

Rest and analgesics constitute therapy for back injuries in cattle. A clumsy animal should be moved to a box stall until healing occurs. Keeping the cow isolated from others will prevent further injury from riding behavior. Dexamethasone or NSAID therapy greatly aid the affected

animal and should be used for 3 days to 2 weeks, depending on severity and pregnancy status. Improvement is suggested when the stance becomes less arched and the gait more normal.

Dealing With Recumbency and Downer Cows

Recumbent adult cattle remain a challenge for veterinary practitioners, especially because the resources available on the farm to reach an accurate diagnosis and establish optimal therapy are frequently very limited. Determining the prognosis for each case is always very challenging because it requires a definitive diagnosis, something that may only come after necropsy, or might require ancillary diagnostics such as imaging and blood work. Over the past 20 to 25 years, systems to lift down cows have advanced and diversified; in particular, flotation tanks designed to float cows have become popular because of their effectiveness and their ability to prevent secondary problems, facilitate examination, and provide comfort to the cow.

The list of conditions that can potentially cause an adult cow or first lactation heifer to become recumbent is lengthy, however, they can be summarized within a few broad categories:

1. **Electrolyte imbalance:** Calcium, potassium, magnesium, and phosphorus are the most commonly incriminated. Although hypoglycemia is an important cause of weakness and recumbency in calves, it is a rare cause in adults. Hypoglycemia can accompany severe clinical ketosis, but unless complicated by other metabolic, musculoskeletal, or toxic conditions, it is very unusual for ketosis to be the sole reason for recumbency.

2. **Dystocia related:** Especially in first-calf heifers. Pelvic, back, and soft tissue injuries associated with assisted fetal extraction and compounded by exhaustion are common causes of recumbency.

3. **Musculoskeletal injuries:** Coxofemoral subluxation or luxation, femoral injuries (femoral neck fracture), gastrocnemius rupture, and non–calving-related traumatic back and pelvic injuries can all incur sufficient damage to cause recumbency.

4. **Systemic inflammatory illness:** Peracute coliform mastitis is the most important and common example, but recumbency can also be seen with other septic conditions such as peritonitis and, occasionally, metritis.

5. **Peripheral or central neuropathy:** This category includes sciatic, obturator, or spinal paresis. Peripheral neuropathy develops as a common sequela to recumbency, so it can be challenging to determine which came first. Spinal lymphosarcoma, usually located epidurally as a compressive mass in the lumbosacral spine, is a potential central nervous system cause of recumbency in adult dairy cattle.

6. **Miscellaneous:** Toxic and infectious causes such as organophosphate poisoning and botulism complete the differential list but are uncommon compared with those listed above.

In the teaching hospital at the University of Wisconsin over the past 25 years, the most common medical history in dairy cattle referred for recumbency has been one of clinical hypocalcemia in an adult cow whose response to symptomatic treatment has been partial or only transient. The second most common reason for presentation has been presumed or witnessed musculoskeletal trauma, often in an individual that had been struggling to rise before the traumatic event. Continued recumbency after dystocia represents the third most common reason for referral. Undoubtedly, the alacrity with which these cases are referred, specifically for flotation, has improved over this time frame.

Myopathic and Neuropathic Events Associated with Recumbency

It is evident to all bovine veterinarians that no matter what the primary reason for a cow to be down, the risk of complications increases with time, and with this, the chances of recovery decrease. As long ago as 1969, Fenwick demonstrated that the incidence of problems related to recumbency after milk fever increased with time elapsed between onset of recumbency and treatment with calcium. For recumbency lasting less than 6 hours before the first treatment, the proportion that went on to become down cows was negligible. For 7 to 12 hours, he estimated the complication rate to be 26%; for 12 to 18 hours, it was 32%; and for more than 18 hours, it reached 38%. These numbers appear roughly applicable to individuals that are recumbent because of hypocalcemia in our hospital, but one should always remember that secondary complications hugely impact any attempt at prognosis, and the veterinarian's challenge often comes in both the prevention and diagnosis of such.

In 1981, Cox revealed how a pathological condition recognized in human medicine and recognized in horses also affects down cows. This condition is known as compartment syndrome, and it is perhaps the most important complication of primary metabolic, neurologic, or musculoskeletal diseases that result in prolonged recumbency in adult cattle. Ischemia will occur because of prolonged pressure on a limb during recumbency. Consequent to an increase in external pressure on soft tissues, vascular permeability increases, producing an extracellular accumulation of fluid and swelling. If the fascia that surrounds the muscle prevents distention, the internal pressure will increase dramatically, even beyond the external pressure that initiated the problem. Tissue anoxia leads to cell damage and inflammation, which in turn induce further increases in pressure within the tissue. These pressure changes and localized anoxia cause not only muscle necrosis but also implicate local nerve branches running through the affected soft tissues.

Direct experimental evidence for damage to the major nerve branches in the hind limbs of recumbent cattle also came from Cox and colleagues in 1982. Sixteen adult cows were kept in sternal recumbency on rubber mats for 6, 9, or 12 hours with the right hind limb under the body, mimicking what happens frequently in clinical patients. Swelling and stiffness were evident in the right hind limbs of the eight cows that could not stand at the end of the experiment, and at necropsy, the most obvious lesions were those of the sciatic nerve in the caudal region of the femur. The nerve was grossly discolored as well as inflamed histologically, and the surrounding musculature of the caudoproximal thigh was damaged; specifically, the semitendinosus was very pale and necrotic, and the gluteal musculature around the greater trochanter was also similarly affected. Clinicopathologically, the serum activity for creatine kinase (CK) was elevated in all animals regardless of outcome from the onset of recumbency to 24 hours but peaked at this time point in animals that stood but continued to elevate in those that did not. Curiously, reevaluation of serum activities for CK 6 days later did not demonstrate any difference between the two groups (able to stand and not able to stand). The potential for involvement of, and injury to, the sciatic nerve and its distal branches, the peroneal (fibular) and tibial nerves, secondary to myopathy appears to be particularly important in recumbent cows in terms of prognosis and outcome.

The pattern of CK elevation after experimentally induced recumbency is repeatable in clinical patients. Most recumbent cattle have some degree of elevated CK and aspartate aminotransferase (AST) values, so slight elevation should not be taken as diagnostic for severe myopathy. The relative level of CK and AST elevation may be a diagnostic-prognostic indicator, but it is also important to realize that CK peaks very quickly after muscular injury and has a short

(4–8 hours) serum half-life, whereas AST peaks more slowly but remains elevated or steady for several days. Therefore CK is a better diagnostic test for the cow recumbent only 24 to 48 hours, but a cow that has been recumbent for 7 days might be better assessed by AST, assuming muscle damage occurred early in her recumbent course. CK values greater than 5000 to 10,000 IU/L are typical in acutely myopathic cattle and frequently exceed 20,000 IU/L if severe heavy muscle damage has occurred. Severe myopathies may cause AST elevations of 3000 IU/L or greater that persist for several days after reaching peak levels. In general, CK values exceeding 100,000 IU/L or AST levels exceeding 10,000 IU/L carry a poor prognosis, but excepting these very severe cases, it is very difficult to correlate prognosis with CK or AST levels. A number of retrospective studies of down cows have examined the prognostic value of CK and AST values at varying points following the onset of recumbency, and the results are conflicting. Perhaps the most appropriate study to consider when discussing the value of muscle enzyme activities for modern bovine practitioners is that by Burton et al. from Cornell University in 2009. This study looked at several potential prognostic indicators in cattle that underwent flotation and found no correlation between CK at admission or the highest value of CK recorded in a patient and survival. Severely myopathic cattle may also have elevated serum potassium levels in the acute phase as a result of muscle cell breakdown and are at risk for myoglobin nephrosis. Metabolic acidosis may be present because of profound lactic acid release from muscle cells or poor perfusion. In cattle with drastic exertional myopathy (e.g., having been trapped in mud, or inadvertently caught by chains or under stall dividers in housing) that destroys many heavy muscle groups, a shocklike state and neurologic signs may be seen secondary to release of lactic acid, potassium, and probably many other products from damaged muscle. This scenario is highly reminiscent of the capture myopathy that can be induced in wild ungulates following attempts to sedate, anesthetize and handle them for veterinary reasons.

In addition to compartmental syndrome caused by recumbency, down individuals typically experience some degree of exertional myopathy as they struggle to rise, either of their own accord or after encouragement from humans. Exertional myopathy can be significant and is potentially caused by; struggling; uncoordinated efforts to rise; being entangled in mud, manure, wires, or equipment; or repeated attempts to rise on treacherous footing such as ice or wet concrete. Such repeated muscular exertion results in microscopic or gross muscle injury with breakdown of cells, edema, hemorrhage, release of lactic acid, and eventual necrosis or fibrosis. Various muscle groups may be involved, depending on the patient's position, weight, or environment, but the hind limb musculature again is most commonly affected. Adductor musculature may be involved if cattle have split their hind limbs secondary to calving paralysis or splayed their legs on slippery flooring. The quadriceps may be involved in "creeper cows" that struggle to move or rise with their

hind limbs extended behind the body. The gastrocnemius or semimembranosus-semitendinosus musculature in the caudal thigh may be involved when the patient repeatedly struggles to rise but is too weak to do so. In most instances, a primary disease (e.g., hypocalcemia, nerve dysfunction after dystocia or injury, hypokalemia) has caused recumbency, and myopathy follows in patients that struggle excessively or that are left on slippery footing.

The clinical result of compartmental syndrome or exertional myopathy is limb dysfunction characterized by the inability to rise or bear weight normally on affected limbs. Signs may include limb swelling, muscular swelling, rigid extension of the limb, inability to rise, and flexion of the limb with knuckling, among others. Obviously, the exact posture and signs will vary based on the muscle groups involved and any concurrent skeletal injuries or neuropathies. Muscle swelling in acute myopathy may be firm, but in some cases, the muscle will be relatively flaccid or soft. Physical diagnosis relies on detection of muscular swelling, asymmetry, and characteristic signs when the patient is standing, lying in recumbency, or attempting to rise. Simple ancillary data confirmation may be obtained by using test reagent strips on the patient's urine. In the most severe myopathies, frank myoglobinuria will be apparent as distinctly brown or deep red urine that is also cloudy. In less severe cases, the urine may be clear and brown or clear and yellowish but show a strong positive reaction to the hemoglobin and protein reagents on the multiple test strips. Because the m-orthotoluidine reagent used in the hemoglobin test also responds to myoglobin, it is useful for detection of myoglobin in a field setting.

Taking a Systematic Approach to the Recumbent Individual

A systematic approach by the veterinarian to a recumbent animal is suggested in terms of history taking, physical examination, and monitoring response to therapy. The following are meant as general guidelines.

History

1. **Age:** The age of the cow is relevant. First-calf heifers will not be suffering from hypocalcemia, but cows older than 4 or 5 years of age will not only be more likely to experience hypocalcemia but will also be stronger candidates for spinal lymphosarcoma (if the individual is bovine leukemia virus [BLV] positive).

2. **Parturition history:** Recent dystocia or forced fetal extraction can lead to pelvic inflammation and peripheral nerve injury. Recumbency associated with dystocia is not always immediate; time is sometimes needed for swelling and peripheral nerve impairment to develop.

3. **History of musculoskeletal trauma or fall:** Recumbent cattle that are not postparturient have often sustained trauma that may or may not have been seen by farm

personnel. This can be a challenging definitive diagnosis to reach if unwitnessed but is often suggested by exclusion of other causes and location of the individual at the time she was found. A history of recent estrus can also be suggestive since normal mounting behavior is a common cause of trauma leading to recumbency.

4. **Sequence of events after onset of recumbency but before veterinary attention:** It can be especially valuable to obtain a detailed account of what has happened since the animal was first observed to be recumbent: Has there been an initial attempt at treatment, and what was the response? Has the patient stood briefly or not at all, and if standing, what was her posture at that time (e.g., knuckled, weight bearing in three limbs, creeping)? Was the cow moved to her current position by farm personnel, and if so, how – was she dragged forcibly or placed on a gate or mat that was then moved with her on it?

5. **Specific treatment history:** A detailed account of drugs administered along with their doses and frequencies is relevant and important. Repeated, overzealous calcium administration can lead to cardiac disasters. Steroidal and nonsteroidal types and doses used are also critical to record so as to avoid toxicity, particularly with regard to NSAID-induced abomasal ulceration.

Physical Examination and Ancillary Diagnostics

The physical examination of a recumbent cow requires extra effort and usually a degree of discomfort for the veterinarian; one is typically working in a confined space surrounded by a mixture of wet bedding, feces, and urine, on top of concrete, squatting on one's knees or lying down for much of the examination. Nonetheless, time and energy should be directed toward this first, important task.

1. **Temperature, pulse, and respiration:** Although pivotal parts of most clinical examinations, there are limitations to the diagnostic value of these baseline parameters in down cattle. The rectal temperature is only very rarely helpful, but if markedly increased (>104°F), it indicates systemic illness (e.g., coliform mastitis) or potentially exertional efforts if the animal has been in direct sun and struggling. Hypothermia may indicate hypocalcemia or systemic shock (as would be seen in a moribund patient with septic peritonitis from a perforated abomasal ulcer). The pulse rate of down cows is most commonly influenced by pain (usually myopathic or musculoskeletal), systemic toxemia (coliform mastitis), and treatment effect (especially parenteral calcium solutions; these may also cause arrhythmias). Respiratory rate and lung sounds are rarely informative; the rate tends to increase with exertional effort and pain in synchrony with the pulse rate. Occasionally, pneumonia may be diagnosed in down cows, typically as a complicating health issue rather than as a primary problem. Hypocalcemic individuals are at risk for aspiration and particular care must

be taken in the oral drenching or orogastric intubation of such patients in order to avoid more severe pulmonary disease. Abnormal lung sounds may signal further evaluation by thoracic ultrasound examination.

2. **Rumen motility and abdominal auscultation:** These are rarely of great value in recumbent cattle; poor rumen motility is anticipated and nonspecific. The recumbent position makes ventral abdominal auscultation and ballottement impossible.

3. **Musculoskeletal evaluation:** Examination of all four limbs is very important, although the emphasis should be on the hind limbs. Palpation of all limb joints is relevant, alongside particular attention to palpation during manipulation of the coxofemoral and stifle joints. The stifle joints should be evaluated for swelling, effusion, and symmetry and coxofemoral joints evaluated during protraction and abduction on both sides; this requires the patient to be moved from one side to the other or can be alternatively done while in a sling. Simultaneous manipulation of the hind limb by an assistant while performing rectal palpation of the pelvis and the obturator foramen on that side can be highly informative in the case of hip joint and proximal femur injuries. Both gastrocnemius tendons and muscles should be palpated for swelling and symmetry, and the entire caudal thigh and gluteal musculature should also be evaluated for swelling and symmetry. The angle of the hock can be a useful guide to gastrocnemius (hyperflexed) or peroneus tertius (hyperextended) injury. Palpation of the thoracic and lumbosacral spine for crepitation, swelling, and instability should also be performed.

4. **Neurologic evaluation:** A brief examination of mentation and cranial nerve function can be performed, but it is rare for adult cattle to have encephalitis or selective cranial nerve deficits associated with recumbency. Specific exceptions include rabies (rapidly progressive over a 24- to 48-hour period) and botulism (pupil dilation and dysphagia alongside generalized flaccid weakness). Evaluation of perineal sensation, anal and tail tone and bladder function is relevant, and if loss of distal sacral or cauda equina function is noted, it usually denotes either lymphosarcoma in a lumbar location or caudal spinal (lumbosacral) trauma.

5. **Mammary evaluation:** Under all circumstances, the veterinarian is remiss unless a proper examination of the udder and secretions from all quarters is performed in a recumbent dairy animal. Toxic mastitis, often accompanied by marked electrolyte abnormalities and dehydration, is the commonest systemic illness associated with recumbency. After milk has been expressed from each quarter the teat end should be dipped because environmental contamination through an open teat sphincter and streak canal is more likely in recumbent animals.

6. **Rectal examination:** This is of some, but limited, value in a recumbent individual but is reliably the least comfortable part of the examination for the veterinarian. The veterinarian should incorporate palpation of the

pelvis for crepitation, the presence of the femoral head in the obturator foramen (see earlier), and an evaluation of the uterus in a recently parturient cow. Prior bladder evacuation by perineal stimulation or sterile catheterization may be helpful because many recumbent cattle will be reluctant to void normally. In an individual in whom septic peritonitis is suspected, attention should be paid to the presence of diffuse pneumoperitoneum (gives a sensation of tightness around the hand and sleeve, more reminiscent of palpating a horse than a cow), which suggests rupture of the abomasum. Iliac and caudal abdominal lymph node palpation for notable enlargement can occasionally increase one's suspicion of lymphosarcoma in a mature animal deemed a candidate for spinal lymphosarcoma. For recumbency associated with a known history of dystocia, a vaginal examination is indicated, but this procedure is otherwise unnecessary.

After the initial physical examination, the clinician must decide whether a primary cause of the recumbency can be pinpointed and initiate therapy accordingly. In many instances, there may already have been some form of treatment administered; in such circumstances, further therapeutic interventions must be considered carefully. Occasionally, an obvious, catastrophic cause for recumbency will be identified at the time of the initial examination, and humane euthanasia should be performed; down cattle with no hope of recovery can suffer miserably, and veterinarians are obligated to prevent this to the best of their ability.

Ancillary diagnostics are limited, particularly on farm, but may include:

1. **Serum biochemistry profile:** This is most useful for electrolyte measurement and assessment of renal and hepatic function. As mentioned previously, serum activities for CK and AST provide insight on the extent of muscle damage, but one has to be mindful of when the sample has been obtained relative to the onset of recumbency. The conflicting literature regarding prognostic accuracy of CK values implies that adamant conclusions regarding the implications of either a low or high value should be avoided, but the higher the CK value in the immediate 24- to 36-hour period after recumbency, the more pessimistic many clinicians will be. However, there are many animals with mild to moderate elevations that do not recover. Calcium (ionized or total), potassium, magnesium, and phosphorus levels should be the most carefully followed, and serum betahydroxybutyrate (BHBA) levels can provide an accurate assessment of ketosis status. Although uncommon, hypoglycemia related to ketosis may be responsible for recumbency. Care needs to be taken with the interpretation of serum potassium levels if the sample was not rapidly analyzed or at least separated by centrifugation; falsely elevated potassium levels will be obtained because of leakage from erythrocytes within just a few hours. Assessment of electrolytes is a key step because imbalances need to be addressed before the animal can be expected to stand. Moreover, efforts to stand by a patient

whilst obvious deficiencies in electrolytes such as calcium and potassium persist may lead to catastrophic injury due to weakness that may have been avoidable.
2. **Complete blood count:** This is generally less informative than the biochemistry profile in terms of guiding therapeutic interventions, but it may reveal an acute inflammatory response with mastitis or metritis associated with endotoxemia. Severe anemia from abomasal ulceration or persistent lymphocytosis in a BLV-positive individual may provide further helpful information.
3. **Ultrasound examination:** The increasing availability of variable frequency probes means that transabdominal, thoracic, rectal, and musculoskeletal ultrasound examination will be increasingly used in the future and not just as a teaching hospital modality. Muscle, joint, and tendon imaging with high-frequency probes (such as are used for reproductive use) can be helpful when the physical examination has left some doubt about the integrity of the coxofemoral joint, gastrocnemius muscle or tendon, or other large muscle groups. Abdominal ultrasonography can reveal peritoneal effusion and guide diagnostic abdominocentesis in the occasional case of recumbency associated with diffuse peritonitis or abdominal neoplasia.
4. **Radiographic examination of the pelvis and upper limb:** This is likely to remain the province of referral hospitals because of the equipment needed and the practical challenges involved. It is most useful for further evaluation of patients suspected to have coxofemoral injury (full luxation or subluxation), pelvic fractures, or femoral injury based on the initial physical examination. Heavy sedation and a significant number of personnel are usually needed to complete this procedure in adult cattle.

On farm, it is critically important to assess the producer's attitude to the individual case because if one's perception is that the owner already believes the battle is lost or that continued effort is pointless, no amount of veterinary effort will compensate. As farm veterinarians, our contribution is typically circumscribed by the duration of the visit, any specific diagnosis we reach, and by the treatment plan we instigate; however, the overall quality of care that the animal receives rests on the shoulders of farm personnel. It is clear from experience, as well as from the literature, that small details matter with respect to nursing care and persistence with down cows.

Cattle that are bright, alert, and willing to attempt to rise and in whom the primary problem has been resolved are undoubtedly the best patients with whom to work. Unfortunately, the neuropathic and myopathic consequences of continued recumbency are often the biggest obstacles to recovery; therefore moving the animal to a flooring surface other than concrete should be an absolute priority. Ideally, the cow should have a large area, such as an individual stall, where she can turn around and move without difficulty. A dirt floor covered with a deep layer of straw is ideal, or approximately 30 cm of sand with a gentle slope for good drainage can be an excellent alternative. Sand has the added benefit of not retaining water or urine, which can help prevent skin maceration; it also conforms to the cow's body to provide better weight distribution. A deeply bedded pack,

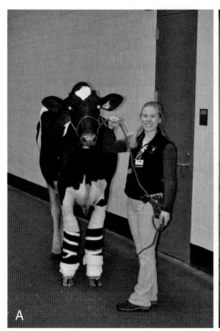
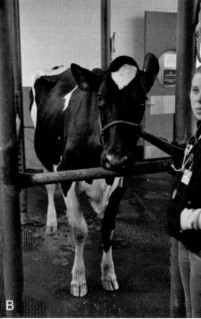

• **Figs. 12.76 A,** Bandage placement on the carpus of a Holstein cow that could not rise on her own for 2 weeks but eventually made a full recovery with nursing care and use of the flotation tank. **B,** Same cow showing evidence of pressure necrosis that had occurred over the carpi.

such as that provided by a dry cow pen, may also work well for this purpose on many farms. If the cow is unable to change sides independently, then she will need to be rolled, beginning as early in the course of the recumbency as possible. Ideally, this should be at least every 4 to 6 hours to minimize pressure on muscles and nerves. When the cow has been rolled, it is prudent to pay attention to the posture of the down-side limb; it is important that it is in a normal resting and sleeping position and not extended or stretched out underneath the body.

Useful Treatments for Recumbent Cows

1. **Nursing care:** Be sure to have the recumbent animal on good footing with a nonslip surface. This may be a manure pack, dirt box stall, well-bedded box stall, or solid ground outside. Cows lunge forward when rising, and straw bales can be placed around the inside of the stall to prevent the cow from lying down with her head near the wall. The cow also should be fed and watered where she lies; preventing other cows sharing the same pen from eating the downer cow's feed seems a regular challenge on larger dairies. Cows with a tendency to abduct the hind limbs because of calving paralysis should be hobbled to prevent splitting (see Fig. 13.58). Indeed, some clinicians opt to hobble the back legs of all down cows as a preventive measure. Recumbent cattle should be rolled from one side to the other several times daily to reduce the possibility of compartmental syndrome. Bandages can be placed over the carpal area because cows having difficulty rising often place prolonged pressure over the carpus when trying to do so (Fig. 12.76).

2. **Analgesics:** The administration of analgesics can improve the comfort of the patient and helps maintain appetite;

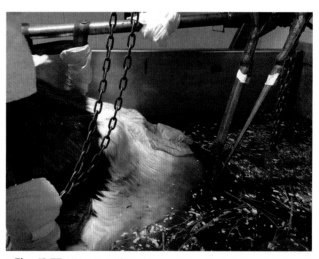

• **Fig. 12.77** Holstein heifer with caudal epidural catheter in place. Morphine was administered through the catheter, two to three times daily for 2 days, to provide analgesia after closed reduction of a coxofemoral luxation.

whether it is by reducing inflammation around muscles and nerves or decreasing the acute inflammatory response associated with endotoxemia, there is ample justification for the use of antiinflammatory drugs. Severely myopathic animals are often in a great deal of pain. The downside, particularly with NSAIDs, is the potential for abomasal ulceration and nephrotoxicity, the former being more likely than the latter with repeated use, in patients that are already highly stressed and painful. Strategic administration of flunixin, meloxicam, or dexamethasone can be critical in the management of inflammation and pain. We have also used epidural analgesia (5 mg of dexamethasone or morphine [0.1-0.2 mg/kg Q 12 hrs]) in many cases of pelvic pain and possible nerve root injury (Fig. 12.77).

3. **Fluid therapy:** Recumbent animals are often dehydrated, and fluid replacement should be considered. The signalment of affected individuals and stage of lactation often justify the addition of calcium and potassium to fluids unless blood work indicates that these are within normal ranges. The presence of myoglobinuria obligates volume expansion to prevent renal damage from pigment nephropathy. Some patients with severe myopathy or poor peripheral perfusion associated with dehydration and endotoxemia will also develop profound metabolic acidosis with lactatemia that is best approached with IV balanced electrolyte solutions that are alkalinizing. Blood BHBA or urinary ketone tests are indicated in early lactation animals to direct dextrose administration. The IV route is preferred for fluid therapy, but large-volume oral fluid administration by drench is a less expensive means of addressing volume and specific electrolyte deficiencies. Great care needs to be taken when drenching recumbent cattle so as to avoid aspiration; individuals should be in sternal recumbency, never lateral, and personnel should always check that tube placement is appropriate. Never assume that down, early lactation cattle will reliably cough if a tube is in the trachea. Similarly, one should be aware of the greater potential for regurgitation when large volumes of fluids are administered by orogastric tube to recumbent cattle. Commercial or homemade "fresh cow drenches"—for example 15 to 20 gallons of water containing calcium propionate (500 g), magnesium sulfate (250 g), sodium monophosphate (220 g), and potassium chloride (150 g)—provide an excellent oral fluid alternative to more expensive IV treatment. Small-volume hypertonic solutions (e.g., 2 L of 7× normal saline) can be an excellent resuscitative fluid treatment for dehydrated, endotoxemic, recumbent patients but should always be followed by access to water or orogastric administration as described.

4. **Miscellaneous:** Although most adult cattle have sufficient levels of blood selenium, empirically, it does no harm to administer a single therapeutic dose of vitamin E and selenium to ensure that the cow has an adequate rebuilding capacity for muscle repair. Empiric treatment is used because laboratory evaluation of selenium or glutathione peroxidase values may have a rather long turnaround time, and it may be best to provide these supplements rather than wait for laboratory confirmation or denial of low selenium levels. The use of antibiotics should only be dictated by the presence of a diagnosed indication to do so; the two most common reasons are a primary toxic mastitis and the development or coexistence of pneumonia. A word of caution concerning the diagnosis of pneumonia; many myopathic and painful cattle will be tachypneic, and one should not overinterpret this alone as justification for antimicrobial administration. Exertional efforts, especially in warm and humid weather, may also increase rectal temperature via hyperthermia rather than true pyrexia.

Complications of Recumbency

1. **Coxofemoral injury:** Luxation, subluxation, and femoral neck fractures (Fig. 12.78) are potential consequences of struggling to rise, especially in cattle that hyperabduct when footing is slippery or there exists some degree of joint laxity or prior injury. Furthermore, obturator nerve and partial sciatic nerve paresis are highly relevant predisposing causes of coxofemoral injury because they interfere with normal hind limb adduction as affected individuals struggle to stand. Muscle tearing and ligament and capsular damage add to the pain and reluctance to rise even if complete luxation does not occur.

2. **Abomasal ulceration:** Stress induced by recumbency as well as the inciting primary condition are sufficient to explain the relatively high incidence of this co-morbidity. Unfortunately, iatrogenic influences from antiinflammatory medication can also contribute to the impairment of mucosal blood flow within the abomasum, leading to ulceration with melena.

3. **Myopathy and neuropathy:** As discussed earlier, these are the most common complications to recumbency, and regardless of the primary cause, represent the biggest hurdle to recovery. A physical inability to stand combined with severe pain can combine to create a hopeless prognosis.

Lifting a Recumbent Cow

Several assistive devices are available for use in clinics and on farm. Manual or mechanical devices are subject to individual clinical experience and, of course, availability. The simplest means of assisting a cow to rise is to provide manual help by lifting the cow by her tail as she drives with her hind limbs during her own attempts to get up. It is important to take the time to properly position the limbs beforehand and to change the side the cow is on before giving her a boost in this way in case the limb on which she had been most recently lying is a bit weaker. Manual assistance at the base of the tail is more effective than more distally and is less likely to result in tail fracture.

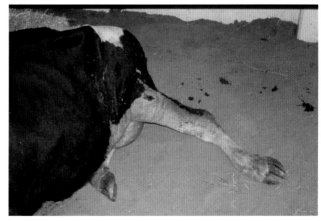

• **Fig. 12.78** Mature Holstein cow demonstrating abnormal hind limb posture caused by a femoral neck fracture. The cow had been treated successfully for hypocalcemia after freshening but had relapsed the following day and sustained the injury while struggling to rise on slippery concrete in an alleyway.

Other mechanical means include the use of hip lifters, cattle walkers, inflatable air bags, or slings.

All mechanical aids must be used judiciously, lest they do more harm than good. Hip lifters, in particular, although still widely used, can cause significant damage to the muscles that attach to the ilium and even disastrous skeletal injury if not used or secured properly. They are especially problematic in modern, larger body frame and body weight Holsteins because of the mechanical principle upon which they depend. Increasingly, we discourage their use in favor of other techniques, principally flotation, but if employed as mechanical aids, hip lifters must be extremely well padded (Fig. 12.79), and should preferentially be used in heifers or smaller body frame cows. Part of their attraction lies in the fact that they are relatively inexpensive, can be used indoors (beam hooks) or outdoors (hydraulic tractor lift), and require fewer people for their use. In areas of the United States where flotation tanks are not available they are still the most commonly used aid to assist recumbent cattle to stand.

The best patient candidates for mechanical aids are those that want to stand, will try to stand, and can stand after they are assisted to their feet. These cattle usually only require mechanical assistance twice daily for 1 to 5 days before being able to rise by themselves. Some recumbent cattle are apprehensive and frightened when raised for the first time and will refuse to bear weight. Therefore the initial attempt should not be overinterpreted but rather thought of as a "training session." The hip lifter should be attached quickly and tightly over the tuber coxae and the cow quickly lifted!! If she does not try to stand immediately, some form of stimulation should be given. The cow must *not* remain hanging in the hip lifter; it should be removed or at least loosened within 1 to 2 minutes after the animal is standing to reduce the amount of pressure necrosis over the skin and deeper tissue on the tuber coxae region (Fig. 12.80). Hip lifters

should *never* be left in place for longer than 5 minutes during any lifting episode, and they always should be heavily padded. If the cow cannot support any weight and needs to be milked, she should be lowered to the ground and milked in lateral recumbency. If repeated lifting with a hip lifter is required, we sometimes apply ice to the area after each use in hopes of decreasing swelling, inflammation, and pain (Fig. 12.81). One author (GF) believes that routine hiplifter use should be discouraged in the treatment of downer cows as they are likely to cause more harm than benefit.

The individual value of the animal and the manpower available for nursing care will dictate the length of time devoted to care of a recumbent myopathic patient. No absolute rules exist regarding the length of time a cow may remain down before the prognosis becomes hopeless. However, each additional day spent in recumbency obviously worsens the prognosis because further musculoskeletal and neurologic damage is more likely to occur. Subtle signs of improvement such as progressively bearing more weight on the affected limb(s) day by day are the keys to an improving prognosis and the decision as to whether to treat for a longer time. Raising a recumbent cow also allows a more thorough

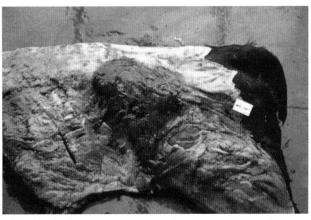

• **Fig. 12.80** Autopsy appearance of the tuber coxae area in a cow that had been repeatedly lifted with a hip sling.

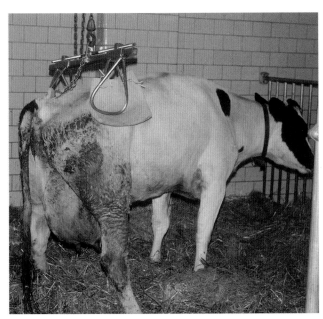

• **Fig. 12.79** Hip slings being used to raise the rear quarters of a cow with exertional myopathy.

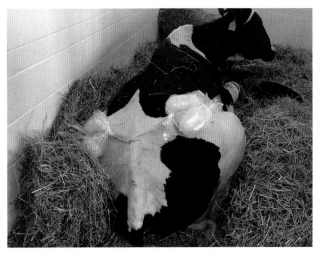

• **Fig. 12.81** Ice packs applied to a valuable cow that required lifting with hip lifters on several occasions before being able to stand.

physical examination, including an easier rectal examination and evaluation of weight-bearing abilities in each limb. This can be an extremely helpful aid to prognosis.

The preferred method for both facilitating an individual to stand and providing physical therapy for a downer cow is a flotation tank. There are commercial units available, including those with the capacity to heat the large volume of water required up to 36°C or 95°F. It is best, although not always possible, to fill the tank quickly to minimize panic on the cow's part. The fact that some cows fear the rising water is supported by the observation that certain individuals, previously abjectly resistant to even the smallest attempt to rise with manual assistance or in a sling, will generate support and stand by the time the water level gets to their dew claws. The means by which the cow is moved into the tank varies; most commercial devices have a winch system attached to a rubber mat on which the individual must first be positioned to be pulled into the tank and then the front and back panels are closed. At the University of Wisconsin, we first place the cow in a sling and then pick her up using a hoist attaching the sling to an I beam in a specially retrofitted stall and slide the cow into the tank. Even the tallest dairy cows can be lifted slightly above the front lip of the floor of the tank via the hoist to safely position them into the flotation tank by this means. Only very rarely is it necessary to sedate a recumbent animal to place the animal into the tank, either for the animal's own safety or that of others, but for obvious reasons sedation is best avoided before flotation.

Periodically, hot water is added to the tank to keep the water temperature as close to the normal thermal range of the cow as possible. In the northern United States and Canada during the winter months, flotation tanks that are used outdoors present a challenge from this perspective. However, several companies that lease flotation tanks in the Upper Mid-West concurrently provide portable hot water tanks with heaters that allow producers to replenish without exhausting the dairy's hot water reserves. In hot ambient temperatures, a shade may also be important outdoors to protect the cow from hyperthermia. Most tanks are equipped with large-diameter drain spigots so that the water can be removed quickly when the decision is made to remove the cow from the tank.

Flotation times are variable according to the individual case and the clinical experience of the clinician or farm. Our most common approach at the University of Wisconsin is to remove the cow twice daily for milking and evaluation but to otherwise maximize the period of time in the flotation tank. Typically, this means that the cow is in the tank for approximately 16 to 18 hours of every day, with two intervals of 2 to 4 hours each outside, when interventions can occur. However, our use of a sling while the cow is in the tank means that there are periods when some cows rest within the tank suspended in the sling with no possibility of falling below the water line; this will not always be the case for different tank setups, so the duration of flotation may have to be adjusted down in those cases. There is little

doubt in our minds that during the early stages of flotation, as cattle attain the ability to stand again, they become tired, and periods of time outside of the tank to lie down and rest are beneficial, if not critical. Some colleagues prefer to place the cow in the tank for only 1 or 2 hours initially, but others leave the cow in the tank for 18 to 24 hours, as long as she is comfortable and eating. At the University of Montreal another of the authors (GF) and his colleagues prefer to leave cattle in the flotation tank for no more than 10 out of each 24-hour period, again believing that the time out of the tank during which cows can lie down is critical for rest and recovery. At the University of Wisconsin we have had a small number of cows develop laminitis after 2 to 3 days of flotation according to our protocol, and it is interesting to theorize that the combination of claw submersion and forced standing for periods that exceed what would be the normal lying-to-standing ratio for a dairy cow have caused this complication. The clinical severity of the laminitis is mild, albeit a nuisance, and has not merely occurred in cattle with primary endotoxemic conditions; still we would rather deal with a moderately footsore, standing, and ambulatory patient rather than one that is persistently recumbent. There is no doubt that with hospital-based supportive care, it is possible to keep a down cow "going" for many days, and with owner persistence and investment, we have continued flotation tank therapy for in excess of 1 week in some instances. However, as a very general guideline, we have found that a continued inability to stand after day 3 carries a poor to grave prognosis. Some sources report successful outcomes for cattle that have been managed in a flotation tank for several weeks but this must be considered unusual and would certainly be expensive. Perhaps the most difficult cases to make decisions on, for owners and veterinarians alike, are those individuals that are able to stand squarely when floated but that are unable, or unwilling, to get up on their own outside the tank. Patience and persistence are justified in these cases, but there are occasional individuals that never progress beyond this point and are euthanized, often for pragmatic, financial reasons.

Twice-daily reassessment of the individual by physical examination, paying particular attention to the musculoskeletal and peripheral nervous system, is important, ideally alongside a daily reevaluation of electrolyte and metabolic status. Food and water must be available to the individual both inside and outside of the flotation tank (Fig. 12.82).

Empirically, cows that have stood squarely in the tank have generally had a better prognosis than those that constantly shift weight (Fig. 12.83 A, and B). There appears to be a small risk of mastitis in cattle remaining in a flotation tank for prolonged periods, and this should be monitored carefully. We commonly use commercial teat sealants in lactating cows and on rare occasions have used these same sealant preparations for cows with surgical incisions that require flotation, although this latter scenario is obviously to be avoided if possible. There is not a great deal of literature examining prognostic indicators for cows in flotation tanks, but the largest published retrospective study from Cornell University identified that cattle

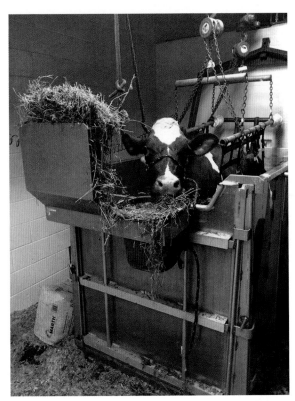

• **Fig. 12.82** Red and White Holstein cow in flotation tank (note the sling used to move the cow into the tank). A homemade, removable addition for feed and water has been attached to the front door.

that were able to walk out of the tank after the first flotation event were almost five times as likely to survive as those that could not, those that could stand squarely within the tank during the first flotation were three times more likely to survive, and cattle that did not eat during first flotation were twice as likely not to survive. Appetite and quickly regaining the ability to stand unassisted and walk are therefore excellent findings in a recently floated cow.

There have been very few disastrous experiences with flotation tanks, but one has to be careful with animals with profound weakness and an inability to support the weight of the head if drowning is to be avoided. Consequently, cattle with botulism or severe hypokalemia are among the poorest candidates for flotation, although we have successfully managed the latter on occasions, with intensive levels of nursing support to ensure the patient does not drown (Fig. 12.84).

As mentioned previously, cattle slings can work very well as a means of moving a cow into and out of a flotation tank when an overhead trolley is available (see Figs. 12.46 and 12.82), but cattle do not tolerate hanging in slings for long periods (Fig. 12.85). Whether used independently or as part of a flotation setup, it is important to position the straps of the sling correctly and use rubber or towel padding to reduce pressure necrosis in the thighs and axillae (see Figs. 12.46 and 12.86). Adult cows with large body frames that hang in slings will develop rub sores and occasionally deep, secondarily infected ulcers in these areas of the body quite rapidly if neglected. But if properly managed, many patients

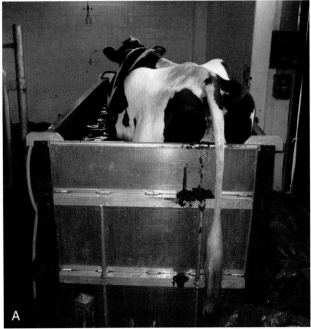

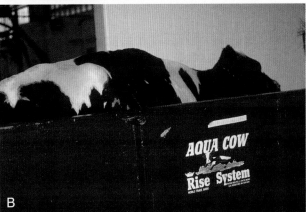

• **Fig. 12.83** Stance of two cows placed in flotation tanks because of an inability to stand. **A,** The cow was recumbent because of a metabolic disease and when placed in the tank stood squarely and recovered. **B,** The cow did not stand squarely, was euthanized after 3 days of treatment, and was found to have a pelvic fracture on necropsy examination.

with mild to moderate myopathies can be saved. Cattle with severe myopathies or cattle with lesser myopathies that are improperly managed have poor prognoses.

White Muscle Disease

Nutritional myodegeneration characterized histologically by Zenker's degeneration was once common in dairy calves in selenium-deficient geographic areas, which constitutes much of the northern United States. The disease can occur in growing animals, and although most common in calves younger than 6 months of age, it can be observed in animals up to 2 years of age. All commercial diets in the United States are now supplemented with the allowable levels of selenium, and hence deficiency has become uncommon. Herds that formulate their own mineral and vitamin

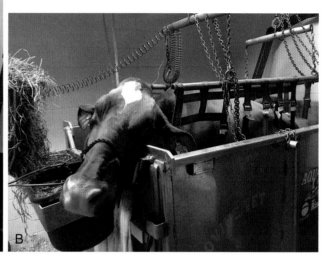

• **Fig. 12.84** Red and White Holstein heifer with severe hypokalemia (serum potassium, 1.8 mEq/L) being managed in a flotation tank. Profound weakness and consequent inability to support the weight of the head (**A**) necessitated constant supervision and use of ropes or the sides of the tank (**B**) by the heifer herself to keep her head above the water. With aggressive oral supplementation, the potassium level normalized within 24 hours, and the heifer made a complete recovery.

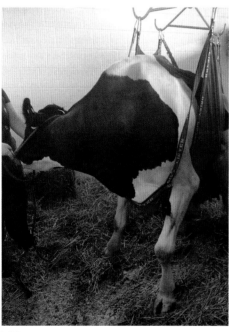

• **Fig. 12.85** Cattle generally do not tolerate being slung for any extended time and often collapse in a sling. The quality of the sling can have some effect on the time of standing. Rigid stabilization bars and focused, balanced lifting of both the hind quarters and front quarters (see image 12.86) would likely offer more support than the sling seen here in Fig. 12.85.

mixtures or have them custom made may be feeding more than allowable levels (which may be necessary to meet requirements because they are based on an allowable concentration and not on milligrams of selenium consumed per

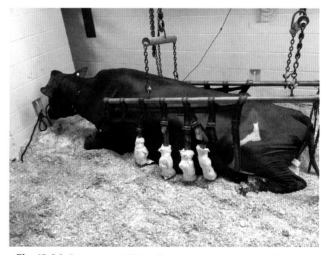

• **Fig. 12.86** Recumbent Milking Shorthorn cow in a sling. Towels and rubber sleeves have been placed on the straps that pass under her body or in between the thighs and her udder—areas that are prone to pressure sores. Similar padding can be beneficial over parts of the sling that pass through the axillae.

day). As a consequence of this widespread use of selenium supplementation, clinical cases of white muscle disease are now mostly seen in calves from hobby farms where commercial diets are not fed.

Deficiency of selenium, vitamin E, or both may play a role in predisposing to the disease. Selenium is an important trace element that plays a role in the defense against the accumulation of hydroperoxides from cellular metabolism. This is accomplished through the selenoproteins such as the glutathione peroxidase family, iodothyronine deiodinases, and the thioredoxin reductases, in which selenium is a structural component of the enzymatic active site. Vitamin E also protects against superoxide damage resulting from the normal oxidation of unsaturated lipids in the diet. Forages and grain should contain at least 0.1 to 0.3 ppm of selenium (on a dry matter basis) to be considered adequate. Aging, fermentation, and other factors may have a negative impact on vitamin E content of stored feeds such that levels of this vitamin are much lower when fed than when originally harvested. Studies in other species suggest that certain dietary minerals may interact with selenium to increase or decrease bioavailability, but this work has not been repeated in cattle.

Signs of white muscle disease may involve any striated muscles, including those in the pharynx (see Figs. 13.66A and B), larynx, tongue, respiratory muscles, heart, neck, or limb musculature. In newborn calves, the tongue may be the only tissue affected, such that the animal may be unable to nurse. The tongue feels slightly flaccid, and the calf wants to eat, but the tongue merely lolls when a finger is inserted into the calf's mouth to evaluate the sucking reflex. Inhalation pneumonia may develop in several calves within a group, or obvious dyspnea may appear when pharyngeal, laryngeal, and respiratory muscles such as the intercostals and diaphragm are affected. Indeed, in recent years, the few cases that one of the authors (SP) has seen have commonly had tachypnea or dyspnea (or both) as the major presenting signs, erroneously, but understandably, perceived by the client as being attributable to pneumonia. Unfortunately, because weakness caused by selenium deficiency so easily leads to aspiration, the two may go hand in hand.

Classic signs of a stiff gait may be observed early in the course, especially in calves that have just moved from close confinement to a large area where more exercise occurs. A stilted gait may be apparent in just the hind limbs, just the forelimbs, or all limbs. When present, this sign requires differentiation from laminitis, polyarthritis, and tetanus. Diffuse muscle degeneration leads to weakness, and this is a common sign in young calves (Fig. 12.87). When lifted to a standing position, these calves will have muscular tremors within seconds of trying to support their own weight, and then within a short time, the head will drop as a result of cervical musculature weakness. If made to stand longer, the limbs may collapse, or the animal may show obvious dyspnea. Severe diffuse muscular degeneration can lead to complete collapse, and affected individuals may appear paralyzed at first glance. The worst cases are depressed and dyspneic and may show apparent neurologic signs secondary to metabolic acidosis associated with high levels of lactic acid released from damaged musculature. Gross myoglobinuria usually is present in these severely affected animals. Pigment nephropathy may also lead to secondary renal failure.

When the myocardium is affected, arrhythmias, heart murmurs, dyspnea associated with pulmonary edema, or sudden death with no premonitory signs may be observed. Exercise accentuates the signs in affected animals, and stimulation or handling may precipitate the signs in apparently normal but deficient animals.

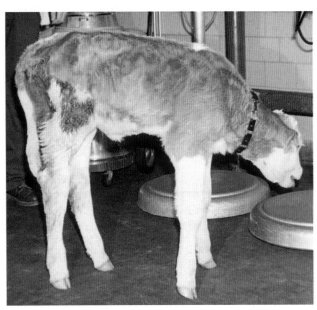

• **Fig. 12.87** A 1-week-old calf with diffuse white muscle disease. After being raised, the calf could only support itself for a few seconds before collapsing. The calf was unable to raise its head because of neck musculature weakness. Open-mouth breathing is apparent as a result of myopathy involving the muscles of respiration.

In acute cases with localized Zenker's degeneration in heavy muscle groups, the muscle may be firm and swollen when palpated. In most instances, however, and certainly in those with severe diffuse Zenker's degeneration, the affected muscles are soft when palpated. Chronic cases that have been recumbent for days may show obvious muscle atrophy and fibrosis.

Clinical signs, especially if more than one animal is affected, coupled with myoglobin in the urine often suffice for clinical diagnosis. Gross myoglobinuria is more common in diffuse degeneration or in older calves that have heavy skeletal musculature affected. Less obvious myoglobinuria should be suspected when urine dipstick evaluation confirms a positive blood (this can be triggered by hemoglobin, red blood cells [RBCs], or myoglobin) and protein reaction. Laboratory findings of very elevated CK and AST values help confirm the diagnosis. Values for CK increase quickly and, because of the short half-life of this enzyme, may decrease within 2 to 4 days unless continued muscle destruction occurs. Values for AST tend to increase slowly over 1 to 2 days and then reach a plateau for nearly 1 week. Therefore the history coupled with enzyme values can be helpful in interpretation. CK values will be greater than 1000 IU/L and frequently exceed 10,000 IU/L. Values for AST usually exceed 500 IU/L. These values tend to be much higher in older animals in which the sheer mass of affected musculature tends to elevate the enzymes far more than in a young calf, for example, that has only myocardial involvement or muscles of deglutition affected. Final confirmation of the diagnosis rests on laboratory assessment of whole-blood selenium (heparinized sample) or glutathione peroxidase (ethylenediaminetetraacetic acid sample). Postmortem tissue levels, specifically those in liver or kidney, can also

TABLE 12.1	Ranges for Selenium and Glutathione Peroxidase	
	Whole Blood Selenium (µg/dL)	Glutathione Peroxidase (U/g Hb)
Normal	>12.0	>30
Marginal	8.0–12.0	20–30
Deficient	<8.0	<20

be used for selenium quantitation in animals suspected to be deficient. Selenium is incorporated in glutathione peroxidase in erythrocytes, and this enzyme facilitates cellular breakdown of peroxides. Because selenium must be incorporated into RBC glutathione peroxidase during erythrogenesis, an increase in measured glutathione peroxidase requires 4 to 6 weeks. Therefore glutathione peroxidase can be evaluated even if an affected or suspected calf has recently received supplemental selenium, although selenium values from the same calf may not be as valuable. In untreated calves, whole-blood selenium usually is assessed. Ranges for selenium and glutathione peroxidase are listed in Table 12.1, even though individual laboratories may establish slightly different normal ranges.

White muscle disease is a "selenium-responsive" disease, so that, regardless of the exact etiology (selenium, vitamin E, or binding of selenium by other minerals), treatment and prevention require supplementation with selenium products through injection or feeding.

Affected calves require injection of selenium and vitamin E at manufacturers' recommended dosages, and these injections may be repeated up to three to four times at 3-day intervals.

Overtreatment with selenium and vitamin E preparations by injection is dangerous because selenium toxicity may develop, with subsequent death of the patient. Therefore it is important to adhere strictly to label dosage recommendations when treating with commercial vitamin E and selenium preparations.

Suggested Readings

Adams, S. B. (1985). The role of external fixation and emergency fracture management in bovine orthopedics. *Vet Clin North Am Food Anim Pract, 1*, 109–129.

Anderson, D. E., St-Jean, G., Morin, D. E., et al. (1996). Traumatic flexor tendon injuries in 27 cattle. *Vet Surg, 25*, 320–326.

Apley, M. D. (2015). Clinical evidence for individual animal therapy for papillomatous digital dermatitis (hairy heel wart) and infectious bovine pododermatitis (foot rot). *Vet Clin North Am Food Anim Pract, 31*(1), 81–95.

Bentley, V. A., Edwards, R. B., III, Santschi, E. M., et al. (2005). Repair of femoral capital physeal fractures with 7.0 mm cannulated screws in cattle: 20 cases (1988-2002). *J Am Vet Med Assoc, 227*, 964–969.

Berg, J. N., & Loan, R. W. (1975). Fusobacterium necrophorum and Bacteroides melaninogenicus as etiological agents in foot rot in cattle. *Am J Vet Res, 36*, 115.

Bergsten, C. (1994). Haemorrhages of the sole horn of dairy cows as a retrospective indicator of laminitis: an epidemiological study. *Acta Vet Scand, 35*, 55–66.

Bicalho, R. C., Cheong, S. H., Warnick, L. D., et al. (2006). The effect of digit amputation or arthrodesis surgery on culling and milk production in Holstein dairy cows. *J Dairy Sci, 89*, 2596–2602.

Blood, D. C. (1956). Arthrogryposis and hydrancephaly. *Aust Vet J, 32*, 125–131.

Bouckaert, J. H., & DeMoor, A. (1966). Treatment of spastic paralysis in cattle: improved denervation technique of the gastrocnemius muscle and postoperative course. *Vet Rec, 79*, 226.

Burton, A. J., Nydam, D. V., Ollivett, T. L., et al. (2009). Prognostic indicators for non-ambulatory cattle treated by use of a flotation tank system in a referral hospital: 51 cases (1997-2008). *J Am Vet Med Assoc, 234*, 1177–1182.

Colam-Ainsworth, P., Lunn, G. A., Thomas, R. C., et al. (1989). Behaviour of cows in cubicles and its possible relationship with laminitis in replacement dairy heifers. *Vet Rec, 125*, 573–575.

Cox, V. S. (1981). Understanding the downer cow syndrome. *Compend Contin Educ Pract Vet, 3*, S472–S478.

Cox, V. S., McGrath, C. J., & Jorgensen, S. E. (1982). The role of pressure damage in pathogenesis of the downer cow syndrome. *Am J Vet Res, 43*, 26–31.

Crawford, W. H. (1990). Intra-articular replacement of bovine cranial cruciate ligaments with an autogenous fascial graft. *Vet Surg, 19*, 380–388.

Dermirkan, I., Walker, R. L., Murray, R. D., et al. (1999). Serological evidence of spirochaetal infections associated with digital dermatitis in dairy cattle. *Vet J, 157*, 69–77.

Desrochers, A., Anderson, D. E., & St.-Jean, G. (2001). Lameness examination in cattle. *Vet Clin North Am Food Anim Pract, 17*, 39–51.

Desrochers, A., & Ducharme, N.G. (2017). Cranial cruciate rupture. In S. L. Fubini, & N.D. Ducharme (Eds.), *Farm Animal Surgery* (2nd ed.). St. Louis:Elsevier.

Desrochers, A., & Francoz, D. (2014). Clinical management of septic arthritis in cattle. *Vet Clin North Am Food Anim Pract, 30*(1), 177–203.

Desrochers A., Steiner A., Anderson D. et al. (2017). Surgery of the Bovine Musculoskeletal System in Farm Animal Surgery (2nd ed.) Fubini SL and Ducharme NG (editors) St.Louis: Elsevier.

Ewoldt, J. M., Hull, B. L., & Ayars, W. H. (2003). Repair of femoral capital physeal fractures in 12 cattle. *Vet Surg, 32*, 30–36.

Fenwick, D. C. (1969). Parturient paresis of cows. I. Response to treatment and the effect of the duration of symptoms. *Aust Vet J, 45*(4), 111–113.

Fenwick, D. C. (1969). The downer cow syndrome. *Aust Vet J, 45*(4), 123–126.

Ferguson, J. G. (1982). Management and repair of bovine fractures. *Compend Contin Educ Pract Vet, 4*, S128–S136.

Ferguson, J. G. (1985). Principles of application of internal fixation in cattle. *Vet Clin North Am Food Anim Pract, 1*, 139–152.

Ferguson, J. G. (1985). Special considerations in bovine orthopedics and lameness. *Vet Clin North Am Food Anim Pract, 1*, 131–138.

Firth, E. C., Kersjes, A. W., Kik, K. J., et al. (1987). Haematogenous osteomyelitis in cattle. *Vet Rec, 120*, 148–152.

Foditsch, C., Oikonomou, G., Machado, V. S., et al. (2016). Lameness prevalence and risk factors in large dairy farms in upstate New York. Model development for the prediction of claw horn disruption lesions. *PLoS One, 11*(1), e:0146718.

Francoz, D., Desrochers, A., Fecteau, G., et al. (2005). Synovial fluid changes in induced infectious arthritis in calves. *J Vet Intern Med, 19*, 336–343.

Frankena, K., van Keulen, K. A. S., Noordhuizen, J. P., et al. (1992). A cross-sectional study in prevalence and risk indicators of digital haemorrhages in female dairy calves. *Prev Vet Med, 14*, 1–12.

Frei, S., & Nuss, K. (2015). Intermittent upward fixation of the patella in 12 cows: a retrospective study of treatment and long-term prognosis. *Schweiz Arch Tierheilkd, 157*(10), 553–558.

Gangl, M., Grukle, S., Serteyn, D., et al. (2006). Retrospective study of 99 cases of bone fractures in cattle treated by external coaptation or confinement. *Vet Rec, 158*, 264–268.

García-Muñoz, A., Vidal, G., Singh, N., et al. (2016). Evaluation of two methodologies for lameness detection in dairy cows based on postural and gait abnormalities observed during milking and while restrained at headlock stanchions. *Prev Vet Med, 128*, 33–40.

Garrett, E. F., Nordlund, K. V., Goodger, W. J., et al. (1997). A cross-sectional field study investigating the effect of periparturient dietary management on ruminal pH in early lactation dairy cows. *J Dairy Sci, 80*(Suppl. 1), 169 (abstract).

Gilhuus, M., Kvitle, B., L'Abée-Lund, T. M., et al. (2014). A recently introduced Dichelobacter nodosus strain caused an outbreak of footrot in Norway. *Acta Vet Scand, 56*, 29.

Gilliam, J. N., Streeter, R. N., Papich, M. G., et al. (2008). Pharmacokinetics of florfenicol in serum and synovial fluid after regional intravenous perfusion in the distal portion of the hind limb of adult cows. *Am J Vet Res, 69*(8), 997–1004.

Greenough, P. R., MacCallum, F. J., & Weaver, A. D. (1997). *Lameness in cattle* (3rd ed.). St. Louis: WB Saunders.

Grubelnik, M., Kofler, J., Martinek, B., et al. (2002). Ultrasonographic examination of the hip joint region and bony pelvis in cattle. *Berl Munch Tierarztl Wochenschr, 115*, 209–220.

Gütze, R. (1932). Spastic paresis of the hindquarters of calves and young cattle. *Dtsch Tierärztl Wochenschr, 40*, 197.

Hull, B. L., Koenig, G. J., & Monke, D. R. (1990). Treatment of slipped capital femoral epiphysis in cattle: 11 cases (1974-1988). *J Am Vet Med Assoc, 197*, 1509–1512.

Hum, S., Kessell, A., Djordjevic, S., et al. (2000). Mastitis, polyarthritis and abortion caused by Mycoplasma species bovine group 7 in dairy cattle. *Aust Vet J, 78*, 744–750.

Jones, M. L., Washburn, K. E., Fajt, V. R., et al. (2015). Synovial fluid pharmacokinetics of tulathromycin, gamithromycin and florfenicol after a single subcutaneous dose in cattle. *BMC Vet Res, 11*, 26–30.

Krull, A. C., Shearer, J. K., Gorden, P. J., et al. (2016). Digital dermatitis: natural lesion progression and regression in Holstein dairy cattle over 3 years. *J Dairy Sci, 99*(5), 3718–3731.

Leonard, F. C., O'Connell, J., & O'Farrell, K. (1994). Effect of different housing conditions on behaviour and foot lesions in Friesian heifers. *Vet Rec, 134*, 490–494.

Livesey, C. T., & Fleming, F. L. (1984). Nutritional influences on laminitis, sole ulcer and bruised sole in Friesian cows. *Vet Rec, 14*, 510–512.

Logue, D. N., Offer, J. E., & McGovern, R. E. (September 1998). The housing effects of first calving Holstein Friesian heifers separately or with the adult herd on claw conformation and lesion development. In C. J. Lischer, & P. Ossent (Eds.), *10th International Symposium on Lameness in Ruminants* (pp. 60–62). Lucerne: Department of Veterinary Surgery, University of Zurich.

Maas, J. P. (1983). Diagnosis and management of selenium-responsive diseases in cattle. *Compend Contin Educ Pract Vet, 5*, S393–S399.

Madison, J. B., Tulleners, E. P., Ducharme, N. G., et al. (1989). Idiopathic gonitis in heifers: 34 cases (1976-1986). *J Am Vet Med Assoc, 194*, 273–277.

Manson, F. J., & Leaver, J. D. (1988). The influence of concentrate amount on locomotion and clinical lameness in dairy cattle. *Anim Prod, 47*, 185–190.

Marchionatti, E., Fecteau, G., & Desrochers, A. (2014). Traumatic conditions of the coxofemoral joint: luxation, femoral head-neck fracture, acetabular fracture. *Vet Clin North Am Food Anim Pract, 30*(1), 247–264.

Martens, A., Steenhaut, M., Gasthuys, F., et al. (1998). Conservative and surgical treatment of tibial fractures in cattle. *Vet Rec, 143*, 12–16.

Maton, A. (1987). The influence of the housing system on claw disorders with dairy cows. In H. K. Wierenga, & D. J. Peterse (Eds.), *Cattle housing systems, lameness, and behaviour: Proceedings of Commission of European Communities, Brussels, June 1986* (pp. 151–158). Dordrecht: Martinus Nijhoff Publishers.

McDuffee, L. A., Ducharme, N. G., & Ward, J. L. (1993). Repair of sacral fracture in two dairy cattle. *J Am Vet Med Assoc, 202*, 1126–1128.

Mehdi, Y., & Dufrasne, I. (2016). Selenium in cattle: a review. *Molecules, 21*, 545–549.

Metz, J. H. M., & Wierenga, H. K. (1987). Behavioural criteria for the design of housing systems for cattle. In H. K. Wierenga, & D. J. Peterse (Eds.), *Cattle housing systems, lameness, and behaviour: Proceedings of Commission of European Communities, Brussels, June 1986* (pp. 14–25). Dordrecht: Martinus Nijhoff Publishers.

Murphy, P. A., Hannan, J., & Monaghan, M. (1987). A survey of lameness in beef cattle housed on slats and on straw. In H. K. Wierenga, & D. J. Peterse (Eds.), *Cattle housing systems, lameness, and behaviour: Proceedings of Commission of European Communities, Brussels, June 1986* (pp. 67–72). Dordrecht: Martinus Nijhoff Publishers.

Nelson, D. R. (1983). Surgery of the stifle joint in cattle. *Compend Contin Educ Pract Vet, 5*, S300–S306.

Nelson, D. R., & Kneller, S. K. (1985). Treatment of proximal hind-limb lameness in cattle. *Vet Clin North Am Food Anim Pract, 1*, 153–173.

Nuss, K., & Weaver, M. P. (1991). Resection of the distal interphalangeal joint in cattle: an alternative to amputation. *Vet Rec, 128*, 540–543.

Offinger, J., Herdtweck, S., Rizk, A., et al. (2013). Postoperative analgesic efficacy of meloxicam in lame dairy cows undergoing resection of the distal interphalangeal joint. *J Dairy Sci, 96*(2), 866–876.

Pejsa, T. G., St. Jean, G., Hoffsis, G. F., et al. (1993). Digit amputation in cattle: 85 cases (1971-1990). *J Am Vet Med Assoc, 202*, 981–984.

Peterse, D. J., Korver, S., Oldenbroek, J. K., et al. (1984). Relationship between levels of concentrate feeding and incidence of sole ulcers in dairy cattle. *Vet Rec, 115*, 629–630.

Potter, M. J., & Broom, D. M. (1987). The behaviour and welfare of cows in relation to cubicle house design. In H. K. Wierenga, & D. J. Peterse (Eds.), *Cattle housing systems, lameness, and behaviour: Proceedings of Commission of European Communities, Brussels, June 1986* (pp. 129–147). Dordrecht: Martinus Nijhoff Publishers.

Rajkondawar, P. G., Liu, M., Dyer, R. M., et al. (2006). Comparison of models to identify lame cows based on gait and lesion scores, and limb movement variables. *J Dairy Sci, 89*, 4267–4275.

Read, D. H., Walker, R. L., Castro, A. E., et al. (1992). An invasive spirochete associated with interdigital papillomatosis of dairy cattle. *Vet Rec*, *130*, 59–60.

Rebhun, W. C., Payne, R. M., King, J. M., et al. (1980). Interdigital papillomatosis in dairy cattle. *J Am Vet Med Assoc*, *177*, 437–440.

Rebhun, W. C., de Lahunta, A., Baum, K. H., et al. (1984). Compressive neoplasms affecting the bovine spinal cord. *Compend Contin Educ Pract Vet*, *6*, S396–S400.

Reiland, S., Stromberg, P., Olsson, S. E., et al. (1978). Osteochondrosis in growing bulls. *Acta Radiol*, *358*, 179–196.

Scholz, R. W., & Hutchinson, L. J. (1979). Distribution of glutathione peroxidase activity and selenium in the blood of dairy cows. *Am J Vet Res*, *40*, 245–249.

Studder, E., & Nelson, J. R. (1971). Nutrition related degenerative joint disease in young bulls. *Vet Med*, *66*, 1007–1010.

Thomas, H. J., Remnant, J. G., Bollard, N. J., et al. (2016). Recovery of chronically lame dairy cows following treatment for claw horn lesions: a randomised controlled trial. *Vet Rec*, *178*(5), 116.

Thyssen, I. (1987). Foot and leg disorders in dairy cattle in different housing systems. In H. K. Wierenga, & D. J. Peterse (Eds.), *Cattle housing systems, lameness, and behaviour: Proceedings of Commission of European Communities, Brussels, June 1986* (pp. 166–178). Dordrecht: Martinus Nijhoff Publishers.

Toussaint-Raven, E. (1989). *Cattle footcare and claw trimming*. Ipswich, UK: Farming Press.

Toussaint-Raven, E. (1985). The principles of claw trimming. *Vet Clin North Am Food Anim Pract*, *1*, 93–107.

Trent, A. M., & Plumb, D. (1991). Treatment of infectious arthritis and osteomyelitis. *Vet Clin North Am Food Anim Pract*, *7*, 747–778.

Trott, D. J., Moeller, M. R., Zuerner, R. L., et al. (2003). Characterization of Treponema phagedenis-like spirochetes isolated from papillomatous digital dermatitis lesions in dairy cattle. *J Clin Microbiol*, *41*, 2522–2529.

Tulleners, E., Divers, T. J., & Evans, L. (1985). Bilateral bicipital bursitis in a cow. *J Am Vet Med Assoc*, *186*, 604.

Tulleners, E. P. (1986). Metacarpal and metatarsal fractures in dairy cattle: 33 cases (1979–1985). *J Am Vet Med Assoc*, *189*, 463–468.

Tulleners, E. P., Nunamaker, D. M., & Richardson, D. W. (1987). Coxofemoral luxation in cattle: 22 cases (1980–1985). *J Am Vet Med Assoc*, *191*, 569–574.

van Amstel, S. R., & Shearer, J. K. (2006). Review of pododermatitis circumscripta (ulceration of the sole) in dairy cows. *J Vet Intern Med*, *20*, 805–811.

Van Pelt, R. W. (1972). Idiopathic septic arthritis in dairy cattle. *J Am Vet Med Assoc*, *161*, 278–284.

Van Vleet, J. F. (1982). Amounts of eight combined elements required to induce selenium-vitamin E deficiency and protection by supplements of selenium and vitamin E. *Am J Vet Res*, *43*, 1049–1055.

Verschooten, F., Vermeiren, D., & Devriese, L. (2000). Bone infection in the bovine appendicular skeleton: a clinical, radiographic, and experimental study. *Vet Radiol Ultrasound*, *41*, 250–260.

Walker, R. L., Read, D. H., Loretz, K. J., et al. (1995). Spirochetes isolated from dairy cattle with papillomatous digital dermatitis and interdigital dermatitis. *Vet Microbiol*, *47*, 343–355.

Wenzinger, B., Hagen, R., Schmid, T., et al. (2012). Coxofemoral joint radiography in standing cattle. *Vet Radiol Ultrasound*, *53*(4), 424–429.

White, S. L., Rowland, G. N., & Whitlock, R. H. (1984). Radiographic, macroscopic, and microscopic changes in growth plates of calves raised on hard flooring. *Am J Vet Res*, *45*, 633–639.

Zinicola, M., Higgins, H., Lima, S., et al. (2015). Shotgun metagenomic soequencing reveals functional genes and microbiome associated with bovine digital dermatitis. *PLoS One*, *10*(7): e0133674.

Zinicola, M., Lima, F., Lima, S., et al. (2015). Altered microbiomes in bovine digital dermatitis lesions, and the gut as a pathogen reservoir. *PLoS One*, *10*(3): e0120504.

13

Neurologic Diseases

THOMAS J. DIVERS AND ALEXANDER de LAHUNTA

Bovine Neurologic Examination

There are five components of a neurologic examination: sensorium, gait, postural reactions, spinal reflexes, and cranial nerves (CNs). The order and degree to which these can be performed depend on the clinician's choice and the size and attitude of the patient respectively.

Sensorium

This is best assessed by observing the patient before it is handled. Abnormalities that reflect intracranial interference with the ascending reticular activating system (ARAS) include (in increasing severity) depression, lethargy, obtundation, semicoma (stupor), and coma. Behavioral changes occur with prosencephalic disorders, especially those that affect the limbic system and include propulsive pacing and circling, head pressing, agitation, excessive licking, charging, and mania. Occasionally, head pressing may be demonstrated as a nonspecific sign of pain, particularly abdominal pain, but sometimes it provides evidence of headache or meningitic pain. When it is associated with abdominal pain, the behavior is intermittent, and the patient demonstrates an otherwise normal sensorium when distracted from the activity.

Gait

If the patient is ambulatory, its gait should be observed in a closed area, ideally while being led. Observation from the side is the most informative and while the patient is being walked in small circles in each direction. The quality of the deficits observed with the various anatomic sites of lesions will be described at the beginning of each anatomic area that is covered in this chapter. For difficult cases, it helps to video the gait abnormality so it can be studied repeatedly and with slow motion. With recumbent animals, it is essential to try to sling the animal to determine which limbs are affected, how much voluntary limb movement is present, and the quality of the paresis or paralysis. Be aware that compression of a large muscle mass in heavy animals that are recumbent can reduce the accuracy of your assessment. Animals with

a lower motor neuron (LMN) disorder have difficulty supporting their weight and walk with short strides, but they know where their extremities are located. If they can move their limbs, postural reactions can be performed. Animals with brainstem or spinal cord lesions that interfere with upper motor neuron (UMN) and general proprioceptive (GP) pathways exhibit a delay in the onset of protraction as well as an overreaching of the affected limb, and its course and placement may be abnormal (ataxic). Postural reactions will be delayed, if able to be performed.

Postural Reactions

In calves and young stock that are cooperative, you can assess their ability to hop on each limb by holding up the opposite limb and pushing the patient laterally on the limb being tested. Difficulty in supporting weight with rapid attempts to do so suggests neuromuscular disease. Brainstem or spinal cord disorders that interfere with descending UMN and ascending GP pathways will cause a delay in the hopping response or none at all. (Despite what has been written about neurologic examinations, there is *no* test that is specific for conscious proprioception, and that misconception should be discarded.)

Spinal Reflexes: Muscle Tone and Size

Denervation atrophy is best observed in a standing animal. Realistically, spinal reflex testing is only of value in a recumbent patient, and it is influenced by the extent of muscle compression secondary to recumbency. The limbs can be manipulated to assess muscle tone, but in adult animals, hypotonia can be difficult to determine. The only reliable tendon reflex is the patellar reflex (femoral nerve: L4, L5 spinal cord segments, roots, and nerves). Withdrawal (flexor) reflexes can be done in each limb to assess the integrity of the respective spinal cord intumescence and the nerves that arise from each.

The spinal reflexes are influenced by how much nociception and voluntary movement are still present in the patient. Tail and anal tone and the associated reflexes are readily assessed either in a standing or recumbent animal. In animals with severe nerve or spinal cord disease, the determination of nociception has prognostic importance. Using forceps to produce a noxious stimulus may not be adequate in the recumbent patient, and it may be necessary to use an electric (hot shot) stimulus. This is *not* a pain stimulus. Pain is not a sensory modality. Pain is the subjective response of the patient to a noxious stimulus and varies considerably among individual animals.

Differentiating "superficial and deep pain" as is often described is not only a misnomer but also superfluous and of no practical value in localizing lesions even if one thought he or she could determine the difference.

Cranial Nerves

In most animals and especially young calves, this part of the examination is best done initially without handling the patient and consists of the following:

Assess the menace response with your hand (eye – II – central visual pathway – VII).

Assess the symmetry of the pupils and the pupillary light reflex (eye – II – rostral brainstem – III – ciliary ganglion – iris).

Look for strabismus (III, IV, and VI – vestibular).

Look for resting nystagmus – jerk nystagmus (vestibular VIII), pendular nystagmus – ocular tremor (idiopathic).

Look for the size of the palpebral fissure (VII, III, sympathetic), ear position, and movement (VII).

All of the above can be done without handling the animal.

Move the head side to side for normal physiologic nystagmus (vestibular VIII – brainstem – III, VI).

Hold the head to each side and in extension, and look for development of a positional nystagmus (vestibular VIII).

Evaluate the palpebral reflex (V-brainstem-VII), lip tone (VII), and the response to stimulating the nasal mucosa with your finger (V – brainstem – prosencephalon). Palpate the size of the muscles of mastication, and assess for jaw tone and movement (motor V). Assess the tongue for its strength and size (XII). The ability to swallow is the only way to realistically check the function of the pharyngeal branches of IX and X.

Brain

Clinical Signs of Brain Dysfunction

Prosencephalic signs include all forms of seizure disorders and behavioral changes that range from mild alterations in the animal's relationship with its environment to profound changes in its habits, propulsive pacing and circling, head pressing, and extreme aggression and mania. Changes in the animal's sensorium range from depression to lethargy to obtundation to semicoma (stupor) and to coma. The most profound of these (obtundation to coma) most often

reflect disorders involving the ARAS in the diencephalon (e.g., pituitary abscess). Cerebral disorders cause blindness with normal pupillary light reflexes. Lesions of the eyeballs, prechiasmatic optic tract (optic nerve) or chiasm will cause blindness with abnormal pupillary light reflexes.

There are three features of the neurologic examination that localize lesions in the prosencephalon. All three are contralateral to a unilateral prosencephalic lesion. (1) A normal gait with postural reaction deficits: In animals too large to hop, this may be reflected by observing limbs on one side slide out on a slippery surface or seeing hooves scuff or drag when going over rough ground or a curb; (2) loss of the menace response; and (3) cutaneous or nasal mucosal hypalgesia.

Cranial nerve deficits help localize brainstem lesions: II, diencephalon; III and IV, mesencephalon; V, pons; and VI to XII, medulla.

Gait abnormalities usually occur with lesions caudal to the diencephalon from involvement of the UMN and GP pathways. With unilateral lesions, these deficits are usually ipsilateral.

Vestibular system signs (e.g., balance loss, head tilt, and abnormal nystagmus) occur with lesions in the pons, medulla, and cerebellum. Involvement of the brainstem ARAS results in depression, lethargy, or obtundation. Severe mesencephalic or pontine lesions may cause semicoma or coma.

Cerebellar lesions usually cause a dysmetric gait with a delay in the onset of protraction, followed by an over response creating a sudden burst of flexor activity that is poorly directed. Balance loss often accompanies this gait, as well as an abnormal nystagmus and a head tilt if the lesion is asymmetric. Severe rostral cerebellar lesions may cause opisthotonos.

Malformation of the Brain
Cerebellar Hypoplasia and Atrophy

This is the most common brain malformation observed in the northeastern United States and is most commonly the result of an in utero infection with the bovine viral diarrhea virus (BVDV) agent, usually between 100 and 200 days of gestation. The inflammation peaks about 14 days after infection and resolves before birth. The small malformed cerebellum seen at birth reflects atrophy of the already differentiated cerebellar parenchyma at the time of the infection and hypoplasia from the destruction of the embryonic precursor cells primarily in the external germinal layer (Fig. 13.1). In most affected calves, the cerebellum is largely absent with only a few remnants of cerebellar folia remaining. Clinical signs vary (see Video Clips 13.1 to 13.3). Some calves are unable to stand and often thrash around in their attempts to get up, and they exhibit periods of opisthotonos and sometimes abnormal nystagmus. Others can stand and walk but have a wide-based posture, stagger, and weave from side to side with a hypermetric gait and balance loss (Fig. 13.2).

In some calves, the retina and optic tracts are affected, resulting in blindness. In these calves, the optic nerves, chiasm, and tracts are less than one half their normal size. Cataracts can also occur. Occasionally, there are cavities in the

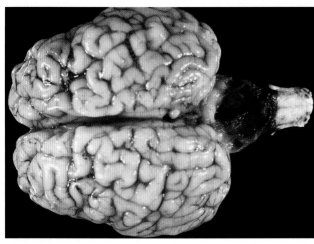

• **Fig. 13.1** Brain from a 3-week-old calf with cerebellar hypoplasia and atrophy caused by in utero bovine viral diarrhea virus infection. Amazingly, the calf was able to stand.

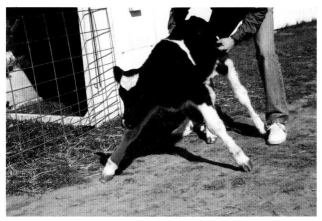

• **Fig. 13.2** A 3-week-old calf with severe cerebellar hypoplasia and atrophy (see Fig. 13.1) that was able to stand; notice the wide-based stance and lowered head position.

cerebrum (porencephaly), which do not contribute to recognizable signs. It is important to obtain a necropsy diagnosis for these calves because their clinical signs do not differ from a possible genetically induced cerebellar malformation. The latter has been observed in Angus and Scottish Highland calves with a symmetrically reduced cerebellar size but no gross or microscopic evidence of any destructive process. In addition, there is no trapezoid body on the ventral surface of the rostral medulla, but there is an abnormal band of parenchyma passing across the fourth ventricle just caudal to the cerebellar peduncles with a nucleus at each end. This may be the trapezoid body and the cochlear nuclei in an abnormal position that cannot be explained by an in utero viral infection. The fourth ventricle is remarkably reduced in size in such cases.

Congenital Cerebellar Function Disorder

On a few occasions, we have seen Holstein calves unable to get up at birth that exhibit opisthotonos and extensor rigidity on attempts to rise. If the calves are assisted, voluntary movements are delayed and overreactive. These calves

are unable to balance and have abnormal nystagmus but are alert, responsive, and visual. Their anatomic dysfunction is primarily cerebellar. At necropsy, there are no gross or microscopic lesions anywhere in the nervous system. This is presumed to be a functional cerebellar disorder that may be inherited, but the latter remains unproven.

Hydranencephaly

This is primarily a cerebral abnormality in which the neopallium is reduced to a thin transparent membrane of pia and glial tissue as a result of complete destruction of the cerebral parenchyma. The lateral ventricle, containing a huge volume of cerebrospinal fluid (CSF), expands to take up the space vacated by the parenchymal loss. This is compensatory hydrocephalus. The hippocampus and olfactory bulb and peduncle and the basal nuclei are usually spared. The skull has a normal shape because CSF circulation is not obstructed in these calves. In utero infection with Akabane or bluetongue virus at around 125 days of gestation are recognized causes of this lesion. BVDV has also been reported as a cause of this cerebral abnormality, but this has not been seen in the northeastern United States where the BVDV-induced cerebellar lesion is common. The Aino and Chuzan viruses have also been implicated. The lesion is probably the result of the destruction of mitotically active progenitor germinal cells, as well as a vasculitis of the branches of the arterial circle that compromises the blood supply to the developing cerebrum. If the lesion is limited to cerebral hydranencephaly, the clinical signs are prosencephalic, and the animal will be able to ambulate but will be obtunded and blind.

Schmallenberg, Akabane, bluetongue and Aino viruses may cause congenital malformations of the brain and appendicular skeleton (e.g., arthrogryposis). Intrauterine infection of the fetus during the susceptible periods of development, i.e. around gestation days 60-180, by these viruses may also cause malformations in the central nervous system, especially in the brain.

Congenital Obstructive Hydrocephalus (Hypertensive)

Inherited forms are described in numerous breeds, including Hereford, Charolais, Dexter, Ayrshire, and Holstein. The obstructive hydrocephalus is often accompanied by other brain malformations, which will influence the character of the clinical signs. A common cause of the obstruction is a failure of the mesencephalic aqueduct to develop normally. The latter may be associated with the presence of a single structure representing the rostral colliculi. The cause of this mesencephalic malformation is unknown in cattle but is inherited in laboratory rodents. Clinical signs will be prosencephalic, but brainstem and cerebellar signs may be present if there is significantly increased intracranial pressure.

Meningoencephalocele

This malformation occurs along the midline of the calvaria through an opening referred to as a cranioschisis or cranium bifidum. The size of the extracranial accumulation of CSF may be extensive, producing a soft, fluctuant, pendular

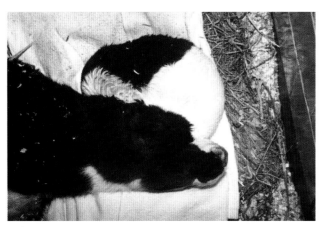

• **Fig. 13.3** A newborn calf with a large fluctuant swelling of the head (meningoencephalocele).

skin-covered structure (Fig. 13.3). Although it is possible that some of these malformations may just be meningoceles, microscopic study of the tissues containing the CSF usually reveals a thin layer of brain parenchyma associated with the meninges immediately beneath the skin, and therefore these are more accurately called meningoencephaloceles.

Lipomeningocele

These also can occur along the midline of the calvaria or vertebral column through a cranioschisis or spina bifida, respectively. They consist of fat-filled meningeal tissue continuous with the falx cerebri in the head or the dural surface in the vertebral canal. With no associated neural tube malformation, there are no neurologic signs in these animals. The cause is unknown.

Complex Nervous System Malformation

A unique multifocal bone and neural tube malformation described in calves has been called an Arnold-Chiari malformation, presumably because of an assumed similarity to a human malformation given this eponym. Although there are some similarities, the distinct differences in the bovine disorder make use of this eponym incorrect. These calves are usually born recumbent and unable to coordinate their limb and trunk function to stand. They often exhibit opisthotonos and abnormal nystagmus. There is a sacrocaudal spina bifida with a meningomyelocele, a malformed tail, and associated loss of tone and reflexes in the anus and tail. At necropsy, the meningomyelocele consists of sacrocaudal nerves connecting from their spinal cord segments in the exposed vertebral canal into the skin-covered swelling over the spina bifida. The ganglia for these nerves are located in this skin. Myelodysplasia is present in the sacrocaudal segments. In the head, the cerebellum is flattened and elongated into a cone-shaped structure, and it is displaced into the foramen of the atlas and cranial axis along with the medulla. The associated CNs are elongated to extend back into the cranial cavity to exit through their respective foramina. There is a bilateral abnormal extension of each occipital lobe into

the caudal cranial fossa space vacated by the cerebellum. These abnormal extensions of the otherwise normal occipital lobes pass ventral to the tentorium, which results in a groove on the lateral side of each of these extensions. These are not herniations of the normal occipital lobes. This malformation has been sporadically recognized in calves since the early 1900s.

Partial Diprosopus and Dicephalus

Occasionally, calves are born with partial duplication of the face (diprosopus). This usually consists of varying degrees of two separate nasal regions; therefore, four nares, parts of two lower jaws, and three orbits with the central one enlarged to accommodate two separate or fused eyeballs. The cranial region is broad, but there are two normal ears and a single normal atlantooccipital joint. These calves have four cerebral hemispheres (one for each naris formed from the embryonic olfactory placode, which gave rise to the olfactory nerves). Each cerebral hemisphere has a normal olfactory bulb, which resides in the cribriform plate related to each nasal cavity. There are four ethmoid bones. Two diencephalons are present (one for each set of eyes, two pairs of prechiasmatic optic tracts [nerves], and two optic chiasms). The brainstem usually becomes single somewhere in the mesencephalon. The pons, medulla, and cerebellum are single structures. This is a partial dicephalus. These calves are usually born alive but are typically recumbent and unable to stand.

Prosencephalic Hypoplasia with Telencephalic Aplasia

Calves with this sporadic, unique malformation are alive at birth and unable to stand. The cranium is flattened between two normal orbits with normal eyeballs. A dorsal midline skin defect is present at the level of the caudal aspect of the orbits. There usually is a slight bloody discharge from this opening, which probably contains CSF. The skin tissue surrounding the opening is continuous caudally with a malformed diencephalon at the rostral portion of the brainstem. There are no cerebral hemispheres, just a malformed brainstem and cerebellum. There are no recognizable geniculate nuclei, no mesencephalic colliculi, and the cerebellum is elongated. With the exception of the olfactory nerves, all of the remaining CNs are present, including the optic nerves that extend to the two eyes. In humans, this defect is called anencephaly, which is inappropriate because a brainstem and cerebellum are present. There is no adequate term for this combination of malformations, and we have chosen to call this prosencephalic hypoplasia with telencephalic aplasia. The cause is unknown in cattle but has been blamed on maternal folic acid deficiency or hyperthermia in humans.

Congenital Tremors
Hypomyelinogenesis

Failure to develop normal central nervous system (CNS) myelin can be the result of an inherited defect in oligodendroglial function or an in utero infection of the fetus that interferes with this process. Some strains of BVDV have been implicated. Diffuse myoclonus (tremors), ataxia, and nystagmus have also been reported (and seen by one author, TJD) in newborn calves persistently infected in utero with BVDV. Diffuse neuraxial hypomyelination is the predominant lesion with occasional cerebellar dysgenesis. The diagnosis is reached by clinical signs, histopathologic findings, and detecting noncytopathic BVD virus antigen in white matter glia or in blood. There does not seem to be a breed predilection or a BVD-specific strain (although most reports have involved type 1 genotypes) associated with the disease, but it is associated with early (<90 day) in utero infection. Occasionally, calves affected by an in utero BVDV infection at later stages of gestation will improve over a few weeks, suggesting that some CNS myelination is possible after recovery from infection. Tremors in newborn calves may be a result of in-utero viral infection or inherited disorders. (see Video Clips 13.4 to 13.6).

An inherited hypomyelinogenesis has been reported in Jersey calves. Calves are usually recumbent at birth, and any muscular activity elicits diffuse whole-body tremors. The more excited the calf becomes and struggles to move, the worse the tremor. It disappears when the calf is completely relaxed. These calves are usually alert, responsive, and visual.

Axonopathy

We recently studied a group of related Holstein calves that at birth were consistently able to stand and walk but had a constant coarse tremor primarily of the trunk and pelvic limbs (see Video Clip 13.5). At necropsy, they all had a diffuse primary axonopathy throughout the spinal cord with secondary demyelination. The condition is of unknown etiopathogenesis.

Inflammation of the Brain

Meningitis

Etiology

Meningitis is inflammation of one or more of the three covering layers of meninges (dura mater, arachnoid, pia mater) in the CNS. Gram-negative septicemia with neuroinvasion in neonates is the most common cause of meningitis in dairy cattle. Calves given inadequate amounts of high-quality colostrum have insufficient levels of passively acquired immunoglobulins to fend off opportunistic organisms. Septicemia may originate in umbilical infections or more commonly via oral inoculation of pathogens. Gram-negative organisms such as *Escherichia coli*, *Klebsiella* spp., and *Salmonella* spp. predominate, with *E. coli* being the most common organism to infect the nervous system of neonatal calves. A summary of four studies on bacterial causes of septicemia in calves found that *E. coli* was the offending isolate in more than 50% of the cases in each study. There may be specific *E. coli* virulence factors that overcome host defense mechanisms, permitting neuroinvasion of the organism. *E. coli* isolates cultured from calves with meningitis are reported to be nonhemolytic, express the 31a surface antigen, and exhibit fimbriation. In colostrum-deficient calves, *Streptococcus* spp. may also cause bacteremia with meningitis, endophthalmitis, and peritonitis. Although any opportunistic or environmental organism may infect a calf with inadequate amounts of passively acquired immunoglobulins, only extremely pathogenic organisms will cause meningitis in a calf having adequate immunoglobulin supplies. Bacteria that gain entrance to the meninges can easily proliferate in the CSF because of low levels of antibody and complement.

Although meningitis is a sporadic disease on well-managed farms, endemic problems may develop when calf husbandry is poor. Certain strains of causative gram-negative or less commonly gram-positive bacteria seem to result in meningitis in a high percentage of calves that develop septicemia. The owner may report similar signs in other calves that have subsequently died. We have identified an unusual strain of *E. coli* as the cause of endemic meningitis in a "baby beef" Holstein calf operation. Affected calves were 2 to 5 months of age. This outbreak represented the first time that we have seen *E. coli* meningitis in calves of this age that are immunocompetent. Another recent report identified *Mannheimia haemolytica* as the cause of acute fibrinosuppurative meningoencephalitis in a 5-month-old Holstein calf. The calf also had bronchopneumonia and was BVDV positive, suggesting that immunosuppression played a role in the co-morbidities of severe meningitis and pneumonia.

Acute bacterial meningitis in adult dairy cattle is not common, and most cases are sporadic. Confirmed sporadic cases of meningitis in adult cows are associated with septicemic spread of bacterial organisms from acutely infected organs such as the mammary gland or uterus, or foci of chronic infection such as traumatic reticuloperitonitis abscesses. Coliform mastitis may be the most common predisposing cause of sporadic bacterial meningitis in adult cattle in our practice area. Mycotic encephalitis has also been observed as a sequela to mycotic mastitis and mycotic rumenitis with subsequent embolic septicemia. Direct extension of chronic infections such as pituitary abscesses and chronic frontal sinusitis may also result in meningitis in adult dairy cattle. When multiple cases of acute meningitis occur within a herd of adult cattle, *Histophilus (Haemophilus) somni* infection should be suspected. It should be emphasized that *H. somni* may cause meningitis rather than thromboembolic meningoencephalitis (TEME) in adult dairy cattle. TEME is rarely observed in dairy heifers in the U.S. between 6 and 24 months of age.

Clinical Signs

Signs of meningitis in neonatal calves may be overt, with classical fever, somnolence, intermittent seizures, head pressing, and blindness, or may be masked by hypovolemic shock and collapse in overwhelming septicemias. When meningitis precedes other major organ dysfunction, signs of fever, depression, head pressing or "headache" appearance, seizures, hyperesthesia, and cerebral blindness signal the diagnosis (Fig. 13.4) (see Video Clip 13.7 and 13.8). If ambulatory, the patient's gait is stiff and the head is often held straight, with the muzzle extended.

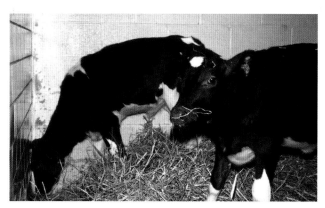

• **Fig. 13.4** Two calves with meningitis. The calf on the left is head pressing into the wall. The calf on the right is unaware of its surroundings and has hay in its mouth but is not chewing. Both calves are blind.

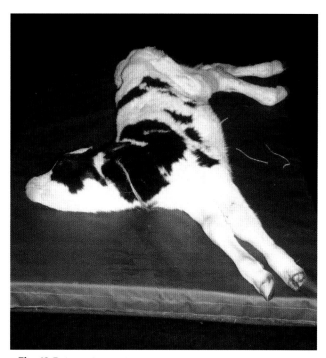

• **Fig. 13.5** A 10-day-old Holstein calf with bacterial meningitis causing severe opisthotonos. The cerebrospinal fluid was grossly abnormal.

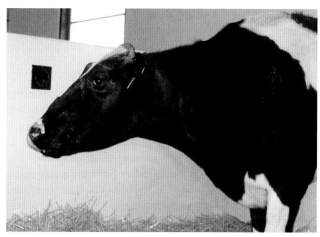

• **Fig. 13.6** An adult cow exhibiting depression with a rather rigid "stargazing" appearance. The cow had a fractured skull, bacterial sinusitis, and meningitis.

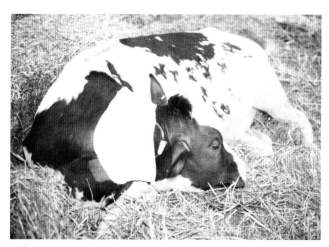

• **Fig. 13.7** A 13-month-old recumbent red and white Holstein heifer with *Histophilus somni* meningoencephalitis. The heifer was treated with ampicillin and supportive treatment and recovered in 1 month. This favorable outcome is unusual in such a severely affected animal.

The condition is painful, and the animal may appear to have a "headache" with the eyelids partially closed and the head and neck extended. However, when meningitis coexists with other organ infection and signs of uveitis, septic arthritis, and omphalophlebitis are apparent, it may be difficult to recognize specific signs of meningitis. Overwhelming septicemia results in rapid deterioration of the neonate such that shock may also mask clinical signs of meningitis. Some calves affected with meningitis have opisthotonos—perhaps caused by cerebral inflammation and edema exerting pressure on the cerebellum and caudal brainstem (Fig. 13.5). Affected calves are generally between 2 and 14 days of age, with the mean being 6 days of age.

Adult cattle affected with meningitis usually have fever and profound depression. A stiff, stilted gait and "headache" appearance (stargazing or continually pressing the head or muzzle against an object) are common (Fig. 13.6), but seizures are less common than in calves. Inflammation of the visual cortex can result in blindness but normal pupillary function will be present.

Meningitis caused by *H. somni* is acute, with affected cattle becoming extremely depressed over just a few hours. Fever usually is present and may be as high as 106.0°F (41.11°C). The depression progresses over 12 to 24 hours to total inappetence and somnolence, and the affected cow may be unable to rise (Fig. 13.7). Depression is so severe that the presence or absence of vision may be difficult to determine, and occasional seizures are observed in some patients. Affected cows typically die within 24 to 48 hours of onset unless treated specifically for *H. somni*. Herds experiencing *H. somni* meningitis often have multiple cases over a period of several months until appropriate diagnostics and preventive measures are used. TEME caused by *H. somni*, although rare, does occur in growing dairy heifers over 4 months of age and causes acute severe neurologic disease that may be accompanied by retinal lesions (Fig. 13.8).

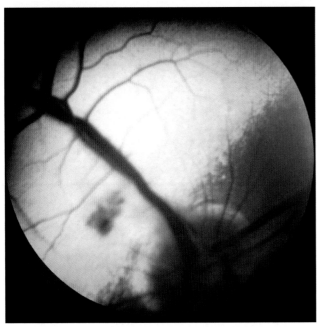

• **Fig. 13.8** Focal chorioretinitis with hemorrhage dorsal to the optic disc in a Holstein yearling with thromboembolic meningoencephalitis. *Histophilus somni* was cultured from a cerebrospinal fluid tap obtained from this patient.

Diagnosis

Clinical signs coupled with CSF analysis confirm the diagnosis of meningitis. Increased values for protein (normal ≤40 mg/dL) and white blood cells (WBCs) (normal ≤6 nucleated cells/μL) are present in the CSF of meningitis patients, and the WBCs are mostly neutrophils in acute cases (Table 13.1). In subacute cases, macrophages may predominate. The fluid can appear normal on visual examination, or it can be grossly discolored (red to orange). Neonatal calves showing neurologic signs that also have omphalophlebitis, uveitis, or septic arthritis should be suspected of having meningitis.

Bacterial cultures of the CSF and blood are indicated to determine the exact causative organism. Serum protein and immunoglobulin levels should be evaluated in neonatal calves to investigate adequacy of passive transfer of immunoglobulins and thereby assess the effectiveness of preventive calf management procedures.

The diagnosis may be more difficult in adult cattle with meningitis secondary to acute or chronic infections elsewhere in the body. These cattle have been ill for variable lengths of time, and the developing signs of meningitis may be mistakenly assumed to be progressive systemic illness associated with failure to respond to therapy for the primary condition.

TABLE 13.1	Cerebrospinal Fluid Results in 66 Cattle with Infectious Central Nervous System Disease, Grouped by Disease Diagnosis*							
Disease Diagnosis	Patients (*n*)	Protein (mg/dL)	RBC/μL	TNCC/μL	Mean Differential Cell Count (%) NEUT	Mean Differential Cell Count (%) LYM	Mean Differential Cell Count (%) MONO	Mean Differential Cell Count (%) EOS
Listeriosis	23	72 (16–371)	50 (0–18,310)	25 (2–328)	2	20	78	0
Neonatal meningitis	11	414 (61–1236)	600 (5–160,000)	2900 (425–30,000)	83	2	15	0
Older calf meningitis	4	255 (46–971)	4045 (430–64,500)	1225 (405–12,800)	33	29	38	0
Otitis with meningitis	4	118 (17–565)	202 (2–83,200)	329 (2–1200)	19	21	60	0
TEME	3	(156–818)	(38–2916)	(90–462)	(0–94)	(0–100)	(0–86)	0
Abscess	12	85 (34–425)	74 (0–10,170)	13 (2–5100)	4	11	85	0
Rabies	2	(68–97)	(1–219)	(7–14)	(0–1)	(50–54)	(46–49)	0
Malignant catarrhal fever	2	(36–98)	(26–70)	(17–40)	(0–1)	(23–51)	(48–77)	0
Parelaphostrongylus tenuis	5	86 (24–101)	133 (0–522)	406 (113–1026)	0	71	10	19

*Cerebrospinal fluid results expressed as single number = mean or percentage for differential count and ( ) = range.

EOS, eosinophils; *LYM,* lymphocytes; *MONO,* monocytes; *NEUT,* neutrophils; *RBC,* red blood cell; *TEME,* thromboembolic meningoencephalitis; *TNCC,* total nucleated cell count.

Adapted from Stokol T, Divers TJ, Arrigan JW, et al: Cerebrospinal fluid findings in cattle with central nervous system disorders: a retrospective study of 102 cases (1990-2008). *Vet Clin Pathol* 38(1):103-112, 2009.

Depression, an extended head and neck, head pressing, blindness with intact pupillary light responses, and seizures are all possible signs that may exist in individual patients. To repeat, CSF evaluation is necessary for diagnosis and will yield increased protein and WBCs, primarily neutrophils in acute cases and macrophages in more chronic cases.

Treatment

Broad-spectrum antibiotics constitute the primary treatment for meningitis in calves and adult cattle. Although the blood–brain barrier normally interferes with effective CSF levels for most antibiotics, the barrier is compromised by inflammation in meningitis patients. Therefore most antibiotics enter the CSF in higher levels than would be possible in the healthy state. Antibiotics should be chosen based on the likely causative organism. For example, in neonatal calves, the anticipated cause would be a gram-negative organism such as *E. coli*, and ceftiofur, florfenicol or enrofloxacin would be appropriate antibiotics. Enrofloxacin use in dairy calves in the United States is only permitted for respiratory disease so this is an obstacle to its use unless pneumonia and meningitis exist as co-morbidities. Furthermore, ceftiofur and enrofloxacin should only be administered at doses and via the route of administration as specified by the label instructions and these might not result in adequate or sustained levels in the CSF. In very valuable calves or when the cultured organism is resistant to commonly used antibiotics, aminoglycosides (amikacin 20 mg/kg once daily), could be considered. If amikacin is used, fluids should be given and proper meat withdrawal time advised. In valuable calves, one of the authors (TJD) has also administered a single dose of 125 mg preservative free amikacin intrathecally at the LS site to supplement parenteral antibiotic therapy when amikacin treatment has been indicated. Ampicillin (5 mg/kg IM twice daily or 10–20 mg/kg IV three times daily – these constitute an extralabel dose) or trimethoprim/sulfa 30 mg/kg orally twice daily are alternative treatments to those antibiotics listed above. These antibiotics have both gram negative and gram positive activity and are appropriate choices in those cases of calf meningitis where a *Streptococcus* spp. is the causative agent. In adult cattle with secondary meningitis, the likely cause of the primary disease (e.g., mastitis, metritis) should be considered when choosing a systemic antibiotic. Gram stain evaluation of CSF may be rewarding in some cases and thereby guide antibiotic selection. When *H. somni* is suspected, ampicillin (5 mg/kg twice daily or 10-20 mg/kg IV three times daily) and florfenicol (20 mg/kg in replacement heifers) are reasonable antibiotic choices. Without early treatment, the prognosis for recovery is grave. Some calves that are aggressively treated too late, even with appropriate antibiotics, may live for several days but never regain reasonable mentation. Such cases often have necrotic lesions in the brain or gross suppurative meningitis at necropsy (Fig. 13.9).

Supportive treatment with a single dose of corticosteroids (5–10 mg of dexamethasone) and mannitol (0.5 mg/kg slowly intravenously [IV]) may help decrease life-threatening inflammation and cerebral edema associated with meningitis. Some practitioners administer nonsteroidal antiinflammatory drugs (NSAIDs) instead of corticosteroids. If the inflammation cannot

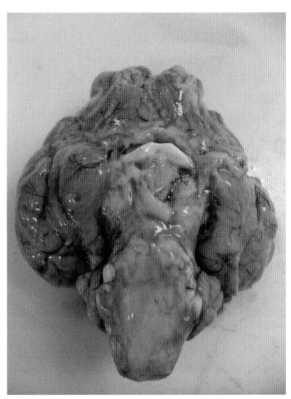

• **Fig. 13.9** The brain from a 10-day-old Brown Swiss calf (seen in Video Clip 13.7) showing gross suppurative meningitis. There was a heavy growth of *Escherichia coli* from the cerebrospinal fluid.

be immediately controlled, the calf will probably die despite proper antimicrobial therapy. Seizures may be controlled with 5 to 10 mg of diazepam in neonatal meningitis patients.

Prevention

Adequate passive transfer of immunoglobulins through well-managed colostrum feeding of each newborn calf is the most important method of prevention. Dipping navels and providing a clean, dry environment will minimize opportunities for navel infection, septicemia, and meningitis. Herd vaccination against *H. somni* is indicated whenever meningitis or TEME are found to be caused by this organism.

Brain Abscesses and Pituitary Abscesses
Etiology

Brain abscesses, similar to abscesses affecting the spinal cord, usually arise from embolic spread of bacteria from distant sites of infection or during septicemic episodes. Calves develop brain abscesses most commonly from umbilical sepsis, pneumonia, and by extension from otitis media or interna, but in adult cattle they are usually associated with chronic infections, such as hardware disease, chronic musculoskeletal abscesses, or rumenitis. In addition, direct extension from chronic frontal sinusitis and bacterial seeding associated with nose rings in bulls or other infections of the head are other potential causes of brain abscesses in adult cattle. Although the relationship with frontal sinusitis is obvious, the inferred higher risk of cattle or bulls with nose rings for brain or pituitary abscesses is very interesting. Theories to explain this phenomenon center around

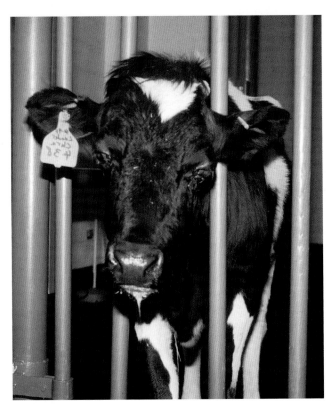

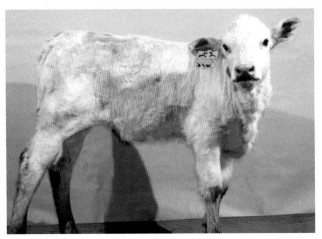

• **Fig. 13.11** Calf with a brain abscess. The calf is profoundly depressed, is unaware of its surroundings, has a "stargazing" head carriage with the head and neck turned to the right (pleurothotonos), and has right-side hemianopsia and right hopping deficits. A left cerebral abscess was identified at necropsy.

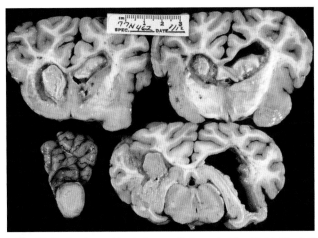

• **Fig. 13.12** Sections of brain from calf shown in Fig. 13.11. The left side of the photo illustrates the left side of the brain.

• **Fig. 13.10** A heifer with exophthalmos, swollen conjunctivae, excessive salivation, and depression caused by a brain abscess. Cerebrospinal fluid was normal.

the complex rete mirabile circulation that encircles the pituitary region suspended within the cavernous sinuses which receives venous drainage from the nasal cavity. Also see the description of cavernous sinus syndrome in Chapter 14. *Trueperella pyogenes* is the most common organism isolated from brain abscesses in cattle.

Clinical Signs

Signs vary tremendously, depending on the neuroanatomic location of the brain abscess. Initial signs such as mild depression, dysphagia, hemiparesis, and hemianopsia may be subtle and frequently go undetected by the owner. As the abscess enlarges, varying degrees of visual disturbance, paresis, ataxia, profound depression, and CN signs become apparent. Head pressing may be observed (see Video Clips 13.9 and 13.10). Calves tend to be affected between 2 and 8 months of age, thereby being past the typical age for neonatal meningitis. If the abscess becomes sufficiently large, it will interfere with venous return of blood from the orbital region and cause exophthalmos (Fig. 13.10). Adult cattle with brain abscesses can be of any age. Depression and a stargazing attitude have been observed in some cattle with cerebral abscesses. Bradycardia coupled with depression and a stargazing attitude have been described to indicate a pituitary abscess (Fox FH, personal communication, 1985, Ithaca, NY), but other signs such as blindness, dysphagia, or CN deficits are possible. A review of pituitary abscesses found that approximately 50% had bradycardia in addition to other neurologic signs. The bradycardia may result from both involvement of the hypothalamus and the

accompanying anorexia. Cranial nerves that arise from the medulla oblongata may be affected by a pituitary abscess causing tongue paresis (CN XII), dropped jaw (motor CN V), dysphagia (CNs IX & X), in addition to signs of facial (CN VII) or vestibular (CN VIII) nerve dysfunction.

Abscesses localized to one cerebral hemisphere usually cause blindness with intact pupillary function in the contralateral eye (hemianopsia) as a result of optic radiation or cerebral cortical injury (Figs. 13.11 and 13.12). Similarly, contralateral abnormal postural reactions would be anticipated with a normal gait in animals light enough to be hopped or a scuffing of the limbs would be evident when walked in a tight circle or over rough ground. Propulsive tendencies may also appear with large cerebral abscesses. Anorexia secondary to severe depression may be accentuated by specific CN dysfunction (CNs V, VII, IX and X) that interferes with eating, if the cerebral abscess directly or indirectly damages the brainstem. Unilateral involvement of these brainstem nuclei will be ipsilateral to an abscess in one cerebral hemisphere. Some affected cattle continue to eat despite extensive space-occupying abscesses.

Neurologic signs worsen and become more numerous as the abscess (or abscesses) enlarges. Antiinflammatory or antibiotic therapy may stabilize or transiently improve the animal's signs, but regression coincides with stoppage of medications. Eventually, locomotion is affected, and tetraparesis and ataxia followed by recumbency occur as the caudal brainstem becomes compromised. Occasionally, a pituitary abscess will rupture, and the inflammation will spread caudally in the meninges, where it can involve and compromise numerous CNs. Caudal brainstem abscesses are common in calves secondary to suppurative otitis media or interna. In addition to loss of palpebral reflex, head tilt, loss of balance, and abnormal nystagmus, these calves have difficulty standing and if ambulatory, exhibit UMN paresis and GP ataxia at first on the side of the otitis and then in all four limbs before recumbency. Postural reactions are deficient in calves that are still able to stand and walk. With the increased incidence of otitis in commercial rearing operations, this particular form of CNS disturbance in older calves has become much more common. Indeed, the development of worsening central signs in a calf with a history of otitis should be interpreted very negatively in a prognostic sense.

Diagnosis

Antemortem confirmation of brain or pituitary abscesses may be difficult. The neurologic signs are the most helpful to diagnosis, especially in young animals in whom inflammatory lesions are more common than other intracranial disorders. Serum globulin should be assessed because it frequently is elevated in adult cattle with brain abscesses but may be variable in calves and young cattle. A neutrophilic leukocytosis may intuitively be anticipated, but in fact the hemogram often is normal.

The CSF may or may not be helpful in the diagnosis. The CSF may be normal in early cases but can be profoundly abnormal in advanced cases of abscessation with both protein and WBCs elevated. Generally, a high percentage, but not all, of the WBCs are mononuclear because of macrophage activity instigated by the chronic infection. Erosion of the abscess to cause leptomeningitis incites a neutrophilic pleocytosis in the CSF.

Radiographs of the skull occasionally show fluid lines consistent with gas–fluid interfaces in large, advanced, cerebral abscesses. Computed tomography (CT) and magnetic resonance imaging (MRI) procedures are the most reliable but are expensive and require general anesthesia, or at least very heavy sedation, at this time.

Treatment

Other than long-term antibiotic therapy and potential drainage, therapy is limited, and the prognosis grave. We are unaware of successful surgery for brain abscesses in cattle, although this is occasionally possible in some other species. Symptomatic therapy with antibiotics and antiinflammatories may cause a slight improvement in the animal's neurologic signs but is generally short lived, and death is inevitable for most cattle affected with brain abscesses.

There is a case report of a 22 month old bull with a pituitary gland abscess being treated successfully with medical treatment and in Chapter 14 of this text Dr. Irby describes the successful treatment of an 8 month old bull with a cavernous sinus abscess.

Listeriosis

Etiology

Listeria monocytogenes, a small gram-positive rod that is ubiquitous in soil, vegetable matter, and fecal material from humans and animals, is the cause of the most common meningoencephalitis of adult cattle. Although this facultative intracellular organism occasionally causes septicemia in young calves and abortion in adult cows, it is best known for the neurologic infection of the brainstem that is labeled listeriosis or "circling disease" in adult cattle and other ruminants. The use of gloves when examining a suspect case is advised because humans are susceptible to this infectious agent.

L. monocytogenes type 4b has been demonstrated to be the most common serotype to cause meningoencephalitis in cattle. The organism is present in chopped forages such as corn silage and haylage owing to the presence of both soil and vegetable matter in these feedstuffs. Proper ensiling, wherein fermentation lowers the pH of the silage to less than 5.0, kills or prevents multiplication of *L. monocytogenes.* However, improper ensiling as a result of excess dryness of the forage, lack of fermentation caused by trench ensiling, silage inoculants, and other variables may prevent the silage from achieving a pH of less than 5.0, thereby allowing proliferation of *L. monocytogenes.* Corn silage is most commonly incriminated as the forage source on dairy farms. Other silages, haylages or contaminated large round bales of hay may also be contaminated with *L. monocytogenes.*

Infection is thought to occur after injury to mucous membranes of the oral cavity, nasal cavity, or conjunctiva with subsequent retrograde passage of the organism most commonly via the sensory branches of the fifth CN (CN V) and less commonly via other CNs to the brainstem. *L. monocytogenes* spreads to the ruminant brain by axonal migration along CNs in the vast majority of infected animals and then spreads intraaxonally within the brain along interneuronal connections. A possibility exists that cattle could become infected through the gastrointestinal (GI) tract with hematogenous spread to the brainstem as may occur in rodents and humans, but this route is thought less likely than following the branches of CN V. The incubation time for disease is unknown but may be prolonged (weeks).

When established in the brainstem, the organism proliferates in the pons and medulla but may spread elsewhere. The trigeminal nerve and its neighboring CN nuclei are subject to injury as a result of neuritis, encephalitis, and meningitis. The classical histologic lesions of listeriosis consist of microabscesses subsequent to focal necrosis with abundant neutrophils and perivascular cuffing with mononuclear cells.

Fortunately, and rather inexplicably, given the common exposure of the whole herd to similar feedstuffs, the disease tends to be sporadic with often only one animal in the herd affected. Endemics have been observed in which disease prevalence may approach 10% over a short period of time when several cattle demonstrate clinical signs over a period of a few months, but this is much more rare in cattle than in sheep, in which high flock morbidity is common. Calves are seldom affected, and the disease is seldom confirmed in cattle younger than 12 months of age. This most likely coincides with less relative risk of exposure to feedstuffs containing *L. monocytogenes* in young animals but may also be influenced by increased dental eruption and therefore mucosal injury in young adult cattle. Septicemic listeriosis in the fetus or bovine neonate can be seen as a cause of late-term abortion, stillbirth, or very rarely precocious neonatal meningoencephalitis in the first few days of life. In the case of neonatal meningoencephalitis, the precise pathogenesis is uncertain but may represent true transplacental spread in utero or vertical transmission during parturition caused by fecal–oral contamination from the dam. The fact that asymptomatic shedding by mature dairy cows has now been well established in a number of naturally occurring herd outbreaks leads to the possibility that heavily contaminated maternity pens may also be a means of neonatal infection via the umbilicus or by oral inoculation.

Clinical Signs

Fever may be present, especially during the first few days of illness. The fever is often 103.0° to 105.0°F [39.4° to 40.5°C] but absence of fever certainly does not rule out listeriosis. The median age of affected cattle is 4 years.

Depression coupled with a variable array of CN signs constitute the major clinical signs of listeriosis in cattle. Classically, the disease was known as circling disease because of the frequency of this clinical sign. The anatomic basis for this is unclear. Asymmetric involvement of vestibular nuclei with loss of balance and circling to that side is one explanation. However, the propulsive tendency to circle suggests involvement of extrapyramidal system nuclei such as the substantia nigra or the descending reticular formation. Although propulsion is a common prosencephalic sign, this portion of the brain is much less affected in listeriosis. Patients may circle until they collapse from exhaustion or eventually wander into solid objects. Stanchioned cattle constantly push or propel themselves into the stanchion in an effort to circle (Fig. 13.13).

Anorexia, or perhaps an inability to eat, is present in most cattle affected with listeriosis and may be caused by deficits in CNs V, VII, IX, X, and XII, as well as depression of brainstem origin. An inability to drink frequently accompanies the inability to eat but is not present in all cases. Individual or combinations of CN deficits unique to each patient may occur (Fig. 13.14) (see Video Clips 13.11 to 13.13).

General signs of depression characterize brainstem disease but may be accentuated by dehydration and acid–base deficits in cattle affected with listeriosis.

Lesions of the motor nucleus of CN V and altered mandibular nerve function create weakness in the muscles

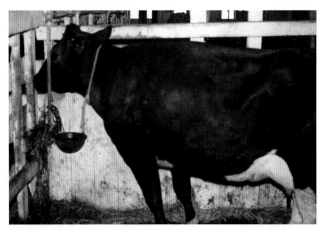

• **Fig. 13.13** This cow with listeriosis would circle constantly to the left until finding respite by securing her muzzle between the water pipe and wall of the box stall.

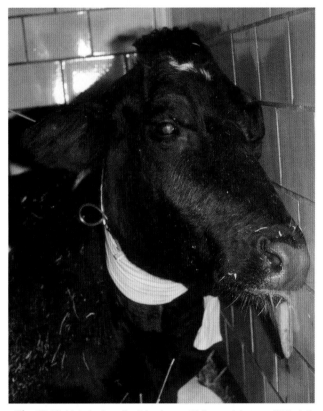

• **Fig. 13.14** Listeriosis patient having multiple cranial nerve (CN) deficits, including left side CN VII and CN VIII, as well as CNs V, IX, X, and XII. The right ear is drooped in the image.

of mastication. When severe and bilateral, a dropped jaw results (Fig. 13.15). When mild, weakness may be appreciated during manual efforts to open the patient's mouth and the tip of the tongue may be seen protruding at the front of the mouth. Although this lesion may be unilateral, it is only obvious clinically when bilateral. Difficulty in prehension and mastication of food results.

Lesions of the abducent nucleus (CN VI) are relatively uncommon but, when present, cause a distinct medial strabismus (Fig. 13.16).

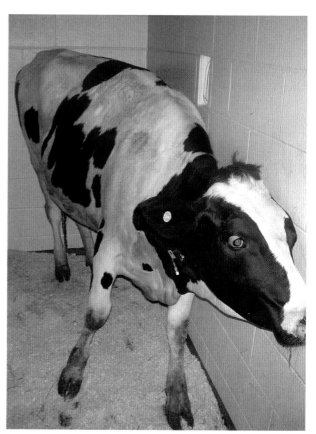

• **Fig. 13.15** Patient with listeriosis with major signs of depression and inability to close her mouth (cranial nerve CN V deficit) and swallow (CNs IX and X deficit). Tongue tone was normal and the slight protrusion of the tongue is common with CN V (mandibular branch) motor dysfunction.

• **Fig. 13.16** Patient with listeriosis demonstrating medial strabismus (see also Video Clip 13.13).

Facial nerve deficits caused by lesions involving the facial nucleus or the intramedullary components of the facial nerve are a very common sign of listeriosis and often are unilateral, causing a drooped ear, ptosis, and flaccid lip (Fig. 13.17). Very early cases or cases recovering from complete facial nerve paralysis occasionally have facial nerve irritability evidenced by eyelid or lip spasticity in response to noxious stimuli. Although unilateral deficits in CN VII are classic for *Listeria* meningoencephalitis of cattle, the deficits may be subtle, incomplete, or bilateral, and therefore require careful evaluation during the neurologic examination. Exposure keratitis is the major ophthalmic complication found in patients with listeriosis and results from facial nerve dysfunction and subsequent failure of tear distribution to prevent corneal desiccation or injury. Additionally, involvement of the parasympathetic facial nucleus may cause a decrease in the aqueous phase of tear secretion. Exposure keratitis can rapidly progress with resultant deep corneal ulceration, uveitis, corneal perforation, and endophthalmitis unless addressed promptly. Endogenous uveitis with hypopyon or endophthalmitis has been suggested as a possible ophthalmic complication by some authors, but in our experience, exposure keratitis and exogenous infection of the eye are the most common ophthalmic complications of listeriosis in cattle (Fig. 13.18). Listeria may also cause corneal disease (silage eye) in cattle without evidence of CN VII signs (see Fig. 14.39).

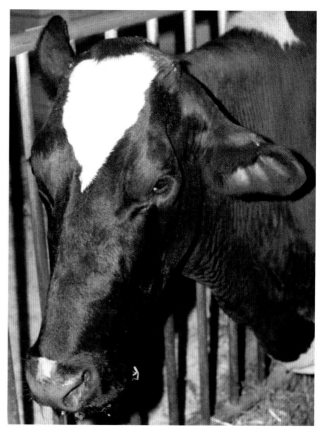

• **Fig. 13.17** Listeriosis. Classical appearance of unilateral cranial nerve VII paralysis with ear droop, ptosis, and a flaccid lip.

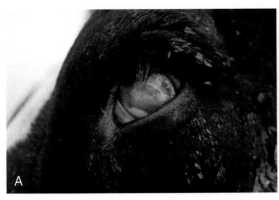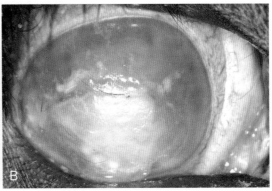

• **Fig. 13.18** Examples of exposure keratitis, hypopyon, and uveitis caused by listeriosis in two patients (**A** and **B**).

Damage to vestibular nuclei affects central vestibular control, leading to head tilt, circling, and vestibular ataxia. Abnormal posture and truncal ataxia also are possible; when these signs are present, the cow's trunk leans toward the affected side and is flexed, so a concavity toward the affected side is seen. When abnormal nystagmus is observed, the direction (fast phase) is variable, as expected with a central vestibular deficit. Adjacent unilateral lesions affecting reticulospinal UMN and spinocerebellar GP pathways may cause ipsilateral paresis and ataxia. Bilateral lesions in this area resulting in spastic tetraparesis and GP ataxia may be severe enough to cause recumbency.

Lesions involving neuronal cell bodies of CN IX and X in the nucleus ambiguus cause dysphagia and excessive salivation. Vomiting or bloat occasionally can be observed (Fig. 13.19) as early signs of listeriosis in cattle and are thought to result from inflammatory irritation of the parasympathetic vagal neurons in the medulla.

Protrusion or weakness of the tongue is associated with lesions in the hypoglossal nuclei or the intramedullary components of CN XII. Tongue protrusion caused by these lesions is accentuated if lesions of the motor nuclei of CN V coexist, thereby allowing a dropped jaw.

Cerebellar signs also have been observed in patients with listeriosis but are not common. Lesions caused by listeriosis are uncommon in the prosencephalon, and therefore blindness is very unusual. Spinal cord lesions are also very rare.

Diagnosis

Anorexia, depression, and possibly fever are the general signs that accompany the more specific CN deficits in cattle having meningoencephalitis caused by *L. monocytogenes*. It is important to remember that "anorexia" may in fact be a result of inability to prehend or swallow food and water. A careful neurologic examination to confirm brainstem disease and identify specific CN deficits is essential when considering a diagnosis of listeriosis. In some cases, the deficits may only be detected on careful clinical examination.

In addition to the clinical signs, CSF analysis is the most valuable ancillary aid to support a diagnosis of listeriosis in cattle. With few exceptions, the CSF from patients with listeriosis has an elevated nucleated cell count and protein level. In one study, 44 of 57 affected cattle had high leukocyte counts in the CSF. In addition,

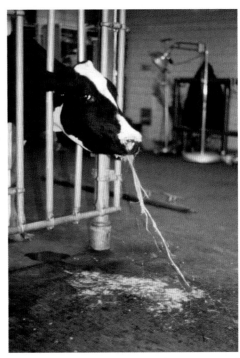

• **Fig. 13.19** An adult Holstein cow with an acute onset of depression, bloat, and vomiting. The cow had listeriosis and recovered with treatment.

at least 50% of the nucleated cells are mononuclear, with macrophages being slightly more common than lymphocytes. In acute disease, neutrophils may comprise 30% to 40% of the WBCs in the CSF, but in more chronic cases, the percentage of neutrophils diminishes, and macrophages increase (see Table 13.1). CSF is usually obtained from the lumbosacral region unless the patient is recumbent and obtunded. The fluid is generally clear on visual inspection. (See Video Clip 2.2).

A complete blood count (CBC) may show mild leukocytosis and monocytosis, which is suggestive, but not absolute, for this disease. Unfortunately, cattle affected with listeriosis do not usually have the peripheral monocytosis that is typically present in other species infected with this organism and that gave *L. monocytogenes* its name.

When loss of saliva is obvious, an acid–base and electrolyte profile may be helpful for subsequent therapy because patients with listeriosis can develop profound salivary loss.

Because the saliva of cattle is rich in buffer, patients so affected may have metabolic acidosis, low bicarbonate values, associated depression, and weakness.

Lactating cattle also may become ketotic because of continued (albeit reduced) milk production in the face of inappetence.

Many differential diagnoses exist for listeriosis, with rabies being the most important from a public health and medicolegal standpoint. Inner and middle ear infections may cause CN VII and VIII signs; affected cattle are more alert and more able to eat and drink than are cows with listeriosis. In general, middle ear infections are common in calves of several weeks to a few months of age, but listeriosis seldom occurs in cattle younger than 1 year of age.

Polioencephalomalacia (PEM), lead poisoning, and other diseases of the cerebral cortex can usually be differentiated from listeriosis unless the patient is recumbent or comatose, which limits the neurologic examination and interpretation of a patient's responses. PEM causes profound depression and bilateral cortical blindness with intact pupillary function, and it may cause a dorsomedial strabismus in calves (not necessarily present in adult cattle). Opisthotonos may develop in advanced cases. Similarly, lead poisoning manifests with bilateral cortical blindness, depression, seizures, and bellowing but no CN signs as seen with listeriosis. In addition, the neurologic form of listeriosis does not result in blindness unless a severe exposure keratitis from facial nerve paralysis leads to uveitis or endophthalmitis in the ipsilateral eye. The lack of a menace response in listeriosis is a result of facial paralysis, which also causes a lack of a palpebral reflex.

Thromboembolic meningoencephalitis or pure meningitis caused by *H. somni* can lead to acute signs of brain disease in young cattle. Although TEME occurs mainly in beef cattle, we occasionally observe this problem in dairy heifers. Signs vary based on the multifocal location of the septic thrombi within the brain, and CN signs are possible, as well as the typical cerebral signs and depression. Fever may be present in the acute phase, and blindness caused by chorioretinal hemorrhages and thrombosis is possible. The CSF, however, helps differentiate *H. somni* from listeriosis because, although protein values are elevated in both diseases, the nucleated cell count with *H. somni* usually is greatly elevated and consists primarily of neutrophils. The fluid may also be grossly discolored on visual inspection.

Nervous ketosis can occasionally be confused with listeriosis in stanchioned cattle that become propulsive or constantly push forward into the stanchion, mimicking the propulsion seen in some patients with listeriosis. However, a lack of CN deficits, positive urinary ketones, history of early lactation, and, if necessary, a normal CSF would rule out listeriosis.

Subtle or mild cases of listeriosis have occasionally been confused with GI disorders such as traumatic reticuloperitonitis. This can easily happen if the patient shows little or no evidence of CN dysfunction but cannot eat or drink.

Subsequent dehydration or lack of water intake causes the rumen ingesta to become very firm and dry. Deep ventral abdominal pressure exerted on the rumen may lead to apparent painful responses that erroneously lead one to suspect peritonitis. In addition, occasional patients with listeriosis show vomiting as one of their initial signs before other CN signs become apparent. Vomiting is more commonly associated with highly acidic diets, indigestion, irritation of reflex centers from ingested hardware, and other GI disorders. Again, a careful neurologic examination is essential, and a CSF analysis should be considered if there is any uncertainty.

Space-occupying lesions in the cerebrum or brainstem (e.g., lymphosarcoma) or parasitic migration can rarely be confused for listeriosis.

Unfortunately, rabies is the most difficult disease to differentiate from listeriosis when dysphagia or other CN signs are present. Because rabies can result in virtually any neurologic sign, it must be considered in the differential diagnosis of listeriosis in endemic areas. In general, CSF obtained from rabies patients has fewer nucleated cells and lower protein than are found in patients with listeriosis. In addition, the high percentage of monocytes and macrophages compared to lymphocytes found in patients with listeriosis is not typical of rabies, in which case small lymphocytes predominate. Because overlap may occur in these values, extreme caution is warranted for handling patients in rabies-endemic areas.

Definitive diagnosis by culture of *L. monocytogenes* from samples obtained antemortem is challenging. Specific cold enrichment culture techniques were historically relied upon, and notoriously difficult, when samples of CSF, blood, milk or feces were used. Polymerase chain reaction (PCR) has offered greater sensitivity and is a valuable research tool in the public health arena for identification and tracking of *Listeria* strains during outbreaks. However, PCR may not be routinely available for veterinarians at this time. At postmortem, culture of tissue from the brainstem can be tried, although demonstration of brain-stem meningoencephalitis with microabcesses alongside a negative rabies fluorescent antibody (FA) test is often relied on for diagnosis.

Treatment

Historically, treatment has usually consisted of intensive antibiotic therapy with either penicillin or tetracycline, although other antibiotics are reported to be more effective in vitro. In a recent study of *L. monocytogenes* isolates from mastitic milk of cattle (including serotype 4b) more than half the isolates were resistant to penicillin and tetracycline; a lower percentage of isolates were resistant to ampicillin, and only one isolate was resistant to erythromycin. Two major therapeutic obstacles exist to antibiotic therapy for *Listeria monocytogenes* that dictate higher dosages than normally used for other susceptible bacteria:

1. *L. monocytogenes* is a facultative intracellular organism that can survive and hide from drugs in macrophages.

2. The blood–brain barrier, although compromised by inflammation, may still impede antibiotic penetration of the brain to some degree.

Therefore, we have historically chosen to use penicillin in an extra-label dose at 44,000 U/kg twice daily, either intramuscularly (IM) or subcutaneously (SC), to treat patients with listeriosis, often with success. This is used for at least 7 days before being reduced to either once daily or 22,000 U/kg twice daily, IM or SC.

Intravenously administered penicillin, 22,000 U/kg four times daily, or ampicillin, 10 mg/kg thrice daily, would likely result in higher concentration in the CSF but are more expensive. Based on recent sensitivity results, ampicillin administered at a dose of 11 mg/kg IM is one recommended treatment. Some clinicians prefer to use oxytetracycline HCl at 10 mg/kg twice daily, IV or SC but without oral or IV fluid administration to prevent dehydration, this may lead to nephrotoxic renal failure. Dosage reduction should only coincide with signs of obvious clinical improvement, such as a return to an ability to eat and drink. Although the exact duration of therapy will vary in each case based on severity of signs and many other factors, the treatment should continue for at least 1 week beyond apparent improvement in neurologic deficits based on appetite, attitude, and other factors. Most affected cows require 7 to 21 days of therapy. Premature reduction in dosage or discontinuation of treatment risks relapse in patients with listeriosis. Some degree of facial paralysis may persist for a long time in recovered patients with listeriosis, and neurologic signs tend to resolve in the opposite order of their original appearance. There may be no improvement in clinical signs for the first 7 to 9 days in some animals that ultimately recover.

Fluid and electrolyte status may be very important to the well-being of patients with listeriosis that lose the ability to drink. Cattle that cannot drink but are not losing saliva excessively can be given water and balanced electrolytes (especially containing sodium and potassium) through a stomach tube. This improves patient hydration, softens the firm rumen contents, and encourages rumen activity. Patients that cannot swallow and have excessive loss of saliva should be monitored for buffer loss and often require bicarbonate replacement therapy and fluids. These may be given IV— although this is a more expensive route—or orally with substantial water to correct dehydration. Replacement therapy is necessary daily until salivary losses stop. The depression and weakness that occur with severe metabolic acidosis may be confused with progression of the disease or lack of response to therapy for listeriosis. Depending on the degree of salivary loss, 4 to 16 oz of sodium bicarbonate may be required daily to compensate. For example, an adult cow with a base deficit of 10 mEq/L bicarbonate will need approximately 125 g or 4.5 oz of baking soda to replace this deficit. Cattle with facial paralysis also require frequent treatment of the ipsilateral eye with topical ointments to prevent keratitis and corneal ulcers.

Nursing care, including a well-bedded box stall with good footing, is essential to survival of cattle affected with listeriosis. Assuming intensive antibiotic therapy, fluid therapy, and supportive care are given, the prognosis for clinical recovery is fair to good for cattle infected with listeriosis that are ambulatory when the diagnosis is made. The prognosis for cattle that are recumbent and unable to rise at the time of diagnosis is very poor.

L. monocytogenes is capable of infecting humans and thus causing meningoencephalitis. This is especially true in very young, very old, and immunocompromised persons. Therefore public health concerns exist. Patients with listeriosis may shed *L. monocytogenes* in their milk, and this fact obligates veterinarians to warn owners and caretakers against the consumption of raw milk under all circumstances but certainly from clinical cases. Milk from affected cattle should be discarded. Even pasteurized milk subjected only to low-temperature pasteurization may contain the organism. Pregnant cattle with the neurologic form of listeriosis may abort during the duration of their disease. The cause of the abortion is generally septicemic spread of *L. monocytogenes* to the uterus. Therefore handling of the fetus, placenta, and so forth should be done carefully.

Rabies

Etiology

Rabies virus is transmitted to cattle and other warm-blooded animals by bites from infected vectors such as foxes, raccoons, skunks, bats, and vampire bats. Cats and dogs are more routinely vaccinated against the disease, but unvaccinated cats and dogs also present a risk to cattle, humans, and other species. The rabies virus is a member of the genus Lyssavirus within the Rhabdoviridae family and is uniformly fatal to infected animals. Therein lies the tremendous fear of the infection that the word "rabies" holds for humans. Public health and medicolegal implications are obvious.

Although aerosol transmission occurs in nature, mainly from infection in bats within caves, people and animals have been infected through aerosols in laboratory settings. Ingestion of infected tissues also may occasionally result in infection of carnivores. However, the primary means of transmission of this neurotrophic virus is through bites from an infected animal that inoculate virus-laden saliva into the tissues of a non-infected individual.

The virus replicates at the site of inoculation in a recently bitten animal. It then travels in retrograde fashion within the axons of peripheral nerves to spinal ganglia in the spinal cord and eventually the brain. The virus is then shed into the salivary and nasal secretions of the infected animal through centrifugal distribution following CN axons to these secretory glands. Therefore, the virus is concentrated in saliva and nasal secretions, making these fluids the most feared source of exposure for uninfected animals or people.

Incubation periods vary widely. Most experts agree that 1 week is the minimum, but the range varies from 1 to 3 weeks, 10 to 60 days, or 3 weeks to 3 months; all authors agree that rare instances exist when the incubation may be as long as 6 months. Infection through bites closer to the brain (i.e., face and neck) may lead to shorter incubation periods than distal limb bites. In the United States, the number of cases of rabies diagnosed in cattle in 2013 was nearly identical to the number diagnosed in dogs.

Clinical Signs

Clinical signs of rabies in cattle, as well as other species, are variable and may include spinal cord signs, brainstem signs including CN deficits, cerebral signs, apparent lameness, genitourinary signs, GI signs, unwillingness to eat or drink, and combinations thereof.

Because of the variation in clinical signs of rabies, veterinarians practicing in endemic areas are more cautious of cattle with overt neurologic signs. Several points are worth remembering as important generalities when discussing signs of rabies in cattle.

1. The signs are progressive; this may mean, for example, that appetite continues to decline or neurologic signs observed on day 1 will be more pronounced by day 3. Most cattle are recumbent in 4 to 5 days.
2. Death usually occurs by day 10 after the onset of signs, with the average being around 5 days from onset of signs to death.
3. In endemic areas, rabies should be on the differential diagnosis for almost every sick cow with nervous system signs examined by a veterinarian.

The clinical signs at the onset usually relate to the area of the body that was bitten and where the virus first entered the central nervous system. Spinal cord signs are seen frequently. These may include subtle hind limb lameness or shifting of weight in the hind limbs that progresses to knuckling at one or both fetlocks. Ataxia and weakness may follow these signs and progress until the cow needs help getting up or becomes completely paralyzed in the pelvic limbs (Fig. 13.20). In some cases, there is a spastic uncontrolled flexion of the limbs (Fig. 13.21 and Video clip 13.14). Associated with these lumbar and sacral signs, constipation, tenesmus, paraphimosis (males), dribbling of urine from bladder paralysis, and a flaccid tail and anus may become apparent. Therefore, progressive signs of spinal cord or spinal nerve dysfunction should raise concern for rabies. With head bites, CN signs may occur initially.

Cerebral signs include signs of progressive depression ("dumb form") or aggression ("furious form"). Few veterinarians would fail to quickly identify any newly aggressive cattle as rabies suspects, but certainly nervous ketosis and hypomagnesemia need to be ruled out. Other accentuated cerebral responses observed in patients with rabies are hypersexuality (e.g., frequent mounting), localized or generalized pruritus that can progress to self-mutilation, seizures, tremors, alert eyes and ears despite paresis or ataxia, head pressing, bellowing, and opisthotonos. Blindness can occur but is not common.

Dysphagia, salivation, and a weak tongue are apparent in some cattle affected with rabies. An inability to drink usually accompanies these signs, which is reflective of pharyngeal paralysis. Bellowing is described as "peculiarly low pitched and hoarse and may progress to bubbly sounds prior to death." Laryngeal paralysis associated with pharyngeal dysfunction may contribute to these sounds.

These are signs reported and observed in past cases, but no sign is pathognomonic for rabies Affected cattle may have all or none of the signs described..

The differential diagnosis is exhausting, but several common diseases should be considered. In the paralytic form with spinal cord signs predominating, lumbosacral injuries from estrus activities or trauma and vertebral canal lymphosarcoma or abscesses should be differentiated from rabies. As discussed earlier, a personality change to furious or aggressive behavior should be differentiated from nervous ketosis, hypomagnesemia, or the occasional cow recently transported to a new location that simply "goes crazy" but has neither rabies nor nervous ketosis. With brain signs, the differential list is too long to consider simply because the spectrum of brain signs possible with rabies is so broad. In our experience, atypical listeriosis that causes dysphagia with or without tongue paralysis but without facial or vestibular nuclear signs is the disease most easily confused with rabies. However, in an advanced rabies case that is approaching

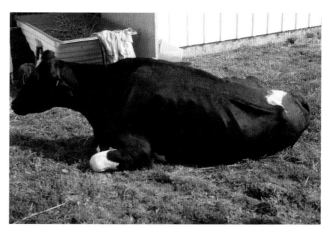

• **Fig. 13.20** A 4-year-old Holstein cow that was first noticed to be abnormal when she buckled on both hind limbs coming into the parlor. Within 2 hours, she was recumbent, would not eat, and began bellowing. Cerebrospinal fluid had a lymphocytic pleocytosis. She tested positive for rabies.

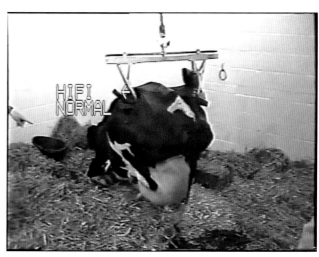

• **Fig. 13.21** A 5-year-old cow with rabies and dramatic and seemingly uncontrolled hyperflexion of both hind limbs when lifted in a hip sling. (See Video Clip 13.14).

coma, many encephalitic and toxic CNS diseases would need to be considered.

Diagnosis

The CSF from rabies patients may be normal, have only elevated protein values, or have both elevated nucleated cells and protein. Most nucleated cells in the CSF of rabies patients are lymphocytes. No other premortem tests are helpful to the practicing veterinarian, and the brain from suspect animals must be submitted to the regional laboratory approved by the respective state health department for rabies testing. Currently, FA-stained sections of brain offer the quickest and most accurate means of diagnosis. The FA test has replaced histologic examination of the brain for Negri bodies and the mouse inoculation tests. In addition, FA tests using monoclonal antibodies to epitopes of the virus can help distinguish the vector source of rabies (i.e., raccoon, fox, and bat) to aid epidemiologic studies and surveillance.

No treatment is possible for rabies patients. However, cattle suffering bite wounds should have the injured soft tissues cleaned vigorously, as well as washed and disinfected, just as is done for people sustaining bite wounds from animals of unknown rabies status.

When rabies is suspected in a cow or calf, gloves should be worn by the handlers and veterinarians during examination and treatment. A minimal number of people should be involved in treatment of the cow, and her milk should be discarded. Obtaining, handling, and analyzing CSF from rabies suspect cases should be performed with the greatest of caution for very obvious reasons. If a cow is confirmed to have had rabies, public health authorities should be consulted for advice on rabies immunoprophylaxis for any humans that worked with the animal and had likely exposure to the virus.

Rabies vaccination of cattle is now being practiced in many endemic areas and is a viable means to counteract the public and private anxiety regarding exposure to rabies while working with livestock. Vaccination also greatly reduces the likelihood of human exposure and subsequent expensive post-exposure prophylaxis and treatment with globulin and human diploid vaccines. An entire herd (small size) of dairy cattle can be vaccinated for less than the cost of one human post-exposure treatment. Therefore vaccination of cattle in endemic areas is worthy of consideration. Veterinarians should be certain to use only vaccines approved for use in cattle because some modified vaccines are inappropriate for herbivores. There are 3 or more vaccines currently available for use in cattle in the United States. Vaccines can be given initially at 3 months of age for primary immunization and thereafter repeated annually.

Pseudorabies (Aujeszky Disease, Mad Itch)
Etiology

This herpesvirus of swine is the cause of pseudorabies. Often a mild disease in swine, this disease is highly fatal in cattle and may cause signs similar to rabies, hence the name pseudorabies. This is a rare disease in dairy cattle because pigs and dairy cows seldom are housed together. However, trends in agriculture change constantly, and diversification that includes swine and dairy cattle operations located on the same premises could occur, thereby risking spread of this virus from swine to cattle.

The virus is shed in the nasal secretions and pharyngeal secretions of infected pigs. Contact with cattle may occur via contamination of feedstuffs, contamination of wounds (because intradermal and SC routes of infection are possible), and nose-to-nose contact. Infected brown rats also have been incriminated in carrying pseudorabies virus from farm to farm. After infection, the incubation period is between 2 and 7 days.

Clinical Signs

Intense pruritus that may be localized or generalized develops, with licking, rubbing, and self-mutilation possible. This pattern has led to the name "mad itch" in cattle. However, many other neurologic signs are possible—similar to rabies—and fever usually is present. Peracute cases may die suddenly or have primary brain signs, which include salivation, pharyngeal or laryngeal dysfunction, dyspnea, bloat, ataxia, paresis, abnormal nystagmus, depression or aggression, and seizures. The course of the disease is 2 to 3 days, and although rare instances of survival have been noted in cattle, most infected individuals succumb. The differential diagnosis must include rabies and many other neurologic diseases, but historical proximity of swine is a key point.

Diagnosis

Serology, viral isolation from the CNS (especially from a spinal cord segment supplying a pruritic area/lesion) or edematous fluid from a localized skin lesion, and FA tests are possible. Tests continue to change and improve for this disease, and if this diagnosis is suspected, it would be best to contact a regional diagnostic laboratory for advice on sample collection. Rabies may need to be ruled out as well. No treatment exists. We are unaware of published CSF values for cattle affected with pseudorabies virus.

Bovine Herpesvirus Encephalitis
Etiology

Both bovine herpesviruses (BHV) 1 and 5 may cause encephalitis in cattle. BHV1, a cause of abortion, infectious bovine rhinotracheitis, and pustular vulvovaginitis, only sporadically causes meningitis in cattle as BHV1 virus rarely advances beyond the neurons located in the trigeminal ganglia. On the other hand, BHV5 has marked neurotrophism, and in some parts of the world, particularly South America, it is a common cause of meningoencephalitis in cattle. BHV5 encephalitis can cause single-animal disease or herd outbreaks, mostly in young replacement heifers, but the incidence in North America appears much lower than in South America. BHV5 meningoencephalitis may result during initial exposure to the virus or from a stress or corticosteroid reactivation at a later time. Clinical signs generally occur approximately 1 week after either initial exposure or reactivation of the virus. The virus invades the CNS via the olfactory mucosa after intranasal infection or reactivation. A trigeminal ganglionitis is found in infected calves, and this is also the anatomic area of persistent infection in some individuals.

Clinical Signs and Diagnosis

Clinical signs of respiratory disease may be concurrent with neurologic signs, especially with BHV1. Prosencephalic signs predominate and are usually accompanied by a fever. Most affected animals remain visual, which helps separate many of the infectious encephalitides from metabolic or toxic diseases affecting the cerebral cortex. One of the authors (TJD) has analyzed CSF on a BHV1 encephalitic calf (Fig. 13.22), and it had a lymphocytic pleocytosis. If BHV-infected cattle survive, they seroconvert in 7 to 10 days. Animals that die with nonsuppurative encephalitis can be confirmed as having BHV1 or 5 by immunohistochemistry. Genomic analysis or PCR can be used to differentiate between the two strains. The CNS lesion consists of a diffuse nonsuppurative meningoencephalomyelitis affecting both the gray and white matter.

Treatment and Prevention

Treatment is supportive and includes control of seizures when necessary in addition to the use of NSAIDs. Corticosteroids are likely to be contraindicated, although this is controversial.

Although complete protection against either strain does not occur with vaccination, the modified live intranasal BHV1 vaccines offer the best efficacy against both strains.

Malignant Catarrhal Fever

Malignant catarrhal fever (MCF) is caused by a gamma herpesvirus and sporadically causes fatal meningoencephalomyelitis in cattle. The virus that causes MCF in cattle in North America and Europe is sheep associated (ovine herpesvirus 2). Most cases of MCF in cattle occur when affected cattle have

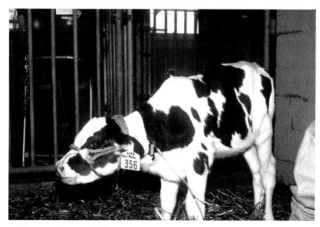

• **Fig. 13.22** A 2-month-old calf with acute onset of fever and depression followed by seizures and respiratory distress. The cerebrospinal fluid had a lymphocytic pleocytosis. Bovine herpesvirus 1 inclusion bodies were identified in the brain at autopsy.

had contact with sheep that are actively shedding the virus. It has been hypothesized that this is most common in postpartum ewes or weaned lambs. Outbreaks in cattle have occurred following exposure to sheep at fairs. There have been some cases of MCF in cattle when direct contact with sheep did not occur, raising the possibility that the virus may circulate within cattle populations including dairy farms. The infection causes a vasculitis and lymphoproliferative reaction in many organs, including the CNS. The incubation period may be several weeks or more in cattle. We have recently identified the disease in pigs in contact with sheep.

Clinical Signs

Clinical signs are most common in cattle 1 to 2 years of age, and sporadic cases are the norm, although outbreaks can occur. There are basically two clinical forms: (1) the head and eye and (2) the intestinal form. Cattle with the head and eye form have a high fever, corneal opacity, nasal discharge, enlarged lymph nodes, hematuria, and diffuse neurologic signs. Similar to keratitis associated with infectious bovine rhinotracheitis (IBR), the corneal lesions often start at the limbus and spread centrally. Recovery with this form of the disease is rare. In the intestinal form, fever and diarrhea are the predominant clinical signs. Outbreaks are more common, as is recovery, compared with the head and eye form. We have collected CSF on only a few MCF head and eye form cases. They had a remarkable mononuclear pleocytosis, and the exact phenotype of some of the mononuclear cells was difficult to determine.

Diagnosis and Treatment

The diagnosis is based on signalment, clinical signs, history of sheep exposure (may be in distant past), and ruling out other diseases that may cause similar clinical signs (e.g., IBR or BVD). Hematuria, lymphadenopathy, and finding bizarre-appearing mononuclear cells in the CSF should help distinguish between these diseases. An antemortem diagnosis can be made by performing PCR on whole blood (ethylenediaminetetraacetic acid [EDTA] anticoagulated sample). Postmortem diagnosis can be made by performing PCR on tissues. Lesions consist of a primary immune-mediated vasculitis with secondary parenchymal degeneration. Treatment is symptomatic.

Other Causes Nonsuppurative Encephalitis of Unknown Etiology

Nonsuppurative encephalitis has been reported in a large number of feedlot-age beef cattle in western Canada, but a specific etiology has not yet been determined. Sporadic bovine encephalitis (SBE or Buss disease), which is a chlamydial infection primarily seen in young beef cattle in the western United States, was ruled out. We have on rare occasion observed a similar nonsuppurative encephalitis or myelitis of unknown etiology in dairy cattle of varying ages. A divergent astrovirus has been recently associated with encephalitis in cattle and future cases of non-suppurative encephalitis should be tested for this virus. Rabies should always be considered in cattle with non-suppurative encephalitis!

Aichivirus B

Recently, an 11-day-old calf with both diarrhea and neurologic signs of diffuse encephalitis associated with Aichivirus B infection was described from the University of Wisconsin. The affected animal had a xanthochromic and lymphocytic CSF analysis and the virus was demonstrated by next generation sequencing (NGS), although confirmation by conventional PCR was not possible. As NGS technology is used increasingly as a tool in infectious disease research it is probable that other novel viruses will be discovered in association with many types of disease in cattle, including heretofore unexplained neurologic conditions.

Thrombotic Meningoencephalitis

Thromboembolic meningoencephalitis (TEME) is caused by *Histophilus somni*, formerly known as *Haemophilus somnus*. This small coccobacillus attacks the vascular endothelium, causing a septic vasculitis with thrombosis. The parenchymal lesions of ischemic and hemorrhagic infarction are secondary to the primary vascular lesions that can occur anywhere in the CNS. In addition, similar vascular lesions can occur in the lungs, heart, skeletal muscle, and joints. Death may occur acutely without evidence of neurologic signs. Pyrexia is present in clinically ill patients. This disease is more common in feedlot cattle than in pastured or dairy animals. In New York state, pulmonary signs and lesions are the most common manifestation of this disease. The diagnosis and treatments for TEME were discussed previously.

Bovine Spongiform Encephalopathy

Although the purpose of this book is not to be all-encompassing as regards exotic diseases but to concentrate on common problems in dairy cattle in the United States, bovine spongiform encephalopathy (BSE) deserves brief mention because of the threat to the United States, the fact that several cases have occurred in the United States, and the ensuing public health concerns. Through August 2017, BSE surveillance has identified 25 cases in North America: 5 BSE cases in the United States (one was Canadian born and a classic case) and 20 in Canada. The abbreviation BSE should not be confused with sporadic bovine encephalitis (SBE or Buss disease), which is a chlamydial infection primarily seen in young beef cattle in the western United States. BSE is not an inflammatory disease but is caused by an unusual infectious agent that is classified as a prion.

Etiology

Bovine spongiform encephalopathy is a fatal neurodegenerative disease that causes spongy degeneration of the brain and spinal cord. It is considered to be a form of scrapie in cattle. Scrapie is a disease of sheep and goats that is one of a group of diseases referred to as the transmissible spongiform encephalopathies (TSEs). These include BSE, chronic wasting disease of deer, mink encephalopathy, and Creutzfeldt-Jakob disease of humans. The cattle disease first emerged in Great Britain in 1986. The infectious agent is an altered host protein referred to as a prion.

One pathogenetic theory holds that BSE was most likely initially caused by scrapie-infected, sheep-origin, meat and bone meal products that were used as part of calf starter rations or adult cattle concentrates. Another theory is that BSE developed de novo in cattle and was exacerbated by feeding the tissues from infected cattle to other cattle. Public health concerns have focused on the similar features of the causative agents of Creutzfeldt-Jakob disease and kuru in humans to the prion-type causative agents found in scrapie and BSE. Because cattle were thought to have acquired this agent through ingestion, fears were raised relative to human consumption of meat products. Because the United States has scrapie and chronic wasting disease as endemic problems in sheep and deer, respectively, the threat of BSE in cattle raised in the United States has been of great concern. However, large differences in the amount of sheep byproducts fed to cattle, as well as differences in rendering procedures, currently make the risk of classical BSE in U.S. cattle small. An atypical strain or variant form has been seen in the four United States–born cattle with BSE in that these cattle were all older than 10 years of age. There is a genetic predisposition to the disease in cattle, as there is in sheep.

In addition to horizontal transmission, presumably from feeding contaminated ruminant tissue, there is the possibility of vertical transmission of TSE agents as well. For example, BSE-infected cattle were three times more likely to have infected offspring than noninfected cows during the British outbreak. After banning the feeding of ruminant meat and bone meal to cattle in the United Kingdom, there has been a dramatic decrease in the incidence of BSE in the past 10 to 15 years and it is now a relatively rare disease.

Clinical Signs

Bovine spongiform encephalopathy (in its classic form) occurs in adult dairy cattle 3 to 6 years of age, or older. The disease is usually slowly progressive over 2 or more weeks. Hyperexcitability, an anxious expression, hypermetric ataxia, and hyperesthesia characterize the clinical signs. Affected cattle have facial and ear twitching, may kick repeatedly, and develop progressive ataxia and paresis that lead to stumbling, falling, and eventually, recumbency. Only a small number of affected cattle display abnormal aggression, an occasional behavioral feature that gave rise to the colloquialism, "mad cow" disease. Loss of weight is a significant sign in cattle clinically affected with BSE.

Diagnosis

Histopathologically, lesions consist of vacuoles in neuronal cell bodies or their processes in the neuropil, sometimes associated with a mild gliosis but no inflammation. There is no serum antibody production, and the CSF is normal.

Immunodetection tests are available for detecting the prion in brainstem tissue. Currently in the United States, the disease has been confirmed in only five cows, with rigorous surveillance efforts having been put into place.

Degenerations: Metabolic and Toxic Brain Diseases

Polioencephalomalacia

Polioencephalomalacia (PEM) describes a degenerative lesion of the gray matter of the cerebral cortex; a cerebrocortical necrosis for which there are many causes. These include thiamine deficiency, sulfur toxicity, lead poisoning, osmolality aberrations associated with salt and water imbalances, and hypoxia.

Despite this, most clinicians equate PEM with thiamine deficiency, which is how it will be used in the following description.

Etiology

Polioencephalomalacia (PEM) or cerebrocortical necrosis is a thiamine-responsive disease that occurs in ruminant calves and less commonly in adult cattle. In dairy calves, the disease usually is sporadic, but in grouped yearling heifers, the morbidity may reach 10% to 25%, similar to herd outbreaks in beef feeder calves or yearlings. The most common age for sporadic PEM in dairy calves is 2 to 8 months of age; calves younger than 3 weeks of age are seldom at risk for PEM. Adult dairy cattle are rarely affected unless associated with acute ruminal acidosis.

The cause of PEM has been the subject of much research regarding thiamine metabolism, thiaminase activity in the rumen, the effect of various feedstuffs on rumen microbial flora related to thiamine production or destruction, and chemicals that alter thiamine levels in ruminants. Thiamine is present in tissue as free thiamine or derivatives of thiamine, with thiamine pyrophosphate (TPP) being the most biologically active form and a coenzyme/cofactor in several key pathways of energy metabolism.

Thiamine must be present in adequate levels to allow production of the coenzyme TPP (also called thiamine diphosphate), which is the active form of thiamine that works as a coenzyme for several enzymatic reactions such as those involving red blood cell transketolase, and both pyruvate and α-ketoglutarate dehydrogenases. Erythrocyte transketolase is important in the pentose phosphate shunt pathway for glucose metabolism in the bovine brain. Thiamine (as TPP) also participates as a cofactor in the production of adenosine triphosphate (ATP) in the Krebs cycle. The brain is at great risk when thiamine is inadequate because of the brain's dependence on aerobic metabolism for which TPP is a critical participant. Within the CNS, specific groups of neurons are more susceptible to this interference with aerobic metabolism than others (i.e., neocortex, lateral geniculate nucleus, and caudal colliculus). It is important to appreciate that in severe cases the clinical signs represent a much more diffuse neuronal dysfunction than the distribution of histologic lesions

seen at necropsy. This is a metabolic disorder that can disrupt neuronal function before causing ischemic-type degeneration or necrosis that is visible with the light microscope. The clinician's objective is to stop this process as soon as possible before the neuronal changes become permanent (i.e., treatment in the edema stage before the development of necrosis).

Cattle normally produce thiamine as a result of rumen microbial activity. However, thiamine deficiency or alterations in normal thiamine production can be induced by a variety of means. High-grain, low-fiber diets are one of the most commonly encountered problems associated with field outbreaks of PEM. Such diets may alter the rumen flora to allow production of thiaminase type 2 by various anaerobes or other organisms. Similarly, feedstuffs that contain thiaminase activity, such as bracken fern ribozyme and horsetail, may alter thiamine levels via thiaminase type 1. Type 2 thiaminase appears to be most important in causing PEM in cattle. Worming with levamisole or thiabendazole and tranquilization with acepromazine have also been incriminated by field experience. Although the feeding of amprolium, a thiamine analogue, has been associated with PEM, experimental cases needed to be fed extremely high levels to reproduce the disease and we have never associated amprolium administration with naturally occurring PEM. Recently, it has been found that cattle fed a high sulfur diet that developed PEM had elevated levels of thiamine in the brain but decreased amounts of TPP. This suggests that high sulfur intake increases the need for TPP.

The exact etiology in sporadic cases usually is impossible to determine, although herd outbreaks warrant close analysis of possible contributing factors, especially concentrate versus roughage ratios.

Clinical Signs

Symmetrical cerebrocortical signs predominate in PEM. Depression and anorexia are present in both calves and adults, but these signs may only be present for a short time before more overt signs of cortical disease become apparent. Blindness with intact pupillary function is one of the first signs observed because of the sensitivity of the visual cortex to the ongoing pathology (see Video Clips 13.15 and 13.16). Pupillary response to light may be lost in some recumbent cases as the disease progresses when presumably the oculomotor nerve becomes compressed. Head pressing and odontoprisis may be observed, or an extended head and neck typical of cattle with "headache"-type pain. A slow, shuffling gait is usually apparent if the animal is able to walk. Vocalization, as observed in some early cases in goats, is usually not observed in calves or adult cattle with PEM. A dorsomedial strabismus, thought to be caused by involvement of the CN-IV nucleus, is common in calves and yearlings, but observed less often in adult cattle. Muscle tremors and excessive salivation also may occur.

If the disease has progressed enough to cause recumbency, opisthotonos frequently is observed, and abnormal nystagmus, seizures, or coma are likely to follow (Fig. 13.23). Untreated cases may die within 24 to 96 hours, depending on the severity of the metabolic dysfunction. CN signs other than dorsomedial strabismus usually are not present (Fig. 13.24). Although optic disc edema has been reported to occur, we have never observed this in any calf or cow affected with PEM. Therefore, in our opinion, blindness is entirely of cortical origin (Fig. 13.25). Associated with either cortical blindness or cerebral edema, cattle may have a stargazing appearance (Fig. 13.26).

The major differential diagnoses are lead poisoning, sulfur toxicity, meningitis, encephalitides including rabies, salt poisoning, nervous ketosis (in adult lactating cows), hepatoencephalopathy, and clostridial enterotoxemia type D (calves only).

Diagnosis

In acute cases, the clinical signs and CSF evaluation usually allow a diagnosis. The CSF in acute PEM is usually clear, has no increase in nucleated cells, and may have a normal or only slightly elevated protein. In chronic cases that have been affected 3 or more days, the CSF may show increased protein and mild to moderate increases in nucleated cells—especially macrophages—as a result of advanced cerebrocortical necrosis. Therefore the CSF helps rule out most meningitic and encephalitic diseases,

except rabies. Blood and tissue lead assays may be necessary to rule out lead poisoning if this disease cannot be completely eliminated by history. In addition, animals with lead poisoning tend to show more seizure activity than patients with PEM, although this is a subjective statement. Blood ammonia can be measured to rule out a portosystemic shunt (see Video Clips 13.17A and B) or other causes of hyperammonemia. Urinary and blood ketones can be assessed in lactating cattle to rule out nervous ketosis. Comparative assessment of serum and CSF sodium levels would be necessary if salt toxicity or water deprivation were considered.

Many specific laboratory tests have been suggested to confirm PEM, but they all suffer from the disadvantages of unavailability to the practicing veterinarian, expense, and the limited number of more research-oriented laboratories that offer the service. These tests include those measuring erythrocyte transketolase levels (should be decreased with PEM), blood pyruvate, blood lactate, pyruvate kinase, and fecal and ruminal thiaminase (all may be high with PEM). In herd outbreaks of PEM,

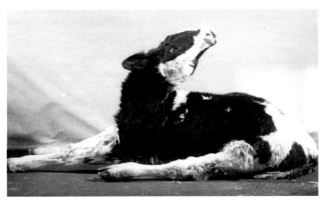

• **Fig. 13.23** Profound opisthotonos in a calf with polioencephalomalacia.

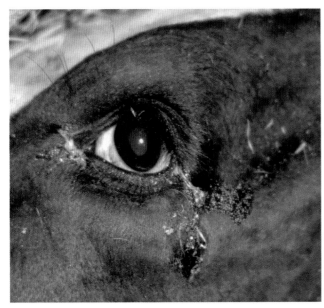

• **Fig. 13.24** Dorsomedial strabismus in a yearling Holstein recumbent as a result of polioencephalomalacia. The strabismus was bilateral.

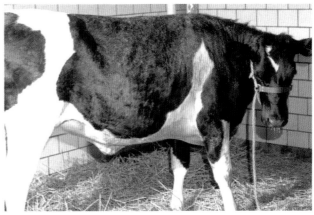

• **Fig. 13.25** Two-year-old Holstein heifer that was blind with intact pupillary light responses and profoundly depressed as a result of polioencephalomalacia.

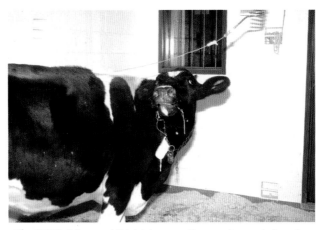

• **Fig. 13.26** A 3-year-old Holstein cow with an acute onset of cerebrocortical blindness and a stargazing appearance. The cow was treated with thiamine and intravenous crystalloids and appeared normal within 72 hours. The diagnosis was thiamine-responsive polioencephalomalacia, which is uncommon in adult cows.

the attending veterinarian may wish to contact regional laboratories as to the availability, practicality, turnaround time, and expense of these tests.

On a practical basis, necropsy becomes the most reliable means of diagnosis in cattle that die or do not respond to therapy for PEM. Gross postmortem examination may reveal a slight yellow discoloration of neocortical gyri as a result of cortical edema. If brain edema is extensive, herniation of the caudal cerebellar vermis at the foramen magnum (cerebellar coning) may occur. An ultraviolet light may cause fluorescence of the cerebral cortex because of mitochondrial changes that occur in the affected cortex. Microscopic lesions vary from cytotoxic edema and ischemic-type degeneration to complete necrosis of the neocortex and selective brainstem nuclei. This depends on the severity and duration of the disorder. Response to specific therapy often is used as a clinical confirmation of PEM in the field. In many cases, the microscopic lesions are difficult to differentiate from those caused by lead poisoning and sulfur toxicity.

Treatment

Specific treatment for PEM requires thiamine hydrochloride administered slowly at 10 to 20 mg/kg IV as an initial bolus and then repeated at 10 mg/kg IM or SC 2-4 times daily for 3 to 10 days, depending on the severity of signs and response to treatment. Mannitol has been used in some valuable calves, but its efficacy is unproven. This is administered as a 20% solution IV slowly over 20 to 30 minutes at 0.5 to 2.0 g/kg. This may be repeated once or twice at 3- to 4-hour intervals. Corticosteroids are generally not used.

In acute cases, improvement is apparent within hours, but subacute cases respond gradually over 24 to 96 hours. Blindness is usually the last sign to disappear, and we have observed one young animal that did not show evidence of vision until the ninth day of treatment. Rarely, blindness may be permanent despite resolution of all other neurologic signs. A high-sulfur diet (feed or water) associated PEM is less responsive to thiamine such that high sulfur feeds should be considered when outbreaks of PEM occur and the response to thiamine is poorer than expected. Lead poisoning cases can have some response to thiamine treatment alone and thiamine should always be used in such cases but systemic chelation and oral binding agents are the primary treatments.

Prevention

The diet should be assessed in all patients with PEM. This is especially true when multiple individuals within a group have been affected. When all grain or mostly grain diets are identified, adding fiber in the form of long-stem hay at 5 to 10 lb/head/day should stop further incidence of PEM. Other possible nutritional factors discussed in the etiology section may be addressed when necessary. The addition of thiamine to the diet at a rate of 5 to 10 mg/kg of feed may help prevent further incidence. For group outbreaks in calves, injections of thiamine hydrochloride at 10 mg/kg

IM may be given to unaffected animals and repeated weekly in the hope of deterring further cases.

Sulfur Toxicity

Diets or water high in sulfates may also cause a condition similar to classical PEM. Sulfur is metabolized to sulfide ions, which appear to be the toxic form. Sulfur, sulfates, and even sulfites (e.g., preservative in pretzels) may be found in feeds, water, or minerals. The clinical signs are the same as those seen with PEM caused by classical thiamine deficiency. Elevated levels of hydrogen sulfide gas can be determined from trocharization of the ruminal gas cap. Cattle with sulfur toxicity and PEM have normal ruminal and blood thiamine concentrations, and brain levels may even be elevated. In contrast, brain TPP is decreased in high-sulfur diet–associated PEM cases. This would suggest that high dietary sulfur either increases the metabolic demand for, or inhibits the synthesis of, TPP and when sufficiently low levels of the enzyme occur in the brain, PEM may develop. The treatment is the same as for PEM resulting from thiamine deficiency. The response to treatment is often poor and should emphasize the need to locate a possible source of sulfur to prevent other cattle from developing the same, rarely reversible, lesions.

Lead Poisoning
Etiology

Accidental or malicious exposure to materials containing lead predisposes cattle to lead poisoning or plumbism. Lack of discrimination in eating habits, coupled with the species' tendency for licking objects and ingesting odd-tasting foreign materials, also predisposes cattle to lead poisoning. Although modern housing tends to reduce the likelihood of lead toxicity in dairy cattle, ample opportunity still exists in many geographic areas where pasturing and other management techniques allow cattle to roam, escape from fences or enclosures, and thereby gain access to areas where lead-containing chemicals or materials may exist. Used motor oils, certain roofing materials, lead- and aluminum-based paints, lead arsenate sprays, lead shot, linoleum, solder, used batteries, and weather-worn lead sheeting comprise some of the more common sources of lead to which cattle may be exposed. Environmental contamination caused by industrial production of lead or lead wastes is possible in certain areas. Lead absorption from the GI tract depends on the form ingested and the age and nutritional status of the animal. Metallic lead is the least well absorbed form and can remain in the rumen and reticulum for many months. Mature animals only absorb 1% to 3% of ingested lead, but young milk-fed animals can absorb up to 50%.

As a consequence, although all ages of animal are susceptible, calves are more susceptible than adult cattle and calves fed milk may be more susceptible than calves fed hay and grain. The dose of lead necessary to cause toxicity to cattle varies tremendously because single time point exposure to a massive quantity (1 g/kg body weight) could induce acute lethal signs, but exposure to 2 to 3 mg/kg body weight daily

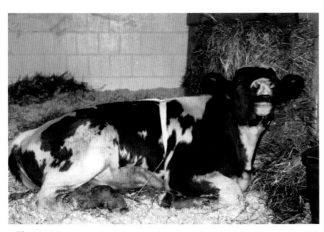

• **Fig. 13.27** Lead poisoning causing recumbency, blindness, and bellowing. There also were uncontrolled jerking actions in this 16-month-old heifer.

might require 1 month or longer before clinical signs appear. Other factors, such as age, diet, ruminal pH, previous or ongoing lead levels in diet before exposure, and many other details may influence the amount of lead required to cause clinical signs. It is simplest to remember that the incubation period is shortened, the clinical signs accentuated, and the mortality elevated by increasing dosages.

Clinical Signs

Neurologic signs predominate in cattle poisoned with lead, but GI signs also may appear. Early signs induced by low levels of lead in the diet include excessive salivation (ptyalism) and teeth grinding (bruxism), muscle tremors, tongue wallowing, inability to prehend food and hyperesthesia (see Video Clips 13.18A and B). More advanced cases or animals that have ingested higher concentrations show classical signs of cerebrocortical disease, including blindness with normal pupillary function, propulsive activity, seizures, abnormal posture, facial spasticity, head pressing, vocalization, bruxism creating foamy saliva at the mouth, and aggression as possible signs (Fig. 13.27). Acute death without premonitory signs also is possible. Although various theories exist as to the cellular effect of lead on the CNS, the exact cellular pathophysiology is unknown.

Gastrointestinal signs, including ruminal stasis, bloat, dark colored manure, diarrhea, or constipation occur in some cases. Abdominal pain characterized by colic also has been described and is thought to result from irritation of the bowel by the toxic material. Mild to moderate levels of exposure may result in both cerebrocortical and GI signs. Such animals are noticed to be depressed and blind, sometimes wander aimlessly or head press, and have ruminal stasis. The clinical signs can look nearly identical to thiamine deficiency PEM. Occasionally during the clinical examination of the patient, the odor of used motor oil or some other suggestive chemical will be detected and can aid greatly in the diagnosis.

Normocytic, normochromic anemia, basophilic stippling, reticulocytosis, and mild elevation of blood urea nitrogen (BUN) and creatinine have been found in some

patients with chronic lead poisoning but are not common enough in bovine lead poisoning to be reliably diagnostic.

Diagnosis

The clinical signs coupled with a thorough search of the premises on which affected cattle have been housed or turned out constitute the principal means of diagnosis. Laboratory confirmation usually is essential.

Blood or tissue lead levels must be obtained to confirm the diagnosis of lead poisoning. Although references vary greatly, most laboratories use 0.05 to 0.25 ppm as reference ranges for normal blood lead (heparinized sample) levels and indicate that any values above 0.30 ppm (0.30 mg/L) are abnormal. Kidney and liver lead values above 10 ppm on a wet basis are considered toxic levels. Low-grade, chronic exposure may not generate greatly elevated blood lead levels.

Although blood and tissue lead values are the most practical means to confirm lead toxicity in cattle, other specific tests are available at some laboratories. These tests measure the effect of lead on porphyrin and heme metabolism. Specifically, lead inhibits activity of delta-aminolevulinic acid dehydrase, which is essential to heme synthesis. Resultant low levels of delta-aminolevulinic acid dehydrase in blood and high levels of delta-aminolevulinic acid in urine may be measured to diagnose lead toxicity. These changes may occur before clinical signs are pronounced and thus may offer an early monitoring technique. These levels also offer a more sensitive means than blood lead analysis to monitor remaining tissue lead values after treatment. However, these tests are not widely available to veterinarians at present.

Cerebrospinal fluid analysis generally reveals normal protein and nucleated cell counts in acute cases. Subacute cases showing obvious neurologic signs may have mild protein and cellular elevations caused by cerebrocortical necrosis and consequently be indistinguishable from PEM.

Gross necropsy offers little help unless oil, grease, or a particular suspect material such as paint is found in the rumen. Subacute cases may have enough cerebrocortical necrosis to be detectable as gross cortical swelling and yellow discoloration. Microscopic examination of the neocortex will reveal patches of cerebrocortical degeneration that vary with the severity and duration of the disorder. In the first 72 hours, these consist of cytotoxic edema, ischemic degeneration of neuronal cell bodies, and reactive blood vessels with increased and enlarged endothelial cells. In more prolonged lesions, necrosis is more extensive, and macrophages will accumulate. These lesions are similar to those caused by thiamine deficiency. Mild liver and kidney changes also have been described in chronic cases. These include acid-fast intranuclear inclusion bodies in the renal proximal tubular epithelium.

The major differential diagnosis to lead poisoning in dairy cattle is PEM resulting from thiamine deficiency or sulfur toxicity, with salt poisoning, hepatic encephalopathy, vitamin A deficiency, rabies, and other causes of meningitis or meningoencephalitis, such as *H. somni*, also requiring consideration. In general, acute lead toxicity patients have more of a tendency to have seizures, vocalize, and appear irritable (e.g., facial twitching, hyperesthesia) than do cattle with thiamine deficiency PEM, but these signs may occur with either disorder. Both diseases cause cortical blindness with intact pupillary function, and both may lead to depression, head pressing, bruxism, and other signs. Dorsomedial strabismus may be more common in PEM. It may be difficult in a single patient to appreciate these differences, but in herd outbreaks, the pattern of clinical signs may be more obvious. Also, whereas in PEM ruminal activity may be unaltered, lead poisoning tends to depress ruminal activity. In cases of suspected acute metallic lead ingestion in young or smaller cattle (e.g., lead shot), abdominal radiographs can identify x-ray–dense metallic material within the forestomach.

Meningitis or meningoencephalitis is characterized by inflammatory CSF, fever, or other clinical and clinicopathologic signs indicative of inflammation. Rabies must be considered in all differential diagnoses, but blindness is not common with rabies.

Treatment

Unless history confirms the source of lead, prevention of further exposure must be the primary concern of the veterinarian. This may require removal of all suspect feedstuffs, confinement of cattle heretofore pastured, or other measures. When the history confirms that the only affected cow is the one who "got loose and was found in the machinery shed," then the mystery of exposure is usually solved. Much more difficult are herd outbreaks with multiple cattle affected and no known means of exposure. Much detective work may be necessary to find the source in feed, water, or on the premises. Suspect feed material should be sent to toxicology laboratories for confirmation.

Specific treatment requires calcium disodium EDTA (CaNa$_2$-EDTA) given parenterally. Suggested doses for IV CaNa$_2$-EDTA vary between 62 and 110 mg/kg body weight given once or twice daily. Some clinicians recommend dividing the dose and giving half of the total daily dose twice daily. SC administration also is acceptable. During IV administration, CaNa$_2$-EDTA should be given very slowly because reactions (e.g., increased heart and respiratory rates, trembling, hair elevation) may occur if the drug is administered rapidly. The mechanism of action of CaNa$_2$-EDTA is chelation of lead held in bone, thereby allowing solubilization and urinary excretion. It does not chelate lead in soft tissue, and continued effectiveness depends on soft tissue lead equilibrating with the decreasing bone levels. Therefore, treatment with CaNa$_2$-EDTA is designed to be intermittent. One well-controlled study used 62.0 mg/kg body weight CaNa$_2$-EDTA IV twice daily for 4 days, skipped 4 days, and then treated again for 4 days. In summary, a twice-daily IV treatment with 60 to 110 mg/kg of CaNa$_2$-EDTA should be used to treat lead poisoning in cattle. The exact number of days is not likely to be important, but a period of 3 to 5 days seems reasonable. This initial therapy should then be repeated after a lag time of 3 to 5 days, during which time soft tissue accumulation of lead may be shifted to bone and thus again, subjected to chelation by CaNa$_2$-EDTA. Unfortunately, CaNa$_2$-EDTA labeled for use in cattle for treating lead poisoning is no longer available, and use of a more expensive product labeled for small animals may be necessary or the product can be purchased from some compounding pharmacies.

Thiamine should be administered as well at a dose of 10 mg/kg body weight or higher. Thiamine does not protect against, nor remove, lead that has accumulated in tissue but does seem to improve clinical signs in lead-poisoned cattle. In fact, whereas treatment with CaNa$_2$-EDTA alone may worsen the clinical signs, treatment with thiamine or thiamine and CaNa$_2$-EDTA in combination improves the clinical signs in lead-poisoned cattle. Thiamine's exact mechanism is unknown. However, because the cerebrocortical lesions of PEM and lead toxicity are so similar, it has been theorized that lead interferes with thiamine or thiamine pyrophosphate levels and therefore energy metabolism to some degree and that some of the cerebrocortical lesions are in fact the result of relative thiamine deficiency. Intravenous mannitol as described for PEM resulting from thiamine deficiency is the treatment of choice for cytotoxic edema but is seldom used in bovine practice in the treatment of lead poisoning.

When recent ingestion of a known lead-containing material has occurred, a rumenotomy offers the best opportunity to remove the material, wash out the rumen, and institute supportive therapy. Magnesium sulfate laxatives are indicated to cause formation of insoluble lead sulfides that can be passed in the feces. If the rumen contents are fluid from drinking used motor oil, ororumenal gavage may be possible.

The prognosis is best for those cattle with mild neurologic deficits or GI signs. Cattle that are having seizures or showing opisthotonos, blindness, and dementia have a poorer prognosis. Anticonvulsants are not of great use in adult cattle, but diazepam (5–10 mg IV) has been used in calves. Lactating cows or pregnant heifers that recover from lead poisoning should have milk lead levels tested before the milk is used for consumption. It may be necessary to test the animal multiple times because blood and milk lead levels can change depending on the stage of lactation and metabolic demand for bone calcium. It is likely that milk lead levels may remain high for several months following successful treatment of a cow for lead poisoning. If other lactating cows are exposed, bulk tank samples should be monitored for lead. Recent author experience suggests that definitive proof of lead poisoning in commercial dairy cattle can have profound and lengthy consequences for dairy farmers because of the obvious public health concerns regarding commercial milk or meat consumption from animals exposed to lead on affected premises.

Salt Intoxication

Etiology

Salt intoxication (water deprivation) or hypernatremia is a frequent cause of neurologic signs in calves but is uncommon in adult cattle. Its occurrence in preweaned dairy calves is frequent enough to retain it as an important differential for acute neurologic signs in this age of animal, especially if there is a recent history of treatment for diarrhea or if free choice water is not available to milk replacer–fed calves. Sodium imbalances may be caused by dysfunction in either sodium or water regulation. Failure to properly dilute electrolyte solution or milk replacers for calves may result in hypernatremia because calves seem willing to drink solutions containing excessive sodium chloride. Failure to provide access to water for milk replacer–fed calves is probably the most common cause of salt intoxication. Sodium containing feed additives or medications such as lasalocid when added to milk replacers may predispose to the disease. On rare occasions, high-salinity water used to mix milk replacer may be the culprit.

Adult cattle have suffered salt intoxication primarily as a result of water deprivation that was accidental or brought on by natural disasters or droughts. We have observed an outbreak of salt poisoning in replacement heifers during freezing weather when both their water source and walkways were covered with ice; salt was sprinkled on the walkways to melt the ice, resulting in the cattle drinking the surface water, which contained very high amounts of salt. Consumption of salt water also has caused the disease in beef cattle. We have observed one instance of salt poisoning in heifers fed liquid whey that contained excessive amounts of sodium chloride. Excessive salt in the ration generally is not a problem as long as plenty of fresh water is available to cattle. However, excessive salt in the water (>0.25%) may also decrease milk production in dairy cattle. Feeding errors that allow excessive sodium chloride in the diet and dilutional errors when compounding large quantities of IV fluids for cattle may also be responsible for some salt poisoning cases.

Although both sodium and chloride levels are greatly elevated in the serum and CSF, sodium is of more concern because hypernatremia apparently inhibits glycolysis in cerebral neurons. Hypernatremia causes plasma osmolality to increase relative to tissue osmolality. This causes neurons to shrink as water is lost to the extracellular space in an attempt to equilibrate the osmotic gradient between the intracellular and extracellular spaces. A partially protective mechanism occurs with accumulation of amino acids, sugars, and alcohols in neuronal cells in an attempt to balance the intra- and extracellular osmolality. Neurons are damaged from the hypernatremia and fluid shifts associated with these osmolality changes. The neurons are further damaged by neuronal edema if rapid correction of the hypernatremia occurs. Beware that signs of cerebrocortical degeneration may follow the consumption of excessive quantities of water after a period of hypernatremia. This rapid effect of the hypo-osmolar serum can result in cytotoxic brain edema. Sudden restoration of ad libitum access to water for cattle previously deprived of it due to frozen pipes is a potential cause of the syndrome.

Clinical Signs

In calves, depression, diarrhea, and weakness are the major signs, but seizures may occur in advanced cases (see Video Clip 13.19). Serum and CSF sodium levels usually are above 160 mEq/L, and neurologic signs tend to be directly proportional to sodium level elevations. Diarrhea caused by saline catharsis and enteric pathogens in calves contributes to dehydration, which worsens the electrolyte problems. Seizures may occur spontaneously or after administration of IV fluid intended to correct dehydration. Rapid administration of isotonic IV fluids to hypernatremic patients or excessive intake of water orally decreases intracellular osmolarity in the brain cells, causing subsequent neuronal edema, and worsening neurologic signs such as seizures.

Adult cattle that are water deprived tend to show GI signs, including anorexia, and sometimes diarrhea. Neurologic signs initially reflect the prosencephalic cerebrocortical lesion—depression, blindness, and seizures. More severe lesions will involve the brainstem and cerebellum, causing vestibular and cerebellar ataxia.

Ancillary Aids and Diagnosis

Definitive diagnosis requires laboratory confirmation of hypernatremia in the serum of patients showing typical clinical signs. Most cases in calves go undiagnosed in the field because of lack of laboratory data. Groups of calves or cows that are affected usually stimulate greater diagnostic efforts. Most calves with salt poisoning have a moderate to severe azotemia. Measurement of serum osmolality can also be revealing in suspect cases. If the calf has died and salt poisoning without water intoxication is suspected, then sodium concentration of CSF or aqueous humor fluid can be tested, with normal CSF and aqueous levels being approximately 130 mEq/L. Sodium concentrations in brain tissue >2000 ppm suggest salt poisoning.

Rations and water should be analyzed for salt content when adult dairy cattle or heifers are affected with hypernatremia. When calves are affected, investigation into feeding protocols such as dilution rates of milk replacer as fed or oral electrolyte solutions, and the availability of ad libitum access to fresh water, are required. It is important to remember, however, that the ad libitum availability of fresh water is a preventive measure, *not* a therapeutic one, for affected individuals! Measuring total solids by Brix refractometer can be done as an initial screening for high sodium in the milk replacer.

The differential diagnosis in calves may include acid–base electrolyte abnormalities associated with neonatal infectious enteritis, meningitis, metabolic conditions such as D-lactic acidosis and PEM in fully ruminant calves. In adult cattle, PEM, lead poisoning, and rabies may be considered.

Treatment

Treatment should be designed to produce a slow, gradual decrease in serum and CSF osmolarity. For adult animals, this means allowing access to small amounts of fresh water at regular intervals. Free-choice water would likely create cerebral edema as previously discussed because ECF osmolarity decreases much more rapidly than brain intracellular osmolarity, which may then cause a "rush" of water into neurons with resultant cerebral edema. Before making a treatment plan for hypernatremia, a clinicopathologic assessment of hydration status should be performed. For example the use of diuretics such as furosemide at a low dose (0.50 mg/kg) may be indicated if the patient's hydration status is adequate and the hypernatremia is a result of acute sodium toxicosis.

Conversely, if the hypernatremic calf has diarrhea and is dehydrated, administration of isotonic saline or sodium bicarbonate should be provided to correct dehydration and acid–base disorders and then the water deficit should be replaced slowly. This can often be accomplished in calves having hypernatremia by administering a slow-drip IV therapy with low percentage dextrose solutions containing half-strength to normal saline until serum sodium values return to normal. Some clinicians have also enjoyed success using gradually diminishing concentrations of hypertonic saline in the treatment of hypernatremic neonates. An alternative therapeutic fluid regimen has successfully used hypertonic (8.4%) sodium bicarbonate solution by slow IV infusion in addition to isotonic dextrose (5%) infusion. Ideally, correction of hypernatremia should occur at less than 1 mEq/hr. Therapy is complicated if severe dehydration exists because the patient needs intensive fluid therapy for dehydration but will likely suffer neurologic complications if administered low sodium concentration fluids too rapidly. Generally, the azotemia resolves, and calves with sodium concentration as great as 201 mEq/L have completely recovered. Calves that have received a high sodium electrolyte solution and have acute salt toxicosis are easier to manage and have a better prognosis than calves with chronic hypernatremia caused by a high sodium milk replacer and lack of free water. Supportive therapy with thiamine may be of benefit and is unlikely to be harmful. If the sodium has returned to normal but the calf has not responded appropriately, an I.V. dose of mannitol (0.5 mg/kg) can be given.

D-Lactic Acidosis

Etiology

D-lactate is a product of bacterial overgrowth in the GI tract and commonly occurs in calves with either abnormal rumen or hind gut fermentation. The normal closure of the calf's esophageal groove during nursing allows most of the consumed milk to bypass the forestomachs and go directly to the abomasum. Some calves, especially bucket-fed and older milk-fed calves, have less than ideal function of the esophageal groove, leading to increased amounts of milk spilling into the rumen followed by abnormal bacterial carbohydrate fermentation in the rumen or reticulum. Esophageal groove dysfunction is also common in calves with a preexisting disease such as pneumonia, otitis, or thrombophlebitis. Adverse consequences to the calf from the ruminal fermentation of milk include abnormally low rumen pH (<6), improper development of, or damage to, rumen papillae, diarrhea, ill thrift, ruminal bloat, and both D- and L- lactic acidosis. Marked neurologic signs in affected calves have been shown to be principally due to the elevated D-lactate. The physiologic events and clinical signs of D-lactic acidosis have also been experimentally produced by tube feeding milk, milk replacer, or some electrolyte and glucose products. Calves with small intestinal malabsorption (e.g., rotavirus diarrhea) fed even "normal" amounts of milk or milk replacer may also develop D-lactic acidosis because excessive milk is presented to the hindgut and abnormal bacterial fermentation occurs at that site. The ruminal and hindgut D-lactic acidoses would be expected to be more common in older (>7 days of age)

milk-fed calves because they would have a larger and more functional rumen, cecum, and colon. It should be noted that young calves (<7 days of age) frequently have diarrhea and metabolic acidosis, but in these calves, the acidosis is mostly a result of L-lactate accumulating from dehydration, poor perfusion, and anaerobic cellular metabolism.

Clinical Signs and Diagnosis

A severe clinical syndrome with marked depression or advanced neurologic signs may occur in calves with markedly elevated concentrations of D-lactate (>6 mmol/L). Calves with ruminal or hindgut D-lactic acidosis demonstrate variable degrees of depression, loss of blink (palpebral) reflex, and ataxia. Some are obtunded. In one study, determining the degree of loss of the palpebral reflex was identified as the best clinical tool for diagnosing an increase in serum D-lactate concentrations. The more advanced neurologic signs caused by D-lactic acidosis are believed to be a result of impaired energy production centrally in neurons. D-lactate is not only a poor substrate for energy production in the brain when compared with pyruvate and L-lactate (the brain can readily use L-lactate as a source of energy), but its presence also impairs energy production from pyruvate and L-lactate. The diagnosis is based on the neurologic signs and laboratory finding of marked metabolic acidosis. D-lactate is not measured in commercial laboratories or by any point-of-care test equipment, but a calf with severe metabolic acidosis, markedly elevated anion gap, and normal or only mildly increased L-lactate (which can be readily measured by point-of-care testing) and without severe azotemia, can be assumed to have an elevated D-lactate level. It must be emphasized that not every dehydrated calf with metabolic acidosis has increased concentrations of D-lactate and that calves with D-lactic acidosis are not necessarily dehydrated.

Treatment

Treatment of clinical cases of D-lactic acidosis mostly involves administration of sodium bicarbonate either intravenously or orally. When clinical signs are less severe, orally administered fluids with bicarbonate are appropriate but when base deficit is greater than 10 mEq/L, IV fluids are likely required. When calculating the amount of bicarbonate needed for replacement in calves with D-lactic acidosis, replacement should be determined by; base deficit × weight in kilograms × 0.6 = mEq of bicarbonate required for replacement. The extracellular fluid:body weight multiplier (0.6) is higher than that used for treatment of dehydration with increased L-lactate associated acidosis in which fluid volume therapy is most important. Treatment with sodium bicarbonate may rapidly (within a few hours) decrease D-lactate by both increased renal elimination and decreased intestinal production of D-lactate following alkalization of the intestinal lumen.

Prevention of D-lactate syndromes includes;
1. not tube feeding milk to calves after a few days of age,
2. feeding properly mixed milk replacers with a consistent total solids value,
3. feeding milk or milk replacer near or at body temperature,

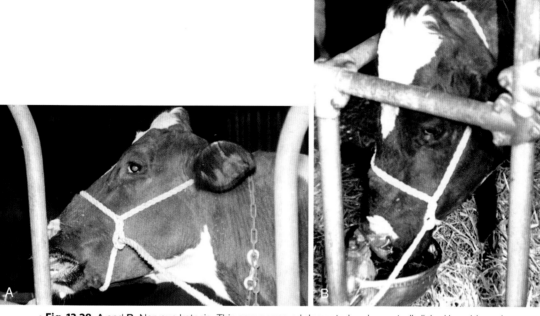

• **Fig. 13.28** **A** and **B,** Nervous ketosis. This cow appeared demented and repeatedly licked her side and stall pipes and bit the water cup.

4. preventing or properly treating predisposing primary diseases,
5. more frequent feeding of smaller amounts of milk or milk replacer to calves with diarrhea or malabsorption, or mixing lactase tablets with the milk, and
6. bottle feeding rather than bucket feeding calves at risk.

Nervous Ketosis

Etiology

Nervous ketosis is simply an encephalopathic form of conventional metabolic ketosis and may occur at any time during the first 8 weeks of lactation. The pathophysiology of ketosis is discussed in Chapter 15. Metabolic derangements such as hypoglycemia, elevated free-fatty acids and ketonemia are associated with negative energy balance and likely cause the clinical signs associated with the wasting and neurologic forms of the condition. In severe ketosis, the relative energy imbalance causes extreme ketonemia. The reasons for the neurologic signs in nervous ketosis are not known but may simply be a combination of hypoglycemia and elevated acetoacetic acid or acetone levels that are toxic to the brain. Alternatively, the production of isopropyl alcohol from acetoacetic acid breakdown in the rumen may play a role. A degree of hepatic encephalopathy could contribute to neurologic signs in some cattle, but we are unaware of studies to confirm or deny this theory.

Clinical Signs

Signs observed in cattle affected with nervous ketosis vary from recumbency to aggression. Many cows having nervous ketosis act demented, constantly licking one or more spots on their own body or on inanimate objects. Some cows bite objects such as drinking cups and have been known

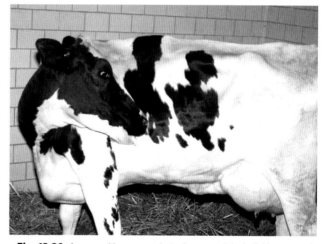

• **Fig. 13.29** A cow with nervous ketosis compulsively licking on only one side of the thorax.

to break cups off water pipes (Fig. 13.28). Other cows, if confined, show propulsive tendencies by constantly leaning into a stanchion or tie stall. Cattle not confined to tie stalls may wander about, circle, appear ataxic and sometimes blind, and will head-press. Sometimes hyperesthesia is observed. Some severely affected cattle become recumbent as their degree of hypoglycemia worsens. When recumbent, the patient may appear similar to hypocalcemic or hypomagnesemic patients. Signs of constant licking or depraved appetite in recumbent cattle suggest nervous ketosis (Fig. 13.29). Overly fat periparturient cows may develop severe ketosis and signs of nervous ketosis within days after calving. Therefore, if recumbent, these cows are often assumed to be hypocalcemic or hypomagnesemic but may have nervous ketosis or combined metabolic problems. In conventional housing, cattle with severe ketosis may walk short distances after release for exercise and then collapse because of hypoglycemia or have difficulty rising.

Cattle showing irritation or aggression are obviously more dramatic and can be dangerous to handlers, veterinarians, and themselves. Irritability resulting from hypoglycemia, just as in people, can worsen if the patient is stressed. Therefore, uncontrolled activity, including aggression, wild running, bellowing, and a wild-eyed appearance, may be seen by the clinician. Usually this form is observed after attempts to capture or restrain the patient.

Blindness is observed only occasionally in cattle having nervous ketosis. Cattle with blindness due to nervous ketosis regain vision after treatment, which has caused many authors to describe this blindness as "transient" or "apparent." However, blindness may persist and be permanent in some nervous ketosis patients, even though all other signs have resolved with treatment. This bilateral blindness, first described by Dr. F.H. Fox, is a cerebrocortical blindness with intact pupillary function and is most likely caused by permanent damage to the visual cortex. The visual cortex is extremely sensitive to metabolic derangements, such as severe hypoglycemia, making this the most likely cause. The retinas and optic nerves are normal in appearance in such patients.

Diagnosis

The diagnosis depends on identification of ketonuria in cattle showing bizarre neurologic signs. Ketonemia and ketonuria are usually dramatic, and test tablets or reagent strips quickly turn purple. However, not all patients have strongly positive reaction for urine ketones. There may be a dilutional effect if the cow has been drinking large quantities of water or chewing on a salt block because of a depraved appetite. Therefore some variation in the degree of ketonuria exists in nervous ketosis patients. Reagents to detect ketones in urine, blood, or milk also vary in their accuracy and can give rise to false negatives. Many of the tests detect only acetoacetate and do not detect acetone or β-hydroxybutyric acid.

Clinical signs of constant licking, chewing, or biting objects in a "ketotic" cow make this diagnosis likely (see Video Clips 13.20 and 13.21). More bizarre signs cause the clinician to consider a wider differential diagnosis, including other metabolic diseases (e.g., hypocalcemia, hypomagnesemia) when recumbent. Aggression brings the fear of rabies into consideration. Blindness, if present, requires a wide-ranging differential diagnosis, including PEM and lead poisoning, among others. Leaning into a stanchion or propulsive activity by the patient requires consideration of listeriosis. Despite the broad differential diagnosis, the triad of early lactation, positive (usually strongly so) urine, blood or milk ketones, and nervous signs, generally allow accurate diagnosis.

Occasionally, cows with other neurologic diseases such as listeriosis, and especially those with dysphagia, may become ketotic secondary to continued milk production. However, in these instances, neurologic signs have usually preceded ketosis by several days.

Overly fat periparturient cows with nervous ketosis require further workup, including acid–base and electrolyte status, serum calcium, serum magnesium, and serum biochemistry to evaluate liver function.

Treatment

Intravenous dextrose (300–500 mL of 50% dextrose) is the initial therapy for nervous-ketosis patients. In aggressive or demented patients, it may be necessary to sedate the animal with xylazine (20 mg IM or IV) before IV dextrose. Dextrose should be repeated in 6 to 12 hours in field settings. If possible, slow constant administration of 20 L of 5% dextrose over a 24-hour period provides superior follow-up to initial concentrated dextrose. If this is not practical, repeated administration of dextrose should be suggested at 12-hour intervals for at least three treatments. A single treatment is rarely sufficient to correct the underlying metabolic derangement. In addition to dextrose, low-dose corticosteroids have been used as therapy for ketosis. An initial dose of 10 to 20 mg of dexamethasone is followed by 10 mg daily for 3 to 4 additional days. Dexamethasone treatment is contingent on the fact that the patient has no contraindications to use of this drug.

Other supportive measures for treating nervous ketosis are controversial and vary greatly. Most clinicians use oral propylene glycol or glycerol at 6 to 8 oz, usually twice daily, as a supplemental energy source. It is important not to use these products in excessive doses because they may contribute to decreased ruminal activity and diarrhea. Therefore they are most useful in patients that have good ruminal activity. On some farms, propylene glycol may be the only treatment required for ketosis. Oral calcium propionate (1–1.5 lb in several gallons of water by drench) may be a useful, alternative 3-carbon energy source to propylene glycol for some farms. It has the advantage of also supplying bioavailable oral calcium to what is usually an early lactation animal.

Chloral hydrate (30 g orally in gelatin capsules) may be extremely helpful as initial therapy in very agitated patients because of the sedative properties of the drug. It may also contribute to starch metabolism in the rumen and aid glucose production in some unknown ways. It is currently difficult to acquire chloral hydrate in the United States.

Periparturient patients with nervous ketosis have a fair prognosis. However, these patients may require repeated treatments. The prognosis for nervous-ketosis patients, other than those that are periparturient, is good with therapy as directed. With the exception of the rare permanent blindness observed in some patients, most cattle fully resolve the neurologic signs within hours and only relapse if maintenance therapy is neglected.

Vitamin A Deficiency
Etiology and Clinical Signs

An absolute or relative deficiency of vitamin A may cause a multitude of abnormalities in growing cattle. Poor growth, blindness, inappetence, seizures and other neurologic signs, dermatitis, diarrhea, xerophthalmia, and pneumonia have been observed in young dairy cattle experimentally deprived of vitamin A. Mature cattle may show blindness and GI, neurologic, and reproductive abnormalities.

Most natural outbreaks of vitamin A deficiency involve growing or feedlot beef cattle, but much experimental work has been completed with dairy animals. Because natural occurrence in dairy animals is now rare, discussion of this deficiency will be brief and primarily useful because it is a differential diagnosis for PEM and lead poisoning.

Clinical signs are the result of (1) increased intracranial pressure secondary to meningeal thickening and altered arachnoid villi that interfere with CSF absorption and (2) abnormal bone growth with deficient bone resorption contributing to compression of the prechiasmatic optic tract (nerve). The meningeal fibroplasia and narrowing of the caudal cranial fossa and foramen magnum result in caudal cerebellar vermal herniation.

Neurologic signs, in both experimental and natural outbreaks, include blindness, seizures, circling, disorientation, opisthotonos, depression, and elevated head carriage. Blindness is a classic finding and is primarily caused by progressive optic disc edema from increased CSF pressure in adult cattle. Optic disc edema must be severe to result in blindness because many deficient cattle remain visual despite mild-to-moderate edema. In growing cattle, optic disc edema and blindness are caused by both elevated CSF pressure and dural fibroplasia in the optic canals with resultant optic nerve compression. In severe cases, this causes dilated pupils with deficient pupillary responses to light. These pupillary abnormalities help to differentiate this form of blindness from that which occurs in PEM, in which they are normal. Nyctalopia or night blindness also is associated with vitamin A deficiency and, although it is one of the earliest signs, may be difficult to assess in field settings. Vitamin A is essential for rhodopsin regeneration required for photoreceptor activity during dark adaptation. Rod photoreceptors may be more affected than cones, thus contributing to nyctalopia.

Diets consisting of aged feed material, all-grain diets that have not been supplemented with vitamin A, diets in which vitamin A may have been destroyed by heat, or diets completely devoid of green forage can lead to natural outbreaks of vitamin A deficiency. Similarly, animals pastured during extreme drought conditions or only offered coarse roughage in addition to pasture may become deficient.

Diagnosis

Optic disc edema with associated retinal edema and hemorrhages are present in vitamin A–deficient animals (Figs. 13.30, 14.57 and 14.58). The finding of optic disc edema in a group of animals showing signs of blindness with abnormal pupillary light responses and other neurologic signs is pathognomonic for vitamin A deficiency. Although optic disc edema has been reported in lead toxicity and PEM in cattle, it rarely, if ever, occurs in these diseases. Therefore

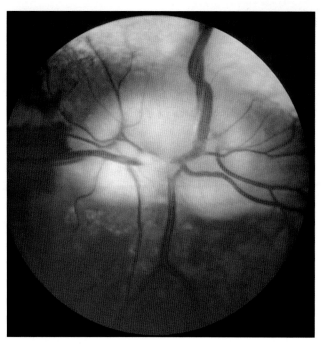

• **Fig. 13.30** Optic disc edema, peridiscal retinal edema, and hemorrhage in a vitamin A–deficient heifer.

optic disc edema, especially in multiple animals, should make vitamin A deficiency the most likely diagnosis.

Rations and blood from affected animals should be assessed for vitamin A or carotene levels. Normal values for vitamin A in serum range from 25–60 µg/dL. The severity of clinical signs is inversely proportional to the level of vitamin A when serum levels decrease to less than 20 µg/dL.

Histopathology from active cases in growing animals reveals prechiasmatic optic tract degeneration resulting from dural fibrosis within the optic canal, squamous metaplasia of parotid salivary ducts, and many other changes.

Treatment

Normally, vitamin A deficiency is prevented by feeding green forage or a diet supplemented with vitamin A. However, if the disease occurs, all animals in the group should receive 440 IU/kg body weight of vitamin A by injection. This may be repeated, and dietary supplementation should begin immediately with sufficient levels of vitamin A in the diet to provide 40 IU/kg body weight/ day for the cattle.

Hepatic Encephalopathy

Hepatic encephalopathy (HE) is a metabolic disorder that most commonly results from a diffuse liver disease that causes hyperammonemia along with other circulating toxic factors that interfere with neuronal function. In calves, HE is usually caused by a portosystemic shunt (PSS). In older cattle, HE is usually secondary to diffuse liver disease caused by the consumption of pasture grasses that contain large quantities of plant species that produce a pyrrolizidine alkaloid. Species of *Crotalaria* and *Senecio* are most commonly implicated. The chronic consumption of these alkaloids causes liver degeneration that can result in HE. Most clinical signs are prosencephalic in origin with changes in behavior and seizures. Calves with a PSS may seem normal for the first couple of weeks of life until the rumen becomes functional; then the increase in blood ammonia causes waxing and waning signs of both cerebral and spinal cord disease (Fig. 13.31) (Video Clips 13.17 A and B). The diagnosis of liver failure and HE can be made by serum chemistry changes that reflect liver disease (elevated aspartate aminotransferase, sorbitol dehydrogenase, and gamma glutamyltransferase) and organ failure, including hyperammonemia, bilirubinemia, and abnormal clotting function test results. A PSS will cause increased serum blood ammonia without bilirubinemia, elevated hepatic derived enzymes, or abnormal clotting function tests. When blood ammonia is high and a shunt is suspected, it can be diagnosed by ultrasonography and contrast radiography or advanced imaging (CT or MRI). Microscopic examination of a biopsy piece of liver may reveal proliferating small arterioles but hypoplastic to absent portal veins. Ascites is not a feature of congenital PSSs, but with acquired shunts from chronic liver disease and fibrosis, high-protein ascites is common. One calf has been surgically corrected, but the surgery is difficult even when there is a single extrahepatic shunt. If surgery is being contemplated, medical management would include thiamine and fluids administered IV and vinegar given per os to lower the ruminal pH. If the calf is eating, it should continue to be fed a low-protein diet because removing all feed will elevate ruminal pH and may actually increase blood ammonia. The CNS lesions that accompany hyperammonemia, including astrocyte proliferation alongside altered and dilated myelin sheaths, are reversible.

Pyrrolizidine alkaloid toxicity can be diagnosed by liver biopsy to demonstrate a triad of fibrosis, megalocytosis, and bile duct proliferation. Pyrrolizidine toxicosis

is usually fatal but can be prevented by avoiding pastures or hays containing these plant species. In general, hyperammonemia in cattle is much less common than in horses. In addition to pyrrolizidine toxicity and shunts, we have also seen hyperammonemia accompany rare cases of hepatobiliary neoplasia in which both significant hepatic parenchymal involvement as well as bile duct obstruction have occurred.

Nervous Coccidiosis

Neurologic signs in calves infected with intestinal coccidia are rare in the northeastern United States and most common in the northwestern states and western Canada. Coccidiosis in calves is discussed in detail in Chapter 6. Neurologic signs are more common in heavily infected feedlot beef cattle in severe winter weather. The pathophysiology of these neurologic signs is unknown and assumed to be both neurotoxic and metabolic in nature because there are no brain lesions. Clinical signs include partial or generalized seizures, tremors, and recumbency with opisthotonos and abnormal nystagmus. The mortality rate is high.

Additional Toxins and Deficiencies Causing Signs of Brain Dysfunction

Mycotoxicosis is rare in cattle in the northeastern and midwestern United States. The toxins are produced by fungal agents that contaminate various grass species consumed by cattle. A list of these tremorgenic neurotoxins, along with other miscellaneous toxins that can cause neurologic signs, can be found in table form in Chapter 17.

Calves that are administered excessive lidocaine can develop seizures. If the lidocaine is being given by infusion (as for intestinal ileus), stopping the infusion and the administration of a single dose of diazepam generally results in recovery within a few hours. Nutritional deficiencies that cause seizures in adult cattle are mostly caused by the combination of hypomagnesemia and hypocalcemia. Careful treatment with magnesium- and calcium-containing fluids intravenously is often curative.

Injury

Intracranial injury from external causes is uncommon. Newborn calves are most susceptible because of their less dense calvarium and less resistant brain at this age. Most injuries relate to falls and striking their heads on concrete within their environment. Brain swelling from hemorrhage and edema can lead to herniation.

Neoplasia

Brain neoplasms are uncommon in cattle, which may relate to their short life span. Intracranial lymphosarcoma is the most common (Fig. 13.32). Intracranial lymphosarcoma is usually not caused by the bovine leukemia virus (BLV). Gliomas have

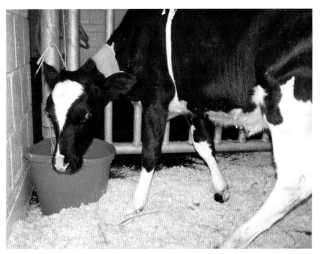

• **Fig. 13.31** A 3-month-old calf with intermittent depression, falling, and a shuffling gait (which can be seen by the tracks in the shaving) caused by a portosystemic shunt.

also been reported. One of us (TJD) has seen two calves (both ≈2 months of age) with medulloblastomas causing opisthotonos (Fig. 13.33). It should be remembered that opisthotonus may also be seen with many other cerebral and cerebellar diseases, including cerebellar abiotrophy (Fig. 13.34).

Uncommon Causes of Brain Signs

For ease of presentation and completeness a list of uncommon causes of brain signs in calves and adult cattle are summarized in Table 13.2.

Spinal Cord

Clinical Signs of Spinal Cord Dysfunction

Based on clinical signs, the spinal cord can be divided into four regions: C1 to C5, C6 to T2, T3 to L3 and L4 to the coccyx. Lesions that interfere with the gray matter of the intumescences (C6–T2, L4–S2) will cause a gait quality that reflects LMN paresis accompanied by loss of tone, spinal reflexes, and denervation atrophy. The posture and gait reflect degrees of inability to support weight, and if the patient is ambulatory, there will be short strides, sometimes accompanied by trembling. Lesions that spare the intumescence gray matter but affect the white matter tracts that connect with the gray matter will result in a gait quality that reflects interference with the UMN and GP systems. The UMN tracts are descending from nuclei in the caudal brainstem and function to maintain normal muscle tone and to influence the central pattern generators in the intumescences to generate the limb movements for the gait. Interference with these pathways will result in UMN quality paresis. The cranial projecting GP pathways function to provide the sensory information necessary for smooth, coordinated limb movements. Interference with these pathways results in a GP quality ataxia. The resultant gait abnormality is a reflection of the loss of function in the pathways of both

of these two systems, which are adjacent to each other at every level of the spinal cord. It is not possible, nor necessary, to distinguish between the signs because of interference within these two systems. The clinician's goal is to recognize the signs and locate the region of the spinal cord involved such that specific diagnostics can be applied.

Sacrocaudal lesions cause a loss of tail and anal tone, reflexes, and nociception. S1 and S2 contribute primarily to the tibial nerve component of the sciatic nerve. Loss of their function will result in an overflexed tarsus, "dropped hock," and a unique dorsal buckling of the fetlock seen only in cows with tibial paresis. Incontinence with dribbling of urine and rectal impaction or pneumorectum may occur. L4 to L6 (femoral nerve) lesions cause varying degrees of

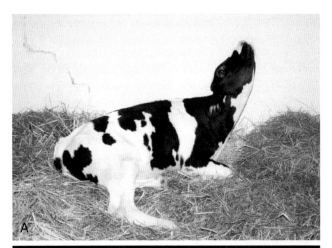

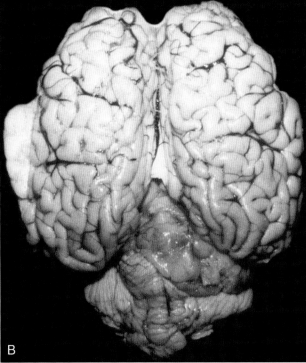

• **Fig. 13.33** A, A 2-month-old calf with severe opisthotonos caused by a medulloblastoma. The clinical signs of opisthotonos often suggest brainstem or cerebellar dysfunction and can look identical to other diseases such as the calf in Fig. 13.34 with cerebellar abiotrophy. **B,** Gross appearance of the medulloblastoma.

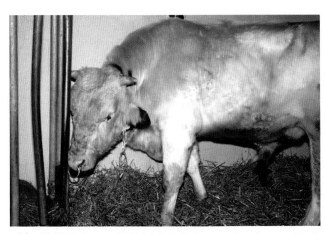

• **Fig. 13.32** A 3-year-old Holstein bull depressed and compulsively circling to the left. The bull was blind in the right eye but had normal pupillary response to light. A large mass (BLV negative lymphosarcoma) was found in the left cerebral hemisphere.

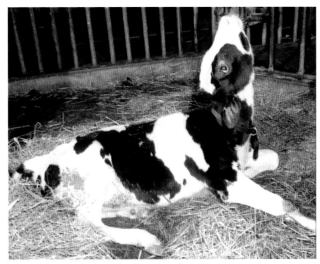

• **Fig. 13.34** Inherited cerebellar abiotrophy in a 6-month-old Holstein heifer. When standing, the heifer had a wide-based stance and a hypermetric gait. Searching head movements and tremor were observed.

difficulty in supporting weight in the pelvic limbs with a very short stride if the patient is ambulatory. There will be a tendency to collapse when weight is placed on the limb and the patella reflex will be diminished. L6 primarily contributes to the peroneal component of the sciatic nerve. Loss of its function will cause the animal to stand on the dorsal surface of the digits (this is more dramatic than the mild overflexion seen with tibial paresis). Depending on the severity of the lesion, there will be varying degrees of loss of tone, spinal reflexes, and nociception.

T3 to L3 lesions on both sides of the cord cause a delay in the onset of protraction of the pelvic limbs, a longer hindlimb stride with inaccurate placement of the hooves, a swaying of the trunk and limbs, an excessive adduction or abduction of the hind limb as it is protracted, and a scuffing of the hooves at the onset of protraction or landing on their dorsal surface at placement. Severe lesions can cause complete pelvic limb paralysis. With caudal thoracic and cranial lumbar lesions, the recumbent patient may use its thoracic limbs and cranial trunk muscles to sit up like a

TABLE 13.2	Uncommon or Additional Causes of Brain Signs				
Disease	**Etiology**	**Clinical Signs**	**Differential Diagnoses**	**Diagnosis**	**Treatment**
Bovine "hysteria" or "bonkers"	Anhydrous ammonia	Intermittent wildness, aimless wandering, bellowing, seizures, recumbency, aggression	Rabies Lead poisoning	History of feeding good-quality forage treated with anhydrous ammonia	Stop feeding ammoniated forage; toxic agent not known—but may be substituted imidazole
Sporadic bovine encephalomyelitis (Buss disease)	Chlamydial organisms have been incriminated, as has paramyxovirus	Fever, depression, respiratory signs, ataxia, weakness; mostly adult cattle with a subacute to chronic course	Malignant catarrhal fever	Rare, nonsuppurative encephalomyelitis on histopathology, culture of organisms, serology	Oxytetracycline
Hypomagnesemia	Magnesium deficiency	Tremors, seizure-like activity, recumbency (See Video Clip 15.1)	Toxicities Vitamin A deficiency Rabies	Low serum and CSF magnesium and absence of magnesium in the urine	Magnesium and calcium, which is also low in most cases
Hypoglycemia	Low blood glucose; most common in young calves, although occasionally seen in adults with overwhelming sepsis or ketosis	Mostly depression and weakness, rarely seizures	Metabolic diseases	History and very low blood glucose from a sample measured within 2 hours of collection	50% glucose initially followed by continual administration of 5%-10% glucose
Nervous coccidiosis	High levels of coccidia; often complicated by inclement weather	Convulsions, recumbency, hyperesthesia, diarrhea, high mortality	Toxicities. PEM	Usually beef calves. Not blind; usually associated with high levels of coccidia in feces but direct cause-and-effect relationship not established	Check serum electrolytes, Mg++, Ca++, glucose, treat if necessary. Coccidiostats and supportive therapy

TABLE 13.2   Uncommon or Additional Causes of Brain Signs—cont'd

Disease	Etiology	Clinical Signs	Differential Diagnoses	Diagnosis	Treatment
Neosporosis	*Neospora caninum*	Mostly abortion with early fetal infection but a few clinically affected calves will be born; most calves infected after 30 weeks' gestation are normal; both brain and spinal cord signs may exist	Cerebellar hypoplasia and other congenital anomalies	Necropsy and histopathology	No proven treatment
Sarcocystis infection	Ingestion of *Sarcocystis* spp. from carnivore feces in contaminated feeds	Poor growth, fever, "rat tail," weakness, GI signs; many possible neurologic signs depending on site and severity of lesion in CNS	Broad	Serology or histopathology	Prevent contamination of cattle feeds by carnivore feces
Pyrrolizidine alkaloid poisoning	Hepatic encephalopathy	Depression, head pressing, aggression, seizures, tenesmus, jaundice rarely detected	Encephalopathies Rabies	Elevated serum liver enzymes and blood ammonia values. Gross and microscopic pathology. Multiple animals affected	Supportive; usually fatal Removal or replacement of causative feedstuff
Portosystemic shunt; patent ductus venosus	Hepatic encephalopathy (See Video Clips 13.17 A and B)	2- to 3-month-old calf; poor growth; intermittent neurologic signs such as ataxia, weakness, depression; bruxism and tenesmus also noted	Encephalitis	Rare Elevated blood ammonia Normal liver enzymes	Surgical repair if valuable
Enterotoxemia	Epsilon toxin of *Clostridium perfringens* type D	Acute death or convulsions, mania, and coma in well-grown and well-fed calves	PEM Lead poisoning Rabies	Culture of organism or toxin assay on fresh postmortem gut specimen	Prevent by vaccination
Grass staggers	Rye grass, Dallisgrass (*Claviceps paspali*)	Mostly tremors, hypermetria, ataxia, and change in behavior	Other toxicities (e.g., organophosphates) Hypomagnesemia	History, detection of fungi on plants	Remove from suspect pastures, diazepam may calm excitable cattle
Cerebellar hypoplasia (See Video Clips 13.1–13.4)	BVDV infection of fetus during midtrimester of pregnancy	Strong but uncoordinated calf with intention head tremor; if standing, has wide-based stance and hypermetric gait. May have ocular or visual signs such as cataracts, retinal scarring, optic nerve lesions, microphthalmia	Other congenital cerebellar disease	Pre-colostral antibody or viral tests for BVDV; suggestive farm history of BVDV infection. Post mortem examination to show grossly small cerebellum	No treatment – some may actually adapt to ataxia and compensate
Cerebellar abiotrophy	Inherited in Holstein breed	Acute onset of cerebellar signs at 3 to 8 months of age; intention head tremor, wide-based stance, hypermetric, ataxia (see Fig. 13.34)	Brain abscess PEM	Acute onset of cerebellar signs that progress Cerebellum may be grossly normal size at necropsy but histopathology shows distinct loss of Purkinje cell layer	None

Continued

TABLE 13.2	Uncommon or Additional Causes of Brain Signs—cont'd				
Disease	**Etiology**	**Clinical Signs**	**Differential Diagnoses**	**Diagnosis**	**Treatment**
Blue-green algae toxicosis	Ponds contaminated with blue-green algae (microcystin toxin)	Multiple cattle with muscle tremors, ataxia, overresponse to stimuli, bloody diarrhea, profuse salivation	Other toxicities	Culture of blue-green algae from pond	Supportive Activated charcoal Copper sulfate to pond water (0.0001% concentration in pond water desired)
Hydrocephalus	Congenital lesion, can be due to in utero viral insult	Newborn calf with gross abnormality of skull or profound neurologic deficits		Consider pre-colostral blood for viral isolation and serology (BVDV, bluetongue, akabane)	None; congenital
Hydranencephaly	Viral insults in utero	Profound and diffuse neurologic deficits		Consider pre-colostral blood for viral isolation and serology (BVDV, bluetongue, akabane)	None; congenital
Encephalocele	Toxic insults in utero				
Hypomyelinogenesis (See Video Clip 13.5)	Inherited in Jersey breed	Neonatal calf; head and body tremors that worsen when the calf tries to move; spastic gait—possible cerebellar signs	Hereditary neuraxial edema (Herefords) BVDV infection	Precolostral blood for viral isolation and titers to rule out viral causes Histopathology	None; congenital

BVDV, Bovine viral diarrhea virus; *CNS, central nervous system; CSF,* cerebrospinal fluid; *GI,* gastrointestinal; *PEM,* polioencephalomalacia.

dog (dog-sitting posture). In all situations, the pelvic limb tone and spinal reflexes will vary from normal to hyperactive. Severe transverse lesions will cause complete paralysis and analgesia caudal to the lesion.

C6 to T2 lesions cause the same signs in the pelvic limbs as a T3 to L3 lesion, but LMN quality paresis will be seen in the thoracic limbs with difficulty supporting weight and short strides if the animal is ambulatory. Muscle tone and spinal reflexes will be diminished in the thoracic limbs, and normal to increased in the pelvic limbs.

C1 to C5 lesions cause the same signs in all four limbs that were described for the pelvic limbs with a T3 to L3 lesion. The longer strides seen in the thoracic limbs appear similar to an overreaching movement with the limb in extension, sometimes referred to as a "floating" movement.

Malformation

Malformations of the spinal cord are occasionally encountered in calves and are almost always confined to the thoracolumbar and sacrocaudal segments. In most of these myelodysplasias, the gray matter of the lumbosacral intumescence is normal or not depleted of neurons, and usually considerable voluntary movement can be generated. However, there may not be enough interaction of the long tracts (UMN-GP) and the ventral gray columns to permit the animal to stand. Most of

these calves exhibit some limb movement when supported in a standing position. A few can walk unaided. However, as is characteristic of nearly all myelodysplasias, the flexor responses to advance the limb or in response to a noxious stimulus in the recumbent calf occur simultaneously in both pelvic limbs. The common description of these simultaneous voluntary movements is "bunny hopping." Nociception is usually normal unless an aplasia has occurred. These are very consistent clinical signs regardless of the more specific nature of the myelodysplasia in most instances. In all cases, the clinical signs are present at birth and do not get progressively worse.

Severe myelodysplasias in which there is a failure of the lumbosacral intumescence to develop cause a dramatic pelvic limb deformity. Joint and muscle development are dependent on the muscle being innervated. If this does not occur, the muscle remains undeveloped, and the joints are abnormal in their development and position and cannot be moved. This joint fixation is often referred to as "contracture" or "arthrogryposis."

A common clinical finding in calves with myelodysplasia is the presence of a vertebral column malformation such as kyphosis, scoliosis, spina bifida, absence of one or more vertebra or their arches, and shortened or crooked caudal vertebrae in the tail. Simultaneous malformation of the spinal cord and vertebral column is common because of the close relationship of the development of the somitic sclerotomes and the neural tube. Both are influenced by the growth factors elaborated from the adjacent notochord.

Although a variety of myelodysplasias can affect the T3 to caudal spinal cord segments, the neurologic signs are usually the same. Examples include segmental hypoplasia of one or more segments;

1. syringomyelia, which often consists of numerous cavities but with no specific gray or white matter location; abnormal gray matter formation without apparent dorsal or ventral gray column differentiation;
2. diplomyelia, which is a duplication of the spinal cord all within one meningeal sheath; and
3. diastematomyelia, which is a duplication of the spinal cord with each spinal cord in its own meningeal sheath and in which the two spinal cords are usually separated by a bony partition.

The latter two conditions can both occur in the same calf at different levels of the spinal cord. Diplomyelia is the most common myelodysplasia seen in our experience (see Video Clips 13.22 to 13.24). Perosomus elumbis is a congenital disorder characterized by the lack of the lumbar, sacral and coccygeal spinal cord and the corresponding vertebrae. Most malformations are diagnosed at necropsy, although there is a recent report of ultrasonographic identification of syringomyelia and segmental hypoplasia of the lumbar spinal cord in a calf. This 4-day-old Holstein calf had clinical signs suggestive of LMN dysfunction of the hind limbs. By placing the calf in lateral recumbency and performing an ultrasound examination using a high-frequency probe and an acoustic window between the intervertebral junctions, lumbar hypoplasia and syringohydromyelia were observed at L4 to L5 and L3 to L4, respectively. Additionally, segmental (lumbar) spinal cord hypoplasia was diagnosed in an 8-day-old Holstein calf by myelography and MRI. The calf had exhibited signs of spastic paresis in its hind limbs since birth.

Segmental aplasia is uncommon. One Simmental calf was presented recumbent with remarkable rigidity of the pelvic limbs. Neurologic function was normal in the head, neck, and thoracic limbs. Pelvic limbs were held in rigid extension, but any stimulus caused a rapid simultaneous flexion of both limbs. Nociception was absent caudal to the midlumbar level. When supported by the tail, any contact of the hooves with the floor elicited flexion movements at the hips and a short limb advancement. Forceps stimulation of the tail, anus, or pelvic limbs elicited the same response. The cranial lumbar region was depressed where no vertebral spines could be palpated.

At necropsy there was no spinal cord (segmental aplasia) from the T13 segment through the L3 segment and no vertebral arches over T13 through L2. All the pelvic limb "hopping movements" represented the uninhibited activity of the lumbosacral intumescence and would classify as an example of spinal reflex walking. This case exemplifies the major role of the UMNs in the inhibition of motor neuron activity, especially that of extensor motor neurons to the antigravity muscles. Alternate limb movements are dependent on a subset of commissural interneurons within the intumescences. Because the lack of these alternate movements is so common in these myelodysplasias, a lack, or abnormality of,

development of these commissural interneurons may be the basis for this unique but consistent clinical sign.

In contrast to the above description, a severe myelodysplasia with diplomyelia and large syrinx formation in the lumbosacral segments was observed in a 2-year-old Holstein bull with just a very slight ataxic gait and no loss of alternate limb movements. Observations like this tend to keep the clinician humble!

Inflammation

Myelitis is uncommon in cattle as a primary lesion. Occasionally, a vertebral epidural abscess will invade the meninges, causing a suppurative leptomeningitis and myelitis. Newborn calves infected in utero with *Neospora caninum* may rarely be born alive with a diffuse myelitis caused by this protozoal agent.

Abscesses
Etiology

Although most common in calves, epidural abscesses also occasionally occur in adult cattle. These abscesses may originate either within vertebrae as areas of osteomyelitis or adjacent to the vertebrae in the epidural space. Calves with acute or chronic septicemia secondary to umbilical infections are at risk for vertebral abscesses. These same calves may have polyarthritis, meningitis, uveitis, pneumonia, or other sites of infection as well. Pneumonia and coughing may predispose to the bacteremic organism localizing in the vertebral vessels because there are significant pressure changes and bidirectional flow of blood in those blood vessels associated with the coughing. Adult cattle with vertebral abscesses generally have suffered septicemic spread of bacterial organisms from areas of acute or chronic infection such as lung abscesses. *Trueperella pyogenes* remains the most common organism isolated from vertebral abscesses, but other organisms, such as *Pasteurella* sp., *Fusobacterium necrophorum*, *Streptococcus* spp., *Pseudomonas aeruginosa*, and strain 19 *Brucella abortus*, have also been isolated. Although bacteria reach the vertebrae or epidural location through embolic spread (endogenous) in most cases, we have observed several cows that developed exogenous origin abscesses from external trauma to the lumbosacral region and subsequent large subcutaneous abscesses. Cauda equina neuritis and abscessation can occur from tail docking, and clostridial organisms are often the infective agent. This problem had become more common since the first edition of this book because of the widespread practice of tail docking dairy cattle but that has now thankfully declined in popularity. A similar condition of cauda equina neuritis with soft tissue infection and ascending myelitis can also occur as an occasional complication of repeated epidural anesthesia with poor-quality aseptic technique. Genetically valuable dairy cattle may currently undergo a frequency of epidural administration that exceeds what was previously performed, particularly for in vitro fertilization procedures, emphasizing the need for careful attention to cleanliness, equipment usage, and technique, lest a valuable animal be rendered incontinent or develop hind limb paresis.

Clinical Signs

Fever, a painful stance, and stiff gait constitute the initial signs observed in cattle with epidural/vertebral abscesses. Fever may be low grade and does not occur in all cases but is very helpful to the diagnosis when present. When cervical vertebrae are involved, the discomfort causes the animal to have a "weather vane" neck, resist attempts at neck movement or flexion, and tend to hold the head and neck extended or in unusual positions (Figs. 13.35 and 13.36). If the abscess is in the caudal cervical or cranial thoracic vertebrae, the animal may refuse to lower its head and eat from the ground. When thoracic or lumbar vertebrae are involved, the animal assumes an arched stance. A more remarkable arched stance and contracted flexor tendons may be present if polyarthritis coexists or if prolonged recumbency has occurred. Palpation of the vertebrae may cause a painful response when pressure is exerted over the affected bone. Neurologic signs consistent with spinal cord disease are present as the vertebral or epidural abscess progressively exerts pressure on the spinal cord. Paresis, ataxia, and paralysis occur as the lesions progressively damage the spinal cord. Occasionally, the infection invades the meninges and spinal cord, causing a focal meningitis and

myelitis. Paraparesis and "dog sitting" would be expected with severe thoracolumbar lesions (Fig. 13.37) and tetraparesis and ataxia with cervical abscesses. Abscesses located in the lumbosacral region, which seems to be quite a common location in calves, or the sacrum, may cause difficulty in urination, defecation, tail paresis, and progressive sciatic nerve dysfunction that usually is bilateral. Therefore a neurologic examination is essential to identify the neuroanatomic location of the lesion. Peracute spinal cord signs may occur associated with a fracture of the infected vertebral body (see Video Clip 13.25). Cauda equina neuritis following tail docking often results in a rapidly progressive ascending disease. Initially, tail, anal, and bladder function become hypotonic, but there can be rapid progression to pelvic limb LMN paresis and recumbency in addition to marked swelling of the gluteal area.

Radiography is the most definitive means of confirming a diagnosis of vertebral abscessation (Figs. 13.38 and 13.39). Radiographic studies are more easily accomplished in calves than adult cattle because of their smaller size. CSF may be normal or have slight elevation in protein values unless the abscess has extended into the subarachnoid space, resulting in both increased numbers of WBCs (neutrophils and macrophages) and more markedly elevated protein values. A case series of five vertebral body abscesses reported that only one of the five had abnormal CSF values, but another more recent report found six of six vertebral body or spinal abscess patients had grossly elevated nucleated cell (macrophage and neutrophil) counts and protein values.

Epidural and vertebral body abscesses must be differentiated from congenital vertebral malformations, degenerative vertebral conditions, white muscle disease, spinal cord trauma, tumors, and vertebral fractures. Radiography, CSF analysis, serum biochemistry to assess creatinine kinase and aspartate aminotransferase, and blood selenium values provide ancillary data when necessary. Adult cattle with abscesses frequently have elevated serum globulin levels that support the diagnosis, but calves with this disease may not. Rectal examination only rarely identifies the site of the lesion when the abscess has created detectable swelling ventral to an affected caudal vertebral body. This is most

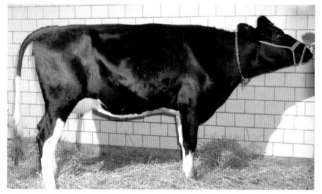

• **Fig. 13.35** Cervical vertebral abscess that was in the vertebral body of C4. Note the anxious expression and the stiff "weather vane" neck.

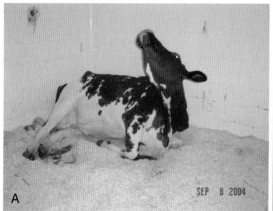

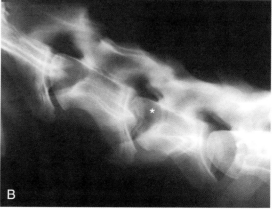

• **Fig. 13.36** **A,** A 5-year-old Red and White Holstein cow with fever of 2 weeks' duration. Increased respiratory rate was observed alongside a tendency to hold the head and neck in an unusual position. **B,** Cervical radiographs were suggestive of subchondral bone lysis and irregular cranial epiphyseal margin at C4 *. Surgical removal of the diseased bone was successful, and *Trueperella pyogenes* was cultured from the blood.

likely to be helpful if the neurologic examination suggests a lumbosacral lesion.

Clinical signs coupled with radiographic or more advanced imaging studies alongside CSF analysis remain the most reliable diagnostic tools.

Treatment

The causative organism is usually unknown unless a culture from a suspected primary focus of infection, blood culture, or other secondary area of infection has been obtained. *T. pyogenes* is in the authors' experience the most commonly isolated organism. Surgical decompression, drainage of the abscess, and curettage of infected bone followed by antimicrobial therapy have been successfully performed in a small number of cattle after identification of the lesion by radiography or advanced imaging. Appropriate antibiotics and analgesics constitute the main therapy for vertebral abscesses. Penicillin, tetracycline, and cephalosporins have been used. Tetracycline (8-11 mg/kg twice daily) is a good choice because this antibiotic maintains good penetration in bony tissues. Treatment needs to be long term (minimum of 2 to 4 weeks) and should be directed by cultures when possible. If tetracycline is used long term attention should be paid to renal function. Analgesics such as flunixin meglumine or other NSAIDs at standard dosages encourage patient mobility and appetite. Recently, surgical curettage of a cervical abscess was successful (see Fig. 13.36). Clinical signs of improvement include resolution of fever, improved appetite, and increased range of mobility (cervical lesions) or lessening of the arched stance (thoracolumbar lesions).

The prognosis is poor, but cattle without detectable septicemia, severe spinal cord signs, or other sites of infection have the best chance for recovery. Acute lesions obviously carry a better prognosis than chronic ones.

Parasitic Causes

Etiology

Several parasitic diseases may cause spinal cord compression or inflammation in cattle, but all are rare except for sporadic cases of *Parelaphostrongylus tenuis*. *P. tenuis* is a common, predominately nonpathogenic, nematode parasite of white-tailed deer *(Odocoileus virginianus)* with a complex life cycle involving intermediate terrestrial gastropod hosts. Naturally occurring aberrant migration of *P. tenuis* causes neurologic disease in various mammals, including young cattle. Affected calves develop clinical signs of *Parelaphostrongylus* spp. infection because of the ingestion of large numbers of infective larvae that are deposited by snails around cattle feeding areas. After ingestion, the larvae migrate to the spinal cord and cause disease. The inflammatory reaction to the parasite is mostly eosinophilic and lymphocytic.

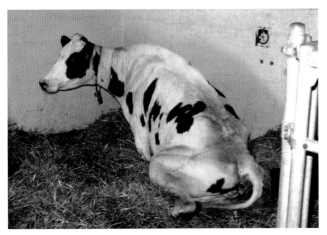

• **Fig. 13.37** Vertebral body abscess of T12 in an adult Holstein cow causing severe pelvic limb paresis and a dog-sitting position.

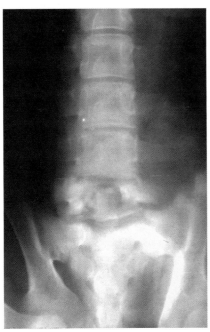

• **Fig. 13.38** Radiograph of a calf with L6 vertebral body abscess. The calf had no tail tone, dribbled urine, and was paretic in the pelvic limbs.

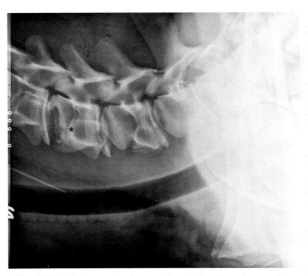

• **Fig. 13.39** Radiograph of a yearling bull with osteomyelitis and abscessation of the cranial aspect of the vertebral body of C5.* Note additional soft tissue gas shadowing dorsal to the spinous processes of C5 and C6.

Clinical Signs

The clinical signs of *P. tenuis* are mostly ataxia and paresis of the hind limbs, although in some cases the front limbs can also be involved. Neurologic examination reveals signs consistent with UMN spinal cord disease in most cases. Signs of LMN disease (hyporeflexia of the limbs, loss of tail tone, and dribbling urine) can be seen in approximately 50% of cases. The CSF analysis shows marked pleocytosis and increased total protein in all calves in whom analysis has been performed. More acute cases show an eosinophilic (>20% eosinophils) pleocytosis, but chronic cases have a lymphocytic (>70% lymphocytes) pleocytosis with a lower percentage of eosinophils. *Hypoderma bovis* may very rarely cause posterior paresis in a cow associated with death of the larvae near the dural membrane and the accompanying inflammatory reaction.

Treatment

Calves can be successfully treated for *P. tenuis* parasite migration with ivermectin (0.2 mg/kg SC for 5 days), fenbendazole (10 mg/kg orally for 5 days), and dexamethasone (0.05 mg/kg). Management changes should also be implemented on the farm to decrease deer, snail, and slug exposure.

Compressive Neoplasms

Etiology

Extradural compression of the spinal cord by neoplasia is one cause of focal or multifocal spinal cord injury that may result in spinal cord signs in the pelvic limbs or all four limbs. Lymphosarcoma is the most common neoplasm identified, but nerve sheath neoplasms occasionally cause similar spinal cord compression. Lymphosarcoma is usually located in the epidural space and may occur at any level of the vertebral canal, although involvement of the lumbosacrocaudal spinal cord and spinal nerves seems most common. Lymphosarcoma lesions usually, but not always, can be identified in other target organs in cattle affected with spinal cord compressive lymphosarcoma, especially at post mortem, although it is common for cattle with spinal lymphosarcoma to have paresis as their major presenting clinical sign.

Clinical Signs

Progressive spinal cord signs in a cow that is bright, alert, responsive, and eating are the major clinical signs of extradural tumor compression of the spinal cord. The history may be acute, subacute (5–14 days), or chronic (>2 weeks) and indicate progression from mild paresis and ataxia to recumbency. Signs usually are bilaterally symmetric. Neurologic examination frequently allows neuroanatomic localization of the mass or masses (see introductory description of spinal cord signs). Lesions from T3 to L3 cause spastic paresis and ataxia in the

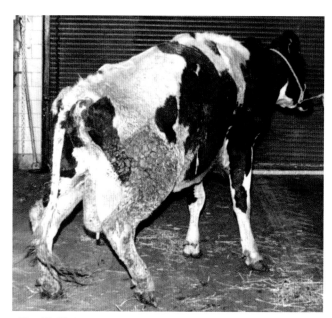

• **Fig. 13.40** Pelvic limb ataxia and paresis in a cow with thoracolumbar spinal cord compression caused by lymphosarcoma.

pelvic limbs because of white matter compression (Fig. 13.40 and Video Clip 13.26). These patients tend to "dog sit" with the forelimbs bearing weight as observed in distal lumbar and sacral lesions (Fig. 13.41). Pelvic limb reflexes and tone are judged normal or exaggerated.

Lesions from C6 to T2 lead to greater paresis in the forelimbs, and the forelimbs may lose tone and reflexes but the pelvic limbs remain normal or exaggerated as regards reflexes. We have seen a Holstein cow with subacute to chronic bloat and bilateral forelimb weakness and muscle atrophy that was progressive due to massive neurofibromatosis of the brachial plexus, heart, and other spinal nerves. A large neoplastic lesion in the thoracic inlet interfered with effective eructation. Lesions from C1 to C5 will cause spastic paresis and ataxia in all four limbs. Rarely, lymphosarcoma may occur diffusely in the subarachnoid space.

As mentioned, the history may indicate great variation in the duration of clinical signs. Owners often notice the cow developing progressive weakness or difficulty in rising; she may require manual assistance to rise for some time before recumbency. Overt ataxia and paresis usually ensue within days or weeks (Figs. 13.42 and 13.43). Treatment with corticosteroids by the owner or veterinarian may temporarily alleviate the signs, but the effect is short lived, and obvious paresis returns within days of discontinuing corticosteroids. Cattle with compressive neoplasms affecting the spinal cord that have acute histories must be differentiated from cattle with injuries from bulling or riding activities, metabolic diseases such as hypocalcemia, *Hypoderma* larvae migration, and chute or stall divider injuries. Those with subacute or chronic histories must be differentiated from patients with vertebral or epidural abscesses, ascending meningitis from tail injuries or epidural injections, rabies, musculoskeletal injuries, and other conditions.

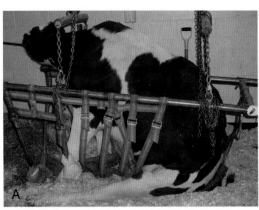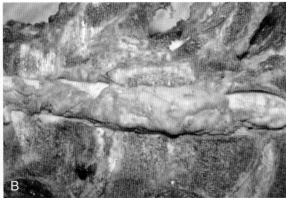

• **Fig. 13.41** **A,** Dog-sitting posture in 4-year-old Holstein with lymphosarcoma in a caudal lumbar location. Exfoliated neoplastic cells were obtained by lumbosacral spinal tap. **B,** Extradural lymphosarcoma identified at post mortem in the caudal lumbar spine from cow in *A.*

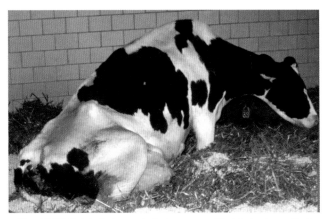

• **Fig. 13.42** Pelvic limb paralysis in a cow still able to rise with the thoracic limbs but affected with compressive lymphosarcoma subsequently identified in the lumbar and sacral epidural region.

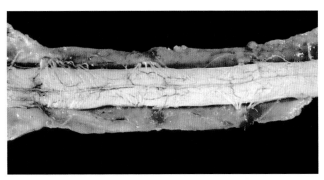

• **Fig. 13.43** Cranial lumbar spinal cord from the cow in Fig. 13.42 showing lymphosarcoma infiltrates in the meninges surrounding the cord.

Diagnosis

Physical examination must be thorough both to rule out other causes of paresis and to seek out other evidence of neoplasia in the patient. Limbs and joints must be manipulated to rule out musculoskeletal causes of paresis or recumbency. Peripheral nerve injuries must be assessed and their status as either a primary problem or a secondary consequence of recumbency determined. Peripheral and abdominal lymph nodes palpable per rectum should be assessed for enlargement

consistent with lymphosarcoma. Cardiac arrhythmias occasionally are present if the heart is affected with either lymphosarcoma or neurofibromatosis lesions. Muffling of heart sounds caused by myocardial, epicardial, or pericardial lymphosarcoma masses also may occur. Melena may indicate abomasal infiltration with subsequent ulceration. Palpation of the uterus may reveal masses consistent with lymphosarcoma, and unilateral or bilateral exophthalmus may indicate retrobulbar infiltration with this neoplasm.

Because cattle affected with extradural neoplasms usually are bright and appetent, many diseases that include anorexia as a prominent sign can be ruled down. If no other target organ infiltration is identified during the physical examination, ancillary data will be helpful. CSF should be evaluated. In one review of 14 cattle with spinal cord compression caused by neoplasia, 10 cattle had CSF evaluations. Elevated protein levels (>40 mg/dL) were found in 5 of 10, but only 1 of 10 had elevated nucleated cell counts. If pleocytosis occurs, macrocytic and neutrophilic responses would be expected because of chronicity of the disease. In another study involving cattle with lymphosarcoma, CSF values were abnormal in three of four patients. Therefore, as with epidural abscesses, the CSF may not be specifically diagnostic but tends to rule out some other diseases. On several occasions, we have attempted lumbosacral puncture to obtain CSF from recumbent cattle suspected to have extradural lymphosarcoma only to be unable to obtain any fluid after feeling the characteristic "pop" associated with needle entrance into the lumbosacral subarachnoid space. On these occasions, aspiration with a syringe attached to the spinal needle allowed neoplastic cells to be recovered that were made into smears on microscopic slides, stained, and used to confirm a diagnosis of lymphosarcoma.

Serum globulin values are usually normal in cattle affected with tumors, as opposed to cattle with epidural or vertebral abscesses in which serum globulin may be elevated. Similarly, systemic fever and neutrophilia in the peripheral blood usually are absent in patients with tumors. Metabolic diseases may be ruled out by serum evaluation of major organ function, as well as magnesium, calcium, and potassium values.

Rectal examination helps to rule out recent sacral or caudal injury and allows the reproductive tract to be examined to determine whether the cow is in heat or just past heat; this is useful primarily in cases of acute pelvic limb paresis in which bulling injuries from being ridden by other cows must be ruled out. The iliac lymph nodes should be carefully palpated because these are frequently enlarged if the lymphosarcoma involves the caudal spinal cord.

A CBC will very rarely confirm a diagnosis of lymphosarcoma but may raise the index of suspicion if lymphocytosis is present. Similarly, assessment of the patient's serum for antibodies against BLV or identification of BLV infection by PCR does not confirm the diagnosis (because many cows are infected but never do develop clinical tumors), but proof of infection raises the index of suspicion. Most cattle with lymphosarcoma masses causing extradural compression will test positive for BLV unless they have the juvenile form of lymphosarcoma, as did a single 5-month-old calf in one of the retrospective case series. Calves with the juvenile, thymic, or skin form usually test negative for BLV antibodies or proviral DNA.

Treatment

No effective treatment exists for the great majority of these patients, and necropsy frequently reveals multifocal masses in the epidural region of the vertebral canal. Symptomatic improvement that is temporary and short lived has been observed in some cattle treated with dexamethasone or other corticosteroids. This treatment is usually reserved for nonpregnant cattle and when the owner has a short-term goal such as embryo transfer from an extremely valuable patient. We have used isofluprednone acetate in late-pregnant cows to improve the clinical signs long enough to allow delivery of the calf. However, the calf may be infected with BLV. L-asparaginase has also been used successfully as short-term therapy but is expensive.

Injury

Spinal cord injury can be external in origin from trauma or internal from compressive lesions such as a tumor or abscess causing a compressive myelopathy, as just described.

Traumatic (External) Injury: Vertebral Fractures

Etiology

Trauma is the most common cause of vertebral fractures in adult cattle. Nutritional factors must be considered in calves and growing heifers when vertebral fractures or multiple instances of long bone and vertebral fractures occur within a group of calves. Riding injuries either caused by a great weight discrepancy between mounted and mounting cows or the mounted cow slipping on a slippery surface may predispose to thoracolumbar vertebral fractures. Cattle traumatized by automatic chutes or that fall while caught in chutes or even stanchions may fracture cervical vertebrae. The latter is more likely if the head is restrained in the chute or stanchion when the animal falls. Cattle trapped under divider bars in tie stalls or free stall barns may struggle excessively and fracture

the thoracolumbar vertebrae. Mature bulls with ankylosing spondylosis eventually may fracture a vertebral body if forced to mount despite showing early signs of spondylosis.

Vertebral fractures or displacements of the sacral and caudal vertebrae are usually a result of cows being mounted during normal estrus activity or being repeatedly ridden because of cystic ovaries. Dystocia also may be a cause of sacral and caudal vertebral injury or fracture. Self-induced trauma from being caught under pipe partitions also may injure the sacral-caudal vertebrae. We have even observed this as a "herd problem" on dairies where new free-stall construction has occurred with remarkable ignorance regarding stall dimensions and design. Malicious or sadistic handlers often fracture caudal vertebrae by excessive force applied to the tail during tail restraint. Excessive traction, especially rotational traction, during dystocias can fracture the thoracolumbar vertebrae of a newborn calf.

Calves or heifers with metabolic bone disease such as vitamin D deficiency or calcium-deficient diets may experience vertebral compression fractures. With nutritional causes, frequently more than one animal in the group will suffer either long bone or vertebral fractures within a period of a few weeks to a month. A nutritional secondary hyperparathyroidism occurs in calves or heifers fed a diet extremely low in calcium, such as poor-quality or aged grass hay, Sudan grass, or high-phosphorus, low-calcium diets (Fig. 13.44). As mentioned earlier, cattle with vertebral body abscesses may develop acute spinal cord signs if the diseased bone acutely fractures.

Clinical Signs

Clinical signs are sudden in onset and not obviously progressive unless the patient struggles excessively or is handled too vigorously (i.e., a nondisplaced fracture becomes displaced). The clinical signs will reflect the fracture site and the neuroanatomic diagnosis (see introductory section on spinal cord signs) (see Video Clip 13.27). Cattle with cervical fractures may lie in lateral recumbency, have an anxious expression, and be unable to right themselves into sternal recumbency. Physical examination may raise suspicion of the fracture location based on observation and palpation of dorsoventral or lateral deviation of the vertebral spines. This is most helpful in calves and heifers but more difficult in heavily muscled or fat

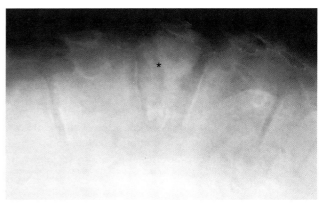

• **Fig. 13.44** Compression fracture of L1 * in an 8-month-old Holstein calf that had been fed a calcium-deficient diet. Several other calves in the group sustained long bone or vertebral fractures over a period of 4 weeks.

adult animals. In severe cases, nociception and the cutaneous trunci reflex may be reduced caudal to the site of the fracture, and these are easily performed tests during the neurologic examination. A cow with even severe thoracolumbar spinal cord injury seldom demonstrates the Schiff-Sherrington syndrome with thoracic limb extension and hypertonia coupled with paraplegia and hypotonia in the pelvic limbs.

Cattle with acute sacrocaudal or caudal vertebral fractures usually have obvious swelling at the site, demonstrate extreme pain when the affected area is palpated or the tail moved, and show a crushed tail head if the injury was caused by being mounted. Affected cattle may have reduced tail mobility and varying degrees of perineal anesthesia. Cattle having sacral fractures may show evidence of sciatic nerve dysfunction, as well as bladder atony; tail paresis; hypalgesia or analgesia of the anus, perineum, or vulva; and an atonic anus allowing pneumorectum (Figs. 13.45 and 13.46).

The acute onset and nonprogressive course helps differentiate fractures from vertebral abscesses and neoplasms, both of which tend to have a progressive course that begins as paresis but progresses to paralysis.

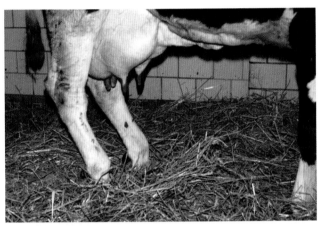

• **Fig. 13.45** Sacrocaudal injury with crushed tail head and associated bilateral overflexed hocks, fetlock dorsal buckling, and weakness in the hind limbs caused by injury of the spinal nerve roots that contribute to the tibial nerves. The cow was in heat on the day the injury occurred.

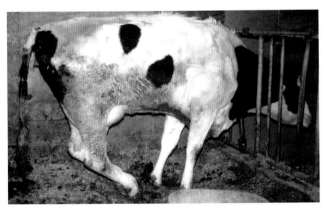

• **Fig. 13.46** Sacrocaudal spinal injury with partial sciatic (tibial) nerve paralysis in a first-calf Holstein heifer that had forced extraction of a large calf 1 month earlier. Initially, the heifer could not stand with her pelvic limbs. Now, with assistance, she can support weight. Tail and bladder paralysis also are present. The sacrocaudal vertebrae are elevated dorsally from the lumbosacral junction caudally.

Pain is a pronounced feature of most vertebral fractures, and cattle with fractures may show anorexia and increased heart and respiratory rates. Certainly, patients with vertebral or epidural abscesses also show pain, but cattle with compressive neoplasms usually do not.

Diagnosis

The history, neurologic examination, and radiography are key components for diagnosing vertebral fractures. The CSF usually is normal unless spinal cord injury from a displaced fracture is severe enough to cause bleeding, in which case the CSF may be xanthochromic and have increased numbers of red blood cells and protein. Radiographs, if available, are diagnostic. Special equipment may be necessary to perform diagnostic radiography of adult animals, but calves and younger cattle may be radiographed easily. Particular attention should be directed to bone density if nutritional causes are considered in young cattle or bony proliferation is observed with spondylitis in older cattle (see Fig. 10.26).

Treatment

Treatment is symptomatic and may include corticosteroids (dexamethasone; 0.10 mg/kg body weight) and supportive care. The use of large doses of corticosteroids is no longer considered to be efficacious and should not be used in pregnant cows or cattle thought to be at high risk of infection. Neck braces may be indicated for nondisplaced cervical fractures. The prognosis is guarded to poor for all cattle with vertebral fractures, but younger animals with nondisplaced fractures have the best chance of recovery. Extremely valuable calves may be candidates for referral to orthopedic specialists. It may also be possible to surgically repair crushed tail heads associated with sacral and caudal vertebral injuries or displacements. If orthopedic repair is performed promptly, neurologic deficits may be minimized and cosmetic appearance improved.

Assessment and correction of dietary inadequacies must be performed whenever multiple animals are involved.

Vertebral Malformation

Vertebral malformations without a spinal cord malformation are uncommon. They usually involve thoracic vertebrae and slowly compress the spinal cord secondary to a progressive kyphosis that develops at the site of the malformation as the calf grows. Progressive T3 to L3 signs occur at a few months of age (see Video Clips 13.28 and 13.29). Diagnosis can be made by observation and palpation of the kyphosis and radiographs (Figs. 13.47 to 13.49). Surgical repair has not been attempted.

Degeneration

Degenerative Myeloencephalopathy of Brown Swiss Cattle (Weaver Syndrome)
Etiology

Degenerative myeloencephalopathy is an inherited disorder in Brown Swiss cattle that causes progressive neurologic signs. It is commonly called Weaver syndrome because of the layperson's impression of a weaving gait that some affected animals show.

Clinical Signs

The disease causes bilateral pelvic limb paresis and ataxia that appear in affected animals at 6 to 18 months of age and slowly progress to total loss of hind limb control by 3 to 4 years of age. Clinical signs most commonly become apparent at 5 to 8 months and continue to worsen until the animals become unable to rise, usually between 18 and 36 months of age. The earliest signs reflect a T3 to L3 spinal cord lesion with UMN/GP signs of spastic paraparesis and ataxia. As the degeneration progresses, thoracic limbs will be similarly affected, and these cattle will fall if turned quickly or if they attempt to run. There are no signs of brain involvement.

Diagnosis

The progression of neurologic signs with no evidence of associated discomfort tends to rule out trauma or vertebral fracture. Vertebral or epidural abscesses would likewise cause pain and perhaps fever and might lead to evidence of chronic inflammation (e.g., neutrophilia, monocytosis) in the hemogram or an elevated serum globulin. In contrast, animals with Weaver syndrome are not expected to have an abnormal hemogram or increased globulin values. In addition, the CSF should be normal in cattle with Weaver syndrome, but it may or may not be in cattle with an abscess. Spinal cord compression from neoplasia such as lymphosarcoma also may be a differential for cattle with Weaver syndrome, but neoplasms generally progress quickly to cause recumbency; those with Weaver syndrome are more slowly progressive.

Ruling out other diseases and spinal cord histopathology are the only means to confirm a diagnosis. Histopathology of the spinal cord from cattle with Weaver syndrome has shown a primary axonal degeneration and secondary demyelination. Lesions appear more severe in the thoracic region.

Weaver syndrome is a progressive neurologic disease thought to be due to an inherited recessive trait, and bulls that may carry this trait have been identified and a diagnostic test based on microsatellite markers is commercially available.

Motor Neuron Disease

A congenital motor neuron disease occurs in Brown Swiss calves that is heritable and associated with an autosomal recessive gene. It is also often referred to as bovine spinal muscular atrophy. Affected homozygote calves exhibit a progressive neuromuscular disorder at birth or within the first few weeks of life. When ambulatory, their gait is very short strided, and they fatigue rapidly and collapse. They progress over a short period to recumbency with loss of muscle tone and reflexes and develop severe muscle atrophy. At necropsy, the spinal cord ventral gray columns contain neuronal cell bodies in various stages of degeneration or glial scars where neurons have been lost. Secondary Wallerian degeneration occurs in the intramedullary axons and throughout their distribution in the peripheral nerves. Both North American and European bulls have been identified as carriers.

A similar syndrome of progressive weakness beginning at approximately 2 weeks of age and progressing to tetraparesis by just a few months of age has been described in Holstein-Friesian calves and is referred to in the literature as spinal muscular atrophy.

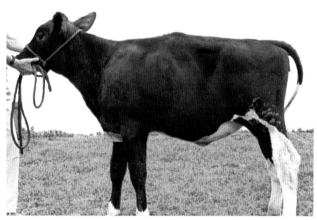

• **Fig. 13.47** Vertebral malformation causing a kyphosis visible as a focal arch in the topline of an 8-month-old Holstein heifer. Although the vertebral malformation was present since birth, overt signs of ataxia and paresis did not become obvious to the owner until the heifer was 6 months old and the kyphosis was first appreciated.

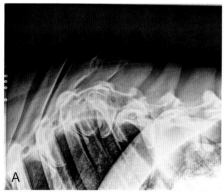
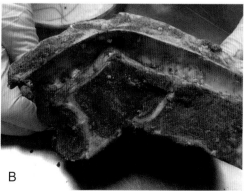

• **Fig. 13.48** Radiographs (**A**) and postmortem specimen (**B**) from 2-year-old Holstein heifer with vertebral malformation of T9 and T10 associated with kyphosis and paraparesis. (Also Video Clip 13.28).

Delayed Organophosphate Toxicity

Cattle that have consumed some forms of organophosphate may develop a diffuse primary axonopathy of the spinal cord and exhibit a slowly progressive UMN/GP gait abnormality. This will begin with a spastic paresis and ataxia in the pelvic limbs which progresses to involve the thoracic limbs. The most commonly incriminated form of organophosphate is one of the many triorthocresyl phosphates, which are often a component of machinery lubricants. There is usually a delay of a few weeks between the period of consumption and neurologic signs. The toxicity affects the ability of neurons to maintain their axons, which results in a dying-back axonopathy. This pathologic pattern is observed in spinal cord funiculi at necropsy.

Postanesthetic Poliomyelomalacia

A rare spinal cord ischemic disorder has been observed in a calf that was anesthetized for surgery to evacuate the contents of the abomasum. Postsurgically, this calf was unable to stand in the pelvic limbs and exhibited a mixture of LMN signs with some loss of nociception along with UMN/GP signs that were asymmetric. After 2 weeks, there was no change in the neurologic signs. At necropsy, there was a severe asymmetric ischemic degeneration in the lumbosacral segments centered in the ventral gray column with varying degrees of extension into the adjacent dorsal gray column and white matter (Fig. 13.50). This lesion is similar to what has been described in horses that have been anesthetized for various surgical procedures that require a period of dorsal recumbency. It is hypothesized that during surgery, altered organ position compresses the blood supply in those lumbar spinal arteries that would normally be responsible for perfusion of the areas of ischemic spinal cord.

Functional Disorders

Spastic Paresis

Spastic paresis is a progressive, presumed spinal cord disorder, that causes overextension of the pelvic limbs secondary to severe contraction of the gastrocnemius muscles. One or both pelvic limbs can be involved, and affected cattle have very straight pelvic limbs with overextension of the hock. In Holstein calves, spastic paresis has also been called Elso heel because the condition tends to appear in animals whose genealogy dates back to a Friesian bull in Europe called Elso II. An overactive stretch reflex has been proposed by De Vlamynck to be responsible for the clinical signs of spastic paresis. Although this disorder is called spastic paresis in the veterinary literature, it is a misnomer as paresis is not a component of the disorder.

Calves usually begin showing signs between 2 and 10 months of age. Affected calves have extremely straight pelvic limbs and a stiff gait. When forced to stand, the affected limb (or limbs) is often held extended caudally with only the tips of the claws contacting the ground (Fig. 13.51). The gait is awkward and stiff because of the difficulty advancing the limb. In the early stages, the limb may relax or intermittently relax after the gastrocnemius contraction that occurs once the calf rises (see Video Clip 13.30). The calf may also raise its head and neck dorsally while simultaneously showing overextension of the limb. In some calves, the back is arched, and the tail head elevated. Because of the progressive nature of the problem, the calf will be in extreme discomfort if both pelvic limbs are affected because of the excessive prolonged gastrocnemius contraction and "cramping." The calf will prefer lying down to standing and will eventually lose weight. When the calf is lying down, the affected limb can be readily flexed. Palpation of the gastrocnemius muscle in the standing calf confirms a tense contracted muscle in the affected limb. Epidural

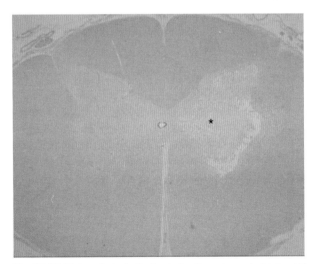

• **Fig. 13.50** Histopathologic finding in the thoracic cord of a 3-week-old calf that had ischemic myelopathy after anesthesia for surgical drainage of the abomasum because of severe abomasitis. The entire gray matter * on one side of the cord was degenerate with complete necrosis at the periphery, which included the adjacent white matter. All of the parenchyma was replaced with lipid-filled macrophages.

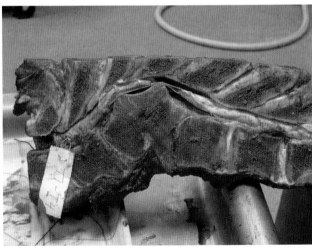

• **Fig. 13.49** Cranial thoracic spine from an 8-month-old Holstein bull with malformation of T1 to T4 with marked cord compression at this location but remarkably mild clinical signs of paraparesis. (Also Video Clip 13.29).

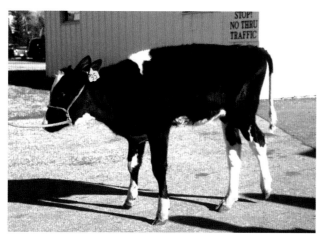

• **Fig. 13.51** A Holstein calf with spastic paresis. Notice that although the calf is standing still, she keeps the left pelvic limb extended caudally, only touching the hooves to the ground.

injection with local anesthetic has been reported to temporarily resolve the clinical signs, but we have no experience with this as a diagnostic test. The condition occurs in many beef and dairy herds, but Holsteins and Guernseys are the most commonly affected of the dairy breeds. Abnormalities of muscle groups other than the gastrocnemius may be implicated in an atypical form of spastic paresis. In these calves, there may be a bilateral swaying gait with cranial, lateral, and caudal movement of the limb while the hock remains fully extended.

A similar syndrome that occurs in adult cattle, especially confined bulls at sire centers or older cows that are kept in box stalls, has been called spastic syndrome or "crampiness," with the first signs appearing between 2 and 6 years of age (see Figs. 10.23 and 10.24). Holsteins and Guernseys are the most frequently affected dairy breeds. Preexisting "post leggedness" (straight pelvic limbs) may be observed as a conformational defect in most animals before the onset of signs. Signs in adult animals are slowly progressive over a period of years. Initially, affected cattle show crampiness as they attempt to rise and subsequently extend the affected pelvic limb caudal to their bodies. In confined cattle, this results in the animal standing off the curb or placing the hooves in the manure drop. The pelvis is lowered, and the head and neck may be raised. Within minutes, the muscles relax, and the animal may assume a more normal stance except for the conformationally straight pelvic limbs. As the condition progresses, the affected cattle become more consistently and more severely spastic when they attempt to rise, and after rising may extend their pelvic limbs caudally and shake them as if attempting to relieve the gastrocnemius muscle contraction. The same caudal pelvic limb extension and shaking may occur intermittently in the standing animal. If severely affected cattle are confined without exercise for several days, they may experience such severe muscle cramping as to be unable to rise.

No microscopic lesions have been observed in the spinal cord or peripheral nerves that are involved in the innervation of the caudal crural muscles of affected calves or adults with this disorder. In calves, experimental studies have determined that the clinical signs are caused by uninhibited ventral gray column gamma neuron activity. The cause of the hyperactivity within gamma neurons is unknown and presumed to be at a neurochemical or membrane channel level.

Diagnosis is based on the physical signs and palpation of the affected gastrocnemius muscles. A tibial nerve block may improve hock flexion and the gait.

Treatment of calves with spastic paresis is popular in Europe, where the animals may be raised only for meat production. Treatment involving tenotomy of the gastrocnemius tendon or gastrocnemius tendon plus a portion of the superficial digital flexor tendon has yielded improvement in most but not all cases. Neurectomy of branches of the tibial nerve supplying the gastrocnemius muscle has also been successful. In the United States, at least in dairy cattle, the probable heritability of the condition makes it unwise to treat affected calves, and slaughter should be recommended. Surgical procedures on either the gastrocnemius tendon or tibial nerve would not be effective for atypical spastic paresis animals.

Treatment of adult cows and bulls with spastic syndrome is generally not practiced except for occasional suggestions for the use of muscle relaxants or analgesics such as flunixin to help make an individual cow or bull more comfortable. Unfortunately, this is a commonly observed condition in bull studs, and affected bulls have been used extensively for artificial insemination, thereby possibly propagating the condition within the affected breeds.

See Table 13.3 for a list of uncommon causes of spinal cord disease.

Peripheral Nerves

Injury

Peripheral nerve injuries are very common in dairy cattle. Frequently, peripheral nerve injuries accompany myopathy in recumbent cattle and in cattle that develop exertional myopathy from metabolic weakness or repeated attempts to rise on slippery surfaces. Peripheral nerve injuries may be confused with musculoskeletal lameness in dairy cattle, so it behooves the veterinary practitioner to be well versed in the variable gaits and stances that accompany them.

Spinal cord root and nerve injuries from vertebral injury may create peripheral nerve dysfunction in the limbs, especially the hind limbs in cattle. Therefore, it is best to consider the entire course and origin of the peripheral nerves when attempting to localize the neuroanatomic site of injury, especially in the more commonly affected pelvic limb.

Thoracic Limb

Suprascapular Nerve Injury

Etiology

The suprascapular nerve is a motor nerve to the supraspinatus and infraspinatus muscles. Because of its location and origin (C6–C7), it is subject to occasional injury caused by chutes or other objects cattle run into forcefully or are abruptly stopped by, as pressure is placed against the caudal cervical or shoulder area. The suprascapular nerve winds

TABLE 13.3 Uncommon Causes of Spinal Cord Disease

Disease	Clinical Signs	Differential Diagnosis	Diagnosis	Treatment
Hemivertebrae	Spinal cord signs; pelvic limb paresis and ataxia May progress or be more obvious after calf is several months of age (see Video Clips 13.28 and 13.29)	Trauma, abscess, tumor, white muscle disease	Obvious deviation of vertebral column Radiography	None; congenital
Myelodysplasia	Spinal cord signs at birth; ataxia, paresis, or paralysis	Trauma, myelitis, white muscle disease	Radiography	None; congenital
Fibrocartilaginous emboli	Rare in cattle but may cause acute, nonprogressive spinal cord dysfunction	Iliac thrombosis, fracture	Histopathology	Might improve with time and supportive care
Protozoan myelitis	Spinal cord signs at birth with paresis or tetraparesis and ataxia; may be more than one individual involved	Trauma, white muscle disease	Histopathology (toxoplasmosis, sarcocystosis, *Neospora caninum*) Serology of dam	None
Degenerative myelopathy	Holstein or Holstein - Gir crossbred calves; both sexes with progressive gait disturbances beginning by 3 months of age	Abscess, trauma, rarely copper deficiency, delayed organophosphate toxicity	Histopathology	None
Delayed organophosphate toxicity	Tetraparesis—may be progressive	Abscess, tumor	Histopathology (diffuse axonal degeneration)	None
Hypoderma bovis larvae-induced spinal cord disease	Pelvic limb paresis and ataxia within 2 to 3 days of administration of larvicidal anthelmintics More than one animal may show signs	Trauma, abscess, tumor	History Usually normal or slightly abnormal CSF; eosinophils *not* typical. (Signs may be from toxins. Larvae are extradural and do not usually cause direct spinal cord injury.)	Antiinflammatories such as steroids, nonsteroidals; do not use grub treatments or other larvicidal anthelmintics after October in northern climates and August or September in southern climates
Motor neuron disease (spinal muscular atrophy)	Holstein-Friesian calves with progressive paraparesis or tetraparesis within first 1–2 months of life	Trauma, abscess, rarely copper deficiency	Age, breed, genetics, and histopathology demonstrating degeneration and loss of motor neurons in the spinal cord; EMG is consistent with denervation atrophy	None

CSF, Cerebrospinal fluid; *EMG,* electromyography.

around the neck of the scapula and can be injured at this site. Inadvertent injections of irritating material into the caudal neck or cellulitis secondary to SC injections may inflame the nerve. Working oxen of dairy breeds occasionally may be at risk, depending on the type of yoke or collar used for pulling.

Clinical Signs

Cattle with suprascapular nerve paralysis abduct the shoulder when placing weight on the affected side and may circumduct when advancing the limb. The stride is shortened. The affected limb tends to jut out at the shoulder joint when bearing weight, and this appearance becomes more prominent if permanent nerve injury has occurred because of neurogenic atrophy involving the supraspinatus and infraspinatus. In working draft horses, this has been called "Sweeney" when the collar is too tight and compresses the suprascapular nerve at the neck of the scapula (Sweeney was a brand of horse collar).

In severe cases, loss of the lateral rotatory function of the infraspinatus muscle at the shoulder may cause the elbow to rotate laterally on weight bearing. In acute cases, a reluctance to bear weight on the affected limb may be apparent and will require differentiation of suprascapular nerve injuries from radial paralysis, scapulohumeral fractures, or bicipital bursitis.

Treatment

Treatment of suprascapular nerve injuries is symptomatic. Acute injuries may be treated with hydrotherapy, if possible. Antiinflammatory drugs such as dexamethasone (10–40 mg IM) or appropriate dosages of NSAIDs (see the section on the fibular [peroneal] nerve that follows) are indicated. Best results are found in cases that are witnessed and treated immediately such as a suprascapular nerve injury resulting from a cattle chute injury. Chronic or neglected cases have obvious signs of muscle atrophy and excessive shoulder laxity as seen in horses with Sweeney and are far less amenable to therapy.

Radial Nerve Injury

Etiology

Complete or partial injury to the radial nerve may result from direct trauma, humeral fractures, or chute injuries but most commonly occurs secondary to recumbency on tilt tables for surgery or foot trimming. The latter may result in direct pressure on the nerve or, more likely, a compartmental syndrome that involves the radial nerve as it courses laterally over the distal humerus proximal to the elbow joint.

Clinical Signs

Signs of radial nerve injury proximal to the innervation of the triceps brachii involve loss of extensor muscle function of the entire forelimb. Collapsing on the limb caused by the inability to extend the elbow to bear weight is the most obvious sign of paralysis. In addition, there is an inability to advance the lower forelimb and digit by extending the carpus, fetlock, and digits (Fig. 13.52). The hooves may be dragged, thus leading to abrasions on the dorsum of the digit, or the limb may be

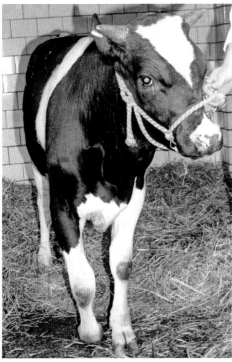

• **Fig. 13.52** Radial nerve paralysis after tabling of a yearling Holstein bull.

carried off the ground. The elbow may be "dropped" or carried lower than in the normal opposite limb, but this does not become as dramatic or severe as when brachial plexus paralysis exists. Analgesia of the dorsum of the digits and metacarpus may be present. With partial lesions proximal to the innervation of the triceps muscle, the patient will walk "lame"—short strided—because of the partial loss of weight support, and occasionally, the hooves will drag from partial inability to extend the fetlocks and digits. Partial injuries at the level of the elbow joint may be associated with the ability to support weight and no elbow drop but less ability to readily extend the carpus, fetlock, and digits causing the digits to be dragged. This reflects an injury distal to the nerve supply to the triceps brachii muscle where the radial nerve courses over the lateral surface of the brachialis muscle. Adult cattle with radial nerve injury may have difficulty rising.

Most acute radial nerve injuries respond to therapy or improve spontaneously but should be attended promptly for best results.

Treatment

When acute radial paralysis is detected as a cow recovers from surgery or comes off a tilt table, the cow should be encouraged to stand and walk a few steps on good footing. Many mild cases spontaneously recover function within minutes. If the paralysis is still present after 5 minutes, it is better to overtreat than to neglect the injury. If there are no contraindications (e.g., pregnancy) for corticosteroids, dexamethasone (20–50 mg IV or IM usually single dose) and a NSAID (aspirin, 240–480 grains orally twice daily or flunixin meglumine, 0.5–1.1 mg/kg every 24 hours) are given. Hydrotherapy by hosing is especially helpful when a concurrent myopathy or compartment syndrome exists. If the affected animal has great difficulty standing or rising, which may be the case in some adult cows, they can be placed in a float tank for as many days as necessary to give the nerve a chance to return to full function. Float tanks are generally better for muscle diseases but have helped save the lives of some cows with nerve paresis that could not stand otherwise. If the cow cannot place the limb in the proper position in the tank, which is sometimes the case with severe radial paralysis, the tank flotation is usually not very successful. After these initial treatments, antiinflammatory drugs are continued for 2 to 3 days and then discontinued or tapered. The prognosis is good in most cases when therapy can be instituted quickly after the onset of signs. However, the prognosis worsens in direct proportion to the length of time the cow was recumbent or tabled. Humeral fractures causing radial nerve paralysis have a guarded to poor prognosis for return of nerve function.

Neglected or chronic cases have no specific therapy, but hydrotherapy and NSAIDs for analgesia may help slightly. Spontaneous healing may take 3 to 6 months in some severe cases. The prognosis in chronic cases is better for younger and light animals. Multiparous cows or adult bulls do poorly because of the stress placed on the opposite forelimb and secondary injuries. Chronic, disproportionate, contralateral limb load bearing does not seem so closely associated with laminitis in the "sound" feet as in horses but can certainly result in suspensory and flexor tendon injury at the level of the fetlock or distal cannon, especially in large bulls.

Prevention

Prevention of radial paralysis involves using adequate padding for the shoulder and elbow region of recumbent cattle. It is best if extra padding is built into, or added to, existing tilt tables. If tables are not supplied with extra padding, each animal tabled should have a shoulder pad inserted to protect the area from the scapula distal to the carpus on the down side. At least an 8- and 12-in-thick pad should be used for cows and bulls, respectively. Similarly, cattle in lateral recumbency for surgery should have the down forelimbs padded heavily. The down forelimb should be pulled forward as well.

Brachial Plexus

Etiology

Injury to the brachial plexus is rare in dairy cattle, but it has been associated with severe lacerations of the axilla, excessive traction on the forelimbs of a calf during dystocia, and severe abduction of a forelimb.

Clinical Signs

Signs of brachial plexus injury are profound with complete inability to advance the forelimb or support weight. The limb is dragged on the dorsum of the digit and fetlock and is dramatically limp. The elbow is "dropped" below the level of the sternum, and the affected animal may assume a stance with the hind limbs more cranial than normal and the opposite forelimb extended forward to support weight. Severe lesions are associated with extensive loss of nociception in the affected limb distal to the elbow.

The prognosis for brachial plexus injury is guarded and depends on the cause and extent of injury as regards permanence of paralysis.

Treatment

Medical treatment for brachial plexus injury is identical to that described for radial nerve injury. Wounds in the axilla, if present, should be treated as indicated. The prognosis is guarded, and the condition must be differentiated from fractures of the olecranon and humerus.

Pelvic Limb

Femoral Paralysis

Etiology

Unilateral or bilateral femoral nerve paralysis is most commonly observed in calves after dystocia—especially those requiring forced traction due to a "hip-lock"—and is thought to occur because of overextension of the hip and tearing of the femoral nerve where it emerges from the iliopsoas muscle and enters the proximal portion of the quadriceps femoris. In a necropsy of a 3-month-old Hereford calf with femoral paralysis since birth, the L4 and L5 spinal nerve roots were torn from the spinal cord. Traction trauma to the quadriceps femoris muscle may also contribute to the inability to support weight. Severe lesions cause analgesia in the autonomous zone of the saphenous nerve when tested on the medial side of the crus. Loss of nociception suggests a poor prognosis for recovery. Femoral nerve injury or paralysis in adult dairy cattle is most common in cattle that struggle to rise when their hind limbs are retracted caudally. Cattle that are positioned on slippery footing and have metabolic diseases such as hypocalcemia or that are trapped may struggle excessively and repeatedly until direct femoral nerve injury or quadriceps femoris muscle damage and compartmental damage to the femoral nerve occur. Frequently, the femoral nerve injury is bilateral in adult cattle. In dairy cattle, "creeper" cows that have had hypocalcemia are most at risk for femoral nerve injury. Slippery concrete surfaces in some free stalls also contribute to possible femoral nerve injury because it is not at all rare to see cows fall in free-stall alleys with their hind limbs extended caudally. Such cows are lying on the ventral abdomen, udder, and cranial surface of the stifles. Occasionally, these animals have difficulty getting their hind limbs back under them as they struggle to rise and risk femoral nerve injury.

Clinical Signs

The femoral nerve supplies motor innervation to the quadriceps femoris to extend the stifle and a portion of the iliopsoas muscle to help flex the hip. The femoral nerve also gives rise to the saphenous nerve, which supplies skin sensation to the medial aspect of the limb from the midthigh to the tarsus. The major clinical sign of femoral nerve paralysis is an inability to support weight on the affected hind limb. Loss of extensor and reciprocal apparatus function causes the stifle and all joints distal to the stifle to be flexed (Fig. 13.53). However, there is no loss of muscle function distal to the stifle. With complete paralysis, attempts to bear weight will lead to collapse. The limb can still be advanced by hip flexion due to the complex innervation of the iliopsoas group by the ventral branches of all the lumbar spinal nerves. With partial paralysis, the limb will be flexed, be lowered, and struggle to bear weight. The stride will be shortened, creating a "lame" gait. Trembling is obvious in the quadriceps femoris muscles (see Video Clip 13.31 and 13.32). In bilateral partial paralysis, affected cows struggle to rise with all joints in the hind limbs flexed. Consequently, they bear weight on the dorsal surface of the digits, and assume a "squatting" posture. The forelimbs are placed caudal to their normal position in order to assume greater weight bearing.

Calves with femoral nerve paralysis have been studied extensively. Complete bilateral paralysis results in recumbency, and unilateral paralysis still carries a guarded prognosis in calves. Neurogenic muscle atrophy involving the quadriceps femoris appears within 10 days and worsens dramatically over the next several weeks. Associated with this muscle atrophy, the patella becomes freely moveable, and the cause of limb dysfunction may be misdiagnosed as patellar luxation.

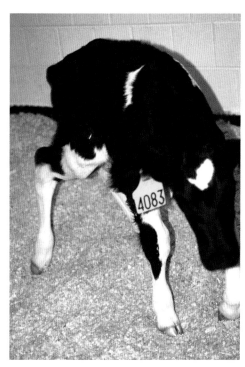

• **Fig. 13.53** A calf with femoral nerve paresis of the right pelvic limb. This was believed to have been caused by a difficult delivery and "hip lock" while passing through the maternal pelvis. (See Video Clip 13.32).

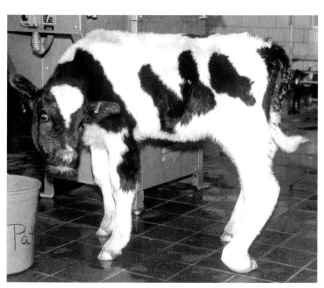

• **Fig. 13.54** Complete sciatic paralysis secondary to intramuscular injection of an irritating drug into the gluteal muscle in a calf.

Treatment

Medical therapy for femoral nerve paralysis should be instituted immediately on recognition of the problem. Dexamethasone and NSAIDs (see the earlier section on radial nerve injuries) should be administered. The cow should be moved to a well-bedded box stall or an area where good footing is available. Slippery floors must be avoided, lest the condition be worsened or the cow experience further musculoskeletal injury. Placing the cow's hind limbs in proper position and rolling her onto her opposite side helps. Warm compresses applied to the quadriceps femoris may be helpful, as may massage. Appropriate dosages of vitamin E and selenium are recommended empirically. Assistance in rising should be given. The cow may only need manual assistance by tail lifting or judicious use of mechanical aids, such as well-padded hip slings. When mechanical aids are used, it is important not to further damage the quadriceps femoris muscles. If the cow is affected unilaterally, the prognosis is fair. If bilateral femoral nerve paralysis has occurred in an adult, the prognosis is guarded to poor, but some cows so affected can be slowly nursed back over a 2- to 3-week convalescence with assistance in rising. Cattle that are improving gradually return to a full-standing position rather than the flexed, squatting and trembling posture of the hindlimbs typical of partial femoral nerve injury.

Antiinflammatory and analgesic therapy is continued as long as necessary. Corticosteroids usually are a one-time treatment but may be tapered over 3 to 4 days in severely affected cattle.

Calves with femoral nerve paralysis after forced traction have a poor prognosis. Symptomatic therapy should be intense as outlined for adult cattle, and vitamin E and

selenium should be given at recommended dosages. Good bedding and footing are especially important to avoid decubital sores in calves. If muscle atrophy and patellar laxity develop, the prognosis is very poor.

Sciatic Nerve Paralysis
Etiology

Injuries to the sciatic nerve and its branches are the most common peripheral nerve injuries affecting limb function in dairy cattle. When the characteristic clinical signs are observed, the neuroanatomic diagnosis includes the origin of the sciatic nerve from spinal cord segments L6, S1, and S2; the nerve roots and spinal nerve ventral branches of the fibular (L6, S1) and tibial (S1, S2) nerves that innervate the caudal thigh and all areas distal to the stifle.

Damage to the sciatic nerve proper most commonly results from iatrogenic injury following injection of irritating drugs in the gluteal region or too close to the course of the nerve near the hip joint between the greater trochanter and the tuber ischium. These reactions or injuries seldom cause complete or permanent loss of sciatic function in adult cattle but may do so in calves. Calves are particularly at risk for sciatic nerve injury from injections made in the gluteal or caudal thigh regions. Although irritating injectable products are most risky, direct injury through needle puncture is possible because of the paucity of gluteal and caudal thigh musculature in dairy calves.

Pelvic fractures involving the ilium or femoral fractures may also cause severe damage to the sciatic nerve. In a prolonged dystocia, compression of the ventral branch of the L6 spinal nerve where it courses caudally over the ventral surface of the sacrum may cause a fibular nerve dysfunction in the dam.

Clinical Signs

Complete sciatic nerve paralysis results in slight lowering or "dropping" of the hip and hock with overflexion of the fetlock (Fig. 13.54). The animal can advance the limb by hip flexion and may still support weight, but the

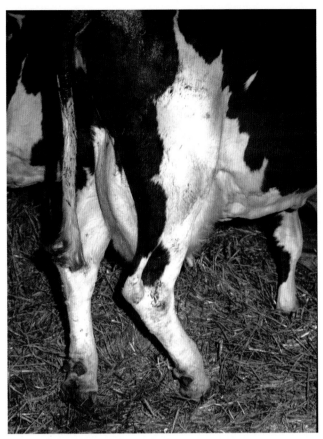

• **Fig. 13.55** Partial sciatic nerve injury in an adult Holstein cow that received repeated intramuscular injections in the gluteal region. Note the dropped hock and dorsal buckling of the fetlock.

digit may drag as the limb is advanced, and the animal usually stands on the dorsum of the digit and fetlock with the hock overflexed, or "dropped." Analgesia of the limb is present distal to the stifle with the exception of the medial surface. When incomplete or partial sciatic nerve paralysis exists, the cow can support weight but has overflexion (dorsal buckling) of the fetlock and a slightly dropped hock compared with the unaffected hind limb. Tell-tale swelling or "blood tracks" in the gluteal region of the affected limb allow diagnosis of iatrogenic injury from injections and should be looked for because laypeople may not always volunteer such information in the history (Fig. 13.55). Sciatic nerve injuries must be differentiated from tibial nerve injury, fibular (peroneal) nerve injury, partial rupture of the gastrocnemius tendon or muscle, and sacral root and sacral nerve injuries associated with vertebral and spinal cord diseases.

Treatment

Treatment for acute sciatic nerve injury is symptomatic. Fortunately, most sciatic nerve injuries are partial rather than complete. Educating clients to avoid giving injections in the gluteal region of adult dairy cattle is imperative. There is a distinct difference between dairy and beef cattle in that beef cattle have more gluteal mass, are moved through chutes where gluteal injection is safer and easier, and injections in the hamstrings of beef cattle are contraindicated, lest meat

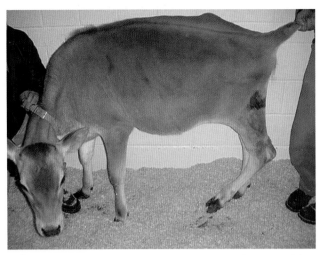

• **Fig. 13.56** Tibial nerve paresis, as part of partial sciatic nerve injury, of a heifer caused by an injection abscess in the hind limb.

quality be compromised at slaughter. Dairy cattle, on the other hand, have a "dished-out" gluteal area with little muscle protection for sciatic nerve branches. If an abscess has formed at the site of a gluteal injection, drainage is indicated to relieve pressure on the sciatic branches. Direct injury through needle laceration or indirect injury through an irritating drug placed adjacent to nerve branches are both possible.

In dairy calves, the giving of gluteal injections constitutes malpractice. Even well-placed injections into the caudal thigh muscles occasionally cause sciatic or tibial nerve injury in calves.

Acute injuries may be treated symptomatically with antiinflammatory drugs and hydrotherapy. A support wrap or gutter-pipe splint may need to be applied to the lower limb if buckling and walking on the dorsum of the fetlocks occurs. Further injections into the affected limb should be avoided, and the animal should be placed on the best footing available to minimize further complications.

Tibial Nerve Injury

Etiology

Injury to the tibial nerve in dairy cattle and calves may result from injection of an irritant drug or a large volume of drugs distally in the caudal thigh muscles. This is more of a risk in calves than in adult cattle. Abscesses, hematomas, and seromas in this region also may compress the nerve. "Downer" cows may develop compartmental syndrome involving this nerve and associated musculature. Be aware that sacral fractures can injure the ventral branches of S1 and S2 that contribute to the tibial nerve and also cause a tibial nerve paralysis.

Clinical Signs

The tibial nerve supplies motor innervation to the gastrocnemius, popliteus, superficial digital flexor, and deep digital flexor muscles. Therefore tibial nerve paralysis or partial injury will affect function of these muscles, causing a dorsal buckling of the fetlock and reduced extension or increased flexion of the hock (Fig. 13.56). The hock does not appear as "dropped" or lowered as with sciatic nerve paralysis, but this is often difficult to assess because of fetlock buckling (see Video Clips 13.33 and 13.34). The cow is not observed to stand on the dorsum of the digit nor does she drag the digit when walking, as in peroneal or complete sciatic paralysis. The limb bears full weight during walking but may be favored slightly at rest.

The skin of the plantar metatarsal area and digits may be analgesic because the tibial nerve supplies sensation to this region.

Tibial nerve injury or paralysis must be differentiated from partial sciatic nerve injury (and doing so may be difficult), partial rupture of the gastrocnemius or superficial digital flexor tendon or muscle, and peroneal paralysis.

Treatment

Treatment of tibial nerve paralysis is symptomatic and similar to sciatic nerve injury. Tibial nerve injury may, in some instances, be a manifestation of a partial unilateral sciatic nerve injury. If present, abscesses, hematomas, or seromas in the distal thigh area should be treated accordingly.

Fibular Nerve Injury

Etiology

Fibular (peroneal) nerve injury is common in downer cows, including milk fever patients, because of the superficial location of this nerve where it crosses the lateral surface of the lateral head of the gastrocnemius muscle and the fibula to enter the craniolateral crural muscles.

Prolonged recumbency with the hind limbs in a normal position allows pressure injury to the nerve at this site. The anatomic location of this injury is often highlighted by abrasions or decubital sores just distal to the stifle on the lateral surface of the limb in cows with prolonged recumbency. Even relatively short periods of recumbency on hard surfaces or when the cow is recumbent with the stifle region resting on the edge of a concrete platform may produce fibular nerve injury.

Clinical Signs

The fibular nerve supplies motor function to the flexor muscles of the hock and the extensor muscles of the digit. Therefore, paralysis of the fibular nerve results in straightening or overextension of the hock, and the affected limb may bear weight on the dorsum of the flexed fetlock and digits (Fig. 13.57). Because the hock cannot flex normally, the limb is advanced with the hock extended and the limb stiff. The dorsum of the metatarsus, fetlock and digits may show analgesia because of loss of sensory function of the fibular nerve.

Treatment

Recumbent cattle should be bedded heavily and kept on good footing to minimize direct pressure to the fibular nerve or the development of compartment syndrome to affect this nerve indirectly. These nursing recommendations apply to both prevention and treatment. In addition, recumbent cattle should be rolled to the opposite side every two to four hours to minimize pressure damage to muscles and nerves on the down limb. Physical therapy, including warm compresses, massage, and vigorous manipulation of the limb, may be helpful to cattle with fibular nerve paralysis.

Systemic therapy with corticosteroids (10–40 mg of dexamethasone) and NSAIDs (aspirin 240 to 480 grains orally twice daily or flunixin meglumine 0.5–1.1 mg/kg every 24 hours for lactating dairy cows) may be helpful, especially in acute cases, assuming there are no contraindications to the use of these drugs.

Encouraging the cow to stand and assisting her in rising by manually lifting the tail promotes circulation in the limb if the cow can support weight on the opposite limb and can stand for short periods.

The prognosis is fair to good for acute unilateral cases diagnosed promptly. An affected cow should be managed individually, preferably in a well-bedded box stall or one with a dirt or sand surface, and nursed accordingly. The prognosis is guarded when recumbency persists or in bilateral fibular nerve paralysis because cattle so affected are extremely prone to other musculoskeletal injuries. Hip luxations, fractures of the femoral head or neck, and exertional myopathy are all possible complications if the cow falls or

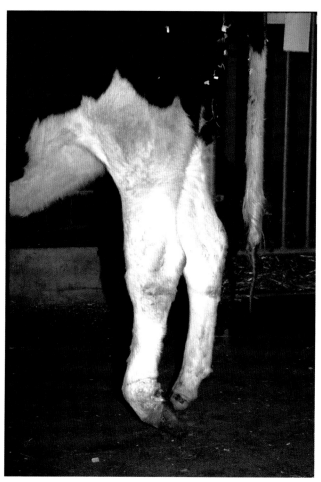

• **Fig. 13.57** Fibular (peroneal) nerve paralysis caused by trauma in a heifer.

struggles to rise in an awkward fashion. Owner education regarding management of down cows and prompt attention to individuals with signs of fibular nerve damage are important in the successful treatment and prevention of this condition.

Obturator Nerve Injury (Calving Paralysis)

Etiology

The classical description of obturator nerve paralysis causing unilateral or bilateral inability to adduct the hind limbs after calving may or may not be explained simply by obturator nerve dysfunction. Experimental studies in calves and cows have shown that both the obturator nerve and the L6 lumbar nerve root of the sciatic nerve are probably involved in the clinical signs previously described as "calving paralysis." These studies demonstrated that bilateral obturator neurectomy did not produce lasting recumbency and total adductor failure but did predispose the animal to slipping and abduction on slippery footing. Dystocia, especially in first-calf heifers or dams with an oversized fetus, may compress the obturator nerve as it courses ventrally on the medial shaft of the ilium. In addition, the sixth lumbar spinal nerve passes ventral to the prominent ridge of the sacrum and is vulnerable to compression and injury during dystocia. Whereas the obturator nerve supplies motor function to several adductor muscles of the hind limb, the sixth lumbar spinal nerve contributes to the sciatic nerve branches to the semitendinous and semimembranosus muscles, as well as contributing to the peroneal nerve, which innervates the cranial crural muscles.

A syndrome similar to calving paralysis may occur in cattle that "split" on slippery floors or ice and tear adductor musculature in the hind limbs.

Clinical Signs

Cattle with unilateral or even bilateral damage to only the obturator nerves will be able to rise and support weight, assuming they have good footing. They may show a tendency for abduction when standing, and this tendency is accentuated on slippery surfaces.

Cattle with true calving paralysis caused by simultaneous damage to the sixth lumbar nerve component of the sciatic nerve as well as the obturator nerve may have unilateral or bilateral signs. Unilateral signs include an inability to adduct the affected hind limb and standing on the dorsum of the pasterns and digits. These latter two signs correlate well with sciatic nerve damage, especially that involving fibers supplying the fibular nerve. Depending on the cow's weight and agility, unilateral cases may be able to rise with assistance and support weight. Cattle with bilateral damage to both the sciatic nerve and obturator nerve are unable to rise; frequently lie in a froglike position on the ventral abdomen with the hind limbs flexed but abducted; and may, in the worst cases, have the hind limbs split and extended perpendicular to the body's long axis.

Adductor muscle myopathy frequently accompanies calving paralysis in a limb and complicates the condition. Cattle

with calving paralysis are also at extremely high risk of developing hip and femoral complications, including hip luxation, femoral head or neck fractures, and femoral shaft fractures.

Cattle recumbent because of calving paralysis must be differentiated from those with pure adductor muscle myopathy, pelvic fractures, femoral fractures, hip luxations, metabolic disorders, and severe septicemia or endotoxemia. The prognosis is fair for unilateral cases and poor to guarded for bilateral calving paralysis associated with recumbency. First-calf heifers generally have a better prognosis than multiparous cows because of their size, their smaller abdominal visceral mass, and their overall agility.

Treatment

Therapy is most successful when started immediately on recognition of signs indicating calving paralysis after dystocia. Otherwise, muscular damage is likely to complicate the already serious neuropathy. Initially, dexamethasone (20–40 mg) parenterally and a NSAID at the discretion of the veterinarian (see the previous discussion in the section on the fibular nerve) should be administered. The hind limbs should be hobbled together in the metatarsal region with 24 to 30 in (61–76 cm) allowed between the hobbles, depending on the size of the individual (Fig. 13.58). A soft connecting rope can be connected to nylon or rope straps applied to the metatarsal region when constructing the hobbles. The hobbles should be fashioned to minimize trauma and so as not to compromise circulation at their attachments

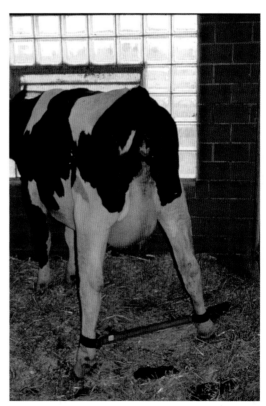

• **Fig. 13.58** First-calf heifer with calving paralysis leading to a tendency to limb abduction after assisted delivery. Canvas hobbles are in place to prevent injury.

to the metatarsal areas. The cow must be placed on the best footing available, such as a well-bedded, dirt-based, or manure-packed box stall, or outside on grass with a quickly constructed fence to prevent excessive room for movement.

It should be determined whether the cow can rise with assistance provided by one or two people lifting the tail as she attempts to get up. If she can stand, albeit briefly, the cow should be milked out; standing also promotes circulation to the hind limbs. A rectal examination should be done to rule out pelvic fractures, coxofemoral luxation or separation of the pelvic symphysis.

Any associated metabolic or infectious diseases should be treated, and analgesic therapy with NSAIDs should be continued for several days at least; dexamethasone may be administered for 1 to 2 days.

Cattle unable to rise with manual assistance should be assessed daily as to the benefits of slings, cattle walkers, or hip lifters that might be mechanical aids used to assist the animal in standing. Well-padded hip lifters can be used judiciously to lift the cow to a standing position in order to assess her ability to support weight when standing. If the cow can support weight, these should be removed quickly and the cow allowed to stand for as long as she is comfortable. Because many cows are frightened or "give up" when initially lifted by slings or other mechanical aids, the usefulness of these devices should not be ruled out until at least a second or third attempt is made at 8- to 12-hour intervals. Flotation tanks should also be considered when available.

Recumbent cattle should be rolled to the opposite side as often as practical and kept in well-bedded areas. Other symptomatic therapy may include vitamin E and selenium injections according to the manufacturer's recommendations. Recumbent cattle require daily reassessment to detect complications that may alter the prognosis. Severe adductor muscle damage usually appears as obvious muscular swelling between the medial thigh and rear udder attachment (Fig. 13.59). Hip

and femoral complications are possible, as well as gastrocnemius injuries (Fig. 13.60). Neglected cases or cattle with previous severe adductor myopathy have a poor prognosis.

Animals that regain the ability to rise require at least 10 to 14 days or longer before they can be safely moved to milking facilities. Decisions regarding removal time for hobbles and allowable exercise must be made on an individual case basis.

Cranial Nerves VII and VIII

Otitis Media and Interna
Etiology

Middle ear infections are common in dairy calves from 3 weeks to 6 months of age. Although exogenous infections from otitis externa are possible, the great majority of cases arise from ascending endogenous infections from the nasopharynx via the eustachian tube to the middle ear. Extension of endogenously acquired otitis media to otitis interna is common. Exogenous infections from filthy surroundings, manure contamination, and ear sucking by penmates cause malodorous, purulent otitis externa. Endogenous infections, unless very chronic, seldom show signs of otitis externa. *Mycoplasma bovis* is currently the predominant endogenous cause of acute otitis media or interna. This organism is a common inhabitant of the upper respiratory tract and has become an endemic problem on an increasing number of dairies and heifer-rearing facilities. Herds that have *Mycoplasma* mastitis appear to also have a high incidence of otitis media/interna. *Pasteurella multocida* and *H. somni* occasionally have been isolated from acute otitis media or interna cases as well. In chronic cases, *Mycoplasma* spp. may be joined, or replaced, by *T. pyogenes* or *Corynebacterium pseudotuberculosis*. Exogenous infection generally results in a mixed infection with *T. pyogenes* eventually predominating. Pneumonia may also be commonly present in calves with otitis media/interna and *M. bovis* in addition to *P. multocida*

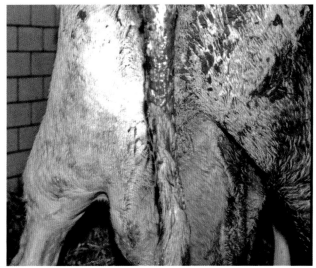

• **Fig. 13.59** Left adductor muscle myopathy causing filling of the normal space between udder and medial thigh in a cow with calving paralysis. The cow cannot stand and is being supported by hip slings.

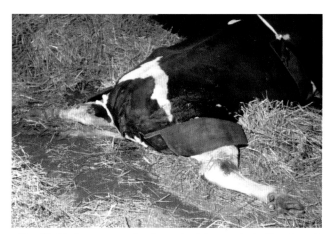

• **Fig. 13.60** Severe complications of calving paralysis. Despite suffering calving paralysis, this cow was allowed on a slippery floor. Bilateral femoral neck fractures and massive adductor myopathy are present.

are common isolates from such cases. It is not common for concurrent joint infection with *Mycoplasma* spp. to accompany mycoplasmal otitis media/interna.

Clinical Signs

Acute unilateral or bilateral signs of dysfunction in CNs VII and VIII occur with acute otitis media/interna. If the clinical signs are unilateral, the syndrome is easily diagnosed because there is often a head tilt toward the affected side

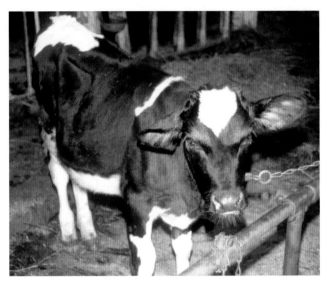

• **Fig. 13.61** Facial paralysis and drooped ear as a result of a middle and inner ear infection in a 3-month-old Holstein calf.

with ipsilateral drooped ear, reduced palpebral reflex, and hypotonic lip present (Fig. 13.61) (see Video Clips 13.35 and 13.36). Low-grade fever (103.0° to 105.0°F [39.44° to 40.56°C]) may occur, but the calf remains fairly bright and does not show signs of brainstem disease. In some cases, dysphagia with cud leaking onto the chin and depression are present. The dysphagia presumably is associated with inflammation extending beyond the boundaries of the tympanic bulla to involve CNs IX and X as they course near the tympanic bulla (Fig. 13.62). Mild balance loss with drifting to the affected side and circling may accompany the head tilt, but the animal remains strong. Hopping is normal. If abnormal nystagmus is present, the fast phase is away from the side of the lesion. Acute bilateral otitis media/interna is difficult to diagnose because an observable head tilt is absent. With bilateral vestibular lesions, wide head excursions to both sides may be exhibited, especially when the calf is blindfolded (Fig. 13.63). Deafness may also be apparent in severe bilateral lesions. The gait may be awkward, and the head may be carried low. Partial or complete facial nerve paralysis may be present bilaterally in this instance and may only be determined by a careful clinical examination. Bilateral disease without asymmetric neurologic signs is often interpreted by calf handlers as a mere "poorly" calf because of the symmetrically droopy ears (see Fig. 13.62, A), low-grade fever, and partial feed refusal. Recognition and treatment of the otitis may be delayed in these cases compared with an obviously asymmetric unilateral case with vestibular signs. Because of accompanying respiratory tract

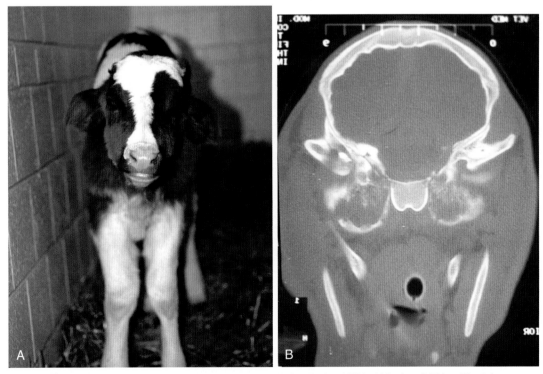

• **Fig. 13.62 A,** Bilateral purulent otitis interna and media in a Red and White Holstein calf. This calf had dysphagia and was depressed. **B,** Computed tomography scan of the calf showed distention and destruction of the bony areas surrounding the bullae and exudates within. Antibiotics were not effective in this calf, but surgical drainage was.

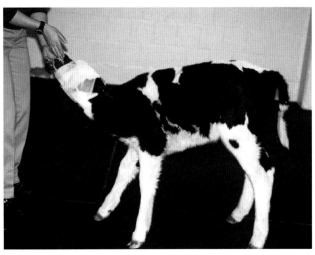

• **Fig. 13.63** Blindfolding a calf with otitis interna and media, which exacerbates the abnormal head carriage of an affected individual.

inflammation in many calves, calves may also demonstrate concurrent nasal and lachrymal discharges. Chronic cough and nasal discharge often accompany otitis interna/media.

Chronic or neglected cases may have pronounced head tilt, other vestibular signs, complete facial paralysis, and exposure keratitis. These same patients may have purulent otitis externa from rupture of the tympanic membrane. Purulent otitis externa may be observed occasionally in the external canal on the affected side when exogenous infection has caused the disease but generally is absent with endogenous infections.

Diagnosis

Clinical signs and farm history suffice for diagnosis in most cases. Oblique or dorsoventral skull radiographs of the tympanic bullae would be helpful but are seldom necessary. Radiographs sometimes, and CT always, will demonstrate the fluid-filled tympanic bulla and bony destruction, if present (see Fig. 13.62, B). A CSF analysis will be normal unless, as in many chronic cases, there is intracranial extension of the inflammation with either mononuclear or neutrophilic pleocytosis. Ultrasound imaging of tympanic bullae can be used to help provide an onsite diagnosis, but the sensitivity of the test may be low.

Treatment

Rigorous therapy is required to prevent this infection from extending into the cranial cavity and causing meningitis and a brain abscess. The response to appropriate antibiotic therapy is commonly thought to confirm a diagnosis of acute otitis. Because *Mycoplasma* spp. is the usual causative organism for acute endogenous infections and pneumonia is often concurrent, tetracycline (11 mg/kg) IV or IM, once or twice daily, is one possible initial therapeutic choice as long as the calf is well hydrated. Unfortunately, a significant number of *Mycoplasma* organisms are resistant to tetracycline and increasingly to most other approved antibiotics for dairy cattle. Almost all strains remain

sensitive to enrofloxacin, but in the United States, this drug is not approved for use in young dairy animals unless they also have pneumonia. Fortuitously, this is often the case for many calves with otitis media/interna, making this antibiotic an excellent choice under such circumstances. Tulathromycin is another acceptable initial treatment and has been shown to be effective in treating the disease. Most opportunistic *P. multocida* and *T. pyogenes* isolates are sensitive to tetracycline, cephalosporins, and even penicillin (22,000 U/kg twice daily). However, β-lactam antibiotics are not sound choices when *Mycoplasma* spp. may be present. Acute infections typically respond within 5 to 7 days, so even longer acting antibiotics may require more than one treatment. Treatment early in the disease process is important to prevent caseous exudation, bony lysis, and "superinfection" with *T. pyogenes*. In addition to antimicrobial therapy, non-steroidal antiinflammatory treatment with flunixin meglumine may be considered for 1-2 days in acute cases. Unfortunately, because of subtle, bilateral clinical signs, many cases are not treated early enough for a good prognosis. If facial paralysis is obvious, antibiotic or protective ophthalmic ointments should be applied to the ipsilateral cornea to prevent exposure keratitis, although calves seem much more resilient regarding this sequela than horses.

Chronic or neglected cases require longer term therapy, and the possibility of *T. pyogenes* infection should be considered. Therefore, long-term penicillin administration may be indicated in chronic cases. Surgical drainage may be required in cases that are not responsive to antibiotics. The prognosis is good for acute cases and fair to poor in chronic disease. Removal of cows shedding *Mycoplasma* in the milk should occur or at least the *M. bovis* contaminated milk should not be fed to calves. Pasteurization of whole milk should remove *Mycoplasma* spp. infectivity when waste milk is being fed back to calves.

Facial Nerve Injuries

Etiology

Peripheral injuries to the facial nerve usually are caused by halters or collars that become excessively tight over facial nerve branches. Animals that struggle in lateral recumbency or that are tightly held with ringed halters on tilt tables may also develop signs of facial nerve paralysis. Mass lesions such as abscesses, granulomas, or rarely, tumors in the area of the stylomastoid foramen may also injure the facial nerve.

Frightened or nervous cattle held in stanchions often pull back violently to escape the stanchion if approached from the front. This occasionally results in a cow becoming trapped caudal to the orbital rim along the zygomatic arch. If the cow remains trapped this way in the stanchion for a period of time, bilateral traumatic injury to the auriculopalpebral nerve occurs as the cow tries to move back or forward or tilts her head to escape. The resultant bilateral auriculopalpebral nerve injury, often referred to as "stanchion paralysis," causes loss of palpebral response and occasionally is severe enough to also cause a bilateral ear droop.

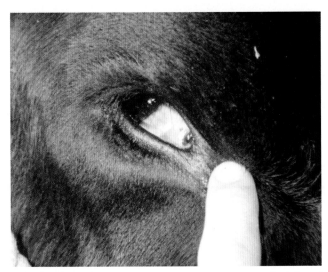

• **Fig. 13.64** Inability to close the eyelids in response to stimulation of the palpebral reflex in a Holstein cow with "stanchion paralysis." The condition was bilateral.

Clinical Signs

Signs of ptosis, loss of palpebral response, and flaccid ipsilateral lip are most apparent with traumatic facial nerve injuries. Deeper or more extensive lesions may injure the nerve where it emerges from the stylomastoid foramen, resulting in a drooped ear as well. Exposure keratitis may be present in chronic cases and should be anticipated, and treated prophylactically, in acute cases.

The auriculopalpebral nerve, a branch of the facial nerve, carries motor function to the orbicularis oculi muscle and muscles of the ear. The palpebral branch is more commonly injured by stanchion trauma than the auricular branch, but both may be. The key to diagnosis of stanchion paralysis is observation of bilateral ptosis, tearing, loss of palpebral response (Fig. 13.64), and possible bilaterally drooped ears. Exposure keratitis evidenced by bilateral central corneal ulcers may be apparent in subacute or chronic cases. Close examination of the head may reveal obvious swelling along the zygomatic arch caudal to the orbits and may aid diagnosis. Cattle may be slightly off feed as a result of pain associated with temporomandibular joint movement; the owner's complaint is that the cow looks "droopy" and may be tearing bilaterally. Stanchion paralysis must be differentiated from bilateral middle ear infections and brainstem disease. Lack of vestibular signs, normal gait and strength, and usually the ability to eat help rule out other causes. The same signs could occasionally occur in animals run through a chute with a head catch, but this is less common because the aberrant catch location is apparent immediately, unlike a stanchion in which a trapped cow may remain unobserved for hours.

Treatment

Symptomatic therapy with topical and systemic antiinflammatories is indicated for traumatic lesions. Topical application of cold compresses may help reduce soft tissue edema at the site of acute injury. The cornea must be treated prophylactically with lubricant or broad-spectrum antibiotic ointments to prevent exposure keratitis until nerve function returns. The prognosis is good for injuries and poor for other causes (i.e., neoplasia).

For auriculopalpebral nerve injury caused by a stanchion, intially cold and then warm compresses and topical antiinflammatory drugs may suffice for therapy. The corneas need to be protected with ophthalmic lubricants or broad-spectrum antibiotic ointments three to four times per day. If there are no contraindications to the use of dexamethasone, one IM injection of 20 to 30 mg in an adult cow may quicken resolution of the problem. Careful evaluation of the cornea for evidence of ulceration should always be performed before systemic corticosteroids are used at these doses.

Cranial Nerves IX and X

Retropharyngeal abscesses or cellulitis may involve the pharyngeal branches of CNs IX and X, resulting in varying degrees of dysphagia. One cause of such infection is the trauma secondary to excessively vigorous use of a balling gun or other oral device. Treatment of the primary infection is necessary to resolve the dysphagia.

Sympathetic Nerves

Although not a CN, the function of the sympathetic nerves that innervate the head should be examined during the CN examination. The preganglionic sympathetic axons in the cervical portion of the sympathetic trunk are at risk of injury when needles are placed in the external jugular vein for drug injection or for obtaining blood samples. The sympathetic trunk is in the carotid sheath associated with the vagus nerve (vagosympathetic trunk) and the common carotid artery. Although this sheath is deep to the sternomastoideus muscle, which separates it from the external jugular vein, occasionally it is injured during a difficult venipuncture. This results in a unique paralysis referred to as Horner's syndrome.

The most obvious clinical signs are ipsilateral ptosis and a dry muzzle only on the paralyzed side. There will be slight miosis and a very slight elevation of the third eyelid on the paralyzed side (see Video Clip 13.37). The skin will be slightly warmer on that side of the face, which is best felt in the ear. This is because of the cutaneous vasodilation that occurs, which also causes a nasal mucosal congestion and a decreased airway diameter through that nasal cavity (see Figs. 4.6 and 4.7). On a cold wintry day, an astute observer will see less mist at this nostril during expiration (see Fig. 4.7). Usually this sympathetic paralysis will resolve spontaneously over a few days if it is only because of some local hemorrhage at the needle puncture site. Some drugs and calcium solutions that are injected inadvertently into the perivascular connective tissues at this site will result in an inflammation that can involve the components of the carotid sheath and produce a longer lasting sympathetic paralysis, which may be more difficult to treat and resolve.

Neuromuscular Junction

Botulism

Etiology

Signs of botulism in cattle may follow the ingestion of toxin produced by various strains of *Clostridium botulinum*. This organism is a gram-positive spore-forming rod that is an obligate anaerobe and has been subdivided into types based on antigenic variation of the potent exotoxin produced. The neurotoxins that result in the clinical disease of botulism are extremely potent blockers of acetylcholine release at neuromuscular junctions and other cholinergic nerve endings. Currently, at least eight toxin types are recognized: A, B, Ca, Cb, D, E, F, and G. *C. botulinum* is ubiquitous in soil and decaying plant and vegetable material. In general, type B is the most common cause of botulism in the eastern United States; type A is much more common west of the Rocky Mountains. Types C and D are found in the intestinal tract of many animals and birds. Therefore contamination of feedstuffs or water supplies with carrion or dead animals may increase the risk of botulism in cattle subsequently ingesting this feed or water. Poultry litter applied to pastures is a risk factor for types C and D in cattle grazing those fields. Similarly, phosphorus deficiency may create pica in cattle, so decaying carcasses become attractive food sources for these cattle. This phenomenon of botulism in phosphorus-deficient cattle is well described in South Africa where the disease has been called "lamziekte." Types other than C and D usually are saprophytes of soil and water that proliferate in stagnant or decaying vegetable matter.

   C. botulinum releases the neurotoxin during its vegetative growth phase, and ingestion of preformed toxin followed by intestinal absorption is the most common route of entry, but occasional cases of toxicoinfectious botulism and wound botulism may be encountered. Toxicoinfectious botulism implies vegetative growth of *C. botulinum* spores in an anaerobic or necrotic region of the GI tract of the patient with subsequent systemic absorption of the toxin. Wound botulism—similar to tetanus—implies that a necrotic wound that provides an anaerobic environment may allow the vegetative growth of *C. botulinum* spores and subsequent absorption of the toxin into the bloodstream of the patient. However, ingestion of preformed toxin in feedstuffs such as silages and brewer's grains contaminated with *C. botulinum* and, more importantly, its toxin, has caused most outbreaks of this disease in cattle. Improperly ensiled forages that never reach a pH less than 4.5 may be at much greater risk of harboring both live *C. botulinum* and toxin. An increased incidence of botulism caused mostly by *C. botulinum* type B has been seen in association with the use of silage bags and round bales for forage storage, and feeding improperly fermented haylage. Cattle may be slightly less sensitive to botulinum toxin and therefore less clinically susceptible to the disease than horses.

Clinical Signs

Clinical signs usually occur within 1-3 days of ingestion of the toxin. Anorexia and weakness predominate as clinical signs of botulism. Affected cattle that can still stand may tremble, stumble, or hang their heads because of weakness in the neck musculature. Salivation, pharyngeal paralysis, and mild tongue weakness are the major signs that indicate an inability or reduced ability to prehend and swallow food or water. Affected animals may continually chew the same bite of food without swallowing it. Animals that retain the ability to drink and eat—albeit reduced transiently—may have a better chance for survival. A recumbent cow may lie with the head tucked in the flank and her muzzle resting on the ground (Fig. 13.65). Although tongue tone seems preserved better in cattle than horses, the tongue may protrude from the mouth in severe cases, and drooling of saliva is common.

   Ruminal contractions are weak or absent and feces may vary from excessively dry (lack of water intake, hypocalcemia) to diarrhea (perhaps associated with spoiled feed materials that contained toxin). Reported heart rates in affected cattle usually are normal or elevated, although Dr. Fox always taught that bradycardia is typical (Fox FH, personal communication, 1985, Ithaca, NY).

   Urine dribbling may be observed, resulting from atonic distention of the urinary bladder and loss of tone in the urethralis muscle. Tail tone is also lost. Ptosis and a mild mydriasis with slower than normal pupillary response to direct light have been detected in some patients.

   The severity of disease is directly proportional to the amount of toxin ingested. Unfortunately, the amount is impossible to assess clinically. In general, recumbency and an inability to rise are bad prognostic signs. Severely affected cattle may die within 1 to 3 days. Cattle that show signs of botulism but can still rise from recumbency, eat, and drink, have a much better chance of survival.

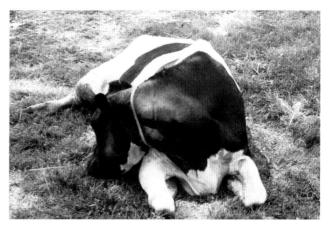

• **Fig. 13.65** An adult cow with generalized weakness from botulism. She was one of several that became affected when a new grass silage that had not been properly fermented was fed. The cow was recumbent for nearly 30 days but recovered with supportive care.

Diagnosis

Although the clinical signs can be highly suggestive, identification of toxin in the ruminal contents, feces, wound, or suspected feed or water is the only means possible to definitively diagnose botulism. Unfortunately, the amount of toxin necessary to cause toxicosis in animals is often very small and may be difficult to detect. Mouse inoculation with extracts of feed or intestinal contents is the standard laboratory test. Both susceptible mice and mice passively immunized with antitoxin are used in these methods. Few laboratories provide this service, and the attending veterinarian will need to contact diagnostic laboratories if confirmation is essential. PCR for detection of the neurotoxin gene of *C. botulinum* type B has been found to be very sensitive and specific. Necropsy reveals no diagnostic lesions. A differential diagnosis list for botulism could include selenium deficiency (white muscle disease). This condition can closely mimic botulism; for example, we recently diagnosed an adult Holstein bull with the highly suggestive clinical signs of dysphagia, persistent displacement of the soft palate and aspiration pneumonia with white muscle disease due to a near absence of selenium in the blood. With selenium treatment the bull made a complete recovery (Fig. 13.66).

Severely hypokalemic cattle (serum potassium <2.2 mEq/L) share some of the clinical features of botulism, specifically, recumbency with marked flaccid paralysis. Simple bloodwork can be used to rule out this differential, but one should be aware of the need to process and measure serum for potassium quantitation promptly so as to avoid falsely elevated results caused by erythrocyte lysis.

Treatment and Prevention

Treatment is largely supportive because toxin already fixed to neuromuscular receptors is irreversibly bound until natural deterioration occurs. Antitoxin may be indicated, as in tetanus, as an immediate treatment to counteract circulating toxin not yet bound to receptors. Polyvalent equine origin antitoxins for *C. botulinum* are available and have been used occasionally in the treatment of bovine botulism patients. Although certainly indicated, polyvalent antitoxins may not be readily available, are expensive, and do not ensure efficacy because the exact type (e.g., A, B, C, or D) of *C. botulinum* toxin affecting the patient may not be known. If available and indicated based on geographic probability of toxin type (type B in the eastern United States), they may be of use as an initial treatment.

If ingestion of feedstuffs containing toxin is the suspected source, cathartics and oral medication to prevent further absorption are indicated. Mineral oil and high-volume saline cathartics administered through a stomach tube may be helpful in this regard. Magnesium products should be avoided because they may further neuromuscular weakness. Similarly, antibiotics such as procaine penicillin, tetracycline, and aminoglycosides should be avoided. Cholinergic drugs have been used but are of little clinical use, may serve to excite the animal, and subsequently contribute to respiratory failure. Obviously, feeding of forage or water suspected to be the source of the toxin should be stopped.

In individuals suspected of having wound origin botulism or toxicoinfectious botulism, crystalline penicillin, drainage and aeration of wounds, and supportive therapy are indicated.

Dehydrated patients or those that cannot eat or drink may be given water, alfalfa pellet gruels, or rumen transfaunates through a stomach tube.

Prophylactic vaccination with toxoid may be administered when the type of botulinum toxin is known and the cattle continue to have risk of exposure. This should be repeated two to three times at 2-week intervals. Yearly boosters are then recommended. In one type B outbreak, this allowed the contaminated forage to be fed rather than destroyed after cattle had been fully immunized. The authors

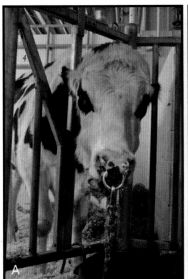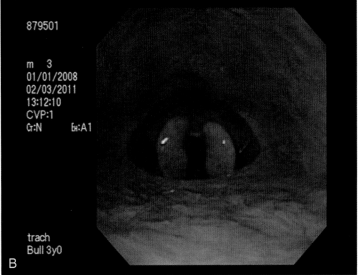

• **Fig. 13.66** A 3-year-old Holstein bull with weight loss, dysphagia (**A**), and persistent displacement of the soft palate (**B**) caused by selenium deficiency.

also recommended not using the manure from affected or recovering cattle for fertilization of gardens or fields that will contain forage crops for at least 8 weeks. *C. botulinum* spores could contaminate milk products, although most are killed by pasteurization.

Vaccination of affected animals with toxoid is indicated if risk of toxin exposure is high regardless of apparent recovery because the dose of toxin required to cause disease is so minute that it may not induce lasting humoral antibody production against *C. botulinum*.

Myasthenia Gravis

Myasthenia gravis is rare in cattle. There is no description of the acquired immune-mediated form. A congenital form occurs in Brahman calves, and the gene defect responsible for the inability to form functional acetylcholine receptors on the muscle cell membrane has been determined. This is an autosomal recessive inherited disorder in Brahman calves but has also been seen in a Holstein calf that "outgrew" the condition (see Video Clip 13.38). Affected calves have difficulty standing; prefer to lie in sternal recumbency; walk with very short strides; and quickly fatigue, tremble, and collapse. They show immediate brief improvement after IV anticholinesterase treatment using edrophonium (Tensilon). The defect is permanent.

Muscle Disorders

Myotonia

A form of inherited congenital myotonia has been recognized in a breed of buffalo cattle in Brazil that is similar to what has been seen since the late 1800s in goats. This is a disorder of the muscle cell membrane that permits episodes of continuous contraction of muscle cells without relaxation. The limb extensor muscles are primarily affected. The myotonic episodes can be elicited by sudden, exciting events. Affected cattle suddenly develop extensor rigidity of their limbs and often fall onto their sides. If left alone, they will relax in a few minutes, stand and walk with a mild stiffness, and then be normal for a short period in which they are refractory to further episodes. The diagnosis can be supported by electromyographic studies. In goats, a chloride channel defect in the muscle cell membrane has been described. Whether or not such a channel defect exists in affected cattle remains to be determined.

Metabolic Disorders

Diffuse neuromuscular signs occur acutely in cattle with hypokalemia, hypocalcemia, and hypomagnesemia. Hypokalemia leading to severe paresis and recumbency may occur because of overzealous treatment with mineralocorticoid drugs used for treating ketosis or mastitis. The clinical signs of severe neuromuscular paresis mimic those seen with hypocalcemia. Occasionally, cattle are found dead. Affected cattle generally have plasma potassium levels below 2.2 mg/dL and

are recumbent. They may be confused for botulism cases as described earlier. Treatment is generally unsuccessful in larger cattle because of secondary muscle damage from being down. Potassium chloride (½–1 lb) given via oral-rumen tube is the best treatment.

Sporadic cases of hypomagnesemia occur in dairy cattle, and the reason for these is rarely proven. Clinical signs are generalized hyperexcitability, leading to recumbency and constant flashing of the third eyelid and seizure-like activity. Plasma magnesium is usually below 0.4 mg/dL (see Video Clip 15.1), CSF levels are similarly low, and there is an absence of measurable magnesium in the urine. Plasma calcium is also moderately decreased. Treatment is an IV magnesium and calcium preparation, best followed by an oral magnesium salt to prevent relapse. Postparturient hypocalcemia (milk fever) is discussed in Chapter 15. Myopathy and myositis are described in Chapter 12.

Diffuse Central Nervous System Disorders

Tetanus

Etiology

Tetanospasmin, a powerful exotoxin of *Clostridium tetani,* is the cause of tetanus in humans and animals. Although not a strict anaerobe, *C. tetani* is a spore-forming gram-positive rod that is commonly found in soil and the intestinal tracts of some animals. Both soil contamination and GI flora containing *C. tetani* may be more prevalent in some geographic regions than others and may be increased following flooding. Soil containing livestock feces is more likely to harbor *C. tetani.* The vegetative growth of *C. tetani* eventually will result in spore formation. Spores are viable in soil for years and are not easily destroyed. In addition to tetanospasmin, *C. tetani* produces two other exotoxins; tetanolysin and a peripherally active nonspasmogenic toxin. Of these, tetanolysin seems to contribute greatly to the pathogenicity of *C. tetani* in vivo by promoting local tissue necrosis at sites of vegetative growth, thereby lowering oxygen tension in tissue.

After gaining access into soft tissue, *C. tetani* spores convert to vegetative forms when tissue necrosis, relative or absolute anaerobic environments, and other favorable microbial growth requirements are present. Washed spores of *C. tetani* placed in healthy oxygenated tissue may never vegetate. Therefore puncture wounds, deep wounds with substantial tissue necrosis, heavy purulence within a wound, and mixed infections that produce many exotoxins and endotoxin that damage adjacent tissue, create the greatest risks for *C. tetani* growth.

In cattle, the most common infection sites associated with tetanus are umbilical infections in neonatal calves, dehorning wounds, castration wounds, castration by elastrator bands, nose rings, overly tight neck chains, tail docking with elastrator bands, sole abscesses, ear-tag wounds, chronic sinus infections, deep necrotic wounds of any location, necrotic lesions in the vulva or vagina secondary to dystocia, and severe metritis in recently calved cattle. Other sites of infection certainly have been observed, and in some cases, the location of the infection cannot be found.

Dr. Francis Fox suggested considering infection at the site of deciduous teeth about to be lost in younger cattle as a possibility in such instances (Fox FH, personal communication, 1970, Cornell University). However, it appears that overgrowth of massive numbers of *C. tetani* in the forestomach may occasionally result in tetanus, thereby explaining sporadic cases without obvious wounds or infection sites. This is an attractive theory, albeit difficult to prove.

After becoming established at the site of infection, *C. tetani* produces tetanospasmin, which seeks local vasculature and nerve endings. The toxin is thought to bind to the axons of alpha motor neurons at the neuromuscular junction and pass in a retrograde fashion via these axons to the neuronal cell body in the ventral horn of the spinal cord. Here, the toxin passes into the presynaptic inhibitory neurons (Renshaw cells) within the ventral gray column and inhibits function of these neurons. The toxin inhibits glycine release from the Renshaw cells, a neurotransmitter normally responsible for limiting the duration and intensity of motor neuron discharge. Within the brainstem tetanospasmin also inhibits the release of γ-aminobutyric acid from inhibitory interneurons; collectively, therefore, tetanospasmin "inhibits the inhibition" of alpha motor nerves, resulting in a continuous contraction producing the rigidity defined as tetanus. By definition, tetanus is the clinical sign of continuous contraction of antigravity-extensor muscles that is not intermittent. Somewhat confusingly, in classical medical literature *tetany* has been a term used to describe brief but continuous contraction of these extensor muscles in an intermittent pattern such as can be seen with a variety of endocrine and metabolic diseases. Most veterinary clinicians use the term *tetanus* for the disease caused by the toxins of *C. tetani*.

Clinical Signs

Clinical signs may be mild or severe, with rapid progression indicating a guarded prognosis. A stiff gait is classic for tetanus in cattle, but many confined animals are never observed walking. The stiffness may initially appear as lameness in just one limb, especially if that limb contains the source of infection (i.e., sole abscess), but this is rare. A sawhorse stance is typical because of extensor muscle rigidity and tetany in the major limb muscles. Bloat and an anxious expression characterized by the ears held back, eyelids held open widely, head extended, and nostrils flared are typical in cattle (Figs. 13.67 and 13.68) (see Video Clip 13.39). Bloat probably results from failure of eructation because the complex act of eructation requires interaction of striated muscles in the larynx, pharynx, and proximal esophagus—all muscles that could be affected by the toxin. The tail head is raised away from the perineum, and this response is often apparent when the animal's temperature is taken. Rather than having the tail snap back down over the anus, the tail remains elevated and should raise the clinician's index of suspicion for tetanus. The muscles of mastication are involved and give rise to the layperson's term "lockjaw." Attempts to open the mouth are met with extreme rigidity of the mandibles and only serve to upset the patient.

Affected cattle usually lose the ability to eat because efforts to chew result in tetany. They frequently, at least transiently, lose the ability to drink and thus may become progressively dehydrated. Prolapse of the nictitans is apparent in most, but not all, cattle. Passive prolapse of the nictitans results from the disinhibited retractor oculi muscles. Prolapse of the nictitans and other clinical signs can be accentuated by provoking muscular activity through visual, auditory, or touch stimuli applied to the patient.

Clinical signs are unmistakable in cattle with advanced tetanus but may be more subtle in milder and earlier cases.

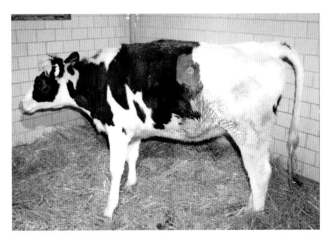

• **Fig. 13.67** Patient with tetanus showing an anxious expression with the ears held caudally, raised tail head, and sawhorse stance. A temporary indwelling ruminal trocar has been placed because of chronic bloat. A rumen fistula is a more useful technique than trocharization for treatment of bovine tetanus.

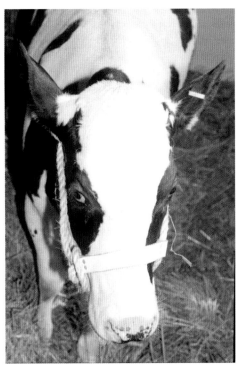

• **Fig. 13.68** Passive protrusion of the nictitans and anxious expression with ears retracted caudally in a patient with tetanus.

On many occasions, veterinarians have been embarrassed by misdiagnosing tetanus; the usual mistake is to concentrate on bloat as a sign of GI disease with resulting erroneous diagnoses such as traumatic reticuloperitonitis or indigestion. Because not all patients show all of the classical signs described, there are two physical examination techniques that will help the physician avoid overlooking tetanus in mild cases:

1. If the animal is confined (i.e., stanchion, tie stall), release her and make her move so the gait can be observed.
2. Look at the animal's face, and if necessary, attempt to open the mouth.

These two procedures may sound simple, but they are frequently not performed, especially on stanchioned cattle.

Depending on the severity of clinical signs and the ease of treatment for the site of infection, affected cattle have a highly variable prognosis. Severely affected animals or cattle with rapidly progressive signs may be unable to rise, continue to struggle to rise, and eventually die from respiratory failure as the muscles of respiration suffer from tetany during exertion. Regarding recumbency in tetanus patients, cattle are more fortunate than horses because they tend to lie in sternal recumbency, whereas horses prefer to lie in lateral recumbency. When an animal of either species with tetanus lies in lateral recumbency, it may "self-destruct" because the initial attempt to raise the neck and flex the extended limbs provokes tetany, and a vicious cycle of lateral recumbency, extensor rigidity, pain, panic, and exertion ensues.

Most cattle that die from tetanus do so because of exertion and respiratory failure. Bloat also can result in death as can aspiration pneumonia. Musculoskeletal injuries such as fractures of the femur and hip luxations are other common reasons for the demise of tetanus patients. Affected cattle housed on slippery floors are at much greater risk of musculoskeletal injury or difficulty in rising and resultant respiratory failure.

Diagnosis

The diagnosis is usually based on the clinical signs shown by the patient. These signs disappear immediately after death in patients with tetanus, so confirmation of tetanus antemortem is based on ruling out other diseases, hoping to find the site of growth of *C. tetani*, and demonstrating the organism through Gram stain or cultures. Similarly, if the site of infection is found in a patient showing signs of tetanus, pus or necrotic tissue from the site may be examined microscopically or cultured to confirm *C. tetani*. However, failure to find *C. tetani* organisms should never rule out tetanus in a patient with obvious clinical signs.

Treatment

Tetanus is one of the most frustrating diseases to diagnose in any species because there is no way for the clinician to offer an accurate prognosis for patients with the condition. Myriad complications are possible. Empathy for the patient is essential because the disease causes exquisite pain, and

therapeutic exuberance by neophyte clinicians often results in further patient suffering rather than cure.

Firstly, the infection that has resulted in tetanus must be addressed. If the wound or site of infection can be identified readily, it should be cleaned, debrided, and drained after sedation and providing analgesia for the patient. The wound should be aerated as well as possible to minimize further vegetative growth and toxin production in an anaerobic environment. Tetanus antitoxin should be administered at least once and may be repeated at 12-hour intervals for three or four total treatments even when the site of infection is not apparent. Tetanus antitoxin obviously cannot counteract toxin already bound to receptors but may bind any circulating toxin or toxin not yet fixed. Treatment with antitoxin is empiric, and dosages suggested vary from 1500 to 300,000 U. We usually administer 15,000 U once or twice parenterally as initial therapy. Intrathecal administration of tetanus antitoxin of equine origin should not be performed.

Penicillin should be used to kill vegetative *C. tetani* at the wound site. If no wound is obvious then penicillin should be administered parenterally. Usually procaine penicillin at 22,000 to 33,000 U/kg body weight twice daily is used for this purpose. In calves or extremely valuable cows, crystalline penicillin administered through a jugular catheter at the same dose but four times daily provides less discomfort for the patient and decreased excitement associated with the IM or SC injections.

Tetanic episodes, excitement, and the pain associated with tetanic episodes should be minimized. Therefore cotton should be packed into the patient's external ear canals to muffle sound stimuli; the animal should be kept by itself in a darkened box stall in as quiet a location as possible. All treatments should be performed by a single concerned caretaker, and footing and bedding in the stall should minimize any slippery floor conditions. Tranquilization is very helpful in most cases. Acepromazine is used for this purpose, and the dosage should be adjusted to the individual patient. Most adult patients receive 20 to 40 mg of acepromazine two to four times daily. This can be given IV through an indwelling catheter or IM. Sedation helps the animal remain calm, and most cows continue to be able to rise from sternal recumbency at this dosage. Milking machines should be brought to the cow, or she should be hand milked. Judicious use of analgesics may be indicated at the veterinarian's discretion.

A ruminal fistula via rumenotomy should be established in tetanus patients that have sufficient free-gas bloat that would otherwise require stomach tubing. Because stomach tubing and other therapeutic measures about the head cause tremendous patient anxiety, it is best to sedate the patient; use analgesics; and, following standard surgical preparation of the left paralumbar fossa and with the use of local anesthesia, surgically create a ruminal fistula of 2.5 to 5.0 cm in diameter. The fistula allows free gas to escape until the patient regains the ability to eructate and allows a portal for water and alfalfa pellets to be placed in the rumen of patients unable to eat or drink. The fistula thus avoids stressful procedures that otherwise may be required two or more times daily.

In most cases tetanus patients should be considered to be in critical condition for 14 days after the diagnosis. Mild cases may respond within 1 week, but this is unusual. Patients that continue to deteriorate despite therapy and become recumbent or cannot rise or develop other complications usually die. Patients that stabilize within 24 to 48 hours of the onset of therapy have a chance for recovery. Many patients stabilize only to develop unforeseen complications resulting in death or necessitating euthanasia up to 5 to 10 days after the initial diagnosis. Regaining the ability to drink is one of the most encouraging signs of improvement and tends to occur 3 to 5 days after the onset of treatment in cattle that initially could not do so. All possible complications must be anticipated and avoided. Cattle that assume lateral recumbency usually self-destruct. In our experience, mechanical support aids such as slings are worthless in this situation because they tend to further excite cattle that already are in severe tetanus. Patients that survive 14 days generally make a full recovery.

Prevention

Although cattle are thought to be less susceptible to tetanus than horses and other farm animals, there is no reason to tolerate blatant risks such as filthy surgery, neglected wounds, and the use of elastrator bands in unvaccinated animals. Cattle at risk or in certain geographic areas with a high incidence of tetanus can be vaccinated easily and inexpensively with tetanus toxoid twice during the first year of life and once yearly thereafter. As with botulism, the amount of toxin associated with clinical signs of tetanus may not be adequate to create sufficient, protective humoral antibodies in the patient. Therefore cattle affected with tetanus should be vaccinated twice at a 2- to 4-week interval to ensure future protection against the disease.

Congenital Tetany

An inherited congenital tetany has been reported in newborn polled Hereford calves. This has been described in the literature both as congenital myoclonus and hereditary neuraxial edema. Neither of these terms is correct. The clinical sign exhibited is tetany, a continuous contraction of antigravity muscles that is mildly intermittent. Myoclonus is a sudden contraction of muscles followed by immediate relaxation. When myoclonus is continuous, a tremor results. There are no microscopic lesions in the CNS, and therefore neuraxial edema is not present in this disorder. These calves have an abnormality in the gene responsible for the normal development of the glycine receptors on neuronal cell membranes (see Video Clip 13.40). Therefore, the glycine released from inhibitory interneurons, the Renshaw cells, cannot bind to alpha motor neurons of extensor muscles, resulting in their lack of inhibition. Cranial motor neurons are not affected. Calves are born recumbent and unable to get up. Tetany is

exacerbated by stimulation of the calf, such as just tapping it on the muzzle. The intermittent periods of mild relaxation never are enough to allow the calf to stand. This disorder is similar to an inherited glycine receptor deficiency in humans that causes episodic tetany, referred to as startle syndrome or hyperekplexia.

Suggested Readings

Abeye, S., Naylor, J. M., Wassef, A. W., et al. (2007). D-lactic acid-induced neurotoxicity in a calf model. *Am J Physiol Endocrinol Metab, 293*, E558–E565.

Abtutarbush, S. M., & Petrie, L. (2007). Treatment of hypernatremia in neonatal calves with diarrhea. *Can Vet J, 48*, 184–187.

Agerholm, J. S., Hewicker-Trautwein, M., Peperkamp, K., et al. (2015). Virus-induced congenital malformations in cattle. *Acta Vet Scand 24, 57*, 54–68.

Amat, S., McKinnon, J. J., Olkowski, A. A., et al. (2013). Understanding the role of sulfur-thiamine interaction in the pathogenesis of sulfur-induced polioencephalomalacia in beef cattle. *Res Vet Sci, 95*, 1081–1087.

Aschenbroich, S., Nemeth, N., Rech, R., et al. (2013). Mannheimia haemolytica A1-induced fibrinosuppurative meningoencephalitis in a naturally-infected Holstein-Friesian calf. *J Comp Pathol, 149*, 167–177.

Behling-Kelly, E., Kim, K. S., & Czuprynski, C. J. (2007). Haemophilus somnus activation of brain endothelial cells: potential role for local cytokine production and thrombosis in central nervous system (CNS) infection. *Thromb Haemost, 98*, 823–830.

Bernier Gosselin, V., Babkine, M., Gains, M. J., et al. (2014). Validation of an ultrasound imaging technique of the tympanic bullae for the diagnosis of otitis media in calves. *J Vet Intern Med, 28*, 1594–1601.

Bertin, F. R., Baseler, L. J., Wilson, C. R., et al. (2013). Arsenic toxicosis in cattle: meta-analysis of 156 cases. *J Vet Intern Med, 27*, 977–981.

Bertone, I., Bellino, C., Alborali, G. L., et al. (2015). Clinical-pathological findings of otitis media and media-interna in calves and (clinical) evaluation of a standardized therapeutic protocol. *BMC Vet Res, 11*, 297.

Binanti, D., Fantinato, E., De Zani, D., et al. (2013). Segmental spinal cord hypoplasia in a Holstein Friesian calf. *Anat Histol Embryol, 42*, 316–320.

Bischoff, K., Higgins, W., Thompson, B., et al. (2014). Lead excretion in milk of accidentally exposed dairy cattle. *Food Addit Contam Part A Chem Anal Control Expo Risk Assess, 31*, 839–844.

Bischoff, K., Thompson, B., Erb, H. N., et al. (2012). Declines in blood lead concentrations in clinically affected and unaffected cattle accidentally exposed to lead. *J Vet Diagn Invest, 24*, 182–187.

Borges, A. S., Mendes, L C., Luvizotto, M. L., et al. (2003). Myelopathy in Holstein x Gir calves in Brazil. *J Vet Intern Med, 17*, 730–731.

Bratton, G. R., Zmudzki, J., Bell, M. C., et al. (1981). Thiamin (vitamin B1) effects of lead intoxication and deposition of lead in tissue: therapeutic potential. *Toxicol Appl Pharmacol, 59*, 164–172.

Braun, U., Malbon, A., Kochan, M., et al. (2017). Computed tomographic findings and treatment of a bull with pituitary gland abscess. *Acta Vet Scand, 59*(1), 8–14.

Braun, U., Feige, K., Schweizer, G., et al. (2005). Clinical findings and treatment of 30 cattle with botulism. *Vet Rec, 156*, 438–441.

Butler, J. A., Sickles, S. A., Johanns, C. J., et al. (2000). Pasteurization of discard mycoplasma mastitic milk used to feed calves: thermal effects on various mycoplasma. *J Dairy Sci, 83,* 2285–2288.

Cascio, K. E., Belknap, E. B., Schultheiss, P. C., et al. (1999). Encephalitis induced by bovine herpesvirus 5 and protection by prior vaccination or infection with bovine herpesvirus 1. *J Vet Diagn Invest, 11,* 134–139.

Constable, P. D. (2004). Ruminant neurologic diseases. *Vet Clin N Am Food Anim Pract, 20,* 185–434.

Coppock, R. W., Wagner, W. C., Reynolds, J. D., et al. (1991). Evaluation of edetate and thiamine treatment of experimentally induced environmental lead poisoning in cattle. *Am J Vet Res, 52,* 1860–1865.

Cox, V. S. (1981). Understanding the downer cow syndrome. *Compend Contin Educ Pract Vet, 3,* S472–S478.

Cox, V. S., & Breazile, J. E. (1973). Experimental bovine obdurator paralysis. *Vet Rec, 93,* 109–110.

Cox, V. S., Breazile, J. E., & Hoover, T. R. (1975). Surgical and anatomic study of calving paralysis. *Am J Vet Res, 36,* 427–430.

Davis, T. E., Krook, L., & Warner, R. G. (1970). Bone resorption in hypovitaminosis A. *Cornell Vet, 60,* 90–119.

de Lahunta, A. (2014). *Veterinary neuroanatomy and clinical neurology* (4th ed.). Philadelphia: Elsevier.

De Vlamynck, C., Pille, F., & Vlaminck, L. (2014). Bovine spastic paresis: current knowledge and scientific voids. *Vet J, 202,* 228–235.

Del Médico Zajac, M. P., Ladelfa, M. F., Kotsias, F., et al. (2010). Biology of bovine herpesvirus 5. *Vet J, 184,* 138–145.

Del Médico Zajac, M. P., Puntel, M., Zamorano, P. I., et al. (2006). BHV-1 vaccine induces cross protection against BHV-5 disease in cattle. *Res Vet Sci, 81,* 327–334.

DeMeerschman, F., Focant, C., Detry, J., et al. (2005). Clinical, pathological and diagnostic aspects of congenital neosporosis in a series of naturally infected calves. *Vet Rec, 157,* 115–118.

Divers, T. J., Bartholomew, R. C., Messick, J. B., et al. (1986). Clostridium botulinum type B toxicosis in a herd of cattle and a group of mules. *J Am Vet Med Assoc, 188,* 382–386.

Divers, T. J., Blackmon, D. M., Martin, C. L., et al. (1986). Blindness and convulsions associated with vitamin A deficiency in feedlot steers. *J Am Vet Med Assoc, 189,* 1579–1582.

Divers, T., Sweeney, R., Rebhun, W. C., et al. (1992). Cerebrospinal fluid evaluation in cattle: a retrospective study. *Proceedings: Societé Francaise de Buiatrie,* 207–214.

Dyer, J. L., Yager, P., Orciari, L., et al. (2014). Rabies surveillance in the United States during 2013. *J Am Vet Med Assoc, 245,* 1111–1123.

Fecteau, G., Smith, B. P., & George, L. W. (2009). Septicemia and meningitis in the newborn calf. *Vet Clin North Am Food Anim Pract, 25,* 195–208.

Figueiredo, M. D., Perkins, G. A., & Opsina, P. A. (2004). Case report: discospondylitis in two first calf heifers. *Bovine Pract, 38*(1), 31–35.

Goeckmann, V., Rothammer, S., & Medugorac, I. (2016). Bovine spastic paresis: a review of the genetic background and perspectives for the future. *Vet J, 216,* 64–71.

Hemboldt, C. F., Jungherr, E. L., & Eaton, H. D. (1953). The pathology of experimental hypovitaminosis A in young dairy animals. *Am J Vet Res, 14,* 343–354.

Henke, D., Rupp, S., Gaschen, V., et al. (2015). Listeria monocytogenes spreads within the brain by actin-based intra-axonal migration. *Infect Immun, 83,* 2409–2419.

Jamali, H., & Radmehr, B. (2013). Frequency, virulence genes and antimicrobial resistance of Listeria spp. isolated from bovine clinical mastitis. *Vet J, 198,* 541–542.

Johns, J. T., LaBore, D., & Evans, J. K. (1984). Ammoniated forages and bovine hysteria. *J Am Vet Med Assoc, 185,* 215.

Johnson, A. L., Sweeney, R. W., McAdams, S. C., et al. (2012). Quantitative real-time PCR for detection of the neurotoxin gene of Clostridium botulinum type B in equine and bovine samples. *Vet J, 194,* 118–120.

Kaneps, A. J., & Blythe, L. L. (1986). Diagnosis and treatment of brachial plexus trauma resulting from dystocia in a calf. *Compend Contin Educ Pract Vet, 8,* S4–S6.

Kelch, W. J., Kerr, L. A., Pringle, J. K., et al. (2000). Fatal Clostridium botulinum toxicosis in eleven Holstein cattle fed round bale barley haylage. *J Vet Diagn Invest, 12,* 453–455.

Konold, T., Gone, B., Ryder, S., et al. (2004). Clinical findings in 78 suspected cases of bovine spongiform encephalopathy in Great Britain. *Vet Rec, 155,* 659–666.

Kretschmar, A., Kaiser, M., Brehm, W., et al. (2016). Peripheral-limb pareses in cattle. Part 1: General causes and specific pareses of the fore- and hindlimbs. *Tierarztl Prax Ausg G Grosstiere Nutztiere, 44*(6), 388–388.

Kretschmar, A., Kaiser, M., Brehm, W., et al. (2017). Peripheral limb pareses in cattle. Part 2: Diagnostics, prognosis and therapy. *Tierarztl Prax Ausg G Grosstiere Nutztiere, 45*(1), 47–59.

Lee, K. J., Kishimoto, M., Shimizu, J., et al. (2011). Use of contrast-enhanced CT in the diagnosis of abscesses in cattle. *J Vet Med Sci, 73,* 113–115.

Li, L., Diab, S., McGraw, S., et al. (2013). Divergent astrovirus associated with neurologic disease in cattle. *Emerg Infect Dis, 19,* 1385–1392.

Lindström, M., Myllykoski, J., Sivelä, S., et al. (2010). Clostridium botulinum in cattle and dairy products. *Crit Rev Food Sci Nutr, 50,* 281–304.

Lorenz, I., & Gentile, A. (2014). D-lactic acidosis in neonatal ruminants. *Vet Clin N Am Food Anim Pract, 30*(2), 317–331.

Marin, M. S., Quintana, S., Leunda, M. R., et al. (2014). Toll-like receptor expression in the nervous system of bovine alpha-herpesvirus-infected calves. *Res Vet Sci, 97,* 422–429.

Maunsell, F. P., Woolums, A. R., Francoz, D., et al. (2011). Mycoplasma bovis infections in cattle. *J Vet Intern Med, 25,* 772–783.

McClure, M., Kim, E., Bickhart, D., et al. (2013). Fine mapping for Weaver syndrome in Brown Swiss cattle and the identification of 41 concordant mutations across NRCAM, PNPLA8 and CTTNBP2. *PloS One, 8,* e59251.

McDuffee, L. A., Ducharme, N. G., & Ward, J. L. (1993). Repair of sacral fracture in two dairy cattle. *J Am Vet Med Assoc, 202,* 1126–1128.

Mitchell, K. J., Peters-Kennedy, J., Stokol, T., et al. (2011). Diagnosis of Parelaphostrongylus spp. infection as a cause of meningomyelitis in calves. *J Vet Diagn Invest, 23*(6), 1097–1103.

Moore, D. A., Kohrs, P., Baszler, T., et al. (2010). Outbreak of malignant catarrhal fever among cattle associated with a state livestock exhibition. *J Am Vet Med Assoc, 237*(1), 87–92.

Moreira, A. S., Raabis, S. M., Graham, M. E., et al. (2017). Identification by next generation sequencing of Aichivirus B in a calf with enterocolitis and neurologic signs. *J Vet Diagn Invest, 29*(2), 208–211.

Morgan, J. H. (1977). Infectious keratoconjunctivitis in cattle associated with Listeria monocytogenes. *Vet Rec, 100,* 113–114.

Oevermann, A., Di Palma, S., Doherr, M. G., et al. (2010). Neuropathogenesis of naturally occurring encephalitis caused by Listeria monocytogenes in ruminants. *Brain Pathol, 20,* 378–390.

Ollivett, T. L., & McGuirk, S. M. (2013). Salt poisoning as a cause of morbidity and mortality in neonatal dairy calves. *J Vet Intern Med, 27*, 592–595.

Otter, A., Welchman Dde, B., Sandvik, T., et al. (2009). Congenital tremor and hypomyelination associated with bovine viral diarrhoea virus in 23 British cattle herds. *Vet Rec, 164*, 771–778.

Oyster, R., Leipold, H. W., Troyer, D., et al. (1991). Clinical studies of bovine progressive degenerative myeloencephalopathy of Brown Swiss cattle. *Prog Vet Neurol, 2*, 159–164.

Parish, S. M., Maag-Miller, L., Besser, T. E., et al. (1987). Myelitis associated with protozoal infection in newborn calves. *J Am Vet Med Assoc, 191*, 1599–1600.

Paulsen, D. B., Noordsy, J. L., & Leipold, H. W. (1981). Femoral nerve paralysis in cattle. *Bov Pract, 2*, 14–26.

Payne, J. H., Hogg, R. A., Otter, A., et al. (2011). Emergence of suspected type D botulism in ruminants in England and Wales (2001 to 2009), associated with exposure to broiler litter. *Vet Rec, 168*, 640.

Pearson, E. G., & Kallfelz, F. A. (1982). A case of presumptive salt poisoning (water deprivation) in veal calves. *Cornell Vet, 72*, 142–149.

Perdrizet, J. A., Cummings, J. F., & deLahunta, A. (1985). Presumptive organophosphate-induced delayed neurotoxicity in a paralyzed bull. *Cornell Vet, 75*, 401–410.

Perdrizet, J. A., & Dinsmore, P. (1986). Pituitary abscess syndrome. *Compend Contin Educ Pract Vet, 8*, S311–S318.

Porter, B. F., Ridpath, J. F., Calise, D. V., et al. (2010). Hypomyelination associated with bovine viral diarrhea virus type 2 infection in a longhorn calf. *Vet Pathol, 47*, 658–663.

Pringle, J. K., & Berthiaume, L. M. M. (1988). Hypernatremia in calves. *J Vet Intern Med, 2*, 66–70.

Pumarola, M., Anor, S., Majo, N., et al. (1997). Spinal muscular atrophy in Holstein-Friesian calves. *Acta Neuropathol, 93*, 178–183.

Raisbeck, M. F. (1982). Is polioencephalomalacia associated with high sulfate diets? *J Am Vet Med Assoc, 180*, 1303–1305.

Rebhun, W. C., & deLahunta, A. (1982). Diagnosis and treatment of bovine listeriosis. *J Am Vet Med Assoc, 180*, 395–398.

Rebhun, W. C., et al. (1984). Compressive neoplasms affecting the bovine spinal cord. *Compend Contin Educ Pract Vet, 6*, S396–S400.

Reimer, J. M., Donawick, W. J., Reef, V. B., et al. (1988). Diagnosis and surgical correction of patent ductus venosus in a calf. *J Am Vet Med Assoc, 193*, 1539–1541.

Ricardo, P., Dell Armelina, R., Lomonaco, S., et al. (2013). Ruminant rhomboencephalitis-associated Listeria monocytogenes strains constitute a genetically homogenous group related to human outbreak strains. *Applied Environ Micro, 79*, 3059–3066.

Sánchez, S., Clark, E. G., Wobeser, G. A., et al. (2013). A retrospective study of non-suppurative encephalitis in beef cattle from western Canada. *Can Vet J, 54*, 1127–1132.

Saunders, L. Z., Sweet, J. D., Martin, S. M., et al. (1952). Hereditary congenital ataxia in Jersey calves. *Cornell Vet, 42*, 559–611.

Schuijt, G. (1990). Iatrogenic fractures of ribs and vertebrae during delivery in perinatally dying calves: 235 cases (1978-1988). *J Am Vet Med Assoc, 197*, 1196–1202.

Schweizer, G., Ehrensperger, F., Torgerson, P. R., et al. (2006). Clinical findings and treatment of 94 cattle presumptively diagnosed with listeriosis. *Vet Rec, 158*(17), 588–592.

Selimovic-Hamza, S., Boujon, C. L., Hilbe, M., et al. (2017). Frequency and pathological phenotype of bovine astrovirus CH13/NeuroS1 infection in neurologically-diseased cattle: towards assessment of causality. *Viruses, 9*(1), E12.

Sherman, D. M., & Ames, T. R. (1986). Vertebral body abscesses in cattle: a review of five cases. *J Am Vet Med Assoc, 188*, 608.

Smith, J. S., & Mayhew, I. G. (1977). Horner's syndrome in large animals. *Cornell Vet, 67*, 529–542.

Stokol, T., Divers, T. J., Arrigan, J. W., et al. (2009). Cerebrospinal fluid findings in cattle with central nervous system disorders: a retrospective study of 102 cases (1990-2008). *Vet Clin Pathol, 38*, 103–112.

Stuart, L. D., & Leipold, H. W. (1985). Pathologic findings in bovine progressive degenerative myeloencephalopathy ("weaver") of Brown Swiss cattle. *Vet Pathol, 22*, 13–23.

Testoni, S., Mazzariol, S., Daniele, D. P., et al. (2012). Ultrasonographic diagnosis of syringohydromyelia and segmental hypoplasia of the lumbar spinal cord in a calf. *J Vet Intern Med, 26*, 1485–1489.

Trefz, F. M., Lorch, A., Feist, M., et al. (2012). Metabolic acidosis in neonatal calf diarrhea—clinical findings and theoretical assessment of a simple treatment protocol. *J Vet Intern Med, 26*, 162–170.

Tryphonas, L., Hamilton, G. F., & Rhodes, C. S. (1974). Perinatal femoral nerve degeneration and neurogenic atrophy of quadriceps femoris muscle in calves. *J Am Vet Med Assoc, 164*, 801–807.

Tsuka, T., Yamamoto, N., Saneshige, M., et al. (2016). Computed tomographic images of discospondylitis in a calf. *J Vet Med Sci, 77*(12), 1689–1691.

Van Biervliet, J., Perkins, G. A., Woodie, B., et al. (2004). Clinical signs, computed tomographic imaging, and management of chronic otitis media/interna in dairy calves. *J Vet Intern Med, 18*, 907–910.

Vaughan, L. C. (1964). Peripheral nerve injuries: an experimental study in cattle. *Vet Rec, 76*, 1293–1301.

Wallis, A. S. (1963). Some observations on the epidemiology of tetanus in cattle. *Vet Rec, 75*, 188–191.

White, M. E., Whitlock, R. H., & deLahunta, A. (1975). A cerebellar abiotrophy of calves. *Cornell Vet, 65*, 476–491.

Wiedmann, M., Bruce, J. L., Knorr, R., et al. (1996). Ribotype diversity of Listeria monocytogenes strains associated with outbreaks of listeriosis in ruminants. *J Clin Microbiol, 34*, 1086–1090.

Zani, D. D., Romanò, L., Scandella, M., et al. (2008). Spinal epidural abscess in two calves. *Vet Surg, 37*, 801–808.

14

Ocular Diseases

NITA L. IRBY AND JOHN A. ANGELOS

Introduction

Exactly how much a dairy cow's vision contributes to the quality of her life cannot be fully comprehended by her caretakers, but good vision and comfortable, pain-free eyes are surely a right of every animal and something that we as their caretakers should try to provide whenever possible. Diseased eyes can cause a great deal of pain to patients, as those who have personally experienced corneal erosions or other painful ocular conditions will attest. In caring for cattle, our treatments should be directed at preventing ocular disease whenever possible, instituting treatment for diseases as soon as they occur, and providing pain relief as part of all treatment plans. Table 14.1 lists the most common ocular disorders of cattle.

Examination of the Eye

A general inspection of the globe, orbit, conjunctiva, and pupil size alongside a quick assessment of cranial nerves associated with the eye should be part of every physical examination because many systemic diseases manifest in the eye (see Figs. 3.51, 3.56, 3.57, and 3.58 A). A detailed ophthalmic examination is indicated any time the eye is the primary complaint, whenever vision is a concern, and as a component part of every detailed physical examination.

Proper restraint of the head of the cow is needed, or a complete ophthalmic examination is not safe for the patient or the examiner; a stanchion, head gate, or squeeze chute combined with proper haltering and tying of the head are critical. Nose tongs may be used but are not usually needed for tractable dairy cattle. When tying the cow's head for examination of one eye only, tie the head to the side of the cow with the nose in a neutral or lower position rather than with the nose elevated to avoid the normal downward movement of the eyes that occurs when the head is elevated (a normal vestibular reflex). When tying the head to examine both eyes, tying with two halters is recommended (see Fig. 4.32). Sedation with 0.01 to 0.03 mg/kg of xylazine intravenously may be used if needed, but is rarely required.

Most dairy cattle can be examined with minimal restraint and without eyelid blocks. However, when the eye is painful, bovine eyelids are sufficiently strong as to preclude a complete examination, and the eyelids may need to be temporarily paralyzed to facilitate a complete ophthalmic examination, or to permit certain diagnostic or therapeutic procedures. In these cases, akinesia of the eyelids may be achieved by placing a local anesthetic such as lidocaine hydrochloride perineurally around the palpebral branch of the auriculopalpebral nerve (Fig. 14.1). The nerve can be palpated midway along the zygomatic arch between the lateral canthus and the base of the ear, and 2 to 3 mL of local anesthetic should be placed adjacent to the palpable nerve. If the nerve cannot be palpated, 2 to 3 mL of local anesthetic can be deposited 3 to 5 cm caudal to the lateral canthus. If excisional or incisional biopsies of the cornea or conjunctiva or other such procedures are to be performed, it is helpful to carefully instill 0.5 to 1.0 mL of local anesthetic into the adjacent eyelid margin so that the patient does not feel instruments placed in contact with its eyelids.

As for any other species, a complete ophthalmic examination begins with a general assessment of the size and the position of the globe within the orbit. In cattle especially, globe position reflects the hydration status of the animal, with dehydrated cattle becoming enophthalmic proportional to their degree of dehydration (Fig. 14.2). Enophthalmos, exophthalmos, convergent or divergent strabismus, nystagmus, buphthalmos, gross ocular defects, or tumors are all noted at this stage of the examination. Before the head rope is tied, the vestibular eye reflexes in both eyes should be assessed (the normal movements of the globe that change with head position). Ideally, every bovine ocular examination should include a Schirmer tear test at this point, but if the globe appears moist and a visible meniscus of moisture is present between the eyelids and the globe, then this test can be skipped. Next, but *only* if the globes appear grossly normal *with no* evidence of corneal or scleral ulcerations or lacerations, the eyelids of both eyes should be closed, and the examiner should gently push both globes posteriorly into the orbit (retropulsion of the globes) to ensure that no space-occupying orbital masses are present (the eyes of most dairy cattle will retropulse at least 5 cm into the orbit). Next, as the globes are retropulsed again, the examiner should open the eyelids while pushing caudally on the globe to carefully

TABLE 14.1	The Most Common Ocular Disorders in Cattle in the United States	
Disorder	**Most Common Presenting Signs**
Infectious bovine keratoconjunctivitis	Afebrile, otherwise healthy animal Unilateral or bilateral ocular disease Central corneal ulcer or focal edema progressing to ulcer Occurs as outbreak or rarely may be single animal Most common in young or new additions to herd Resolves in 4–6 wks
Infectious bovine rhinotracheitis	Sick animal (nasal discharge, fever) Bilateral ocular disease Conjunctivitis (chemosis with white plaques), peripheral corneal edema 5–7 days later in disease Occurs as outbreak High morbidity, low mortality Most animals recover in 1–2 wks
Malignant catarrhal fever	Sick, febrile animal Bilateral ocular disease Peripheral keratitis with straight, deep intracorneal vessels starting at ≈5 days Hypopyon Panuveitis, panophthalmitis Low morbidity, high mortality
Squamous cell carcinoma	Otherwise healthy animal Unilateral or bilateral ocular disease Affected animals 5-10 yrs of age Painless until advanced Classic presentation; raised, pink-white, cauliflower-like mass at temporal limbus or chronic, nonhealing scabs or ulcers on eyelids Distribution of lesions; temporal limbus (75%), eyelids (15%), nictitans (10%)

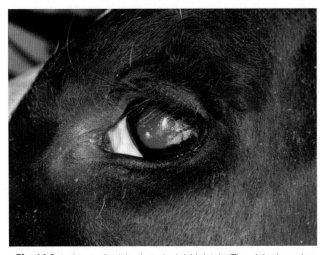

• **Fig. 14.2** Left eye of a dehydrated adult Holstein. The globe is sunken (note the space between the upper medial eyelid and the globe); the nictitans has prolapsed secondarily; and the cornea has a dry, lackluster appearance. (Courtesy of Dr. Mary Smith, Cornell University.)

inspect the free margin of each membrana nictitans (third eyelid) to ensure no masses or defects are present. The eyelids should be inspected to ensure that the eyelid margins are normal with no inflammation, masses, or defects present and that the eyelid margins are in the normal position (i.e., no entropion is present).

Next, a brief cranial nerve examination should be performed. The medial and lateral commissures of the eyelids should be gently tapped to elicit a blink or palpebral reflex. If the blink reflex is absent, then a defect in eyelid sensation (maxillary and ophthalmic branches of cranial nerve V) or a defect in motor control of the eyelids (facial nerve VII), or both, is present. Interestingly, it has recently been found that a reduced palpebral reflex in calves is highly specific for elevated D-lactate levels, likely caused by skeletal muscle weakness. However, one should be cautious regarding overinterpretation of an absent menace or blink response in neonatal calves during the first week of life because this reflex does not appear to be reliably present in true neonates. If a cranial nerve VII deficit is suspected, the examiner should assess ear position and lip and cheek tone in an effort to localize the lesion (see Figs. 13.14 and 13.17). Vision should be assessed historically and by performing a careful menace response to assess the retina and cranial nerve II (optic nerve tract), ensuring that the threatening hand gesture does not create air currents that the patient may feel and thus blink in response. (If air is felt, the ophthalmic branch of cranial nerve V may be being stimulated instead of the retina.) The pupils should be examined next; their shape should be a horizontal ellipse, and small brown protuberances should be present in the dorsal and ventral central pupillary margins (corpora nigra or granula iridica). To assess the pupillary light reflex (PLR), a bright light should be held *very close to the eye*, directed temporally in the eye, and the pupil should constrict in response (the pupil reflex being slower

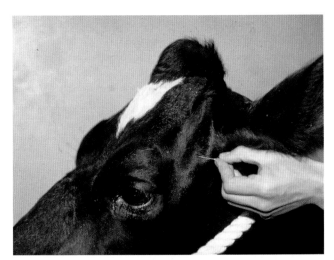

• **Fig. 14.1** Location for administration of local anesthetic for an auriculopalpebral nerve block in an adult cow. (Courtesy of Dr. Gareth Jones, UK.)

TABLE 14.2	Differential Diagnosis for Blindness in Cattle Based on Pupillary Light Reflexes
Blind; PLR present in both eyes	Polioencephalomalacia associated with thiamine deficiency
	Polioencephalomalacia associated with excess sulfur
	Lead or other heavy metal toxicity
	Sodium ion or salt toxicity or water deprivation
	Hepatic encephalopathy (PLR can be variable)
	Ketosis (rare)
	Hypoglycemia (rare)
	TEME or *Histophilus somni*–related vasculitis, thrombosis, hemorrhage or other lesions in the cerebral cortex
	Other causes of cerebrocortical disease (e.g., hemorrhage, trauma, abscess, necrosis)
	Some rabies cases
Blind; PLR absent in both eyes	Vitamin A deficiency (in young calves caused by optic canal stenosis; in all ages caused by widespread retinal degeneration secondary to impaired rhodopsin formation)
	Locoweed toxicity
	Male fern toxicity (*Dryopteris filix-mas*)
	Moldy corn (fumonisin mycotoxin)
	TEME or *Histophilus somni*–related vasculitis, thrombosis, retinal hemorrhage or other lesions in the retinas, optic nerve, optic chiasm, proximal optic tracts
	Other toxins or chemicals
	(Consider polioencephalomalacia because PLR may be absent in rare cases)

PLR, pupillary light reflex; *TEME,* thromboembolic meningoencephalitis.

in ungulates than in carnivores). After this direct PLR has been generated, the light should very quickly be directed into the opposite eye. If that pupil is already constricted and remains so (or constricts only slightly) with the light in place on the second eye, then both PLRs can be considered normal (this is called the swinging-flashlight test). If the patient is blind with absent PLRs, then the blindness is usually due to disease in the retina, optic nerve, optic chiasm, or proximal optic tracts. If the patient is blind and pupillary responses are normal, then in most cases, the blindness is due to cerebrocortical disease. Table 14.2 lists possible causes of blindness with and without intact PLRs.

Next, in *every* animal with eye pain or a complaint of eye pain, a strip containing fluorescein dye should be moistened, a drop should be applied to each eye and the cornea, and the conjunctiva should be assessed for abrasions or ulcerations. (This can be followed 2 to 15 minutes later by an inspection of the nares to ensure fluorescein has passed through the nasolacrimal system.) Fluorescein staining should be performed in a darkened area whenever possible. Corneal disease is the most common ocular problem in veterinary medicine, and the cornea should be examined carefully as part of every eye examination using direct, focal illumination followed by focal illumination directed from the sides of the cornea to retroilluminate

any abnormal areas. The pneumatic otoscope head (Part #20260), available as a component of the Welch Allyn Veterinary Diagnostic Set (Part #96220, Welch Allyn, Inc., Skaneateles Falls, NY; phone: 800-535-6663), is an excellent focal light source. After corneal and conjunctival ulcers and abrasions have been ruled out, topical anesthesia should be applied and intraocular pressure (IOP) readings obtained from both eyes, although this procedure is unfortunately rarely performed in dairy cattle (and may be the reason glaucoma is rarely diagnosed in this species). Decreased IOP readings support a diagnosis of uveitis, and increased IOPs are consistent with glaucoma.

After these components of the external ocular examination, a more detailed examination of the intraocular structures is always warranted. Again, this should be performed in a darkened area because it is challenging to accurately assess intraocular structures in a brightly lit environment. Using the instrument discussed earlier and looking through the magnifying lens, the anterior chamber, iris, and anterior lens should be examined. The vitreous, retina, and optic nerve should be examined subsequently using the otoscope head with the magnifying lens moved out of the line of the examiner's sight. All findings should be recorded.

Diseases of the Orbit

Inflammatory Orbital Diseases

Inflammatory diseases of the orbit, regardless of species or etiology, are usually acute to peracute in onset, accompanied by malaise, fever, difficulty opening the mouth, reluctance to eat, and discomfort when gentle backward pressure on the ipsilateral globe is applied through the closed eyelids (globe retropulsion).

Orbital Cellulitis
Etiology
Puncture wounds and lacerations of the periocular area, eyelids, or conjunctiva that allow opportunistic bacteria to invade orbital soft tissue are the most common causes of orbital cellulitis. Hooking the eyelid on a sharp object or stanchion lock can result in deep puncture wounds; migration of plant-origin fibrous foreign bodies from the oral cavity also may result in orbital cellulitis. Severe ocular infections that progress from endophthalmitis to panophthalmitis may then infect orbital soft tissue. Chronic inflammation in the orbit from cellulitis or foreign bodies may allow orbital or retrobulbar abscess formation.

Signs
Acute orbital cellulitis patients have rapid onset of a warm, painful swelling of the orbital region, eyelids, and nictitans; chemosis of the conjunctiva; and mild to severe exophthalmos (Fig. 14.3). The nictitans, variably prolapsed, may almost completely cover the cornea if the abscess is localized to the medial orbital region. Fever is usually present and, as a result of the exophthalmos, corneal ulceration caused by exposure

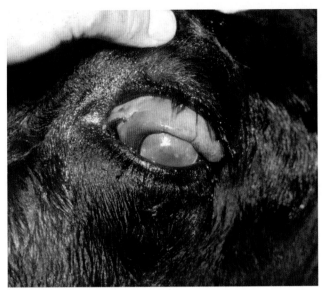

• **Fig. 14.3** Swelling of the orbit, eyelids, conjunctival chemosis, and exposure keratitis secondary to orbital cellulitis and conjunctival laceration. Note fibrin medially, covering the site of a presumed penetrating injury.

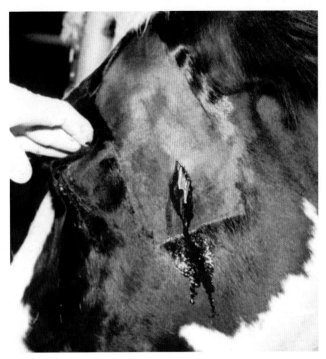

• **Fig. 14.4** Drainage of a chronic retrobulbar abscess.

keratitis often occurs as the globe is pushed outward to such an extent that the eyelids no longer protect the central cornea. Patients are often reluctant to eat or are totally off feed because of pain created in the retrobulbar tissues as the coronoid process of the mandible displaces these tissues during chewing. Furthermore, patients with acute orbital cellulitis will resent any attempts to manually displace the globe into the posterior orbit (retropulsion of the globe).

Chronic orbital cellulitis or abscessation results in a more insidious but painful exophthalmos with soft tissue swelling that may be more localized. Fever is inconsistent. As discussed later, if the major presenting sign is exophthalmos in an otherwise healthy cow that seems nonpainful when the globe is retropulsed, then lymphosarcoma should be considered. Exophthalmos caused by orbital lymphosarcoma usually is chronic in onset and mild to severe with attendant ocular inflammation (see following discussion). However, some cases of ocular lymphosarcoma appear to have an acute to peracute onset and may be confused with orbital cellulitis.

Diagnosis

Acute to peracute ocular and periocular signs coupled with fever, anorexia, and resistance to retropulsion suggest acute orbital cellulitis. Definitive diagnosis is potentially aided by finding an entry wound in the eyelid, conjunctiva, or periocular tissues (see Fig. 14.3), but in many cases, no entry wound can be found. Differential considerations include periorbital fractures with or without orbital hemorrhage (see Fig. 3.58), chronic sinusitis (see Figs. 4.10 and 4.11), orbit neoplasia or extension of a neoplasia from other areas into the orbit (see Fig. 4.6), brain abscesses (see Fig. 13.10, and discussion of cavernous sinus syndrome below). Physical examination (including sinus percussion and deep palpation of the topically anesthetized conjunctival sac), plus

radiographs, may help rule out periocular fractures; orbital ultrasound evaluation helps rule out neoplasia or the presence of a foreign body. Orbital and periocular tissue aspirates with or without ultrasound guidance may reveal large numbers of neutrophils. Computed tomography (CT) with contrast may be needed to rule out cavernous sinus syndrome and provides the most diagnostically useful images of this region in cases where physical diagnostics have been inconclusive as to a cause (see following discussion). A complete blood count (CBC) is worthwhile, but results may be normal in peracute cases or show only mild neutrophilia.

Chronic orbital cellulitis or abscessation must be differentiated from orbital neoplasia and chronic frontal sinusitis. A complete physical examination, percussion of sinuses, orbital ultrasonography, radiography or CT may be required in confusing cases. Serum globulin levels may be elevated to greater than normal reference ranges in cases that last longer than 2 weeks, suggesting chronic inflammation or abscessation.

Treatment and Prognosis

If physical examination, ultrasonography, or tissue aspirates suggest a localized abscess (uncommon) rather than diffuse cellulitis (common), then the abscess should be opened, and latex drains should be placed for 3 to 5 days. The recommended location for drain placement is caudal to the globe, ventral to the zygomatic arch (Fig. 14.4). Before performing any surgical procedures, a careful review of bovine skull and orbit anatomy is mandatory to avoid damaging the many critical structures located within, or adjacent to, the orbit, especially when attempting to lance a deep orbital abscess (Fig. 14.5). In addition to any other specific therapies provided, treatment protocols for acute orbital cellulitis should always

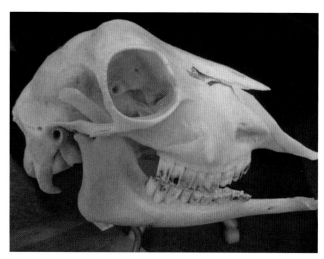

• **Fig. 14.5** Normal bovine skull. Note the thin shelf of bone in the floor of the orbit. This is a caudal extension of the maxillary sinus, easily breached during enucleation surgery if the surgeon is not careful.

include systemic broad-spectrum antibiotics. Although penicillin (22,000 U/kg once daily for 2 weeks) may be effective because *Trueperella pyogenes* is a likely causative organism, ampicillin may be a better choice because of its broader spectrum. Nonsteroidal antiinflammatory agents (NSAIDs) should be used. Flunixin meglumine is the recommended NSAID for the first 1 to 3 days in most cases (1.1 mg/kg slowly intravenously every 12-24 hours). Aspirin (240 to 480 grains orally, twice daily) provides mild analgesia and mild antiinflammatory action, as does meloxicam (1 mg/kg orally once daily for two days and then every other day (EOD)).

Warm compresses or gentle hosing of the tissues with warm water two or three times daily for 5 to 15 minutes may aid in reducing orbital and eyelid swelling and thereby lessen the degree of exophthalmos. Eyelid massage and eyelid manipulations plus gentle globe retropulsions (if the patient allows) aid in return of normal eyelid function.

Topical antibiotic ointment or lubricant should be applied liberally to the cornea to prevent exposure keratitis and should be repeated at least six times daily until the eyelids are again completely covering the exposed cornea. If no ulceration of the cornea is present and the axial cornea appears healthy, sterile ocular lubricating ointments may be used prophylactically three to four times daily. (Ocular lubricants with a petrolatum base are preferred for their longer contact time.) If exposure ulceration has occurred or if the cornea looks at all irregular but has not yet ulcerated, then the eye should be treated topically, ideally at least every 6 hours, with a broad-spectrum antibiotic ointment to control infection and 1% atropine ointment to provide cycloplegia and thus pain relief.

If an abscess cavity is found, gentle flushing may be performed once or twice daily if the cavity is not adjacent to the optic nerve, optic canal, or other posterior orbital foramina. Recurrent orbital abscesses or chronic cellulitis dictate more intensive diagnostic workup, especially if a penetrating wound was found, and surgical exploration may be indicated focused on finding occult foreign bodies. Further

workup usually includes ultrasonography, radiography, and culture-sensitivity testing to rule out resistant organisms. CT studies or magnetic resonance imaging may be indicated in valuable animals.

The prognosis for acute orbital cellulitis is good if medical and nursing care can be provided; most cases resolve within 5 to 7 days with the aforementioned therapy, and some improve almost immediately after antibiotic therapy is initiated. Do not, however, discontinue antibiotic therapy any sooner than 10 to 14 days, even if the patient improves immediately, because disease signs will usually recur when treatment duration is inadequate.

Inflammation of the Tissues Adjacent to the Orbit
Etiology
Chronic frontal sinusitis in dairy cattle may lead to inflammatory bony expansion of the frontal sinus with ipsilateral exophthalmos that may be mild to moderate (see Figs. 4.10 and 4.11). Chronic sinusitis most commonly results from previous (months to years) dehorning or ascending respiratory infections of the sinus. *T. pyogenes* or mixed infections usually are found after dehorning, but *Pasteurella* spp. are most common in ascending respiratory tract infections.

Sporadic infections of the maxilla and other bones of the skull caused by *Actinomyces bovis* may occasionally cause bony expansion into the orbit, resulting in an exophthalmos.

Maxillary sinusitis also may be so severe as to expand into the ventral orbit, causing apparent ocular disease and exophthalmos. (Note the caudal expansion of the maxillary sinus that forms the floor of the orbit in Fig. 14.5). Infected tooth roots are the most common cause of maxillary sinusitis in adult dairy cattle.

Neoplasia of the frontal sinus, maxillary sinuses, or nasopharynx may expand adjacent structures such that the orbit is compromised and ipsilateral exophthalmos with orbital swelling results. Carcinomas, fibrosarcomas, and adenocarcinomas have been diagnosed (see Fig. 4.6).

Signs
Mild to marked unilateral exophthalmos that is usually slowly progressive and sometimes associated with bony expansion of the ipsilateral frontal or maxillary sinus, depression, and mild ocular discharge, with or without fever, constitute the major signs in chronic sinusitis (see Chapter 4 and Figs. 4.10 and 4.11). Fever may be absent, transient, or intermittent, usually depending on the patency of frontomaxillary-nasal drainage. When purulent material cannot escape, bony expansion of the sinus and fever are more consistent findings. Purulent material can escape through sinus openings into the nasal cavity and cause unilateral purulent nasal discharge. Chronic infection causes extreme softening of the bones surrounding the sinuses and variations in the normal contours of the skull. The caretaker may report that the animal's skull appears swollen on some days but normal on others.

When orbital swelling is obvious, exophthalmos, eyelid swelling, and chemosis usually are also present. Serous ocular discharge may be present initially but may become mucopurulent with time. Affected cattle show signs of "headache" and may be seen head pressing or holding the head extended with eyelids partially closed. Affected sinuses sound duller than normal on percussion.

Actinomyces bovis lesions that impinge or extend into the orbit establish obvious bony swellings that eventually ulcerate and form draining tracts.

Sinus or skull tumors that compromise the orbital space usually lead to exophthalmos, ocular discharge, ipsilateral nasal discharge, and fetid breath. Inspiratory dyspnea is more common with neoplasia than infection; fever is less common with neoplasia. Retrobulbar lymphosarcoma is especially common in dairy cattle and should be considered in every case of exophthalmos, whether peracute or chronic.

Diagnosis

The diagnosis may be obvious after physical examination or may require radiography, ultrasonography, aspirates for cytology, cultures, or biopsy to confirm specific diseases.

Radiographs are useful to confirm sinusitis, and aspirates for cytology and culture allow appropriate antibiotic selection in some cases and may confirm lymphosarcoma in others (there are no normal lymphoid aggregations within the orbit). Biopsies are essential when the presence of neoplasia is suspected. Radiographs are very useful to detect cheek and tooth root abnormalities in patients with chronic maxillary sinusitis.

Treatment

Frontal Sinusitis. Trephining of the skull in at least two areas is necessary to provide adequate drainage and lavage of chronic frontal sinusitis in adult cattle. Trephine holes should be 1.75 to 2.5 cm in diameter and drilled at the cornual area (former area of horn) and 3.75 to 4.50 cm off the midline of the skull along a transverse line drawn through the caudal bony orbit (see Figs. 4.14 and 4.15). Some references suggest a third opening dorsocaudal to the orbit, but in Dr. Rebhun's experience, this was associated with complications such as entering the orbit. The frontal sinus expands in size with age such that calves and heifers *do not* have an extensive frontal sinus except at the cornual region; therefore, trephining the frontal sinus of heifers younger than 15 to 18 months of age may lead to invasion of the calvarium, something to be avoided.

Purulent material in the sinus should be cultured so that an appropriate antibiotic may be selected for systemic use. The most common isolates from adult cattle and bulls are *T. pyogenes* and *Pasteurella* spp. In extremely chronic cases, fluid pus may be replaced by a pyogranulomatous semisolid mass of tissue that fills the sinus. When the sinuses cannot be flushed, these patients have an extremely poor prognosis and may develop fatal meningitis. Lavage of the sinus should be performed daily to flush away discharges and maintain the patency of trephine holes. Saline, dilute iodine solutions, and other nonirritating lavage solutions may be used. Analgesics such as flunixin meglumine, meloxicam, or aspirin are indicated to alleviate the pain associated with sinus headache.

Successful treatment usually requires at least 2 weeks of local therapy, lavages, systemic antibiotics, and analgesics.

Maxillary Sinusitis. Treatment of maxillary sinusitis varies depending on whether the cause is a primary sinusitis, tooth root infection, sinus cyst, or neoplasia. In dairy cattle, bad teeth that result in sinusitis usually are grossly abnormal, and can be identified as fractured, loose, or missing on careful oral examination. Diseased teeth should be removed, and a trephine hole should be drilled into the sinus to allow lavage into the nasal or oral cavity (depending on cause). Because the maxillary sinus has less of a labyrinth-like anatomy than does the frontal sinus, a single hole may be drilled using a 1.0- to 2.0-cm trephine or a large Steinmann pin to allow placement of polyethylene or plastic tubing into the sinus to facilitate daily flushing. Culture of the purulent material found in the sinus is essential for selection of appropriate systemic antibiotic therapy. Analgesics as discussed earlier may relieve some of the pain associated with eating and thus improve appetite.

Nothing other than palliative treatment is practical for most large sinus tumors in cattle.

Actinomycosis (lumpy jaw) is best treated with sodium iodide and very long-term antibiotic therapy with penicillin (20,000 U/kg once or twice daily). Organic iodides, although commonly used in practice, are of unproven efficacy.

Neoplastic Orbital Diseases

Neoplastic diseases of the orbit, regardless of species or etiology, are usually slow in onset (the exception being some cases of bovine lymphosarcoma) and are rarely accompanied by malaise, fever, or difficulty opening the mouth. The patients usually maintain a good appetite and show no discomfort when gentle backward pressure on the ipsilateral globe is applied through the closed eyelids.

The most common orbital tumor in dairy cattle is lymphosarcoma. It may be unilateral or bilateral and eventually causes progressive exophthalmos. The exophthalmos may be peracute in onset or more chronic and insidious. Mild to severe exposure keratitis and corneal ulceration usually occur if the disease is not detected early; proptosis may result (Fig. 14.6).

Because some Jersey, Ayrshire, and Holstein cows have "normal" bilateral conformational exophthalmos (i.e., they are "bug-eyed"), detection of abnormal exophthalmos may be difficult for new caretakers or owners of these individuals. All "bug-eyed" cows should be retropulsed on initial examination to ensure the orbits are normal; the globes in these animals will easily sink deeply in the orbit such that the corneal limbus (and in some cases, the entire cornea) will align with the orbital rim when gentle backward pressure on the globe is applied through the closed eyelids. Because of the capacious nature of the bovine orbit, cattle with space-occupying orbital masses rarely display exophthalmos until these masses are quite large. If, upon retropulsion, the eye of a cow does not sink into the orbit 4 to 5 cm, or the approximate axial length of the globe, then an orbital mass should be suspected. If in doubt, retropulse a few normally conformed herdmates.

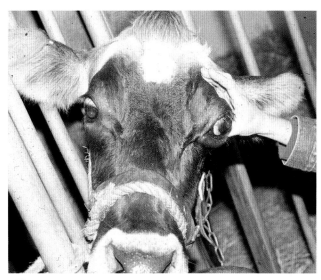

• **Fig. 14.6** Six-year-old Jersey, late gestation, with severe exophthalmos of the left eye that developed over a 3-day period.

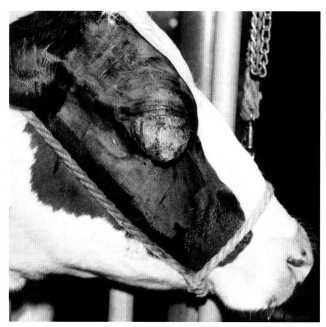

• **Fig. 14.7** Exophthalmos and chemosis, with very severe exposure keratopathy secondary to retrobulbar lymphosarcoma.

History is an important and helpful consideration in most lymphosarcoma cases. A slowly progressive onset of exophthalmos is typical, but do not rule out lymphosarcoma in cases presenting acutely! Affected patients may have unilateral or bilateral disease, are usually in mid to late gestation, are in good health otherwise, and are afebrile. Unless the cornea is severely ulcerated, the patient shows no signs of pain. A thorough physical examination to detect other neoplastic target areas is indicated (heart, uterus, gastrointestinal tract, and central nervous system [CNS]). Even though the retrobulbar lymphoid masses may have been present and enlarging for some time before pathologic exophthalmos, the pathology may appear acutely when exophthalmos prevents the eyelids from completely protecting the central cornea, and severe ulcerative corneal disease develops. Exposure damage and desiccation of the central cornea are variable according to the degree and duration of the exophthalmos. Corneal disease may be accompanied by blepharospasm, chemosis, and eyelid swelling, all of which dramatically worsen the appearance of the eye and rapidly cause great discomfort to the patient (Fig. 14.7). When examining what appears to be a mildly affected animal (Fig. 14.8), bear in mind that a visual eye with moderate exophthalmos but without exposure keratopathy may change to a blind, proptosed eye with complete corneal desiccation in less than 48 hours; thus all patients with suspect orbital masses should be provided immediate topical lubrication and frequent observation.

Diagnosis is aided by finding other evidence of lymphosarcoma in the patient, for which a thorough physical examination and abdominal palpation per rectum are always indicated. Enlarged lymph nodes, melena, cardiac abnormalities, uterine masses, or neurologic signs may be present. However, in many patients, the retrobulbar mass or masses are the sole clinical abnormality detected, with other lesions absent or undetectable. A CBC and bovine leukemia virus

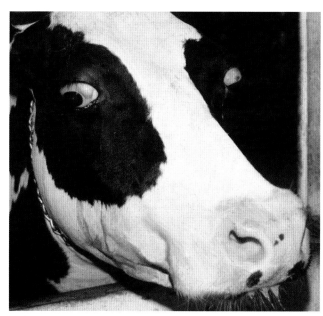

• **Fig. 14.8** Bilateral pathologic exophthalmos caused by retrobulbar neoplasia in a cow with widespread lymphosarcoma. Orbital fat prolapse is evident beneath the bulbar conjunctiva bilaterally, presumably caused by anterior displacement of the normal orbital fat by the tumor masses.

(BLV) agar gel immunodiffusion, enzyme-linked immunosorbent assay or polymerase chain reaction (PCR) test may be indicated to add supportive data. Most cattle with clinical lymphosarcoma test positive for BLV infection. Such test results are supportive but not conclusive because most BLV-positive cattle never develop tumors. Definitive diagnosis is via biopsy. Unlike orbital abscess cases, serum globulin concentration and inflammatory markers are often normal in cattle with lymphosarcoma.

As part of the physical examination, the retrobulbar tissues should be palpated through the posterior conjunctival sac (conjunctival fornix) after topical anesthesia has been achieved following the administration of topical agents such as 0.5% proparacaine (Akorn Inc., Lake Forest, IL; phone: 800-932-5676). If a mass is felt deep to the fornix at any point, the examiner should stabilize the mass, and a needle can be directed along the examiner's digit to obtain one or more fine-needle aspirates. Aspirates may provide a diagnosis if *any* lymphoid tissue is obtained because there is no solid lymphoid tissue in the orbit. If a distinct mass cannot be felt by this means, abnormal tissue detected with ultrasound can be aspirated via ultrasound guidance.

In questionable cases where a diagnosis cannot be confirmed and where the cornea is already severely diseased such as in Fig. 14.7, the globe should be enucleated to alleviate the cow's pain and allow collection of tumor material from the orbit for histopathologic confirmation of the diagnosis. The lymphoid masses are often palpated along the periorbita and in the orbital cone at the time of surgery. The globe itself usually is free of lymphosarcoma, but rare cases have also had conjunctival, corneal, eyelid, or scleral involvement.

In confirmed cases, the only indication for treatment occurs in extremely valuable cattle that are in the last trimester of pregnancy or candidates for embryo transfer or oocyte recovery in the near future. In these cases, the prime consideration is alleviating or preventing patient discomfort for a relatively short period of time. In patients in whom exophthalmos is not severe and the cornea is not severely diseased (patients with no or only mild corneal ulceration), the eyelid margins may be excised and a permanent tarsorrhaphy performed, taking care that sutures used to close the eyelids are split thickness and do not penetrate the eyelids, or iatrogenic corneal ulceration will result. In other cases, and always when the cornea is significantly diseased, enucleation is required to relieve the cow's pain and reduce the possibility of progressive disease (e.g., panophthalmitis and orbital cellulitis). At the time of enucleation, as much of the orbital mass as possible should be excised, along with the eye. Surgical and anatomy texts should be consulted before performing this procedure. Cattle with confirmed orbital lymphosarcoma usually die within 3 to 6 months as a result of diffuse lymphosarcoma; therefore further treatment is usually not warranted. Pregnant cattle with confirmed lymphosarcoma seldom live through more than 2 to 3 additional months of gestation. Embryo transfer attempts in cows with confirmed lymphosarcoma frequently are unsuccessful if the cow is in a catabolic state.

Squamous cell carcinoma (SCC) may occur in the bovine orbit, but because this is a tumor of epithelial origin, orbital involvement is usually preceded by eyelid, third eyelid (nictitans; see Fig. 7.14), conjunctival, or corneal SCC. Orbital SCCs are locally invasive, tend to recur locally, may metastasize, and carry a grave prognosis. Carcinomas of respiratory epithelial origin also have been observed in aged dairy cattle (older than 8 years of age). These tumors are slow- growing over months to years; cause progressive unilateral exophthalmos, inspiratory stridor, and reduced airflow in the ipsilateral nasal airway; and may cause ipsilateral Horner's syndrome (see Figs. 4.6 and 4.7). Although the prognosis for recovery with any form of treatment is poor, affected cattle may still be productive for 1 to 3 years with these slow-growing tumors.

Cattle sent to slaughter with severe ocular or orbital neoplasia are condemned whenever the eye is destroyed; when the eye is heavily infected, maggot laden (see Fig. 7.37), or draining pus; when the eye is obscured by neoplasia; when the tumor has invaded bone; or when there is associated lymph node enlargement or emaciation. Carcasses found to have localized neoplasia may pass inspection after removal of the diseased parts unless there is evidence that the general health has been impaired.

Exophthalmos Due to Vascular and Other Causes

As noted earlier, unilateral or bilateral exophthalmos in cattle is usually secondary to infection or neoplasia in the orbit, but other causes should always be considered. Townsend et al (2003) reported on six Holstein calves receiving daily dexamethasone injections as part of a metabolic study that developed mild to severe progressive exophthalmos. Virtually identical to the orbital fat changes seen commonly in horses with Cushing's disease, these calves were found on necropsy examination to have marked deposition of retrobulbar adipose tissue, presumably the cause of the progressive exophthalmos. Lamb and Naylor reported an Ayrshire calf with a fluctuant swelling dorsal to the orbit in which pulsations, a palpable thrill, and a machinery-like bruit were noted on auscultation over the swelling. On postmortem examination, the frontal bone was eroded by a mass of tortuous vessels found connecting an enlarged superficial temporal artery with a branch of the maxillary vein.

Cavernous sinus syndrome has also been diagnosed on necropsy of a young Holstein bull presenting with unilateral exophthalmos, a dilated and unresponsive pupil, and deficits in cranial nerves III to VI. That bull had been recently treated for an abscess at the base of the ipsilateral ear. Cavernous sinus syndrome was also diagnosed in a 10-month-old Holstein bull calf presented for an acute onset of nonpainful unilateral exophthalmos; a resolving abscess and mild cellulitis along the facial crest were noted (Fig. 14.9 *A*). Deficits in cranial nerves II, III, IV, V, and VI were found on physical examination, and cavernous sinus disease was diagnosed via contrast computed tomography (Fig. 14.9 *B* and *C*). In the latter case, long-term empirical antibiotic therapy resulted in complete resolution of clinical signs (NI, personal communication). All facial venous drainage in cattle is through the cavernous sinus (A. Delahunta, personal communication). Based on these cases, cavernous sinus disease should be considered in cattle presenting with nonpainful exophthalmos accompanied by deficits in cranial nerves II to VI.

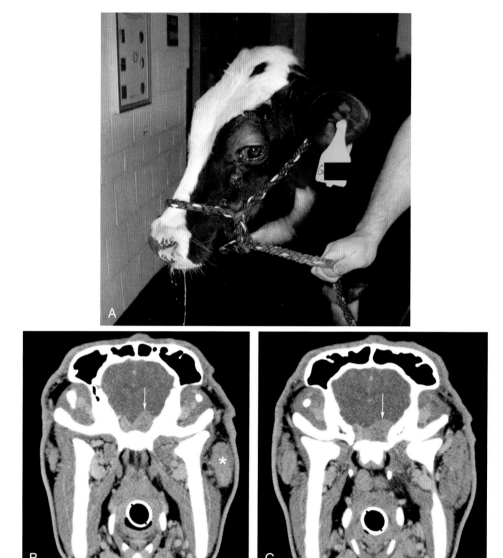

• **Fig. 14.9 A,** Ten-month-old Holstein bull with acute onset of nonpainful exophthalmos, hyperemia, epiphora, chemosis, vision deficits and inability to move his left eye; a small resolving abscess was present over the rostral aspect of the left facial crest. Septic cavernous sinus syndrome was suspected, confirmed via computed tomography (CT) and successfully treated with long-term antibiotic therapy. **B** and **C,** Transverse head CT scan (soft-tissue window) at the level of the cavernous sinus. Image B is obtained rostral to image C. The left (L) cavernous sinus has a large space occupying lesion (arrows) with a slight hypoattenuating center and dorsal convexity that compresses the overlying brain. The left parotid lymph node (*) is enlarged. (Images courtesy Dr. Pete Scrivani, Cornell University).

Neurologic Diseases

Pendular nystagmus was first reported in 15 of 2932 mature dairy cattle surveyed by McConnon et al in 1983 and is seen several times a year in our clinics. The bilateral, rapid, constant, pendular (horizontal) nystagmus develops by a few months of age and persists throughout life. Affected cattle appear to have functional vision, and their caretakers report no apparent visual deficits. Affected cattle occasionally show subtle, abnormal twitching movements of the eyelids and, upon close inspection of the eyes, markedly rapid, back-and-forth oscillations are noted (nystagmus). The nystagmus does not change with head position but may stop during head movement. Complete ophthalmic examination of affected animals performed by one

of the authors (NI) has found no accompanying ocular abnormalities. The heritability or mode of inheritance is unknown. No treatment is recommended (Video Clip 14.1).

Horner's syndrome is occasionally seen in dairy cattle and is usually unilateral. The clinical signs of Horner's syndrome include ptosis, miosis, ipsilateral conjunctival hyperemia, and ipsilateral facial warmth, as well as ipsilateral dryness of the normally moist muzzle, nares, and nasal passage. Because of the ipsilateral nasal mucosal vascular congestion, secondary to the Horner's syndrome–induced vasodilation, there is reduced airflow from the nostril and, in cold climates, a reduced "cloud" of warm breath from the affected nostril may be apparent (Fig. 14.10). Horner's syndrome in cattle is most commonly caused by iatrogenic injury to the cervical vagosympathetic

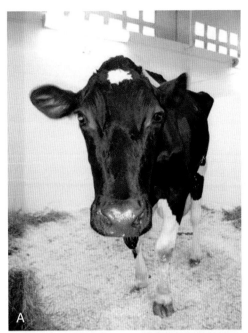

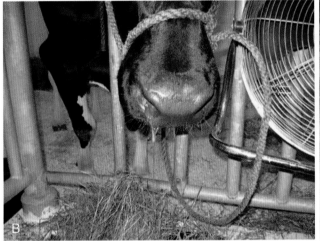
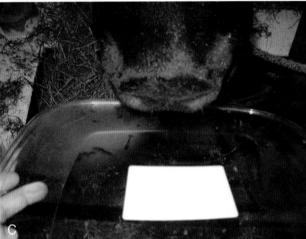

• **Fig. 14.10** **A,** Adult Holstein cow with left sided Horner's syndrome. Ptosis and miosis were obvious in the left eye in this image. **B,** None of the normal mucoid nasal discharge is seen from the left nostril. **C,** No airflow if present from the left nostril. Moisture accumulates below the right nostril on a cold plastic tray held under the muzzle, but no moisture appears on the tray below the left nostril.

trunk associated with direct injury by traumatic venipuncture of the jugular vein (Fig. 14.11) but is also seen with cervical trauma, carotid artery hematomas, cellulitis of the neck, and so on. Other causes are rare, but the syndrome has been observed with skull tumors (e.g., SCC, other carcinomas, and adenocarcinoma), causing upper respiratory dyspnea and decreased airflow from one or both nostrils as well as other signs of Horner's syndrome. If a patient presents with bilateral signs, then the cranial thorax should be carefully examined by palpation of the thoracic inlet and by cranial thoracic ultrasonography performed with the limbs alternately protracted cranially or pulled caudally as far as possible.

Treatment for unilateral idiopathic Horner's syndrome or Horner's secondary to vagosympathetic trunk injury is symptomatic with topical and systemic antiinflammatory drugs. The prognosis is good for return to function within 6

to 8 months. Horner's syndrome secondary to tumors carries a grave prognosis.

Bilateral dorsomedial strabismus with blindness and opisthotonus of the head are commonly seen with polioencephalomalacia (Fig. 13.24). Medial strabismus caused by lesions in the brainstem nucleus of the abducens nerve may be seen with listeriosis (see Fig. 13.16).

Diseases of the Globe

Developmental Diseases of the Globe
Etiology and Signs

Developmental malformations of the globe commonly result in megaglobus or microphthalmos. Anophthalmos, absence of all ocular tissue, is rarely an appropriate term

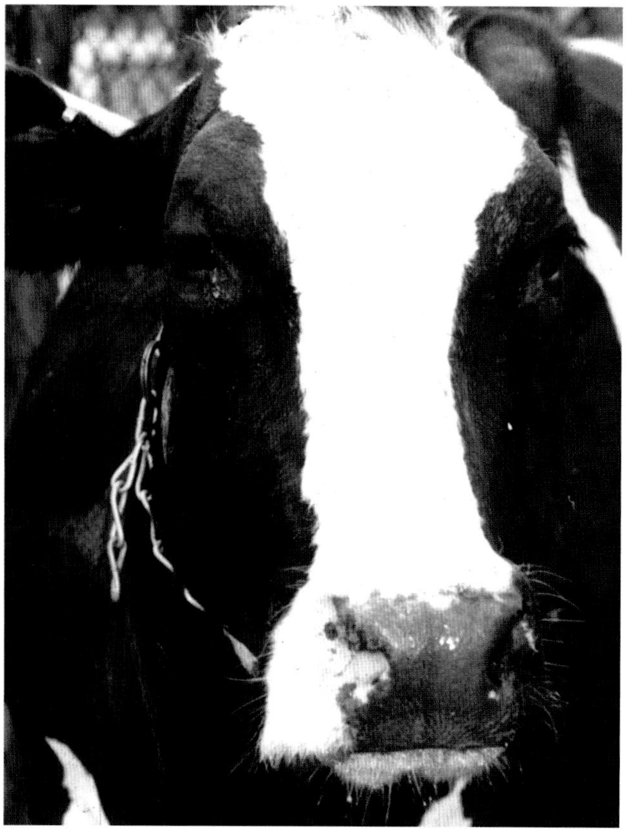

• **Fig. 14.11** Right-sided Horner's syndrome in a cow secondary to a perivascular reaction in the right jugular vein region. Note the ipsilateral ptosis and dryness of the right half of the muzzle.

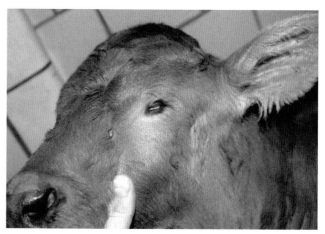

• **Fig. 14.12** Microphthalmia in a Guernsey calf. The calf also had congenital absence of the tail and a ventricular septal defect.

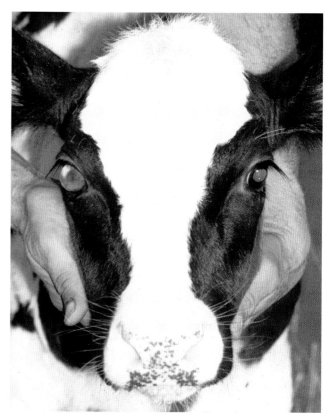

• **Fig. 14.13** Congenital buphthalmos and glaucoma in the right eye of a calf caused by an anterior segment dysgenesis similar to Peter's anomaly in humans.

because histologic sectioning of tissue from suspected anophthalmos cases almost always produces some evidence of ocular tissue, thus making microphthalmos the proper term. Congenital microphthalmos may be unilateral or bilateral in calves. Physical, toxic, and infectious causes have been suggested but seldom are confirmed to explain sporadic microphthalmia. In utero infection with bovine viral diarrhea virus (BVDV) during the middle trimester (days 125–175) has resulted in microphthalmos, as well as retinal dysplasia and other ocular defects.

Genetic causes of microphthalmia may occur in dairy cattle. In Guernsey and Holstein calves, the defect has been linked with cardiac and tail anomalies (Fig. 14.12). These calves commonly have a ventricular septal defect and wry tail, as well as unilateral or bilateral microphthalmia. Tail defects other than wry tail have been observed in some Guernsey and Holstein calves with microphthalmia or ventricular septal defect. These include absence of a tail, short tail, absence of some sacral vertebrae in addition to coccygeal vertebrae, and atresia ani coupled with absence of vertebrae. In Guernseys, these malformations may be recessive, but in Holsteins, the exact mode of inheritance remains unknown.

Congenital megaglobus results from anterior cleavage abnormalities or multiple congenital ocular anomalies producing glaucoma in utero. Dr. Rebhun observed several calves with anterior cleavage anomalies in which the lens placode had not separated from the surface ectoderm during development. Subsequent influx of mesodermal tissue in an attempt to form the corneal stroma, endothelium, Descemet's membrane, and iris surrounding the lens, had resulted in the absence of an anterior chamber causing congenital glaucoma and secondary buphthalmos (Fig. 14.13).

All cases of congenital megaglobus seen by the author (NI) to date have been unilateral, and the affected eye is noticeably buphthalmic at birth, with corneal edema, central dense opacity (often a definable lens in the cornea) (Fig. 14.14), grossly enlarged corneas (megalocornea), and no discernible anterior chamber. The grossly enlarged globe

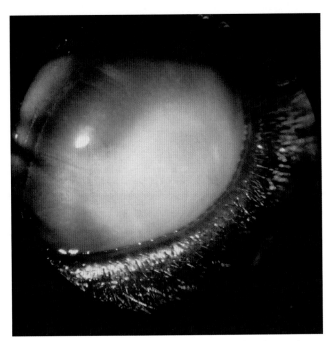

• **Fig. 14.14** Congenital megaglobus; the lens can be observed as a dense circular opacity within the cornea. Corneal edema radiates from the lens opacity.

suggests glaucoma, but the IOP is normal in some cases (Fig. 14.14 and 14.15 *A*). Affected eyes are often enucleated to ensure patient comfort (Fig. 14.15 *B*).

Convergent strabismus with or without associated relative exophthalmos has been described as an autosomally inherited trait in Jersey and Shorthorn cattle. It also has been observed occasionally in Ayrshire, Holsteins, and Brown Swiss cattle. Progressive bilateral convergent strabismus with exophthalmos (BCSE) is widespread in some breeds and can progress to blindness when the degree of rotation is sufficiently severe that the pupils are hidden behind the medial orbital rim (Fig. 14.16). German animal welfare laws forbid breeding affected animals. Fink et al. have associated genes on bovine chromosome 18 with BCSE in German Brown cattle or Braunvieh. Bilateral relative exophthalmos without strabismus ("bug-eyed cows") is a condition that has been observed in several dairy breeds and is likely a genetic trait. Exophthalmos can be profound in the affected cows but does not always progress to a pathologic state (i.e., development of exposure keratitis and corneal ulceration) because the eyelids continue to cover the cornea adequately, aided by retractor bulbi action in some affected animals (NI, personal observation). However, pigmentation of the exposed bulbar conjunctiva and peripheral cornea develops in almost all affected animals, presumably as a result of exposure of the globe to dust, air, or debris.

Congenital nystagmus (discussed earlier) has been observed in several breeds and is common in Holsteins.

Treatment

Enucleation is indicated for calves with unilateral congenital megaglobus because the affected eyes become grotesque and soon sustain exposure damage (see Fig. 14.15 *A*). Enucleation has been successful in these cases, and the

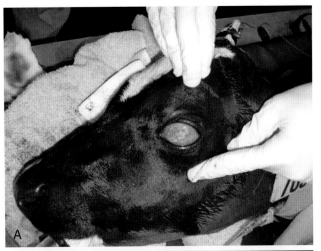

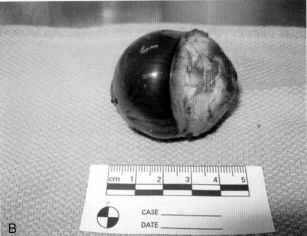

• **Fig. 14.15 A,** Congenital megalocornea in a calf at the time of enucleation. The central cornea is densely opaque with a connective tissue–like appearance; this area contained lens-like tissue when examined histologically. **B,** The enucleated globe showing the dramatic megalocornea. The grossly enlarged cornea is to the left, sclera is to the right, and a small optic nerve to the far right. Histopathology showed no iris or other definable anterior segment structures; the retina was markedly dysplastic.

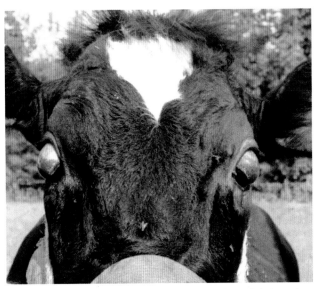

• **Fig. 14.16** Severe, convergent strabismus and exophthalmos in a Holstein cow. The exposed bulbar conjunctiva has become mildly pigmented as a result of its chronic exposure. Courtesy of Dr. Kit Blackmore.

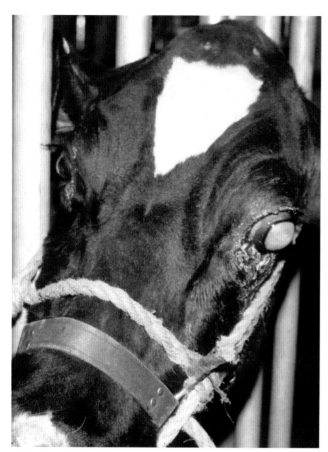

• **Fig. 14.17** Enlarged globe (buphthalmos) after severe pinkeye infection in a Holstein cow. Enucleation of this eye resulted in rapid improvement in appetite and production as a result of resolution of pain and irritation caused by the enlarged globe.

relatively rare incidence rules against simple Mendelian inheritance. Microphthalmic globes usually are not treated; if no other anomalies exist, the owner may elect to raise and breed a calf with unilateral microphthalmos. Chronic conjunctivitis occurs in some microphthalmic patients and if persistent and severe dictates enucleation to eliminate the chronic discharge and fly irritation, thereby aiding patient comfort.

Acquired Diseases of the Globe

Acquired secondary glaucoma and buphthalmos may follow severe intraocular inflammation of either an exogenous or endogenous cause. Infectious bovine keratoconjunctivitis (IBK), trauma, and uveitis are the usual causes of the anterior or posterior synechiae, lens luxation, and adhesions that disturb aqueous outflow, thereby creating glaucoma. Endophthalmitis and panophthalmitis secondary to septic uveitis or ocular perforation are other causes. If globe enlargement is severe enough to cause any degree of exposure keratitis, the affected globe should be enucleated to prevent eventual perforation and panophthalmitis. Adult dairy cattle with severely enlarged globes treated by enucleation become comfortable and return to anticipated production within several days (Fig. 14.17). It is important that acquired buphthalmos is not diagnosed erroneously as retrobulbar

neoplasia; the clinician must differentiate an enlarged globe from a pathologically exophthalmic one.

Less frequently, globe enlargement accompanies intraocular neoplasia or granulomatous infections of the uveal tract. SCC is the most frequent tumor to invade the globe, and tuberculosis must be considered any time a granulomatous infection of the globe is diagnosed.

Phthisis bulbi (shrinking of the globe) often follows ocular perforations, chronic uveal inflammation, and complications of severe pinkeye such as corneal perforation and iris prolapse. If a phthisical globe is sterile and nonpainful, it may be ignored or treated as for a microphthalmic globe (discussed earlier). However, if chronic conjunctivitis, irritation, facial dermatitis from discharges, fly irritation, or other problems are noted or the cow's production diminishes, enucleation should be performed.

Diseases of the Eyelids, Nictitating Membrane, and Nasolacrimal System

Congenital and Acquired Nasolacrimal Diseases

Supernumerary (aberrant) nasolacrimal duct (NLD) openings have been reported in related Brown Swiss cattle and are also seen in Holstein-Friesians (Fig. 14.18 *A* and *B*). Affected animals have a constantly wet face ventral to the eye, and teardrops may be seen falling from the face when pan feeding is introduced. Closer inspection will disclose one or multiple, unilateral or bilateral, round or slitlike, pigmented or nonpigmented, haired or hairless openings located anywhere from a few to 5 to 8 cm medial or rostromedial to the medial canthus (see Fig. 14.18 *A* and *B*). The fistulae may be pinpoint to 10 mm or greater in diameter. The examination for abnormal fistulae should begin at the medial commissure of the eyelids and continue along a curved line drawn between the medial commissure and lateral alar fold of the nostril (the line along which the embryonic fusion of the frontonasal prominences and the maxillary processes of the face occurs, forming the ectodermally lined NLD). In some cases, the medial canthus itself may be abnormally formed. Aberrant openings are usually in addition to the normal puncta found in the upper and lower eyelid margins. If fluorescein dye is applied to the affected eye(s), fluorescein exits the aberrant opening(s) onto the face within moments (Fig. 14.18 *C*). The condition is likely to be inherited in Brown Swiss cattle. If treatment is elected, attempt to preplace an indwelling nasolacrimal catheter that is secured proximally near the normal upper eyelid puncta and distally near the lateral alar fold. A portion of the aberrant opening(s), including all hairs, can be excised and an ectodermally lined duct re-formed over the indwelling stent catheter using 6-0 absorbable suture. The stent catheter should be left in place for 3 weeks.

Congenital NLD atresia occurs uncommonly in cattle but should be considered any time chronic epiphora is present in a young or very young animal. In affected animals, the medial upper and lower eyelids should be inspected to ensure that the normal eyelid punctae are present. After application

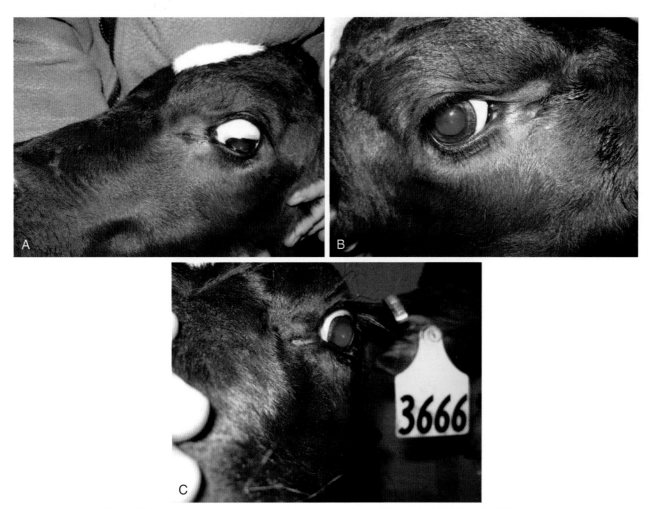

• **Fig. 14.18** **A,** Supernumerary nasolacrimal duct opening in the left eye of a Holstein calf (slit-like opening approximately 1.5 cm medial to the medial eyelid commissure). Not easily seen in this image is an abnormal adhesion between the medial eyelid commissure and the nictitating membrane. **B,** Supernumerary nasolacrimal duct openings in the right eye (moisture apparent medial to the opening; another pinpoint orifice was found farther down the face). **C,** Fluorescein applied to affected eyes appears almost instantly on the face.

of topical anesthetic, an 18- or 20-gauge Teflon intravenous (IV) catheter (without stylet) is attached to a 20-mL syringe filled with warm tap water and used to flush the system, first establishing patency from one eyelid puncta to the other and then, while occluding the opposite puncta, gently attempting to flush to the nose (Fig. 14.19). If patency is not established via normograde flushing, then the nasal vestibule should be examined for the presence of a normal nasal opening. In cattle, the NLD opening is located *dorsally* within the nasal vestibule in the mucosa at the rostral edge of the medioventral surface of the lateral alar fold (Fig. 14.20). It is easily seen if the examiner looks dorsally in the nasal vestibule while pulling the alar cartilage laterally. This orifice is most easily cannulated (after the application of a topical anesthetic gel) using a 3.5- to 5-Fr polypropylene canine urinary catheter and the system flushed retrograde using warm tap water in a 20-cc syringe (cattle hate cold water in their NLDs) or sterile saline if cultures are indicated. If patency cannot be established, additional diagnostic procedures such as dacryocystorhinography could be considered but rarely are performed in cattle except in extremely valuable animals.

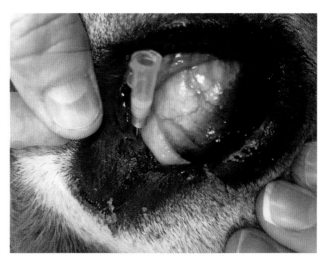

• **Fig. 14.19** An 18-gauge Teflon intravenous catheter has been placed in the upper nasolacrimal puncta prior to normograde flushing of the nasolacrimal duct.

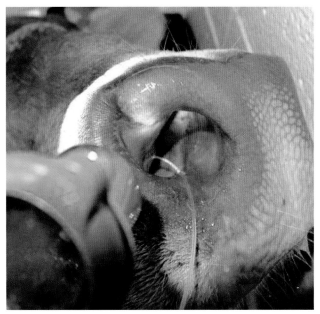

• **Fig. 14.20** Right nasal vestibule of an adult Jersey cow (green light source visible at the bottom left). An 18-gauge Silastic tube has been placed in the distal opening of the nasolacrimal duct before retrograde flushing of the duct.

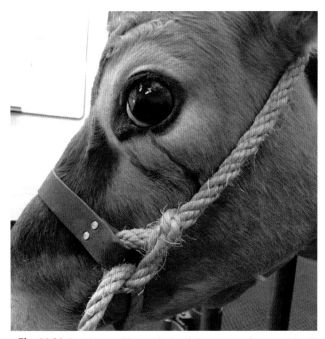

• **Fig. 14.21** A pet cow with constant epiphora, normal eyes, and patent nasolacrimal ducts. Conformational exophthalmos with pressure on the nasolacrimal puncta is the presumed cause of many cases of functional, nonobstructive nasolacrimal drainage failure.

If normal tear drainage cannot be established, then chronic facial dermatitis and fly problems are to be expected.

Acquired NLD obstruction is a common incidental finding with chronic epiphora in otherwise normal eyes of cows presenting to our hospital for other conditions, but NLD obstruction in cattle seems to receive little attention otherwise. An individual cow's conformation seems to be the cause of some bilateral epiphora complaints (Fig. 14.21) because

many exophthalmic bovine globes appear to be tightly apposed to the eyelids, and this may result in failure of the lacrimal pump mechanism. However, a complete ophthalmic examination to rule out other causes of excess tearing is always indicated. After a careful ophthalmic examination to rule out any painful condition or ocular irritant causing increased lacrimation, fluorescein should always be applied. Failure of fluorescein to pass to the nose after 5 to 15 minutes indicates some defect in NLD drainage. After the patient is adequately restrained and the NLD openings located, the NLDs in adult cattle are usually very easy to flush, as described in the previous paragraph. If the ducts do not flush easily, then foreign bodies, neoplasia, and other acquired obstructions may be present, and standard ophthalmology texts should be consulted for further recommendations.

Neurologic Diseases

Unilateral facial nerve palsy causing ptosis and exposure keratitis is common in calves affected with otitis media or interna and in adults affected with listeriosis (see Figs. 13.17, 13.61 and 13.62). Trauma may cause facial nerve injuries resulting in neuroparalytic keratitis in bovine patients of any age. The most common cause of bilateral eyelid paralysis in cattle is "stanchion trauma" wherein a cow pulls back against a stanchion with her head trapped, applying pressure along the zygomatic arch midway between the ears and orbit. The result is a bilateral traumatic palpebral nerve paralysis that may be temporary or permanent (see Fig. 13.64).

Signs of neuroparalytic keratitis include lacrimation, ptosis, absence of palpebral response, and progressive corneal exposure damage (e.g., ulceration) (see Fig. 13.18), although cattle with facial nerve paralysis appear to be slower to develop corneal ulcers than many other species, likely because of their strong retractor bulbi muscles. Treatment requires therapy for the primary disease and protection of the cornea with application of antibiotic ointments every 4 to 6 hours. A more practical and recommended solution is to carefully place a temporary tarsorrhaphy (see Fig. 4.6) to close the paralyzed eyelids for 2 to 3 weeks, during which time *most* cases will have return of eyelid function. Additional treatments include warm compress application several times daily to the area(s) of nerve injury, systemic and topical antiinflammatories, and treatment of any corneal ulceration with antibiotic ointment.

The palpebral reflex may be weak in calves with elevated D-lactate levels. Trefz et al. noted that skeletal muscle weakness caused by hyperkalemia with hypovolemia might produce a clinical picture similar to that of calves with marked D-lactic acidosis. The latter group, however was noted to have weak to absent palpebral reflexes. Therefore, if a strong palpebral reflex is present in a calf having trouble standing, the weakness in that calf is more likely to be due to hyperkalemia than increased D-lactatemia. This was confirmed experimentally by Lorenz and Gentile.

Flashing or intermittent protrusion of the nictitating membrane is common in patients with tetanus. This is a passive motion secondary to globe retraction rather than active movement of the nictitans, as tetany of the retractor oculi muscles pulls the globe caudally in the orbit, displaces other contents therein, and affects passive prolapse of the nictitans (see Fig. 13.68).

Traumatic and Inflammatory Diseases

Etiology and Signs

In dairy cattle, trauma to the eyelids occurs from blows to the head by other cattle or handlers; from the cow crashing into feed troughs, stanchions, and chutes; or when the eyelid is hooked over a heavy or immovable object and then torn or avulsed as the cow pulls away her head. Infection of the eyelids can result from neglected lacerations or puncture wounds from similar causes. The eyelids often become severely swollen as a result of hemorrhage or inflammation because cattle have abundant eyelid skin with a great deal of loose subcutaneous tissue and tissue elasticity. This elasticity affords the surgeon a great deal of tissue to work with if surgical or plastic repair is necessary.

Signs of trauma or laceration are obvious. Cellulitis of the eyelids and secondary orbital cellulitis are possible in neglected or dirty wounds. Eyelid swelling and ocular discharge accompany most traumatic injuries. Less common causes of eyelid inflammation include Actinobacillosis granulomas appearing at the site of previous eyelid injury and demodectic mite infestation.

Allergic reactions commonly result in eyelid swelling and conjunctival edema (chemosis). These signs are usually, but not always, accompanied by other systemic signs such as urticaria, skin wheals, facial swelling, and other mucocutaneous junctional swellings. Allergic reactions may occur secondary to administration of antibiotics, IV fluids, blood transfusions, and biologics. Similar reactions accompany individual animal sensitivities to various feedstuffs, plants, and milk allergy (see Chapter 7).

Bacterial diseases of the eyelids such as dermatophilosis have been reported in cattle, and *Moraxella bovoculi* has been reported to cause eyelid ulcerations (as well as the much more common keratoconjunctivitis). Ringworm as well as sarcoptic and other forms of mange should be considered any time eyelid alopecia, crusting, and scaling are noted and appropriate precautions and isolation steps taken while the diagnosis is confirmed (see Figs. 7.5, 7.6 and 7.36).

Treatment

Crushed, lacerated, or torn eyelids should be surgically repaired if at all possible and as soon as possible or lifelong ocular irritation and recurrent ulcerations may occur secondary to the deformed eyelid. Farm animal surgery or ophthalmology texts should be consulted for detailed repair recommendations. Lacerations of the eyelid may be closed using a two-layer technique with absorbable sutures (2-0 or 3-0) preplaced to appose the margins perfectly and then to close the deep tissues (the connective tissue layer or tarsus), *all the while ensuring that sutures do not penetrate the conjunctiva at any point.* Finally, absorbable sutures (2-0 or 3-0) are placed in the skin, with the ends closely trimmed to ensure they cannot reach the cornea. *Conjunctiva should never be (nor does it need to be) sutured.* Topical and systemic antibiotics for 5 to 7 days are indicated postoperatively to help prevent infection and subsequent wound dehiscence.

Conservative measures such as cold or hot compresses, cleaning and débridement of damaged tissue, local and systemic antibiotic therapy, drainage of abscesses, and protection of the cornea with topical antibiotic ointments may suffice in cases in which the eyelid is damaged but the damage is neither full thickness nor disruptive to the eyelid margin. NSAIDs may be used judiciously for control of inflammation; corticosteroids are not typically necessary and contraindicated in pregnant cattle.

Actinobacillosis granulomas should be debulked, and the cow may be treated with 20% sodium iodide (30 g/1000 lb body weight IV) followed by 30 g of oral organic iodide powder once daily for 14 days, or until such time as signs of iodism develop. Currently, iodide use is not permitted in lactating cows in the United States.

Allergic reactions require treatment and subsequent avoidance or correction of the primary cause; antihistamines, antiinflammatories, or epinephrine (see Chapter 7), as well as topical lubrication to protect the cornea if tissue swelling prevents normal eyelid function are appropriate therapies depending on severity.

Neoplastic Diseases

Etiology and Signs

Fibropapillomas, "warts," "horns," and other proliferative epithelial lesions caused by bovine papillomaviruses are the most common tumor to involve the eyelid of calves and young cattle. In most instances, the tumors are raised, firm masses with gray crusty coverings (Fig. 14.22) (see also Figs. 7.1, 7.2 and 7.3). The problem is self-limiting in most cases.

Lymphosarcoma rarely infiltrates the eyelids, but when it does, it manifests as a diffuse eyelid swelling with conjunctival chemosis (Fig. 14.23).

Squamous cell carcinomas are the most common tumor to affect the eyelids and nictitating membrane (nictitans or third eyelid) of one or both eyes of adult cattle (Figs. 14.24 and 14.25), but other neoplasias are also seen occasionally in the eyelids of cattle. White-faced beef cattle and Holsteins that are mostly white or have nonpigmented eyelid margins or nictitans are at risk, but SCC can be seen in any breed. In a predominantly dairy practice, most bovine patients with SCC ("cancer eye") are Holsteins. The tumors are classically pink, raised or ulcerated, cobblestone in appearance, and most commonly appear in middle-aged (5–10 year-old) cows. Squamous cell carcinomas can also present as chronic eyelid ulcerations; flat, scablike lesions; nonhealing wounds, or ulcers; or wartlike growths on the eyelid or eyelid margins (epitheliomas, keratomas, keratoacanthomas, papillomas, carcinoma in situ) (Fig. 14.26 *A*). Histopathology is recommended to confirm the diagnosis; cytology may be used but is not definitive because reactive, inflamed epithelial cells may be confused with neoplastic cells in some cases.

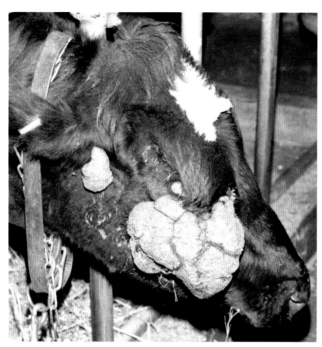

• **Fig. 14.22** Atypically large fibropapilloma growing from the upper eyelid of a Holstein heifer.

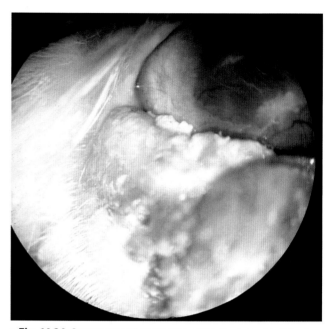

• **Fig. 14.24** Squamous cell carcinoma of the lower eyelid. This classic tumor is pink, raised, ulcerative, and has a white necrotic surface (abnormally exfoliating epithelial cells). Chronic superficial keratitis is present, a result of tumor irritation of the cornea.

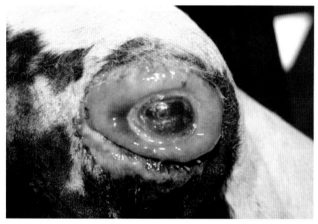

• **Fig. 14.23** Mature Holstein cow with ocular lymphosarcoma infiltrating both upper and lower eyelids. Note exposure keratitis caused by an inability to close the orbital fissure.

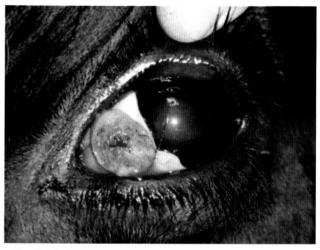

• **Fig. 14.25** Squamous cell carcinoma of the nictitans in a Holstein cow.

Treatment

Fibropapillomas normally are self-limiting within 4 to 6 months and do not require treatment. Persistent or large fibropapillomas (see Fig. 14.22) may interfere with eyelid function or cause corneal injury and require surgical treatment via cryosurgery or sharp dissection.

Squamous cell carcinomas may be locally invasive, locally recurrent and may metastasize, particularly in neglected cases. However, cattle treated when lesions are small almost always do very well and have a normal life expectancy. Early recognition and removal is critical—do not "just monitor" these! This tumor requires aggressive, early therapy to prevent progression, or the cow will be lost.

Many therapeutic options exist for early, small SCCs of the eyelids, but enucleation, radical exenteration, or culling may be required for large eyelid lesions. Recognition of early tumor formation when the mass is smaller than 2.0 cm in diameter allows removal using cryosurgery, radiofrequency hyperthermia, radiation (if available), (Fig. 14.26 *B*), sharp surgical excision, immunotherapy, or combinations of these treatment modalities. Large eyelid masses (>5.0 cm in diameter) are more complicated to treat surgically, requiring minor to major plastic procedures, and may have no response to other therapies. Destruction or removal of a large amount of eyelid margin may lead to ocular exposure damage and chronic irritation. These large tumors also are more likely to invade adjacent adnexal tissue, orbital ligaments, periorbita, and bones of the skull.

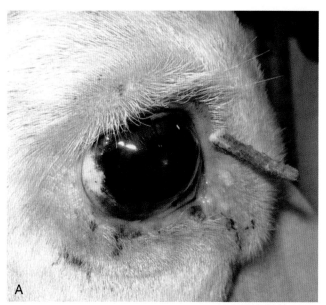

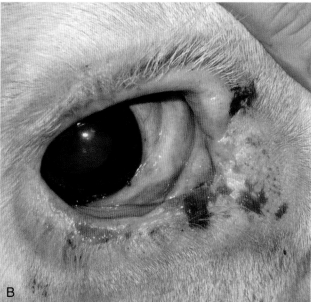

• **Fig. 14.26** **A,** A cutaneous horn, two lower eyelid ulcerations, and several dysplastic epithelial changes in the right eye of a 9-year-old, pet, mixed breed dry cow. **B,** Tissue erythema, swelling, and chemosis after excision and irradiation of all abnormal areas with strontium-90. The eye remained tumor-free for 3 years of follow-up.

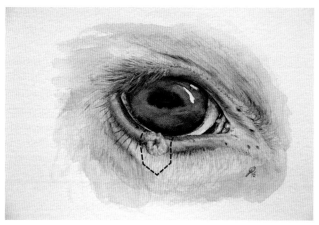

• **Fig. 14.27** Tent-shaped, pentagonal-shaped incisions are preferred for removal of small eyelid masses because of the amount of eyelid margin they conserve when compared with V-shaped excisions. (Courtesy of Dr. Laurie Peek.)

Tumors at the medial canthus are extremely concerning because they need to advance only 2.0 cm along the medial orbital ligament before entering the bony orbit and, anecdotally, carry a greater likelihood of metastasis. If possible, in nonpregnant cattle, 10 to 14 days of topical steroid before surgical excision allows the surgeon better definition of tumor margins.

Treatment options include:

1. *Sharp surgery*: This is the most accepted option, best performed on lesions smaller than 2.5 cm in diameter for which en bloc removal or tent-shaped eyelid margin excision (Fig. 14.27), including a 2- to 3-mm or more rim of normal tissue, is possible. Sharp excision is indicated for SCCs of the third eyelid that are smaller than 3 cm in diameter (see Fig. 14.25), and the best treatment is surgical removal of the entire third eyelid. See farm animal surgical texts for detailed descriptions, but briefly, after sedation of the patient with xylazine, a palpebral nerve block is performed. Liberal topical anesthesia is applied to the eye and conjunctiva using 0.5% proparacaine (lidocaine can be used if ocular anesthetics are not available). The free edge of the nictitans then is grasped with forceps, and 3 to 5 mL of 2% lidocaine is injected into the base of the nictitans, taking care while doing so that the needle is directed away from the globe. Dr. Rebhun recommended removing the entire nictitans using heavy serrated scissors. The author (NI) prefers to place Kelly hemostats dorsal and ventral to the cartilage, cutting along the jaws of the hemostats and leaving them on the patient for 10 to 15 minutes to aid hemostasis and prevent orbital fat prolapse (this is especially important in obese animals). At a minimum a 5-mm margin of normal tissue should be removed with the tumor. If possible, all of the cartilage within the nictitans should be removed because if a sharp cartilaginous stump remains in the medial canthal region, it may incite painful corneal ulcer formation. Topical antibiotics are applied to the eye three or four times daily for 7 days, and systemic penicillin (22,000 U/kg body weight) is given intramuscularly or subcutaneously once daily for 3 days postoperatively. If the tumor extends beyond the borders of the third eyelid, then more aggressive treatment is indicated.

2. *Cryosurgery*: This is perhaps the best therapy for moderate-sized lesions because the "freeze" can be adjusted to the size of the tumor, and cosmetic results at the eyelid margin tend to be good, thereby preventing subsequent exposure keratitis from loss of eyelid margin. The cow is restrained, sedated and topical anesthetic drops are applied to the ocular surface. Furthermore, the tumor site should also be blocked by regional anesthesia. If a freeze spray device is used, tissue peripheral to the lesion should be shielded with petroleum

jelly. In all cases, Styrofoam or other insulating material should be placed to cover the entire cornea before freezing commences. The tumor is frozen by free spray or by use of any of a number of probes or cups until the periphery of the tumor adjacent to normal skin reaches −40°C. The tissue is allowed to thaw and then is refrozen. Cryodestruction is maximum when a quick freeze, slow thaw, and quick refreeze routine is used. Frozen tissue necroses and sloughs over the next 7 to 14 days and is gradually replaced by granulation tissue followed by epithelialization of the wound. Frozen tissue and adjacent normal tissue often may remain depigmented, and returning hair will be white in most instances. Topical protective ointments should be applied to the eye daily, the eye examined, and all dead tissue cleaned away until the necrosed tissue has completely sloughed from the eyelid. The only complication Dr. Rebhun observed with this technique was corneal ulceration in one cow caused by a large scab that was not cleared away from the eyelid margin.

3. *Radiofrequency hyperthermia (RH)*: This is an older treatment option reported for small tumors or tumors with a small base that can be debulked before application of the device. Cancer cells are usually more susceptible to heat damage than normal body cells and so are preferentially killed. RH uses a localized current between its two probes to heat tissue up to 50°C but penetrates to a depth of only 3 to 5 mm. High temperatures have been found to alter cancerous tissue with minimal damage to surrounding normal tissue; tissue sloughing and necrosis occur subsequently. Treatment duration and temperature are important. Note that hyperthermia only penetrates to a maximum depth of 0.5 cm, so large lesions are not candidates for this technique, but multiple applications may be attempted. Instructions are supplied with the instrument which is still available at the current time (LCF MegaTherm, Western Instrument Co., a subsidiary of the Colorado Serum Company, Denver, CO; phone: 800-525-2065 or 303-295-7527).

4. *Radiation*: This is another older, but very effective, treatment option for small tumors or tumors with a small base that can be debulked before radiation is applied (see Fig. 14.26 *B*). SCC is a very radiosensitive tumor. Lesions smaller than 2 mm in depth (or large lesion beds after removal of the primary mass) are treated with 10,000 rad of beta-radiation per site using a strontium-90 applicator. At the time of this publication, the author (NI) is not aware of any commercially available strontium-90 probes. More radical radiation (e.g., radon, gold, iridium, and other radioactive seeds) has been used successfully for therapy of SCC, but radiation safety laws in many countries limit their use. External-beam irradiation is available at some university-affiliated hospitals.

5. *Immunotherapy*: Many attempts at immunotherapy, including autogenous vaccines made from tumor tissue and injections of Bacillus Calmette Guérin (BCG), have been used to treat ocular SCC previously. Although fair results have occasionally been reported, many questions remain regarding these techniques. BCG (a mycobacterium cell wall product) should not be used in dairy cattle because it can cause false positives with future tuberculin testing.

6. *Enucleation*: Enucleations in cattle can be performed using subconjunctival or transpalpebral approaches. Before planning surgery, assess the patient carefully for obvious metastasis (palpate the parotid and mandibular lymph nodes and along the jugular furrow for evidence of lymphatic enlargement). Also be sure to assess for obvious neoplastic bony invasion by tumor (palpate the bony orbital rim), and most importantly, assess for abnormal nasal discharge. If excess purulent discharge is present from the ipsilateral nostril, there is a high likelihood of tumor having already invaded into the sinuses or nasal cavity, in which case euthanasia may be a consideration (Fig. 14.28). Subconjunctival enucleation is recommended for noninfected globes; the procedure is less invasive, results in minimal bleeding, and can be performed in 30 minutes or less. However, most bovine eyes to be enucleated are already infected or contaminated, so a transpalpebral approach is more appropriate and therefore most commonly performed. Details of both approaches are found in *Farm Animal Surgery* by Fubini and Ducharme (2017). In brief, the cow is restrained in a chute or stanchion and sedated with xylazine (20 mg IV) before routine clipping and preparation of the orbit and periocular tissues. A circumferential infiltration of the eyelids approximately 5 cm from the eyelid margins is performed using 2% lidocaine. Next, 15 to 30 mL (according to the patient's size) of 2% lidocaine is deposited within the periorbital

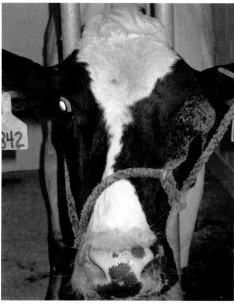

• **Fig. 14.28** Adult Holstein cow presented for enucleation. Because of the purulent, fetid, ipsilateral nasal discharge, skull radiographs were obtained showing extensive bony destruction, and the cow was euthanized.

cone via a 8.75-cm (3.5-in), 18-gauge needle, or alternatively a four-point block can be used. The classic Peterson block can be used, but the periorbital block is safer and provides more effective analgesia. Note: If the cow moves or vocalizes excessively during the enucleation, it is usually because pain is being felt. If this occurs, STOP the procedure and administer additional anesthetic.

The orbital area is surgically prepped again after the blocks and draped with a fenestrated drape that can be clamped to the halter with sharp towel clamps. (It is helpful to tape back the ipsilateral ear before draping.) Recently, fully self-adhesive sterile plastic sheet drapes have been used instead of cloth drapes, with excellent results because the drapes remain in place when the cow moves. The eyelid margins are clamped or sewn together. A circumferential incision is made at the point where hair starts to appear, approximately 1.0 to 1.5 cm from the eyelid margin, through the skin and subcutaneous tissues *but not through the palpebral conjunctiva.* Keeping this dissection close to the eyelid margins helps avoid cutting the several large vessels found farther back in the eyelids. Dissection continues using scissors. The lateral and medial canthal ligaments connecting the eyelids to the bones of the orbit are severed using a blade, and dissection continues around the globe, remaining external to the conjunctiva all the while. When possible, the extraocular muscles should be severed at their attachments on the sclera to reduce bleeding. When all muscles are severed, gentle medial traction of the globe will allow palpation of the optic nerve stalk. Directing scissor tips between the globe and the surgeon's fingertip placed on the optic stalk will allow relatively precise cutting of the now-stabilized nerve and will avoid the uncontrolled cutting that occurs with inexperienced hands. After the optic nerve is severed, the globe can be rolled out of the orbit as remaining attachments are severed. The orbit is packed with gauze and pressure maintained as the excised globe is examined to ensure completeness of excision. Note: *It is not necessary, and in fact is harmful in some cases, to clamp the optic stalk!* The author (NI) has never clamped the optic stalk in any enucleation, in any species, with no untoward bleeding occurring. Excess bleeding during enucleation occurs when infection or severe orbital inflammation is present, when some orbital tumors are incised, when muscles must be severed through their bellies, or when cutting tissues blindly severs one or more of the major vessels found in the deep orbit. After removal of the globe, the entire nictitans and lacrimal gland are removed. (Additional local anesthetic may be required to remove the lacrimal gland.) The orbit is then inspected to ensure all secretory tissue has been removed; this includes conjunctival remnants, the lacrimal caruncle at the medial canthus, the gland of the third eyelid (attached to the nictitans cartilage), and the main lacrimal gland deep to the dorsotemporal orbital rim.

Meticulous attempts at hemostasis while closing only serve to prolong the procedure. The orbital fascia and a subcutaneous continuous suture of 2-0 absorbable material close the orbit; absorbable or nonabsorbable interrupted sutures may be used to close the skin. Preoperative followed by postoperative systemic antibiotics should be administered for 5 days in routine cases but may be prolonged in infected globes or orbits. Drains are not used unless the orbital tissues appear infected or contaminated.

Schulz and Anderson reported postoperative infection in approximately 19% of enucleations and that recurrence of SCC after enucleation was uncommon.

7. *Exenteration*: Surgical removal of all orbital tissue is recommended if any suspected neoplastic tissue is found behind the globe. Closure is similar to that for enucleation.

Diseases of the Conjunctiva

Conjunctiva and the Systemic State

The normal palpebral conjunctiva and the conjunctiva overlying the nictitans are pink and free of inflammation. The bulbar conjunctiva is thin, colorless, but appears white because the underlying sclera is white. As every veterinary student learns, various systemic states may be reflected in the conjunctiva and subsequently it should be evaluated during every physical examination. Chemosis, or edema of the conjunctiva, is observed most commonly in allergic reactions, urticaria, or with hypoproteinemia. Extreme pallor of the conjunctiva (Fig. 14.29) suggests anemia, and anemia coupled with hypoalbuminemia results in extreme pallor plus chemosis. A yellow tint to the conjunctiva and sclera suggests jaundice or icterus but should not be confused with the yellow eyelid and skin discoloration known as carotenoderma seen in cattle with excess carotene intake or metabolism (Fig. 14.30). Conjunctival hemorrhages are common in healthy newborn calves after normal parturition and especially so after dystocia. In newborn calves, either direct trauma to the globes or severe passive congestion resulting from a prolonged stay of the head in the vagina or protruding from the vagina may lead to severe subconjunctival hemorrhage. Septicemia is the most common serious

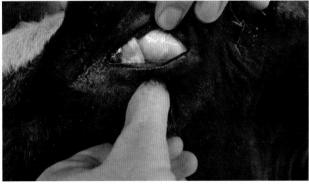

• **Fig. 14.29** Extreme pallor of the bulbar and nictitans conjunctivae.

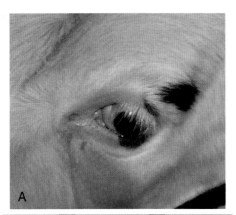

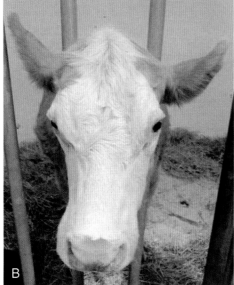

• **Fig. 14.30 A,** Yellow discoloration of the nose, eyelids, and poll caused by carotenoderma, a condition associated with excess carotene consumption or metabolism that should not be confused with icterus. Icterus manifests as yellow discoloration of the mucous membranes only, including the conjunctiva; carotenoderma discolors only the skin, but the conjunctiva appears normal. **B,** The yellow skin discoloration is evident in many body regions.

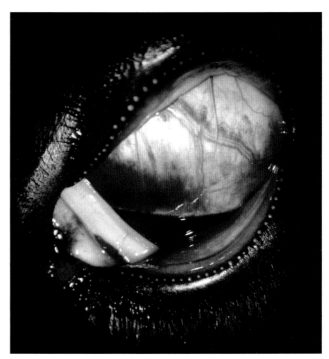

• **Fig. 14.31** Conjunctival hemorrhage caused by thrombocytopenia in a Holstein cow.

cause of conjunctival hemorrhage in neonatal calves and has been associated with thrombocytopenia or other coagulopathies. In older cattle, trauma, septicemia, thrombocytopenia (e.g., BVDV, bracken fern intoxication), disseminated intravascular coagulation, and other coagulopathies may result in conjunctival hemorrhages (Fig. 14.31 and Fig. 3.56).

Developmental Diseases

Dermoids of the conjunctivae cause irritation because of the hair growth on the dermoid and require surgical removal in all cases when hairs are present. Careful examination should be performed to ensure that dermoids move freely and are not attached to deeper ocular tissues in which case referral to a specialist may be indicated. A full-thickness resection of the involved conjunctiva has given excellent results. Closure of the conjunctiva is not needed in most cases. Topical antibiotics should be administered three to four times a day for 7 to 10 days post operatively. Dermoid treatment is also discussed in the section on diseases of the cornea that follows.

Inflammatory Diseases

Etiology and Signs

Moraxella bovis, the cause of IBK (i.e., pinkeye), is the most important bacterial disease of the conjunctiva and cornea in cattle. The organism and IBK are discussed extensively later in the chapter.

Pasteurella spp. and other bacteria may also cause mucopurulent conjunctivitis in cattle. *Pasteurella* conjunctivitis sometimes occurs in conjunction with severe *Pasteurella* pneumonia or septicemia in calves. The organisms are normal inhabitants of the upper respiratory tract in cattle and therefore can easily gain access to the conjunctiva. *Neisseria* spp. have also been isolated from cattle with conjunctivitis and infectious keratitis. Atypical (winter) outbreaks of IBK-like endemics have been blamed on these other bacteria, but overwhelming evidence supports *Moraxella bovis* as the most likely causative organism in these cases. Calves with respiratory infections caused by *Histophilus somni* may have conjunctivitis, rhinitis, laryngitis, and pneumonia. Cattle affected with simple bacterial conjunctivitis have a serous or mucopurulent ocular discharge and conjunctival injection and do not appear to have ocular pain.

Mycoplasma spp. and *Ureaplasma* spp. have been isolated from the eyes of cattle during herd epidemics of conjunctivitis. Affected cattle do not appear ill, but 10% to 50% of the animals may have unilateral or bilateral ocular discharge and conjunctival hyperemia. The ocular discharge is serous initially, becoming mucopurulent after 1 to 4 days. No keratitis is associated with this problem.

Infectious bovine rhinotracheitis (IBR) virus, the herpes virus 1 of cattle, may cause a severe endemic conjunctivitis in nonvaccinated cattle. Conjunctivitis may be the only sign observed in sick cattle or may occur in conjunction with the typical respiratory form of IBR. The disease has been observed in both heifers and adult cattle.

Typical lesions of ocular IBR include severe conjunctival hyperemia, heavy ocular discharge that converts from serous to mucopurulent over 48 to 72 hours, and the presence of multifocal white plaques in the perilimbal palpebral conjunctiva (Figs. 14.32 *A* and 4.51). The lesions may be unilateral or bilateral and affect 10% to 70% of the herd. The plaque lesions are pathognomonic for IBR. Affected adult cattle have high fever (105.0° to 108.0°F [40.56° to 42.22°C]), depression, and decreased milk production. Adult milking cattle with the conjunctival form of IBR appear ill regardless of whether the respiratory form coexists. Heifers with the conjunctival form of IBR may have fever and mild systemic illness but seldom appear as sick as adult milking cattle. The reason for this difference is not known but may be related to the stress of lactation in older cows.

Five to nine days after the onset of disease, the white conjunctival plaques begin to coalesce and slough, and the conjunctiva becomes very chemotic. During this same time, peripheral corneal edema develops in some of the more severely affected cattle (see Fig. 14.32 *B*). The corneal edema with IBR is circumferential edema that usually leaves the central cornea clear compared with IBK in which the central cornea is cloudy.

Occasionally, extremely severe cases develop complete corneal opacity with severe edema and peripheral vascularization. These corneal opacities may cause confusion with pinkeye (IBK), but no primary corneal ulceration occurs in IBR conjunctivitis. The early pathognomonic lesions persist for only a few days, and the virus usually cannot be recovered from the eyes for longer than 7 to 9 days after the onset of disease (see Table 14.1). Cytology of the plaques yields mononuclear cells.

Although other viral diseases of cattle may cause conjunctivitis experimentally, none appear to be important clinically in the United States at this time.

Foreign bodies may result in persistent conjunctivitis in one or both eyes. Animals that are shipped in open trailers, kept in areas where wind is likely to raise foreign bodies, or those in lateral recumbency are at risk for foreign body conjunctivitis. Generally, causative material is of plant origin. Signs include persistent epiphora, blepharospasm, conjunctival hyperemia, and chemosis. Corneal ulceration may occur in neglected cases or when the foreign body lodges in the eyelids. Conjunctival foreign bodies may be trapped in edematous folds of palpebral conjunctiva, in the conjunctival fornix, or, in or on, the bulbar conjunctiva, or may be positioned on the bulbar surface of the nictitans.

Parasitic conjunctivitis caused by the eye worms *Thelazia skrjabini* and *Thelazia gulosa* has been found to be prevalent in some regions of the United States.

Diagnosis

With the exception of IBR conjunctivitis and when *Thelazia* spp. can be found, the clinical appearance seldom identifies the cause of conjunctivitis in cattle. After a careful clinical examination to rule out foreign bodies, viral diagnostics,

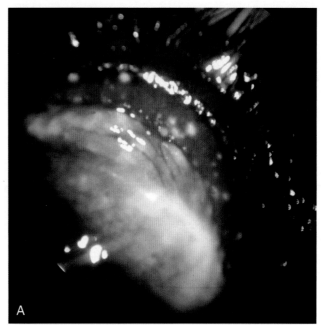
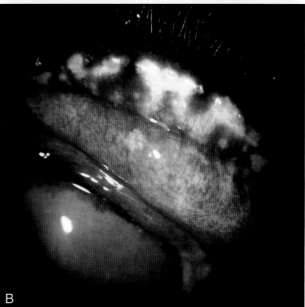

• **Fig. 14.32 A,** Multifocal white plaques on the palpebral conjunctiva as a result of acute infectious bovine rhinotracheitis virus conjunctivitis. **B,** Infectious bovine rhinotracheitis conjunctivitis in a cow that has been affected for 7 to 10 days. The white plaques have coalesced into nonpigmented areas of necrosis. Chemosis is severe, and corneal edema is present.

bacterial culture of the conjunctival discharge and cytologic examination of conjunctival scrapings are the most useful diagnostic procedures, especially when faced with a herd epidemic of conjunctivitis in calves or adult cattle. These samples should be submitted to established state or national diagnostic laboratories familiar with bovine infectious diseases and not submitted to laboratories specializing in human or small animal diseases. Cytology and culture will identify bacterial causes, as well as *Mycoplasma* and *Ureaplasma*, provided organism-specific media are requested or the laboratory is familiar with the most current diagnostic techniques such as PCR for these more unusual organisms.

Infectious bovine rhinotracheitis can be diagnosed in acute cases by fluorescent antibody tests applied to heavy conjunctival smears, virus isolation or PCR detection of viral nucleic acid. Alternatively, serology using acute and convalescent (14 days apart) sera may be attempted.

Treatment

Viral conjunctivitis, including IBR conjunctivitis, resolves without therapy. Nursing procedures such as cleansing the discharge from the patient's eyes and face certainly aid healing and patient comfort but seldom are practical because of the labor involved in handling large numbers of cattle. The conjunctival form of IBR resolves after a clinical course of 14 to 20 days. Severe cases benefit from nursing care and topical treatment with broad-spectrum antibiotics to deter secondary bacterial infection. Corticosteroids of any type or route of administration are contraindicated during this time.

Bacterial conjunctivitis should be treated with appropriate broad-spectrum ophthalmic ointments approved for use in cattle. Mastitis ointments may be excellent, affordable choices and usually do not irritate the eye. The dose of any ointment is a ¼-inch strip. Although dairy farmers tend to have difficulty using small tubes of ophthalmic ointment without wasting a great deal of the ointment, it sometimes is necessary to use these when a specific ophthalmic antibiotic is indicated. Partially used tubes should not be left uncapped in the barn because fungal agents may contaminate the ointment.

The presence of foreign bodies should be ruled out by a thorough ophthalmic examination when an individual cow has persistent bacterial conjunctivitis unresponsive to antibiotic therapy.

Mycoplasma or *Ureaplasma* may cause an insidious herd epidemic of conjunctivitis with a few initial cows having mucopurulent ocular discharge followed by several new cases during the ensuing 7 to 10 days. Caretakers report a slow spread of conjunctivitis through 10% to 50% of the cows in a typical outbreak. Most cases resolve without therapy, but cleansing of the ocular discharge coupled with topical tetracycline ophthalmic ointment speeds recovery.

Neoplastic Diseases

The most common tumor of the conjunctiva is SCC. This tumor may arise from bulbar conjunctiva, palpebral conjunctiva, or conjunctiva of the nictitating membrane. Treatment has been discussed in the section on eyelid neoplasia.

Lymphosarcoma rarely involves the conjunctiva but may appear as a diffuse, pink-tan, firm swelling within or deep to the conjunctiva of the eyelids, nictitans, globe, or perilimbal tissues or invading the cornea in one or both eyes. Ruggles et al. reported a Holstein cow with corneoscleral lymphangiosarcoma that lived at least 2 years after enucleation.

Orbital fat prolapse deep to the bulbar conjunctiva may be confused with neoplasia. Subconjunctival orbital fat prolapse (Fig. 14.33) usually develops in or adjacent to the third eyelid or on the surface of the globe (deep to the conjunctiva) medially or laterally. It appears as a pale yellow or yellow, mildly lobulated, soft mass that is freely moveable

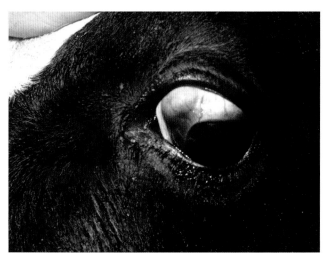

• **Fig. 14.33** Subconjunctival fat in a Holstein cow that was affected bilaterally. The condition seems painless, and no treatment is required unless fat protrudes from the closed eyelids or interferes with blinking.

if manipulated after applying topical anesthesia. It occurs most commonly in older, overconditioned cattle but may be seen at any age, especially after blunt trauma. Treatment is not usually required unless affected cattle show signs of ocular irritation or have trouble blinking over exposed tissue. In no case should the fat be excised without careful planning and preparation for orbit septal suturing; patient sedation and restraint are critical during excision, or additional orbital fat may erupt from the wound, which can result in permanent enophthalmos of the globe if not corrected. In these cases, consultation with a specialist is recommended before treatment. If orbital fat prolapse is diagnosed, the veterinarian should retropulse the eye to ensure that the fat prolapse is not attributable to a space-occupying lesion behind the globe.

Diseases of the Cornea

Developmental Diseases

Corneal dermoids, normal skin in an abnormal location on the globe or adnexa, occur commonly in cattle, may be unilateral or bilateral, usually originate at or near the corneoscleral junction, and extend a variable distance across the cornea (Figs. 14.34 and 14.35). They may be single, multiple, or complex, with complex dermoids involving multiple, surface tissues (cornea, conjunctiva, nictitans, lacrimal caruncle, or eyelids). They may extend full thickness through the eyelids, nictitans, cornea, or sclera. Removal is always indicated to prevent persistent corneal and conjunctival irritation caused by the hairs growing from the dermoid but only after a complete ocular examination is performed because although removal of most dermoids is relatively simple, removal of a full-thickness lesion is best performed by a specialist. A keratectomy is necessary to remove tissue on the cornea, and permanent corneal scarring is anticipated subsequent to keratectomy. Valuable calves with deep lesions should be referred to specialists. There

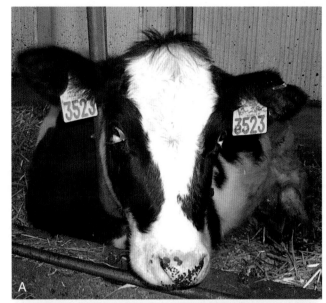

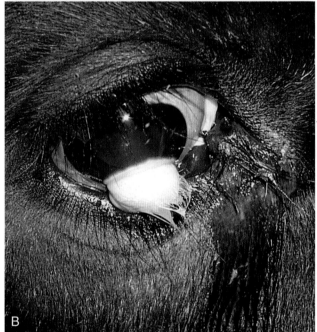

• **Fig. 14.34** **A,** Holstein calf with bilateral dermoids. A simple, small dermoid in the left eye was located in the ventral cornea. **B,** Complex dermoid in the right eye. A large white full-thickness dermoid is present in the ventral cornea. Smaller black dermoids are present at the medial canthus (the long hairs visible there are abnormal), on the palpebral face of the nictitans, on the free margin of the nictitans, and in the ventral conjunctival fornix (not visible). (Courtesy of Dr. Mary Smith, Cornell University.)

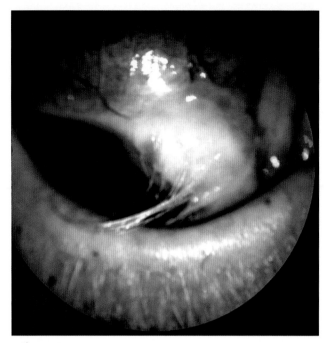

• **Fig. 14.35** Corneoscleral dermoid in a calf. Dermoids may be pigmented or, as in this case, depigmented but usually produce hair that irritates the eye.

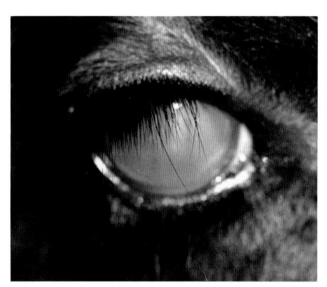

• **Fig. 14.36** Congenital endothelial dystrophy in a Holstein calf. The lesion was bilateral.

is no scientific evidence proving that dermoids are hereditary, but breeding of affected animals is discouraged.

Congenital bilateral corneal opacities have been described in Holsteins as a recessive condition. The basic lesion is an endothelial plaque or dystrophy; corneal edema develops secondarily and leads to a nonpainful, milky-white corneal opacity (Fig. 14.36). Although partially or completely blind secondary to the corneal edema, these cattle appear otherwise normal, and some have been raised for production purposes. Breeding affected animals is discouraged. No successful treatment has been reported.

Failure of the front portions of the eye to separate normally embryologically, called anterior cleavage anomalies or anterior segment dysgenesis, results in a severe corneal opacity present at birth that usually precludes intraocular ophthalmic examination, but the ensuing glaucoma and megaglobus aid in identification of the basic lesion. This condition is discussed in the earlier section on the globe.

Although not a true developmental disease, Holzhauer et al. reported recently on calves in the Netherlands with low birth weight and "blue eyes" caused by corneal edema associated with in utero bluetongue infection.

Toxic Injury

Toxic injury to the cornea most commonly results from accidental exposure of the cornea to exogenous chemicals. Chlorhexidine is extremely toxic to the corneal epithelium and stroma in all species, including humans; thus, chlorhexidine disinfectants, soaps, and teat dips must be handled with great care, or permanent corneal opacities may result. Insecticide and other chemicals, including organophosphate fly repellents, are toxic to the corneal epithelium and should not be sprayed in the periocular region of cattle. Most chemical toxicities cause acute, widespread, corneal epithelial loss and ulceration.

Anhydrous ammonia, a commonly used fertilizer and silage additive, is especially dangerous to the eyes and respiratory tracts of both humans and animals. Leaks from broken hoses or tanks may result in exposure to this very dangerous chemical. Peracute respiratory distress and corneal opacity occur almost immediately because the anhydrous chemical "seeks" water and desiccates the tissues from which it has extracted the water. Severe and permanent corneal opacity develops as a result of epithelial necrosis and stromal injury. Chlorine bleach or gas exposure results in similar clinical signs.

Phenothiazine toxicity is the classic example of endogenous chemical corneal toxicity in cattle. Although less common today because of reduced use of phenothiazine, this toxicity still is encountered, and the diagnosis is made most easily by observing the ophthalmic manifestations. Excessive levels of phenothiazine metabolites, such as phenothiazine sulfoxide, circulate in the bloodstream and enter the aqueous humor. Normally, these metabolites are detoxified in the liver. The presence of phenothiazine metabolites in the aqueous, coupled with exposure to sunlight (ultraviolet [UV] radiation), results in a photochemical reaction in the aqueous that releases energy and heat, thereby injuring the inner corneal layer, the so-called corneal endothelium. Damage to the corneal endothelium results in development of irreversible corneal edema because the Na^+K^+-ATPase pump of the endothelium has been affected. Clinical signs include bilateral corneal edema, usually located in the ventral two-thirds of the cornea. The dorsal cornea usually is unaffected because the upper eyelid protects it from UV radiation (Fig. 14.37).

Inflammatory and Traumatic Disorders

Diseases Other Than Infectious Bovine Keratoconjunctivitis

Etiology

Traumatic injuries that cause abrasions, lacerations, or ulceration of the cornea may be caused by feedstuffs, conjunctival foreign bodies, restraint devices such as stanchions or chutes, and tail switching. Infection of corneal wounds occurs commonly because most are neglected until they appear severely diseased.

Opportunistic bacterial organisms from the conjunctival flora or inoculants carried by the offending object that caused the trauma can foster infection of any corneal wound.

Corneal foreign bodies (Fig. 14.38), often consisting of plant material, may be embedded to variable depths in the cornea after strong winds, from blowers or fans forcing

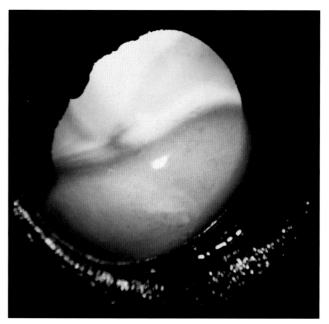

• **Fig. 14.37** Phenothiazine toxicity. The ventral half of the cornea is edematous secondary to photochemical damage to the corneal endothelium in this area.

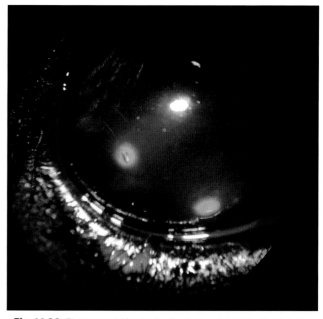

• **Fig. 14.38** Plant material foreign bodies in the cornea of a Holstein cow. Fluorescein dye has been applied to the eye to highlight the lesions.

feed and bedding into the eyes, or secondary to accidental trauma from feed or bedding material.

Exposure keratitis (see Figs. 13.18 and 14.23) secondary to diseases of the orbit or globe or neurologic diseases of the eyelids results in corneal desiccation and subsequent ulceration. When the corneal tear film is no longer spread to protect the epithelium, rapid desiccation followed by necrosis occurs in the central to ventral, paracentral epithelium and underlying stroma. The result is a deep, slow-healing ulceration of the cornea that may progress to perforation if unattended.

Intrastromal abscesses in the cornea of cattle affected with the neurologic form of listeriosis have been described

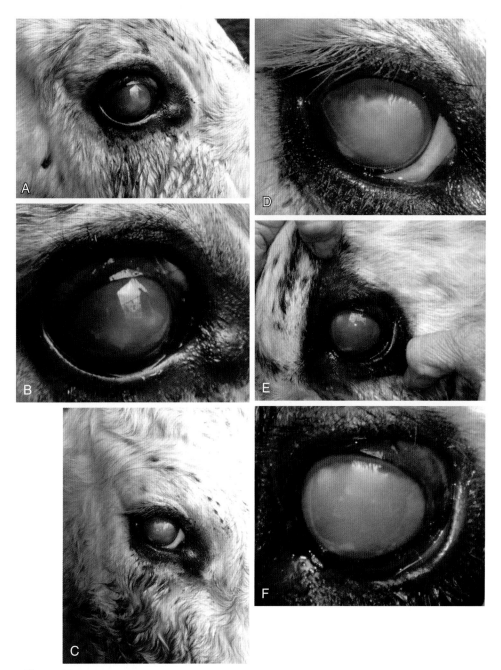

• **Fig. 14.39** Lesions consistent with "silage eye" or *Listeria monocytogenes* infection developed acutely in all eyes of a group of Randall cattle shortly after introduction to round bale feeding. *Listeria monocytogenes* and a few *Moraxella bovoculi* were cultured. Affected cattle were acutely blind with cloudy eyes; all but one regained vision over 3 to 4 weeks after systemic antibiotic treatment. No topical medications were administered. (Courtesy of Dr. Jadene Patch, Riverbend Veterinary Clinic, Plainfield, NH.) Figures A to F show varying degrees of corneal edema, non-ulcerative keratitis and severe uveitis with hypopyon and stromal abscessation. Note prominent corneal neovascularization originating from the limbus in D and F.

and exposure keratitis secondary to unilateral facial nerve paralysis may also be present in these cases; Dr. Rebhun believed the latter to be the most common ocular lesion seen in cattle with neurologic listeriosis.

A more common ocular condition associated with *Listeria monocytogenes* (but without accompanying neurologic signs) is the disease known as "silage eye," a unilateral or bilateral keratouveitis seen in many parts of the world that has been associated with *Listeria* spp. and may affect between 25% to 100% of animals in a group.

The condition most commonly occurs in cattle that are otherwise stressed or poorly managed and that are eating from improperly prepared "big bales" of silage. Silage eye takes many forms, from mild epiphora and conjunctivitis to severe, nonulcerative keratitis with marked, blinding corneal edema (an edema that acutely begins peripherally and progresses centrally very quickly), intrastromal abscess formation and other severe corneal changes, with or without hypopyon and other signs of uveitis (Fig. 14.39). The problem may be unilateral or bilateral. The diagnosis is based on history, management and feeding, clinical signs, and positive *L. monocytogenes* cultures or PCR testing from affected eyes. IBK, most commonly caused by *Moraxella bovis,* should be ruled out (by culture whenever possible), but the history and character of this corneal disease accompanied by severe uveitis make it clinically distinct. No single, approved, antibiotic regimen has been reported more effective than another; in some cases, the disease has been reported to run its course in about 2 weeks, with or without treatment. Topical atropine (once or twice daily) should always be used to improve patient comfort and reduce the sequelae associated with uveitis. Topical dexamethasone three or four times daily will improve signs of uveitis and patient comfort as well as shorten the clinical course but should be used with caution in pregnant cattle. Penicillin, oxytetracycline, ampicillin, erythromycin, oxytetracycline–polymyxin B sulfate ointment and neomycin–polymyxin–bacitracin ointment have all been reported efficacious (topically or parenterally according to the drug). Fluoroquinolones are very effective when used topically three or four times daily, but their use in the eyes of cattle is not approved in the United States. Guyot and others have suggested that the presence of ocular listeriosis may serve as a sentinel sign of concerning levels of *Listeria* infection in herds. In addition to abortions, weight loss, and ocular signs in adult cattle in two herds, one report also noted a large number of calves in one herd that were being fed milk containing large amounts of *Listeria* spp presenting with hypopyon without neurologic signs.

Deep interstitial keratitis characterized by diffuse corneal edema and circumferential vascular ingrowth from the limbus is occasionally observed in cattle with uveitis associated with septicemia, endotoxemia, malignant catarrhal fever (MCF) (see Figs. 6.59 and 6.60), and other systemic diseases. The conjunctival form of IBR also may result in a nonulcerative stromal keratitis that is primarily limbal in its distribution.

Signs and Diagnosis

Lacrimation, blepharospasm, and photophobia are almost always present when ulcerative corneal disease or corneal foreign bodies exist. Severe blepharospasm in cattle quickly leads to eyelid swelling and is associated with conjunctival injection and ocular pain. Corneal ulcers or opacities associated with ulceration may be apparent on inspection of the cornea, but the best means of diagnosis is via staining of stroma underlying the epithelial defects with fluorescein dye (Fluor-I-Strip, Ayerst Laboratories, New York, NY). The stroma deep to the epithelial defects will stain green and may be further highlighted with an UV light source (this is particularly helpful in detecting small lesions). Bear in mind that ulcerative stromal disease may occur deep to the intact epithelium, and eyes with stromal abscesses may *not* stain with fluorescein. Reflex uveitis (evidenced by pain, aqueous flare, and secondary miosis) is present in almost all bovine eyes affected by corneal ulceration. Blocking the palpebral nerve with 2% lidocaine, thereby interrupting the motor supply of the facial nerve (cranial nerve VII)

to the orbicularis oculi muscle, greatly facilitates examination of the painful bovine eye. In addition, downward rotation of the animal's head should be used to better expose the cornea (i.e., downward rotation facilitates examination of the cornea).

Corneal ulcers associated with facial nerve paralysis tend to be located in the central or lower central cornea (see Fig. 13.18). Absence of the palpebral response makes the diagnosis of exposure keratitis in such cases.

Infected corneal ulcers may be bacterial or fungal in origin and usually have necrotic or melting adjacent stroma alongside more dramatic corneal edema, and may have peripheral vascularization if more than 5 days in duration. A mucopurulent ocular discharge, severe miosis, and hypopyon or fibrin in the anterior chamber may be present. In general, signs of pain such as lacrimation, photophobia, and blepharospasm are more pronounced when infection complicates traumatic corneal injuries.

Most corneal foreign bodies can be identified by inspection with a focal light source, but magnification may occasionally be necessary to locate very small foreign bodies. Signs of ocular pain, conjunctival hyperemia, and eyelid swelling are present when a foreign body is located in the cornea. Initial serous ocular discharge will change to mucopurulent with chronicity or secondary infection associated with the foreign body. If a foreign body is suspected, the third eyelid should be examined after topical anesthetic application in every case by lifting it so that the conjunctiva behind the eyelid can be thoroughly examined, using magnification if possible.

Interstitial keratitis is a nonulcerative condition in which corneal edema and circumferential vascular influx from the limbus co-exist. Depending on severity, the vascular influx may be superficial (branching vessels) or deep (straight "paintbrush" vessels), and edema may vary in severity. Rather than a specific diagnosis, interstitial keratitis usually accompanies uveitis in cattle and is therefore accompanied by blepharospasm, lacrimation, photophobia, ciliary and conjunctival hyperemia, severe miosis, and cellular-protein accumulation in the anterior chamber. A primary systemic disease should be sought to explain the uveitis. Neither *Mycoplasma* nor *Chlamydia* have been identified as causes of stromal keratitis in dairy cattle despite the frequency of keratoconjunctivitis caused by these organisms in sheep and goats.

Treatment

Corneal abrasions, ulcers, or nonperforating lacerations that are acute and not infected are best treated with topical broad-spectrum antibiotic ointments as prophylaxis against bacterial infection. Corticosteroids are usually contraindicated because they reduce the eye's inherent ability to resist infection. Subconjunctival antibiotics may be administered deep to the bulbar conjunctiva as an adjunct to topical antibiotics or as sole antibiotic therapy when it is impossible to catch the cow routinely for topical treatment. Veterinarians should be aware, however, that subconjunctival antibiotics are not deposit-type residual medications and are absorbed

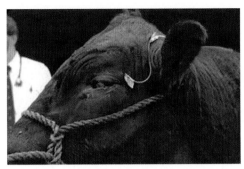

• **Fig. 14.40** Silastic palpebral lavage apparatus in a bull placed to aid in safe treatment of a deep ulcer in the left eye and for safety of his handlers. Infusion pumps were used and changed once daily.

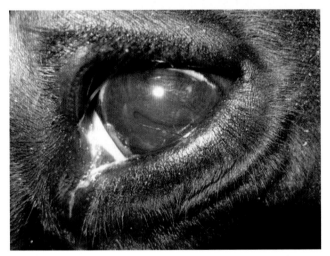

• **Fig. 14.41** Nonspecific bilateral miosis without other signs of uveitis in a toxemic cow with septic metritis.

into the eye within 12 hours of administration. It is also important to utilize the bulbar conjunctiva and not perform an "eyelid injection" because absorption of drug from the eyelid does nothing for the eye. The only possible benefit from eyelid injections is leakage of drug from the eyelid puncture site onto the cornea. Topical antibiotics should be applied as frequently as practicality and labor allow. In fractious patients, an eyelid lavage catheter may be used, inserted as for equine patients (Fig. 14.40).

Topical 1% atropine ophthalmic preparations are indicated (1 drop of solution or 2–3 mm of ointment, one to three times daily, to effect) in any eye that is painful due to corneal disease whenever miosis is present to relieve ciliary spasm and dilate the pupil secondarily (Fig. 14.41). A single dose usually results in dramatic improvement in patient comfort within 3 or 4 hours, and at least one dose should be used topically in almost every ulcer. When the patient is more comfortable, treatments often become easier to administer.

Infected corneal ulcers and wounds require more aggressive antibiotic therapy. Very painful eyes with obvious deep ulcers or ulcers with necrotic edges should be assumed to be infected. Ideally, scrapings should be obtained from the ulcer edges for Gram staining, cytology, and culture and susceptibility, to identify the causative organism(s). In practice, this is seldom done with cattle, but for valuable animals, this diagnostic step is appropriate to more accurately direct the initial treatment. Therapy may be compromised because of restraint difficulties with cattle, but this should not discourage frequent treatment of the eyes of valuable calves or cows because the frequency of treatment with appropriate antibiotics is directly proportional to the speed of resolution of infection. Topical and sub-bulbar conjunctival antibiotics comprise the major therapeutic weapons but are limited in some countries because of restrictions on legal drug use in food animals. Subconjunctival injections of penicillin (150,000–300,000 U), administered under the bulbar conjunctiva, establish high but short-lived antibiotic levels in the cornea and anterior segment of the eye. These injections can be repeated daily if necessary. Topical antibiotics (optimally based on Gram stain and culture of scrapings or smears from the ulcer) should be applied as frequently as possible. Systemic antibiotics usually are not helpful. In milking cattle, antibiotic residues need to be considered and withdrawal times observed.

With any infected ulcer, in any species, ocular and periocular hygiene are critical to maintain patient comfort and reduce contaminants around the eye. Discharges should be cleared away from the eyelids and face at least once daily to prevent secondary dermatitis and to remove debris.

Corneal foreign bodies need to be removed as gently as possible to prevent further penetration of the object into, or through, the cornea. The easiest means to remove most foreign bodies is via sharp saline lavage. After blocking the palpebral nerve and applying topical anesthetic (0.5% proparacaine or lidocaine) to the eye, a stream of saline is directed at the corneal foreign body through a 12-mL syringe and attached to the hub of a 25-gauge needle, *with the needle broken from the needle hub.* Most foreign material, even that which is embedded in stroma, will flush free with this technique. If flushing fails to resolve the problem, sedation of the animal, further anesthesia of the eye, and surgical manipulation of the lesion may be necessary. After the foreign body is removed, topical or subconjunctival antibiotics are applied to the eye as prophylaxis against infection until the lesion epithelializes.

Stromal keratitis usually indicates underlying uveitis, and therapy of uveitis is indicated and discussed later. One exception is stromal keratitis secondary to IBR conjunctivitis. This keratitis resolves spontaneously 2 to 4 weeks after the onset of the viral conjunctivitis.

Exposure keratitis secondary to facial nerve lesions should be treated with topical ocular lubricants –four to six times daily, and prophylactic antibiotics even when little or no ulceration exists. If central exposure damage and ulceration are present, the dried central cornea should be flushed gently with saline to remove dried crusts, hairs, necrotic corneal tissue, and other foreign material. Topical antibiotics should be applied as frequently as possible, and 1% atropine should be applied one to four times daily to improve the animal's comfort. A temporary tarsorrhaphy (see Fig. 4.6) is indicated in every case of exposure keratitis and should be performed immediately or as soon as possible after the diagnosis is made unless topical ointment lubrication can be provided a minimum of four to six times daily. A temporary partial tarsorrhaphy is performed by placing half-thickness sutures in the temporal third of the upper and lower eyelids using size 3-0 or 4-0 mattress sutures that split the eyelid thickness. Sutures *must not* penetrate the full thickness of the eyelid, to the level of the palpebral conjunctiva, or corneal ulceration will occur. Consult the Farm Animal Surgery textbook edited by Drs. Fubini and Ducharme for further details. Depending on the anticipated healing time for the primary neurologic deficit, a tarsorrhaphy is more or less mandatory. For example, acute otitis interna or media in a calf may result in facial nerve paralysis, but prompt treatment of the primary condition may improve facial nerve function within a few days. Therefore a tarsorrhaphy would be less necessary than in a listeriosis patient with severe facial paralysis requiring prolonged healing time. Eyelids with partial nerve function are less likely to require a temporary tarsorrhaphy than eyelids in which paralysis is complete. Although cattle may be less susceptible to corneal ulceration after facial paralysis than horses, exposure keratitis lesions are slow to heal compared with traumatic or infected ulcerations and must be prevented whenever possible. The best and least labor-intensive way in the longterm to prevent exposure keratitis is by means of a *properly placed* temporary tarsorrhaphy. Eyelid paralysis of longer duration is best treated with a reversible, split-eyelid tarsorrhaphy, somewhat similar to a Caslick's operation in brood mares, which can be removed, restoring full eyelid function when nerve function returns months to years later. Specialist phone consultation and eyelid anatomy review, as well as very small instrumentation and sutures, are recommended before performing this procedure for the first time.

Infectious Bovine Keratoconjunctivitis

Overview

Infectious bovine keratoconjunctivitis, or "pinkeye," is the most common eye disease of cattle and is present in dairy and beef cattle populations throughout the world. Less severely affected cattle can recover with or without corneal scarring; however, severely affected animals can develop permanent blindness after corneal rupture and lens or iris prolapse. The disease is more common in young stock and typically affects one eye; however, both eyes can become affected. Disease estimates of annual incidence vary depending on herd, but it is possible to have severe outbreaks, in which case attack rates can reach nearly 90% to 100% of animals. Although most economic impact studies have evaluated losses from IBK in beef cattle breeds, outbreaks of the disease in dairy heifer raising and dairy beef operations occur and can result in significant economic losses to producers. Along with economic impacts, the disease can lead to individual animal pain and suffering and therefore negatively affects animal welfare. Although any breed can be affected, a higher incidence has been reported in Herefords and a lower incidence in Brahmans and cattle with increased periocular pigmentation. More recent research has also identified genetic susceptibility to the disease.

Etiology

Moraxella bovis is the only organism for which Koch's postulates have been fulfilled with respect to IBK; however, other bacteria and viruses have also been associated with IBK, including IBR virus, *Moraxella bovoculi* and *Mycoplasma* spp., which probably increase the risk for IBK by enhancing opportunities for corneal injury as well as by increasing ocular and nasal discharge that may facilitate spread of *Moraxella bovis* in a herd. In some outbreaks, *Mycoplasma bovoculi* and *Mycoplasma bovis* have been isolated from affected animals in the absence of *Moraxella bovis*.

During the summer of 2002 in northern California, the majority of bacteria isolated from IBK-affected calves were found to be hemolytic gram-negative cocci. Genetic and biochemical characterization of these isolates later (in 2007) identified the organisms as being distinct from *Moraxella bovis* and *Moraxella ovis* (*M. ovis*), and the isolates were named *Moraxella bovoculi*. It is likely that *Moraxella bovoculi* has circulated within cattle populations for many years, and until this gram-negative coccus had been shown to be distinct from *Moraxella ovis*, it may have been misidentified by diagnostic laboratories as *Moraxella ovis*, *Branhamella ovis*, *Moraxella ovis*–like, or *Branhamella ovis*–like. Although recent reports have demonstrated that *Moraxella bovoculi* is now the most commonly isolated organism from IBK sample submissions to diagnostic laboratories and is also the *Moraxella* species most highly correlated with occurrence of acute IBK, a challenge study has failed to demonstrate keratoconjunctivitis in *Moraxella bovoculi* infected calves. Although it is possible that *Moraxella bovoculi* does not play a direct causal role in IBK, it is also possible that similar to *Moraxella bovis*, loss of certain pathogenic factors such as pili during frequent laboratory passage may have diminished infectivity of the challenge *Moraxella bovoculi* strain used in that study. Therefore, similar to *Mycoplasma* spp. and IBR, *Moraxella bovoculi* might also act as a risk factor for IBK.

In addition to bacterial ocular infections, other risk factors that are important in IBK pathogenesis include flies, solar irradiation, and mechanical trauma from plant awns. Outbreaks of IBK typically occur in summer months when heat and dust are present and fly populations are greatest. *Moraxella bovis* survives up to 3 days on the external surface and 2 days in the gut of face flies (*Musca autumnalis*). IBK can be experimentally induced in cattle exposed to face flies fed on *Moraxella bovis* cultures. Associations between solar irradiation and IBK have also been documented. Plant awns are also associated with IBK because these can cause mechanical injury to the cornea thereby facilitating ocular infections with *Moraxella* spp.

Pathogenesis

Moraxella bovis expresses many hydrolytic enzymes that may be important in facilitating ocular injury; however, only two proteins have been linked to pathogenicity: pilin and cytotoxin.

Pilin proteins (expressed on the surface of filamentous bacterial pili) of *Moraxella bovis* enable bacteria to adhere to the corneal epithelium and colonize the ocular surface. Pilus-based vaccines reduce the incidence and the severity of IBK; however, the presence of multiple pilus serogroups coupled with the potential for pilin gene inversions increases antigenic variability and may account for antigenic switching that is hypothesized to enable *Moraxella bovis* to evade a host immune response in animals vaccinated with pilus based antigens.

The *Moraxella bovis* cytotoxin (cytolysin/hemolysin) is a pore-forming protein that lyses bovine erythrocytes, neutrophils, lymphoma cells, and corneal epithelial cells in vitro. The lytic activity of this cytotoxin occurs through calcium-dependent formation of transmembrane pores in target cell membranes. Eye lesions induced by purified hemolytic and cytolytic fractions of *Moraxella bovis* are identical to ocular lesions observed in naturally occurring IBK.

An association between the *Moraxella bovis* cytotoxin and the RTX (repeats in the structural toxin) family of bacterial exoproteins followed the discovery that *Moraxella bovis* cytotoxin induces the formation of pores in target cell membranes. The *Moraxella bovis* cytotoxin gene (mbxA) is contained within an RTX operon (mbx operon) that encodes activation and export proteins; this operon is absent in nonhemolytic *Moraxella bovis*. The mbx operon defines a pathogenicity island, and acquisition or loss of mbx genes may help explain the historical observation that *Morxella bovis* could switch from a hemolytic to nonhemolytic phenotype. *Moraxella bovoculi* and *Moraxella ovis* have also been shown to encode RTX toxins that reside within classical RTX operons. Near complete identity within the deduced amino acid sequences of cytotoxin genes between geographically diverse *Moraxella bovis* isolates has been reported and demonstrates that there is a high degree of conservation in the gene encoding this important pathogenic factor.

Signs and Diagnosis

Clinical signs of IBK include conjunctivitis, corneal ulceration, corneal edema, photophobia, blepharospasm, and lacrimation. Initial signs of conjunctivitis include redness and serous to mucopurulent ocular discharge. In herd settings, multiple animals are often affected. Within 1 to 3 days of initial infection, a circular corneal ulcer develops in the central or lower central cornea (Fig. 14.42). Although early ulcers may go unnoticed, affected animals are more easily identified with the onset of more severe blepharospasm, lacrimation, photophobia, and tear staining, or accumulation of dirt and ocular discharge on the facial region. Focal light ophthalmic examination often then reveals a central, circular, and crater-like ulcer with corneal edema, deep peripheral vascularization at the limbus, and miosis (Fig. 14.43).

After these classic early signs, the eye may deteriorate and reach a variety of endpoints, depending on management and success of treatment. Most affected cattle show progression of the circular central ulcer to a less circular, deep crater-like ulcer with melting edges that appear necrotic.

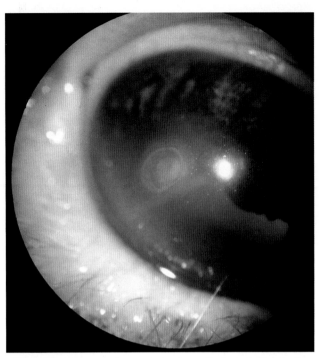

• **Fig. 14.42** Early central corneal ulcer in a calf affected with infectious bovine keratoconjunctivitis.

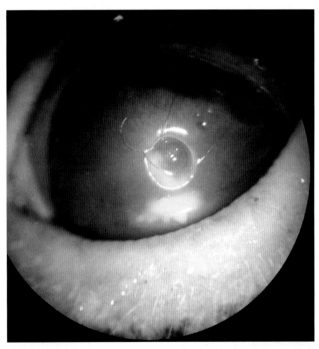

• **Fig. 14.43** Deeper crater-like corneal ulcer in a heifer with infectious bovine keratoconjunctivitis of 1 week's duration. Corneal edema surrounds the ulcer, and peripheral corneal vessels are present. Hypopyon is present in the anterior chamber as a result of secondary uveitis.

The center of the ulcer may appear clear or dark in color as Descemet's membrane is approached (Fig. 14.44). Corneal edema intensifies through the cornea peripheral to the ulcer, and deep corneal vascularization advances inward from the limbus to the edge of the ulcer. These vessels provide metabolic and cellular components for completion of the healing process. At this stage, the animal suffers severe pain, resulting in loss of appetite and bodyweight. Deep ulcers that begin to heal, with or without therapy, will fill in the crater with granulation tissue as the corneal vascularization reaches the ulcer bed. The vessels provide capillaries, and the corneal stroma contributes fibroblasts for granulation tissue. Much clinical variation exists in the appearance of infected eyes. Blue (edema), red (vessels, granulation tissue), and yellow (necrosis, stromal abscesses) are the predominant colors that can be observed.

Superficial ulcers epithelialize whereas deep ulcers first fill with granulation tissue and then epithelialize during the healing process. After epithelialization is complete, ocular pain resolves. Central corneal granulation tissue changes color from red to pink and finally to white as the corneal stroma reorganizes and healing progresses. Corneal edema resolves from the periphery first and clears progressively toward the central lesion. Corneal deep straight vessels recede, leaving only superficial branching vessels. Complete corneal remodeling requires weeks to months. Most recovered cattle have central nebulas, maculas, or leukomas but little visual loss, which is a testament to the amazing healing ability of the bovine cornea. Eyes that are unattended may progress to descemetoceles, corneal perforation, or panophthalmitis. During an outbreak in a herd, all degrees of severity can often be observed across affected cattle. Secondary uveitis in severe pinkeye cases may cause residual posterior synechiae and cataract formation.

The clinical signs and herd morbidity often suffice for accurate diagnosis of IBK in most instances. Aerobic culture of ocular swabs from affected eyes can provide evidence for the presence of *Moraxella* spp.; however, cases that are refractory to therapy with β-lactam drugs warrant consideration of other potential causes of corneal lesions such as *Mycoplasma* spp.

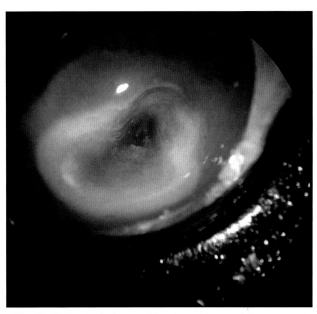

• **Fig. 14.44** Extremely deep melting ulcer with central descemetocele *(dark central area)* in a heifer with infectious bovine keratoconjunctivitis of 1 week's duration.

Treatment

Infectious bovine keratoconjunctivitis has been treated successfully through both local (subconjunctivally administered), as well as parenterally administered antibiotics. Because *Moraxella bovis* is susceptible to a variety of antimicrobials, many have been shown prospectively to be effective in treating IBK, including subconjunctival penicillin, and parenteral oxytetracycline, florfenicol, ceftiofur, and tulathromycin. Only two of these, oxytetracycline and tulathromycin, are specifically labeled for treatment of IBK in the United States. It is worth noting that the use of a 1-mL (300,000 U) subconjunctival dose of penicillin in lactating dairy cows has been shown to result in detectable milk penicillin residues for 22 hours after treatment. Susceptibility patterns for *Moraxella bovoculi* are generally similar to those for *Moraxella bovis*.

Other elements of therapy to consider besides either subconjunctival or parenteral antibiotics include topical atropine to maintain cycloplegia and NSAIDs to reduce inflammation and pain. Unfortunately, restraint difficulties and limited labor can affect availability and feasibility of frequent treatment application.

Several treatment regimens are listed below; the suitability of one over another depends on facilities and feasibility of repeat treatments for affected animals.

1. 300,000 U of penicillin G administered subconjunctivally
2. Topical application of gentamicin, erythromycin, or tobramycin ointments several times daily to affected eyes. Ophthalmic ointments or mastitis tubes may be used for this purpose. Appropriate milk and meat withdrawals should be considered before their use
3. Topical 1% atropine ointment twice daily
4. Confining the animal so as to avoid sunlight, cleansing discharges from the eye, and using fly control to discourage fly irritation on the animal's face

A less intensive therapeutic plan could include:

1. Initial subconjunctival injection of penicillin
2. One application of topical antibiotic and atropine
3. Repeat topical treatments daily
4. Parenteral oxytetracycline or tulathromycin dosed per manufacturer's label

With increased recent scrutiny by veterinarians, consumers, regulatory officials and the industry regarding prudent antibiotic use in food-producing animals, it is important for practitioners to educate producers on how to recognize a healed IBK lesion to avoid unnecessary antibiotic administration to animals with white-appearing eyes that have already fully healed.

Other adjunctive treatments to the above include NSAID administration and, when possible, frequent topical administration of patient serum. More invasive surgical therapies that can be considered include tarsorrhaphy or third eyelid flaps. Topical or subconjunctival corticosteroids, although often practiced, have not been shown to improve healing. Such drugs may weaken defense mechanisms of the infected cornea and possibly exacerbate disease. Although antibacterial sprays designed for ophthalmic use also are advocated, practitioners should evaluate the contents before recommending their use. Furazolidone sprays, although effective against IBK, are illegal to use in the United States. Irritating sprays and powders should be avoided, especially when applied to an already painful eye.

No controlled studies have evaluated the use of eye patches in cattle affected with IBK. It is likely that these patches provide relief from bright light; however, producers should regularly check (at least two or three times weekly) to make sure that eyes are not deteriorating under a patch. Neglected eyes that perforate or develop severe keratoconus with endophthalmitis or panophthalmitis may require enucleation to prevent continuous pain, irritation from flies and discharges, worsening infection, and failure to thrive.

Prevention

Efforts at IBK prevention should focus on reducing risk factors for the disease, optimizing immune responsiveness in animals, and minimizing iatrogenic infections. To reduce fly populations, insecticide-impregnated ear tags placed on calves and topical insecticides with back and face rubbers are recommended. Cutting mature grasses before cattle are turned out may help minimize risks associated with direct mechanical corneal injury from plant awns. In areas where trace mineral deficiencies are prevalent, it is important to pay attention to supplementation of trace minerals such as copper and selenium that are important for maintaining a healthy immune system.

To enhance immune responsiveness to ocular *Moraxella* infections, vaccination with commercially available *Moraxella bovis* bacterins should be considered. Unfortunately, such bacterins are not universally effective. Variability in results from vaccination is likely related to differences between antigenic composition of vaccinal strains and the *Moraxella* strains that may be circulating in a herd. Recently, a commercially available *Moraxella bovoculi* bacterin (Addison Laboratories, Fayette, MO, 65248) has become available that could provide another option for immunoprophylaxis against IBK.

With the increase in reporting of *Moraxella bovoculi* from clinical samples after the initial speciation of that organism in 2007, producers and veterinarians have also sought to improve vaccination coverage by using autogenous *M. bovoculi* (or *Moraxella bovis*) vaccines in prevention programs. Studies investigating the efficacy of autogenous *Moraxella bovis* or *Moraxella bovoculi* vaccines for the prevention of IBK have reported these vaccines to be ineffective; however, anecdotal reports by veterinarians in support of the use of such *Moraxella bovis* or *Moraxella bovoculi* bacterins do exist, and the topic of vaccination to prevent IBK remains contentious. When owners are considering vaccination, it is important to discuss timing of vaccination to optimize immune responses in vaccinated animals. In general, a vaccine series should be initiated at least 4 weeks before seasonal outbreaks of disease would be predicted to occur based on prior experience.

To avoid iatrogenic spread of infective bacteria between animals, use of disposable gloves is recommended along with plastic aprons and obstetrical sleeves when handling pinkeye-affected cattle. Protective clothing, halters, and instruments should be changed or at least disinfected between animals. An inexpensive disinfectant is 10% household bleach made by mixing one part of regular strength household bleach to nine parts water (or ≈1–1.5 cups regular strength bleach per gallon of clean water). With concentrated bleach, only about 1/2 cup per gallon of clean water is needed. Producers who attend affected animals on their own without their herd veterinarian should be reminded that diluted bleach should be made fresh daily to maintain effectiveness and that it becomes less effective when heavily soiled with dirt, manure, or other organic material. For this reason, it should be refreshed frequently, depending on use and working conditions.

Corneal Neoplasms

Squamous cell carcinoma and its precursors (e.g., actinic keratosis, acanthosis, carcinoma in situ, epitheliomas, keratomas (Fig. 14.45)) are the most frequent tumors of the bovine cornea. Holsteins appear to have the highest incidence among dairy breeds. Corneal SCC usually originates at or near the temporal limbal area and then extends circumferentially, affecting adjacent corneal tissue and bulbar conjunctiva (Fig. 14.46). Early recognition of abnormal lesions is key! Treating small lesions allows effective, often curative, therapy using cryosurgery, radiofrequency hyperthermia, radiation, or keratectomy. Large or neglected tumors may require enucleation. Owners should bear in mind that regardless of size, any SCC can metastasize, but the likelihood of metastasis increases with duration. Histopathology should be performed on all excised masses to more reliably predict the likelihood of metastasis (e.g., vascular or lymphatic

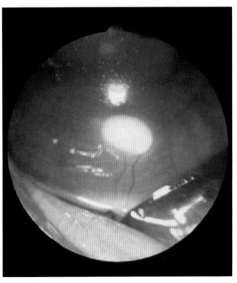

• **Fig. 14.45** Keratoma in a 7-year-old bull.

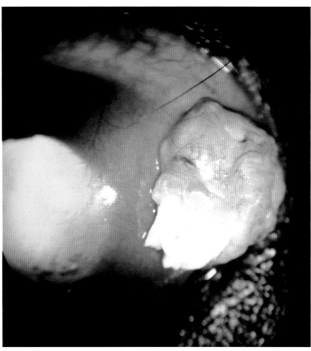

• **Fig. 14.46** Corneoscleral squamous cell carcinoma originating from the temporal limbus in an 8-year-old Holstein cow.

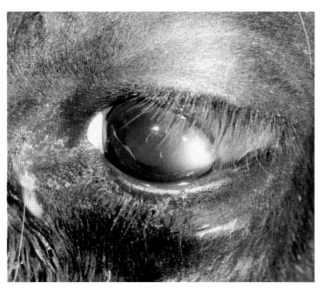

• **Fig. 14.47** Ocular lymphosarcoma that appeared as temporal conjunctival thickening and a white mass in the temporal cornea of a cow with multifocal lymphosarcoma.

invasion, mitotic index). Metastasis usually occurs first to regional lymph nodes, especially the parotid nodes and smaller nodes along the jugular furrow; lung metastasis has been seen in neglected cases.

Lymphosarcoma has been observed in the bovine cornea and globe, but only infrequently (Fig. 14.47). In these cases, the corneal lesion was not a solitary tumor but rather was one of many tumors involved in diffuse lymphosarcoma. Ocular lymphangiosarcoma has also been confirmed as a cause of corneoscleral neoplasia in a Holstein cow.

Corneal Lacerations

Partial-thickness (nonperforating) corneal lacerations should be treated as noninfected corneal injuries (see the earlier discussion), with excision of the partial-thickness flap as the first step in treatment. Flaplike lesions may be reattached surgically but unless repair is performed in the first few hours most flaps become dramatically edematous and dehiscence is usual. Perforating corneal lacerations with iris prolapse require specialized ophthalmic instrumentation, ophthalmic suture material, and general anesthesia for effective cosmetic repair. In valuable and show cows, referral is recommended. If the cow's value does not warrant referral or when the initiating trauma has caused massive intraocular injury (i.e., lens or vitreous prolapse), the affected eye should be enucleated.

Diseases of the Uveal Tract

Inflammatory Diseases of the Uveal Tract
Etiology and Signs

The iris, ciliary body, and choroid constitute the uveal tract, which is the vascular layer of the inner eye. The vascular nature of the uveal tract predisposes to proteinaceous and cellular exudates accumulating intraocularly when these tissues are inflamed from any cause such as trauma, septicemia, severe corneal ulceration, or immune-mediated disease. The iris is the most easily examined portion of the uveal tract, making iritis more obvious and easier to diagnose than inflammation of the ciliary body and choroid even though these tissues also may be involved.

The cardinal signs of uveitis in any species are miosis (see Fig. 14.41), aqueous flare ("headlights in fog" effect caused by protein and/or cells in the aqueous humor), and decreased IOP. Accompanying, nonspecific signs that develop at varying times include conjunctival and ciliary injection, peripheral corneal edema and vascularization, edema of the iris, and cellular and fibrinous exudates accumulating in the anterior chamber. Inflammation of the uveal tissues results in vasodilation with the consequence that fibrin, white blood cells and red blood cells may extravasate from the inflamed iris vasculature. When white blood cells and fibrin predominate and accumulate in the ventral anterior chamber it is referred to as hypopyon (Fig. 14.48); if red blood cells and fibrin predominate, hyphema is described (Fig. 14.49). Exudates from the choroid may also accumulate between the retina and choroid, resulting in chorioretinal inflammation, serous detachment of the retina, or both.

Uveitis is common in any animal with septicemia, particularly in neonates. This uveitis may be caused by direct endogenous bacterial spread to the uveal tract or by secondary endotoxemia acting on the uveal vasculature. Painful eyes with variable degrees of hypopyon, iris swelling, and miosis appear as predominant signs in these calves (see Fig. 14.48). Signs of uveitis are an extremely important diagnostic clue in a comatose neonatal calf because they indicate septicemia, possible meningitis, and correspondingly a poor prognosis.

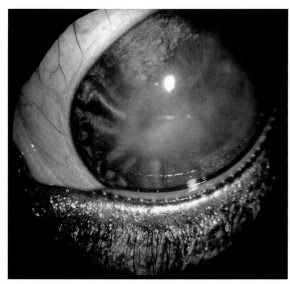

• **Fig. 14.48** Uveitis in a neonatal calf with septicemia. The iris is thickened and has a corrugated appearance. A fibrin clot obscures the markedly miotic pupil.

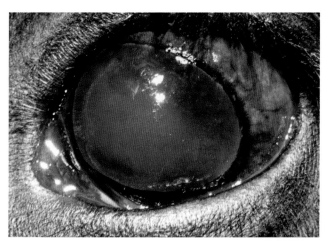

• **Fig. 14.49** Uveitis in an adult cow with septic metritis. A large fibrin clot and hyphema occupy the anterior chamber and obscure a miotic pupil.

Adult cattle with septicemia associated with gram-negative septic mastitis, septic metritis, endocarditis, and other causes occasionally develop unilateral or bilateral uveitis (see Fig. 14.49). Again, either true septicemia or endotoxemia may trigger the intraocular inflammation.

Idiopathic unilateral or bilateral uveitis occasionally occurs in otherwise healthy cattle. Affected cattle may lose vision temporarily or permanently. Various causes have been theorized but none proven. *Leptospira* spp., *H. somni,* toxoplasmosis, *Borrelia burgdorferi,* and other infectious organisms have been suspected. Immune-mediated uveitis also may exist in adult cattle, and the European disease known as specific ophthalmia bears resemblance to recurrent uveitis in horses and is thought to have a viral cause.

The acute form of MCF causes a severe anterior uveitis and vasculitis that involves virtually every part of the eye except the choroid (see Fig. 6.59). Corneal opacity resulting from edema and peripheral vascularization may be sufficiently severe as to prevent intraocular examination, but

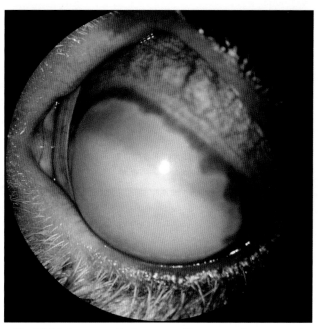

• **Fig. 14.50** Severe uveitis in a cow with acute malignant catarrhal fever (MCF). The lesions were bilateral and consisted of severe conjunctival and scleral vascular engorgement ("scleral injection"), corneal edema, dense hypopyon filling the ventral two-thirds of the anterior chamber, and peripheral corneal stromal vascularization. The hypopyon in MCF is composed of mononuclear cells.

severe anterior uveitis and hypopyon are present in almost all cases (Fig. 14.50 and 6.59). The uveitis associated with MCF is always bilateral and is characterized by massive influx of mononuclear cells into the anterior uveal tract. Chronic MCF or a mild form of MCF may result in more subtle signs of bilateral uveitis such as mild corneal edema, mild iritis, fibrin or hypopyon in the anterior chamber, and peripheral corneal vascularization, or the original inflammation may leave severe, permanently blinding changes in the eye (Fig. 14.51). Zemljic et al. reported on a group of cattle with sheep-associated MCF in which the degree of corneal edema at presentation had no prognostic significance for survival but the progression of corneal edema and persistence of uveitis were negative prognostic indicators.

Historically, granulomatous uveitis resulting from tuberculosis was observed commonly before the disease was controlled. Subsequently, tuberculosis should remain in the differential diagnosis when granulomatous uveitis coexists with weight loss and chronic respiratory disease, and the public health implications of the disease cannot be overemphasized.

Nonspecific bilateral miosis is observed commonly without other signs of uveitis in "toxemic" cattle. These cattle usually have overwhelming infections, and the miosis likely reflects subclinical uveitis associated with a systemic inflammatory response (see Fig. 14.41).

Uveitis secondary to trauma to the globe occurs from head butts, stanchion and chute trauma, and rough handling of cattle by humans. Signs of traumatic uveitis are similar to those found with other types of uveitis except that hyphema tends to be a prominent finding; periocular lesions and corneal ulceration or other signs of head trauma may also be present.

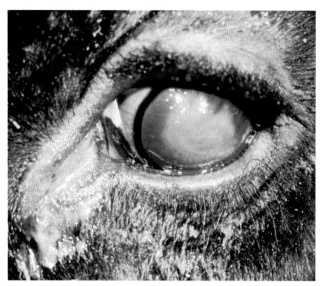

• **Fig. 14.51** Left eye of a Holstein calf with chronic malignant catarrhal fever. Both eyes had chronic uveitis and chronic keratitis with edema and vascularization of the cornea.

Secondary uveitis may occur following any serious corneal inflammatory disease, especially pinkeye, and can cause sequelae that limit future vision (e.g., synechiae, cataracts); therefore such cases of secondary uveitis should always be treated.

Diagnosis

Primary uveitis is diagnosed by observation of the ophthalmic lesions described earlier, coupled with absence of corneal injury or fluorescein dye uptake. Causes of secondary uveitis may be obvious when facial trauma is observed or septic foci such as severe septic mastitis or metritis are identified during the physical examination. Septicemia should be obvious in neonatal calves with depression, fever, diarrhea, a swollen navel, or other signs consistent with diffuse bacterial sepsis.

Non-ocular, primary sites of infection should be sought in any adult cow presenting for uveitis. When no primary sites of infection exist and fever is absent, idiopathic uveitis should be considered. Although causes of idiopathic uveitis currently are nebulous, future efforts should be directed toward diagnostic investigations that might uncover specific etiologies. When more than one cow in a herd experiences uveitis of unknown cause, acute and convalescent serology or advanced molecular diagnostics for *Listeria* spp., *Leptospira* spp., *H. somni*, toxoplasmosis, *B. burgdorferi*, and other diseases may be considered. Mucosal lesions, nasal discharge, high fever, nervous system signs, lymphadenopathy, hematuria, and other physical abnormalities are usually present in addition to uveitis in MCF patients.

Secondary uveitis may be obscured by severe primary corneal inflammation such as pinkeye, but miosis and hypopyon usually are apparent during a careful examination.

Treatment

If uveitis appears to be secondary to a septic condition (i.e., calf septicemia, septic mastitis, metritis, or endocarditis), treatment should address both the primary disease and the possibility that bacterial pathogens have entered the uveal tract. Antibiotics administered topically and subconjunctivally, as well as systemically, may be indicated. Whenever possible, the antibiotics should be the same antibiotics as those best suited for systemic treatment of the primary disease. For example, when a coliform mastitis is present and suspected to be the primary infection, ceftiofur may be used locally in the quarter and perhaps systemically as well if the cow appears severely ill. If this cow also develops uveitis, neomycin–polymyxin B–bacitracin topical ophthalmic ointment several times daily and subconjunctival antibiotics would be indicated. Similarly, a neonatal calf with probable gram-negative septicemia that has uveitis may be treated with similar drugs but a lesser dose of subconjunctival antibiotics would be used compared to an adult. Penicillin and ampicillin might be appropriate choices for subconjunctival and topical use when a gram-positive organism is suspected as the cause of uveitis—as for a cow with endocarditis in which gram-positive organisms are likely to be causative.

Cycloplegia is an important adjunct therapy (to control pain and establish pupillary dilation in order to prevent synechiae or pupil occlusion because of fibrin and inflammatory cells in the anterior chamber), and atropine sulfate ophthalmic ointment (1%) should be applied three or four times daily to the affected eye(s) until the pupil dilates and thereafter once or twice daily.

When cattle appear to have idiopathic uveitis in one or both eyes but otherwise appear clinically normal, topical therapy includes 1% atropine several times daily to establish cycloplegia and pupil dilatation, as well as topical antibiotic and steroid preparations to counteract the presumed nonseptic uveal inflammation. Similar therapy is indicated for traumatic uveitis unless corneal abrasions or ulcers are present. If no corneal injury exists, traumatic uveitis is treated with 1% atropine ointment to effect, dexamethasone ophthalmic ointment applied several times daily, or topical NSAIDs such as diclofenac or flurbiprofen four times daily in pregnant patients. Systemic NSAIDs are helpful in the treatment of idiopathic (nonseptic, probable immune-mediated) and traumatic uveitis.

Hemorrhage into the anterior chamber (hyphema) may occasionally occur from trauma or the many potential causes of thrombocytopenia (e.g., BVDV, bracken fern intoxication, idiopathic) or other clotting abnormalities. Hyphema without obvious hypopyon may occur in septic patients with thrombocytopenia associated with disseminated intravascular coagulation (see Fig. 3.57). Cycloplegics and topical antiinflammatory treatments can be used, but the therapeutic focus is usually on the primary disease and the other affected organ system(s).

Diseases of the Lens

Developmental Diseases
Etiology and Signs

Hereditary cataracts, including nuclear cataracts in Holsteins and a recessive microphakia with cataract, ectopia lentis, and aniridia

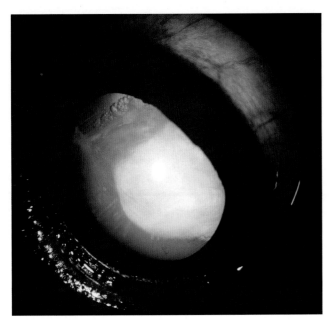

• **Fig. 14.52** Holstein calf with a dense nuclear cataract plus additional lens cortex abnormalities. Intralenticular balloon cells can be seen in the equatorial lens at 10 o'clock position, suggesting additional, progressive cataract change is likely.

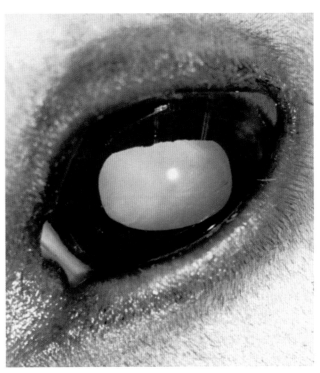

• **Fig. 14.53** Diffuse cortical cataract in a Jersey calf.

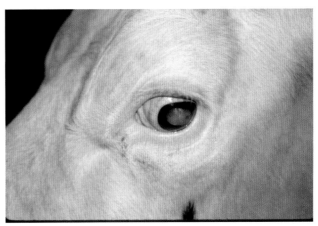

• **Fig. 14.54** Diffuse, congenital cataract in a 4-month old Holstein heifer, bilateral and complete cataracts had been present in this calf since birth.

in Jerseys, have been described. Krump recently reported on a herd in which 26% of 110 pedigreed Ayrshire cattle had cataracts. Sporadic cases of microphthalmia were also identified in this herd. As in other species, a newborn calf with cataracts may represent either an inherited condition or simply an embryological accident during development of the eye, and differentiation is usually impossible based solely on clinical signs. If similar cataracts are found in other age-matched calves from different genetic lines, a gestational accident such as toxicity, bovine viral diarrhea virus (BVDV) infection during the midtrimester (days 125–175) of pregnancy, or other common exposure should be investigated. A 2009 report by Hassig et al., for example, noted a statistically significant increase in nuclear cataracts in Swiss veal calves raised near mobile telephone towers!

When the only affected calves are from a common genetic line, heredity should be suspected. Otherwise, the cause of cataracts in a single affected calf is generally impossible to determine unless other signs of in utero BVDV infection (e.g., cerebellar hypoplasia or brachygnathism) are present. Unless inheritance can be disproven, any bull calf with cataracts should not be considered for use as a stud. When BVDV is suspected as the cause of cortical cataracts in newborn calves, precolostral titers should be assessed for evidence of prenatal BVDV infection, and viral isolation or PCR from whole blood may be attempted to rule out persistent infection (although this would be unlikely given the timing of in utero BVDV exposure associated with congenital eye defects).

Signs of congenital cataracts may be sufficiently subtle as to require slit-lamp biomicroscopy for observation of nuclear or cortical opacities (Fig. 14.52). Other cases are obvious with the lens being completely opaque as a result of a cataract (Figs. 14.53 and 14.54). Congenital cataracts that involve only parts of the lens may progress very slowly,

if at all. When offering a prognosis, the veterinarian always should caution the owner that any cataract may progress and may eventually cause blindness.

Occasionally, diseases in the vitreous (discussed later) may be confused with cataracts; additionally some primary vitreal diseases can result in cataracts.

Acquired Diseases
Etiology and Signs

Acquired cataracts in cattle usually occur from either intraocular inflammation or previous trauma to the eye. Ocular inflammation associated with uveitis or severe IBK may result in posterior synechiae formation and fibrin coating the anterior lens capsule. Damage to the anterior lens capsule alters normal lens metabolism, resulting in capsular and cortical cataract formation. Cataracts formed by these mechanisms usually develop slowly after the initiating inflammation. Therefore the eye may appear "quiet" or free of inflammation at the time cataracts first are observed, but with close observation, telltale markers of the previous inflammation are usually present. These markers include posterior synechiae, iris pigment "rests" that appear as brown or black spots on the anterior lens capsule (from previous iris adhesions), and corneal scarring from previous IBK.

Similarly, traumatic uveitis may allow fibrin, hemorrhage, and iris adhesions to damage the lens capsule. Trauma may initiate lens luxation or a lens rupture in addition to uveitis and thereby further predispose to cataract formation.

Treatment

Bovine cataracts are rarely removed surgically, primarily because of economic concerns, but cataract removal in cattle is usually successful at restoring vision; a veterinary ophthalmologist should perform this surgery.

One of the simplest and best means of preventing acquired cataracts in cattle is the routine usage of topical atropine sulfate in ophthalmic injuries, with all IBK infections, and with uveitis from any cause because by dilating the pupil, iris adhesions (posterior synechiae) and their lens sequelae are much less likely to occur.

Diseases of the Vitreous and Fundus

Developmental Diseases

Persistent hyaloid arteries are visible in virtually all newborn calves examined by ophthalmoscopy; the remnants of this artery are detectable in 25% to 50% of yearling cattle. In adult cattle, the fibrosed proximal end of the vessel (Bergmeister papilla) is usually visible floating in the posterior vitreous just anterior to the optic nerve head and attached at the center of the optic disc (Fig. 14.55). Occasionally, the primary vitreous is malformed or fails to regress, and affected patients may be blinded if this occurs bilaterally (Fig. 14.56).

Inflammatory Diseases

Vitreal abscesses and endophthalmitis occur on rare occasions in septicemic calves. Vitreitis also may be associated with MCF or embolic septic uveitis in cattle. Treatment is similar to that discussed for septic uveitis.

Congenital Inherited Diseases

Although many congenital retinopathies, retinal dysplasias, and retinal detachments may represent inherited defects in other species, the paucity of reported cases in dairy cattle reflects either a low incidence, or a failure of recognition of these disorders. Retinal detachments have been observed in association with multiple congenital anomalies in four related Irish Friesian cattle.

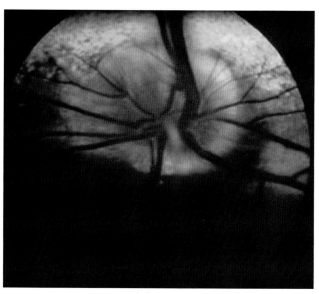

• **Fig. 14.55** Normal optic nerve head and peripapillary fundus in a Holstein cow. A soft pink-white, out-of-focus strand at the point of vessel confluence is a remnant of the hyaloid artery (normal finding persisting into adulthood).

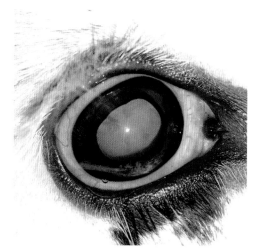

• **Fig. 14.56** Presumed persistent hyperplastic primary vitreous in one of two twin 3-month old Holstein heifers. The iris, anterior lens capsule and lens cortex were normal (Courtesy of Dr. Tom Linden, Homestead Large Animal, Auburn, NY).

Because dairy cattle are seldom surveyed for fundic lesions unless they appear blind, subtle retinal lesions likely go undetected.

Nutritional Causes

Hypovitaminosis A

Etiology and Signs
Increased cerebrospinal fluid (CSF) pressure has been confirmed in experimental studies of vitamin A deficiency and is thought to be responsible for the neurologic signs observed. Increased CSF pressure results from failure of proper resorption of CSF through the abnormal arachnoid villi and thickened dura mater. The pathophysiology of visual loss is more complex. Although papilledema is a classical finding in both adult and growing vitamin A–deficient cattle (Figs. 14.57,

14.58 and 13.30), the mechanism by which papilledema occurs differs in these two age groups. In adult cattle, papilledema is thought to be secondary to chronic elevation of CSF pressure. Papilledema by itself does not lead to blindness unless it becomes chronic enough to result in vascular ischemia, interference with axonal transport, and secondary optic nerve degeneration. Increased CSF pressure probably also contributes to the papilledema observed in growing cattle. However, in this younger age group, dural fibrodysplasia and altered bone metabolism resulting in decreased bone resorption in the optic canals causes direct optic nerve damage and this may also lead to papilledema. This decreased bone resorption leads to dorsoventral compression of the canals. Resultant vascular compromise, ischemic necrosis of the nerve, and direct interference with axonal transport through the optic nerve lead to more severe papilledema, edema in the nerve fiber layer of the retina, and retinal or vitreal hemorrhages as congested vessels rupture. The pathophysiology within the optic canals is irreversible in growing animals, and when present, blindness is usually permanent.

Nyctalopia, or night blindness, has been reported as the earliest sign of visual disturbance in experimental hypovitaminosis A but seldom is observed in field outbreaks. Vitamin A is required for regeneration of the rhodopsin necessary for photoreceptor activity during dark adaptation. Rod dysfunction and subsequent loss have been shown to be greater than cone dysfunction and loss in chronic vitamin A deficiency in rats. Photoreceptor dysfunction, especially of rods, probably contributes to nyctalopia and visual loss in both adult and growing cattle. Therefore visual alterations in adult cattle are caused by photoreceptor abnormalities and papilledema. In growing calves, the same physiologic and biochemical problems occur, but additive insult occurs as a result of anatomic optic nerve compression and vascular ischemia.

Physical disruption and ischemic necrosis of the optic nerves in the stenotic optic canals is followed chronically by their replacement with mature dense sheets of collagen. Destruction of optic nerve axons at this site leads to orthograde (Wallerian) degeneration in the optic tracts and secondary astrogliosis.

Male animals seem to be less tolerant of hypovitaminosis A than females. Rations persistently low in vitamin A are rare but have been found when growing cattle or feeder beef rations were formulated using either feedstuffs that had been stored for an excessive time or were composed primarily of feedstuffs (cereal grains) inherently low in vitamin A. Deficient rations must be fed for months before clinical signs of hypovitaminosis A occur. Clinical signs include blindness with dilated, nonresponsive pupils, optic nerve changes (see Fig. 14.57), and diffuse retinal pathology beyond the optic nerve, best visualized in the nontapetal fundus (Fig. 14.58).

Ophthalmic examination confirms papilledema; retinal edema; and, in some cases, retinal hemorrhage as congested retinal vessels leak blood into the retina or vitreous (see Figs. 14.57, 14.58 and 13.30). Although there are variations in the degree of visual loss and the fundic lesions seen,

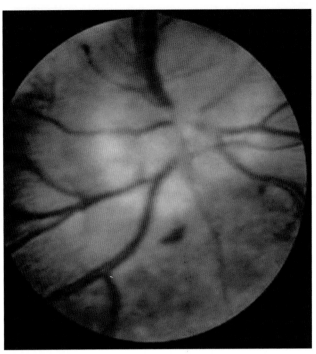

• **Fig. 14.57** Optic nerve swelling (papilledema), peripapillary retinal edema, and preretinal hemorrhages in a Holstein steer with vitamin A deficiency. (Courtesy of Dr. Tom Divers.)

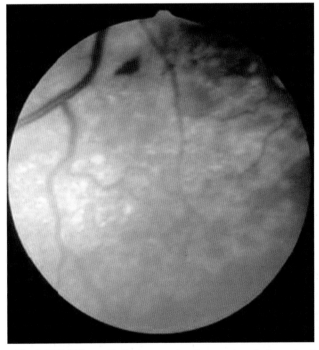

• **Fig. 14.58** Diffuse retinal edema and cotton wool spots throughout the non-tapetal fundus from the same animal as Fig. 14.57.

papilledema is present in almost all animals showing neurologic or ophthalmic signs.

Diagnosis. Although clinical signs often create a strong suspicion of hypovitaminosis A (e.g., neurologic plus ophthalmic signs, plus failure to grow), evaluation of serum or plasma vitamin A must be done to confirm the diagnosis.

Serum levels less than 20 µg/100 mL (200 ng/ml) support the diagnosis, and the severity of visual lesions is inversely proportional to levels less than 20 µg/100 mL. Normal values range from 25 to 60 µg/100 mL.

Treatment

Correcting the deficient diet so that it provides a minimum of 40 IU of vitamin A/kg body weight daily is essential. Further, treatment with up to 440 IU/kg body weight for several days is indicated as initial therapy. The prognosis is poor for growing animals that are blind because permanent damage to the optic nerves as they traverse the optic canals is already likely.

Male Fern Poisoning (Dryopteris filix-mas)

European workers have reported optic neuropathy in cattle secondary to ingestion of male fern. Variable degrees of retrobulbar optic neuritis, indigestion, and constipation are the observed signs. Papillitis, papilledema, and peripapillary hemorrhage may appear. Blindness may be temporary or permanent, depending on the amount of fern ingested.

The only treatment is removal from contaminated pasture and symptomatic support to include laxatives.

Inflammatory Lesions

Etiology and Signs

Bovine viral diarrhea virus infection between 75 and 150 days of gestation may cause inflammatory damage to the retina and optic nerve of the fetus. Resultant visual loss may be partial or complete depending on the degree of optic nerve damage. Retinal atrophy appearing as hyperreflective areas in the tapetal area or depigmented lesions in the nontapetal portion of the fundus, retinal hemorrhages, and optic nerve degeneration have been observed in affected calves at birth (Figs. 14.59 and 6.56). If cataracts coexist, the fundic lesions may be hidden from ophthalmoscopic view (Fig. 6.55). Other congenital aberrations such as brachygnathism (Fig. 6.54) or cerebellar hypoplasia may or may not be observed in affected calves and in other calves born about the same time in the herd.

Septicemia probably causes multifocal chorioretinal inflammation more commonly than we realize because many adult cattle have evidence of multifocal chorioretinal scarring. Ophthalmoscopic examination in acute cases shows round fluffy lesions ("cotton wool spots") of active chorioretinitis, always best recognized in the nontapetal portion of the fundus. These lesions later appear as scars with depigmented peripheral zones and central hyperpigmented zones which have been subsequently called "bullet hole" lesions (Fig. 14.60). Calf septicemia or adult septicemia caused by mastitis, metritis, and endocarditis may also cause similar lesions, as, it is also presumed, may some viral respiratory infections. It is possible that the cow is asymptomatic or shows only vague illness when these fundic lesions develop because most lesions are quiescent when discovered. Unless the cow loses all vision, retinal lesions are neither suspected nor investigated clinically. Subclinical infections with *H. somni* or other pathogens may also be involved, but this has not been proven.

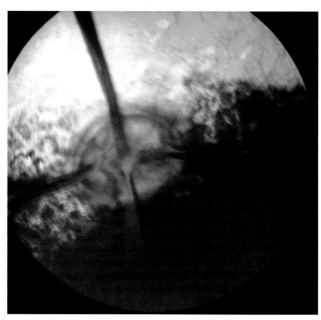

• **Fig. 14.59** Optic nerve degeneration, retinal vascular attenuation, peripapillary chorioretinal scarring, and tapetal hyperreflectivity in a calf that was born blind as a result of in utero bovine viral diarrhea virus infection.

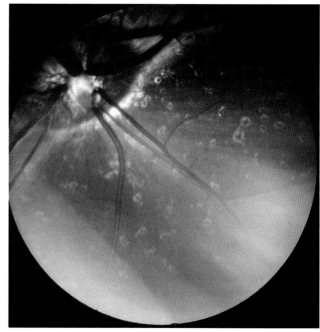

• **Fig. 14.60** Multifocal chorioretinal scars in the nontapetal portion of the fundus of a Holstein cow with reduced vision in the eye. The lesions are depigmented peripherally and have a hyperpigmented center and are known as "bullet hole" scars.

Treatment and Prevention

Therapy and prevention of inflammatory lesions are possible only when a direct cause and effect can be determined. For example, in utero BVDV infection may be confirmed by precolostral antibody determination. In a majority of cases, the ocular manifestations of in utero BVDV exposure occur after fetal immunocompetence has been reached, so affected calves will not be persistently

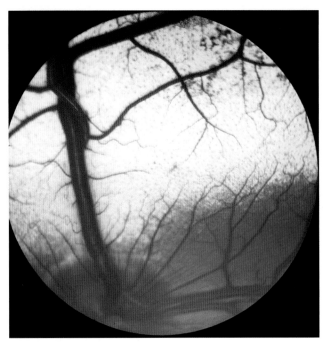

• **Fig. 14.61** Engorged retinal veins in a calf with polycythemia secondary to a tetralogy of Fallot (compare with normal vasculature in Fig. 14.56).

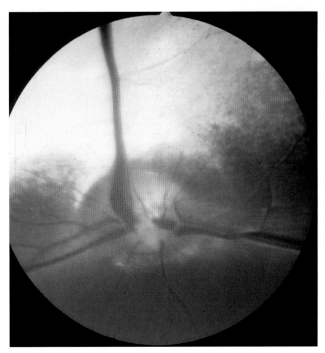

• **Fig. 14.62** Diffuse tapetal hyperreflectivity and vascular attenuation in a Holstein cow with retinal degeneration.

infected BVDV individuals. Control of BVDV is discussed in Chapter 6.

Vascular Lesions of the Fundus

Severe compression of the jugular veins through prolonged neck entrapment in a tight chute or accidental choking occasionally results in papilledema, retinal edema, and peripapillary retinal hemorrhages secondary to greatly increased venous pressure. Blindness with bilateral, dilated and nonresponsive pupils is present. Treatment consists of freeing the trapped animal and administering dexamethasone (in nonpregnant animals) at 20 to 50 mg IV once or twice at 12-hour intervals. Most animals diagnosed with this condition by Dr. Rebhun and colleagues remained blind, but none were treated during the acute phase. The ophthalmoscopic lesions are identical to those observed in vitamin A deficiency (see Fig. 14.57) but can be differentiated easily by a history of entrapment and the fact that only one animal is affected.

Polycythemia, as observed in some congenital cardiac anomalies such as tetralogy of Fallot, may cause the retinal vasculature to appear grossly enlarged (Fig. 14.61). Primary and secondary causes of polycythemia should be considered. Primary polycythemia was reported by Dr. Tennant as a recessive trait in Jersey cattle.

Retinal Degeneration and Blindness

Sporadic retinal degeneration with clinical features and ophthalmoscopic findings similar to those observed with progressive retinal degeneration in other species has been observed in cattle. Several unrelated cows in a Friesian herd in England developed clinical signs of retinal degeneration. The signs, ophthalmoscopic findings, and histopathology of these animals formed the basis for two reports. There appeared to be no exposure to known toxins or any evidence of a genetic relationship in this herd.

Dr. Rebhun observed several sporadic instances of retinal degeneration in adult Holstein dairy cattle and one herd that had two cases in unrelated cattle at the same time. Invariably, the affected cows were reported to appear clumsy and behave erratically until they were ultimately recognized as blind by the caretakers. Affected animals may be reluctant to move from their stalls or may behave in an unruly and anxious manner—running into people or doors or through fences. These signs only appear when the retinal degeneration is well advanced. The pupils are dilated and either completely unresponsive or poorly responsive to direct light stimulation. Fundus examination confirms generalized hyperreflectivity of the tapetal fundus, vascular attenuation, and optic atrophy (Fig. 14.62). Evidence of a possible inherited retinal degeneration was found in another herd in which the condition was diagnosed in a cow and her daughter. Both animals acquired the retinal degeneration during the first 2 years of life. Histopathology demonstrated photoreceptor degeneration and retinal thinning in the absence of inflammatory lesions.

Cortical Blindness

Cortical blindness is defined as visual loss with intact pupillary light responses in the absence of retinal or optic nerve lesions to explain the blindness; diffuse lesions of the cerebral cortex should be suspected when this combination of findings is identified.

TABLE 14.3	Differential Diagnosis for Central Nervous System Dysfunction and Blindness in Cattle*		
Disease	**Signs**	**Disease**	**Signs**
Hepatoencephalopathy (e.g., portosystemic shunts in calves, severe hepatopathy in calves or adults)	Dilated pupils Tenesmus is a common sign Photosensitization may occur with hepatopathy Bizarre behavior	Malignant catarrhal fever	Nasal, oral, and ocular lesions Endophthalmitis Deep peripheral keratitis Pyrexia
Hypomagnesemia	Lactating animals affected first Low serum Mg—response to therapy Tetany symptoms Hyperesthesia Incoordination	Plant toxicity (e.g., locoweed, male fern, rape)	Optic neuritis, papillitis Retinal degeneration, dry eyes
		Polioencephalomalacia	Autopsy findings (Wood's Lamp), possibly papilledema
Hypovitaminosis A	(Mainly Calves) Exophthalmos Papilledema Gait abnormalities Seizures	Salt poisoning	Often normal but variable light reflexes May progress to seizures
		Prussic acid toxicity	Bright red mucosa, dyspnea Plant exposure, numerous animals affected
Ketosis	(Nervous form) Ketonuria Usually in high-producing cows Bizarre behavior but convulsions and tetany rare	Rabies	Blindness rare Bellowing, mania, ascending paralysis Salivation, anesthesia
Lead toxicity	Muscle tremors of head and neck Mydriasis Mania History of environmental exposure High lead levels in blood, kidney, liver, and feces	Ruminal acidosis	Fluid-filled rumen, dehydration, acidosis
		Sporadic bovine encephalomyelitis	Pyrexia, respiratory signs Lameness, sporadic occurrence
		Thromboembolic meningoencephalitis	Retinal hemorrhages, retinitis Cold-climate occurrence, somnolence, acute death
Listeriosis	Dummy syndrome and convulsions (calves) Head deviation Facial paralysis Endophthalmitis Sporadic circling	Urea poisoning	Colic, bloat Excitement

*Cattle with some of these diseases may also show, nystagmus, strabismus, or nictitans proptosis in addition to blindness, especially during convulsions.
Table extrapolated and revised from Slatter D: *Fundamentals of Veterinary Ophthalmology,* 3rd ed, St. Louis, 2001, Saunders.

Polioencephalomalacia in calves and adult cattle, lead poisoning, salt poisoning, and severe cerebral trauma should be in the differential diagnoses. Other less common causes include severe meningitis in calves and brain abscesses in the cerebral cortex. This latter cause may result in hemianopsia (vision is present from only one half of the visual field) if the abscess resides in the cerebral cortex contralateral to the blind eye.

One unusual cause of cortical blindness in adult cattle is severe ketosis. Dr. Francis Fox observed an occasional severely ketotic cow that appeared suddenly blind and remained so despite therapy that corrected acetonemia and reestablished normal appetite. Severe hypoglycemia or other metabolic factors may trigger cerebral cortical dysfunction in the visual cortex in these cows. Fortunately, the syndrome is rare. Although treatment usually is futile with respect to restoration of vision, low-percentage IV dextrose infusions and corticosteroids can be tried. Table 14.3 lists the rule-outs for CNS dysfunction and blindness in cattle.

Acknowledgment

We would like to thank Dr. Ron Riis, Professor Emeritus, Cornell University, for his contribution in the previous edition of Diseases of Dairy Cattle.

Suggested Readings

Abeynayake, P., & Cooper, B. S. (1989). The concentration of penicillin in bovine conjunctival sac fluid as it pertains to the treatment of *Moraxella bovis* infection. (I) Subconjunctival injection. *J Vet Pharmacol Ther, 12,* 25–30.

Allen, L. J., George, L. W., & Willits, N. H. (1995). Effect of penicillin or penicillin and dexamethasone in cattle with infectious bovine keratoconjunctivitis. *J Am Vet Med Assoc, 206,* 1200–1203.

Anderson, W. I., Rebhun, W. C., deLahunta, A., et al. (1991). The ophthalmic and neuroophthalmic effects of a vitamin A deficiency in young steers. *Vet Med, 86,* 1143–1148.

Angelos, J. A., Hess, J. F., & George, L. W. (2003). An RTX operon in hemolytic *Moraxella bovis* is absent from nonhemolytic strains. *Vet Microbiol, 92,* 363–377.

Angelos, J. A., Dueger, E. L., George, L. W., et al. (2000). Efficacy of florfenicol for treatment of naturally occurring infectious bovine keratoconjunctivitis. *J Am Vet Med Assoc, 216,* 62–64.

Angelos, J. A., Ball, L. M., & Byrne, B. A. (2011). Minimum inhibitory concentrations of selected antimicrobial agents for *Moraxella bovoculi* associated with infectious bovine keratoconjunctivitis. *J Vet Diagn Invest, 23,* 552–555.

Angelos, J. A., Spinks, P. Q., Ball, L. M., et al. (2007). *Moraxella bovoculi* sp. nov., isolated from calves with infectious bovine keratoconjunctivitis. *Int J Syst Evol Microbiol, 57,* 789–795.

Angelos, J. A., & Ball, L. M. (2007). Relatedness of cytotoxins from geographically diverse isolates of *Moraxella bovis. Vet Microbiol, 124,* 382–386.

Angelos, J. A., Ball, L. M., & Hess, J. F. (2007). Identification and characterization of complete RTX operons in *Moraxella bovoculi* and *Moraxella ovis. Vet Microbiol, 125,* 73–79.

Annuar, B. O., & Wilcox, G. E. (1985). Adherence of *Moraxella bovis* to cell cultures of bovine origin. *Res Vet Sci, 39,* 241–246.

Arends, J. J., Wright, R. E., Barto, P. B., et al. (1984). Transmission of *Moraxella bovis* from blood agar cultures to Hereford cattle by face flies (Diptera: Muscidae). *J Econom Entomol, 77,* 394–398.

Ashton, N., Barnett, K. C., Clay, C. E., et al. (1977). Congenital nuclear cataracts in cattle. *Vet Rec, 100,* 505–508.

Barnett, K. C., Palmer, A. C., & Abrams, J. T. (1970). Ocular changes associated with hypovitaminosis A in cattle. *Br Vet J, 126,* 561–577.

Beard, M. K., & Moore, L. J. (1994). Reproduction of bovine keratoconjunctivitis with a purified haemolytic and cytotoxic fraction of Moraxella bovis. *Vet Microbiol, 42,* 15–33.

Bistner, S. I., Shaw, D., & Sartori, R. (1980). Ocular manifestation of low level phenothiazine administration to cattle. In *Transactions: 11th Annual Scientific Program of College of Veterinary Ophthalmologists* (pp. 85–94).

Bistner, S. I., Robin, L., & Aguirre, G. (1973). Development of the bovine eye. *Am J Vet Res, 34,* 7–12.

Blood, D. C., Radostits, O. M., & Henderson, J. A. (2007). *Veterinary medicine, a textbook of the diseases of cattle, sheep, pigs, goats and horses* (10th ed.). London: Saunders.

Booth, A., Reid, M., & Clark, T. (1987). Hypovitaminosis A in feedlot cattle. *J Am Vet Med Assoc, 190,* 1305–1308.

Bradley, R., Terlecki, S., & Clegg, F. G. (1982). The pathology of a retinal degeneration in Friesian cows. *J Comp Pathol, 92,* 69–83.

Braun, U., Jacober, S., & Drogemuller, C. (2014). Congenital nasolacrimal duct fistula in Brown Swiss Cattle. *BMC Vet Res, 10,* 44.

Carter-Dawson, L., Kuwabara, T., O'Brien, P. J., et al. (1979). Structural and biochemical changes in vitamin A-deficient rat retinas. *Invest Ophthalmol Vis Sci, 18,* 437–446.

Clare, N. T. (1947). The metabolism of phenothiazine in ruminants. *Aust Vet J, 23,* 340–344.

Clare, N. T., Whitten, L. K., & Filmer, D. (1947). Identification of the photosensitizing agent in photosensitized keratitis in young cattle following use of phenothiazine as an anthelmintic. *Aust Vet J, 23,* 344–348.

Clegg, F. G., Terlecki, S., & Bradley, R. (1981). Blindness in dairy cows. *Vet Rec, 109,* 101–103.

Clinkenbeard, K. D., & Thiessen, A. E. (1991). Mechanism of action of *Moraxella bovis* hemolysin. *Infect Immun, 59,* 1148–1152.

Collor, J. S. (1994). Safety and efficacy of Gram-negative bacterial vaccines. *Bov Pract, 29,* 13–17.

Cook, N. (1998). Combined outbreak of the genital and conjunctival forms of bovine herpesvirus 1 infection in a UK dairy herd. *Vet Rec, 143,* 561–562.

Davis, T. E., Krook, L., & Warner, R. G. (1970). Bone resorption in hypovitaminosis A. *Cornell Vet, 60,* 90–119.

Deas, D. W. (1959). A note on hereditary opacity of the cornea in British Friesian cattle. *Vet Rec, 71,* 619–620.

Den Otter, W., Hill, F. W., Klein, W. R., et al. (1995). Therapy of bovine ocular squamous cell carcinoma with local doses of interleukin-2. *Cancer Immunol Immunother, 41,* 10–14.

Divers, T. J., Blackmon, D. M., Martin, C. L., et al. (1986). Blindness and convulsions associated with vitamin A deficiency in feedlot steers. *J Am Vet Med Assoc, 189,* 1579–1582.

Dueger, E. L., George, L. W., Angelos, J. A., et al. (2004). Efficacy of a long-acting formulation of ceftiofur crystalline-free acid for the treatment of naturally occurring infectious bovine keratoconjunctivitis. *Am J Vet Res, 65,* 1185–1188.

Dueger, E. L., Angelos, J. A., Cosgrove, S., et al. (1999). Efficacy of florfenicol in the treatment of experimentally induced infectious bovine keratoconjunctivitis. *Am J Vet Res, 60,* 960–964.

Eastman, T. G., George, L. W., Hird, D. W., et al. (1998). Combined parenteral and oral administration of oxytetracycline for control of infectious bovine keratoconjunctivitis. *J Am Vet Med Assoc, 212,* 560–563 comment 212:1365, 1998.

Eaton, H. D. (1969). Chronic bovine hypo- and hypervitaminosis A and cerebrospinal fluid pressure. *Am J Clin Nutr, 22,* 1070–1080.

Edmondson, A. J., George, L. W., & Farver, T. B. (1989). Survival analysis for evaluation of corneal ulcer healing times in calves with naturally acquired infectious bovine keratoconjunctivitis. *Am J Vet Res, 50,* 838–844.

Erb, C., Nau-Staudt, K., Flammer, J., et al. (2004). Ascorbic acid as a free radical scavenger in porcine and bovine aqueous humour. *Ophthalmic Res, 36,* 38–42.

Evans, K., Smith, M., McDonough, P., et al. (2004). Eye infections due to Listeria monocytogenes in three cows and one horse. *J Vet Diagn Invest, 16,* 464–469.

Fox, F. H. (1956). The eyes. In M. G. Fincher, W. J. Gibbons, K. Mayer, et al., (Eds.), *Diseases of cattle* (pp. 385–398). Evanston, IL: American Veterinary Publications.

Frank, S. K., & Gerber, J. D. (1981). Hydrolytic enzymes of Moraxella bovis. *J Clin Microbiol, 13,* 269–271.

Frisch, J. E. (1975). The relative incidence and effect of bovine infectious keratoconjunctivitis in Bos indicus and Bos taurus cattle. *Animal Prod, 21,* 265–274.

Funk, L., O'Connor, A. M., Maroney, M., et al. (2009). A randomized and blinded field trial to assess the efficacy of an autogenous vaccine to prevent naturally occurring infectious bovine keratoconjunctivis (IBK) in beef calves. *Vaccine, 27,* 4585–4590.

Garcia, M. D., Matukumalli, L., Wheeler, T. L., et al. (2010). Markers on bovine chromosome 20 associated with carcass quality and composition traits and incidence of contracting infectious bovine keratoconjunctivitis. *Anim Biotechnol, 21,* 188–202.

Gearhart, M. S., Crissman, J. W., & Georgi, M. E. (1981). Bilateral lower palpebral demodicosis in a dairy cow. *Cornell Vet, 71,* 305–310.

George, L. W. (1984). Clinical infectious bovine keratoconjunctivitis. *Compend Contin Educ Pract Vet, 6,* S712–S724.

George, L., Mihalyi, J., Edmondson, A., et al. (1988). Topically applied furazolidone or parenterally administered oxytetracycline for the treatment of infectious bovine keratoconjunctivitis. *J Am Vet Med Assoc, 192,* 1415–1422.

George, L. W., & Kagonyera, G. (1988). Pathogenesis and clinical management of infectious bovine keratoconjunctivitis. *Bov Pract, 20,* 26–32.

George, L. W., Ardans, A., Mihalyi, J., et al. (1988). Enhancement of infectious bovine keratoconjunctivitis by modified-live infectious bovine rhinotracheitis virus vaccine. *Am J Vet Res, 49,* 1800–1806.

George, L. W., Borrowman, A. J., & Angelos, J. A. (2005). Effectiveness of a cytolysin-enriched vaccine for protection of cattle against infectious bovine keratoconjunctivitis. *Am J Vet Res, 66*, 136–142.

Gillespie, J. H., & Timoney, J. H. (1981). *Hagan and Bruner's infectious diseases of domestic animals* (7th ed.). Ithaca and London: Comstock Publishing Associates.

Glass, H. W., Jr., Gerhardt, R. R., & Greene, W. H. (1982). Survival of *Moraxella bovis* in the alimentary tract of the face fly. *J Econ Entomol, 75*, 545–546.

Gokhan, N., Sozmen, M., Ozba, B., et al. (2010). Meibomian carcinoma of the eyelid in a Simmental cow. *Vet Ophthalmol, 13*, 336–338.

Gould, S., Dewell, R., Tofflemire, K., et al. (2013). Randomized blinded challenge study to assess association between *Moraxella bovoculi* and infectious bovine keratoconjunctivitis in dairy calves. *Vet Microbiol, 164*, 108–115.

Grahn, B., & Wolfer, J. (1995). Diagnostic ophthalmology (orbital emphysema in a calf). *Can Vet J, 36*, 388–399.

Grier, R. L., Brewer, W. G., Jr., Paul, S. R., et al. (1980). Treatment of bovine and equine ocular squamous cell carcinoma by radiofrequency hyperthermia. *J Am Vet Med Assoc, 177*, 55–61.

Grimes, T. D. (1986). Retinal detachment with associated intra-ocular abnormality in related Irish Friesian cattle. *Transactions: 17th Annual Meeting of the American College of Veterinary Ophthalmology and Scientific Program of the International Society of Veterinary Ophthalmologists.*

Guard, C. L., Rebhun, W. C., & Perdrizet, J. A. (1984). Cranial tumors in aged cattle causing Horner's syndrome and exophthalmos. *Cornell Vet, 74*, 361–365.

Guyot, H. (2011). Two cases of ocular form of Listeriosis in cattle herds. *Cattle Practice, 19*, 61–64.

Hässig, M., Jud, F., Naegeli, H., et al. (2009). Prevalence of nuclear cataract in Swiss veal calves and its possible association with mobile telephone antenna base stations. *Schweiz Arch Tierheilkd, 151*, 471–478.

Hayes, K. C., Nielsen, S. W., & Eaton, H. D. (1968). Pathogenesis of the optic nerve lesion in vitamin A deficient calves. *Arch Ophthalmol, 80*, 777–787.

Heider, L., Wyman, M., Burt, J., et al. (1975). Nasolacrimal duct anomaly in calves. *J Am Vet Med Assoc, 167*, 145–147.

Henson, J. B., & Grumbles, L. C. (1960). Infectious Bovine Keratoconjunctivitis. I. Etiology. *Am J Vet Res, 21*, 761–766.

Hess, J. F., & Angelos, J. A. (2006). The *Moraxella bovis* RTX toxin locus mbx defines a pathogenicity island. *J Med Microbiol, 55*, 443–449.

Hoffmann, D., Jennings, P. A., & Spradbrow, P. B. (1981). Immunotherapy of bovine ocular squamous cell carcinomas with phenol-saline extracts of allogeneic carcinomas. *Aust Vet J, 57*, 159–163.

Holzhauer, M., & Vos, J. (2009). 'Blue eyes' in newborn calves associated with bluetongue infection. *Vet Rec, 164*, 403–404.

Hughes, D. E., Pugh, G. W., & McDonald, T. J. (1968). Experimental bovine infectious keratoconjunctivitis caused by sunlamp irradiation and *Moraxella bovis* infection: resistance to re-exposure with homologous and heterologous *Moraxella bovis*. *Am J Vet Res, 29*, 829–833.

Hughes, D. E., Pugh, G. W., Jr., & McDonald, T. J. (1965). Ultraviolet radiation and *Moraxella bovis* in the etiology of bovine infectious keratoconjunctivitis. *Am J Vet Res, 26*, 1331–1338.

Irby, N.L. Surgery of the eyes. (2017). In S.L. Fubini and N.G. Ducharme (Eds), Farm Animal Surgery (2nd ed), St. Louis, Elsevier, 145–173.

Jacob, S., Drees, R., Pinkerton, M. E., et al. (2015). Cavernous sinus syndrome in a Holstein bull. *Vet Ophthalmol, 18*, 164–167.

Jayappa, H. G., & Lehr, C. (1986). Pathogenicity and immunogenicity of piliated and nonpiliated phases of *Moraxella bovis* in calves. *Am J Vet Res, 47*, 2217–2221.

Jeffrey, M., Duff, J. P., Higgins, R. J., et al. (1994). Polioencephalomalacia associated with the ingestion of ammonium sulphate by sheep and cattle. *Vet Rec, 134*, 343–348.

Kagonyera, G. M., George, L. W., & Munn, R. (1989). Cytopathic effects of *Moraxella bovis* on cultured bovine neutrophils and corneal epithelial cells. *Am J Vet Res, 50*, 10–17.

Kagonyera, G. M., George, L. W., & Munn, R. (1988). Light and electron microscopic changes in corneas of healthy and immunomodulated calves infected with Moraxella bovis. *Am J Vet Res, 49*, 386–395.

Kagonyera, G. M., Miller, G. L., & Miller, M. (1989). Effects of *Moraxella bovis* and culture filtrates on ^{51}Cr-labeled bovine neutrophils. *Am J Vet Res, 50*, 18–21.

Kahrs, R. F., Scott, F. W., Delahunta, A., et al. (1970). Congenital cerebellar hypoplasia and ocular defects in calves following bovine viral diarrhea-mucosal disease infection in pregnant cattle. *J Am Vet Med Assoc, 156*, 1443–1450.

Kataria, R. S., Tait, R. G., Jr., Kumar, D., et al. (2011). Association of toll-like receptor four single nucleotide polymorphisms with incidence of infectious bovine keratoconjunctivitis (IBK) in cattle. *Immunogenetics, 63*, 115–119.

Killinger, A. H., Valentine, D., Mansfield, M. E., et al. (1977). Economic impact of infectious bovine keratoconjunctivitis in beef calves. *Vet Med Small Anim Clin, 72*, 618–620.

Kizilkaya, K., Tait, R. G., Garrick, D. J., et al. (2011). Whole genome analysis of infectious bovine keratoconjunctivitis in Angus cattle using Bayesian threshold models. *BMC Proc, 5*(Suppl. 4), S22.

Kleinschuster, S. J., & Rapp, H. J. (1977). Immunotherapy of bovine ocular carcinoma with BCG cell wall vaccine. *Proceedings: 68th Annual Meeting American Association of Cancer Researchers*, 85.

Kopecky, K. E., Pugh, G. W., Jr., & McDonald, T. J. (1981). Influence of outdoor winter environment on the course of infectious bovine keratoconjunctivitis. *Am J Vet Res, 42*, 1990–1992.

Krump, L. (2014). Congenital cataracts in an Ayrshire herd: a herd case report. *Ir Vet J, 25*, 67 2.

Ladouceur, C. A., & Kazacos, K. R. (1981). Eye worms in cattle in Indiana. *J Am Vet Med Assoc, 178*, 385–387.

Lamb, C. R., & Naylor, J. M. (1985). Arteriovenous fistula in the orbit of a calf. *Can Vet J, 26*, 105–107.

Lane, V. M., George, L. W., & Cleaver, D. M. (2006). Efficacy of tulathromycin for treatment of cattle with acute ocular *Moraxella bovis* infections. *J Am Vet Med Assoc, 229*(4), 557–561.

Langford, E. V., & Dorward, W. J. (1969). A mycoplasma isolated from cattle with infectious bovine keratoconjunctivitis. *Can J Comp Med, 33*, 275–279.

Lehr, C., Jayappa, H. G., & Goodnow, R. A. (1985). Serologic and protective characterization of *Moraxella bovis* pili. *Cornell Vet, 75*, 484–492.

Lepper, A. W., & Barton, I. J. (1987). Infectious bovine keratoconjunctivitis: seasonal variation in cultural, biochemical and immunoreactive properties of *Moraxella bovis* isolated from the eyes of cattle. *Aust Vet J, 64*, 33–39.

Lepper, A. W. (1988). Vaccination against infectious bovine keratoconjunctivitis: protective efficacy and antibody response induced by pili of homologous and heterologous strains of Moraxella bovis. *Aust Vet J, 65*, 310–316.

Lepper, A. W., Elleman, T. C., Hoyne, P. A., et al. (1993). A *Moraxella bovis* pili vaccine produced by recombinant DNA technology for the prevention of infectious bovine keratoconjunctivitis. *Vet Microbiol, 36*, 175–183.

Lepper, A. W., Atwell, J. L., Lehrbach, P. R., et al. (1995). The protective efficacy of cloned *Moraxella bovis* pili in monovalent and multivalent vaccine formulations against experimentally induced infectious bovine keratoconjunctivitis (IBK). *Vet Microbiol, 45*, 129–138.

Levisohn, S., Garazi, S., Gerchman, I., et al. (2004). Diagnosis of a mixed mycoplasma infection associated with a severe outbreak of bovine pinkeye in young calves. *J Vet Diagn Invest, 16*, 579–581.

Liljebjelke, K. A., Warnick, L. D., & Witt, M. F. (2000). Antibiotic residues in milk following bulbar subconjunctival injection of procaine penicillin G in dairy cows. *J Am Vet Med Assoc, 217*, 369–371.

Lorenz, I., & Gentile, A. (2014). D-lactic acidosis in neonatal ruminants. *Vet Clin N Am Food Animal Pract, 30*(2), 317–331.

Loy, J. D., & Brodersen, B. W. (2014). *Moraxella* spp. isolated from field outbreaks of infectious bovine keratoconjunctivitis: a retrospective study of case submissions from 2010 to 2013. *J Vet Diagn Invest, 26*, 761–768.

Marolt, J., Burdnjak, Z., Vekelic, E., et al. (1963). Specific ophthalmia of cattle. *Zentralbl Veterinärmed, 10A*, 286–294.

Marrs, C. F., Ruehl, W. W., Schoolnik, G. K., et al. (1988). Pilin-gene phase variation of *Moraxella bovis* is caused by an inversion of the pilin genes. *J Bacteriol, 170*, 3032–3039.

Mason, C. S., Buxton, D., & Gartside, J. F. (2003). Congenital ocular abnormalities in calves associated with maternal hypovitaminosis A. *Vet Rec, 153*, 213–214.

McConnel, C. S., & House, J. K. (2005). Infectious bovine keratoconjunctivitis vaccine development. *Aust Vet J, 83*, 506–510.

McConnon, J. M., White, M. E., Smith, M. C., et al. (1983). Pendular nystagmus in dairy cattle. *J Am Vet Med Assoc, 182*, 812–813.

McKenzie, R. A., Carmichael, A. M., Schibrowski, M. L., et al. (2009). Sulfur-associated polioencephalomalacia in cattle grazing plants in the Family Brassicaceae. *Aust Vet J, 87*, 27–32.

Mohanty, S. B., & Lillie, M. G. (1970). Relationship of infectious bovine keratoconjunctivitis virus to the virus of infectious bovine rhinotracheitis. *Cornell Vet, 60*, 3–9.

Momke, S., & Distl, O. (2007). Bilateral convergent strabismus with exophthalmus (BCSE) in cattle: an overview of clinical signs and genetic traits. *Vet J, 173*, 272–277.

Moore, L. A. (1941). Some ocular changes and deficiency manifest in mature cows fed a ration deficient in vitamin A. *J Dairy Sci, 24*, 893–902.

Moore, L. A., & Sykes, J. F. (1941). Terminal CSF pressure values in vitamin A deficiency. *Am J Physiol, 134*, 436–439.

Moore, L. J., & Lepper, A. W. (1991). A unified serotyping scheme for *Moraxella bovis*. *Vet Microbiol, 29*, 75–83.

Morgan, J. H. (1977). Infectious keratoconjunctivitis in cattle associated with Listeria monocytocytogenes. *Vet Rec, 100*(6), 113–114.

Moritomo, Y., Koga, O., Miyamoto, H., et al. (1995). Congenital anophthalmia with caudal vertebral anomalies in Japanese Brown Cattle. *J Vet Med Sci, 57*, 693–696.

Neilsen, S. W., Mills, J. H. L., Woelfel, C. G., et al. (1966). The pathology of marginal vitamin A deficiency in calves. *Res Vet Sci, 7*, 143–150.

O'Connell, K. A. (1995). The development and testing of a vaccine for the prevention of infectious bovine keratoconjunctivitis. *Thesis, University of California, Davis.*

O'Connor, A. M., Brace, S., Gould, S., et al. (2011). A randomized clinical trial evaluating a farm-of-origin autogenous *Moraxella bovis* vaccine to control infectious bovine keratoconjunctivis (pinkeye) in beef cattle. *J Vet Intern Med, 25*, 1447–1453.

O'Toole, D., Raisbeck, M., Case, J. C., et al. (1996). Selenium induced "blind staggers" and related myths: a commentary on the extent of historical livestock losses attributed to selenosis on Western U.S. rangelands. *Vet Pathol, 33*, 104–116.

Paulsen, M. E., Johnson, LaR., Young, S., et al. (1989). Blindness and sexual dimorphism associated with vitamin A deficiency in feedlot cattle. *J Am Vet Med Assoc, 194*, 933–937.

Pugh, G. W., Hughes, D. E., & Schulz, V. D. (1976). Infectious bovine keratoconjunctivitis: experimental induction of infection in calves with mycoplasmas and Moraxella bovis. *Am J Vet Res, 37*, 493–495.

Pugh, G. W., Jr., Hughes, D. E., & Packer, R. A. (1970). Bovine infectious keratoconjunctivitis: interactions of *Moraxella bovis* and infectious bovine rhinotracheitis virus. *Am J Vet Res, 31*, 653–662.

Pugh, G. W., Jr., & Hughes, D. E. (1972). Bovine infectious keratoconjunctivitis: Moraxella bovis as the sole etiologic agent in a winter epizootic. *J Am Vet Med Assoc, 161*, 481–486.

Raisbeck, M. F., Dahl, E. R., Sanchez, D. A., et al. (1993). Naturally occurring selenosis in Wyoming. *J Vet Diagn Invest, 5*, 84–87.

Rebhun, W. C., King, J. M., & Hillman, R. B. (1988). Atypical actinobacillosis granulomas in cattle. *Cornell Vet, 78*, 125–130.

Rebhun, W. C. (1984). Ocular manifestations of systemic diseases in cattle. *Vet Clin North Am Food Anim Pract 68*, 623–639.

Rosen, E. S., Edgar, J. T., & Smith, J. L. S. (1969). Male fern retrobulbar neuropathy in cattle. *Trans Ophthalmol Soc UK, 89*, 285–299.

Rosenbusch, R. F., Kinyon, J. M., Apley, M., et al. (2005). In vitro antimicrobial inhibition profiles of *Mycoplasma bovis* isolates recovered from various regions of the United States from 2002 to 2003. *J Vet Diagn Invest, 17*, 436–441.

Rosenbusch, R. F. (1983). Influence of mycoplasma preinfection on the expression of *Moraxella bovis* pathogenicity. *Am J Vet Res, 44*, 1621–1624.

Ruehl, W. W., Marrs, C., Beard, M. K., et al. (1993). Q pili enhance the attachment of *Moraxella bovis* to bovine corneas in vitro. *Mol Microbiol, 7*, 285–288.

Ruehl, W. W., Marrs, C. F., George, L., et al. (1993). Infection rates, disease frequency, pilin gene rearrangement, and pilin expression in calves inoculated with *Moraxella bovis* pilin-specific isogenic variants. *Am J Vet Res, 54*, 248–253.

Ruggles, A. J., Irby, N. L., Saik, J. E., et al. (1992). Ocular lymphangiosarcoma in a cow. *J Am Vet Med Assoc, 200*, 1987–1988.

Sandmeyer, L. S., Vujanovic, V., Petrie, L., et al. (2015). Optic neuropathy in a herd of beef cattle in Alberta associated with consumption of moldy corn. *Can Vet J, 56*, 249–256.

Saunders, L. Z., & Rubin, L. F. (1975). *Ophthalmic pathology of animals.* Basel, Switzerland: S. Karger.

Saunders, L. Z., & Fincher, M. G. (1951). Hereditary multiple eye defects in grade Jersey calves. *Cornell Vet, 41*, 351–366.

Schulz, K. L., & Anderson, D. E. (2010). Bovine enucleation: a retrospective study of 53 cases (1998-2006). *Can Vet J, 51*, 611–614.

Shryock, T. R., White, D. W., & Werner, C. S. (1998). Antimicrobial susceptibility of *Moraxella bovis*. *Vet Microbiol, 61*, 305–309.

Slatter, D. (2001). *Fundamentals of veterinary ophthalmology* (3rd ed.). St. Louis: Saunders.

Smith, J. S., & Mayhew, I. G. (1977). Horner's syndrome in large animals. *Cornell Vet, 67*, 529–542.

Snowder, G. D., Van Vleck, L. D., Cundiff, L. V., et al. (2005). Genetic and environmental factors associated with incidence of infectious bovine keratoconjunctivitis in preweaned beef calves. *J Anim Sci, 83*, 507–518.

Stehman, S. M., Rebhun, W. C., & Riis, R. C. (1987). Progressive retinal atrophy in related cattle. *Bov Pract*, 195–197. November.

Steve, P. C., & Lilly, J. H. (1965). Investigations on transmissability of *Moraxella bovis* by the face fly. *J Econ Entomol, 58*, 444–446.

Stewart, R. J., Masztalerz, A., Jacobs, J. J., et al. (2006). Treatment of ocular squamous cell carcinomas in cattle with interleukin-2. *Vet Rec, 159*(20), 668–672.

Stewart, R. J., Masztalerz, A., Jacobs, J. J., et al. (2005). Local interleukin-2 and interleukin-12 therapy of bovine ocular squamous cell carcinomas. *Vet Immunol Immunopathol, 106*, 277–284.

Sykes, J. A., Kmochowski, L., Grey, C. E., et al. (1962). Isolation of a virus from infectious bovine kerato-conjunctivitis. *Proc Soc Exp Biol Med, 111*, 51–57.

Tennant, B., Harrold, D., Reina-Guerra, M., et al. (1969). Arterial pH, PO_2 and PCO_2 of calves with familial bovine polycythemia. *Cornell Vet, 59*, 594–604.

Townsend, W. M., Renninger, M., Stiles, J., et al. (2003). Dexamethasone-induced exophthalmos in a group of Holstein calves. *Vet Ophthalmol, 6*, 265–268.

Trefz, F. M., Lorch, A., Feist, M., et al. (2013). The prevalence and clinical relevance of hyperkalaemia in calves with neonatal diarrhoea. *Vet J, 195*(3), 350–356.

Van der Woerdt, A., Wilkie, D. A., & Gilger, B. C. (1996). Congenital epiphora in a calf associated with dysplastic lacrimal puncta. *Agric Pract, 17*, 7–11.

Voelter-Ratson, K., Monod, M., Braun, U., et al. (2013). Ulcerative fungal keratitis in a Brown Swiss cow. *Vet Ophthalmol, 16*, 464–466.

Ward, J. K., & Neilson, M. K. (1979). Pinkeye (bovine infectious keratoconjunctivitis) in beef cattle. *J Anim Sci, 49*, 361–366.

Whittaker, C. S. G., Gelatt, K. N., & Wilkie, D. A. (2007). Food animal ophthalmology. In K. N. Gelatt (Ed.), *Veterinary Ophthalmology* (4th ed.). Philadelphia: Lippincott, Williams & Wilkins.

Whitten, L. K., & Filmer, D. B. (1974). A photosensitized keratitis in young cattle following the use of phenothiazine as an anthelmintic. *Aust Vet J, 23*, 336–340.

Willoughby, R. A. (1968). Congenital eye defects in cattle. *Mod Vet Pract, 49*, 36.

Zemljič, T., Pot, S. A., Haessig, M., et al. (2012). Clinical ocular findings in cows with malignant catarrhal fever: ocular disease progression and outcome in 25 cases (2007-2010). *Vet Ophthalmol, 15*(1), 46–52.

15

Metabolic Diseases

JESSICA A.A. McART, THOMAS J. DIVERS, AND SIMON F. PEEK

The common metabolic problems of early lactation, milk fever, and ketosis, are really management diseases. At the herd level, disease does or does not occur as a function of how cows are fed and handled during the late dry period and during transition to the nutrient-dense rations needed to support high milk production in early lactation. Because infectious diseases can be more effectively controlled by sound immunization, the economic importance of these common metabolic disorders and their prevention by sound nutritional and herd management has assumed ever-greater relevance for modern dairies. Feeding management includes sources, storage, preparation, ration formulation, delivery, and access. Good feeding management must be coupled with providing an environment as comfortable as possible to facilitate maximal feed consumption. In investigating herd problems of excessive metabolic disease rates, all of these factors must be considered. Individual cows may be predisposed to metabolic problems as a result of improper body conditioning, concurrent illness, genetics, and any other events that may decrease dry matter intake (DMI). In addition to calcium, the other macrominerals of relevance in dairy cattle are potassium, magnesium, and phosphorus, and although disorders involving these elements are of far lesser importance than hypocalcemia, they are also considered in this chapter.

Ketosis: Causes, Classification, and Pathophysiology

Normal dairy cattle undergo a shift in their energy metabolism and its regulation as parturition approaches and the dam transitions from nutrient accrual to rapid mobilization of lipid and protein in readiness for high milk production. There is a decrease in lipogenesis and esterification and a simultaneous increase in hormone-sensitive lipase activity, leading to the release of increased amounts of nonesterified fatty acids (NEFAs) into the bloodstream. The process is initiated by prolactin and precedes the onset of lactation. Insulin secretion declines in preparation for lactation. The mammary gland of dairy cows does not require insulin for glucose uptake, and this lowering of insulin results in greater amounts of glucose being used by the udder for milk lactose production and less being used via peripheral sites. A normal cow in energy equilibrium will reesterify serum NEFAs in the liver and resecrete them as very-low-density lipoproteins (VLDLs). When energy deficits occur and NEFAs are produced in excess of liver capacity for esterification, they are oxidized to ketone bodies. This pattern of regulation of energy metabolism may persist until about 8 weeks into lactation, when DMI increases to a level at which energy intake promotes lipid synthesis. The system is also sensitive to "stress," which through sympathomimetic pathways may lead not only to excessive lipid mobilization but also to pathologic hepatic fat accumulation.

Negative energy balance is a normal occurrence during the transition period because of reduced DMI and increased demand for milk production. In the last weeks of gestation, in addition to hormonal factors increasing lipolysis, a decreased rumen capacity may also cause a decrease in nutrient intake. In part, the decreased rumen capacity is an expected consequence of the enlarging uterus within the caudal abdomen, but this is exacerbated by twin fetuses, or the "space-occupying effect" of increased intraabdominal fat in overconditioned multiparous cows or heifers. At parturition, milk production becomes the major energy demand, such that negative energy balance is exacerbated. Ketosis occurs when cows are in excessive negative energy balance. This most commonly occurs in the last 2 weeks of pregnancy or in the first 2 to 3 weeks of lactation, almost exactly coinciding with the transition period referred to for management purposes (3 weeks before parturition to 3 weeks after). Although the volume of milk production and lactose formation is the predominant demand for energy, there is also a secondary (or possibly primary in some cows) lipid demand for milk fat synthesis. It appears obvious to the authors that our ability to feed cows in the 2 weeks before freshening to 4 weeks after calving has not kept up with our advancements in genetics for milk production. There are many categories of ketosis in cattle, but most involve a similar pathophysiology of lipolysis; excessive release of NEFAs; inadequate hepatic metabolism of increased amounts of NEFAs (incomplete oxidation results in production of ketone bodies); increased fatty acid storage as triacylglycerols in the liver (kidney and muscle to a lesser extent); and, in some cows, decreased hepatic secretion of VLDLs. Certain cows may be genetically predisposed to hepatic lipidosis because of their inability to properly remove triglycerides from the liver.

The severity of ketosis, or hyperketonemia, can be most accurately assessed by measurement of blood or plasma β-hydroxybutyrate (BHB) concentrations because this ketone body is more stable in blood than either acetoacetate or acetone. The threshold for hyperketonemia in dairy cattle has been set at a BHB concentration of 1.2 mmol/L (12.5 mg/dL). Subclinical ketosis denotes "clinically normal" cows in the first weeks of lactation that have BHB values greater than this threshold value (1.2 mmol/L). Subclinical ketosis may be present in 30% to 50% of early lactation cows in some herds and accounts for 80% to 90% of ketotic cows in a herd. Although not clinically abnormal, cows with mild hyperketonemia have been found to be at a higher risk of developing subsequent postpartum diseases such as metritis and displaced abomasum, more likely to leave the herd in early lactation, produce less milk, and may have decreased reproductive performance compared with their nonketotic herdmates. *Clinical ketosis* is the term used to describe cattle with both hyperketonemia and abnormal clinical signs. Acutely, these are typically appreciated by producers as a diminished appetite and decreased milk production, but in time, there is progression to include rapid weight loss and impaired reproductive performance. Many primiparous and multiparous cattle with clinical ketosis have profound hyperketonemia with blood BHB concentrations greater than 3.0 mmol/L (31.25 mg/dL). However, from having performed BHB measurements on several thousand occasions in recent years in both sick and apparently healthy dairy cattle, it is apparent to the authors that there are many mildly hyperketonemic cattle (BHB concentration >1.2 mmol/L but <3.0 mmol/L) that have clinical signs of ketosis alongside a smaller number of cattle with severe hyperketonemia (BHB >3.0 mmol/L) that have no outward clinical abnormalities at all.

In addition to these severity distinctions of hyperketonemia, many periparturient cows experience some degree of hepatic lipidosis. Hepatic lipidosis can take at least three forms: (1) clinically silent in subclinical ketosis, (2) chronic adipose tissue mobilization after early-onset periparturient clinical ketosis with an individual susceptibility as a result of either genetics or periparturient overconditioning, and (3) periparturient clinical ketosis in an obese cow with massive lipid accumulation in the liver within the first days of lactation. Cows with clinical hepatic lipidosis are often referred to as having "fat cow" or "fatty liver" syndrome, the typical example of which is a cow that becomes ill just before or at parturition and has marked anorexia, relapsing milk fever, retained placenta, myopathy, and sepsis.

Clinical Signs and Diagnosis of Ketosis

Negative energy balance–related ketosis is most common in the first month of lactation, with the majority of cases occurring during the first and second weeks of lactation. Cows with either clinical ketosis early (first week) in lactation or cows with persistent clinical ketosis beyond 4 weeks of lactation are most likely to have more marked hepatic lipidosis. Ketones may be detected in the breath, urine, milk, or blood. Some sensitive individuals can easily recognize

the odor of acetone on the breath, although this method of detection is only about 50% sensitive. A urine test for acetoacetate is widely available and is a moderately sensitive test, although typically only half of all cows can be induced to urinate at any one time. A color change to purple indicates the presence of acetoacetate (Fig. 15.1, *A*). The rate and intensity of change are indicative of acetoacetate concentration, but the urine acetoacetate test may be affected by the hydration status of the cow and the concentration of the urine. Many cows with clinical ketosis give a strong purple color on the urine test, although the urine of individuals with hepatic lipidosis may only cause a lighter purple coloration. Milk ketone tests are more expensive than urine tests and suffer from poor sensitivity; however, specificity is high. These tests come as either powder or strips to measure milk BHB or acetoacetate concentrations, respectively. The most accurate test for cow-side diagnosis of ketosis is through use of a handheld ketone meter that uses blood to quantitatively determine BHB concentrations. These types of meters are highly sensitive and specific and very easy to use on farms (Fig. 15.1, *B*). It is to be hoped that there is greater adoption of blood BHB testing in the future because of its greater comparative accuracy. Surveys of dairy producers involved with the University of Wisconsin ambulatory

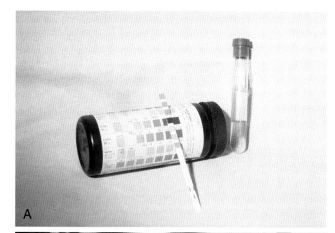

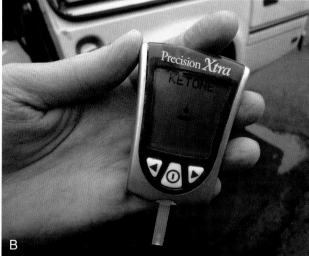

• **Fig. 15.1 A,** Urine ketostrip with urine-positive reaction to acetoacetate from a cow with primary ketosis. **B,** Handheld point-of-care monitor for testing β–hydroxybutyrate.

practice scheme in recent years reveal a surprising number of farms where ketosis is still a diagnosis based on the odor of the breath or nonspecific signs of diminished appetite for grain with lowered production. Confirmatory urine tests for acetoacetate are still popular and attractive to fresh cow pen workers for economic reasons and their perceived ease of use compared with obtaining a blood sample from the coccygeal vessels. A number of recent publications from Europe and North America have validated cut-off points for subclinical ketosis of between 1.1 and 1.4 mmol/L for blood (plasma or serum) using several handheld, cow-side devices. Greater research in the near future will hopefully provide more precise guidelines for large dairies (see later section) for the use of BHB testing as both a diagnostic and screening tool, not just for individual sick cows but also for herd-level testing. The increasing evidence that clinically normal or only subtly and nonspecifically abnormal cattle with subclinical ketosis have increased risk for other common postparturient diseases emphasizes the value of metabolic testing.

Cows with clinical ketosis have reduced feed intake of total mixed rations (TMRs) and may prefer forages over concentrates if component fed. Temperature, pulse, and respiration rarely deviate from normal reference ranges unless other concurrent conditions exist. The exception is the classic, severe "uncomplicated" clinical ketosis case that may be mildly hypothermic. The manure is drier in consistency than herdmates at the same stage of lactation. Affected cows appear dull with a dry hair coat and piloerection. Neurologic signs such as persistent licking at herself or inanimate objects, aggressive behavior, unusual head carriage, and even blindness may be seen with nervous ketosis. The pathogenesis of nervous ketosis is unknown. An inability to rise or ataxia resulting from weakness may be seen in some cows with clinical ketosis, and these signs are directly related to hypoglycemia. Metabolic acidosis may occur in some cows and, although unpredictable, can be severe (bicarbonate of as low as 12 mEq/L) in a few cows.

Ketosis at other stages of lactation can occur because of underfeeding (lack of energy substrates for level of milk production) or secondary to another disease. Secondary ketosis can also occur during the high-risk period for clinical and subclinical ketosis. Cows with secondary ketosis have clinical signs related to the primary disease. Severe, clinical ketosis appears to be rare in cows with systemic disorders such as peritonitis, septic mastitis, and salmonellosis, especially in mid to later lactation when milk production may have naturally waned somewhat and DMIs have already increased in the period before the onset of illness. Subclinical secondary ketosis is more common in the first month of lactation when high-producing cattle are affected with one of several common conditions such as mastitis and metritis, but it is challenging to know which came first. In all cases of secondary ketosis, therapy should correct the primary problem, and the ketosis will normally resolve, with or without specific ketosis treatments.

Cows with persistent ketosis for 1 to 7 weeks usually have hepatic lipidosis. Ultrasound examination and biopsy of the liver in the dorsal right tenth or eleventh intercostal space (Fig. 15.2) can be used to confirm hepatic lipidosis, but this is seldom required because the clinical diagnosis is easy. The appearance of swollen liver edges on transabdominal ultrasonography should be anticipated in recently fresh cattle and should not be overinterpreted, however. If biopsy material is obtained either by ultrasound guidance or during a laparotomy, then a rough guide to the hepatic fat content can be provided by seeing if the biopsy sample will float or sink in a solution of water or two varying solutions of copper sulfate with specific gravities of 1.025 and 1.055, respectively. If the tissue floats in all three, then lipidosis is severe (>35% fat weight wet). If it sinks in water but floats in the two copper sulfate solutions, then the hepatic lipid content is marked at 25% to 35%, and if it only floats in the copper sulfate solution with a specific gravity of 1.055, then the fat level is milder, between 15% and 25%. Clinical signs tend to be seen in the 25% to 35% range and are

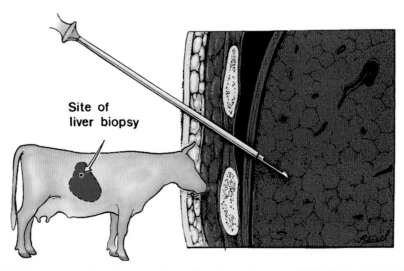

Site of liver biopsy

• **Fig. 15.2** Drawing depicting site and method of liver biopsy in a cow. Neither liver biopsy nor ultrasonography is required for the diagnosis of hepatic lipidosis in most cows. The diagnosis is based mostly on history, clinical examination, and laboratory findings.

more severe in the greater than 35% range, but one cannot reliably use these categories to prognosticate. Some cattle in the higher category will survive with treatment. Unfortunately, treatment of persistent ketosis can be difficult. Cows with chronic ketosis or fat mobilization and hepatic lipidosis lose considerable amounts of weight and have a poor appetite, but they continue to produce moderate amounts of milk considering their poor feed intake (Fig. 15.3). Affected cows may appear weak, which could be caused by hypoglycemia, muscle weakness from fatty accumulation in muscle, or hypokalemia. Some cows may die, be sold, or have complications caused by frequent treatment (e.g., phlebitis from glucose administration, oral trauma from forced feeding). Serum concentrations of hepatic-derived enzymes (aspartate aminotransferase [AST], gamma glutamyl transferase [GGT], and sorbitol dehydrogenase [SDH]) are often elevated, and serum cholesterol is frequently low in cows with hepatic lipidosis. They are also commonly hyperbilirubinemic. However, these parameters are not consistently abnormal enough to be helpful diagnostically or prognostically. Serum cholesterol generally returns toward normal concentrations as the cow begins to eat better.

Cows that are overconditioned (body condition score ≥4.0 out of 5.0, see appendix) before parturition and that have severe periparturient ketosis can rapidly develop hepatic lipidosis and have life-threatening illness (Figs. 15.4 and 15.5). These cows often also have recurrent hypocalcemia and recumbency and, because of their heavy weight, often develop fatal myopathy (Fig. 15.6). Most of these obese, periparturiently ketotic, hepatic lipidosis cows will

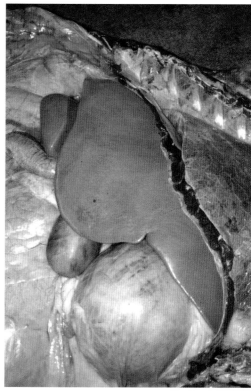

• **Fig. 15.5** Postmortem image of a swollen, fatty liver from a 3-year-old Holstein cow that was euthanized for septic metritis and recumbency 10 days into lactation associated with an excessively long dry period.

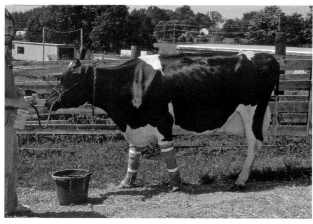

• **Fig. 15.3** A 4-year-old Holstein cow with chronic ketosis, chronic fat mobilization, weight loss, and hepatic lipidosis. The cow recovered after 3 weeks of medical treatments.

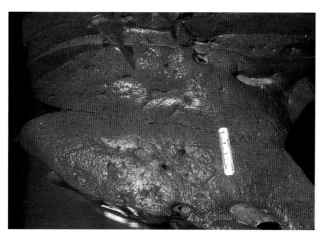

• **Fig. 15.4** Severe hepatic lipidosis observed at necropsy. The liver was from a recently fresh and obese cow.

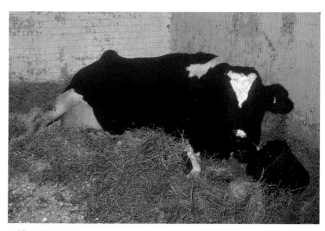

• **Fig. 15.6** A large, overconditioned cow with ketosis and recurrent milk fever that resulted in a severe myopathy. The cow survived but required considerable therapy, including flotation.

have a retained placenta and may die of septic metritis even without a fetid-smelling discharge (Fig. 15.7). Their predisposition to sepsis with mild to moderate metritis may be caused by excessive fat deposition in the liver and diminished hepatic macrophage (Kupffer cells) function. Additionally, elevated concentrations of NEFAs and BHB impede normal immune function. Affected cows may also develop septic mastitis with repeated episodes of recumbency. Although cattle affected with severe hepatic lipidosis obviously have greatly impaired liver function, it is quite uncommon for them to show signs of fulminant liver failure. Usually, as previously stated, they die of sepsis or are euthanized for recumbency. However, on rare occasions, one may see profound jaundice terminally (Fig. 15.8).

Occasionally, cows in late pregnancy can become ketotic, although this is rare. This usually occurs with multiple fetuses and is triggered by some other illness or external event that restricts access to feed. Early signs are identical to early lactation ketosis. Without prompt treatment, the signs progress to extreme constipation followed by recumbency, renal failure, and death. Cows do not commonly become blind as do sheep with pregnancy toxemia.

Predisposing factors to development of ketosis include the herd of origin (management factors are discussed later), advanced parity, increased body condition score (≥3.75 of 5.0), and difficulty calving. Cattle with extended dry periods or long intervals between calving, such as an individually valuable cow that is used as an embryo or oocyte donor, seem to be particularly susceptible.

Treatment

Treatment for ketosis is aimed at restoring energy metabolism to normal for milk production. The most commonly used treatments include oral propylene glycol (doses range from 250 mL twice a day to 300 mL once a day, for up to 5 days), intravenous (IV) 50% dextrose solution (typically 500 mL by rapid infusion) and IV vitamin B_{12} injections (1.25–2.5 mg/day), the latter either being given in the form of a stand-alone, or combination, vitamin B product. One of the authors (JM) has recently reported that a combined treatment with both glucose and propylene glycol is most effective in decreasing BHB concentrations. It is still common on farms for cows with clinical ketosis to receive glucocorticoids, most commonly in the form of dexamethasone, although a commercial preparation of isoflupredone acetate also has widespread use in the United States. The metabolic effects of dexamethasone in ketotic dairy cattle, and its benefit or potential detrimental impact have been the subject of much debate as well as quite a bit of research and remain controversial without high-level proof of efficacy. Frequently, discussion of its use provokes strong clinical and personal opinion. Dexamethasone is

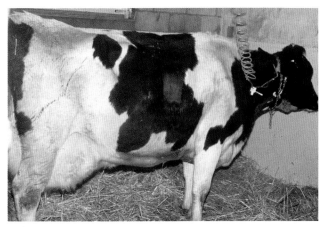

• **Fig. 15.7** An overconditioned, fresh cow with ketosis that died of septic metritis. There was no obvious smell from the rear of the cow, and the metritis did not appear to be severe enough to make most cows systemically ill. The severe hepatic lipidosis most likely predisposed the cow to the fatal toxemia from a relatively moderate metritis.

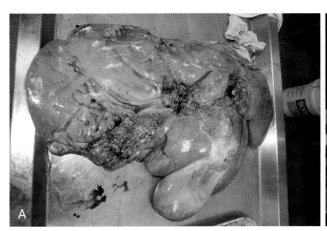
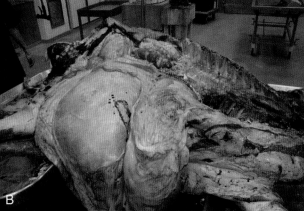

• **Fig. 15.8** Postmortem appearance of the swollen liver (**A**) and icteric thorax and abdomen (**B**) from a 5-year-old Holstein cow that had died after 2 weeks of intensive treatment for refractory ketosis. The cow had freshened 12 days previously with a body condition score of 5 and was profoundly jaundiced for 36 hours before death.

approved for the treatment of ketosis at doses of 5 to 20 mg either intramuscularly or intravenously in the United States. There is evidence that glucocorticoids increase blood glucose concentration and some belief that BHB concentrations are then decreased in cows with clinical ketosis. The mechanism by which they increase blood glucose is uncertain; most likely it is through hepatic gluconeogenesis rather than lipolysis or muscle breakdown. The scientific evidence in support of dexamethasone as a means of combatting clinical ketosis in early lactation by virtue of suppressing milk production is "uneven" to say the least. It is undoubtedly true to say that the drug will decrease milk production in non-ketotic cows during early lactation, but this effect is less repeatable in studies examining ketotic individuals at the same stage of lactation. Studies that have described a depressive effect on milk production in ketotic cows have tended to do so only in higher-producing cattle (higher by 30-year-old standards at least; the effect was seen in cattle producing >60 lb a day). Any discussion of the negative consequences of dexamethasone administration has always involved reference to the potential immunosuppressive effect on both cellular and humoral immune function. The current literature on the effect of dexamethasone on bovine lymphocyte subpopulation numbers, cytokine production, and lymphocyte function is heavily based on in vitro studies and hard to extrapolate into the clinical setting. However, the negative effect of the drug on neutrophil function, despite the reliable peripheral neutrophilia that it induces, is a quite compelling reason to be cautious about its use. Corroborative literature for the use of isoflupredone acetate in the treatment of ketosis is even harder to find; indeed, some literature suggests that its use in healthy early lactation cows actually increases the chances of subclinical ketosis. So what does all this mean? In the author's opinion (JM), current recommended treatments for clinical ketosis should not include the routine use of glucocorticoids. One of the authors (SP) does occasionally use a single (10–15 mg) dose of dexamethasone for cases of severe clinical ketosis (BHB >3.0 mmol/L), most commonly in a high-producing multiparous cow making a great deal of milk, in whom appetite is fair to good and the client is prepared to accept a reduction in yield as part of the treatment. On these occasions, such cattle are usually on a constant rate infusion of 10% dextrose in a hospital setting, to which they have already proven refractory as an initial treatment for ketosis. This idea that dexamethasone treatment should be combined with glucose administration is a sound one from the available literature that demonstrates lower relapse rates when the two treatments are combined. Excessive administration of isoflupredone can cause life-threatening hypokalemia because of its strong mineralocorticoid effect.

Propylene glycol should be given as a drench and not mixed in the feed. In recent years, it has also become quite common to use alternatives to propylene glycol as oral energy precursors on many dairies. For example, in an effort to address both the potential calcium and energy needs of off-feed dairy cows, several commercial drench formulations contain 1 to 1.5 lb of calcium propionate. When mixed with 5 to 10 gallons of water, these drenches can be a very good way of addressing either confirmed or suspected subclinical ketosis and hypocalcemia. In cases of clinical ketosis and milk fever, they can be a valuable adjunct to more specific IV therapy with either dextrose or calcium, specifically to reduce relapses. Care must be taken when drenching cattle, especially when performed by non-veterinarians, that such large volumes are delivered into the rumen (by stomach tube placed through an oral speculum) or into the esophagus (via McGrath pump or equivalent) and never into the airway. Homemade or commercial fresh cow drench mixtures often also contain magnesium sulfate (200 g), monophosphate sodium (220 g) and potassium chloride (50–100 g) as further supportive aids for poorly appetent fresh cows. Full recovery from ketosis requires a return to normal feed intake, and supportive therapy may need to be continued for several consecutive days to allow time for the cow to maintain normoglycemia. Offering a choice of feedstuffs (i.e., brewer's yeast) may help in restoring the cow's appetite. Cows with nervous ketosis can been treated successfully with IV glucose and orally administered chloral hydrate (40 g daily), which serves as both a sedative and as a substrate for glucogenic bacteria.

Cows with ketosis and marked hepatic lipidosis or "fatty liver disease" are challenging cases to treat. Cows with chronic fat mobilization, ketosis and hepatic lipidosis are often the "best cow in the herd" and genetically predisposed to produce a high milk volume. These cows do not get better overnight with any treatment and in fact may have already been treated with the aforementioned traditional therapies for ketosis on several occasions for 1 to 3 weeks before veterinary attention is sought. Treatment in such cases needs to be more aggressive. The experience of many clinicians in referral hospitals supports the use of a constant rate infusion (CRI) of 5% to 10% dextrose, often combined with a balanced electrolyte solution containing supplemental KCl added to a final concentration of 40 mEq/L of fluid administered. With such aggressive dextrose supplementation as a means of maintaining normoglycemia, it is very important to add potassium chloride in this way to help prevent hypokalemia. Periodic assessment of blood BHB level, aiming to keep below 1.2 mmol/L, alongside potassium and calcium measurement is important to fine-tune therapy as needed. Confirmation that blood glucose is not rising to levels in excess of renal threshold and consequently not "spilling" into the urine is prudent, either by specific blood glucose measurement (aiming for <150 mg/dL) or by urine reagent strips. Even in severe cases, it has been our experience that although 10% dextrose CRIs are quite often necessary to reduce BHB levels into the required range, this only rarely causes severe hyperglycemia and glucosuria in such cattle. The bigger challenge is what happens when the IV dextrose support is withdrawn. On occasions with marked hepatic lipidosis, the patient will relapse into a ketotic state within 1 to 3 days. This propensity to relapse has inevitably led to the use of adjunct treatments such as parenteral insulin and force feeding. Theoretically, insulin should promote glucose uptake in peripheral sites, inhibiting further lipolysis such that it is intuitively appealing to administer it to these patients. Interestingly however, the mammary glands and brains of dairy cows do not require insulin for glucose uptake. A protocol for insulin administration to refractory ketosis cases involves the subcutaneous administration of 200 IU of long-acting insulin (typically protamine zinc insulin [PZI]) every 24 to 36 hours combined with a continuous dextrose infusion. Although many doses of insulin have been administered to chronically ketotic cattle without concurrent glucose provision, the authors do not recommend it. The use of insulin in this way would, of course, constitute extralabel drug use, and at the current point in time, the only PZI source available in the United States is a recombinant human protein; indeed, it is increasingly difficult to obtain any animal-sourced insulin for large animal use. There has been some research validating the beneficial antiketogenic effects of exogenous insulin in dairy cattle, but there is a significant risk of hypoglycemia when it is administered without concurrent dextrose treatment. Inducing hyperglycemia by infusions of 250 mL of 50% dextrose solutions several times daily seems an appealing alternative to insulin injection or a CRI, particularly on farms, the theory being that cows respond to the transient hyperglycemia by endogenous insulin secretion. There are downsides to this approach in that repeated hyperglycemia seems to predispose to abomasal displacement and increases the risk of glucosuria, sepsis, and enhanced fluid losses in urine. Furthermore, many of the more severe hepatic lipidosis and chronic ketosis cases, especially obese individuals, have some degree of insulin resistance and highly abnormal and unpredictable endogenous glucose homeostasis. Niacin (12g orally daily) also inhibits lipolysis and is frequently administered daily to cows with chronic ketosis. Vitamin B_{12} is also commonly administered on a daily basis.

The most important treatment of cows with chronic fat mobilization and hepatic lipidosis is forced feeding. Alfalfa meal, 4 oz of KCl, and rumen transfaunation from a healthy donor cow is our traditional gruel, given twice daily.

If these treatments do not appear to be effective after 3 to 5 days, then it may be necessary to reduce the cow's milk production by milking for 1 minute twice daily until the negative energy balance cycle is broken. Cows should test negative on the California mastitis test to qualify for this controlled milking approach. Usually the limited milking is required for 4 to 7 days before ketosis is permanently resolved. Over the years, we have performed this on many cows with chronic fat mobilization, and such an approach, along with previously mentioned treatments, has been successful in a majority of cases. Additionally, owners have reported the subsequent milk production for the remainder of the lactation was very good. Although cows with chronic fat mobilization have delayed time of estrus and their production is diminished during the first 6 weeks of lactation, their prognosis for complete recovery is excellent. Time to recovery is variable, but most cows are well by 6 to 8 weeks into lactation. The most frequent complication associated with treatment of these cows is thrombophlebitis caused by multiple IV administrations of dextrose if a catheter has not been used.

Although the clinical cure rate is high with such intensive treatment, there are some periparturiently obese cows with severe ketosis at freshening or immediately after in whom the hepatic lipidosis will be life threatening or fatal. Cows affected at this extreme end of the spectrum need to be hospitalized and administered IV fluids to combat hypotension, lactic acidosis, sepsis, myopathy, and numerous mineral and electrolyte imbalances. Dextrose and calcium are often added to the fluids, although baseline blood glucose levels may already be high in some of these cows. The cows should be force fed as described earlier and have only limited milk removed. (If there is mastitis in a quarter, it should be stripped out and intramammary antibiotics administered.) Insulin therapy can be used as described previously for these individuals. Reduced neutrophil and hepatic macrophage function in these cows may allow merely mild metritis or mastitis to overwhelm the patient through sepsis, therefore appropriate systemic antibiotics should be given. If metritis is present, which is commonly the case, the uterus should be lavaged gently and oxytocin administered for days 1-3 following parturition. Fresh feed, clean water, and salt should be available, and the cow should be housed in a large well-bedded box stall with excellent footing, a deep sand or recycled manure solids bedded pack, or a grass paddock.

Along with sepsis, musculoskeletal injury is another common reason for euthanasia of overweight cows with severe periparturient hepatic lipidosis. Every effort should be made to maintain calcium levels within normal limits by either slow continuous infusion or subcutaneous (SC) administration; ideally, ionized calcium should be closely monitored and the cow housed in an area that will provide the best comfort for standing up and lying down. If there has been any difficulty in rising and resultant soft tissue trauma, the cow should be administered flunixin meglumine (500 mg once or even twice daily if needed). The knees should be wrapped with soft cotton bandages to provide protection to the carpus area, which is often the first anatomical site to be adversely affected in cows that have difficulty rising. Although lipotropic medications such as choline and methionine are used by some clinicians for cattle with hepatic lipidosis, their therapeutic value is probably not significant. If lipotropic medications are used, rumen-protected choline is preferred. Electrolyte imbalances also should be addressed if laboratory facilities exist that allow easy assessment of these values.

Ketosis as a Herd Problem

Ketosis can be considered a herd problem when more than an acceptable incidence occurs in the cows at greatest risk—that is, cows in early lactation. In traditional, individually housed, component-fed cattle, ketosis cases can occur slightly later in lactation (up to 6 weeks), but in group-housed TMR-fed cattle, the majority of cases tend to occur earlier, during the first 2 to 3 weeks. It is impractical to determine the true incidence of ketosis (number of new cases of blood BHB >1.2 mmol/L during the risk period in question divided by the total number of cows that completed the risk period) in the commercial dairy setting because this would require repeated measures of blood BHB throughout early lactation. Ideally, because the median time period for resolution of subclinical ketosis is about 5 days, one would have to test all cattle twice a week during the risk period, an impractical expense for most dairies. However, when Duffield and colleagues looked at both ketosis incidence (performing blood BHB tests at 1, 2, 3, and 6 weeks after calving) and average early lactation ketosis prevalences in a large field study, they found that the cumulative incidence of ketosis (45%) was approximately 2.2 times the average prevalence of ketosis (20%). It is worth noting that the farm-reported incidence of clinical ketosis in this study was only 1.5%, providing further evidence of the underdiagnosis of the condition in the clinical setting. Based on this research, and experience, the average cumulative incidence in early postpartum cows (<6 weeks in lactation) of subclinical and clinical ketosis has been approximated at 40%. The prevalence of ketosis (testing cows in a cross-sectional fashion once in the first 2 weeks of lactation) averages 20%, with a large range between herds (0% to >70%). The prevalence of ketosis provides a "snapshot" by measuring BHB levels at only one particular point in time; therefore, the measurement of ketosis prevalence is more practical on farm, and one can use the 2.2 multiplier to convert from prevalence to incidence if so desired. To categorize and identify herd problems with ketosis, our colleague Dr. Gary Oetzel at the University of Wisconsin has historically recommended testing a minimum of 12 individuals for blood BHB levels (using the 1.2 mmol/L cut-off point). If 3 or more individuals out of the 12 have elevated BHB levels, then there is a problem. There is no upper limit to the number of cows that can be tested; greater statistical power and accuracy will be generated by a larger sample size, but a sample size of 12 should be the minimum (20 is a useful number on large dairies). The alarm level should be set at 15% if larger numbers are sampled, and 10% or less is a reasonable goal for the best-managed herds. Individuals chosen for sampling may need to be carefully selected based on farm type and management system. Dr. Oetzel recommends choosing cows that are considered healthy at the time of sampling. Most sick cows will have already decreased their milk production and be non-ketotic, and their inclusion in herd-level testing will falsely decrease the herd's prevalence of ketosis. Interestingly, the peak incidence of subclinical ketosis in a large field study involving four large commercial dairies occurred at only 5 days in milk (DIM), suggesting that at least for large free-stall farms, one should choose individuals very early in lactation. However, on stanchion and tie-stall farms, particularly if the feeding system is component based, one might extend the sampling period to as far out as 50 DIM. In small herds, the data may need to be accumulated over more than one sampling time point. Increasingly, some DHI processing centers in the United States are now offering routine milk ketone testing, thereby providing a monthly monitor of the herd's ketosis prevalence and another tool by which producers and veterinarians can evaluate transition cow management. A ketosis monitoring system for U.S. dairy herds was introduced by AgSource in January 2015 that reports the herd-level ketosis prevalence based on predicted blood BHB levels from milk sample results and other milk test result data. This method of predicting blood BHB is much more accurate than that based on milk fat:protein ratios or milk ketones alone. It is not a tool to be used for identifying individuals with ketosis but can be a valuable herd-level monitor.

The impact of underappreciated ketosis in modern dairying is borne out by the observation that the average herd prevalence in North America is about 20%, and there is compelling evidence that herds with a prevalence in excess of 15% (hence this being chosen as the alarm level) are more likely to have high disease risks, lower milk production, higher cull rates, and reduced reproductive performance. The underlying circumstances leading to herd-level problems with ketosis are not fully understood in all situations, but some specific examples of predisposing causes are known. Important risk factors include increased body condition score, increased parity, giving birth to a male calf, increased calving ease score, stillbirth, and elevated precalving NEFAs. When a greater than 10% to 15% herd prevalence has been established, further efforts should be undertaken to investigate the ketosis problem.

Prevention

Probably all cows with ketosis have greater than physiologically necessary accumulation of lipid in hepatocytes. Some are more severely affected than others. Prophylactic medical treatments to prevent ketosis are limited but one author (JM) has reported that in herds with 25% or greater incidence of hyperketonemia, treatment of all fresh cows with propylene glycol for 5 days is economically beneficial. Feeding strategies to prevent ketosis constitute really no more than generally recommended practices of nutrition and feed bunk management. In many herds with a high incidence of ketosis, the problems originate with nutritional mistakes during the dry period, especially in the "close-up" cows, 1 to 2 weeks before calving.

The DMI of a cow frequently declines by up to 30% in late gestation up to the day of calving. This decline (often from ≈15 kg/day DMI to ≤12 kg/day for an adult Holstein cow) in intake is accompanied by an increasing rate of lipid mobilization from body fat stores. The serum concentration of NEFAs correspondingly increases. Consequently, NEFA concentrations in cows destined to develop pathologic hepatic lipidosis, when measured in the prepartum period, are above those of normal cows at their peak in early lactation. When NEFAs are measured between 14 days before calving and 3 days before calving, they can be useful in predicting the development of ketosis and, to some extent, displaced abomasum and metritis. Ideally, NEFA concentrations would remain at 0.3 mmol/L or less during this period. The week before calving is the proper time to measure NEFAs because their measurement can be used to determine whether energy balance in the late dry period may be responsible for a high incidence of ketosis in a herd. In contrast, BHB should be used postcalving to monitor the amount of ketosis in a herd. Values greater than 1.2 mmol/L suggest ketosis, and many of these cows, if monitored and traced back, were only ingesting 12 kg or less DMI the week before calving and had elevated NEFAs. Milk component testing has also been used to monitor energy consumption in lactating cows. A milk fat:milk protein ratio more than 1.5 has also been associated with ketosis development.

Because all cows undergo physiological accumulation of lipid in the liver during the periparturient period, conditions that lead to excessive lipid mobilization are most likely to result in severe hepatic lipidosis and ketosis. Both obesity and other primary diseases that restrict feed intake during the immediate prepartum period are potential causes. Long dry periods per se appear to put cows at increased risk for ketosis whether obesity develops or not. Many individual cows with severe ketosis that was refractory to routine treatments have been discovered to have preceding dry periods of 3 or more months. In recent years, we have particularly noticed this to be common in cows used for embryo transfer. The pathophysiology of this phenomenon has not been described, but many practitioners have made the same observation.

Most data suggest that an attempt should be made to feed a controlled-energy, high-roughage diet throughout the entire dry period, and this has been shown to decrease adipose tissue mobilization and decrease NEFA and BHB concentrations postpartum while sustaining normal milk production. Mismanagement of dry cow diets has occurred both through incorrect diet formulation and restricting physical access to feed, leading to outbreaks of postpartum ketosis. Dr. Charles Guard describes a herd with a ketosis problem that offered its close-up cows an appropriate ration. There were the recommended 30 inches of bunk space per cow for 15 to 25 cows; however, the area in front of the bunk was a deep mudhole, limiting access. In addition, there was an electric fence surrounding the bunk and strung across the top to prevent cows from stepping into the feed. Creating a new feed bunk away from mud and electricity appeared to solve the ketosis problem. Although unlikely under modern management practices, Dr. Guard also describes simple starvation resulting in death from hepatic failure of about half of the periparturient cows during a 4-week period in a 300-cow herd. The manager was so concerned about fat dry cows that intake was limited to 5 kg of poor quality grass hay. The dying cows were thin with body condition scores of 2 to 2.5 but had severe hepatic lipidosis. The late dry period is not a time to try to get cows to lose weight! Cows

that lose condition during the dry period have higher rates of not only ketosis but also of abomasal displacements, milk fever, and metritis.

Undersupply of protein during the dry period and, in particular, during the last 3 weeks before calving, has also been shown experimentally to predispose cows to ketosis. In one experimental study the treatment group was supplemented with animal-source protein to increase the bypass fraction and total crude protein intake. General discussion of this work with nutritionists has suggested that simply increasing the crude protein in the diet of close-up dry cows probably has the same benefit as using the more expensive animal-source ingredients. If diets higher in non-fiber carbohydrate (NFC) are fed to the close-up cows, this would provide the opportunity to increase microbial protein yield. The minimum requirement for metabolizable protein for close-up cows and heifers is 1300 g/day. For lactation, this increases to approximately 3000 g/day. Lysine and methionine in particular should be adequate and balanced in the diet. Unfortunately, ration formulation must be performed mindful of the fact that excess dietary protein in any form, but particularly nonprotein nitrogen or readily soluble protein, may also lead to herd problems with ketosis. Several outbreaks of ketosis affecting animals in many stages of lactation have occurred after the on-farm experimental addition of urea to the diet. Urea has been added for reasons varying from incomplete digestion of the corn grain in corn silage to just trying something because cows were not milking as expected. In all known cases of urea-feeding ketosis outbreaks, recovery was spontaneous when the urea was removed from the diet.

Niacin supplementation has undergone experimental evaluation as a possible means of ketosis prevention and has become particularly popular in the management of individually valuable, overconditioned embryo transfer donor cows that have experienced protracted dry periods. In one study, niacin was supplemented at 6 g/day to cows beginning 2 weeks prepartum and continued at 12 g/day postpartum for 12 weeks. Cows receiving extra niacin had higher blood glucose and lower blood BHB than control animals. In a second experiment evaluating dose response, niacin was fed at 0, 3, 6, or 12 g/day for 10 weeks' postpartum. There was no observable effect of feeding at the 3-g level. Cows receiving 6 or 12 g/day had slightly higher milk production and blood glucose than those receiving 0 or 3 g/day. Despite these seemingly impactful and relevant observations, the feeding of niacin to prevent ketosis has not been widely adopted. Cost and the inconvenience of providing a feed ingredient only to early lactation cows have both contributed to the lack of adoption. The most effective periparturient use of niacin may be in herds with a high incidence of ketosis (clinical or subclinical) or in individual, overconditioned periparturient cows.

The permitted use of ionophores in close-up and lactating cow diets now provides a strong management tool for the prevention of ketosis in many countries. Their action is to reduce acetate production and enhance propionate production by rumen bacteria. Because propionate is converted to glucose by the liver, an increase in its supply diminishes the likelihood of hypoglycemia and excessive lipid mobilization from fat stores. Administration of monensin by rumen-controlled release during the periparturient period has been shown to decrease the incidence of ketosis by 50% and decrease both BHB and NEFA concentrations during this period. Intraruminal controlled release capsules are more effective than when the monensin is simply added to the feed. One of the particular problems with monensin incorporation into the ration is that if DMI decreases for any reason, the concentration of monensin may be too low to have the needed effect on the rumen microorganisms, hence the value of controlled-release boluses. Feeding of monensin and diets with high starch levels postpartum has additionally been found to improve milk production and energy status of early lactation cows.

No discussion on prevention of ketosis would be complete without considering cow comfort. Adequate space for both feeding and some exercise is critically important for periparturient cows in addition to ad libitum access to palatable water. Additionally, proper space and a comfortable environment for resting are critical if cows are expected to ruminate properly. During hot weather, misting and fans should be used to improve cow comfort and feed intake. Frequent pen moves during the late dry period must be avoided because they have a negative impact on DMI, as the time taken to repeatedly establish and reestablish social hierarchy and familiarity with new surroundings distracts the cows from feed consumption.

Currently, investigations of metabolic disease problems in commercial herds at the University of Wisconsin far more frequently identify management errors in the last 2 to 3 weeks of gestation rather than ration formulation mistakes. Common issues include overcrowding (<30 inches of bunk space for every cow if they all chose to eat simultaneously), inadequate stall numbers or inappropriate stall design for lying time and comfort, and pen moves during the last 2 to 3 weeks of gestation (we typically recommend a prefresh pen stay of at least 10 days with no movement into maternity area until "feet are showing"). In addition, first-lactation heifers should be housed in a separate fresh pen from multiparous animals to reduce social stresses that decrease DMI. The fresh pen should also be kept at a stocking density of less than 85% to encourage adequate DMI and rest.

Hypocalcemia

Pathophysiology

The normal blood calcium concentration in adult cows is between 8.5 and 10 mg/dL, which translates into a total plasma pool of only about 3 g in a 600-kg individual. Furthermore, only 45% of the calcium ($\approx$4.5 mg/dL or 1.1 mmol/L) is in the active or ionized form if albumin concentration is normal. It is evident that to meet the calcium needs of colostrum production, fetal maturation, and incipient

lactation at the end of gestation (collectively, these requirements may reach 30 g total calcium/day for late pregnant cows and 50 g/day for lactating cows), adult cows need to mobilize substantial amounts of calcium from bone, which as a total pool contains as much as 8 kg of calcium, and increase the efficiency of gastrointestinal (GI) tract absorption. Intestinal absorption of calcium is heavily dependent on the production of 1,25-dihydroxyvitamin D_3 by the kidney in response to parathormone (PTH) secretion, although a separate means of paracellular absorption can be significant when luminal calcium is high. The third component of calcium homeostasis, namely enhanced renal absorption of calcium in response to PTH, is quantitatively small in terms of its contribution to increased calcium availability in the transitioning adult cow. The action of PTH is considered a common denominator in the skeletal, renal, and intestinal regulation of calcium homeostasis, aiming to keep plasma levels within a range that maintains critical muscular, nervous, and other cellular functions. The normal physiologic response to decreasing ionized calcium levels is to produce PTH, which acts to increase osteoclastic bone resorption (direct PTH effect), increase intestinal absorption (via 1,25-dihydroxyvitamin D_3), and enhance renal tubular resorption of calcium. PTH secretion is exquisitely sensitive to small decreases in plasma ionized calcium, but the response can be blunted by hypomagnesemia, partly explaining the well-documented link between clinical hypomagnesemic tetany and hypocalcemia, even in nonlactating cattle.

There are several other important factors that interfere with PTH activity at a tissue level that can serve to blunt the individual's ability to respond efficiently to the increased demands of lactation, despite appropriate PTH secretion. Perhaps the most important factor, and one that has been the subject of a great deal of interest and research, is the role that acid–base status plays. Metabolic alkalosis predisposes to both milk fever and subclinical hypocalcemia principally because it interferes with skeletal calcium resorption by decreasing readily available calcium in bone fluid as well as lessening intestinal absorption by conformationally altering the PTH–receptor interaction at the tissue level. In addition, alkalosis increases albumin binding of serum calcium, hence lowering ionized, biologically available, serum calcium. By altering these interactions, downstream signaling events that should result in increased plasma calcium may not occur despite high-PTH secretion. The first observations that dietary acidification could reduce the incidence of hypocalcemia by Ender and Dishington in 1971 and the subsequent exploitation of this paradigm by many researchers such as Oetzel and Goff have led to the widespread practice of anionic salt supplementation to the diets of dry cows. In this way, milk fever and subclinical hypocalcemia rates can be reduced via the relative acidification of cattle in late gestation. It is worth noting that strong univalent cations, such as potassium and sodium, probably increase the propensity for milk fever via their alkalinizing effects and subsequent diminished tissue responsiveness to PTH far more than does calcium in the diet during the late dry and early lactational period. Low-calcium diets can theoretically be fed as a means of reducing milk fever incidence because prolonged exposure to high PTH levels can overcome some of the negative effects of alkalinization on tissue responsiveness; however, these prolonged and low-calcium diets are often impractical to formulate and deliver. A more detailed discussion on cation–anion diets and the manipulation of pH in transition cows can be found in a later section in this chapter.

Other factors also contribute to the development of hypocalcemia in dairy cattle, specifically age, breed, and endocrinologic factors such as estrogen levels. With increasing age, there is a reduced pool of calcium available for absorption from bone, and decreased vitamin D receptors predisposing older, high-producing cows, to milk fever. Freshening heifers, that generally give less milk than multiparous cows and have higher osteoblastic activity and calcium availability, rarely suffer from clinical milk fever. Further age-related changes include a reduction in PTH receptors in the peripheral tissues of older cattle alongside decreased intestinal absorption of calcium. It has long been observed by practitioners that the incidence of milk fever is higher in Jersey cattle than in Holsteins, and although an absolute explanation for this is uncertain, two factors that likely contribute to this breed predilection are the higher calcium concentration in colostrum and milk from Jerseys and the lower number of intestinal receptors for 1,25-dihydroxyvitamin D_3 within the breed compared with Holsteins. Although estrogen increases predictably in the last few days of gestation and this hormone has a negative effect on calcium mobilization from bone, it does not appear to be a significant contributor to the incidence of milk fever nor the severity of hypocalcemia.

A high percentage of cows, including some first-calf heifers, have some degree of hypocalcemia (total serum calcium <2.1 mmol/L) at the onset of lactation, and in a substantial number of these individuals, subclinical hypocalcemia may predispose to reduced intestinal motility, abomasal displacements, and a decreased appetite. Conversely, lameness may predispose to having early lactation hypocalcemia. Taken together, these all increase the concurrent risk of ketosis and even hepatic lipidosis. Hypocalcemia may also predispose to mastitis and metritis because of decreased smooth muscle contraction of the teat sphincter and uterus and by decreased neutrophil function. Subclinical hypocalcemia is therefore an important health hazard to fresh cows and can represent a significant potential economic loss for the farm. Serum calcium in normal cows tends to stabilize on day 3 or 4 of lactation, but this subclinical hypocalcemia may persist longer in some cows, especially multiparous ones or those with diminished feed intakes.

Clinical Signs

Parturient hypocalcemia or milk fever mostly occurs from about 24 hours before to 72 hours after parturition with a majority of cases occurring within 24 hours after calving. Historically, texts have divided hypocalcemia into three stages, with stage 1 characterized by the cow still being able to stand, stage 2 by recumbency, and stage 3 by coma and

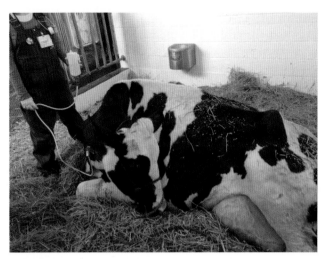

• **Fig. 15.9** A 5-year-old Holstein cow, fresh 1 day, with milk fever and common appearance of flaccid recumbency and head turned into the body.

unresponsiveness. The initial signs are restlessness, excitability, and anorexia. Many cows at this stage protrude their tongues when stimulated around the head. This activity otherwise only occurs in cows as a displacement activity when they would rather kill you or run away but cannot. As hypocalcemia progresses, the ability to regulate core temperature is gradually lost. Therefore rectal temperature will typically be normal in stage 1 but low in stage 2 and 3 depending on ambient temperature. Cutaneous circulation is depressed, leading to cool extremities when the ambient temperature is less than 68.0°F (20.0°C). Rumen contractions deteriorate from weak to absent. Skeletal muscle weakness develops over several hours. Cows may stagger or fall but more commonly are found down with their heads turned to the thorax (Fig. 15.9) or extended in an S fashion and are unable to rise. In stage 3, cows may be obtunded and unable to move and may die quickly. The heart rate increases during the progression of hypocalcemia with rates often 80 to 100 beats/min in stage 2 and even greater in stage 3, yet cardiac output decreases as a result of reduced venous return and weaker cardiac muscle contractions. Bloat occurs because of failure to eructate. Cows recumbent because of milk fever often have decreased corneal responses; Dr. Francis Fox, upon observing flies on the corneas of milk fever cattle, would tell students to observe the fly hockey match occurring on the cornea. Death may occur within 12 hours of the onset of signs caused by suffocation secondary to bloat, aspiration of ruminal contents, or cardiovascular collapse. True tetany does not occur with milk fever in dairy cows likely because magnesium levels are not sufficiently low. It is important to note that, as mentioned earlier, a large proportion of hypocalcemic cows are subclinically hypocalcemic and so will not express the overt clinical signs associated with milk fever.

Treatment

Parenteral administration of calcium borogluconate has been the most common treatment of hypocalcemia for many years worldwide. Concentrations of calcium, calcium salt formulations, and other elemental and carbohydrate components within the infusion solution vary widely according to personal preference and the perceived needs of the cow. There is no doubt that treatment with calcium borogluconate solutions IV leads to rapid recovery of skeletal muscle tone and smooth muscle function in the GI tract. Cows often eructate, defecate, or urinate during the IV administration of calcium, and many cows with truly uncomplicated stage 2 hypocalcemia are capable of standing before or shortly after the infusion is finished.

Individuals with stage 3 hypocalcemia may take longer to generate the ability to stand unassisted but are still frequently able to stand within minutes of receiving IV calcium. Cattle that are recumbent on slippery surfaces such as concrete free-stall alleyways should be moved or slid to good footing before any attempts to stand. This procedure may help prevent exertional myopathy and other musculoskeletal injuries such as coxofemoral luxations common to hypocalcemic cows that struggle to rise on slippery surfaces.

Serum total calcium concentration is normally between 8.5 and 10 mg/dL (2.1–2.5 mmol/L). The degree of hypocalcemia that develops at parturition is not perfectly correlated with the clinical signs. At a level of 6 to 7 mg/dL, cows are often still able to stand but may have moderate weakness, bloat, and anorexia. At a level of 5 mg/dL or lower, most cows will be down, and at a total calcium level of less than 4 mg/dL, most cows will be comatose. When using an i-STAT and measuring ionized calcium, values below 0.7 or 0.8 mmol/L are typically associated with recumbency.

A standard 500-mL bottle of 23% calcium borogluconate contains approximately 10 g of calcium. A mature Holstein cow in good condition weighing 700 kg will have about 210 L of extracellular fluid. If her total plasma calcium level is 5 mg/dL, her calcium deficit is 10.5 g. Thus, one standard bottle of calcium will frequently increase serum calcium to 10 mg/dL in a typical stage 3 milk fever case. Most practitioners will administer all or part of a second bottle of calcium, perhaps giving it subcutaneously (SC), to provide extra calcium for anticipated ongoing losses and to prevent relapse. The heart rate normally decreases to some degree during infusion of IV calcium solutions to hypocalcemic cows. A sudden increase in heart rate or arrhythmia that develops during infusion may require slowing or stopping the infusion, as would severe bradycardia. Calcium solutions to be administered IV should be warmed to body temperature before administration. Subcutaneous calcium treatment alone is inadequate for down cows because of the slow rate of absorption due to impaired circulation. Conversely, IV calcium should not be administered, or at the very least used with great caution in standing cows. Calcium-containing fluids for SC administration should always be checked to be sure that they do not contain dextrose.

Oral boluses and liquids have become increasingly available and used by producers for treatment or prevention of hypocalcemia. Among the simple calcium salts, only calcium chloride and calcium propionate have proved to be adequately bioavailable for therapy of clinical milk fever via the oral route. Calcium chloride, when given as a drench or paste to down cows, tends to be highly caustic and has caused aspiration pneumonia and death. Calcium propionate is less caustic but when aspirated will also cause pneumonia. More recently, Bovikalc (Boehringer Ingelheim Vetmedica Inc, Duluth, GA, 30096), a calcium chloride (quick absorption) and calcium sulfate (slow absorption) bolus coated with fat, has been marketed as a preventive treatment for milk fever in dairy cattle. When given to fresh cows with lameness or higher than mean herd average milk production in the previous lactation, this product was shown to be of clinical and economic benefit; administration within 2 hours of calving and again the next day is recommended if administration of a second bolus 12 hours after calving is logistically unfeasible. The use of oral calcium supplements requires functional swallowing reflexes to prevent these caustic materials from entering the trachea such that the severity of hypocalcemia and muscle weakness should be assessed in an individual before their use. Alternatively, soluble solutions of these calcium salts can be given via stomach tube directly into the rumen, thereby bypassing the direct risk of aspiration. Excessive amounts of oral calcium can cause fatal hypercalcemia, as indeed can overzealous and repeated IV calcium borogluconate administration (or combinations of the two). Calcium propionate has been the most commonly used product for oral or orogastric administration because it is less caustic and also provides a glucogenic precursor (propionate). Calcium propionate, 50 to 90 g, is often used alone or as a supplement to IV calcium therapy for milk fever. Evidence-based research suggests that the relapse rates and clinical response of true milk fever cases to oral calcium administration compare favorably with those seen with conventional IV therapy. However, personal clinician and farm experience often dictate that IV calcium administration is elected for the treatment of recumbent milk fever cases, but on many dairies, calcium administration to anorectic cows that may only be mildly hypocalcemic has moved completely to the oral route. Calcium propionate gel administered orally has also been used successfully for subclinical hypocalcemia and as a routine treatment for fresh cows in some herds. One of the authors (JM) has shown that the routine postpartum oral administration of calcium boluses to multiparous cows can be cost effective, with the highest net impact when the calcium is routinely administered to cows with high milk yield in the previous lactation or to postpartum multiparous lame cows.

In the majority of uncomplicated cases of milk fever, a single calcium treatment, usually IV calcium borogluconate, is all that is required. If relapse occurs or if serum magnesium is low, consideration should be given to supplementing magnesium in addition to more calcium. It should be noted that most cows with milk fever have normal to high serum magnesium likely associated with high PTH levels and increased renal tubular absorption of magnesium. If magnesium therapy is needed, a convenient method for supplementing magnesium is to use magnesium sulfate

(0.5–1 lb) or one or two magnesium hydroxide rumen laxative boluses or magnesium oxide for a few days after parturition. Excessive use of magnesium hydroxide may cause systemic alkalosis and decrease ionized calcium. Magnesium may also be given IV as a commercially prepared calcium and magnesium product or by administering 10% to 20% magnesium sulfate (see later discussion of hypomagnesemia). The administration of phosphorus, even when serum phosphorus is low, has rarely been shown to be helpful in treating milk fever cows, but some cows may benefit from the combined calcium and phosphorus treatment. Overzealous treatment with phosphorus could result in calcium phosphate complexes and worsen hypocalcemia in addition to promoting soft tissue mineralization!

Practitioners vary in their advice regarding complete milkout of mature cows at risk of milk fever. Partial milk removal may lessen the development of hypocalcemia. However, cows not fully milked out may leak milk and be predisposed to environmental mastitis, and udder engorgement produces unreasonable discomfort. We rarely recommend this except for possibly an "old favorite cow in the herd" with poorly responsive and relapsing milk fever (see later).

Relapsing milk fever is most common in older high-producing cows, some of whom may also have other metabolic abnormalities such as fatty liver. These are frequently large, high-producing cows that may already have chronic musculoskeletal abnormalities because of age and that are at high risk of developing life-threatening myopathy with recumbency. If the cows are valuable, which they often are, we have taken an aggressive therapeutic approach, which may include continual IV calcium drips in addition to force feeding calcium supplements to maintain ionized calcium between 1.2 and 1.5 mmol/L. Intramuscular administration of a single dose of vitamin D to such individuals is also recommended. Although two to three days are required for the conversion of vitamin D_3 to 1,25-dihydroxyvitamin D_3, some of these cows have persistent hypocalcemia for 5 to 7 days. If the ability to measure ionized calcium is not available, greater reliance on oral and subcutaneous administration of calcium is preferred, with IV calcium only being administered when clinical signs (hopefully only stage 1 or 2) are noted. When aggressive calcium supplementation is undertaken in this way, it is advisable to measure blood levels frequently and adjust therapy accordingly to avoid severe hypercalcemia and its attendant risks of cardiovascular fatality. Careful attention to both the calcium and magnesium levels in their diet or ration is also important, but intake in affected individuals is often moderate to poor, and it can be hard to accurately assess the amount of these two elements that are actually being consumed, let alone absorbed. It is of utmost importance to house these cows on an excellent footing material with adequate room for rising and to provide analgesics and support bandages (knee wraps can be especially helpful) in the case of a lame or injured individual. All other potential secondary diseases such as mastitis, metritis, and so on should be given due prophylactic

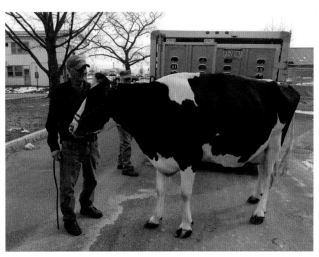

• **Fig. 15.10** An 8-year-old, 92-point, Holstein cow being discharged from the hospital after several days of treatment for recurrent hypocalcemia and renal tubular acidosis.

consideration and treated promptly. Some cases of relapsing hypocalcemia can be aggravated by other metabolic abnormalities such as hypomagnesemia and renal injury. Renal tubular acidosis, likely associated with tetracycline-induced renal injury, was believed to play a role in a 9-day course of relapsing milk fever in one cow. After the azotemia resolved and the serum bicarbonate and chloride returned to normal, the hypocalcemia also resolved (Fig. 15.10).

Milk Fever as a Herd Problem

Results from the 2002 National Animal Health Monitoring System (NAHMS) survey indicated that clinical hypocalcemia incidence in dairy cattle in U.S. herds was 5%, and subclinical hypocalcemia was 25% for primiparous cows and between 41% to 54% for multiparous cows. When the incidence of clinical milk fever exceeds 15% in mature cows, most veterinarians would agree that this is excessive and represents a herd problem. On well-managed dairies, with a cross-section of ages and parities typical of the modern dairy, the incidence of milk fever should not exceed 4%, and many of the better managed herds are able to achieve annual incidence rates for milk fever that are half of this number (≈2%). With the changing distribution of cow ages within modern dairying, such that the proportion of first-calf heifers is becoming much higher on many dairies than was once customary, the relative parity distribution on a farm needs to be carefully considered when judging whether there is a problem with hypocalcemia and milk fever incidence on any given dairy. The most common age distribution of clinical cases of milk fever is twice the rate in third and greater lactations compared with second calvings and none in first calvings. The occurrence of milk fever is dependent on the nutritional management of cows during the dry period and, in particular, during the last 3 weeks before calving. If practitioners wish to investigate parturient hypocalcemia as a subclinical entity, we suggest blood sampling cattle of all ages about 12 to 24 hours after calving and using a cutoff of 30% as an alarm level for parturient hypocalcemia (subclinical and clinical combined) using adult cow reference values from the laboratory in question.

Historically, maintaining low calcium intake during the dry period and then feeding a high-calcium diet after calving was a recommended method of decreasing milk fever in herds. The low calcium diet in the dry period was thought to stimulate PTH, and then when the cow calved and was fed a high-calcium diet, there would be increased absorption of the dietary calcium due to the already high PTH. The physiologic concept was sound, but as reported by Dr. Jesse Goff, it is very difficult to feed low enough calcium (20 g of calcium daily) in a forage-based diet to dry cows such that this actually occurs. Many diets historically formulated for dry cows using conventional forages and grains exceeded minimum requirements for calcium, phosphorus, and potassium, and experiences have illustrated that prevention of milk fever by following these traditional nutritional guidelines often failed because of the high-cationic (particularly potassium containing) forages and the alkalinizing effects of the diet. The maintenance of the late gestation dry cow in a state of mild metabolic acidosis by manipulation of the inorganic cation–anion difference has empirically solved many herd problems with excessive cases of milk fever. This can best be achieved by feeding HCl-containing SoyChlor (West Central, Ralston, IA) to the close-up dry cows. The amount of the product fed (usually 2 to 3 lb/cow/day) and its effectiveness can be easily monitored by checking urine pH. After 5 days of feeding this high-chloride supplement, the urine pH should be between 6.0 and 7.0 (preferably lower in Jerseys), and it should be maintained at this level until parturition. Other nutritional advisors have approached herd problems by concentrating on the potassium-to-magnesium ratio in the dry cow diet to achieve similar results.

The most common problems in formulating dry cow diets to achieve a low incidence of milk fever are the farm-specific necessity to feed legume forages, which have high concentrations of potassium, especially forages grown on soils either fertilized with potash or those with heavy applications of manure. The latter has become more commonplace and significant as liquid manure systems have become the norm. Liquid manure storage and handling is considered environmentally sound because it prevents many soluble nutrients from escaping into surface water around the barnyard and is preferred as both convenient and economical on large dairies. However, as dairies have expanded, the animal units per crop acre have increased with subsequently more manure to dispose of per acre. This manure in liquid form provides more soluble nutrients for plant uptake and recycling to the cows.

Oetzel reviewed the literature on diet and milk fever and found that the incidence was very low at daily calcium intakes of less than 50 g, increased with calcium intake up to about 120 g/day, and then declined at higher calcium intakes. This paradoxical relationship with calcium intake helped refute some of the earlier thinking about calcium intake restriction being of primary importance. In evaluating these experimental diets, the cation minus anion difference was calculated. Measured cations included sodium and potassium (sometimes calcium and magnesium as well); anions included chloride, sulfate, and phosphate. The incidence of milk fever increased as the sum of cations minus anions increased. The equation most predictive for the incidence of milk fever was $(Na + K) - (Cl + S)$ expressed as milliequivalents per kilogram dry matter. Typical dry cow diets are +100 to +250. Further experiments to test this hypothesis relating to the influence of strong ion balance on calcium mobilization and activity have shown that, when the difference is manipulated before calving, serum calcium homeostasis is altered. When cations minus anions was negative (around −100) in prepartum diets, serum alkalinity was reduced, tissue responsiveness to PTH was increased, and serum calcium was increased after calving relative to controls. Acidification of the diet may increase urinary calcium excretion, but this is negated by the increased bone and intestinal absorption at freshening, and discontinuation of the manipulated anionic diet at calving should quickly allow the urine to become alkalinized, as is normal in a herbivore, decreasing the renal loss of calcium.

Salts used to manipulate the diet of dry cows to achieve greater anionic content include ammonium chloride, ammonium sulfate, calcium sulfate (gypsum), calcium chloride, magnesium chloride, and magnesium sulfate (Epsom salts). These salts are relatively unpalatable, and their successful use requires that they be fed in a blended diet such as a TMR. These salts have been mostly replaced by the feeding of more palatable commercial products such as SoyChlor (see the previous discussion on this product). Typically, anionic salts are included in the diet of close-up cows due to calve within 3 weeks. In herds without separate feeding facilities for this group, they may be fed throughout the dry period. Anionic salt feeding is discontinued at calving, with the effect on serum calcium concentration persisting for a few days. There is a delayed rebound hypocalcemia after the discontinuation of anionic salt feeding. In most circumstances, this rebound occurs several days after calving when the DMI of the cow is adequate to provide the calcium necessary to support the current milk production, and no clinical effects are seen. Some herds have had disappointing results with anionic salt supplementation mostly related to over-acidification. Excessive supplementation with acidifying additives can negatively affect palatability to the point where DMIs decrease significantly. Unfortunately, it is common for overzealous anionic salt supplementation to be instituted in the face of a milk fever outbreak, with the undesirable consequence that feed intake decreases dramatically and the metabolic problems on the dairy become confounded by negative energy balance peripartum and clinical ketosis. In addition, there is concurrence that anionic salt supplementation necessitates an increase in the amount of calcium in the diet of close-up cows. For example, National Research Council (NRC) guidelines specify that under conditions of anionic salt supplementation, the amount of absorbable calcium in the diet should be increased to at least 95 g/day (0.98%). Calcium intakes of up to 150 g/day or higher may be necessary in some cases of anionic salt supplementation to prevent milk fever. Occasionally, excessive chloride supplementation will overacidify the diet of transition cows and even cause ruminal acidosis.

Because the success of dietary acidification will be ultimately reflected by urinary pH, measurement and monitoring of the latter are attractive tools for herd monitoring. Therefore, the urine pH of dry cows has been suggested as a parameter to monitor or judge the effectiveness of any anionic salt program. Cows on unsupplemented diets typically have a urine pH of 8 to 8.5. The pH may be as low as 5.5 with excessively heavy anionic salt or HCl acid supplementation. There are studies that suggest that dietary cation–anion difference (DCAD) and milk fever prevention is best served by a target urinary pH of between 6.0 and 7.0. Occasionally, practitioners encounter high urinary pH values (>7.0) in a herd that is supposedly feeding anionic salts. In most instances, this situation will relate to cows not consuming their expected DMI, the TMR not being mixed properly, or improper evaluation and adjustment for other free-choice minerals or forages in the diet. High potassium intake (>150 g/day) during the dry period has been linked to a high incidence of milk fever regardless of dietary calcium level. It is common to find no supplemental magnesium when investigating such herds. The interaction of potassium, magnesium, and calcium is not fully understood and may be separate from the strong ion effect discussed earlier. Potassium is the major cation in forages and cereal grains, and the concentration of potassium in the rumen dictates the transruminal electrical potential. As the amount of ingested potassium increases, ruminal fluid potassium concentration also increases. This reciprocally decreases rumen sodium concentration. The observed transruminal electrical potential increases from about 5 to 60 mV as sodium is isotonically replaced by potassium. The primary site of magnesium absorption in ruminants is across the rumen epithelium via passive carrier-mediated transport. The rate of absorption is inversely related to the transruminal electrical potential. The presence of sodium in rumen fluid is not observed to be important to magnesium absorption because replacement of sodium with lithium has no effect on magnesium uptake. Therefore, high potassium intake in the feed of transition cows directly leads to decreased bioavailability of magnesium and low magnesium should be considered when high-potassium forages are fed prefreshening. Furthermore, low magnesium is an important co-risk factor for hypocalcemia because persistently low serum and intracellular magnesium decrease both the PTH response to hypocalcemia and the tissue sensitivity of PTH for calcium resorption. Supplementing the diet of the dry cow with magnesium in the form of magnesium oxide to provide 1 g of magnesium for every 4 g of potassium up to a maximum of 65 g of magnesium per day has been successful in managing many herd milk fever problems. Alternatively, magnesium sulfate could be fed to address both the K/Mg ratio and the DCAD. Magnesium oxide and magnesium sulfate are relatively unpalatable and must be mixed with other feeds or salt to achieve the desired intake.

It is to be hoped that long-term success in feeding cows to minimize the incidence of milk fever and related magnesium deficiencies will be aided by better understanding of the potassium uptake by forage species. Most grasses and alfalfa respond with greater yields when soil potassium is plentiful. Manure storage systems to control environmental degradation return more potassium to the soil. As purchased grains and concentrates are brought to the farm, there is a net accumulation of potassium. As we inadvertently feed more and more potassium to our dry cows, the occurrence of fresh cow problems may be increasing. Land intentionally underfertilized with potash and not manured, may be set aside for production of dry cow forages. As an alternative strategy, some dairy managers purchase feed from farms with historically low potassium supplementation and no manuring.

Although uncommonly used, a single injection (IV or SC) of 10 million IU of crystalline vitamin D given 8 days before calving is an effective preventive for milk fever. The dose is repeated if the cow does not calve on the due date. Higher or more prolonged treatments should be avoided as life-threatening calcification of soft tissues, including the heart and great vessels, may occur because of the increased absorption of both calcium and phosphorus.

In summary, dry cow diets should be formulated to result in a dietary DCAD of −10 to −15 mEq/100g or −100 to −150 mEq/kg of dietary dry matter. Only the most palatable of anionic mineral supplements should be used, thereby inducing a mild metabolic acidosis verified by confirmation of acidification (pH = 6.0–7.0) of the urine. Jerseys may require a slightly lower urine pH to control the incidence of milk fever. Potassium in the diet should be kept low (1%), and chloride should be kept at a level that is 0.5% less than the potassium. Phosphorus should be 0.35% or less. High serum phosphorus will have an inhibitory effect on renal activation of vitamin D, thereby decreasing both calcium and phosphorus absorption from the intestine. An adequate amount of magnesium (0.35%–0.4%) in the prefresh cow diet is also of utmost importance.

Hypophosphatemia

The clinical relevance of hypophosphatemia in high-producing dairy cattle has long been a matter of conjecture and debate among practitioners and academics. Undoubtedly, many veterinarians include phosphorus supplementation in either oral or IV form in their therapy of repeat milk fevers and persistently recumbent cattle, but convincing scientific evidence for hypophosphatemia as a contributor or absolute cause of recumbency is lacking. The normal reference range for inorganic plasma phosphorus (Pi) in adult dairy cattle is approximately 5.6 to 6.5 mg/dL (1.8–2.1 mmol/L), and it is common for anorectic cattle to demonstrate blood levels below this reference range. Inorganic phosphorus refers to the phosphorus contained in inorganic PO_4 and is the most common laboratory measure of phosphorus in plasma. Most of the phosphorus in plasma is biologically available, with only a small percentage being either protein bound or in complexes.

Measurement of phosphorus levels in blood taken from the jugular vein routinely underestimates phosphorus obtained from the coccygeal vein by up to 0.8 mg/dL. Hypophosphatemia (low Pi) may occur with anorexia, increased mammary gland losses from high milk production, or increased intracellular movement of Pi caused by elevated insulin or alkalosis, the latter being the most common metabolic disturbance in adult dairy cattle. Urinary losses associated with elevated PTH may also occur, but in cattle, these are relatively minor compared with other species; in cattle, salivary gland secretion of phosphorus is the predominant route of excretion. Mild hypophosphatemia (Pi between 2 and 4 mg/dL) is not associated with discernible clinical signs in the absence of other significant macroelement or electrolyte disturbances, and serum phosphorus is a poor predictor of muscle phosphorus. Cattle with severe hypophosphatemia (plasma phosphorus <1 mg/dL) may be recumbent, but the absolute relevance of their hypophosphatemia is clouded by the fact that such individuals are usually hypocalcemic, hypoglycemic, and hypomagnesemic. It should always be remembered that most cows with milk fever will also be hypophosphatemic (cows with plasma calcium <5 mg/dL typically have phosphorus values of <2 mg/dL) likely as a result of increased PTH concentrations and that IV treatment with calcium alone will be followed by normalization of blood phosphorus within a few hours. Although we have never seen hemolysis with hypophosphatemia in early lactation dairy cattle, it has been implicated as a cause of postparturient hemoglobinuria in cattle. Grünberg et al. have recently (2015) demonstrated that cattle with marked serum hypophosphatemia, induced by dietary P depletion, did not have a decline in erythrocyte Pi or decreased osmotic resistance of erythrocytes. They surmised that phosphorus depletion alone is unlikely to cause intravascular hemolysis, and that plasma Pi is an unreliable index for the intracellular Pi of erythrocytes. It has previously been shown that plasma Pi is unsuitable for assessing muscle tissue phosphorus content in cattle.

Treatment

Based on the research currently available, there is strong evidence to recommend supplementing oral P to chronically P-depleted ruminants; however, only moderate evidence exists to justify the treatment of acute hypophosphatemia. Oral phosphorus supplementation has become an integral part of oral drenching solutions administered to nonrecumbent, but anorectic, dairy cattle. Phosphorus treatment, either oral or parenteral, for acute downer dairy cows is also commonly used by some veterinarians. The biologically active form of phosphorus is in the form of inorganic phosphate, and any attempts to therapeutically address real or perceived hypophosphatemia should reflect this. Most phosphorus preparations (except for sodium glycerophosphate in some commercial IV milk fever treatments) have low phosphate availability and therefore have minimal effect on plasma Pi concentration. Sodium monophosphate is the preferred form of phosphorus supplementation either for oral or IV use and should be used for treatment if hypophosphatemia

is thought to be causing a clinical problem. Sterile Fleet solutions are a good source of phosphorus and can be given subcutaneously or intravenously (diluted) in rare cases that might require parenterally administered phosphorus. This preparation is best given over time (20-30 grams IV drip or SC) to have maximal effect and to prevent serum phosphorus from becoming so high that precipitation with calcium and magnesium occur (in blood or soft tissues). High plasma Pi also decreases serum ionized calcium. Likewise, the product should not be mixed in high-calcium or high-magnesium fluids or precipitation may occur. Oral phosphorus supplementation can be given in the form of 200 to 500 g of sodium monophosphate (providing ≈50-100 g of inorganic phosphate), usually combined with other drench components such as calcium, energy sources, and magnesium.

Hypomagnesemia

Hypomagnesemia in dairy cattle very rarely assumes the severe clinical presentation with which veterinarians who work with pastured, spring-calving beef herds will be all too familiar. Normal plasma magnesium concentration is in the range of 1.8 to 2.3 mg/dL, but it should be remembered that blood values are a poor indicator of whole-body magnesium status for this predominantly intracellular cation. However, extracellular magnesium levels are closely linked to nerve and muscle function. Initially, muscle fasciculations followed by hyperexcitability will be seen in some cattle whose magnesium values decrease rapidly to 1.0 mg/dL or less, and untreated, this can progress to convulsions, tetany, and death as levels decrease still lower (Video 15.1). Calcium is also below normal range in hypomagnesemic tetany. Unfortunately, blood magnesium levels, particularly in advanced cases in which convulsions and tetany have led to significant muscle damage and subsequent leakage of magnesium out of cells, may be an unreliable means of definitive diagnosis for hypomagnesemia. Ocular fluids, urine, and cerebrospinal fluid (CSF) (which are normally similar to serum levels) if sampled shortly after death or in a moribund individual will more reliably reflect the antemortem magnesium status of an animal. A low magnesium concentration of less than 1.8 mg/dL (0.75 mmol/L) in the vitreous fluid of a recently deceased cow is indicative of hypomagnesemic tetany when signalment and clinical signs (if observed) are compatible. Cattle with clinical signs of hypomagnesemic tetany will typically have a serum total magnesium (tMg) of less than 0.8 mg/dL (0.33 mmol/L), low tMg in the CSF (<1.0 mg/dL [0.4 mmol/L]), and very little magnesium in the urine. Most of the magnesium in the body is in bone, but with magnesium deficits, this bone source is not readily available (unlike the rapid endocrine mobilization that occurs with calcium from bone in hypocalcemia) because magnesium levels in the serum are mostly regulated by daily intestinal absorption and urinary elimination. Magnesium absorption, which occurs mostly in the rumen in adult cattle, is reduced when the concentration of ammonia or ammonium is high in rumen fluid. The combined effect of a low magnesium and high nitrogen and potassium content in rapidly growing grass causes hypomagnesemia and hypocalcemia, which may result in tetanic signs. The mechanism of high ammonia concentration leading to inhibition of magnesium absorption is not known but may be associated with an ammonia-associated increase in rumen pH, which would hinder magnesium absorption. Dry cow diets based on ammoniated corn silage or the use of urea as the primary non-protein nitrogen supplement may inadvertently lead to secondary magnesium deficiency in dairy cattle. The clinical signs in affected dairy cows can be more similar to milk fever rather than the classic grass tetany of hypomagnesemia and hypocalcemia in pastured beef cattle. On rare occasions, downer cows in early lactation may result if excess non-protein nitrogen or soluble protein is fed without adequate magnesium supplementation.

It is much more common to encounter milder hypomagnesemia with tMg slightly less than 1.5 mg/dL (<0.6 mmol/L) in anorectic dairy cattle in early lactation, and such mild hypomagnesemia is frequently accompanied by mild hypophosphatemia and mild hypocalcemia. Severely hypomagnesemic cattle are also typically mildly to moderately hypocalcemic. The clinical relevance of low-grade hypomagnesemia in lactating dairy cattle is hard to characterize; however, chronically (≥2 days) low magnesium levels are thought to limit productivity and decrease PTH activity and might predispose to hypocalcemia. Sampling of individual, anorectic cows for a herd issue with hypomagnesemia is of dubious value, but the demonstration of plasma magnesium levels of less than 2.0 mg/dL in the majority of cows sampled on a farm within 12 to 24 hours of freshening should be taken as a problem with magnesium availability or absorption in the transition diet. Similar testing can be performed on groups of cows in early lactation. Because dietary magnesium absorbed in excess of requirements for maintenance and lactation is excreted in the urine, a useful measure of herd magnesium status is to evaluate urinary magnesium–creatinine fractional excretion (FEx) ratios for about 10 cows per group. This ratio corrects for the degree of water conservation by the kidney and better reflects magnesium status than serum magnesium concentration alone. Guidelines for target values of this ratio have not been well established in hypomagnesemic cattle, but Mg FEx ratios that average less than 1.0 for a group of cows suggest that the cows are likely magnesium deficient. Magnesium levels in the diet or factors that negatively influence absorption should be examined in response.

Hypomagnesemia should be also considered a likely predisposing cause when "milk fever" cases are encountered in midlactation cattle.

Although fulminant hypomagnesemic tetany is very rare in adult dairy cattle, we have on occasion diagnosed the condition in dairy calves. Affected calves are mostly 2 to 4 months old and are being fed milk and low-magnesium roughage. Magnesium intestinal absorption has been reported to drop appreciably in milk-fed calves after 4 to 5 weeks of age, helping to explain the predisposed age range listed. Chronic diarrhea may also predispose to hypomagnesemic tetany in calves. Clinical signs of tetany are similar to those seen with nervous coccidiosis, lead, strychnine, or organophosphate poisoning. Confirmation of the diagnosis is by finding serum and CSF tMg levels of less than 0.8 mg/dL and negligible or no magnesium in the urine, in addition to a positive treatment response with 100 mL of 10% magnesium sulfate slowly administered IV. Serum calcium will also be decreased if tetany is present.

Hypermagnesemia is rarely encountered, but when present, it usually suggests either compromised renal function or an iatrogenic phenomenon resulting from the overzealous administration of oral magnesium salts. Hypermagnesemia and alkalosis are common in dehydrated cattle receiving Carmalax "pink pills" (magnesium hydroxide), and if magnesium is greater than 5 mg/dL, severe neuromuscular weakness or recumbency may result.

Treatment

Treatment of cattle with hypomagnesemic grass tetany represents an emergency to save the animal's life. Maniacal or convulsing cattle occasionally first need to be sedated before parenteral administration of magnesium. Xylazine, depending on the severity of neurologic signs, can be used. Intravenous magnesium administration is appropriate in such cases, but caution needs to be taken with regard to the speed of infusion because of its potential cardiac and neuromuscular toxicity. Elevating serum magnesium from less than 1.0 mg/dL to within the normal reference range in a severely hypomagnesemic grass staggers cow will require approximately 2 to 3 g of magnesium. If commercial solutions containing multiple macroelements such as calcium, phosphorus, and magnesium are used, their magnesium content should be checked before infusion to verify that there is adequate magnesium present; commonly, these types of solutions contain slightly less than 2 g of magnesium. The infusion should be performed over at least 5 to 10 minutes. To prevent relapses over the next 12 to 24 hours, a further 250 mL of 10% to 20% magnesium sulfate solution can be administered SC divided over at least four sites. It is appropriate to select infusion solutions that also contain calcium because most individuals will be concurrently hypocalcemic, and the relapse rate appears to be lower and the initial response rate greater in cattle that receive both parenteral calcium and magnesium. Many practitioners administer oral magnesium salts (100–200 grams of magnesium sulfate) as further insurance against recurrence, but this requires that the animal has regained good protective upper airway reflexes and also runs the risk of overstimulation and a return to tetany if used prematurely in severe cases. Otherwise, oral magnesium supplementation is a safe and effective way to address less severe hypomagnesemia in cattle. Many drenches, commercial or homemade, that are used as nonspecific supportive enteral fluid therapy in lactating cows now contain 200 to 250 g of magnesium sulfate. Repeated use of magnesium salts will result in catharsis and elevation of serum magnesium above the normal reference range; however, only IV magnesium administration represents a potentially acute cardiotoxic risk. Magnesium oxide is the most palatable magnesium salt for feeding cattle, but the available magnesium may vary considerably among sources.

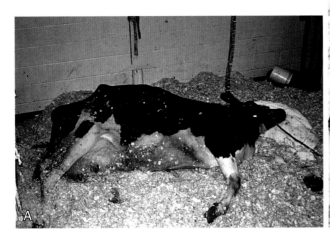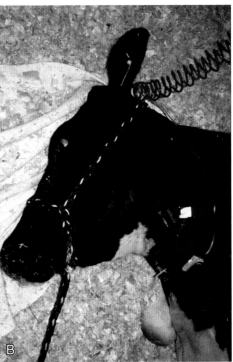

• **Fig. 15.11** **A** and **B,** Cow with severe hypokalemia and recumbency. The cow exhibited flaccid paralysis manifested as an inability to support the weight of the head or maintain herself in sternal recumbency.

Hypokalemia

Potassium homeostasis is a complicated issue in periparturient cows and one that is impacted by numerous factors, including; DMI; concurrent metabolic disease; drug treatments; acid–base balance; and our inability to accurately measure the intracellular K concentration, which constitutes 98% of the total body potassium. Moderate, clinically occult hypokalemia is an anticipated electrolyte disturbance in cattle that are off feed for any reason. Normal plasma potassium is between 3.8 and 5.6 mEq/L, and many cattle with common postparturient diseases such as metritis, left displacement of the abomasum, or ketosis will have measured potassium values slightly below this range. Severely hypokalemic cows in which the plasma potassium has decreased to less than 2.5 mEq/L may demonstrate progressive weakness and become recumbent. Recumbency should be anticipated when the potassium level decreases to less than 2.0 mEq/L. Despite hypokalemia, urine fractional excretion of potassium in even severely hypokalemic individuals is generally normal (27%–120%) or high, indicating an inappropriate renal response to the condition. Typical premonitory signs of obvious muscle fasciculations and increased time lying down will have been noticed by the astute producer, but the progression to being recumbent and unable to stand can be measured in just a few hours. It should be emphasized, however, that severe hypokalemia is a rare cause of recumbency in dairy cattle compared with hypocalcemia or musculoskeletal and dystocia-related trauma. Previously, there has been an observed link between the repeated use of the mixed glucocorticoid–mineralocorticoid isoflupredone

acetate and the occurrence of the severe hypokalemia syndrome. Retrospective clinical observations have been validated by experimental reproduction of severe hypokalemia and weakness after multiple administrations of the drug. The first documentation of hypokalemic recumbency in a group of cows associated with the administration of isoflupredone acetate was in a herd where the farm manager was administering the corticosteroid as a treatment for mastitis in early lactation cows (Dr. Amy Rath, senior seminar, Cornell University, 1994). Isoflupredone acetate is believed to be a risk factor for hypokalemia because of its strong mineralocoid properties and associated renal loss of potassium. It has become evident in recent years that the condition can be seen in the absence of isoflupredone acetate administration. Consistent management, nutritional or other factors in herds experiencing this problem are uncertain; however, many affected cattle have a history of chronic refractory ketosis or at least repeated treatments for presumed ketosis with corticosteroids, IV dextrose preparations, or oral glucogenic precursors that may induce hyperglycemia. Theoretically, the repeated administration of hyperglycemia-inducing agents, such as 50% dextrose, propylene glycol, and glucocorticoids, will act to increase urinary loss and drive potassium intracellularly. This intracellular shifting may be exacerbated by the inevitable metabolic alkalosis that accompanies prolonged inappetence in cattle. Cattle with prolonged anorexia have whole-body potassium depletion caused by inadequate intake in feed, coupled with continued obligate losses in urine and feces. Administration of any drugs with mineralocorticoid or kaluretic action, such as some corticosteroids and diuretics, will further exacerbate urinary losses. The clinical manifestation of severe hypokalemia is a flaccid paralysis (Fig. 15.11) that resembles the profound weakness and flaccidity seen with botulism. Many affected animals are unable to even support the weight of their heads and hence are mistaken for more conventional milk fever cases, but they fail to respond to conventional calcium treatments and become down cows. Aggressive oral treatment with potassium chloride appears to be as, if not more, effective than high-volume potassium-supplemented IV fluid administration in correcting the severe hypokalemia. Recommendations include oral administration of up to 1.0 lb initially and then 0.5 lb of potassium chloride orally twice daily, while monitoring serum potassium, to cattle with confirmed severe hypokalemia (<2.5 mEq/L) and weakness. Administration of such large amounts of potassium to cattle is inappropriate in all but the most severe hypokalemic states and will inevitably lead to catharsis in the following days. However, clinical experience suggests that recumbent individuals with severe hypokalemia do very poorly unless they regain the ability to stand within 24 to 48 hours of the onset of treatment. Some hypokalemic and recumbent cattle develop severe myopathy, which worsens the prognosis further. Devices such as slings, hip lifters, and flotation tanks should not be used until serum potassium returns to normal; severely hypokalemic cattle are potentially difficult to manage in flotation tanks as a result of their marked flaccidity.

Because of the observed risk of worsening hypokalemia in cattle repeatedly treated for ketosis, it is prudent to consider potassium supplementation to such individuals. Indeed, the inevitability of mild hypokalemia in association with anorexia in postpartum cows has led to the inclusion of potassium supplementation by many practitioners to cows that receive oral fluids for whatever reason. Low-level supplementation in the order of 60 to 125 g is well tolerated and safe when large-volume orogastric fluids are administered.

Suggested Readings

Bertics, S. J., Grummer, R. R., Cadorniga-Valino, C., et al. (1992). Effect of prepartum dry matter intake on liver triglyceride concentration and early lactation. *J Dairy Sci, 75,* 1914–1922.

Bhanugopan, M. S., Fulkerson, W. J., Fraser, D. R., et al. (2010). Carryover effects of potassium supplementation on calcium homeostasis in dairy cows at parturition. *J Dairy Sci, 93,* 2119–2129.

Bobe, G., Young, J. W., & Beitz, D. C. (2004). Invited review: pathology, etiology, prevention, and treatment of fatty liver in dairy cows. *J Dairy Sci, 87,* 3105–3124.

Braun, U., Blatter, M., Büchi, R., et al. (2012). Treatment of cows with milk fever using intravenous and oral calcium and phosphorus. *Schweiz Arch Tierheilkd, 154,* 381–388.

Carrier, J., Stewart, S., Godden, S., et al. (2004). Evaluation and use of three cowside tests for detection of subclinical ketosis in early postpartum cows. *J Dairy Sci, 87,* 3725–3735.

Chamberlin, W. G., Middleton, J. R., Spain, J. N., et al. (2013). Subclinical hypocalcemia, plasma biochemical parameters, lipid metabolism, postpartum disease, and fertility in postparturient dairy cows. *J Dairy Sci, 96,* 7001–7013.

Chapinal, N., Leblanc, S. J., Carson, M. E., et al. (2012). Herd-level association of serum metabolites in the transition period with disease, milk production, and early lactation reproductive performance. *J Dairy Sci, 95,* 5676–5682.

Coffer, N. J., Frank, N., Elliott, S. B., et al. (2006). Effects of dexamethasone and isoflupredone acetate on plasma potassium concentrations and other biochemical measurements in dairy cows in early lactation. *Am J Vet Res, 67,* 1244–1251.

Constable, P., Grünberg, W., Staufenbiel, R., et al. (2013). Clinicopathologic variables associated with hypokalemia in lactating dairy cows with abomasal displacement or volvulus. *J Am Vet Med Assoc, 242,* 826–835.

Constable, P. D., Hiew, M. W., Tinkler, S., et al. (2014). Efficacy of oral potassium chloride administration in treating lactating dairy cows with experimentally induced hypokalemia, hypochloremia, and alkalemia. *J Dairy Sci, 97,* 1413–1426.

Curtis, C. R., Erb, H. N., Sniffen, C. J., et al. (1985). Path analysis of dry period nutrition, postpartum metabolic and reproductive disorders, and mastitis in Holstein cows. *J Dairy Sci, 68,* 2347–2360.

Dann, H. M., Morin, D. E., Bollero, G. A., et al. (2005). Prepartum intake, postpartum induction of ketosis, and periparturient disorders affect the metabolic status of dairy cows. *J Dairy Sci, 88,* 3249–3264.

Donovan, G. A., Steenholdt, C., McGehee, K., et al. (2004). Hypomagnesemia among cows in a confinement-housed dairy herd. *J Am Vet Med Assoc, 224,* 96–99.

Drackley, J. K., Veenhuizen, J. J., Richard, M. J., et al. (1991). Metabolic changes in blood and liver of dairy cows during either feed restriction or administration of 1,3-butanediol. *J Dairy Sci, 74,* 4254–4264.

Duffield, T. F. (2004). *Monitoring strategies for metabolic disease in transition dairy cows.* Quebec, Canada: Proc World Buiatrics Cong, 34–35.

Duffield, T. F., LeBlanc, S., Bagg, R., et al. (2003). Effect of a monensin controlled release capsule on metabolic parameters in transition dairy cows. *J Dairy Sci, 86,* 1171–1176.

Dufva, G. S., Bartley, E. E., Dayton, A. D., et al. (1983). Effect of niacin supplementation on milk production and ketosis of dairy cattle. *J Dairy Sci, 66,* 2329–2336.

Elcher, R. (2004). *Evaluation of the metabolic and nutritional situation in dairy herds: Diagnostic use of milk components.* Quebec, Canada: Proc World Buiatrics Cong, 36–38.

Ender F., Dishington I. W., Helgebostad A. (1971). Calcium balance studies in dairy cows under experimental induction and prevention of hypocalcemic paresis puerperalis. *Z Tierphysiol Tierernahr Futtermittelkd, 28;*233–256.

Esposito, G., Irons, P. C., Webb, E. C., et al. (2014). Interactions between negative energy balance, metabolic diseases, uterine health and immune response in transition dairy cows. *Anim Reprod Sci, 144,* 60–71.

Geishauser, T., Leslie, K., Kelton, D., et al. (2001). Monitoring for subclinical ketosis in dairy herds. *Comp Cont Educ, 23,* S65–S71.

Gerloff, B. J. (1988). Feeding the dry cow to avoid metabolic disease. *Vet Clin North Am Food Anim Pract, 4,* 379–390.

Goff, J. P. (2014). Calcium and magnesium disorders. *Vet Clin North Am Food Anim Pract, 30,* 359–381.

Goff, J. P. (2006). Major advances in our understanding of nutritional influences on bovine health. *J Dairy Sci, 89,* 1292–1301.

Goff, J. P. (2004). Macromineral disorders of the transition cow. *Vet Clin North Am Food Anim Pract, 20,* 471–495.

Goff, J. P. (1999). Treatment of calcium, phosphorus and magnesium balance disorders. *Vet Clin North Am Food Anim Pract, 15,* 619–640.

Goff, J. P., Horst, R. L., Jardon, P. W., et al. (1996). Field trials of an oral calcium propionate paste as an aid to prevent milk fever in periparturient dairy cows. *J Dairy Sci, 79*, 378–383.

Goff, J. P., Liesegang, A., & Horst, R. L. (2014). Diet-induced pseudohypoparathyroidism: a hypocalcemia and milk fever risk factor. *J Dairy Sci, 97*, 1510–1528.

Gordon, J. L., LeBlanc, S. J., & Duffield, T. F. (2013). Ketosis treatment in lactating dairy cattle. *Vet Clin North Am Food Anim Pract, 29*, 433–445.

Grünberg, W. (2014). Treatment of phosphorus balance disorders. *Vet Clin North Am Food Anim Pract, 30*, 383–408.

Grünberg, W., Donkin, S. S., & Constable, P. D. (2011). Periparturient effects of feeding a low dietary cation-anion difference diet on acid-base, calcium, and phosphorus homeostasis and on intravenous glucose tolerance test in high-producing dairy cows. *J Dairy Sci, 94*, 727–745.

Grünberg, W., Mol, J. A., & Teske, E. (2015). Red blood cell phosphate concentration and osmotic resistance during dietary phosphate depletion in dairy cows. *J Vet Intern Med, 29*, 395–399.

Grünberg, W., Scherpenisse, P., Dobbelaar, P., et al. (2015). The effect of transient, moderate dietary phosphorus deprivation on phosphorus metabolism, muscle content of different phosphorus-containing compounds, and muscle function in dairy cows. *J Dairy Sci, 98*, 5385–5400.

Hayirli, A. (2006). The role of exogenous insulin in the complex of hepatic lipidosis and ketosis associated with resistance phenomenon in postpartum dairy cattle. *Vet Res Commun, 30*, 479–774.

Head, M. J., & Rook, J. A. F. (1957). Some effects of spring grass on rumen digestion and metabolism of the dairy cow. *Proc Nutr Soc (London), 16*, 25–34.

Holtenius, P., & Hjort, P. (1990). Studies on the pathogenesis of fatty liver in cows. *Bovine Pract, 25*, 91–94.

Horst, R. L., Goff, J. P., & Reinhardt, T. A. (1990). Advancing age results in reduction of intestinal and bone 1,25-dihydroxyvitamin D receptors. *Endocrinology, 126*, 1053–1057.

Idink, M. J., & Grünberg, W. (2015). Enteral administration of monosodium phosphate, monopotassium phosphate and monocalcium phosphate for the treatment of hypophosphataemia in lactating dairy cattle. *Vet Rec, 176*, 494–501.

Iwersen, M., Klein-Jobstl, D., Pichler, M., et al. (2013). Comparison of 2 electronic cowside tests to detect subclinical ketosis in dairy cows and the influence of the temperature and type of blood sample on the test results. *J Dairy Sci, 96*, 7719–7730.

Jenkins, T. C., & Palmquist, D. L. (1984). Effects of fatty acids or calcium soaps on rumen and total nutrient digestibility of dairy rations (Holstein cows). *J Dairy Sci, 67*, 978–986.

Kim, I. H., & Suh, G. H. (2003). Effect of the amount of body condition loss from the dry to near calving periods on the subsequent body condition change, occurrence of postpartum diseases, metabolic parameters and reproductive performance in Holstein dairy cows. *Theriogenol, 60*, 1445–1446.

LeBlanc, S. J., Lissemore, K. D., Kelton, D. F., et al. (2006). Major advances in disease prevention in dairy cattle. *J Dairy Sci, 89*, 1267–1279.

Mahrt, A., Burfeind, O., & Heuwieser, W. (2015). Evaluation of hyperketonemia risk period and screening protocols for early lactation dairy cows. *J Dairy Sci, 98*, 3110–3119.

Mann, S., Leal Yepes, F. A., Overton, T. R., et al. (2016). Dry period plane of energy - effects on feed intake, energy balance, milk production, and composition in transition dairy cows. *J Dairy Sci, 98*, 3366–3382.

Mann, S., Yepes, F. A. L., Behling-Kelly, E., & McArt, J. A. A. (2017). The effect of different treatments for early-lactation

hyperketonemia on blood β-hydroxybutyrate, plasma nonesterified fatty acids, glucose, insulin, and glucagon in dairy cattle. *J Dairy Sci, 100*, ahead of print.

Martens, H., & Blume, I. (1986). Effect of intraruminal sodium and potassium concentrations and of the transmural potential difference on magnesium absorption from the temporarily isolated rumen of sheep. *Quart J Exp Physiol, 71*, 409–415.

Martin-Tereso, J., & Martens, H. (2014). Calcium and magnesium physiology and nutrition in relation to the prevention of milk fever and tetany (dietary management of macrominerals in preventing disease). *Vet Clin North Am Food Anim Pract, 30*, 643–670.

Martinez, N., Risco, C. A., Lima, F. A., et al. (2012). Evaluation of peripartal calcium status, energetic profile, and neutrophil function in dairy cows at low or high risk of developing uterine disease. *J Dairy Sci, 95*, 7158–7172.

Martinez, N., Sinedino, L. D., Bisinotto, R. S., et al. (2014). Effect of induced subclinical hypocalcemia on physiological responses and neutrophil function in dairy cows. *J Dairy Sci, 97*, 874–887.

McArt, J. A. A., Nydam, D. V., & Oetzel, G. R. (2012). Epidemiology of subclinical ketosis in early lactation dairy cattle. *J Dairy Sci, 95*, 5056–5066.

McArt, J. A. A., Nydam, D. V., Oetzel, G. R., et al. (2013). Elevated nonesterified fatty acids and beta-hydroxybutyrate and their association with transition dairy cow performance. *Vet J, 198*, 560–570.

McArt, J. A. A., Nydam, D. V., & Oetzel, G. R. (2012). Dry period and parturient predictors of early lactation ketosis in dairy cattle. *J Dairy Sci, 96*, 198–209.

McArt, J. A., & Oetzel, G. R. (2015). A stochastic estimate of the economic impact of oral calcium supplementation in postparturient dairy cows. *J Dairy Sci, 98*, 7408–7418.

McCarthy, M. M., Yasui, T., Ryan, C. M., et al. (2015). Metabolism of early-lactation dairy cows as affected by dietary starch and monensin supplementation. *J Dairy Sci, 98*, 3351–3365.

Melendez, P., Goff, J. P., Risco, C. A., et al. (2006). Incidence of subclinical ketosis in cows supplemented with a monensin controlled-release capsule in Holstein cattle, Florida, USA. *Prev Vet Med, 73*, 33–43.

Moore, S. J., VandeHaar, M. J., Sharma, B. K., et al. (2000). Effects of altering dietary cation-anion difference on calcium and energy metabolism in peripartum cows. *J Dairy Sci, 83*, 2095–2104.

Morrow, D. A., Hillman, D., Dade, A. W., et al. (1979). Clinical investigation of a dairy herd with the fat cow syndrome. *J Am Vet Med Assoc, 174*, 161–167.

Neves, R. C., Leno, B. M., Stokol, T., Overton, T. R., & McArt, J. A. A. (2017). Risk factors associated with postpartum subclinical hypocalcemia in dairy cows. *J Dairy Sci, 100*, 3796–3804.

Oetzel, G. R. (1991). Meta-analysis of nutritional risk factors for milk fever in dairy cattle. *J Dairy Sci, 74*, 3900–3912.

Oetzel, G. R. (2004). Monitoring and testing dairy herds for metabolic disease. *Vet Clin North Am Food Anim Pract, 20*, 651–674.

Oetzel, G. R., Fetmian, M. J., Hamar, D. W., et al. (1991). Screening of anionic salts for palatability, effects on acid-base status, and urinary calcium excretion in dairy cows. *J Dairy Sci, 74*, 965–971.

Ospina, P. A., Nydam, D. V., Stokol, T., et al. (2010). Association between the proportion of sampled transition cows with increased nonesterified fatty acids and beta-hydroxybutyrate and disease incidence, pregnancy rate, and milk production at the herd level. *J Dairy Sci, 93*, 3595–3601.

Peek, S. F., Divers, T. J., Guard, C., et al. (2000). Hypokalemia, muscle weakness and recumbency in dairy cattle. *Vet Ther Res Appl Vet Med, 1*, 235–244.

Pinotti, L., Baldi, A., Politis, I., et al. (2003). Rumen-protected choline administration to transition cows: effects on milk production and vitamin E status. *J Vet Med A Physiol Pathol Clin Med, 50*, 18–21.

Pravettoni, D., Doll, K., Hummel, M., et al. (2004). Insulin resistance and abomasal motility disorders in cows detected by use of abomasoduodenal electromyography after surgical correction of left displaced abomasum. *Am J Vet Res, 65*, 1319–1324.

Reinhardt, T. A., Lippolis, J. D., McCluskey, B. J., et al. (2011). Prevalence of subclinical hypocalcemia in dairy herds. *Vet J, 188*, 122–124.

Rukkwamsuk, T., Kruip, T. A., & Wensing, T. (1999). Relationship between overfeeding and overconditioning in the dry period and the problems of high producing dairy cows during the postparturient period. *Vet Quart, 21*, 71–77.

Sattler, N., & Fecteau, G. (2014). Hypokalemia syndrome in cattle. *Vet Clin North Am Food Anim Pract, 30*, 351–357.

Seifi, H. A., LeBlanc, S. J., Vernooy, E., et al. (2007). Effect of isoflupredone acetate with or without insulin on energy metabolism, reproduction, milk production, and health in dairy cows in early lactation. *J Dairy Sci, 90*, 4181–4191.

Smith, R. H. (1959). Calcium and magnesium metabolism in calves. 3. Endogenous faecal excretion and absorption of magnesium. *Biochem J, 71*, 306–311.

Sutherland, R. J., Bell, K. C., McSporran, K. D., et al. (1986). A comparative study of diagnostic tests for the assessment of herd magnesium status in cattle. *N Z Vet J, 34*, 133–135.

Teramura, M., Wynn, S., Reshalaitihan, M., et al. (2015). Supplementation with difructose anhydride III promotes passive calcium absorption in the small intestine immediately after calving in dairy cows. *J Dairy Sci, 98*, 8688–8697.

Van der Drift, S. G. A., Houweiling, M., Bocemon, M., et al. (2015). Effects of a single glucocorticoid injection on propylene glycol treated cows with clinical ketosis. *Vet J, 204*, 144–145.

Vernon, R. G. (2005). Lipid metabolism during lactation: a review of adipose tissue-liver interactions and the development of fatty liver. *J Dairy Res, 72*, 460–469.

Wagner, S. A., & Schimek, D. E. (2010). Evaluation of the effect of bolus administration of 50% dextrose solution on measures of electrolyte and energy balance of postpartum dairy cows. *Am J Vet Res, 71*, 1074–1080.

Weich, W., Block, E., & Litherland, N. B. (2013). Extended negative dietary cation-anion difference feeding does not negatively affect postpartum performance of multiparous dairy cows. *J Dairy Sci, 96*, 5780–5792.

West, H. J. (1989). Liver function of dairy cows in late pregnancy and early lactation. *Res Vet Sci, 46*, 231–237.

Body Condition Scoring

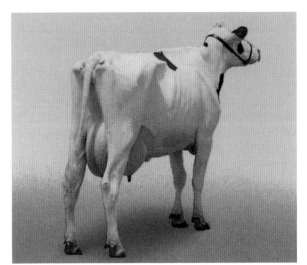

BCS = 1

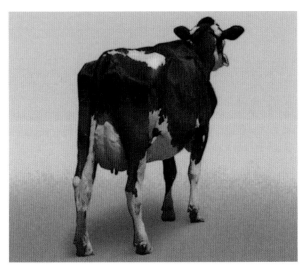

BCS = 2

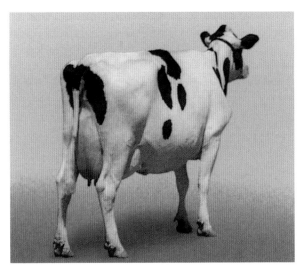

BCS = 3

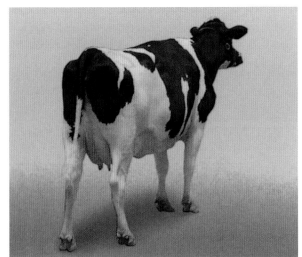

BCS = 4

Appendix images appear courtesy of Elanco Products Company, A Division of Eli Lilly and Company, Lilly Corporate Center, Indianapolis, IN 46285.

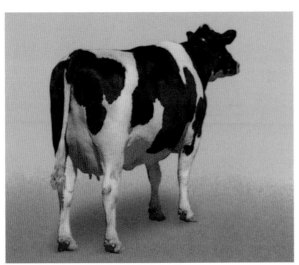

BCS = 5

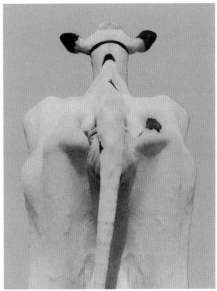

BCS = 1
Deep cavity around the tailhead. Bones of the pelvis and short ribs are sharp and easily felt. No fatty tissue is present in the pelvic or loin area. There is a deep depression in the loin.

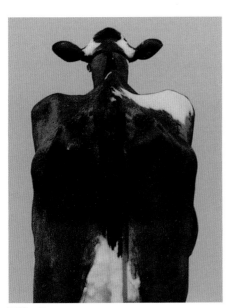

BCS = 2
Shallow cavity around the tailhead with some fatty tissue lining it and covering the pin bones. The pelvis is easily felt. The ends of the short ribs feel rounded, and the upper surfaces can be felt with slight pressure. A depression is visible in the loin area.

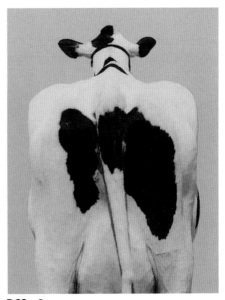

BCS = 3
No cavity around the tailhead and fatty tissue easily felt over whole area. The pelvis can be felt with slight pressure. A thick layer of tissue covers the top of the short ribs, which can still be felt with pressure. There is a slight depression in the loin area.

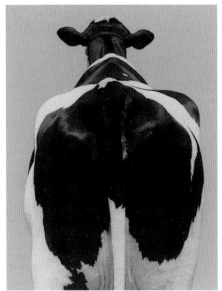

BCS = 4

Folds of fatty tissue are seen around the tailhead with patches of fat covering the pin bones. The pelvis can be felt with firm pressure. The short ribs can no longer be felt. There is no depression in the loin area.

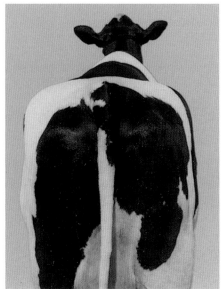

BCS = 5

The tailhead is buried in a thick layer of fatty tissue. The pelvic bones cannot be felt even with firm pressure. The short ribs are covered with a thick layer of fatty tissue.

16

Miscellaneous Infectious Diseases

BELINDA S. THOMPSON AND ERIN L. GOODRICH

Clostridial Myositis

Etiology

Clostridial myositis is a highly fatal disease of cattle caused by the anaerobic spore-forming bacteria *Clostridium septicum, Clostridium chauvoei, Clostridium novyi, Clostridium sordelli, Clostridium perfringens,* and occasionally other opportunistic *Clostridium* spp. For clostridial myositis to develop, both the organism and a suitable anaerobic environment for its vegetative growth must be present. Therefore muscle that has been damaged by trauma, penetrating or puncture wounds, lacerations, surgical incisions, or intramuscular (IM) injections of irritating drugs or chemicals is susceptible.

C. septicum and *C. perfringens* are normal inhabitants of the gastrointestinal (GI) tracts of most warm-blooded animals. The majority of cases of clostridial myositis caused by these two species are associated with injections of the hind limb, the presumption being that the infection has been introduced exogenously (Fig. 16.1). However, the authors have seen occasional cases associated with *C. perfringens* that arose in areas of soft tissue trauma without any detectable break in skin integrity or history of injection suggesting activation of *Clostridium perfringens* type A spores that may normally reside in the muscle. Soil and feces may contain *C. septicum* or *C. perfringens*. Whereas *C. septicum* has been identified specifically as the cause of malignant edema, *C. chauvoei* infections are referred to as "blackleg." It probably is easier to refer to all myopathic clostridial infections as clostridial myositis because clinical differentiation of the species involved is sometimes difficult, and laboratory assistance is usually required. Rather misleadingly, *malignant edema*—implying any clostridial myositis rather than specific *C. septicum* infections—also has been used as a general term for clostridial myositis.

C. chauvoei perhaps has the most confusing pathogenesis. The organism survives in soil, but it is not known whether it survives in both the vegetative and spore forms or only the spore form. Ingestion of *C. chauvoei* by cattle apparently allows the vegetative form to proliferate in the gut and then gain entrance to the lymphatics, bloodstream, and finally seed the muscle and liver. Having reached the muscle and liver, the organism remains innocuously in the spore form unless the surrounding

tissue is injured in some way that creates an anaerobic environment suitable for vegetative growth of *C. chauvoei*. Exogenous infections of muscle also are possible with *C. chauvoei* if soil contamination or inoculation of damaged tissue occurs. Injury may include necrosis associated with selenium deficiency. The authors have investigated one herd with four cases of clostridial myositis caused by *C. chauvoei* primarily affecting the myocardium. Selenium levels were undetectable in the liver of the only animal tested. Farms and soils that harbor *C. chauvoei* create endemic risk of clostridial myositis for cattle grazing this ground or ingesting crops harvested from such soil. Young cattle appear to be at greatest risk for *C. chauvoei* muscular infections, and most cases occur in well-cared-for animals 6 to 24 months of age. However, the authors investigated a herd epidemic of *C. chauvoei* myositis that involved several first-lactation cows that ranged between 2 and 3 years of age. The cows in this outbreak had grazed pastures the previous summer, but the epidemic occurred during the winter months and was triggered by muscle bruising and trauma as a result of crowding through a narrow passage created by a frozen doorway (Fig. 16.2). *C. sordelli* may have a similar pathogenesis because it has been associated with muscle bruising in rapidly growing beef cattle.

Regardless of the species of *Clostridium* causing infection, toxemia, and severe myositis ensue. Clostridial exotoxins promote spread of the infection, are detrimental to host defense mechanisms, and propagate the anaerobic environment essential for vegetative growth. *C. chauvoei, C. septicum,* and *C. perfringens* produce alpha-toxin, which is a hemolytic and necrotizing lecithinase that is also leukocidal and increases capillary permeability. In addition, *C. chauvoei* produces other toxins such as hyaluronidase; *C. septicum* produces beta-toxin (deoxyribonuclease and also leukocidal), gamma-toxin (hyaluronidase), and delta-toxin (hemolysin). *Clostridium perfringens* also may produce toxins other than the alpha-toxin, depending on the serotype involved. Recently, cytotoxin A (CctA) has been identified by genomic sequence analysis as a major toxin of *C. chauvoei*. It is a unique hemolytic and cytotoxic protein found in all isolates of *C. chauvoei* but not in other pathogenic clostridia. As a general statement, *C. chauvoei* and *C. sordelli* are linked with the highest mortality rates, *C. perfringens*

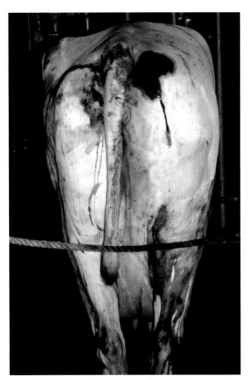

• **Fig. 16.1** *Clostridium perfringens* myositis in the right hind limb of a Holstein cow subsequent to an intramuscular injection of prostaglandin.

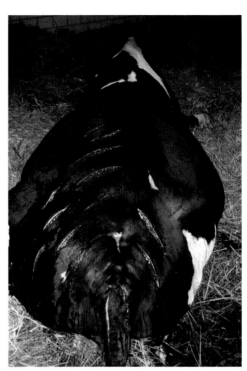

• **Fig. 16.3** Holstein cow with *Clostridium perfringens* infection subsequent to tail docking. Note the extensive surgical fenestrations along the dorsum.

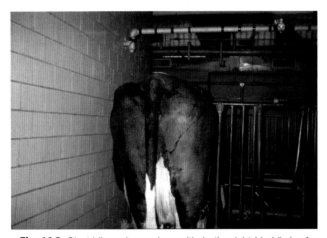

• **Fig. 16.2** *Clostridium chauvoei* myositis in the right hind limb of a 2-year-old Holstein heifer secondary to repeated bruising of the hind limbs by being forced through a narrow passageway.

the lowest, and *C. septicum* in between. Occasional cases or specific geographic areas may encounter clostridial myositis as a result of *C. novyi, C. sordelli, C. fallax,* or other species. *C. novyi* may cause either exogenous or endogenous infections ("black disease") as a result of fluke-induced hepatic activation of spores to vegetative forms.

Regardless of the causative species, most clostridial myositis or cellulitis cases in dairy cattle, other than those associated with *C. chauvoei* (black leg) and some cases of *C. perfringens* type A, occur by exogenous routes. Any procedure that allows feces or dirt to gain entrance to subcutaneous locations constitutes a risk. Minor surgical procedures, tail docking, IM injections, and neglected

wounds predispose to clostridial infections. Clostridial myositis, tetanus, and ascending wound infections caused by other organisms have resulted from dirty tail-docking techniques. An epidemic of *C. perfringens* myositis occurred after tail docking of an entire adult herd (Fig. 16.3). Vaginal tears after calving may lead to severe *C. septicum* cellulitis in the vulva and perineal region.

Another predisposing cause of clostridial myositis in dairy cattle is IM injections. Frequent use of prostaglandin makes this drug the most common offender. However, it may not be so much the drug itself but the fact that some people injecting a drug do not clean, nor discriminate among, injection sites. Nor do some always use sterile needles and syringes. Therefore while injecting a drug, they also inoculate the IM site with clostridial organisms that are present on the hair coat or skin of the cow, present in their multiuse syringe and needle, or present in a contaminated multidose vial. It is also possible that *C. perfringens* type A spores are residing in the muscle, and IM injection of the drug allows the spores to sporulate and release toxins, a pathogenesis similar to that of *C. chauvoei*.

Clinical Signs

The signs of clostridial myositis include fever, depression, inappetence, toxemia, and a progressively enlarging region of swollen muscle. Lameness is severe if the myopathy involves limb musculature. Lameness is not a consistent clinical finding when alternative skeletal muscle groups such as the masseter muscle are the primary disease site. Initially, the skin over the affected muscle is warm and soft and may have pitting edema. However, the primary muscle site eventually becomes firm, and the overlying skin rapidly becomes dark, taut, cool, and necrotic. Crepitus caused by gas formation may be palpable in the infected muscle and overlying subcutaneous tissues. Soft tissue swelling progresses along fascial planes and ascends or descends, depending on anatomic location. Systemic signs are referable to toxemia induced by the potent clostridial exotoxins. Fever usually is present initially, but some patients may become so ill as a result of toxemia that normal or subnormal temperatures are recorded. Heart and respiratory rates are elevated progressively as the pathology worsens. Signs progress rapidly over a 24- to 48-hour course, and few cows survive after 3 days unless therapy is instituted. The clinical course may be so rapid as to be thought a sudden death; "black leg" and other *Clostridium* spp. infections should always be included on the differential diagnosis list for sudden death. Usually, however, progressive swelling, toxemia, and lameness are observed before death with blackleg.

Dehydration, severe lameness or recumbency, apparent neurologic signs, and shock eventually appear in advanced cases. Terminally, some cattle develop disseminated intravascular coagulation (DIC) or multiple organ failure.

Recent tail docking, recent dystocia with vulvar or vaginal lacerations, muscle trauma from herding young stock in a chute, other wounds or evidence of trauma may provide diagnostic clues. Recent injections may be suspected by "needle tracks" or be reported in the history.

Diagnosis

Clostridial myositis must be differentiated from soft tissue cellulitis, phlegmon, abscessation, seroma, or hematoma. In general, the progression of signs is too rapid for consideration of abscessation, and both simple hematoma and seroma can be ruled out by fever and signs of toxemia. In cases of clostridial myositis that result from blunt force trauma (e.g., chute injury or aggressive behavior among young group-housed bulls), there may also be significant hematomas or seromas present concurrently, but the systemic signs and rapidly developing emphysema are distinctive. Clostridial myositis must be considered, as should systemic clostridial diseases in general, in any case of sudden, unexplained death. To ensure that the diagnosis is not overlooked grossly, the entire carcass should be skinned at the time of necropsy to expose any abnormal areas of underlying muscle.

Direct means to ascertain the cause of the infection and differentiate the condition from other causes of cellulitis are indicated immediately. The skin overlying the point of maximal muscular swelling should be clipped and prepared for aseptic aspiration. An aspirate usually reveals serosanguineous or brownish fluid and some gas. Gas may "bubble up" at the needle puncture site following removal of the aspiration needle. Gram staining and culturing the aspirate are indicated. Gram staining can allow a rapid diagnosis because large gram-positive rods are easily found. To perform an anaerobic culture on an aspirate, the fluid must be aspirated aseptically and sampled with a sterile swab. That

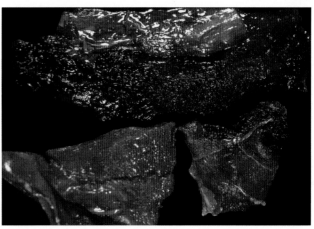

• **Fig. 16.4** Classic blackleg *(Clostridium chauvoei)* lesion in the muscle of a 7-month-old heifer presented for fever and lameness. Two other heifers in this herd had become lame and died the day before.

swab must then be used to inoculate anaerobic transport media. The media must be maintained at room temperature and protected from temperature extremes by enclosing it in insulated packaging material. Alternatively, a portion of the affected muscle (at least 2 cm³) can be surgically obtained, chilled immediately, and submitted within 24 hours or frozen for anaerobic culture. This tissue sample would also be appropriate for fluorescent antibody (FA) identification of clostridial species, Gram stain, or impression smears. Aspirate or biopsy sites do not bleed as healthy tissue would. In fact, incisions into obviously involved muscle ooze serum and serosanguineous fluid, but the blood supply to the most severely affected muscle is greatly reduced or absent. Gram stains and FA preparations provide the most rapid means of definitive diagnosis. Culture or polymerase chain reaction (PCR) are helpful to identify the causative species but usually are completed too late to help an individual patient.

Although generally speaking, *C. chauvoei* produces more gas and *C. septicum* more edema (hence the colloquial name; malignant edema), much overlap exists in the pathology. It is not possible to speciate clostridial organisms accurately based on the clinical signs they produce in affected cattle.

Blood work is not helpful to the diagnosis because neither a complete blood count (CBC) nor serum chemistry panel offer definitive data. The leukogram is extremely variable in patients with clostridial myositis and may be normal despite the patient's overwhelming infection and toxemia. Perhaps even more surprising is the fact that serum creatine kinase and aspartate aminotransferase values are sometimes only mildly elevated. In fact, muscle enzymes released from the region of profound myositis cannot gain access to the peripheral blood because of the self-serving vascular thrombosis and destruction created by clostridial exotoxins. Therefore absorption of enzymes and potassium from affected muscle may be prevented by diminished blood supply to the lesion. Necropsy confirms the presence of black, deep red, or greenish-red necrotic muscle with gas and fluid in *C. chauvoei* infections (Fig. 16.4). Gas also may be present in other types of clostridial myositis, but edema and discolored muscles are the major lesions in *C. septicum* and *C. perfringens.* Serosal hemorrhages also can be observed in many tissues. Dr. John King, veterinary pathologist at Cornell University, likened the odor of affected tissue to the sickeningly sweet odor of rancid butter.

Treatment

Treatment seldom is successful unless the disease is diagnosed early in its course. Penicillin is the antibiotic of choice to kill vegetative *Clostridium* spp., and the drug should be used at very high levels (44,000 U/kg IM or subcutaneously [SC], twice daily). Intravenous (IV) sodium or potassium penicillin given four to six times daily at the same dose is an excellent choice but may be too expensive for use in most dairy cattle. Some clinicians believe it is important to inject some of the penicillin into the region of the infection or proximal to the lesion in an affected limb. Tetracyclines also have been used successfully against clostridial myositis infections and were responsible for some of the earliest successful treatments of grade cattle. Systemic antibiotic therapy kills only those organisms that can be reached by viable circulation. Therefore it tends to counteract spread into new tissue but may not be able to attain inhibitory concentrations in the most severely affected muscle because of loss of blood supply in this tissue.

Fenestration of affected muscle with skin and fascial incisions allows direct oxygenation of the tissue and subsequent interference with the anaerobic environment required for continued replication of the organism. Acute cases should be fenestrated surgically and the wounds lavaged with saline or hydrogen peroxide. Extensive debridement is not necessary or indicated in acute cases but may become necessary if the patient survives the acute infection and the affected area progresses to a sloughing wound.

Analgesics such as nonsteroidal antiinflammatory drugs (NSAIDs) may be used to aid patient comfort, but judicious dosages are necessary if such drugs are used as maintenance therapy, lest toxic GI or renal side effects occur.

Patients that are extremely toxemic or in shock may benefit from IV fluids and a one-time dose of soluble corticosteroids; corticosteroids should not be used repeatedly.

Improvement is signaled by stabilization of the progressive swelling, resolution of fever, reduced depression, and increased appetite. Antibiotic therapy is required for 1 to 4 weeks and can be reduced according to clinical response. Infected muscle frequently sloughs and may necessitate long-term wound care, which can be particularly problematic in the summer months during "fly" season. Lameness may persist in animals that have prolonged wound healing or that suffer fibrosis and contraction of major muscle groups.

Prevention and Control

Client education may help prevent the disease when faulty injection techniques, multiple-dose vials, or dirty syringes and needles are suspected as causes. Similarly, instruction in tail docking may be helpful.

When *C. chauvoei* is identified as the cause, all young animals should be vaccinated against this organism. Although evidence-based medicine surrounding the effectiveness of vaccines against *C. chauvoei* is lacking, at least from an anecdotal perspective, vaccination is highly effective against blackleg and the other causes of clostridial myositis when *C. chauvoei* has been identified or whenever ongoing management conditions may predispose to clostridial myositis caused by any species. Many effective bacterin-toxoids incorporating new adjuvants are available commercially for several clostridial species and should be used according to the manufacturer's recommendations because some vaccines now claim effective immunization with just one dose. In the past, with the exception of *C. chauvoei,* most bacterin-toxoids required two initial doses at a 2- to 4-week interval to protect against most species of *Clostridium* capable of causing myositis. Bacterin-toxoids are best administered after passive maternal antibodies have dwindled. If administered at less than 4 months of age, these vaccines should be repeated at 4 months or older. Herd vaccination programs should include an initial primary course and boosters such that animals have adequate protection before tail docking, if performed. The preventive value of annual boosters in protecting adult dairy cattle against clostridial myositis is uncertain but makes empiric sense for both endemic farms and those with no recent history of the disease.

Bacillary Hemoglobinuria (Redwater)

Etiology

Clostridium novyi type D, an anaerobic organism previously known as *Clostridium haemolyticum,* is the cause of bacillary hemoglobinuria in cattle. This fulminant disease results from peracute proliferation of *C. novyi* in the liver, resulting in a large necrotic infarct. The infarct and systemic signs of hemolysis and toxemia are caused by a potent beta-toxin, phospholipase C, produced by this organism.

C. novyi is endemic in some geographic areas, especially moist or swampy areas that maintain a high soil pH (≈8.0). The spores of *C. novyi* are extremely hardy and remain in contaminated soil for long periods. Ingested spores apparently are transported to liver and other tissue by lymphatics and blood, as happens with *C. chauvoei.* Cattle harboring the organism can shed it in feces and urine but may remain healthy because *C. novyi* is a normal part of the GI flora and can be found in the livers of healthy cattle.

However, livers harboring *C. novyi* are at risk for spores converting to vegetative organisms if hepatocellular damage occurs. Unvaccinated cattle harboring *C. novyi* can have the organism activated to the virulent form by liver lesions associated with flukes, liver abscesses secondary to rumenitis, septicemia, metabolic anoxia of the liver, hepatotoxins, and biopsy. Similar to other clostridia, the organism simply seeks a damaged area of liver with reduced oxygen tension such that anaerobic vegetative growth can occur. Vegetative growth is associated with production of potent exotoxins, including phospholipase C, which then induce hepatic necrosis, hemolysis, and profound toxemia. Liver flukes are the major biologic contributor to disease; therefore bacillary hemoglobinuria is more common in some geographic areas than others and is more common during pasturing of cattle.

Clinical Signs

The disease usually occurs in young mature to adult cattle. Peracute illness with high fever (104.0° to 106.0°F [40.0° to 41.11°C]), elevated heart rate, GI stasis, cessation of milk production, loss of appetite, an arched stance, and evidence of abdominal pain ensue. Intravascular hemolysis causes progressive anemia, eventual dyspnea, and hemoglobinuria that appears after significant lysis of red blood cells (RBCs) has already occurred. Icterus also may be apparent. The course of the disease is rapid, with most patients dying in 12 to 48 hours and some found dead without premonitory signs! It is therefore a differential to be remembered in cases of acute death at pasture.

Diagnosis

The disease must be differentiated from acute leptospirosis (which is seen more commonly in calves), postparturient hemoglobinuria (fresh cows in phosphorus-deficient areas), acute pyelonephritis (hematuria, pyuria), hemorrhagic cystitis associated with malignant catarrhal fever (MCF), and bracken fern toxicity (enzootic hematuria). In certain geographic areas, hemoglobinuria or anemia associated with parasitemic diseases such as babesiosis and anaplasmosis should be considered, but these diseases do not tend to be so peracutely fatal and anaplasmosis does not cause hemoglobinuria. In certain regions, sudden death at pasture without premonitory signs might also obligate the veterinarian to consider anthrax as a differential.

Gross necropsy findings are somewhat pathognomonic in that a large anemic liver infarct and "blackened" kidney are present (Fig. 16.5), and *C. novyi* can be cultured from the lesion with appropriate sample collection and handling. For anaerobic cultures of tissue, a minimum size of about 2 cm^3 is necessary. Identification of clostridial isolates from anaerobic culture has improved with the incorporation of advanced technologies such as 16 S rDNA gene sequencing. Even though *C. novyi* can be cultured from normal livers, the presence of the characteristic infarct associated with the organism usually suffices for diagnosis. Clostridial FA tests also can be helpful but may cross-react with *C. novyi* types B and C. Toxin identification is conclusive but may not be available.

Treatment

Treatment is seldom successful but should include high levels of IV sodium or potassium penicillin (44,000 U/kg four times daily), administration of whole blood, and IV fluids.

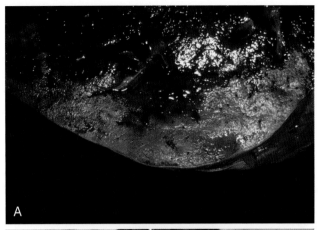

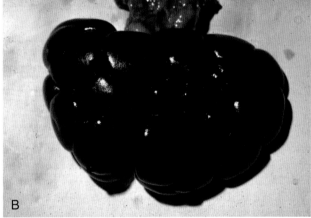

• **Fig. 16.5 A,** Liver infarct caused by *Clostridium novyi* from an adult cow found dead at pasture. **B,** Discolored kidney from the same cow with *C. novyi* infection; the discoloration is caused by hemoglobinemia and hemoglobinuria.

Prevention and Control

When flukes are involved in the pathogenesis of bacillary hemoglobinuria, infected pastures should be kept off limits to cattle, and the animals should be treated with appropriate and approved drugs to kill flukes. Feeding practices that predispose to rumenitis should be corrected.

Vaccination of calves with commercial bacterin-toxoids including *C. novyi* type D is protective if administered twice 3 to 4 weeks apart after maternal antibodies have worn off. Subsequent boosters should be administered twice yearly to cattle at risk.

Leptospirosis

Etiology

The genus *Leptospira* includes at least 21 species that are arranged into three subgroups based on 16 S rRNA phylogeny, DNA–DNA hybridization, pathogenicity, virulence, and in vitro growth characteristics. Two of these subgroups (previously referred to as group I [pathogens] and group II [intermediate pathogens]) contain the 14 species of infectious *Leptospira*; the third group contains the nonpathogenic, saprophytic *Leptospira*. Further division of each species is made into serogroups, serovars (of which there are >250 within the pathogenic *Leptospira*), and types. *Leptospira interrogans* is the most common pathogenic species encountered in cattle, although the host-adapted serovar in the United States actually belongs to a different species, *Leptospira borgpetersenii*. Proper taxonomic nomenclature for these serogroups, serovars, and types is very confusing! Leptospirosis in U.S. cattle is commonly associated with the non–host-adapted serovars of *L. interrogans*, namely *Leptospira interrogans* Pomona, *Leptospira interrogans* Canicola, *Leptospira interrogans* Icterohaemorrhagiae, *Leptospira interrogans* Grippotyphosa, and *Leptospira interrogans* Swajizak. The host-adapted serovar in cattle in North America is referred to as *Leptospira borgpetersenii* Hardjo-bovis. At least two other serovars of *L. interrogans*, Australis and Hebdomadis, have been isolated from dairy cattle in Australia and Japan. A different serovar/type of *L. interrogans* is more common in Europe, specifically referred to *Leptospira interrogans* serovar Hardjo type Hardjoprajitno; it is actually this organism that can be found in several of the multivalent leptospiral vaccines (usually pentavalent products) used commercially in the United States.

The pathogenic leptospires are widely distributed in nature, reflecting maintenance in many wild and domestic hosts. Their natural biology involves shedding in urine, persistence in an ambiently suitable environment, and acquisition by new hosts. Infection occurs by penetration of the organism through the mucous membranes of the conjunctiva, digestive tract, reproductive tract, skin wounds, or moisture-damaged skin. Hematogenous spread of the organism can result in seeding of multiple organs, including the uterus, and establishment of renal infection. Most *Leptospira* spp. colonize the renal tubules and are shed in urine for variable periods of time after infection.

Many natural domestic and wild reservoirs of *L. interrogans* exist that can shed the organism into the environment of cattle. It is difficult to blame any single reservoir species in all instances because most of the serotypes are not host adapted. Dogs, swine, rats, mice, horses, deer, and other wild animals may contaminate the environment of susceptible cattle. Cattle are the maintenance host of *L. borgpetersenii* Hardjo-bovis and appear to be the only reservoir.

After infection and bacteremia, immunoglobulin (Ig) M antibodies that are agglutinins appear within a few days; IgG antibodies with neutralizing activity appear later. Although agglutinating antibodies help clear the bacteremia, they do not result in resolution of residual renal infection. Non–host-adapted *Leptospira* spp. may persist in cattle for 10 days to 4 months.

The clinical consequences of leptospiral infection in cattle include both septicemic and reproductive disorders, but many leptospiral infections are subclinical and are only detected by serologic evidence or by presence of lesions of interstitial nephritis at slaughter. The exact prevalence of leptospirosis is not known, but *L. borgpetersenii* serovar Hardjo-bovis infection seems to be increasing, whereas

L. interrogans serovar Pomona infection rates seem to be decreasing. Some estimates suggest herd infection prevalence in U.S. dairies is between 35% and 50%, mostly attributable to the host-adapted serovar.

Clinical Signs

Both experimental and natural infections with the non–host-adapted serovar *L. interrogans* Pomona have been demonstrated to have an incubation period of 3 to 9 days. Acute, clinical leptospirosis with L. *interrogans* Pomona is most common in calves but can also be seen occasionally in adult dairy cattle. Calves have an acute onset of fever (104.0° to 107.0°F [41.11° to 41.67°C]), septicemia, hemolytic anemia, hemoglobinuria, inappetence, increased heart and respiratory rates, and depression. Petechial hemorrhages and jaundice also are possible. Mortality rates are high in calves less than 2 months of age. Subacute or chronic infections are more common in adult dairy cattle and, unless fever, hemoglobinuria, jaundice, mastitis or epidemic abortions occur, may go undiagnosed. Adult cattle with acute illness will have high fever and a complete cessation of milk flow accompanied by a slack udder with a characteristic thick mastitis secretion that is red, orange, or dark yellow in all quarters. Hemoglobinuria is rare in adults.

Bred heifers or bred cows may abort during the septicemic phase, but it is rather more common for abortion to occur several weeks—on average 3 weeks—after septicemic infection of the placenta and fetus, and a cluster of animals may abort within a few days or few weeks. Aborted fetuses characteristically are in the last trimester of pregnancy but can be anywhere from 4 months' gestation to term. Calves infected in utero during the terminal stages of gestation may be born weak or dead. Because abortion follows infection by such a long time, aborted fetuses are dead and may be somewhat autolyzed. It follows that serum collected from the aborting cow usually will show seroconversion and, in effect, be a convalescent titer because the cow was infected several weeks earlier. A similar pattern of exposure, infection, and abortion can occur with the other non–host-adapted serovars of relevance in the United States.

Certain geographic areas that support *L. interrogans* Pomona or other serovars pathogenic to cattle have a high incidence of leptospiral abortion unless intensive vaccination is practiced. Heifers allowed access to pasture typically abort in late summer or early fall in the northern United States. Failure to establish adequate primary immunity in bred heifers that are pastured is the leading management problem predisposing to leptospiral abortion in this region. A different situation occurs in free stalls, where infection can occur at any time of the year in susceptible cattle exposed to either the host-adapted or non–host-adapted serovars.

Recently, *L. borgpetersenii* Hardjo-bovis has been increasingly associated with epidemic or endemic reproductive problems in cattle in the United States. Definitive proof of a causative relationship between this serovar and abortion in cattle is, however, lacking! This host-associated serovar may have a pathogenesis slightly different from other serovars in cattle in that it primarily infects the uterus and mammary gland after septicemia. Again, it is probably the subacute to chronic form of infection that is most commonly associated with reproductive problems. Studies have demonstrated that cattle naturally infected with *L. borgpetersenii* Hardjo-bovis can shed the organism in their urine for indefinite periods, with the maximal shed occurring early in infection. Acute systemic signs are possible when the disease is introduced into a herd and include fever, depression, inappetence, a sudden drop in milk production, and a flaccid udder that secretes thick yellow to orange milk from all quarters. Most affected cattle will return to normal milk production in 10 to 14 days regardless of whether or not any treatment is administered, with the exception being late gestation cows which may dry off. Abortion is believed to occur most commonly 4 to 12 weeks after initial infection of pregnant cows with the host adapted serovar.

Subclinical disease and possibly abortion are most likely in herds having endemic infection caused by *L. borgpetersenii* Hardjo-bovis. Such endemic herds may have resistant adult cows but persistent reproductive problems in first-calf heifers joining the herd. Infertility and early embryonic death are seen with increased services per conception, prolonged calving intervals, and delayed return to heat. The organism is shed from the reproductive tract for several days after abortion and persists in the oviducts and uterus of infected cows for prolonged periods of weeks to months. In addition, the organism can be cultured from the oviducts up to 3 weeks after abortion or calving. Venereal spread also is possible in bull-bred herds. An association between leptospiral infection and clinically important renal disease has not been documented in cattle.

Diagnosis

For acute infections in young calves showing hemoglobinuria, water intoxication is the major differential, but absence of fever would be expected with the latter. Adult cattle showing acute septicemic disease and hemoglobinuria require differentiation from several diseases, including postparturient hemoglobinuria, bacillary hemoglobinuria, babesiosis, hemorrhagic cystitis associated with MCF, enzootic hematuria, pyelonephritis, and other diseases causing "red urine." However, because hemoglobinuria is rare in adults with acute leptospirosis the differential list is lengthy since it must include a plethora of febrile conditions. Abnormalities in milk secretions as described above may help suggest acute leptospiral septicemia in lactating cattle. In the more common adult scenario of subacute to chronic infection in which abortion is the presenting complaint, the septicemic phase may have passed by the time veterinary attention is sought.

Because many possible cases of leptospirosis are suggested by a history of reproductive failure, sometimes in a group, the differential list must be extended to include the contagious causes of abortion such as neosporosis, salmonellosis, IBR, and bovine viral diarrhea virus (BVDV). Differentiation between these causes relies on diagnostic testing, and confirmation of leptospirosis has been achieved through a variety of techniques

to include serology, PCR assays, and urinary diagnostics. Although antibody tests may be unreliable during the acute phase of the disease, seroconversion as assessed by comparative acute and convalescent titers has been one of the best diagnostic proofs of infection. A fourfold increase in convalescent titer over acute titer is considered significant with most serovars, excluding the host-adapted one. A single high titer after abortion from most serovars would also be strongly supportive of leptospiral disease but should not be expected with *L. borgpetersenii* Hardjo-bovis. Non host-adapted serovars, also called incidental infections, cause abortion several days after initial infection resulting in high titers in the cow at the time of infection and sometimes titers in the aborted fetus.

Vaccination of cattle generally causes a relatively low agglutination titer (1:400 or less), but modern, aggressive vaccination protocols may lead to titers of this magnitude being observed against multiple serovars (Dr. Keith Poulsen, Wisconsin State Diagnostic Laboratory, personal communication). Although several antibody tests are available, the microscopic agglutination test (MAT) and enzyme-linked immunosorbent assay (ELISA) are used most commonly; the ELISA will not provide information on the specific serovar involved. Currently, single time point or paired MAT samples are the most commonly run serodiagnostics, often as a panel of titers against multiple serovars. Cross reaction to multiple serovars may occur with recent infection. Urinary diagnostics have historically been popular using FA techniques or dark-field examination to detect spirochetes in urine during acute leptospiruria. Freshly produced urine from the kidneys is preferred. It is recommended that furosemide be administered per label instructions, then the cow is allowed to urinate twice, and urine is collected from the third urination. However, because of the labile nature of the organism, urine should then be shipped to the diagnostic laboratory to arrive within 24 hours. Ideally, the urine should be submitted in a tube containing commercial urine culture transport media with a preservative to preserve the morphology of the organism and aid in the detection. Increasingly, a PCR assay to detect the DNA of leptospires in the urine is a useful diagnostic tool with superior sensitivity to other urinary diagnostics. However, PCR at this point in time will not identify the offending serovar. Because leptospires need not be viable or intact with this method, the use of the urine culture transport media is less crucial than for other urinary diagnostic testing modalities.

It is worth reiterating that the unique immunologic interaction between the bovine species and the host-adapted serovar *L. borgpetersenii* Hardjo-bovis contrives to produce a greater diagnostic challenge and titers are more difficult to interpret and quite variable. Antibody titers against this serovar, for example, may be low or absent at the time of abortion; similarly, acute to convalescent titers may not be so declarative quantitatively.

Because aborted fetuses are long dead and autolyzed, they generally are not helpful to the diagnosis, although heart blood taken from the aborting fetus should be tested by MAT. Therefore, serology is indicated for abortion epidemics suspected to be caused by *L. interrogans* serovar Pomona or other non–Hardjo-bovis serovars, as would be serology coupled with detection of the organism in placenta, fetal fluids, or urine, in cases of suspected *L. borgpetersenii* Hardjo-bovis abortions. Leptospires or their DNA can also be detected by culture, immunofluorescence or special stains of tissue, and PCR of tissue. Keep in mind that this is a potential zoonotic pathogen and appropriate biosecurity procedures should be used when handling any of these specimens.

Treatment

Acute cases caused by *L. interrogans* Pomona can be treated with tetracycline, beta-lactam antibiotics, or macrolides. Because streptomycin has been withdrawn from the market in the United States and causes prolonged meat residues, this highly successful treatment in cattle no longer can be recommended. Whole blood transfusions and IV fluids may be necessary supportive measures in the treatment of acute septicemic calves or cattle with significant hemolysis.

L. borgpetersenii Hardjo-bovis has been treated successfully with a single dose of long-acting oxytetracycline at 20 mg/kg IM, tilmicosin at 10 mg/kg SC, or multiple injections of ceftiofur sodium (2.2 or 5 mg/kg IM once daily for 5 days or 20 mg/kg IM once daily for 3 days). However, current U.S. Food and Drug Administration regulations regarding cephalosporin use in cattle would strictly limit any ceftiofur administration to approved label dose and duration according to formulation. All of the aforementioned protocols have some efficacy in eliminating urinary shedding of *L. borgpetersenii* Hardjo-bovis. Amoxicillin administered IM at 15 mg/kg, in two doses 48 hours apart, has also been shown to eliminate shedding of *L. borgpetersenii* Hardjo-bovis in urine. After treatment of shedding heifers with a single dose of amoxicillin at 15 mg/kg, no leptospires were isolated from the kidneys at slaughter.

Prevention

Because treatment after illness or abortion does not prevent significant morbidity and economic losses, prevention of infection using vaccination is imperative. Whole-cell bacterins must be serovar specific for protection to occur. Five-way leptospirosis bacterins that are intended to provide protection against five serovars of *L. interrogans* (Pomona, Canicola, Icterohaemorrhagiae, Grippotyphosa, and Hardjo) are most commonly used. Effective prevention against these serovars is possible when primary vaccination of calves is followed by twice-yearly boosters. Calves should be vaccinated after maternal antibodies have diminished at 4 to 6 months of age, and two doses of vaccine are essential to establish primary immunity. Boosters are administered at 4- to 6-month intervals thereafter. The most common mistake that prevents effective vaccination against these serovars of *L. interrogans* is administering a single dose of bacterin to heifers and then not giving them booster shots until 6 to 12 months later, thereby never effecting primary immunization. Effective immunization against *L. borgpetersenii* serovar Hardjo-bovis is more difficult, and only

a few vaccines have demonstrated efficacy against the host-adapted serovar. Monovalent *L. borgpetersenii* Hardjo-bovis vaccines have been shown to protect cattle from infection and urinary shedding, but there is little evidence that currently available pentavalent vaccines do; when *L. interrogans* serovar Hardjo strains are used to prepare these commercial pentavalent products, it appears that the subtle differences between the species and serovar are critical. Currently available monovalent vaccines formulated with *L. borgpetersenii* Hardjo-bovis (Spirovac, Zoetis Animal Health, Kalamazoo, MI, and Leptavoid, Schering Plough, Coopers Animal Health, Wellington, New Zealand) have been demonstrated to induce both humoral IgG responses and cellular immune responses that confer protection against L. *borgpetersenii* Hardjo-bovis infection.

The timing of monovalent vaccine administration for protection against the host-adapted serovar is unusual in that there is increasing concern that modern husbandry is causing heifer calves to be exposed, and potentially become chronic carriers, at a very young age. In an effort to prevent the chronic carrier status, it is now quite commonplace for calves to be vaccinated at or before weaning on many heifer-rearing farms and large dairies. Studies have shown efficacy and safety with these monovalent products as early as 4 weeks of age, even in the face of maternally derived antibody. Although proven disease caused by the host-adapted serovar is controversial, vaccination is recommended because other control measures are not available or at least do not seem to work as well. Isolation of aborting or acutely ill cattle and prompt removal of aborted fetuses may decrease spread of the organism but are seldom a practical means of control. Antibiotic treatment to eliminate the organism in infected cattle should be part of the control strategy because vaccination will not eliminate preexistent or concurrent infection. At the current point in time, vaccine protocols should include use of both the multivalent *L. interrogans* and monovalent *L. borgpetersenii* products.

Tuberculosis

Etiology

Few diseases of cattle (other than perhaps brucellosis) generate the emotional, economic, and public health concerns that tuberculosis (TB) does. The consequences of a positive TB reactor cow or cows may entail depopulation of the herd and economic ruin despite salvage and indemnity or compensation available through regulatory efforts. Few veterinarians in this generation have experience with the disease in dairy cattle and therefore have assumed the disease to be nearly eradicated and of little concern. However, eradication efforts directed toward TB have been hampered by confirmation of the disease in wild and captive Cervidae, exotic imports and zoo animals, and cattle from Mexico. Persistence of TB in wildlife reservoirs is also a challenge to control of the disease throughout the world and in the United States, the principal species of concern are elk, bison, and white-tailed deer. Since 1994, Michigan has recognized bovine TB caused by *Mycobacterium bovis* in wild white-tailed deer, with the re-discovery of TB in cattle populations occurring in 1998. It is highly unusual to have self-sustaining bovine TB in a wild, free-ranging cervid population in North America, and it appears that high deer densities and the focal concentration caused by baiting (the practice of hunting deer over feed) and recreational feeding may have been responsible for this problem. A resurgence in surveillance efforts is currently underway to safeguard dairy cattle in the United States under the cooperative auspices of state and federal regulatory veterinary services. Surveillance programs had been diminished overall in the latter part of the past century because of fiscal cutbacks at both the federal and state levels, but high-risk herds in areas where the disease has been confirmed or where cattle have had contact with infected Cervidae or Mexican cattle are still supported. Research aimed at developing vaccination strategies for wild deer is currently underway as a means of controlling TB in Michigan.

Mycobacterium bovis–infected beef cattle were also detected in northern Minnesota in 2005. A surveillance plan for cattle and deer was initiated in the state, leading to the depopulation of 12 cattle farms. More than 27 positive white-tailed deer were discovered to be infected with *M. bovis* over the course of 3 years. In this instance, baiting of deer was not thought to be associated with the outbreak of TB because it was already outlawed in Minnesota. As a means of control, recreational feeding of deer was also outlawed, and expanded deer hunting programs were initiated. Cattle buyout programs were also initiated to decrease the cattle numbers within the bovine TB management area. Remaining farms instituted increased biosecurity measures such that fencing-in stored feed became a requirement. Minnesota was again classified as TB free as of 2011. Some states and some regions still mandate periodic tuberculin testing of all herds producing or supplying milk to the milkshed. Coupled with the concern for increased risk in certain cattle populations, the resurgence of TB in humans, to include disease associated with multiple drug-resistant strains, has elevated public health awareness of this important zoonosis. At the time of writing (August 2017), Michigan is the only state not characterized as free of bovine TB by the U.S. Department of Agriculture (USDA).

M. bovis is the usual cause of TB in cattle, and the organism is capable of infecting many other species, including humans. *Mycobacterium tuberculosis* is the most common causative species in people and may infect pigs, monkeys, and more rarely cattle, dogs, and parrots. *M. bovis* is very similar to *M. tuberculosis* and can infect cattle, pigs, humans, and rarely cats and sheep. *Mycobacterium avium* is a distinct species that rarely infects cattle, pigs, sheep, or humans. All three organisms are acid-fast, alcohol-fast, gram-positive rods. Growth requirements are stringent, and specific media and laboratory techniques are necessary for culturing. Virulence factors include surface lipids such as 6,6′-dimycolytrehalose or "cord factor" and other factors. The organisms can survive in macrophages as intracellular bacteria, in part as a result of interference with cellular fusion of lysozymes to phagosomes, *M. bovis* also produces proteins (stress or heat-shock proteins) that protect the organism within phagosomes. Metabolic products of *M. bovis* are toxic for neutrophils, and immune responses to the organism eventually recruit cytotoxic T lymphocytes that kill macrophages harboring *M. bovis*.

Infection may occur after inhalation (predominant means) or ingestion by susceptible cattle. Inhalation is thought to be the major route of infection for adult cattle, but younger animals can be infected by ingestion, especially of infected milk. After infection, primary lesions form in the infected organ or lymph nodes draining the area. Therefore inhalation of the organism usually results in small primary lesions in the lung. Because of the small size of early primary lesions, they may be overlooked grossly, but larger lymph node lesions draining the organ typically become more apparent. Lymph nodes may confine or "arrest" the infection for a variable length of time before spread to other lymph nodes and viscera, or generalized spread, which can occur in the most severe cases, immunosuppressed patients, or with extremely virulent strain types. In resistant host species or in highly resistant individuals, the TB organisms may be confined to lymph nodes for extended periods. Genetic resistance, mediated through macrophage killing of intracellular bacteria, may play a role in relative resistance to *M. bovis* in many species. Tubercles are the classic pathologic lesions that evolve in primary lesions and subsequently in lymph nodes that drain the region. Tubercles result from a frustrated, less than fully effective, cellular response by the host and microscopically consist of necrotic centers with a halo of macrophages and other mononuclear cells. Calcification is common, and older lesions are calcareous and caseated. In adult cattle, the lesions are most common in the thorax because inhalation is the major source of infection. Advanced or generalized cases can have diffuse lesions. In calves, for whom ingestion of the organism appears to be a major route of infection, mesenteric and other visceral lymph nodes usually are affected, and the pharyngeal lymph nodes may also develop lesions. However, lesions in the gut itself are uncommon in calves.

Infected cattle shed the organism in sputum, aerosolized tracheal exudates, feces (via ingestion or swallowing of respiratory discharges), and other secretions, depending on the location and extent of their lesions. *M. bovis* may remain infective for weeks in feces and persists for days in moist environments or stagnant water. Reproductive spread, although rare, is possible.

Clinical Signs

Infected individuals that have clinically detectable lesions represent the minority of infected cattle. When present, clinical signs are extremely variable and often nonspecific. Loss of body condition and failure to thrive with progressive emaciation may occur in patients with more advanced disease. Classic respiratory disease with a chronic moist cough and thoracic abnormalities on auscultation may be the most suspicious presentation but this does not occur with great frequency. Lymph node enlargement coupled with chronic respiratory disease may result in a higher index of suspicion. Retropharyngeal lymph node involvement may cause either respiratory signs or difficulty in swallowing or eructation. Apparent forestomach or intestinal obstruction may accompany visceral lymph node enlargement. This is usually painless and may be associated with drainage in advanced cases. Udder infections occur in only a minority of cases but, when present, have drastic public health ramifications if infected unpasteurized milk is consumed by humans or other animals. Fortunately, pasteurization destroys *M. bovis* in milk. Reproductive tract lesions also are rare. Both reproductive and mammary tissue infections usually are accompanied by associated lymph node enlargement.

It is worth remembering that a majority of positive tuberculin reactors have minimal, if any, detectable lung lesions but are more likely to have detectable lymph node lesions. More frustrating is the fact that some severely infected cattle with generalized lesions may occasionally fail to react at all to tuberculin.

Diagnosis

Routine surveillance through intradermal tuberculin tests (antemortem) of herds for milk market regulations and individual cattle for sale (interstate or foreign), and slaughterhouse inspection (postmortem) of carcasses comprise the major means of detection of infected cattle in the United States. Heightened regulatory screening and frequency of tuberculin testing in geographic areas of concern (most recently Michigan, California, and Texas) are also major means of identifying infected but asymptomatic animals. Because *M. bovis* elicits a predominantly cell-mediated immune response during early and intermediate phases of infection, diagnostic techniques have primarily focused on detecting this response. Accredited veterinarians perform intradermal skin testing using 0.1 mL of purified protein derivative (PPD) tuberculin into either of the caudal tail folds. The test is read at 72 hours and interpreted as negative, suspicious, or positive. Any suspicious or positive reactor cattle are retested by regulatory veterinary personnel by means of a comparative (avian and bovine PPD) cervical skin test. Historically, many other tests have been used to include serology and interferon-γ (IFN-γ) release assays, but the intradermal tests are still heavily relied on currently. As the disease progresses, the immune response shifts to the development of a serologically detectable response. This serologic response also increases after an intradermal test has been performed on an animal that has been experimentally infected with *M. bovis,* demonstrating the anamnestic response. In this way, perhaps serologic tests could be used in the future to help detect animals that do not react to the current cell-mediated immunity-based tests. Historically, the sensitivity of serologic assays for detection of *M. bovis* has been very low, but recent approaches have targeted multiple antigens resulting in improved test sensitivity. Slaughterhouse surveillance and subsequent traceback has been the primary large-scale postmortem diagnostic test. Slaughterhouse inspection, however, suffers from a lack of sensitivity because of the small size of lesions in many cattle. Currently, a IFN-γ release assay coupled with tail fold intradermal testing is being used in the El Paso milk-shed area, where endemic TB had existed in several large dairy operations. The IFN-γ assay is an in vitro test that detects specific lymphokines produced by lymphocytes in a whole-blood sample from an infected individual when challenged with PPD. The serologic assays may prove to be useful in combination with intradermal tests in individuals who may not react to the routine skin tests. They are also useful tools in animals with visible lesions. Further studies must be performed to determine the optimal time period after an intradermal test to perform a serologic assay in naturally infected cattle.

Because eradication of TB in cattle remains the goal in the United States, positive tuberculin reactors usually are quarantined, identified, and sent to approved slaughter plants. Owners may collect indemnity and salvage value for these animals. When infection is confirmed in positive reactors, depopulation of the herd is recommended, and traceback measures are instituted to test herds that have sold cows to, or purchased cows from, the infected herd. Large herds, as in the El Paso situation, may undergo a multifaceted quarantine procedure with initial removal of positive reactors followed by at least two negative herd tests at 60-day intervals and finally another test 6 months later. Despite apparent rigor, such quarantine procedures may not always rid the herd of infection. The Veterinary Services arm of the USDA Animal and Plant Health Inspection Service has found that up to 40% of infected large herds remain infected despite testing and quarantine procedures of this type. Unfortunately, this means that depopulation of infected herds is the most helpful procedure when eradication is desired. Inherent errors in the precision and accuracy of skin testing constitute the major reasons for failure of compromise programs. False-positive reaction (no gross lesions) may occur in cattle sensitized to other mycobacteria, including human or avian TB, Johne's disease, and "skin TB." False-negative reactions may occur in advanced cases, recently infected cattle, desensitized cattle, or old cattle. The intradermal tests usually do not result in detectable reactions until 3 to 6 weeks postinfection. The current PPD tuberculin test is considered to have approximately 85% sensitivity and 98% specificity. The IFN-γ test has similar sensitivity and specificity. However, on a herd basis—because of the current low level of TB—skin tests may have a low positive predictive value. In infected herds, however, the positive predictive value increases. In addition, attention to detail and technique by the testing veterinarian also can influence results.

Many states, including New York, no longer support regular tuberculin testing of all cattle but do require testing of cattle in a "high-risk" category. Animals considered at high risk may include herds associated with captive Cervidae or those near exotic animal farms or zoos. High-risk herds obviously also include those found by traceback epidemiology to have a connection with known, infected herds.

Accredited free states have had no known TB herds for 5 years. Such states will have this classification suspended or revoked when one or more cattle or bison herds are identified within a 48-month period. Vaccination using Bacille Calmette Guérin (BCG) as practiced in some areas is not recommended in the United States. Similarly, treatment of infected cattle is not allowed. It is plausible that the increased research effort into safe and effective vaccines for humans may lead to new consideration of animal vaccination as part of a control program, however, this is probably still some way off for now.

Ulcerative Lymphangitis

Etiology

Lymphangitis of the lower limbs occurs sporadically in cattle. The lesion has occasionally been associated with a false-positive tuberculin test result. Although usually present in TB-free cattle, the lesion also has been found in *M. bovis*–infected cattle. The major concern raised by the lesion is the frequency with which affected cattle react as suspicious or positive to tuberculin testing. In the past, such cattle have been labeled as "skin reactors."

Organisms that probably are saprophytic and acid fast have been observed within the lesions, but classification of these organisms and isolation on selected media have not been accomplished. Intradermal transmission of infection through ground tissue samples has been successful in only one report in the literature. The lesions are theorized to develop secondary to front or lower limb injuries that allow seeding of the lymphatics. Affected cattle usually are healthy otherwise.

Similar lesions have been identified in cattle associated with infection by *Corynebacterium pseudotuberculosis*. In these cases, the lesions are restricted to the lower limbs with or without lymph node enlargement. The ulcerative lesions may discharge a clear, gelatinous exudate. Infection of cattle with *C. pseudotuberculosis* can also cause granulomatous cutaneous abscesses, typically located on the exposed lateral face, neck, thorax, and abdomen or less commonly mastitic and visceral infections. Because the clinical signs are

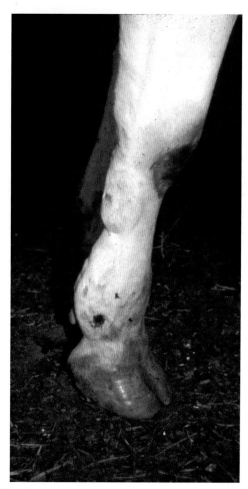

• **Fig. 16.6** Typical lesions of ulcerative lymphangitis involving the right metacarpal area of a Holstein cow.

markedly different to ulcerative lymphangitis, these will be discussed separately later.

Clinical Signs

Multiple subcutaneous nodules in the metacarpal or metatarsal region are the primary lesions. One or more limbs may be affected. The nodules ulcerate periodically and discharge pus that varies from serous to caseous. Mild lameness may be apparent before ulceration and discharge as the nodules swell and become inflamed. Lameness resolves as drainage occurs. Over time, the nodules may coalesce or form knotted cords of tissue that are mainly subcutaneous but may have a dermal component as well (Fig. 16.6). Other than periodic mild lameness and local ulceration, systemic signs are absent.

Diagnosis

Smears of pus or biopsy may allow identification of acid-fast organisms. Culture may be unrewarding, and saprophytic acid-fast bacilli are usually suspected to be the cause, but in some cases, *C. pseudotuberculosis* may be identified. Suspicious tuberculin reactions in such cattle in noninfected herds usually are considered "skin reactors," but a positive reaction may require notification of regulatory veterinarians who may elect a comparative cervical test. Parenteral administration of penicillin or tetracycline, combined with systemic iodides, may be useful in treatment.

Corynebacterium pseudotuberculosis Infection

Etiology

C. pseudotuberculosis is commonly known as the cause of caseous lymphadenitis in sheep and goats and pigeon fever in horses but seldom is mentioned as a cause of disease in cattle. In California and occasionally other areas of the United States, it is sometimes identified as a cause of ulcerative, necrotic skin lesions in cattle. As in small ruminants, the organism tends to become endemic in certain herds, and clinical manifestations occur as sporadic, individual instances. In addition, it is also an occasional, documented cause of mastitis.

The organism survives in soil, the environment, and within infected tissues for long periods. It is generally believed to require an entry site such as a mucosal or skin injury, abrasion, or laceration to infect a host. When it is through the skin or mucosal barrier, the organism travels through lymphatics to lymph nodes or other tissues. In horses, *C. pseudotuberculosis* becomes a facultative intracellular organism that survives in phagocytes and also uses several potential strategies to maintain itself in the host, such as an exotoxin (phospholipase D) that attacks sphingomyelin in erythrocytes and capillary endothelial cells. The organism also possesses a pyogenic factor and surface lipids, which may be toxic to phagocytic cells. All of these factors contribute to chronicity and maintenance of host infection by the organism and are also well recognized in small ruminants.

In cattle, the ulcerative cutaneous lesions exude pus and are typically located on the exposed skin of the lateral face, neck, thorax, and abdomen. Affected cattle do not usually show other signs of disease, and the lesions may heal spontaneously in 2 to 4 weeks, although healing may be enhanced by drainage or surgical debridement. The infection often occurs as a herd problem, and up to 10% of cattle in a herd may be affected. The disease occurs more frequently in adult cattle than primiparous or nulliparous heifers. Spread of infection is apparently enhanced where housing and handling facilities cause abrasions to the lateral body surfaces. It has been assumed that skin trauma and contamination of minor skin abrasions by the organism are causative features of the disease. Affected animals are often culled. The disease has most commonly been seen in dairy cows in the arid western United States and Israel and occurs more frequently in the summer months. It can spread within a herd through movement of cattle from one barn to another or

via mechanical transmission by flies. The incubation period is about 2 months in cattle. The disease can also spread via infected milk, and because of the zoonotic potential, forms a public health concern when raw milk or raw milk products are consumed by humans.

Clinical Signs

In cattle, several forms of the disease exist, including pyogranulomatous reactions, abscesses, ulcerative lymphangitis (see earlier discussion), a mastitic form (less common), a visceral form, an ulcerative dermatitis, and a necrotic lesion of the heel of the foot with swelling and lameness. Signs in cattle most often consist of single or multiple areas of ulcerative lesions on the sides of the face, neck, trunk, tail base, or hip. Necrotic material accumulates in the lesions, and granulation tissue is present deep to the necrotic material. Affected cattle do not otherwise appear ill, although decreased milk production by 4% to 6% may be noted. Sporadic cases may be recognized in endemic herds.

Diagnosis

The lesions must be differentiated from actinobacillosis granulomas, other granulomatous masses, and tumors. Culture confirms the diagnosis, and biopsies differentiate the lesion from tumors and granulomas.

Treatment

Spontaneous cure is common, but some cases benefit from debridement followed by 7 or more days of systemic penicillin or tetracycline therapy.

Babesiosis

Etiology

Babesiosis is a protozoan disease of cattle that has been eradicated from the United States thanks to control of the causative ixodid ticks. The disease is also called Texas fever, redwater, piroplasmosis, or tick fever in cattle. Babesiosis may be caused by seven or more species of *Babesia* that are divided morphologically into large or small types. The major large species is *Babesia bigemina,* and the major small species is *Babesia bovis.* The disease is seen primarily in tropical and subtropical climates around the world and remains a threat to the United States from the Caribbean Islands, Central America and Mexico.

B. bigemina appears as paired, pear-shaped bodies within erythrocytes and is transmitted by *Boophilus* spp., usually *Boophilus annulatus.* Ticks are infected by feeding on infected animals and subsequently infect their larvae through transovarian passage. *B. bigemina* continues to develop in the larvae, nymphs, and eventually adult ticks. Transmission of *B. bigemina* to cattle occurs principally via sporozoites in the saliva of the nymph stage. Other insects and blood-contaminated instruments also may transmit infection, but ticks are the major vector. Infection is most likely to cause clinical disease in cattle older than 6 months of age because calves are thought to have colostral passive protection or unique erythrocyte protective factors (or both) that protect against infection before 6 to 9 months of age. The pathogenesis of *B. bigemina* infection involves direct invasion of host RBCs followed by asexual division via binary fission to produce daughter merozoites that are subsequently released into the circulation following RBC lysis. Intravascular hemolysis, anemia, and hemoglobinuria are therefore hallmarks of the disease.

B. bovis appears as single, multiple, or paired complexes within erythrocytes. Whereas the single and multiple organisms are rounded, pairs may be pear shaped but joined at a more obtuse angle than *B. bigemina*. Erythrocytes infected with *B. bovis* are less numerous and more difficult to identify than in *B. bigemina* infection, and the propensity of *B. bovis* infection to localize in the capillaries of the brain has made microscopic examination of the brain a successful diagnostic test. Multiple *Boophilus* spp., including *B. annulatus* and *Boophilus microplus,* can transmit *B. bovis,* and the larval stage is the major source of infection. Although the pathogenesis and clinical signs caused by infection with *B. bovis* are often highly comparable to those associated with *B. bigemina,* an earlier and more complicated severe reaction associated with cytokine production prior to a hemolytic crisis can sometimes be seen. Furthermore, *B. bovis* has the ability to markedly alter erythrocyte structure and function, causing parasitized RBCs to accumulate in the microvasculature and giving rise to fatal cerebral babesiosis, respiratory distress, and multiorgan failure.

Clinical Signs

Fever, anemia, hemoglobinuria, icterus, weakness, anorexia, depression, and GI stasis are frequent signs of *B. bigemina* infection. Tachycardia, dyspnea, and pallor progress as erythrocyte destruction increases. Abortion sometimes is observed. Intravascular hemolysis occurs as protozoan merozoites emerge from RBCs and rupture cell membranes, with subsequent development of hemoglobinuria and jaundice. The mortality rate may exceed 50%. Examination should include inspection for ticks on affected cattle or herdmates.

B. bovis infections in cattle may be indistinguishable from those caused by *B. bigemina,* but the degree of anemia and hemoglobinuria frequently are less severe with *B. bovis*. Relative host resistance and pathogen differences appear to have an impact on the severity of disease. Neurologic signs, including opisthotonos, seizures, blindness, excitability, aggression, depression, head pressing, or coma, are common in *B. bovis* infections and may explain deaths in cattle that are judged to not have life-threatening anemia. As mentioned earlier, neurologic signs are related to the propensity of infected erythrocytes to accumulate within capillaries in the brain.

Incubation periods of 4 days to 3 weeks (*B. bigemina*) or 10 days to 3 weeks (*B. bovis*) have been reported in experimental and natural disease and appear to depend on the size of the inoculum.

Cattle that survive after the acute signs of babesiosis wane may have chronic disease, remain carriers, have recurrent infections, or die from secondary infections. Recovering cattle experience prolonged production compromise.

Diagnosis

Babesiosis must be differentiated from other causes of hemoglobinuria, hemolysis, fever, and jaundice. Therefore, bacillary hemoglobinuria, theileriosis, leptospirosis, postparturient hemoglobinuria, toxic hepatopathies, plant oxidants, and chronic copper poisoning may be considered in the differential diagnosis. When neurologic signs appear in *B. bovis* infections, differentiation from other diseases of the central nervous system is required. Few other neurologic diseases cause hemolysis and hemoglobinuria, however. Anaplasmosis can lead to similar signs, but hemoglobinuria is absent in anaplasmosis.

Necropsy findings would be expected to include; pale or icteric mucous membranes and tissues; dark urine; watery-appearing blood; a swollen, fleshy spleen; a swollen, orange-red liver; darkened kidneys; and intestinal serosa with a dark pink hue caused by hemoglobin imbibition. For *B. bovis,* there is usually an almost pathognomonic, grossly visible, pink discoloration of the gray matter of the brain. Histologic findings are consistent with severe anemia, intravascular hemolysis, and erythrophagocytosis. Lesions may include widespread extramedullary hematopoiesis, hepatocellular degeneration or necrosis typically associated with hypoxia, and renal tubular changes typical of a hemoglobinuric nephrosis. For *B. bovis* cases, Giemsa staining will often demonstrate parasites within sequestered RBCs in the capillaries of various organs but especially within the cerebral cortex.

Confirmation of babesiosis requires ancillary tests in addition to the suggestive clinical signs. *B. bigemina* is more likely to be observed on Giemsa-stained blood smears than *B. bovis,* and both organisms are more likely to be found in acute infections compared with chronic cases. Antibodies against *Babesia* spp. may appear in the blood of infected cattle within 1 to 3 weeks and are sought by ELISA, complement fixation (CF), or IFA tests. The ELISA test may be more sensitive and can detect antibodies for a longer period after infection than CF, but the CF test result may become positive sooner after infection. PCR tests have proven to be very sensitive for detection of *Babesia* organisms in whole blood samples or blood-rich tissues such as the spleen if the animal has not been treated with imidocarb. Giemsa-stained squash preparations of brain tissue are sometimes used for rapid confirmation of *B bovis* at the time of necropsy.

Treatment and Control

Successful treatment is possible with a number of chemo-therapeutic agents. A dilemma exists in that early effective therapeutic intervention that kills all parasites may deter effective immune responses and leave the patient subject to rapid reinfection.

Trypan blue, an effective treatment for early *B. bigemina* infection, is not effective against *B. bovis* and other small *Babesia* spp. Imidocarb (1–3 mg/kg) successfully treats both infections, as do several other diamidine derivatives such as diminazene diaceturate (3–5 mg/kg) and amicarbalide ise-thionate (5–10 mg/kg). Other successful treatments include quinoline and acridine derivatives.

Tick control is essential and certainly, based on experience in the United States, necessary for eradication of babesiosis. Many effective acaricides currently are available (see Chapter 7). In some countries, tick control rather than complete eradication is practiced in the hopes of maintaining a low level of vectors to effectively immunize cattle but not enough to result in severe or widespread disease.

Vaccines for both *B. bigemina* and *B. bovis* have been used in some areas (e.g., Australia) but are not available commercially in the United States and may require judicious use of chemotherapy when live organisms are used. More effective vaccination strategies combining genomic and proteonomic approaches may be forthcoming.

Tick control and eradication are the ideal control methods when possible.

Anaplasmosis

Etiology

A rickettsial bacterial organism, *Anaplasma marginale,* is the cause of anaplasmosis in cattle; it is considered to be the most prevalent tickborne disease of cattle worldwide and is endemic in North America. The organism parasitizes RBCs after infection of susceptible cattle and is transmitted by ticks and biting insects and introduced mechanically by blood-contaminated instruments that penetrate skin.

Ixodidae ticks, namely *Dermacentor andersoni,* other *Dermacentor* spp., and *Boophilus annulatus,* are the predominant biologic vectors that pass *A. marginale* through their eggs into the next generation of ticks in the United States. Unlike *Babesia* spp., transovarian transmission of *A. marginale* does not occur from one tick generation to another such that establishment of persistent infection within the bovine host is essential for ongoing transmission and survival of the pathogen. Other ticks, tabanids, biting flies, and mosquitoes act as mechanical vectors of the disease as they transfer blood from infected cattle to susceptible cattle while feeding. Needles and veterinary instruments that become contaminated with blood during herd-wide procedures can also transmit the infection. Similarly, blood-contaminated instruments used for reproductive work such as obstetric sleeves, infusion cannulas, embryo transfer instruments, and insemination equipment occasionally can spread the infection.

Cattle younger than 1 year of age tend to show either no clinical signs or have only very mild signs of illness. The opposite is true for adult cattle because susceptible animals more than 2 years of age often have severe acute illness and possible high mortality. The resistance of young animals to infection may be explained partially by passive antibodies obtained from colostrum. However, factors other than maternally derived antibody appear to be important because infection in susceptible cattle between 1 and 2 years of age typically results in mild signs, if any, but infection of susceptible cattle older than 2 years frequently causes acute, severe disease. Fatality is rare in cattle less than 2 years of age but is between 30% and 50% in cattle older than this age. However, sources of stress such as shipment, starvation, weather extremes, and experimental splenectomy apparently can overcome the natural resistance of young cattle to anaplasmosis, thereby resulting in more serious acute disease. Clinical signs of acute illness are an indirect consequence of the presence of the organism, causing potentially massive phagocytosis of erythrocytes by the bovine reticulo-endothelial system and include anemia and icterus *without* hemoglobinuria.

After cattle of any age become infected with *A. marginale,* they remain persistently infected for life regardless of whether clinical disease occurs. After an incubation period of 7 to 60 days, the organism invades erythrocytes and begins cycles of replication, reticuloendothelial system removal, and reinfection of erythrocytes. Depending on strain of the organism and host susceptibility, between 10% and 90% of the entire pool of circulating erythrocytes may be infected acutely; it is estimated that at least 15% of them must be infected for any clinical signs to occur. Throughout the persistently infected animal's life, there are quite consistent cycles over a repeating 10- to 14-day period of increasing, followed by decreasing, numbers of infected circulating erythrocytes. Newly produced erythrocytes are continually reinfected via evasion of the host immune response. In significant part, this is achieved by emergence and replication of antigenic variants of the organism. Each of these cycles represents emergence of one, or multiple *A. marginale* clones expressing a unique hypervariable region encoding two major surface proteins (MSP2 and MSP3). Although the immune response can clear the initial acute parasitemia, it will fail to completely clear the infection because of these antigenic variants. Seroconversion occurs in infected clinical and carrier cattle and may be detected as early as 9 days after infection using a commercially available competitive ELISA (cELISA) assay. Seropositive cattle are assumed to be carriers. Some experimental studies have demonstrated acquired immunity to clinical disease that endures after clearance of infection by chemotherapy regardless of seropositive or seronegative status of the treated cattle. However, in endemic regions harboring anaplasmosis, seronegative cattle within *A. marginale*–infected herds appear susceptible to infection and illness. Therefore, seronegative cows in positive herds have not necessarily developed effective immunity even if they had been seropositive previously and cleared the infection after antibiotic treatment or possible natural clearance. Relative exposure rate, concurrent stresses, vector loads, and length of time between clearance of infection and subsequent reinfection all may influence the susceptibility of seronegative cattle that once had been seropositive.

Chronically infected cattle that are typically asymptomatic act as reservoirs of anaplasmosis, and spread of the disease tends to occur during peak vector seasons or after procedures that result in iatrogenic spread via blood-contaminated instruments.

Transplacental transmission to fetuses in utero, resulting in the birth of carrier calves, has been documented. It is believed to occur infrequently in cattle newly infected during the third trimester of pregnancy. The risk of *A. marginale* transmission in frozen semen is considered negligible.

Clinical Signs

As previously stated, the likelihood of clinical illness associated with *A. marginale* infection is typically proportional to the age of the susceptible animal. Exceptions do occur, especially when extraordinary stress, heavy infective doses, heavy vector parasitism, or concurrent diseases overwhelm the apparent resistance in younger cattle. When present, acute disease is characterized by dramatic signs of fever (104.0° to 107.0°F [40.0° to 41.7°C]), depression, anorexia, GI stasis, anemia, dehydration, and cessation of milk flow. The severity of clinical signs is proportional to the degree of anemia and may include signs of respiratory distress. Icterus is present in many acute cases (Fig. 16.7) but may not appear unless the affected animal survives 2 or more days. Hemoglobinuria *does not* occur. Hemolysis results from erythrocyte

destruction by the reticuloendothelial system and therefore is extravascular. The mortality rate varies but may reach 50% in acute cases in older animals. Infected cattle that survive acute signs may remain weak, anemic, and jaundiced and may lose significant condition. Susceptible adult cattle introduced into endemic herds may have peracute signs and die within 1 to 2 days after onset of signs. Infected animals are assumed to remain carriers of the organism regardless of the extent to which they remain seropositive. Recovery from acute disease may require weeks. Abortion may occur during both the acute and convalescent periods.

Diagnosis

The cELISA and PCR assays have replaced CF and card agglutination assays as the most reliable means of confirmation of infection. These same tests are very useful to detect chronic carrier cattle that may be free of clinical signs. The sensitivity of detection 16 days post-infection in experimental cases was 100% using the cELISA. Because the preclinical period in natural infection is typically longer than 16 days, the use of the serologic assay in acutely ill cattle with clinical signs of anaplasmosis is routinely very useful and can be supplemented with the use of the PCR assay in serologically negative clinical suspects. Diagnosis in acute cases is aided by ancillary tests that verify the severe anemia (low packed cell volume and regenerative) and rule out liver disease as a cause of the jaundice. Microscopic examination of whole blood smears stained by Wright, new methylene blue, or Giemsa stains may allow identification of *A. marginale* in erythrocytes (Fig. 16.8). The organisms appear as one or more spherical bodies in the periphery of erythrocytes and must be differentiated from basophilic stippling and Howell-Jolly bodies.

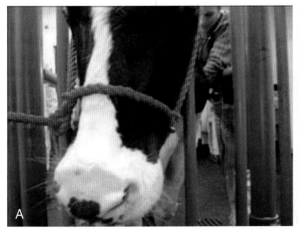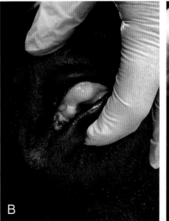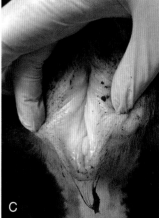

• **Fig. 16.7 A,** A 5-year-old Holstein cow with severe anemia and jaundice caused by *Anaplasma marginale* infection. **B,** Pale and icteric third eyelid and conjunctiva of the cow. **C,** Vulvar membranes of the same cow demonstrating pallor and icterus.

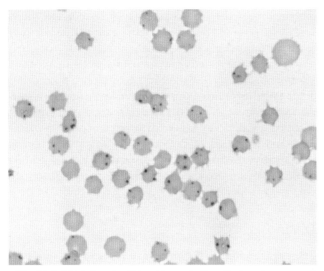

• **Fig. 16.8** Wright's stain of blood from a heifer with *Anaplasma marginale*. The organism can be seen at the margin of several erythrocytes.

Diagnosis in postmortem cases requires confirmation of gross or histologic evidence of clinical anaplasmosis such as pallor and jaundice alongside extravascular hemolysis with hypertrophy and hemosiderin accumulation in lymphoid tissues. Impression smears of blood-rich tissues such as the spleen may allow detection of *A. marginale* in erythrocytes. Although serologic testing of heart blood using the cELISA assay or PCR testing of tissue such as the spleen can confirm infection, chronic carrier animals not currently experiencing clinical anaplasmosis would also be expected to test positive by these assays, so a consistent clinical presentation is important to confirm the interpretation of these tests, especially in endemically infected areas.

Treatment

Treatment with several chemotherapeutic agents is possible but inconsistently effective in clearing the organism. The most current recommendations in North America indicate chlortetracycline or oxytetracycline to be the treatments of choice. In Europe, the fluoroquinolones could be used, but enrofloxacin is not approved for this indication in the United States. Intensity of treatment may dictate whether the organism is eliminated or simply reduced in number within the host. For chemosterilization, oral chlortetracycline at a dosage of 4.4 mg/kg/day for 60 days or injectable oxytetracycline at a dosage of 22 mg/kg at 5-day intervals for five or six injections are the recommended treatments of choice. Imidocarb dipropionate (5.0 mg/kg IM given as two doses at 14-day intervals) will sterilize infected cattle, but this drug is not routinely used in cattle in North America, and no meat- or milk-withholding period has been established. Lesser numbers of injections of long-acting tetracycline may control acute infections but will not eliminate the organism completely. Cattle cleared of infection may eventually be susceptible to infection again. Whole-blood

transfusions also may be necessary when anemia is judged to be life threatening in acutely infected cattle.

Effective clearance of *A. marginale* from either acutely infected or carrier animals should be confirmed with negative PCR assays on ethylenediaminetetraacetic acid (EDTA) anti-coagulated whole blood. Successfully treated cattle should be PCR negative approximately 2 weeks after the end of treatment, but reduction in antibodies to a level below the positive cutoff of the cELISA assay may take an additional 3 months or more. Treatment failures are hypothesized to occur because of failure of the animal's immune system to clear the organisms in the face of bacteriostatic treatments that merely keep the organism from multiplying.

Acaricides and fly control measures always are indicated to reduce the vector population as much as possible, as is the cessation of all husbandry or veterinary practices that could contribute to bloodborne transmission. All treatments and chemical pest control measures must be applied or used in accordance with current regulations related to antibiotic administration and meat and milk withholding.

Prevention

When the incidence of infection is sporadic and low, elimination of infection in acute and asymptomatic carrier cattle (as evidenced by seropositivity) by treatment, coupled with insect control measures, may be sufficient for control. This is the typical scenario in the Northern dairying areas of the United States, where the vast majority of herds are free of any clinical cases, and when it does occur, it is often an individual or a small percentage of the herd that test positive by cELISA or PCR. Chemosterilization followed by confirmation of clearance and careful attention to avoidance of iatrogenic spread are the most relevant parts of prevention in such circumstances. Endemic herds or geographic regions present a more difficult challenge for control measures. In addition to vector control and treatment measures, husbandry practices must be modified. Stress should be minimized, animals from nonendemic areas should not be introduced to the herd, and common use of instruments for veterinary procedures, blood collection, and ear tagging should be avoided unless disinfected between animals.

Vaccinations have been used but require care because no currently available product is completely free of problems. In the United States, a killed product formulated from infected erythrocytes has been used. Therefore, anti–RBC antibodies may develop in vaccinated cattle and predispose to neonatal isoerythrolysis in calves born to vaccinated cows receiving the recommended yearly boosters. Administration of boosters should not be performed during late gestation. Live vaccines are commonly used in many countries, including Australia and countries in Central and South America, but are not licensed in the United States because of concerns regarding pathogen transmission from blood-based vaccines. Currently, no USDA-approved *A. marginale* vaccines are available in the United States. However, autogenous killed products have been variously produced and allowed to be used in multiple states. A product approved in California consists of modified-live irradiated *A. marginale* organisms that is administered to calves younger than 1 year of age to cause immunity associated with persistent infection. This vaccine may cause disease if administered to older animals. The challenges presented by antigenic strain variation and a lack of industry and research support have contributed to the absence of novel anaplasmosis vaccines.

Application of advanced molecular technologies in vaccine development may provide the best hope for future control of anaplasmosis in cattle.

Hemotropic Mycoplasmosis (Eperythrozoonosis)

Etiology

Mycoplasma wenyonii is a gram-negative, eperythrocytic hemotropic *Mycoplasma* that was reclassified from the genus *Eperythrozoon* based on 16 S ribosomal RNA gene sequence analysis, but the former name is also used here for ease of recognition. It appears that infection of cattle with this parasite is common because cattle splenectomized for experimental purposes commonly show parasitemia after splenectomy. However, naturally occurring disease is uncommon, and experimental attempts to reproduce the problem by transfusion of whole blood from infected to apparently uninfected cattle have failed. Clinical disease occurs primarily in dairy heifers in early to midlactation and typically in the summer months, suggesting that there are susceptibility features specific to particular animals, but these have not been identified. The organism can be noted on rare occasions in blood smears of hospitalized nulliparous dairy heifers and young cows that have had blood samples obtained as part of a minimum clinicopathologic database during workup of a condition unrelated to any hematologic abnormality.

Clinical Signs

When specific, attributable clinical disease occurs, it is most commonly described as a syndrome of pitting edema of the distal hind limbs, teats, and udder, coincident with fever, prefemoral lymph node enlargement, decreased milk production, and mild weight loss in dairy heifers. Reports of clinical disease most commonly originate from either North America or Japan. There may be a mild to modest anemia and only rarely, severe anemia. The disease is transient, and acute clinical signs resolve in 7 to 10 days. The pathophysiology linking the organism with erythrocytes and clinical signs of peripheral edema are not understood, but it has been postulated that they relate to immune complex formation and associated immune-mediated illness such as vasculitis. Most commonly, the disease occurs in individual animals in a herd, but it is also occasionally seen as small outbreaks with multiple cattle affected over time. A similar problem has been seen in young bulls, characterized by scrotal and hind limb edema and infertility. These signs are associated with large numbers of *M.*

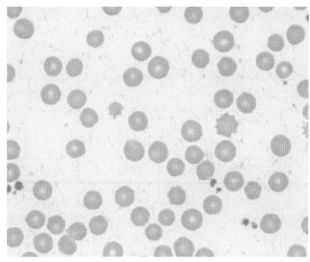

• **Fig. 16.9** Abundant *Mycoplasma wenyoni* organisms can be seen in this blood smear free in the background areas between red blood cells (RBCs) or platelets, as well as overlying the surface of some of the cells. They are basophilic, pleomorphic small rod or coccoid shapes, often in short chains or rings. In vivo, the organisms are thought to be attached to the RBC surfaces, but they quickly detach ex vivo, as seen here.

wenyonii seen in blood smears, and the signs resolve as parasitemia declines. The severe anemia and hemolytic problems identified in swine and sheep with *Eperythrozoon* infection have not been routinely identified in the naturally occurring syndrome seen in cattle, although there are case reports of *M. wenyonii* causing simple anemia as well as severe immune-mediated hemolytic anemia in adult cows in North America.

Diagnosis

Diagnosis is achieved by identifying typical clinical signs in dairy heifers in early to midlactation, verified by identification of the epicellular organisms in dried blood smears (Fig. 16.9). The identity of the organism can be confirmed by PCR assay.

Treatment

Many animals that have remission of signs also experience a decline in parasitemia to undetectable levels over 7 to 14 days. Alternatively, a good response with rapid clearance of the organism and resolution of signs will follow a single dose of parenteral oxytetracycline, and treatment may be indicated when production is significantly affected or signs of illness are more severe.

Theileriosis (Domestic to United States)

Etiology

Theileria parasites can infect a wide range of wild and domestic ruminants, including cattle. Domestic cases of bovine theileriosis are unusual but noteworthy if only because of the transboundary and regulatory relevance of tropical theileriosis (caused by *Theileria annulata*) and East Coast fever (caused by *Theileria parva*), both of which are exotic to the United States and frequently much more severe clinically. The causative agent of domestic theileriosis is *Theileria buffeli,* which is taxonomically included within the so-called benign *Theileria orientalis* group. There has been much debate as to whether this group includes three species—*T. sergenti, T. buffeli,* and *T. orientalis*—or should more correctly be referred to as a single species, usually as *T. orientalis.* Throughout this section, we refer to *T. buffeli* as the North American agent of theileriosis for simplicity.

In the United States, *T. buffeli* infection has been associated with rare, sporadic, sometimes fatal, clinical illness characterized by intravascular hemolysis in dairy cattle. Because of the similarities clinically and morphologically with the aforementioned important high-morbidity and high-mortality transboundary diseases, East Coast fever and tropical theileriosis, these infrequent cases associated with *Theileria buffeli* may result in foreign animal disease investigations in the United States when the *Theileria* organisms are recognized on blood smears of sick cattle. The life cycle of *Theileria* includes two intracellular developmental stages, intralymphocytic schizonts and intraerythrocytic piroplasms. Piroplasms can be identified in the RBCs in stained blood smears (Fig. 16.10) but cannot always be differentiated from other blood parasites such as *Babesia* spp. The disease is vector transmitted, in the case of *T. buffeli* typically by ticks belonging to the *Haemaphysalis* genus, but at this point in time, it is unknown which specific tick species may be capable of infecting cattle with the organism in the United States. No transovarial transmission occurs in ticks and so only by feeding on an infected host can a tick acquire, and subsequently transmit, the infection. Biting

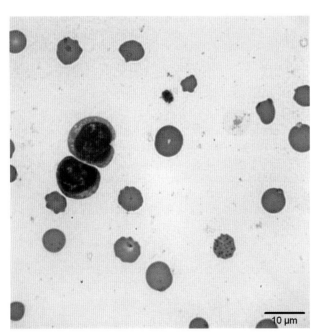

• **Fig. 16.10** *Theileria buffeli* piroplasms seen in the erythrocytes in this blood smear from a cow with clinical theileriosis.

flies and common-use needles or other equipment may spread the infection between cattle, which when infected are considered infected for life.

Clinical Signs

The majority of infections are probably asymptomatic (hence the term *benign theileriosis*); however, there are reports from both the United States and other parts of the world (Australia, New Zealand, and Japan notably) of severe clinical disease associated with *T. buffeli* infection. The organism exerts its major pathogenic effect via its piroplasmic forms causing erythrocyte destruction. The intravascular hemolysis that has been associated with this infection leads to the expected clinical findings of high fever, tachycardia, tachypnea, diarrhea, jaundiced membranes, and dark-colored urine. Lymphadenopathy can also be quite marked, likely associated with the schizont infection. Several hematologic and biochemical changes associated with clinically severe *T. buffeli* infection have been reported, including anemia (regenerative), leukopenia or leukocytosis, neutropenia, lymphocytosis, hypo- or hyperproteinemia, and increased liver enzymes. Hyperbilirubinemia and dark urine are both related to the hemolytic process. Asymptomatic cows may also be in the herd, and the reason why perhaps only one cow develops severe disease is unknown.

Diagnosis

Diagnosis is made by identification of the intraerythrocytic *Theileria* organisms seen on blood smears and by ruling out other *Theileria* spp., or other diseases, especially those associated with different erythrocytic parasites that cause similar signs. Advanced molecular techniques such as specific PCR assays or partial or whole-genome sequencing applied to nucleic acid amplicons can be used on individual cases to speciate the organism and rule out transboundary infections. International reference laboratories use IFA tests for serologic detection of infection, and IFA has been used experimentally for specific *T. buffeli* antibody detection.

Treatment

Treatment with tetracycline and imidocarb has been unsuccessful. Halofuginone, parvaquone, and buparvaquone have been used successfully therapeutically against *Theileria* spp., but their widespread use in cattle may be limited by cost or lack of approval for use in food producing animals, depending upon location.

Control

The *Theileria* spp. associated with benign theileriosis, East Coast fever, and tropical theileriosis are all tickborne, so many of the measures aimed at controlling them are related to vector control, such as zero grazing and application of acaricides. In the United States, acaricide use must conform to Animal Medicinal Drug Use Clarification Act

(AMDUCA) guidelines and after a positive animal is identified should be combined with biosecurity measures to limit spread from an infected animal to susceptible herdmates. Because of its rarity in the United States, the lifelong persistence of infection, and the difficulty in chemosterilization, culling of any positive animal may be worth considering.

Tickborne Fever

Anaplasma phagocytophilum is the causative agent of tickborne fever. Although the organism is present in *Ixodes* spp. ticks in several areas of the United States, to our knowledge, clinical disease in cattle has not been reported in North America. Fever, leukopenia, thrombocytopenia, abortions, ataxia, decreased production, and increased susceptibility to other infections have been reported in cattle and small ruminants in other parts of the world. In dairy cattle, the predominant clinical signs have been abortion and stillbirths alongside a sudden drop in milk yield, usually in naïve, bred heifers or young pregnant cows shortly after introduction to tick-infested pastures. Fever and apparent respiratory signs are also commonly noted in affected cattle in Europe. Observation of morulae within white blood cells or detection of DNA in the blood by PCR are the preferred confirmatory tests. Although the infection is generally self-limiting, oxytetracycline therapy is expected to shorten the clinical course. When infection with *A. phagocytophilum* is suspected as the cause of abortion, maternal whole blood or vaginal fluids should be tested by PCR assay because the organism does not cross the placenta, and fetal tissues remain test negative.

Anthrax

Etiology

Bacillus anthracis, a large gram-positive rod, causes anthrax in humans and animals. Vegetative growth in culture media is characterized by chain formation of tightly packed rods ("Medusa-head" colonies); in vivo growth differs by having short chains, rounded ends to the rods, and well-formed capsules that may surround several adjacent organisms. The organism is a spore former but usually only develops spores when growing aerobically at 15.0° to 40.0°C rather than in vivo. The spores are extremely hardy and may survive in dry alkaline soils that contain high nitrogen levels for decades or more. Therefore discharges or tissue from fatal cases may contaminate soils and can allow the organism to remain in certain geographic pockets where the disease will continue to occur sporadically. Rain or wet conditions, coupled with temperatures greater than 15.5°C, foster germination and vegetative growth that subsequently result in sporulation as dryness returns to contaminated soil. Most clinical cases occur during the grazing season.

Cattle exposed to contaminated ground may ingest the spores either directly from the soil or from plants grown on contaminated soil. The spores then become vegetative in the host. Abrasions of the oral mucosa or digestive tract may allow an edematous localized infection, which then seeds lymphatics and eventually results in bacteremia. Localized infections may occur subsequent to skin wounds and have been called "malignant carbuncle" in humans. Inhalation of spores is a less common means of infection but can occur in humans ("woolsorter's disease") or animals and this form is often fatal. Animal byproducts such as hides, slaughterhouse material, and bone meals from endemic areas may harbor the organism or spores and represent an infectious risk to people and animals exposed to these materials. Insects that feed on blood also may transmit the infection.

Virulence of *B. anthracis* is conferred by a polyglutamic acid capsule that allows evasion of the host immune system by deterring phagocytosis and lysis alongside two potent exotoxins. The organism can grow to very high numbers in the bloodstream, where production of these exotoxins leads to vasogenic shock and vascular collapse. The two anthrax toxins, referred to as lethal factor and edema factor, alongside a third important bacterial protein, named protective antigen, are produced from three bacterial polypeptides. Protective antigen facilitates entry of the two toxins into the cytosol of host cells through pores that it establishes in the cell membrane. These three factors working together frequently form a lethal combination because they kill phagocytic cells, damage capillaries, and interfere with clotting of blood. A vicious cycle of capillary permeability, thrombosis, and tissue edema evolves.

Clinical Signs

Peracute *B. anthracis* infection in cattle may result in death so rapid as to be confused with other causes of sudden death such as lightning, fatal internal hemorrhage, clostridial myositis, bloat, or metabolic conditions. Blood-tinged or dark reddish-black sanguineous discharges from body orifices are common in cattle dying from acute anthrax and may lead to confusion with death resulting from caudal vena caval thrombosis, bleeding abomasal ulcers, jejunal hemorrhage syndrome, arsenic poisoning, or peracute salmonellosis.

Acute anthrax causes fever; complete loss of appetite and production; depression; and evidence of blood in most body secretions, including feces, urine, milk, and nasal discharges. Tachycardia, dyspnea, and possible neurologic signs also are present. Unless treated intensively very early in the course of the disease, affected cattle become recumbent within 1 to 2 days and die. Whenever anthrax is suspected based on signs (or lack thereof) and sanguineous discharges from body orifices, necropsy should *not* be performed until other tests have been performed to rule out the disease.

Localized wound infections with *B. anthracis* are possible in cattle but uncommon and difficult to diagnose. A history of anthrax on the farm or within the locale may add a heightened index of suspicion for fatal peracute or acute cases.

Diagnosis

Blood collected from the jugular vein, mammary vein, or ear vein may provide sufficient diagnostic material for cytologic examination and culture when the carcass is fresh. It is no longer necessary to send an ear from the carcass, and in fact, such procedures may merely increase the risk of human exposure. Carcasses that are rotten or more than 12 hours old may be overgrown by clostridial organisms that confuse attempts at cytologic diagnosis. Fixed blood smears stained with methylene blue (Loeffler or McFadean) have been the traditional rapid diagnostic test for identifying the anthrax bacilli and distinguishing them from clostridial organisms, which lack the characteristic red capsule seen with *B. anthracis.* The vegetative organism is not robust outside of the host, and it will not survive transportation delays of several days; hence, an optimal sample would be an air-dried swab or blood smear that will have undergone sporulation. Before proceeding with diagnostics, it is always prudent to contact local regulatory officials and the nearest reference or diagnostic laboratory for guidance on sample submission and protocol.

Blood samples or smears really should be examined at a qualified laboratory to ensure correct interpretation. Other blood tests, including an FA technique and an ELISA, are available at some laboratories. Inoculation of collected material into guinea pigs has been used to diagnose anthrax in the past, but collected material may contain other opportunistic pathogens, thereby confusing the diagnosis. Additionally, a rapid in-field anthrax immunochromatographic test exists that detects the anthrax toxin in a blood sample within 15 minutes. The published diagnostic sensitivity is estimated to be 93.1%, and the estimated diagnostic specificity approaches 100%. Although necropsy of possible anthrax cases is not recommended, it frequently is performed because other diseases may need to be ruled out. Prosectors should wear gloves, gowns, and masks whenever anthrax has been considered in the differential diagnosis of a dead cow. Rigor mortis is often not present or is incomplete. Splenic enlargement, widespread serosal hemorrhages, sanguineous or serosanguineous body cavity fluids, and dark red or black body orifice discharges are the major necropsy findings. Unfortunately, experience also highlights the possibility that practitioners unaware of the possibility of anthrax in a specific location proceed with a postmortem before subsequently realizing the likelihood of this differential as pathologic details emerge. Under such circumstances or when a diagnosis of anthrax based on a blood smear is made, one must immediately notify state or federal regulatory veterinarians to aid in quarantine management and carcass disposal.

Treatment

Treatment seldom is possible because of the acute or peracute course of illness. Penicillin and tetracycline in high levels should be effective in early bacteremic cases or the less common clinical scenario of a localized wound infection.

Prevention and Control

Prevention and control can be accomplished by the following:
1. Avoid infected pastures. This is seldom possible on a practical basis.
2. Spore vaccines—the Sterne strain of rough, nonencapsulated *B. anthracis* was derived through growth of virulent *B. anthracis* on 50% serum agar in 10% to 30% CO_2. The resulting avirulent organism is used in the spore form as a live vaccine for cattle, sheep, and goats. The vaccine is recommended once yearly before pasture season. Use of any *B. anthracis* vaccine in dairy cattle may require regulatory approval, although there is no evidence that milk contains spores after vaccination of lactating cows.
3. Complete disposal of infected carcasses is done by burning or burial at least 6 feet into the ground and covering carcasses with quicklime. Regulatory veterinarians should be consulted regarding appropriate disinfection techniques.

Younger veterinarians may benefit from consultation with neighboring older colleagues to learn whether and where anthrax has been diagnosed previously in their service territory.

Recently, awareness of the zoonotic potential of this infection has been highlighted by discussion of the "weaponization" of the agent as a terrorist threat. Human cases of anthrax in many parts of the world have become uncommon because of the success of control measures and lack of human exposure to infected livestock. Genetically modified organisms and alternative exposure methods besides livestock have created new concerns for human and animal health. One offshoot is the increase in research to find alternative vaccination strategies, such as DNA vaccines, which may prove useful for animal disease control in the future.

Coxiella burnetii Infection (Q Fever)

Etiology

Coxiella burnetii is an obligate intracellular gram-negative bacterium that is ubiquitous in nature and responsible for the zoonotic illness Q fever in humans. Domestic ruminants are the most common reservoirs of the pathogen, but it also infects many wild animal species and arthropods such as deer and ticks. The infective dose for humans may be as low as just one organism, and recent European outbreaks of zoonotic disease have heightened the awareness and concern over the role that dairy species can potentially play in the spread of the infection to humans. *C. burnetii* can be readily transmitted between hosts and environmental reservoirs principally because it is able to survive in the environment for long periods due to its ability to transition between distinct developmental stages. So-called "small-cell variants" are metabolically inactive and resistant to harsh environmental conditions allowing persistence outside of a host; however, after invasion of host cells and during acidification in phagosomes of host cells, it transitions into a "large-cell variant" that is more metabolically active. One of the principal virulence factors of *C. burnetii* is lipopolysaccharide (LPS), but at this point in time, there is little known about other effectors of pathogenicity. Whereas virulent forms of the organism contain LPS and are referred to as phase I organisms, avirulent forms lack LPS and are referred to as phase II organisms.

Domestic animals, including cattle, sheep, and goats, are the principal reservoirs of *C. burnetii* in North America. Infection in cattle is common based on serologic and bulk tank milk PCR surveys; for example, a study in which more than 300 bulk tank milk samples from dairies predominantly in the Northeastern and Midwestern U.S. were tested over a 3-year period by PCR revealed that more than 90% were positive. This emphasizes yet again the importance of pasteurization for human health. Shedding rates for individual dairy cows on any particular day have been estimated to be approximately 20% to 25% of all lactating cows. There is an uncertain, potentially even paradoxical, relationship in infected cows between shedding patterns and seropositivity, in that the bacterium is not shed continuously, and shedders with high antibody levels tend to shed for longer than those with no antibody. Taken together this would make individual cow monitoring by either serology or PCR challenging.

Ticks may also spread the infection from one animal to another, but the major sources of infectious organisms are; amniotic fluids; placental and fetal membranes of parturient ewes, goats, and cows; and milk, urine, and feces of infected animals. Infected ruminants do not show clinical disease in most instances. High abortion rates are rarely observed, except in some caprine herds. Apparently, the organism concentrates in the placenta and udder of pregnant animals, who then release large numbers of *C. burnetii* at parturition. Aborting animals, but also females with normal parturition, as well as infected cows with metritis, can potentially shed *C. burnetii* for several months. Milk shedding is more frequent and lasts longer in cows and goats than in ewes. Aerosols arising from highly contaminated secretions and tissues allow infection of people and other animals in the vicinity via inhalation. Contaminated environments, hides, wool, and bedding also may allow subsequent aerosol infection of humans. When present in the environment or on inanimate objects, the organism is extremely resistant and persistent. Dust storms may predispose to infection by inhalation in endemic areas. A solution of 1% to 2% chlorine bleach is considered an effective disinfectant.

In humans, Q fever is an occupational disease in agricultural and slaughterhouse workers, veterinarians, and animal researchers. The major reason for concern in dairy cattle is that infection of dairy cattle and subsequent production of milk containing *C. burnetii,* especially in recently fresh cows, is widespread. The frequency of *C. burnetii*–contaminated milk is another reason to avoid unpasteurized milk. Pasteurization temperatures of 62.8°C (145.0°F) for 30 minutes or 71.7°C (161.0°F) for 15 seconds kill the organism; thus, routine pasteurization of milk for retail sale prevents spread of disease to humans through this route. Even though oral ingestion is an infrequent route of infection, it may cause seroconversion, and raw milk may contain enough *C. burnetii* to allow aerosol infection in dairy workers.

Clinical Signs

Infected cattle usually are asymptomatic or subclinical with nonspecific signs. The relevance of Q fever as a disease of dairy cattle is debatable, and as yet there is no clear scientific evidence that infection with *C. burnetti* negatively impacts dairy cow reproductive performance. The disease in humans follows an incubation of 10 to 28 days and is characterized by chills, fever, headache, malaise, and muscle aches. Septicemia is probable based on a high incidence of pneumonitis and hepatitis, as well as lesser incidences of severe endocarditis.

Diagnosis

Serologic testing using an ELISA assay or PCR testing of whole blood, milk, fetal tissues, or vaginal fluids have become the most common means of diagnosis. Infection rates as demonstrated by these assays for cattle vary based on geographic location, herd size, and stage of gestation. In humans, a microimmunofluorescence assay for phase 1 and phase 2 antibodies is the primary diagnostic tool for detection and staging of infection, with some application of PCR assays or cell culture to tissue samples.

Treatment

Treatment is not practiced in cattle, but tetracycline is the primary chemotherapeutic agent for Q fever in humans.

Prevention and Control

Awareness of the zoonotic potential of *C. burnetii* and possible bad press for the dairy industry associated with Q fever mandate concern and respect for this pathogen. Drinking unpasteurized milk should be avoided and could be a problem with organic herds that are not tested! Veterinarians should be aware of the potential for disease so as to protect themselves and farm workers. Considering the potential exposure of veterinarians through obstetric procedures among others, it seems that bovine practitioners are at high risk. Perhaps most have developed immunity, although documentation of this effect is lacking.

Humans deemed at high risk in laboratory or abattoir settings have been vaccinated with apparent success in countries outside of the United States. Vaccination with experimental vaccines in cattle results in seroconversion but does not eliminate shedding.

Brucellosis

Etiology

Brucellosis (Bang's disease) is an infectious cause of reproductive failure in cattle and a disease having profound public health significance. As with TB, brucellosis induces fervent and emotional responses when control and eradication efforts are discussed. Much of the United States is free of brucellosis thanks to testing and control methods fostered by cooperative state and federal efforts. However, the disease persists in cattle in certain states, and bison and wild ruminants (e.g., elk and moose) may carry the disease and could represent a risk to range cattle in certain areas of the western United States. For example, there were 17 documented instances of transmission of *Brucella abortus* from elk to dairy or beef cattle in the Greater Yellowstone Area (portions of Idaho, Wyoming, and Montana) from 2002 to 2012.

In cattle, *B. abortus* is the usual cause of brucellosis, but other *Brucella* spp. such as *B. melitensis* and *B. suis* can also, albeit rarely, infect cattle. *Brucella* spp. tend to have favorite primary hosts but seldom limit infection to only one host species. This discussion will be limited to *B. abortus*.

B. abortus is a short gram-negative rod that is fastidious and grows best in a CO_2-enriched aerobic environment. The organism has many other complex requirements for in vitro growth, and speciation of *Brucella* spp. or identification of biotypes is difficult. Some techniques used for speciation and biotyping include CO_2 requirements, production of H_2S, growth on various dyes, bacteriophage lysis, substrate oxidation, and agglutination tests. Eight biotypes (also referred to as biovars) of *B. abortus* have been identified, but in the United States, biotype 1 is the major type with biotypes 2 and 4 playing smaller roles. Despite the complex growth requirements in vitro, the organism can persist in certain animal products and the environment for prolonged periods under favorable circumstances. In general, the organism likes moisture and cool temperatures but fares poorly in sunlight, dryness, and heat. For example, *B. abortus* may survive in manure at 12°C for 250 days but is killed quickly in manure that is heated. Similarly, infected placental and fetal tissues, refrigerated infected milk and other dairy products, and cool water may support prolonged infectivity. Fortunately, pasteurization kills *B. abortus* in milk.

Infection occurs primarily by ingestion of the organism, but venereal, intramammary, and congenital spread have been documented occasionally. Ingestion of the organism by susceptible cattle is fostered through contamination of feedstuffs, pasture, or fomites by infective placental fluids, tissues, fetuses, or milk. In dairy cattle, large herd size and intensive dairy management conditions predispose to both epidemic infections and the continuation of endemic ones.

After infection has occurred, *B. abortus* exists in the host as a facultative intracellular organism capable of survival in host phagocytic cells. Polysaccharides and LPS-protein components of the cell wall compose the surface antigens that trigger production of agglutinating antibodies by the host. Detection of these antibodies forms the basis for many of the serologic tests used in brucellosis control programs. Cell-mediated immunity, as expected based on the facultative intracellular designation of *B. abortus,* is important but still poorly understood.

B. abortus gains entrance to cattle through mucous membranes of the oral cavity, nasal cavity, and conjunctiva or via broken skin. Because ingestion is the major route of infection, the pharynx is thought to be the primary site of entrance. Calves can be infected by ingesting infected milk, and venereal spread can occur in both cows and bulls. After penetration of the mucous membranes occurs, the organism seeks out and proliferates in regional lymph nodes before causing bacteremia. Similar to *Salmonella* spp., *Listeria* spp., and other facultative intracellular organisms, septicemic spread of *B. abortus* is aided by macrophage circulation. *B. abortus* septicemia results in infection that localizes in the udder, uterus, and associated lymph nodes of these organs. Infection of the pregnant uterus, especially during the second half of gestation in the cow, results in a progressive placentitis involving the chorion followed by an endometritis and fetal placental infection. Interference with fetal blood supply, endotoxemic effects on the fetus, and fetal bacteremia all contribute to subsequent loss of fetal viability and abortion. Most abortions occur from 5 months' gestation to near term. Aborted fetuses have been dead for days but frequently harbor viable *B. abortus* in the lungs and abomasum.

Infected cattle usually remain carriers for life, and subsequent maximal shedding of *B. abortus* in milk and reproductive tract discharges occurs in association with each parturition. Although *B. abortus* abortion is infrequent during subsequent pregnancies in infected cows, the placenta may be infected during pregnancy, and carrier cows may contaminate the environment during calving and through their discharges for variable times following parturition.

Young animals are thought to possess resistance to infection. This resistance is not completely understood but probably is aided by passive, colostral origin antibodies. Cattle appear more susceptible to infection after they reach puberty or become pregnant. This generality regarding age resistance in young cattle is complicated somewhat by the occasional development of so-called latent infections whereby calves that acquire the infection vertically or through ingesting contaminated milk may remain seronegative and not show any overt signs of disease. Such latent infection in heifers can represent a great challenge in terms of control because they can give birth to infected calves of their own and may still abort in maturity.

Latent infections do not result in seroconversion or clinical signs until later in life when these animals are late in gestation, calve, or abort. The exact incidence or prevalence of latency is difficult to determine but appears infrequent based on two generation studies.

Clinical Signs

The organism has a tropism for the uterus, so clinical signs in female dairy cattle are mainly limited to abortion of late term fetuses, usually during the last half of gestation. Abortion storms may occur when the disease has recently been introduced into a herd, but abortion in first-calf heifers or new additions typifies endemic infection. The postabortion uterus will contain variable amounts of a fetid yellow to brown discharge. Abortion is associated with severe placental necrosis, often seemingly randomly distributed such that some placentomes will be relatively normal in appearance while others are severely necrotic and hemorrhagic. On rare occasions, less severe placental lesions may lead to the birth of weak, unthrifty calves that have high neonatal mortality rates. In bulls, the most significant clinical sign associated with *B. abortus* infection is orchitis. Epididymitis and seminal vesiculitis may also be present. Severe illness in people is possible and can be difficult to diagnose unless physicians have an index of suspicion based on historical patient data that indicates occupational risk. In humans, the disease is called undulant fever and is a well-known zoonotic infection. Farm workers, veterinarians, and slaughterhouse workers are at high risk if they handle infected cattle, placentas, fetuses, or milk. Drinking unpasteurized milk or eating unpasteurized cheeses from infected cattle is extremely dangerous for humans. Brucellosis in humans can masquerade as many other more common diseases and may cause fever, myalgia, or joint or eye infection. *Brucella* spp. can infect people through the mucous membranes or breaks in the skin.

Diagnosis

Although culture of *B. abortus* remains the gold standard for positive diagnosis, economics and the need for specialized bacteriologic capabilities limit the use of culture for widespread surveillance and regulatory control programs. Recent development of PCR tests for detection of the agent in aborted fetuses is replacing the need for culture and the difficulties that culturing entails. Serologic testing remains the most common means of diagnosis of infected carrier animals. Many serologic tests are available and are better understood when interpreted in light of normal bovine immune responses to *B. abortus*. Shortly after infection of susceptible cattle, IgM agglutinins appear and peak within 2 weeks. Subsequent IgG antibodies peak by 1 to 2 months and these become the major detectable antibodies in chronic infections. IgG_1 antibodies are nonagglutinating, have no opsonizing activity, block IgM and IgG_2 antibodies, and may aid with the persistence of *B. abortus* in the host. This also may explain why serologic evidence of high humoral antibodies does not correlate with immunity or perhaps effective immunity in clinically infected cattle. Furthermore, protective strain 19 vaccines primarily induce IgM antibodies and lesser IgG_1 responses, suggesting that IgG_1 nonagglutinating antibodies may actually be harmful host responses.

The serum tube agglutination test, the plate (or rapid) agglutination test, and the card test are the most commonly used assays. The serum tube agglutination test and card test tend to detect IgM antibodies, thus facilitating the detection

of recent infection. Historically, it was these serologic tests that would most commonly give false-positive results in animals that had received the strain 19 vaccine. The rivanol and mercaptoethanol tests may be helpful in differentiating antibodies elicited by chronic natural infection (mainly IgG_1) from antibodies subsequent to strain 19 vaccination (mostly IgM). These chemicals remove most IgM from the serum, so a reduction in titer following addition of the chemical to serum suggested that the titer resulted from strain 19 vaccine rather than true infection.

The milk ring test is used widely for surveillance of *B. abortus* infection in dairy cattle. Bulk tank milk samples from each producer are tested at regular intervals by milk plants. A hematoxylin-stained suspension of killed *B. abortus* is added to fresh milk and incubated in a water bath at 37.0°C. Agglutinating antibodies in the milk will be detected by a color change in the cream layer because fat globules cause clumps of agglutinated organisms to rise in the tube, leaving decolorized milk below. A negative test result is confirmed when the milk in the tube remains colored.

None of these tests is completely accurate or foolproof. Statistical probabilities of a positive test result, meaning actual infection, are much lower in areas having little if any brucellosis versus areas with endemic infection. Therefore epidemiologic, surveillance, and control methods are limited by available diagnostic tools, similar to the situation with TB.

The CF test is accurate when testing adults that have never been vaccinated or that were vaccinated as calves. This test only detects IgM and IgG_1, and it is thought that complement fixing antibody levels decrease more rapidly than agglutinating antibodies in calves. Therefore fewer false-positive findings may result from calfhood vaccination when the CF test is used. The accuracy, specificity, and sensitivity of serologic tests may be enhanced in the future by ELISA and other techniques.

The development of new vaccines that do not result in confusing antibody levels in currently available tests has been an exciting development. Strain 19 vaccine has been an extremely helpful tool to control *B. abortus* in cattle but suffers because it produces antibodies in vaccinated cattle, may cause abortion in cattle vaccinated as adults, and can cause illness in people. In calfhood vaccinates, strain 19 origin antibodies present only an occasional problem that leads to frustration for owners when sale, show, or shipment requirements result in a positive serologic test result. However, for adult vaccinates, the resulting antibody levels seriously complicate all current serologic tests and make it extremely difficult to differentiate clinically infected cattle from vaccinates. Therefore vaccines using rough strains of *B. abortus* have been tested. These rough strains lack the outer membrane LPS that is used as the antigenic component in most available tests. Cattle vaccinated with rough forms of *B. abortus* do not give a positive reaction when current serologic tests are used. Consequently, for states still requiring female calfhood vaccination, the RB51 strain has now been adopted as the official calfhood vaccination strain in the United States. The RB51 strain vaccine is also less abortigenic than strain 19 in cattle. However, it is important to use PCR testing capabilities to distinguish field strain from vaccine strain whenever abortions caused by *B. abortus* occur in vaccinated cattle.

Treatment

Treatment currently is not approved for brucellosis in dairy cattle. Similar to therapy in humans, however, experimental treatment of infected cattle supports the use of tetracycline and streptomycin in combination.

Control

Control measures should adhere to current state and federal guidelines. In most areas where brucellosis has been eliminated or minimized, surveillance methods include; regular milk ring tests; serologic tests performed randomly at slaughterhouses for traceback of positive cattle; and serologic tests performed for interstate, international, or private sales. Whenever a positive milk ring test result or individual has been identified, blood testing of the entire herd, removal of reactors, and quarantine usually are carried out. Calfhood vaccination in accordance with regulatory recommendations provides added insurance against epidemic loss. Some states still require calfhood vaccination using strain RB51 vaccine for heifer calves aged 4 to 8 months. Bull calves should not be vaccinated for fear of establishing chronic infection in the reproductive organs.

In endemic large dairy herds located in the southern United States and in range beef cattle, control of infection by test and slaughter may not be possible. Calfhood vaccination and increased efforts in sanitation may minimize or eliminate brucellosis in such herds over a period of years as chronically infected cows are eliminated by attrition. Vaccination of adult cattle has been performed in some areas where heavy infection rates exist, but usually it is discouraged and should only be considered when regulatory veterinary personnel approve the procedure.

In regions (e.g., Greater Yellowstone National Park) where wildlife are potential sources of infection for domestic cattle, control and prevention must necessarily involve a coordinated and collaborative effort between private farmers or ranchers and state or federal fish and game officials. Unfortunately, it is highly likely that sporadic cases of brucellosis test–positive wildlife and domestic cattle and bison will continue to occur as long as there is close proximity between these populations in some western U.S. states.

Bovine Leukemia Virus Infection (Leukosis) (Bovine Lymphosarcoma)

Etiology

Bovine leukemia virus (BLV), a retrovirus, is the cause of most cases of bovine lymphosarcoma. Infection with BLV is referred to as enzootic bovine leukosis (EBL) or simply leukosis of adult cattle. This retrovirus is further classified into the subfamily *Orthoretrovirinae* and genus *Deltaretrovirus* and, similar to other retroviruses, possesses the enzyme reverse transcriptase. Reverse transcriptase enables retroviruses to convert RNA to DNA and then integrate this viral DNA into the chromosomal DNA of the host cell. This mechanism results in lifetime infection of the host and allows viral nucleic acid to be replicated as the host cells replicate. Host antibody production against the virus is continual and lifelong as a result of repetitive viral protein translation and exposure. The host cell for BLV is the B lymphocyte (CD5+, IgM+, B cells are the primary target cell). T cells may also be infected to a lesser degree and may have a role in cell to cell transmission. During initial infection, the encoded viral DNA (provirus) is believed to produce true virions, which escape host cells, and infect other cells. After host antibody production against the virus, however, the virus lives somewhat in limbo within lymphocytes because host antibodies (probably against glycoprotein 51 [gp 51]) outside the cell in the bloodstream may neutralize escaping virions. Infectious virus can escape from lymphocytes, however, if infected lymphocytes are separated from the checking presence of serum antibodies by their removal from the host or dilution of antibody. Therefore horizontal spread of BLV usually requires the transfer of blood containing infected lymphocytes from an infected to a susceptible individual. Infected cells require mechanical aids or compromised surface barriers to bypass intact epithelium or mucosa and be free of neutralizing antibody in a susceptible host. Milk, colostrum, and other body secretions containing infected lymphocytes can therefore also result in horizontal spread of BLV.

Vertical transmission of BLV from infected dams to their fetuses by transfer of virus across the placenta is also possible but probably occurs in fewer than 10% of pregnancies in infected cattle. Higher incidences of in utero infection rates have been observed in herds with an exceedingly high prevalence of cows with persistent lymphocytosis (PL) or in herds with a high incidence of lymphosarcoma. Therefore these cattle represent a higher risk for vertical transmission. Calves infected in utero appear to be infected after establishing immunocompetence because they have both virus and antibody against the virus in their blood at birth, before colostrum ingestion.

Specific references and research data regarding transmission of BLV from infected to susceptible cattle would require an exhaustive and lengthy text and reference list. Some review articles on the subject are included in the bibliography.

Studies of horizontal transmission have used susceptible cattle in natural settings, susceptible cattle in experimental settings, or susceptible sheep, which are very easily infected with BLV. Infective doses of lymphocytes from BLV-infected cattle may be as low as 1000 lymphocytes, although reported dosages vary greatly from several thousand lymphocytes up to 5 or more mL of blood. This can likely be explained by variations in the number of infected lymphocytes in donors; many cows have less than 5% lymphocyte infection, but other cows have greater than 50% lymphocyte infection, most commonly PL cows, who by definition have exceptionally high lymphocyte counts to begin with. In addition, recent work using quantitative PCR techniques has shown that the blood of PL cattle, along with about 40% of nonlymphocytotic cows, consistently contains greater than 10^5 proviral copies per 10^5 peripheral blood mononuclear cells (PBMC). Other nonlymphocytotic cattle may have as few as 10^2 copies per 10^5 PBMC or less. These findings imply higher risks of horizontal transmission of BLV in herds having BLV-positive PL cows or from particular individual animals. Intradermal, SC, IM, and IV parenteral administration of BLV-infected lymphocytes or whole blood have all resulted in infection of susceptible hosts.

Horizontal transmission of blood is frequently iatrogenic by cow handlers and veterinarians through the use or reuse of common needles and syringes, dehorners, ear tattoo instruments, castrating equipment, blood collection needles, IV needles, blood transfusions, and nose leads. Intradermal tuberculin testing also is a possible, although less likely, cause of horizontal spread.

Rectal palpation using a common sleeve for examination of BLV-positive cattle followed by palpation of BLV-negative cattle also can spread BLV horizontally, but conflicting results have evolved in studies designed to assess the relevance and risk of this means of spread. One epidemiologic study in a large dairy failed to detect increased risk of infection for BLV-negative cattle when a common sleeve was used by a single examiner to perform rectal examinations randomly on both BLV-positive and BLV-negative cattle. However, other studies show increased risk of transmission to BLV-negative cows palpated with a common sleeve immediately after BLV-positive cows. This discrepancy may be explained by difference in the number of PL or highly viremic cows in the respective herds. Rectal transmission by unnatural volumes of infective blood and unnatural means of rectal irritation has caused experimental infection of susceptible calves and sheep.

Infection through the use of dehorners and other surgical instruments is much less likely if the instruments are rinsed and disinfected with either chlorine bleach or chlorhexidine between animals. Blood sampling with a common needle is very dangerous, especially for susceptible cattle sampled immediately after BLV-positive cattle. Therefore individual needles are essential for venipuncture and parenteral injections.

The role of insects in horizontal spread of BLV is controversial, and most studies have used completely unrealistic materials and methods, such as injecting mouth parts of various insects that have fed on BLV-positive blood or creating controlled populations of insects that feed on BLV-positive cattle and then are applied to BLV-negative cattle. Tabanids, mosquitoes, and ticks have, in some studies, transmitted infection, but stable flies and horn flies seem less likely to do so. At this time, the role of insects in the spread of BLV is unknown. It is interesting that no studies have assessed the potential for BLV transmission for lice because these parasites constitute a serious parasitic burden for many cattle during the winter months. A higher incidence of BLV infection in beef cattle in the southern states compared with northern states supports the possibility of insects playing a role in BLV transmission.

Epidemiologic studies emphasize that close contact of infected and susceptible cattle enhances the horizontal transmission of BLV. Prevalence within infected herds tends to peak during confinement or with increased cattle density or when BLV-negative cattle are suddenly grouped with BLV-positive cattle. Management procedures that result in increased density or that entail common treatment procedures as heifers come of breeding age or join milking herds seem to facilitate infection. Similarly calves and heifers housed with adult cattle probably have a greater risk of infection. Infected cattle having antibodies to the viral core protein (p24) and those that have PL represent greater risk to susceptible cattle than BLV-positive cattle having only antibodies against the gp 51 surface glycoprotein.

Because infection spreads when BLV-positive cattle are closely confined with BLV-negative cattle, many studies assessing infectivity of various secretions have been performed. Nasal secretions, saliva, bronchoalveolar washes, urine, feces, uterine flush fluid, and semen have been examined. Secretions that are highly cellular are more likely to be infective than those that are relatively acellular. Soluble fractions of secretions are seldom infective because the virus is cell associated, but in one study of urine from BLV-positive cows, BLV p25 antigen was found in the soluble portion in a majority of infected cattle tested. Respiratory secretions may harbor infected cells, but the natural risk of these secretions spreading infection seems low. Similarly, uterine fluid obtained during embryo transfer from BLV-positive donors is most dangerous when cell contamination occurs. Semen presents little risk when artificial insemination is used from reputable commercial sources because highly cellular ejaculates are usually discarded by bull stud services, and bull studs rarely, if ever, keep BLV-positive bulls. However, BLV-positive bulls used for natural service that have reproductive tract infections causing increased numbers of infective cells in the ejaculate could spread infection to susceptible cows and heifers. The relatively low infectivity of secretions fails to explain completely the increased risk of infection observed epidemiologically in closely confined or dense cattle populations. Physical cow interactions and management procedures (e.g., restraint equipment) may play a role. Lymphocytes in milk and colostrum represent a potential source of virus and certainly represent a significant secretory source of virus. The role of milk and colostrum fed to susceptible calves as regards transmission will be discussed later.

In utero transmission of BLV, the implications of BLV infection for donor and recipient during embryo transfer, and the feeding of infected milk or colostrum require consideration. As discussed earlier, in utero spread of BLV from infected dams to susceptible fetuses occurs in a low percentage of cases—probably fewer than 10% in most infected herds. Herds with an extremely high incidence of infected cattle or herds containing many cows with PL or clinical tumors may experience higher in utero infection rates because maternal viral load has been demonstrated to be significantly correlated with the frequency of perinatal infection. In high viral load dams, the risk of vertical transmission may approach 40%. It is always important to remember that such dams represent a risk for viral transmission not just in utero but also during parturition when calves are exposed to maternal blood during delivery. In utero infection appears to represent a direct viral infection through the placenta. Cows that are BLV positive that produce an in utero–infected calf may or may not produce infected calves on subsequent pregnancies.

Embryo transfer is *not* a major means of BLV vertical transmission from donors that are BLV positive; the early stage embryo with an intact zona pellucida being considered resistant to infection with the virus. Embryos from BLV-positive donors neither infect BLV-negative recipients nor result in infected fetuses. Embryos from either BLV-positive or BLV-negative cows, however, would be at risk for in utero infection if implanted into BLV-positive recipients. Therefore the key to successful management of BLV in embryo transfer is the maintenance of BLV-negative recipient stock. Embryo transfer is an authentic way to maximize the genetic potential of valuable BLV-positive donors yet still be able to obtain noninfected progeny. A similar situation exists for oocyte recovery for IVF procedures; the embryos derived from this technique should be negative for BLV infection even from a BLV-positive donor, provided proper technique is observed. Cellular contamination, specifically via those fluids that contain lymphocytes, will always be the biggest risk for acquiring the virus.

Perhaps the area of greatest controversy in transmission of BLV involves the role that feeding infected milk or colostrum may play. As previously stated, the colostrum and milk of BLV-positive cows will contain BLV because lymphocytes constitute a normal cellular component of milk and colostrum. BLV provirus is reliably found in the colostrum of BLV-positive cows such that one should assume that colostrum from BLV-positive cows is likely to harbor infected lymphocytes. In addition to infected lymphocytes, however, the colostrum of BLV-positive cattle contains antibody against the virus, and this antibody is thought to provide some immediate protection against infection. A review of the scientific literature is illustrative of the confusion and debate surrounding this issue: One can read studies from the 1980s that demonstrated both the infective and protective potential of colostrum in experimental studies, but in the 1990s through the early 2000s, the bulk of the evidence was supportive of the fact that colostrum from infected dams was an important risk factor for within-herd transmission, and prevention and control strategies at that time reflected this opinion. More recently (the past decade), epidemiologic studies have shown a reduction in BLV incidence when BLV-positive colostrum is fed to newborn calves. At the time of writing, one would have to say that the role of colostrum in natural transmission is unclear. Paradoxically, the most recent research appears to demonstrate a greater protective effect conferred by high proviral load dams (giving

rise to higher antibody levels in colostrum, too) compared with low proviral load dams whose colostrum accordingly contains lesser antibody titers. Infected lymphocytes given orally to susceptible newborn calves can cause infection experimentally if administered before colostral feeding. It appears that calves are most susceptible to infection by BLV in colostrum or milk from birth to 3 days of age and thereafter may not be as commonly infected by this route. This fact also underscores the risk of feeding blood-contaminated colostrum or milk. Much remains to be learned regarding both colostral transmission of the virus and the duration and extent to which maternally derived antibody will protect neonatal calves. Passive antibodies against BLV can be detected in calves consuming colostrum from BLV-positive cows, and these antibodies persist for as long as 6 months.

Calves fed milk from infected cows up to weaning can become infected with BLV, but the frequency of this occurrence is difficult to determine based on conflicting experimental results. Calves having ingested colostrum with BLV antibodies, as well as those that ingested colostrum without antibodies, may be at some risk. Probably fewer than 10% of calves ingesting infected milk would become infected with BLV in most field settings. Milk containing higher numbers of infected lymphocytes, as might be found in cows with PL or lymphosarcoma, should be considered the most dangerous. Souring milk to reach a pH of less than 4.4 and holding it at 65.0°F (18.33°C) for 24 hours will kill BLV. Freezing followed by thawing will cause lysis of lymphocytes and this or pasteurizing colostrum and milk will destroy BLV in these fluids. The best recommendation regarding colostrum and milk feeding for calves is to feed colostrum from BLV-negative cows to all calves, to use only heat-treated or pasteurized colostrum or milk, or feed previously frozen colostrum and then use a milk replacer or pasteurized milk up to weaning. Such a rigorous approach is unlikely to be adopted by many commercial farms. In addition, there are now colostrum replacement products available that are free of BLV transmission risk. Freedom from passive antibodies should be ascertained from the manufacturer of each specific product in the event that calves without passive antibodies for export markets, for example, are desired. Some of the commercial colostrum replacement products that are available in the United States have been demonstrated to contain proviral DNA by PCR; however, it is unlikely that this represents a significant infectious risk because the BLV detected is likely to have been inactivated during the production process.

Numerous older studies have evaluated the prevalence of BLV infection in dairy and beef cattle in the US. More than 80% of all dairy herds were determined to contain BLV-infected animals in the U.S. National Animal Health Monitoring System (NAHMS) Dairy 2007 study. Individual, within-herd cow prevalence will vary greatly based on geographic area and types of management. In the northeastern United States, it is assumed that 35% or more of all dairy cattle are infected, but rare herds may have no seropositive cattle whilst others have more than 80% positive cattle. Estimates in some southern states reach 50% or greater seropositivity in dairy cattle. Fewer than 5% of all infected (BLV-positive) cattle subsequently develop lymphosarcoma, predominantly in cattle older than 3 years old. This is an important statistic because veterinarians sometimes diagnose lymphosarcoma erroneously when faced with vague illness in seropositive cattle. The risk for lymphosarcoma in a BLV-infected cow is genetically related. Although a number of host genetic factors for susceptibility to infection have been identified within the bovine genome, including ones that permit the monoclonal proliferation of B lymphocytes in tumor-bearing cows, as yet there are no reports of successful selection of BLV-resistant cattle.

Only a small percentage of BLV-positive cattle will demonstrate PL in their peripheral blood. PL has been defined as an absolute lymphocyte count at least 3 standard derivations above the normal mean count that persists for at least 3 consecutive months. PL is the result of benign polyclonal B-lymphocyte proliferation. More than 98% of cattle with PL test positive for BLV, and the tendency for PL in response to BLV infection may be a separately inherited trait. Genetic influences exist on both the occurrence of PL or lymphosarcoma within certain lines of purebred cattle. Evidence for genetic relationships regarding susceptibility or resistance to BLV infection and PL have evolved from studies of bovine lymphocyte antigens (BoLAs). The relative risk of lymphosarcoma in PL cattle versus non-PL, BLV-positive cattle has not been categorically established. A period of PL precedes tumor development in about two thirds of cattle that develop lymphosarcoma, but by no means are all cattle with PL assured of developing tumors; PL can be a stable state that exists for years. One study found no increased risk of lymphosarcoma in PL cows, but further studies are needed because the clinical impression of many clinicians is that a great deal more than 5% to 10% of all individually valuable BLV-positive PL cattle that are followed closely will develop lymphosarcoma over the course of their lifetime.

Another area of considerable debate over the 40 years or so since the virus was discovered has been to what extent chronic BLV infection affects the bovine immune system and whether or not infected cattle are negatively impacted in terms of milk production, reproductive health, or just general susceptibility to disease. There is no doubting the catastrophic effect of lymphosarcoma on the health and productivity of an individually affected cow; rarely do cows live more than a few months after this clinical diagnosis has been made. With individual seropositivity rates in the 35% to 50% range nationwide and more than 80% of all herds having at least some infected cattle, it is obviously of great interest to know whether there is an economic impact at the herd level. A great deal of basic science literature exists examining the interaction of BLV with the bovine immune system, cytokine expression in infected cattle, and the molecular aspects of BLV infection based on elegant in vitro experiments; however, only a very small number of studies have examined the influence of BLV infection on health and productivity in dairy cattle. At least one, fairly large, multivariate study in the United States by Ott and

colleagues revealed that BLV seropositive cattle produced approximately 3% less milk compared with noninfected cohorts, and others have confirmed the negative economic consequences of lymphosarcoma in herds. Recent data also suggest that BLV-positive cattle do not remain in the herd as long as BLV-negative cattle and that this reflects a financial loss for the farmer. The reasons for these observations are not clear. However, at this point in time, many herds largely ignore the disease, partly because the typical age of cattle with tumors is beginning to exceed the average age of cattle on most farms as the national herd becomes younger. Herds with a higher incidence of lymphosarcoma are undoubtedly impacted by the disease via lost productivity, increased susceptibility to other illnesses in cattle with tumors, and reduced cull value when a carcass is deemed unfit for human consumption because of the presence of tumors.

Investigations into the risk of BLV to human health date back to the 1970s, almost since the association of the virus with bovine lymphosarcoma was defined. Communities of people drinking raw milk, cancer patients, farm workers, and bovine veterinarians with a high degree of exposure to potentially infectious bodily fluids have been studied with no definitive link ever made to human illness, including clusters of leukemia, lymphomas, and other cancers, until very recently. Two related studies have defined both the presence of the BLV provirus genome in human breast tissue and an association between human breast cancer and the presence of BLV. These studies are raising new concerns about BLV infection, especially in dairy cattle, even as human-to-human transmission of this virus is also being considered based on a failure to epidemiologically link the presence of the virus in human tissue with behaviors that could account for direct transmission from cattle or consumption of infectious cattle products such as unpasteurized milk by those individuals.

Clinical Signs

Two facts must be emphasized preceding a discussion of signs observed in BLV-infected adult cattle having lymphosarcoma. The first is that fewer than 5% of all BLV-positive cattle develop tumors or illness associated with lymphosarcoma. Most BLV-infected cattle are asymptomatic and immune competent and can be as productive as their seronegative herdmates. Although several classic clinical presentations occur in cattle with lymphosarcoma as a result of specific target organ involvement, the majority require careful differentiation from a multitude of other diseases. The second important fact is therefore that lymphosarcoma can masquerade as a myriad of other inflammatory or debilitating diseases of cattle.

Clinical signs of lymphosarcoma seldom develop before 2 years of age and are most common in cattle between 3 and 6 years of age. Lymphosarcoma occurring in cattle younger than 2 years of age is *rarely* caused by BLV infection. For example, thymic, calf B-cell, juvenile T-cell, and most skin lymphosarcoma patients are younger than 2 years of age. These non-BLV (sporadic) associated forms of lymphosarcoma are discussed later.

Lymphosarcoma may occur in peripheral lymph nodes; internal lymph nodes; and specific target organs such as the abomasum, heart, uterus, retrobulbar space, and epidural region of the central nervous system (see images of lymphosarcoma in other chapters). Any or all of the aforementioned tissues may become neoplastic. In addition, atypical target sites such as the upper and lower respiratory tract, udder, forestomach, kidney, ureter, liver, spleen, and bone marrow may be affected. Chance mixing and matching of lesions in one or more locations is the rule and results in the tremendous variation in clinical signs observed in individual patients.

Most lymphosarcoma patients have nonspecific signs of weight loss, decreased appetite, and decreased production. However, lymphosarcoma cattle with one predominant lesion, such as epidural spinal cord compression, may suffer a rapid onset of clinical signs such as paresis and ataxia despite a normal appetite and body condition. The greater the number of tumors and the more visceral organs involved, the greater is the likelihood of weight loss, inappetence, and reduced production. If cattle with lymphosarcoma lived long enough, they might have neoplasms in many target areas. However, usually a tumor affecting one anatomic region predominates. Fever also may be present in a low percentage of lymphosarcoma patients, thereby confusing the differential diagnosis with inflammatory and infectious diseases. Fever, when present, is a result of tumor necrosis, secondary bacterial infections, or pyrogens associated with various cellular and soluble mediators of inflammation stimulated by neoplastic cells.

Peripheral lymph node enlargement of one or more external lymph nodes is found in approximately 25% of tumorous cows. Superficial cervical (prescapular), superficial inguinal (prefemoral), supramammary, submandibular, or retropharyngeal lymph nodes may be enlarged. Internal lymph nodes such as the sublumbar, mesenteric, or others may be found to be enlarged on rectal examination or laparotomy. Lymph node enlargements sometimes result in clinical consequences such as dyspnea (retropharyngeal) or bloat (retropharyngeal, mediastinal). Bloat occurs as a result of failure of, or interference with, eructation associated with pharyngeal or mediastinal lymph node neoplasia. Similarly, compressive neoplastic lymph nodes may interfere with effective air movement that usually occurs in the pharyngeal or laryngeal region, causing inspiratory dyspnea.

The intestinal tract is a common site for lymphosarcoma tumors. Although the abomasum is the most commonly affected area of the GI tract, the forestomach and intestines can also harbor neoplastic lesions. Abomasal lymphosarcoma can result in melena, signs of vagus indigestion, or simply inappetence and weight loss. Either diffuse infiltration or focal neoplasms can be found in the abomasum (see Figs. 5.75 and 5.76). When a major lymphosarcoma tumor involves the pylorus, abdominal distention typical of vagus indigestion results from interference with abomasal outflow. Bleeding from ulcerative neoplasms or mucosal ulcers resulting from lymphosarcoma infiltrates in the abomasal wall can cause occult fecal blood or obvious melena. Affected cattle also may

grind their teeth because of nonspecific abdominal or abomasal pain. Abomasal lymphosarcoma resulting in melena must be differentiated from primary abomasal ulceration.

Lymphosarcoma tumors in the rumen, reticulum, and omasum cause varying degrees of forestomach dysfunction, weight loss, reduced appetite and production, bloat, or signs of vagus indigestion. Such tumors are difficult to diagnose unless either abdominal fluid cytology or exploratory laparotomy is performed. Focal or diffuse lymphosarcoma masses or infiltrates may rarely involve the small or large intestine.

The uterus and reproductive tract constitute another common "target" location for lymphosarcoma. Neoplasms may be focal, multifocal, or diffuse. Classical uterine lymphosarcoma lesions consist of multifocal firm nodules or masses within the uterine wall (see Fig. 9.14). Palpation of such masses can be compared with palpation of caruncles in that they feel nodular or like raised umbilicated lesions with a central depression. Such lesions may be present in one or both uterine horns. Ovaries and oviducts occasionally are neoplastic as well. Large focal or diffuse tumors may completely involve the uterus or the entire caudal reproductive tract. Reproductive tract neoplasms are much easier to identify in nongravid tracts than in heavily pregnant cows, in which placentomes and the fetus frequently obscure the masses. Routine rectal palpations often uncover reproductive tract lymphosarcoma before development of overt systemic signs, but palpable uterine masses discovered per rectum must first be differentiated from other uterine tumors, as well as uterine and periuterine abscesses and hematomas.

Cardiac abnormalities, including arrhythmias, murmurs, pericardial effusions, muffling of heart sounds, venous distention, and signs of congestive heart failure, are possible consequences of lymphosarcoma affecting the myocardium, epicardium, or pericardium. The right atrium is reported to be the most common site of lymphosarcoma in the heart of cattle, but the tumor may affect any region of the heart or pericardium (see Fig. 3.19). Focal, multifocal, or diffuse neoplasia is possible, thereby explaining the plethora of potential clinical consequences. Cardiac lymphosarcoma may require differentiation from arrhythmias caused by primary electrolyte or GI disturbances, non-neoplastic myocardial lesions, septic pericarditis, cardiomyopathy, and endocarditis.

Respiratory signs associated with lymphosarcoma masses include inspiratory stridor resulting from nasal or upper airway infiltrates, lymph node enlargements, or tumor masses in the upper airway. Dyspnea of lower airway origin may reflect pleural effusions, pulmonary involvement, mediastinal masses, or congestive heart failure.

Ocular signs most commonly reflect involvement of the retrobulbar area as a common target location. Therefore progressive unilateral or bilateral exophthalmos progressing to pathologic exophthalmos and exposure damage to the globe represents the most common ophthalmic manifestation of lymphosarcoma in BLV-positive cattle that develop tumors (see Figs. 14.7 and 14.8). Although the retrobulbar masses or

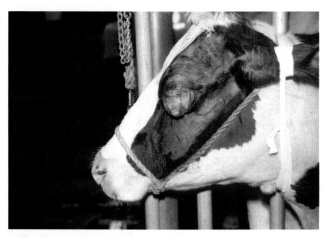

• **Fig. 16.11** Lymphosarcoma in the left retrobulbar region causing pathologic exophthalmos and exposure damage to the globe.

infiltrate usually progress over several weeks, the subsequent appearance of the eye associated with pathologic exophthalmos can appear to be acute as the eyelids lose the ability to completely protect the protruding globe (Fig. 16.11). Corneal exposure damage, desiccation, and profound chemosis generally develop quickly. Although the rate of progression may vary in retrobulbar lymphosarcoma, cattle usually are affected bilaterally if they survive long enough.

Tumors of lymphosarcoma in the epidural region of the spinal cord cause progressive paresis and eventual paralysis consistent with the anatomic location of the tumor. Posterior paresis and paralysis are most common because of the frequency of tumors in the thoracolumbar, lumbar, or sacral areas. However, cervical and cranial thoracic lesions are possible such that tetraparesis may be observed. Tumors in the extradural space may again be focal, multifocal, or diffuse. Lymphosarcoma of the brain also has been observed but is much less common than compressive spinal cord neoplasia and is actually rarely BLV associated. Although not a firm rule, compressive lymphosarcoma affecting the spinal cord frequently causes neurologic signs before the patient's physical status (e.g., appetite, body condition) has deteriorated to such a degree that a neoplastic process would be considered likely. Therefore compressive lymphosarcoma is commonly confused with metabolic conditions or spinal injuries (see Chapters 12 and 13). Cattle with lymphosarcoma masses compressing the spinal cord usually progress from paresis to paralysis within 2 to 7 days. During this time, they may be noticed to have difficulty rising, require manual assistance (lifting them by the tail) to rise or make repeated attempts before being able to rise (see Figs. 13.40 to 13.43). Loss of tail and anal tone and perineal desensitization may also be seen with caudal lymphosarcoma lesions involving the lumbosacral spinal cord and cauda equina. Symptomatic treatment with corticosteroids may result in temporary clinical improvement.

Lymphosarcoma can affect the urinary system by direct or indirect mechanisms. Perirenal lymph node enlargement may result in reduced renal perfusion, renal infarcts, or prerenal azotemia when both kidneys have vascular compromise.

Diffuse lymphosarcoma in one or both ureters may cause hydronephrosis, hematuria, colic, or postrenal azotemia (if bilateral). Neoplasms in the bladder or urethra may cause hydronephrosis, hydroureter, hematuria, tenesmus, dribbling of urine, or colic. Extradural spinal cord compressive neoplasms affecting sacral segments also may cause bladder dysfunction. Renal tumors may result in no outward signs, renal colic, renal azotemia (if bilateral), hematuria, or other signs. Tumors affecting the urinary system frequently are palpable on rectal or vaginal examinations. Enlargement of the left kidney may be appreciated on routine rectal examination, and this should prompt ultrasonographic evaluation of both kidneys transrectally and/or transabdominally. Significant differentials for renal lymphosarcoma include other nonpainful, firm masses such as those encountered with renal carcinomas and renal amyloidosis. The normal shape of the kidney as well as ultrasonographic architecture is often lost with renal lymphosarcoma. Definitive diagnosis may be reached by biopsy.

Lymphosarcoma tumors associated with the mammary gland or mammary lymph nodes may be occult or overt. The mammary lymph nodes are more likely to be clinically affected than the mammary glands, and neoplastic enlargement of the supramammary lymph nodes—unilateral or bilateral—is common (see Fig. 8.10, *A*). Occasionally, mammary lymph node involvement will lead to either asymmetrical or symmetrical udder edema as the first recognized abnormality. Diffuse infiltration or focal lymphosarcoma tumors are possible in one or more mammary glands and are best detected by palpation and ultrasound of the glands. Percutaneous biopsy rather than fine-needle aspirate is the preferred diagnostic procedure for focal or mammary lymph node enlargement suspected to be lymphosarcoma.

Rarely, skin tumors appear in adult lymphosarcoma patients. Such tumors are firm and either nodular or plaque-like. Skin tumors may vary from 5 to 20 cm in diameter. The skin of the trunk or udder is generally involved (see Figs. 7.10–7.12). Enlargement of hemal lymph nodes, most apparent in the region of the paralumbar fossa, is generally a benign finding and is rarely, if ever, associated with lymphosarcoma in dairy cattle. Diffuse splenic neoplasia caused by BLV-positive lymphosarcoma is a form of lymphosarcoma in adult cattle and, although usually accompanied by gross or microscopic neoplasia in other visceral locations, may be the only identifiable lesion. Diffuse splenic lymphosarcoma may result in splenic capsular rupture, subsequent fatal intraabdominal hemorrhage, and acute death. This lesion is observed as the cause of fatal exsanguination approximately once yearly by the Necropsy Service at the Cornell University Veterinary College. Abdominal hemorrhage causing acute death is not rare in adult dairy cattle, most have no proven etiology, but only a few are caused by lymphosarcoma.

Lymphosarcoma masses are possible in virtually any tissue, and cattle with lymphosarcoma in one or more organs may be presented without classical target organ involvement. Visceral or body cavity masses with or without lymphadenopathy can occur. Adult BLV-positive cattle with lymphosarcoma seldom survive more than a few weeks to a few months, and almost all succumb within 6 months. There may be a temporary response to corticosteroids, but treatment is seldom attempted. Occasionally, cattle with lymphosarcoma that are in the last trimester of pregnancy can be successfully treated palliatively in terms of reaching parturition. However, the prognosis beyond palliative treatment for more than a few weeks is hopeless. It is possible to see some success with the use of nonabortifacient corticosteroids in late pregnancy, typically prednisone (1 mg/kg daily) or isoflupredone acetate, in the treatment of cattle with retrobulbar, thoracic, or abdominal visceral tumors. It should be remembered that dexamethasone is highly unlikely to cause abortion in the first 150 days of gestation, so this may be an option for open cows with lymphosarcoma, for which the only goal is to retrieve oocytes or embryos for preservation of genetic merit. However, many of these individuals will be in such a catabolic state that normal cyclicity in unlikely, and their response to superovulation protocols may be muted. Occasionally, severely catabolic cows with lymphosarcoma that are "limped" through to parturition will give birth to very dysmature calves, even if they are term at delivery. These calves are also commonly infected in utero, and bull calves would therefore be of little value. Such calves have high perinatal mortality rates and can be challenging to save. Clinicians at the University of Wisconsin have on occasion used specific chemotherapeutic protocols involving agents such as vincristine, L-asparaginase, and cyclophosphamide in the treatment of individual cows with lymphosarcoma that have extreme genetic and financial merit, but the use of these drugs is obviously prohibited in animals whose milk or meat is intended for human consumption, and the use of such large doses of highly toxic drugs would require hospitalization and careful removal of wastes. L-asparaginase treatment was a very effective "rescue treatment" in a pet farm animal with lymphosarcoma. Palliative treatment of a late pregnant cow with pericardial lymphosarcoma by pericardectomy has also been performed at Cornell.

Sporadic bovine leukosis (SBL) has classically been divided into three forms—the juvenile form, the thymic form, and the skin form. The juvenile form is multicentric and can occur in very young calves up to 6 months of age (sometimes referred to as the calf form), but it may also be seen in cattle up to 24 months of age. It is usually of B-cell origin. The most obvious clinical sign with the juvenile or calf form is diffuse lymphadenopathy that results in obvious and palpable enlargement of peripheral lymph nodes (see Fig. 4.4). Such calves commonly are presented for evaluation because of recurrent or persistent bloat or because of dyspnea. Rare cases of congenital lymphosarcoma are possible (Fig. 16.12). Visceral tumors are possible in calves with juvenile or calf lymphosarcoma, and bone marrow lesions and peripheral leukemia are also common in 4- to 7-month-old calves with the juvenile form. Occasionally, single tumors are found (e.g., in the cerebral cortex). The Milking

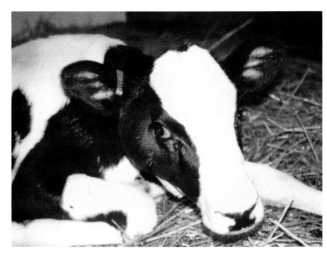

• **Fig. 16.12** Newborn heifer calf with juvenile multicentric lymphosarcoma. Note the huge retropharyngeal lymph node enlargement. The heifer was one of a pair of twins, both of which were born with sporadic lymphosarcoma.

Shorthorn breed seems to have a higher incidence of juvenile or calf lymphosarcoma than the other dairy breeds.

The thymic and skin forms tend to be T cell in origin. Thymic lymphosarcoma usually is observed in 6- to 24-month-old cattle. Progressive enlargement of the thymus occurs in all cases but is most apparent clinically when cervical enlargement develops. In some thymic lymphosarcoma patients, the majority of thymic enlargement remains in the thorax. Most patients, however, develop a caudal cervical swelling, which may progress in a cranial direction to the mid or cranial ventral cervical region. As with juvenile lymphosarcoma patients, the chief complaint for thymic lymphosarcoma heifers usually is either bloat or dyspnea (see Fig. 4.94). External compression of the esophagus interferes with effective eructation, and tracheal compression, pulmonary displacement or compression, pleural effusion, and pulmonary edema contribute to signs of dyspnea. Exceptionally large thymic masses within the thorax or thoracic inlet also may cause jugular vein distention as a result of reduced venous return and thus interfere with cardiac and pulmonary function to such a degree that heart failure may be suspected. A thoracic mass may be suspected based on muffled heart sounds or reduced air sounds in the ventral hemithorax unilaterally or bilaterally. Fever is a common sign, but the exact mechanism of fever in these cases is poorly understood. The presence of fever causes clinical confusion with abscesses, cellulitis, esophageal lacerations, and other inflammatory diseases. Fever may result from tumor necrosis, tumor-induced pyrogens or mediators, or secondary respiratory infections. Palpation of cervical masses resulting from thymic lymphosarcoma can be misleading because the masses may feel soft, fluctuant, or edematous in some patients. In others, the lesions palpate as firm or hard, thus appearing more consistent with neoplasia. Cervical enlargements may be so soft, edematous, or fluctuant as to suggest fluid distention. However, attempts at aspiration reveal little, if any, fluid, but fine-needle aspirates and particularly biopsies confirm the lesions as lymphosarcoma. Tumors may be present in other locations in some patients having thymic lymphosarcoma. One interesting epidemic of thymic lymphosarcoma in BLV-free herds was described in calves 4 to 10 months of age in France during 1987 and 1988. Of the 73 calves affected, 67 were sired by the same bull. Genetic implications have not been described in the United States, possibly because of a lack of cases.

The "skin form" of lymphosarcoma is rare, sporadic, occurs in cattle younger than 30 months of age, and usually affects cattle that are seronegative for BLV. Multiple skin nodules appear on the neck, trunk, and rear quarters (see Fig. 7.11). The lesions become more numerous and enlarge over a period of months. Lymphadenopathy may accompany the skin lesions or appear later in the course of the disease. Lesions may become so numerous that they appear confluent (see Fig. 7.11). Although cattle with skin lymphosarcoma appear otherwise healthy during the early phase of the disease, their body condition and health deteriorate over 6 to 12 months, and eventually these cattle succumb to diffuse neoplasia. Insects severely irritate cattle having skin lymphosarcoma. Insect bites may cause superficial dermatitis or bleeding from the skin nodules, and some lymph nodes may become abscessed. Scores of skin nodules are often present in this form of the disease and allow clinical differentiation from adult lymphosarcoma, in which occasionally an individual or a few skin lesions accompany visceral lesions.

All forms of SBL are rare and mostly occur in cattle younger than 2 years of age. On rare occasion non-BLV associated lymphosarcoma will be found in one or more organs in adult cattle. In the sporadic form, the tumors are not caused by BLV infection, and most, but not all, cattle with SBL are BLV seronegative. Tumor cells of sporadic lymphosarcomas represent immature lineages of T and less commonly B cells. The proto-oncogene, c-myb, is expressed in most sporadic lymphosarcomas but not enzootic lymphosarcomas.

Diagnosis

The diagnosis of BLV infection in cattle has been historically achieved using serologic techniques such as the agar gel immunodiffusion (AGID) or ELISA tests. Recently, PCR tests for identification of the virus in blood have been developed and successfully applied. After infection with BLV virus, most cattle remain persistently infected despite the production of serum antibodies against the virus. Original AGID serologic tests detected antibody to BLV-p24, which is a major core polypeptide that was the first recognized internal protein of BLV, but subsequently, it was discovered that sensitivity was significantly increased when AGID tests that detected antibody to gp 51 were used, principally because antibodies to this glycoprotein are produced earlier in infection and to higher titers overall. The gp 51 antigen is the major external envelope glycoprotein of the virus and plays an important role in viral binding to host cells. The envelope gp 51 antigen may also induce neutralizing activity against BLV, inhibit activity of released virus, and

deter extracellular BLV activity. The most recent iterations of the AGID test incorporate both p24 and gp 51 antigens but have been largely superseded by ELISA tests detecting antibody to gp 51 because the latter offers between 10- and 100-fold greater sensitivity. This means that ELISA tests can be used to examine pooled samples if requested as well as those from individual cows or calves. Furthermore, ELISA assays can also be performed on samples other than blood, to include individual and bulk tank milk samples. Some cattle with lymphosarcoma or PL will have "double-line positive" results when tested by AGID assays that detect antibody to both p24 and gp51. Such results should not, however, be viewed as diagnostic for neoplasia.

After infection of a susceptible cow with BLV, antibodies may be detected by the AGID in 3 to 12 weeks. Although this "lag time" between infection and AGID-detectable levels of antibody has been used to criticize AGID testing, the AGID remains a well-accepted test because of high specificity, high sensitivity, simplicity, and proven ability to provide effective screening to assist in the elimination of BLV infection in cattle populations. The AGID is still required as the test of choice for export testing of cattle to some countries. Because of its greater sensitivity, ELISA has become the industry standard diagnostic serologic test for BLV in the United States and Canada.

A positive AGID or ELISA result would be expected in calves that received colostral antibodies from BLV-positive dams and infection in those young animals could only be confirmed by PCR. However, caution should be used in interpreting negative PCR test results in seropositive animals, based on studies with delayed detection of infection using PCR testing in experimental animals that were infected while vaccine-induced antibodies were present. As previously mentioned, passively acquired maternal antibodies usually decrease to undetectable levels by 6 to 7 months of age, but biologic variation will affect the exact length of time required for passive decay. Therefore, a positive AGID or ELISA result in a calf younger than 6 months of age may either reflect an actual infection or be caused by passive antibodies acquired in colostrum. False-negative findings usually result from failure to detect antibodies during early infection, usually thought to range from 3 to 12 weeks when the AGID test is used. The greater ability of ELISA tests to detect lower levels of antibody to gp 51 means that this technique can be diagnostic as early as 2 weeks after infection and it rarely has a lag interval of more than 6 weeks from initial infection. Some false-negative findings, however, may reflect a decrease in circulating antibody levels in a BLV-infected animal. This most commonly occurs around the time of parturition as maternal antibodies, in effect, "drain" into the udder. The period from 2 weeks before parturition to 6 weeks postpartum may be associated with an overall decrease in antibody levels and is not a recommended time for testing, especially when using the AGID. If this decrease causes antibody levels to fall below detectable AGID levels, a false-negative result may occur. Rarely a false-negative AGID results from failure of host antibody response.

Blood PCR tests may equal or exceed the sensitivity of serologic tests at some future time but will need to become much more economical to displace serologic testing as the method of choice. Pooled serum samples from groups or herds may be surveyed by the ELISA test to detect low levels of infection that may prompt individual testing.

Diagnostic efforts may incorporate ELISA herd screening, milk screening of bulk samples utilizing new ELISA or PCR technology, or other tests and detection of tumor-associated antigens. Tumor-associated antigens are detectable by monoclonal antibodies specific for polypeptides on lymphosarcoma cells. Seropositive BLV cattle commonly do not (≤10%) have detectable tumor-associated antigens. However, lymphosarcoma patients and PL cattle appear almost always to have such antigens.

The diagnosis of lymphosarcoma may require only a physical examination when lymphadenopathy and obvious (or palpable) target organ neoplasia is present. However, most patients with lymphosarcoma require some diagnostic aids. The best aids are cytology or biopsy collected from effusions or target organs. A positive ELISA or other serum-antibody test result adds an index of suspicion but cannot be considered definitive because fewer than 5% of all BLV-positive cattle develop tumors. Peripheral lymphocytosis adds a stronger index of suspicion but again does not equate with lymphosarcoma in all cases.

Taking samples of abdominal and thoracic fluid may be helpful when large tumors are suspected in these body cavities. Cytology of such fluid may sometimes reveal abnormal lymphocytes that confirm a suspected diagnosis. This is most helpful when thoracic effusion, pericardial effusion, or large abdominal (abomasal) tumors are present. Lymph node aspirates or biopsies confirm a diagnosis of lymphosarcoma in some patients that have obviously enlarged lymph nodes. However, it is common to have such lymph node samples interpreted as reactive or hyperplastic rather than definitively neoplastic, although this seems less common when a biopsy is obtained rather than a simple aspirate. Pelvic or reproductive tract masses may be aspirated or biopsied through the vagina in some cattle to confirm a diagnosis of lymphosarcoma. Ultrasound may be helpful in conjunction with aspirates or biopsies for visceral masses within body cavities, the retrobulbar space, or the heart.

Forestomach neoplasia, abomasal neoplasia, and other visceral involvement may require laparotomy to confirm the diagnosis when other ancillary tests have failed to define lymphosarcoma.

Perhaps the two most difficult, yet common, clinical situations in which to confirm suspected lymphosarcoma occur when compressive spinal neoplasia or abomasal infiltration occurs. Unless other target organ lesions or lymph node enlargements are apparent, definitive diagnosis in these anatomic areas can be difficult. When the abomasum is suspected to have lymphosarcoma based on occult or gross melena, weight loss, inappetence, and bruxism, an abdominal paracentesis is indicated. If cytology of this fluid

is not helpful, a laparotomy may be necessary. Compressive lymphosarcoma causing paresis or paralysis in cattle with no other detectable evidence of lymphosarcoma requires a cerebrospinal fluid (CSF) analysis, usually from the lumbosacral region when spinal cord signs predominate. The CSF from such patients often is normal but may have increased protein levels in some instances. In addition, a lesser percentage of these patients will have neoplastic lymphocytes present in the CSF; most likely this occurs as a result of the needle passing through the extradural tumor "en route" to the CSF. When no fluid is obtained from the lumbosacral space but the clinician is confident that the space has been entered with the spinal needle, aspirates should still be attempted because the space occasionally is obliterated by a neoplastic mass (see Figs. 13.41 and 13.43). Although uncommon (<10% of lymphosarcoma patients), true leukemia may be detected by CBCs in some patients with lymphosarcoma. Serum lactic acid dehydrogenase values also may be elevated in some cattle with lymphosarcoma, but this finding is not specific for the disease.

The diagnosis of atypical (sporadic) lymphosarcoma in the juvenile, thymic, calf, and skin forms is relatively easy. Lymph node aspirates or biopsies suffice for the juvenile form, and skin biopsies confirm the skin form. The thymic form may be diagnosed by aspirates, biopsies, thoracocentesis, or ultrasound-guided biopsy.

Control

Control measures for BLV infection in dairy herds may be easy when the prevalence of BLV-positive cattle is low. Under such circumstances serologic testing of all cattle and calves can be performed. Positive cattle and calves older than 6 months could be culled. Seropositive calves less than 6 months of age can be either segregated and retested at 9 months of age or tested by PCR. A positive PCR test result will confirm infection, but a negative test result may not fully exclude infection. Extremely valuable BLV-positive cattle may be superovulated and their embryos placed in seronegative heifers or cows. Infected cattle to be used as embryo donors should have embryos collected without cell contamination and implanted only in noninfected recipients, and recipients should ideally be maintained in a seronegative herd. However, the continued existence of BLV-positive cows is a detriment to eradication of BLV in the herd; this is especially true for PL cows.

If serologic tests are used in a control program, limitations of the test must be recognized. Early infections may yield false-negative results as may some periparturient cows, especially if AGID testing is used. Therefore repeat testing of the entire negative herd is required in 3 to 6 months after a first whole herd–negative result. Several programs have been suggested to eliminate BLV infection from herds, and guidelines were devised by the U.S. Animal Health Association in 1980 to establish BLV-free herds. New York and some other states have also sponsored programs to achieve BLV-free status, but the outcome of such programs has frequently been disappointing. The establishment and maintenance of BLV free herds on a national level has been achieved in a number of European countries.

Stringent culling programs do entail economic losses and are most applicable when a low prevalence of infection exists in the herd. In addition, control measures to deter horizontal spread should be used. These measures include both veterinary and management techniques such as single needle and syringe use, electric dehorning, disinfection of all common instruments between uses (chlorhexidine or chlorine bleach), individual rectal sleeves, stringent insect control, and avoidance of purchasing new animals. Vertical and much of the horizontal transmission can be avoided by culling all PL cattle. Feeding calves colostrum or milk only from BLV-negative cows, pasteurizing or freezing BLV-positive colostrum or milk before feeding, feeding milk replacer to calves after they ingest preferably BLV-negative colostrum, and using only seronegative embryo recipients are other routine recommendations.

If economics disallow test and slaughter, various other plans can be devised such as testing and segregating seropositive cattle away from seronegative cattle. Segregation must be enforced, and facilities such as milking areas must be separate. In addition, management practices to prevent horizontal or in utero spread must be used as outlined earlier. Segregation does allow positive cattle to be productive and culled by attrition over time. When segregation is enforced, the seronegative herd may remain seronegative. Identification and elimination of PL cattle and lymphosarcoma patients should be performed as quickly as possible.

When neither test and slaughter nor test and segregate is feasible because of economic or management factors, control through testing and corrective management procedures may be the only alternative. Corrective practices to reduce horizontal or vertical spread, as outlined earlier, may reduce the prevalence of BLV infection over time. Separation of young stock and adult cows may decrease prevalence when combined with corrective management techniques. Most programs devised to institute corrective measures can reduce but not eliminate BLV infection. Gradual reduction in prevalence over time will require constant vigilance in management practices and may allow the herd to eventually cull positive animals when the percentage of infected animals becomes acceptably low.

Experimental vaccines have been used against BLV, but there are no commercially available products at this time. Inactivated virus, virus components, and lymphoblastoid cell lines from calves with lymphosarcoma have been used to instigate resistance to BLV challenge. Results have been variable and reflect experimental design, antigenic dose of vaccine, and challenge variables. Successful vaccines would require that vaccinates produce specific antibodies that could be differentiated from those antibodies produced by BLV-seropositive, naturally infected cattle. Therefore, for example, if vaccine incorporated only gp 51, diagnostic tests to detect infection would need to detect antibody against p24 or other antigens to differentiate seropositive vaccinates

from infected cows. Alternatively, diagnostic tests might identify proviral DNA in naturally infected cattle by PCR.

Bovine Immunodeficiency Virus

Etiology

Bovine immunodeficiency virus (BIV) is a lentivirus infection of cattle with a worldwide distribution. Serologic and molecular evidence of BIV infection exist in several regions, including the United States, Canada, and Europe. There appears to be great variation regionally and even within herds with respect to the prevalence of infection, but with the advent of more sensitive diagnostic PCR techniques for the identification of proviral BIV sequences, it is evident that some herds may have infection rates of greater than 50%. Previous serologic surveys have only identified seroprevalence rates of between 1% and 6% in Europe and North America. It appears that infection rates are higher in dairy herds compared with beef cattle. The exact mode of transmission for BIV is uncertain, but it is probable that horizontal transmission in body fluids such as blood, milk, semen, and colostrum represents the major means of spread and that very similar risk factors would apply for the transmission of BIV as exist for the transmission of BLV. Natural transplacental infection is possible, and proviral DNA of BIV has been found in frozen-thawed semen.

Clinical Signs

The clinical relevance of BIV infection is uncertain. Although the virus was first discovered in 1969, there have been no compelling experimental studies or reports of naturally occurring disease describing consistent signs in infected cattle. Lymphocytosis and lymphadenopathy have been documented after experimental infection, but the health consequences of BIV infection are not clear. Furthermore, the economic implications of BIV infection are similarly debatable, although trends toward lower milk production and higher incidences of other common diseases are reported in high seroprevalence herds.

Diagnosis

The diagnosis of BIV infection requires either serologic confirmation of an antibody response to the virus by either an IFA or Western blot assay or PCR amplification of proviral DNA sequences. The latter is much more sensitive but not commonly available commercially.

Treatment

Because of its questionable relevance clinically, there are no specific treatment or control measures commonly used for the prevention or eradication of BIV infection. In herds in which diagnostic testing has demonstrated a high prevalence of infection, similar control measures as adopted for BLV may be instituted.

Lyme Disease

Etiology

Lyme disease or Lyme borreliosis is an infectious disease of humans and animals caused by *Borrelia burgdorferi*, a spirochete. The disease is common in humans and dogs in Connecticut and other eastern areas of the United States, the Midwest, Texas, and California. Lyme disease is spread by ticks, especially deer ticks; *Ixodes scapularis* in the east and *Ixodes pacificus* in the west. These ticks have a complicated 2-year life cycle that involves three hosts. Adult ticks feed on vertebrate hosts during warm weather and overwinter in the ground. Adult females lay eggs in the spring, and larvae hatch from these eggs 1 month later. Larvae usually feed once and then become dormant through fall and winter before emerging the following spring as nymphs. Larvae and nymphs commonly feed on white-footed mice from which they obtain *B. burgdorferi*. Nymphs mature to adults and attach to hosts during the warm months. Although deer are the usual hosts for adult ticks, humans and domestic animals may provide suitable alternatives and can therefore be infected with *B. burgdorferi* carried from the white-footed mouse to the new host by nymph or adult ticks. Nymphs of these ticks are extremely small (1–2 mm) and may be difficult to observe on hosts, such that bites may go undetected. At least one study has demonstrated significant numbers of adult ticks in pastures with heifers and dry cows, suggesting a fairly high risk for exposure, but farmhouse yards and forage croplands appear to represent negligible risk.

After infection occurs, several possible consequences may develop in any species including cattle. Subclinical infections with seroconversion are common, and it is likely that only a small percentage of infected animals develop detectable clinical signs. The pathogenetic mechanisms that determine whether infection will produce clinical consequences are poorly understood. In most species, fever, skin rashes (early signs), lameness, neurologic signs, and visceral infections indicate a septicemic spread of the organism after the initial skin infection. A delayed inflammatory response may occur at the site of the original tick bite, and *B. burgdorferi* apparently causes delayed hypersensitivity reactions, immune complexing, and other immunologic factors involved in manifestations of disease in several anatomic areas. Therefore acute local and septicemic consequences can evolve into delayed, immunologically triggered pathology. The acute infection may be mild, inapparent, or misdiagnosed unless a characteristic skin rash is present, the latter being quite unlikely to be noticed in the majority of cattle. Because many infections apparently do not result in clinical disease, diagnostic tests that determine antibody levels are of limited value. In cattle, the organism has been found in blood and urine. Urine may provide a means of transmission because it appears some infected cattle shed *B. burgdorferi* in urine for prolonged periods.

Clinical Signs

The clinical consequences of *B. burgdorferi* infection in cattle have not been well described, and there is little evidence that Lyme disease is a clinically significant entity in cattle. Clinical signs that have been observed in association with *Borrelia* seroconversion include fever, lameness, stiffness, joint distention in one or more joints, swollen lower limbs, and abortions. Cows in a district of Switzerland known to harbor ixodid ticks had *B. burgdorferi* detected in synovial fluid and milk, and signs in these animals included erythematous lesions on the hairless skin of the udder, poor general condition with decreased appetite and milk production, alongside a stiff gait and swollen joints.

Lower limb swelling, distended joints with mononuclear cell inflammation, and other musculoskeletal consequences result in lameness, reluctance to rise or move, and secondary injuries and decubital sores. Therefore, especially when first-calf heifers are affected with these signs, laminitis, "concrete disease" (resulting from poor heifer adaptation to confinement), infection with *Mycoplasma wenyoni*, and vitamin E or selenium deficiency should be ruled out before any consideration is given to Lyme disease! A study from Minnesota and Wisconsin associated high levels of antibody against *B. burgdorferi* with lameness in dairy cattle. Abortion appears to be either a sporadic or endemic consequence of *B. burgdorferi* infection in cattle. In one group of cattle being studied because of persistent urinary shedding of *B. burgdorferi*, 3 of 12 subsequently aborted.

The organism may be found in milk from some infected cattle but is killed by pasteurization.

Diagnosis

Absolute diagnosis of *B. burgdorferi* infection requires a combination of clinical signs, serologic testing or identification of the agent, and judgment. Because serum antibodies do not necessarily indicate disease and may persist for long periods or even for life, diagnosis based only on serology should be avoided. At present, Western blot tests that apply suspect serum to an electrophoresis of *B. burgdorferi* proteins appear to be the most specific diagnostic tests performed on serum from clinical bovine suspects.

When *B. Burgdorferi* is considered as the probable cause of illness in cattle, a specialized diagnostic laboratory capable of isolation techniques, which are very difficult, or PCR in conjunction with Western blot analysis of serum should be contacted for help. The incidence and prevalence of disease caused by *B. burgdorferi* in cattle are unknown. Some reports demonstrate fairly high exposure levels based on serology, but the occurrence of clinical disease is much less frequent.

Treatment

Because the disease is poorly defined in cattle, treatment efficacy is impossible to evaluate. In most species, tetracycline family and beta-lactam antibiotics are used to treat Lyme disease. Whereas antibiotics may or may not successfully clear infection, their role in counteracting immunologically mediated consequences of infection is even less apparent. Tick control may be valuable for cattle in endemic regions for Lyme disease.

Sarcocystosis

Etiology

Infection of ruminant skeletal or cardiac muscle tissue by *Sarcocystis* spp. is extremely common, and although lesions may be present to some degree in more than 75% of cattle, most infections only can be detected histologically rather than grossly. However, sarcocystosis is very much a "dose-related" disease, with lower infective doses causing inapparent infection and massive doses causing acute fulminant disease characterized by anemia, anorexia, fever, neurologic signs, lameness, loss of tail switch (rat tail), or abortion. The occurrence of naturally occurring disease appears to be so low that it is unlikely that modern dairy cattle are exposed to the higher end doses necessary for fulminant illness.

Cattle are a secondary host for three major species— *Sarcocystis cruzi, Sarcocystis hominis,* and *Sarcocystis hirsuta*—whose definitive hosts are dogs, primates, and cats, respectively. Most reports of clinical disease in calves and cows for which speciation was known have been associated with *S. cruzi*. Definitive hosts are infected by eating contaminated bovine tissues harboring the sporozoan. Ingested encysted sporozoites become bradyzoites, undergo sexual reproduction, and form oocysts in the gut lamina propria, and oocysts develop into sporocysts containing sporozoites. Sporulated oocysts are shed for weeks to months by the definitive host, and infection does not preclude reinfection. Cattle are infected by ingestion of feed contaminated by feces containing oocysts from a definitive host. Sporozoites are released in the abomasum and invade capillaries. Merozoites and schizonts remain in blood vessels (usually endothelial cells); more merozoites are produced and spread through the bloodstream to muscle and other organs. This life cycle is extremely complex, and further reproductive cycles may be involved. In any event, eventually *Sarcocystis* cysts are formed in muscle.

Cattle of all ages are susceptible, but infection tends to be more severe in calves or previously naive adult cattle suddenly exposed to great numbers of infective oocysts. Severely infected cattle develop vasculitis and extravascular hemolysis leading to anemia. The hemolysis is likely immune mediated, and DIC has been observed experimentally. Neurologic and reproductive consequences have been described but may require reevaluation and differentiation from *Neospora* spp. since the discovery of *Neospora caninum* (see Chapter 9) as a cause of abortion. Experimental infections with *Sarcocystis* spp. can cause abortion during the second trimester.

Clinical Signs

Clinical signs in cattle may appear approximately 1 to 3 months after ingestion of infective sporocysts. Experimental doses have consisted of 100,000 or more sporocysts. How frequently this level of infection occurs naturally is unknown. However, when clinical signs are observed, fever, anorexia, anemia, weight loss, lameness, lymphadenopathy, salivation, weakness, neurologic signs, and GI abnormalities

may be observed. Hair loss around the eyelids, neck, and tail switch (rat tail) has also been observed. Anemia characterized as a hemolytic extravascular immune-mediated phenomenon may be life threatening, or fatal, and associated with DIC and elevated indirect bilirubin levels. Abortion may occur, especially during the second trimester, and may reflect fetal infection, or maternal stress.

Neurologic signs are associated with inflammatory lesions in the central nervous system, and weakness may reflect the combined effects of myopathy and anemia.

Diagnosis

Although indirect hemagglutination, ELISA, and AGID tests are available for serologic testing of antibody levels against the parasite, these tests are largely limited to specialized laboratories. Early IgM antibody responses appear by 1 month after infection and peak at 3 to 4 months, but IgG increases by 6 weeks and peaks by 3 months. Speciation of *Sarcocystis* organisms is very much a recent, and predominantly research tool, but molecular differentiation of the three species known to infect cattle in North America and Europe can be achieved by PCR of tissue samples from microscopically detected infections.

Clinical signs may be very helpful in severe cases but obviously limited in subclinical or low-grade infections. Postmortem lesions in overwhelming acute infections consist of anemia, multifocal hemorrhages, lymphadenopathy, flaccid edematous striated muscle with alternating light and dark striations, myocardial hemorrhages and myopathy, and a pale liver. Histologically, inflammatory granulomatous encephalomyelitis, intravascular schizonts, or IM schizonts may be observed. Chronic infection may be detected by *Sarcocystis* cysts within striated or cardiac muscle. Frequently, *Sarcocystis* cysts are found in striated or cardiac muscle as incidental findings in cattle dying of other causes.

Treatment

Most references to treatment have described experimental infections, and the efficacy or practicality of therapeutic intervention in field situations is unknown. Amprolium, monensin, and other ionophores may be somewhat effective for prophylaxis, but the effect of these drugs for treatment of infected cattle has not been determined.

Control

Breaking the life cycle of *Sarcocystis* spp. by prompt and complete removal of cattle carcasses and preventing definitive host feces from contaminating cattle feed appear to be the best means of control.

Heat Stroke and Heat Stress

Although certainly not an infectious disease, heat stroke is included within this section because veterinarians are commonly called on to differentiate environmentally induced hyperthermia from true fever associated with infectious disease.

Etiology

High ambient temperatures and humidity predispose to heat stress and, in the most severe instances, heatstroke. The predominant dairy breeds in the United States originate from northern Europe, the British Isles, and western Europe and are well adapted to a temperate climate. In the United States, these animals tend to fare well in the northern states with cold winters and moderate summer temperatures. However, the effects of heat stress can be profound on such animals that are better adapted to milder conditions. High relative humidity exacerbates the impact of ambient temperature, and therefore the potential for heat stress is more closely related to a temperature-humidity index than to environmental temperature alone. Heat stress may be a significant animal welfare challenge facing some dairy herds. The greatest heat stress problems occur in the humid southern and central states. Affected cows show increased core body temperature, altered respiration, abnormal GI function, increased water loss, reduced feed intake, reduced and altered milk production, delivery of low-birth-weight calves, reduced reproductive performance, and other negative effects. The problem can also occur in northern areas of the country but generally is less common and less profound. The means to reduce the impact of heat on cattle include modified shelters, fans that move large volumes of air around the cattle, water-spraying misters, and alterations in diet.

Cattle stressed by handling, shipment, recumbency, or confinement in poorly ventilated areas are prone to heat stroke. Cattle with preexisting respiratory diseases or pyrexia caused by other diseases also are at greater risk. Hypocalcemic cows and cows with hepatic lipidosis that lose thermoregulatory ability can develop heat stroke if recumbent in poorly ventilated areas or in direct sunshine during periods of high ambient temperature and humidity. Dairy cattle that are not ventilated adequately or cooled during times of heat stress frequently have body temperatures of 103.5°F (39.72°C) or more, and minimal additional stress is necessary to increase body temperatures to 106.0°F (41.11°C) or higher. Earlier than anticipated heat and humidity extremes during late spring or early summer may predispose to heat stroke in cattle and heifers that have not fully shed out winter coats and therefore have less efficient heat loss. Most heat loss in cattle occurs from the respiratory tract, and such heat loss may create a vicious cycle of progressive tachypnea, dyspnea, and ultimately pulmonary edema, which interferes with (rather than aiding) heat loss. Heat stroke is relatively common in adult dairy cattle and occasionally occurs in young stock or calves. Fatal DIC has been reported in a calf with exertional heat stress.

Clinical Signs and Diagnosis

Tachypnea (>60 breaths/min) coupled with a rectal temperature greater than 105.0°F (40.56°C) in the absence of an infectious or inflammatory etiology signals heat stroke in cattle exposed to high heat and humidity. Most cows will begin to breathe with an open mouth, exhibit excessive salivation, and have an anxious expression. Tachycardia of 100 beats/min or more is common. Obvious pulmonary edema is apparent as frothy discharge at the mouth or nose in severe cases. Body temperature continues to increase, and prostration, weakness, and recumbency may develop at temperatures greater than 106.0°F (41.11°C). Neurologic damage is possible when core temperature reaches or exceeds 108.0°F (42.22°C).

Clinical signs of tachypnea, tachycardia, hyperthermia, and exertional dyspnea, pulmonary edema, and open-mouth breathing during suspicious environmental conditions suffice for diagnosis, but associated or concurrent diseases also must be suspected, diagnosed, and treated. For example, cattle with septic mastitis, metritis, or pneumonia are already febrile and therefore are more prone to heat stroke. Hypocalcemic cattle that are recumbent in poorly ventilated areas or in direct sunshine require calcium therapy in addition to treatment of heat stroke. Handling or movement of cattle with heat stroke can worsen the condition. Differential causes of extreme pyrexia should be ruled out as much as possible by a complete physical examination.

Treatment

All stress that involves treatment or movement should cease once heat stroke has been diagnosed. If at all possible immediate shade should be provided if the animal is already recumbent in direct sunlight. The animal should be cooled by hosing the entire body with cold water and placing the animal in front of a large fan whenever possible. Concurrent use of a fan facing the animal's head and cold water hosing is the best treatment. Alcohol soaks are not as efficient as cold water because it is impossible to find enough alcohol to adequately cool an adult cow. Cool water administered into the rumen via stomach tube or room temperature crystalloids administered IV may be helpful.

If pulmonary edema is suspected, 0.5 to 1.0 mg/kg of furosemide should be administered systemically. Hypocalcemia should be treated, but great care is required when administering IV calcium because of preexisting tachycardia (often ≥120 beats/min) and the need for restraint of the patient. Excessive restraint must be avoided. NSAIDs and one dose of prednisolone sodium succinate may be helpful in advanced, prostrate patients (those that are not pregnant). Concurrent inflammatory or metabolic diseases should be treated as soon as the patient is stable. Hypocalcemia is an exception to this rule because emergency treatment of hypocalcemia is usually necessary before the animal is moved to an area where cold water is available.

Rectal temperature should be monitored until the temperature falls below 104.0°F (40.0°C) and tachycardia and tachypnea resolve or become less severe. A strong fan should remain in place facing the animal's head. The more air that can be directed at the animal, the better.

Dr. Francis H. Fox of Cornell University had repeated experience with heat stroke in show cattle confined to poorly ventilated stalls during periods of high temperature and humidity at state and county fairs held during the summer months. He had recommended that blocks of ice be placed in feed pans in front of the cow's face and then a strong fan directed at the ice to blow cold air waves at the cow's face. Patients that have not shed out should have the hair coat completely clipped with cow clippers. The prognosis is good unless the cow is recumbent, is prostrate, develops DIC, or cannot be moved to an area where water and fans are available. The prognosis may be poor in patients having rectal temperatures greater than 108.0°F (42.22°C).

Eastern Equine Encephalitis

Etiology

Eastern equine encephalitis (EEE) virus is a *Togavirus* with a wide geographic distribution throughout North America. It is well known for its ability to incite encephalitis in horses (especially those who are unvaccinated for EEE) but has been isolated from several species, including birds, monkeys, humans, rodents, insects, dogs, goats, swine, and both mature and neonatal cattle. Typically, transmission of EEE occurs between reservoir hosts such as birds or rodents via mosquitos with other "dead-end" mammalian hosts such as cattle occasionally becoming infected but not developing levels of viremia necessary for further transmission. There are only three confirmed, documented cases in U.S. cattle in the literature despite the virus being widespread in bird and mosquito populations in several areas of the United States, especially on the East Coast, suggesting that clinical disease is exceptionally rare.

Clinical Signs

Eastern equine encephalitis was diagnosed in two calves in the 1970s by the Veterinary and Investigational Laboratory at Tifton, Georgia. The first calf was 6 weeks old, and the second was 1 week old. Both presented with clinical signs which had begun 2 days earlier. The first had a history of prostration, nystagmus, and opisthotonos. The latter was described as staggering for 2 days before developing convulsions and becoming recumbent. The diffuse encephalomeningitis seen on histopathologic examination in both cases raised suspicions of EEE. Virus isolation was performed on the brain of the first calf, and EEE virus was detected at 72 hours with subsequent confirmation by virus neutralization tests. The cell culture fluid from this virus isolation was later inoculated intracerebrally into a clinically normal 4-month-old calf, and similar clinical signs were noted beginning on day 3. Upon euthanasia, similar microscopic findings were detected along with a very prominent inflammatory infiltration of polymorphonuclear leukocytes.

Since these two initial case reports, EEE has also been diagnosed in a yearling beef heifer submitted to the Mississippi Board of Animal Health Veterinary Diagnostic Laboratory with a 2-day history of recumbency. When assisted to stand, the heifer circled in one direction. No other animals in the herd were affected. The animal was euthanized, and the microscopic examination of the brain yielded similar results to those already discussed except that the inflammatory infiltrate was predominantly lymphohistiocytic rather than neutrophilic. Results of ancillary testing for infectious bovine rhinotracheitis (IBR), BVDV, and rabies were all negative, but IFA testing for EEE antigen detection was positive as was confirmatory electron microscopy.

Diagnosis

Clinical signs of progressive neurologic abnormalities, including abnormal mentation, abnormal gait, opisthotonos, or recumbency in calves or adult cows coupled with evidence of encephalitis (either neutrophilic or lymphohistiocytic in origin) upon necropsy examination should prompt further testing for EEE virus. In horses, cytologic examination of CSF often yields a neutrophilic pleocytosis. Additionally, serologic assays on CSF (preferred) or serum to detect IgM antibodies exist for horses as well but are not currently available for cattle. Neutralizing antibody testing is an option for antemortem testing in horses and cattle, but paired sera samples must be obtained for an accurate diagnosis to be made. Therefore this testing modality would only be possible in animals that recover. Postmortem assays for EEE virus detection may include virus isolation performed on brain tissue or CSF, or PCR on brain tissue or CSF. (Blood is less reliable because clinically affected mammals do not always develop detectable viremic loads.)

Treatment

Treatment for infection with EEE virus involves supportive care in all species. In horses, infection often results in death within 3 to 5 days after the onset of signs. Treatment with interferon-α has been proposed but not yet determined to be effective in any controlled studies. Effective treatment and control of cerebral edema are critical.

Control

In horses, EEE is well prevented with the use of commercial vaccines. No such vaccines exist for cattle at this time.

Cache Valley Fever

Etiology

Cache Valley Fever virus (CVV) is a *Bunyavirus* that is endemic in North America. It is transmitted to a wide variety of mammalian species, including caribou, horses, sheep, cattle, and humans through mosquito vectors (*Anopheles, Aedes, Culex,* and *Coquillitidia*), thereby dictating the seasonality and geographic distribution of the disease.

Clinical Signs

Most CVV infections are subclinical and result in only a transient, asymptomatic viremia. Serologic surveillance of various wild and domestic ruminants in endemic areas, however, has shown that seroprevalence can approach 100% with clinical disease being very rarely observed. If detected, the clinical signs in adult mammalian hosts are often limited to malaise, fever, inappetence, and reluctance to move. Rarely, CVV can cause signs of encephalitis. It has also been discovered in a blood sample from an otherwise healthy cow in a herd with infertility issues. This virus is likely best known, however, for its association with embryonic death, stillbirth, and various congenital malformations in newborn lambs after infection in utero. The clinical signs observed in these lambs are dictated by the timing of infection during gestation. Previously published experimental studies involving sheep have demonstrated mostly subclinical disease (low-grade fevers and some inappetence) in infected adults. Experimental infection of ovine fetuses in utero with CVV has produced pregnancy losses and congenital malformations as seen in natural infection. Similarly, infection of CVV in pregnant cattle appears to also cause fetal mortality and malformations between 30 and 50 days of gestation.

Diagnosis

Diagnosing CVV during an outbreak of fetal loss or malformations can be difficult. The virus is often cleared from the fetus within several weeks and then from the fetal fluids and membranes by the end of the gestation period, making it necessary to rely on serologic techniques for a diagnosis rather than on virus isolation in these cases. Serum from heart blood collected from the fetus at the time of necropsy or precolostral serum collected from live lambs or calves should be submitted for an assay to detect antibodies to CVV (e.g., a serum neutralization test). The presence of an antibody titer to CVV in an adult animal is very common in endemic areas, so simply testing the dam is not enough unless the result is negative for antibodies, indicating that CVV is not the cause of the disease. In adult animals showing signs of disease (fever) or encephalitis, CVV may be isolated from the blood or nervous tissue (brain or CSF), respectively.

Control

There is no vaccine available for CVV, but animals that have been infected seem to remain resistant to future infection. Therefore in most endemic regions where exposure is high, there are often only a few sporadic cases of CVV detected because most pregnant animals have been previously exposed and therefore will not become viremic nor subsequently pass the virus on to their developing fetuses.

Epizootic Hemorrhagic Disease

Epizootic hemorrhagic disease (EHD) is an insect-vectored disease primarily of wild and captive white-tailed and mule deer and pronghorn antelope. The disease tends to be much more clinically severe in cervid populations. It is caused by infection with epizootic hemorrhagic disease virus (EHDV), which is a member of the *Reoviridae* family of viruses in the genus *Orbivirus*. Closely related *Orbivirus* diseases include the equine disease African horse sickness as well as bluetongue, which is a disease of ruminant livestock and Cervidae, and Ibaraki disease, caused by Ibaraki virus, which has been argued to be a variant of EHDV that is associated with more frequent cattle infections and illnesses in parts of Asia. There are at least 10 serotypes of EHDV circulating worldwide, and the strain appears to have an impact on morbidity and mortality rates in cervids as well as the ability of the virus to infect cattle. It is believed that only two strains occur in the United States. Some regions of the world currently are reportedly free of circulating EHDV, so there are transboundary animal movement requirements related to EHDV infection or seropositivity for ruminants and some ruminant products such as semen or embryos.

Insects of the *Culicoides* genus, also called biting midges or "no-see-ums", are usually responsible for the transmission of EHDV. In North America, *C. sonorensis* appears to be the primary vector, but other *Culicoides* spp. may be involved in transmission, and some gnats and mosquitos are also believed to be able to transmit EHDV. This disease occurs seasonally as transmission generally stops after freezing conditions sufficient to kill the vectors have occurred. The disease has been moving eastward within the continental United States in recent years, and outbreaks of disease in wild cervids within a geographic region often herald imminent clinical disease in cattle populations. The disease was seen for the first time in dairy cattle in Iowa and Wisconsin beginning between 2012 and 2014, but clinical cases were sporadic and rare. An unusually large number of cases occurred in the United States in the summer and fall of 2012 with the majority of bovine cases occurring in Nebraska, South Dakota, and Iowa.

Fortunately, infections of EHDV are only rarely associated with clinical illness in cattle in North America and most other parts of the world. Infections in cattle with no clinical manifestations are only apparent because of seroconversion, for example, when tested for export from the United States to countries requiring seronegativity for importation of animals or animal products. When cattle illness does occur because of EHD, although usually self-limiting, it cannot be differentiated clinically from other acute vesicular illnesses, such as foot-and-mouth disease (FMD) or vesicular stomatitis (VS). Therefore outbreaks of EHD in cattle require regulatory reporting and investigation to definitively rule out more serious diseases.

Clinical Signs and Diagnosis

The signs of illness in cattle associated with EHDV infection include fever; anorexia; reduced milk production; swollen eyes; redness and scaling of the nose and lips; nasal and ocular discharge; conjunctival inflammation; ulcers in or on the mouth, muzzle, teats, or coronary bands (Figs. 16.13 and 16.14); excessive salivation; lameness; swelling of the tongue; oral, nasal, teat, or coronary band blisters or vesicles; oral hemorrhages; and labored breathing. Deaths are very infrequent, but unthriftiness may persist related to painful lesions. One of the editors (SP) has noted that some cattle have been presented for dysphagia with remarkable ptyalism when clinical signs occur and that dysphagia can persist for several days to weeks after resolution of fever and oral lesions. The pathogenesis of this dysphagia is uncertain but may be related to esophageal damage rather than a neurogenic process.

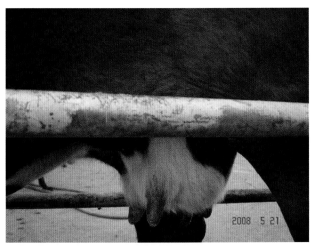

• **Fig. 16.13** Teat lesions associated with epizootic hemorrhagic disease virus infection in a beef cow. (Courtesy of Dr. Lee Torkelson.)

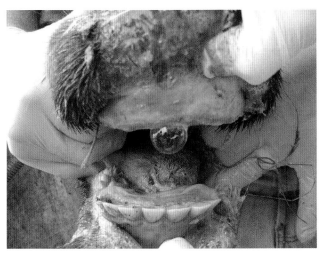

• **Fig. 16.14** Appearance of muzzle and oral lesions associated with epizootic hemorrhagic disease virus infection. (Courtesy of Dr. Roger Dudley.)

The diagnosis is routinely made by PCR assay for virus in tissues, secretions, or EDTA whole blood. Serology with paired acute and convalescent samples demonstrates seroconversion in recovered cattle. In a 2007 outbreak of EHDV in U.S. cattle, large percentages, up to 100%, of animals in herds with clinically ill individuals seroconverted indicating that sub-clinical disease is very common. Virus isolation is also used to confirm the presence of the virus, and in situ hybridization techniques can demonstrate the distribution of virus in frozen tissue sections.

Because of the clinical similarity to other viral vesicular diseases, PCR for bluetongue, VS, and FMD should be performed at the same time, and testing for other diseases in the differential diagnosis may also include BVDV, MCF, and in some cases with primarily respiratory or ocular signs, IBR.

Treatment and Control

There is no practical treatment for EHDV in cattle other than supportive care and management changes to minimize discomfort, such as limiting the need for walking and providing a clean and dry, well-bedded resting space. Cattle usually recover spontaneously. Aggressive insect control could reduce transmission and reduce the negative impact of this disease on the health of the cattle as well as on import–export opportunities for animals or germplasm.

Vaccines have been used to reduce susceptibility to other *Orbivirus* diseases, especially the bluetongue 8 strain that emerged in Europe in 2006. Vaccination could be considered for control of EHDV if clinical disease in cattle becomes more common. However, the impact of seropositivity on trade opportunities may also need to be considered for EHD, as it has been for bluetongue.

Miscellaneous Transboundary Diseases of Dairy Cattle

Contagious Bovine Pleuropneumonia
Etiology

Mycoplasma mycoides subsp. *mycoides* small colony (MmmSC) is the causative agent of contagious bovine pleuropneumonia (CBPP). Based on information from PCR analyses, three main lineages have emerged from Europe, Southern Africa and the rest of Africa. CBPP can be found throughout sub-Saharan Africa, the continent where it is most clinically important. The main hosts for CBPP are cattle, both *Bos taurus* and *Bos indicus;* however, infections in Asian buffalo, captive bison, and yak have also been reported. Sheep and goats can also be infected by the causative agent of CBPP but do not seem to show any associated pathology.

Contagious bovine pleuropneumonia is spread mainly by inhalation of aerosolized respiratory tract droplets from infected animals, and typically requires close and repeated contact. The organism can also be found in saliva, urine, fetal membranes, or uterine discharges from infected individuals, and transplacental transmission is possible. CBPP can manifest as an acute, subacute, or chronic infection. Cattle with chronic infections can form sequestra in lung tissue that can harbor viable organisms for up to 2 years. These nonclinical carrier animals are thought to become active shedders at times of stress and to serve as a major source of infective material. Otherwise, movement of infected animals into naïve herds is thought to be the main method of disease transmission. The organism does not survive in the environment for more than a few days, nor does it survive in meat products, and is readily inactivated by many common disinfectants (i.e., exposure to 1% phenol for 3 minutes). Because of the labile nature of the organism in the environment, fomites are not thought to play a very prominent role in transmission, although there have been a few anecdotal reports. One potential fomite of importance is urine-contaminated hay, which can pose a risk for transmission because infected animals can become septic, leading to renal involvement and subsequent shedding in urine.

Clinical Signs

The incubation period for CBPP ranges from a few weeks to several months. Clinical signs include depression, anorexia, pyrexia, dyspnea, tachypnea, nasal discharge, coughing, and open-mouth breathing. Affected adult animals may stand with their elbows abducted and neck extended. Thoracic auscultation may reveal crepitant sounds, friction rubs, or rales. Depending on the severity of pulmonary involvement and fluid accumulation, lung sounds may also be muffled with dull sounds auscultated upon percussion over more ventral areas of the thorax. Animals that recover from pneumonia may go on to become asymptomatic carriers with persistent shedding. Chronic disease can take the form of recurrent low-grade fever, ill thrift, cough upon exertion, and exercise intolerance. Infected calves less than 6 months of age have a greater tendency to demonstrate arthritis with swollen joints rather than pulmonary involvement. They

will be reluctant to move with discomfort upon rising and lying down and often lie in lateral recumbency with their legs outstretched.

Diagnosis

Gross necropsy examination of affected animals with pulmonary involvement tends to reveal unilateral fibrinous pleuritis with adhesions and copious amounts of straw-colored fluid that can coagulate to form fibrinous clots throughout the affected hemithoracic cavity (Fig. 16.15A). Because of the unilateral appearance, one must be careful not to mistake this for traumatic reticulopericarditis. Other infectious causes of consolidating pleuropneumonia such as *Histophilus somni* and *Mannheimia haemolytica* are potential differentials but have a greater tendency to be bilateral diseases. Lung lobules are consolidated with distended interlobular septa resulting in a characteristic marbled appearance (Fig. 16.15, *B*). In the earlier stages, the interlobular septa are distended by edema, then by fibrin, and later by fibrosis. In recovered animals, pulmonary sequestra may be evident with a fibrous capsule around a necrotic portion of tissue. Calves with arthritis tend to have swollen joints with tenosynovitis and may have intraarticular fibrin and turbid joint fluid upon gross examination of affected joint spaces or aspirates.

Confirmation of CBPP ante-mortem can be performed by isolation of the pathogen from nasal swabs or bronchial alveolar lavage samples. Alternatively, isolation of the organism from lung lesions, lymph nodes, pleural fluid or synovial fluid from arthritic animals can be attempted at necropsy. Besides culture, PCR tests also exist to identify the organism. Histopathology and immunohistochemistry can also be performed on appropriate lesions. In addition, serologic tests including a CF test, competitive ELISA, and immunoblotting test (IBT) can all be performed on serum from live animals. The CF has a low sensitivity and may miss acutely affected animals or those with chronic lesions but is valuable at the herd level for detecting infected groups of animals. The IBT is very specific and sensitive, making it

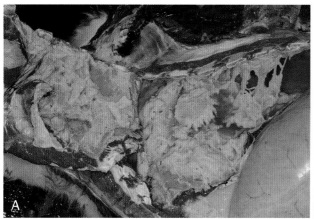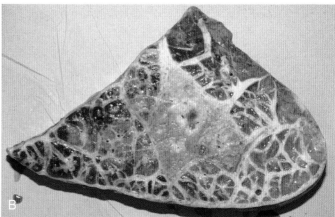

• **Fig. 16.15 A,** Thoracic cavity opened to reveal severe unilateral fibrinous pleuritis with adhesions and copious amounts of straw-colored fluid from a heifer with contagious bovine pleuropneumonia (CBPP). **B,** Distended interlobular septa associated with CBPP resulting in a characteristic marbling appearance to the affected lung. (Courtesy of USDA FADDL, Plum Island, NY.)

a suitable confirmatory test for those testing positive or with questionable results on the CF or ELISA.

Treatment

Although MmmSC is generally susceptible to oxytetracycline, antibiotic treatment is not recommended because it has not been studied extensively and may result in the creation of chronic carrier animals or resistant strains.

Control

Methods for the control of CBPP vary depending on the epidemiologic situation at hand and the available resources. In disease-free areas, serologic screening with slaughter of all positive and in-contact animals is recommended. Controlling the movement of cattle is the most effective method for limiting the spread of disease. In endemic areas, vaccination against CBPP is commonly practiced and pivotal to control. Two strains have been used for producing vaccines against CBPP—T1/44 and T1sr. T1/44 is a mild strain, whereas T1sr is avirulent. T1sr provides a shorter duration of immunity than T1/44 but T1/44 has the added risk of inducing postvaccinal reactions that may necessitate antibiotic treatment following vaccination. In areas where the prevalence is low or the disease does not exist, the use of vaccines must be carefully considered because it can interfere with interpretation of the serologic screening tests.

Heartwater

Etiology

Heartwater is a noncontagious, tickborne disease caused by *Ehrlichia ruminantium,* an intracellular parasite in the order *Rickettsiales. E. ruminantium* is a gram-negative, pleomorphic coccus. It is unable to survive outside of its host for more than a few hours and can only be transmitted through its *Amblyomma* tick vector. Strains of *E. ruminantium* vary greatly in virulence. It is a major cause of livestock loss in sub-Saharan Africa. *Amblyomma variegatum* is the tick species in the Caribbean that can carry the organism but despite the vector's widespread distribution in the region, heartwater cases have only been confirmed on three islands—Antigua, Guadeloupe, and Marie-Galante—likely associated with migration of cattle egrets to the Caribbean from Africa in 1956. Because the spread of disease requires the presence of the *Amblyomma* tick, the epidemiology of disease varies based on the infection rate of host ticks, seasonal effects on tick populations, and the effectiveness of tick control programs. All domestic and wild ruminants living in areas where the *Amblyomma* ticks are present are at risk for heartwater. The organism can also be transmitted vertically and through colostrum of carrier dams. No cases have been recorded in the United States, but there are several species of *Amblyomma* ticks present in the United States.

Clinical Signs

The average incubation period for heartwater is about 2 weeks. *E. ruminantium* multiplies in vascular endothelial cells, especially in the brain and other organs. This results in

cell rupture and release of organisms with increased vascular permeability. Infected cattle can develop high fevers, neurologic signs, hydropericardium, hydrothorax, pulmonary edema, cerebral edema, and death as a result. Disease can manifest as a peracute form in Africa in non-native breeds of sheep, goats, and cattle. This usually results in sudden death with only a brief period of clinical illness, including fever, respiratory distress, hyperesthesia, and diarrhea. Sheep and goats, in general, appear more susceptible to disease than cattle, with Angora goats and Merino sheep being very highly susceptible. More commonly, disease manifests as an acute form in which death typically occurs about 1 week after clinical signs are first seen. In the acute form, nervous signs may be more prominent (especially in cattle), including circling, muscle tremors, head pressing, and opisthotonos. Rarely, subacute forms of the disease can occur. This form typically results in a prolonged fever, coughing, and sometimes mild neurologic signs with either recovery or death within 1 to 2 weeks. White-tailed deer have been experimentally infected. It is also believed that certain species such as the African buffalo and the black wildebeest actually serve as reservoirs for disease with mild or undetectable signs.

Diagnosis

The diagnosis of heartwater is most commonly made based on necropsy findings in combination with a brain smear examination for identification of the organism. Typical gross findings include severe pulmonary edema (often with rib impressions), hydropericardium, hydrothorax, froth in the trachea, coning of the cerebellum, and congested leptomeninges. Affected cattle may also develop congestion of the abomasum. For the brain smear, a small piece of cerebral cortex or hippocampus (<5 × 5 × 5 mm) should be obtained and then placed between two slides and crushed until it is soft and pasty. Next, the top slide should be angled at about 45 degrees, and tissue should be pulled across the lower slide, slightly elevating the top slide every 10 mm. This creates a smear with alternating thick and thin areas. This technique stretches capillaries linearly to aid in the microscopic examination for *E. ruminantium.* The smear should then be air dried, fixed, and stained with Giemsa-type stain and examined for organisms (Fig. 16.16). *E. ruminantium* appears as reddish-purple to blue coccoid organisms in the cytoplasm of endothelial cells, often in close proximity to the nucleus. Other diagnostic techniques such as PCR of blood or target organs and culture of the organism are also available. Serologic tests including IFA, ELISA, and Western blot are available; however, cross-reactions are possible with all of these tests, so serology has limited, accurate, diagnostic value.

Treatment

Treatment with tetracyclines (oxytetracycline or doxycycline) is effective in the early stages of disease when the animal is still febrile. Frequently, animals are not detected early on in the course of illness, and unfortunately, antibiotic

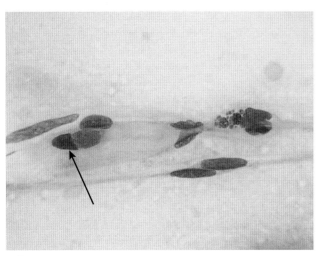

• **Fig. 16.16** Brain smear for *E. ruminatium* (using technique described in the text), Giemsa stain, 100× magnification. Arrow indicates *E. ruminantium* in the cytoplasm of a capillary endothelial cell. (Courtesy of USDA FADDL, Plum Island, NY.)

treatments are often unsuccessful when instituted in the later stages of disease. Eradication of *Amblyomma* ticks by applying acaricides to cattle and small ruminants can be successful in some regions. However, in endemic areas, tick levels are often allowed to remain at levels that allow for reinfection of currently immune animals, offering a boost to their immunity and thereby creating some endemic stability in these regions.

Control

Introduction of heartwater into an area containing naïve cattle can occur through the introduction of subclinically infected animals or by ticks. Animals moving from endemic areas into heartwater-free countries must be tested before importation and must also be inspected thoroughly for ticks. Unfortunately, ticks still may enter these areas via the illegal importation of animals or migrating birds. Quarantine, euthanasia of positive animals, and tick control are all essential methods of control in heartwater-free areas. In endemic regions, tick control, treatment with tetracyclines, and immunization via "infection and treatment" are all used to control the spread of heartwater. Commercial vaccines for heartwater are not available, hence the utilization of the infection and treatment method. This technique involves inoculating animals with blood from infected individuals and then treating them with antibiotics if a fever develops. When this technique is used on young kids, lambs, or calves, treatment is often not required because they possess a degree of nonspecific resistance to infection and therefore do not become febrile.

Rift Valley Fever

Etiology

Rift Valley fever (RVF) virus is a vector-borne *Bunyavirus* (*Phlebovirus* genus) capable of causing disease in sheep, cattle, and goats. Other host species include dromedaries, rodents, wild ruminants, buffaloes, antelopes, wildebeests, and humans as well as some monkeys and domestic carnivores. It is endemic in tropical regions of eastern and southern Africa. Outbreaks have also occurred in periendemic countries throughout Africa and into Saudi Arabia and Yemen when rainfall has been above average and the climatic conditions have been ideal for competent vectors.

Aedes species serve as reservoirs for RVF so that when rainfall increases in dry areas, there is a subsequent increase in the hatching of mosquito eggs followed by an increase in disease among susceptible hosts. Domestic ruminants act as amplifiers of RVF. Aside from exposure through vectors (mosquitos), RVF is also transmitted via nasal discharges, blood, vaginal secretions after abortion, infected meat, aerosols, and possibly through consumption of raw milk from infected individuals.

Clinical Signs

The incubation period varies from one to several days and can be as long as 30 days. The clinical severity of infection with RVF virus varies depending on the species and age of the host. High mortality rates (70%–100%) occur in neonates of several species (lambs, kids, puppies, kittens) as well as mice and hamsters. Slightly lower mortality rates (20%–70%) occur in adult sheep and calves. The "moderately" susceptible species include adult cattle and goats, African buffaloes, domestic buffaloes, Asian monkeys, and humans with death occurring less than 10% of the time. Infection is considered inapparent in several "resistant" species, including camels, equids, pigs, adult dogs and cats, African monkeys, baboons, rabbits, and guinea pigs. Reptiles, birds, and amphibians are not susceptible to RVF virus infection.

Clinical signs can include abortion, fever, depression, inappetence, diarrhea, icterus, nasal discharge, lacrimation, and death. Humans tend to experience influenza-like symptoms with photophobia and nausea, but recovery tends to occur in 4 to 7 days. Rarely, humans can experience complications, including blindness, meningoencephalitis, hemorrhagic syndrome, jaundice, and death.

Diagnosis

Necropsy findings can aid in the diagnosis of RVF and include hepatic necrosis with enlargement and congestion of the liver, icterus (in calves especially) widespread hemorrhages on parietal and visceral serosal surfaces, enlarged lymph nodes with hemorrhages and necrosis, hemorrhagic enteritis, congestion, and hemorrhages of the kidneys.

Additionally, the agent can be identified by various techniques, including; culture of various tissues; immunofluorescence for virus in impression smears of the liver, spleen, and brain; AGID; PCR; and histopathology with immunostaining of the liver.

Several serologic techniques are also available for the diagnosis of RVF. These techniques include virus neutralization (requires live virus and is therefore not recommended for use outside of endemic areas), ELISA, and hemagglutination inhibition (HI) tests. Both the ELISA and the HI tests can result in false-positive results because of cross-reactions with phleboviruses other than RVF.

Control

There are no specific treatments available for RVF, but several control measures exist. Control of animal movement and appropriate precautions within slaughterhouses to minimize exposure are indicated. Minimizing vector populations by draining areas of standing water or spraying with methoprene are also used. An attenuated virus vaccine and a live-attenuated mutant vaccine are also available in some areas.

Acknowledgment

We would like to thank Dr. Franklin Garry, Colorado State University, for his contribution in the previous edition of Diseases of Dairy Cattle.

Suggested Readings

Abt, D. A., Marshak, R. R., Kulp, H. W., et al. (1970). Studies on the relationship between lymphocytosis and bovine leukosis. *Bibl Haemat*, *36*, 527–536.

Aleman, M. R., & Spier, S. J. (2002). Corynebacterium pseudotuberculosis infection. In B. P. Smith (Ed.), *Large animal internal medicine*. St. Louis: Mosby.

Alt, D. P., Zuerner, R. L., & Bolin, C. A. (2001). Evaluation of antibiotics for treatment of cattle infected with *Leptospira borgpetersenii* serovar hardjo. *J Am Vet Med Assoc*, *219*, 636–639.

Animal and Plant Health Inspection Service. (1989). *Bovine tuberculosis eradication*. Washington, DC: United States Department of Agriculture.

Asahina, M., Ishiguro, N., Wu, D., et al. (1996). The proto-oncogene c-myb is expressed in sporadic bovine lymphoma, but not in enzootic bovine leucosis. *J Vet Med Sci*, *58*, 1169–1174.

Behymer, D. E., Biberstein, E. L., Riemann, H. P., et al. (1976). Q fever *(Coxiella burnetii)* investigations in dairy cattle: challenge of immunity after vaccination. *Am J Vet Res*, *37*, 631–634.

Behymer, D., & Riemann, H. P. (1989). *Coxiella burnetii* infection (Q fever). *J Am Vet Med Assoc*, *194*, 764–767.

Bezos, J., Casal, C., Romero, B., et al. (2014). Current ante-mortem techniques for diagnosis of bovine tuberculosis. *Res Vet Sci*, *97*, S44–52.

Bielanski, A., Simard, C., Maxwell, P., et al. (2001). Bovine immunodeficiency virus in relation to embryos fertilized in vitro. *Vet Res Commun*, *25*, 663–673.

Bolin, C. A., & Alt, D. P. (2001). Use of a monovalent leptospiral vaccine to prevent renal colonization and urinary shedding in cattle exposed to *Leptospira borgpetersenii* serovar hardjo. *Am J Vet Res*, *62*, 995–1000.

Bolin, C. A., Thiermann, A. B., Handsaker, A. L., et al. (1989). Effect of vaccination with a pentavalent leptospiral vaccine on *Leptospira interrogans* serovar *hardjo* type *hardjo-bovis* infection of pregnant cattle. *Am J Vet Res*, *50*, 161–165.

Brodie, S. J., Bardsley, K. D., Diem, K., et al. (1998). Epizootic hemorrhagic disease: analysis of tissues by amplification and in situ hybridization reveals widespread orbivirus infection at low copy numbers. *J Virol*, *72*, 3863–3871.

Brown, R. A., Blumerman, S., Gay, C., et al. (2003). Comparison of three different leptospiral vaccines for induction of a type 1 immune response to *Leptospira borgpetersenii* serovar Hardjo. *Vaccine*, *21*, 4448–4458.

Buehring, G. C., Shen, H. M., Jensen, H. M., et al. (2014). Bovine leukemia virus DNA in human breast tissue. *Emerg Infect Dis*, *20*, 772–782.

Buehring, G. C., Shen, H. M., Jensen, H. M., et al. (2015). Exposure to BLV is associated with breast cancer: a case-control study. *PLoS One*, *10*, e0134304.

Burgess, F. C. (1988). *Borrelia burgdorferi* infection in Wisconsin USA horses and cows. *Ann N Y Acad Sci*, *539*, 235–243 Benach JL, Bosler EM, editors [special issue published in conjunction with Lyme Disease and Related Disorders, International Conference held in New York, NY, September 14-16, 1987].

Burgess, E. C., Gendron-Fitzpatrick, A., & Wright, W. O. (1987). Arthritis and systemic disease caused by *Borrelia burgdorferi* infection in a cow. *J Am Vet Med Assoc*, *191*, 1468–1469.

Burgess, E. C., Wachal, M. D., & Cleven, T. D. (1993). *Borrelia burgdorferi* infection in dairy cows, rodents, and birds from four Wisconsin dairy farms. *Vet Microbiol*, *35*, 61–77.

Burridge, M. J., & Thurmond, M. C. (1981). An overview of modes of transmission of bovine leukemia virus. *Proc US Anim Health Assoc*, *85*, 165–169.

Burridge, M. J., Thurmond, M. C., Miller, J. M., et al. (1982). Fall in antibody titer to bovine leukemia virus in the periparturient period. *Can J Comp Med*, *46*, 270–271.

Carstensen, M., O'Brien, D. J., & Schmitt, S. M. (2011). Public acceptance as a determinant of management strategies for bovine tuberculosis in free-ranging US wildlife. *Vet Microbiol*, *151*, 200–204.

Casal, C., Diez-Guerrier, A., Alvarez, J., et al. (2014). Strategic use of serology for the diagnosis of bovine tuberculosis after intradermal skin testing. *Vet Microbiol*, *170*, 342–351.

Catlin, J., & Sheehan, E. (1986). Transmission of bovine brucellosis from dam to offspring. *J Am Vet Med Assoc*, *188*, 867–869.

Cheville, N. F. (2000). Development, testing and commercialization of a new brucellosis vaccine for cattle. *Ann N Y Acad Sci*, *916*, 147–153.

Cheville, N. F., Stevens, M. G., Jensen, A. E., et al. (1993). Immune responses and protection against infection and abortion in cattle experimentally vaccinated with mutant strains of *Brucella abortus*. *Am J Vet Res*, *54*, 1591–1597.

Coetzee, J. F., Apley, M. D., Kocan, K. M., et al. (2005). Comparison of three oxytetracycline regimens for the treatment of persistent Anaplasma marginale infections in beef cattle. *Vet Parasitol*, *127*, 61–73.

Coetzee, J. F., Schmidt, P. L., Apley, M. D., et al. (2007). Comparison of the complement fixation test and competitive ELISA for serodiagnosis of Anaplasma marginale infection in experimentally infected steers. *Am J Vet Res*, *68*, 872–878.

Crawford, R. P., Huber, J. D., & Sanders, R. B. (1986). Brucellosis in heifers weaned from seropositive dams. *J Am Vet Med Assoc*, *189*, 547–549.

Daugschies, A., Hintz, J., Henning, M., et al. (2000). Growth performance, meat quality and activities of glycolytic enzymes in the blood and muscle tissue of calves infected with Sarcocystis cruzi. *Vet Parasitol*, *88*, 7–16.

Daugschies, A., Rupp, U., & Rommel, M. (1998). Blood clotting disorders during experimental sarcocystiosis in calves. *Int J Parasitol*, *28*, 1187–1194.

DiGiacomo, R. F. (1992). The epidemiology and control of bovine leukemia virus infection. *Vet Med*, *87*, 248–257.

DiGiacomo, R. F. (1992). Horizontal transmission of the bovine leukemia virus. *Vet Med*, *87*, 263–271.

DiGiacomo, R. F. (1992). Vertical transmission of the bovine leukemia virus. *Vet Med*, *87*, 258–262.

DiGiacomo, R. F., Hopkins, S. G., Darlington, R. I., et al. (1987). Control of bovine leukosis virus in a dairy herd by a change in dehorning. *Can J Vet Res*, *51*, 542–544.

DiGiacomo, R. F., McGinnis, L. K., Studer, E., et al. (1990). Failure of embryo transfer to transmit BLV in a dairy herd. *Vet Rec*, *127*, 456.

Divers, T. J. (1986). Infectious causes of meningitis and encephalitis in cattle. In J. L. Howard (Ed.), *Current veterinary therapy, food animal practice* (2nd ed.) (pp. 854–855). Philadelphia: WB Saunders Co Ltd.

Divers, T. J., Bartholomew, R. C., Galligan, D. et al. (1995). Evidence for transmission of bovine leukemia virus by rectal palpation in a commercial dairy herd. *Prev Vet Med, 23*, 133–141).

Dubey, J. P., & Fayer, R. (1986). Sarcocystosis, toxoplasmosis, and cryptosporidiosis in cattle. *Vet Clin North Am Food Anim Pract, 2*, 293–298.

Dubey, J. P., Lindsay, D. S., Anderson, M. L., et al. (1992). Induced transplacental transmission of *Neospora caninum* in cattle. *J Am Vet Med Assoc, 201*, 709–713.

Edwards, J. F. (1994). Cache Valley virus. *Vet Clin North Am Food Anim Pract, 10*, 515–524.

Eisinger, S. W., Schwartz, M., Dam, M., et al. (2013). Evaluation of the BD vacutainer plus urine C&S preservative tubes compared with nonpreservative urine samples stored at 4°C and room temperature. *Am J Clin Pathol, 140*, 306–313.

Ellis, W. A. (2014). Animal leptospirosis. *Curr Top Microbiol Immunol, 387*, 99–137.

Ellis, W. A., O'Brien, J. J., Cassells, J. A., et al. (1985). Excretion of *Leptospira interrogans* serovar *hardjo* following calving or abortion. *Res Vet Sci, 39*, 296–298.

Ellis, W. A., O'Brien, J. J., Neill, S. D., et al. (1982). Bovine leptospirosis: serological findings in aborting cows. *Vet Rec, 110*, 178–180.

Enright, J. B., Sadler, W. W., & Thomas, R. C. (1957). Thermal inactivation of *Coxiella burnetii* in milk pasteurization. *Public Health Monogr, 47*, 1–30.

Erwin, B. G. (1977). Experimental induction of bacillary hemoglobinuria in cattle. *Am J Vet Res, 38*, 1625–1627.

Essey, M. A. (1994). The TB challenges—how can we prevent a disastrous comeback? *Large Anim Vet January/February*, 10–14.

Fayer, R., & Johnson, A. J. (1975). Effect of amprolium on acute sarcocystosis in experimentally infected calves. *J Parasitol, 61*, 932–936.

Fayer, R., Johnson, A. J., & Lunde, M. (1976). Abortion and other signs of disease in cows experimentally infected with *Sarcocystis fusiformis* from dogs. *J Infect Dis, 134*, 624–628.

Fernandez, P. J., & White, W. R. (2010). *Atlas of transboundary animal diseases*. OIE (World Organization for Animal Health).

Ferrer, J. F., Marshak, R., Abt, D. A., et al. (1979). Relationship between lymphosarcoma and persistent lymphocytosis in cattle: a review. *J Am Vet Med Assoc, 175*, 705–708.

Ferrer, J. F., & Piper, C. E. (1981). Role of colostrum and milk in the natural transmission of the bovine leukemia virus. *Cancer Res, 41*, 4906–4909.

Fitzgerald, S. D., Hollinger, C., Mullaney, T. P., et al. (2016). Herd outbreak of bovine tuberculosis illustrates that route of infection correlates with anatomic distribution of lesions in cattle and cats. *J Vet Diagn Invest, 28*, 129–132.

Fitzgerald, F. D., & Kaneene, J. B. (2013). Wildlife reservoirs of bovine tuberculosis worldwide: hosts, pathology, surveillance, and control. *Vet Pathol, 50*, 488–499.

Fluegel Dougherty, A. M., Cornish, T. E., O'Toole, D., et al. (2013). Abortion and premature birth in cattle following vaccination with Brucella abortus strain RB51. *J Vet Diagn Invest, 25*, 630–635.

Fox, F. H., & Roberts, S. J. (1949). Recent experiences in the ambulatory clinic. *Cornell Vet, 39*, 249–260.

Frelier, P. F., & Lewis, R. M. (1984). Hematologic and coagulation abnormalities in acute bovine sarcocystosis. *Am J Vet Res, 45*, 40–48.

Galloway, D. R., & Baillie, L. (2004). DNA vaccines against anthrax. *Expert Opin Biol Ther, 4*, 1661–1667.

Gasbarre, L. C., Suter, P., & Fayer, R. (1984). Humoral and cellular immune responses in cattle and sheep inoculated with sarcocystis. *Am J Vet Res, 45*, 1592–1596.

Genova, S. G., Streeter, R. N., Velguth, K. E., et al. (2011). Severe anemia associated with Mycoplasma wenyonii infection in a mature cow. *Can Vet J, 52*, 1018–1021.

Gerritsen, M. J., Koopsman, M. J., Dekker, T. C., et al. (1994). Effective treatment with dihydrostreptomycin of naturally infected cows shedding *Leptospira interrogans* serovar *hardjo* subtype *hardjobovis*. *Am J Vet Res, 55*, 339–343.

Gladden, N., Haining, H., Henderson, L., et al. (2015). A case report of Mycoplasma wenyonii associated immune-mediated haemolytic anaemia in a dairy cow. *Ir Vet J, 69*, 1–8.

Goren, M. B. (1977). Phagocyte lysosomes: interactions with infectious agents, phagosomes, and experimental perturbations in function. *Annu Rev Microbiol, 31*, 507–533.

Grooms, D. L., & Bolin, C. A. (2005). Diagnosis of fetal loss caused by bovine viral diarrhea virus and *Leptospira* spp. *Vet Clin North Am Food Anim Pract, 21*, 463–472.

Gunning, R. F., Jones, J. R., Jeffrey, M., et al. (2000). Sarcocystis encephalomyelitis in cattle. *Vet Rec, 146*, 328.

Gupta, P., & Ferrer, J. F. (1980). Detection of bovine leukemia virus antigen in urine from naturally infected cattle. *Int J Cancer, 25*, 663–666.

Halling, S. M. (2002). Paradigm shifts in vaccine development: lessons learned about antigenicity, pathogenicity and virulence of Brucellae. *Vet Microbiol, 90*, 545–552.

Hatfield, C. E., Rebhun, W. C., & Dill, S. G. (1986). Thymic lymphosarcoma in three heifers. *J Am Vet Med Assoc, 189*, 1598–1599.

Hayes J: Contagious bovine pleuropneumonia, PowerPoint presentation, Veterinary Laboratory Diagnostic Course, Dec 9, 2015.

Henry, E. T., & Levine, J. F. (1987). Rectal transmission of bovine leukemia virus in cattle and sheep. *Am J Vet Res, 48*, 634–636.

Hirsh, D. C., MacLachlan, N. J., & Walker, R. L. (2004). *Veterinary microbiology* (2nd ed.). Oxford: Blackwell Publishing Ltd.

Hopkins, S. G., Evermann, J. F., DiGiacomo, R. F., et al. (1988). Experimental transmission of bovine leukosis virus by simulated rectal palpation. *Vet Rec, 122*, 389–391.

Huber, N. L., DiGiacomo, R. F., Evermann, J. F., et al. (1981). Bovine leukemia virus infection in a large Holstein herd: prospective comparison of production and reproductive performance in antibody-negative and antibody-positive cows. *Am J Vet Res, 42*, 1477–1481.

Ji, B., & Collins, M. T. (1994). Seroepidemiologic survey of Borrelia burgdorferi exposure of dairy cattle in Wisconsin. *Am J Vet Res, 55*, 1228–1231.

Johnson, R., & Kaneene, J. B. (1991). Bovine leukemia virus. Part I. Descriptive epidemiology, clinical manifestations, and diagnostic tests. *Compend Contin Educ Pract Vet, 13*, 315–327.

Johnson, R., & Kaneene, J. B. (1991). Bovine leukemia virus. Part II. Risk factors of transmission. *Compend Contin Educ Pract Vet, 13*, 681–691.

Johnson, R., & Kaneene, J. B. (1991). Bovine leukemia virus. Part III. Zoonotic potential, molecular epidemiology, and an animal model. *Compend Contin Educ Pract Vet, 13*, 1631–1640.

Johnson, R., & Kaneene, J. B. (1991). Bovine leukemia virus. Part IV. Economic impact and control measures. *Compend Contin Educ Pract Vet, 13*, 1727–1737.

Kabeya, H., Ohashi, K., & Onuma, M. (2001). Host immune responses in the course of bovine leukemia virus infection. *J Vet Med Sci, 63*, 703–708.

Kaja, R. W., & Olson, C. (1982). Non-infectivity of semen from bulls infected with bovine leukosis virus. *Theriogenology, 18,* 107–112.

Kanno, T., Ishihara, R., Hatama, S., et al. (2015). Effect of freezing treatment on colostrum to prevent the transmission of bovine leukemia virus. *J Vet Med Sci, 76,* 255–257.

Kim, S. G., Kim, E. H., Lafferty, C. J., et al. (2005). *Coxiella burnetii* in bulk milk tank samples, United States. *Emerg Infect Dis, 11,* 619–621.

King, J. M. (1992). Clinical exposures: bovine splenic lymphosarcoma. *Vet Med June,* 533.

Kocan, K. M., Coetzee, J. F., Step, D. L., et al. (2012). Current challenges in the diagnosis and control of bovine anaplasmosis. *Bovine Pract, 46,* 67–77.

Kocan, K. M., de la Fuente, J., Step, D. L., et al. (2010). Current challenges of the management and epidemiology of bovine anaplasmosis. *Bovine Pract, 44,* 93–102.

Kuckleburg, C. J., Chase, C. C., Nelson, E. A., et al. (2003). Detection of bovine leukemia virus in blood and milk by nested and real-time polymerase chain reactions. *J Vet Diagn Invest, 15,* 72–76.

Kuttler, K. L. Babesiosis. In *Foreign Animal Diseases*. Richmond, VA: United States Animal Health Association, 1998, pp. 81–101.

Langston, A., Ferdinand, G. A., Ruppanner, R., et al. (1978). Comparison of production variables of bovine leukemia virus antibody-negative and antibody-positive cows in two California dairy herds. *Am J Vet Res, 39,* 1093–1099.

Lassauzet, M. L. G., Thurmond, M. C., & Walton, R. W. (1989). Lack of evidence of transmission of bovine leukemia virus by rectal palpation of dairy cows. *J Am Vet Med Assoc, 195,* 1732–1733.

Leonard, F. C., Quinn, P. J., Ellis, W. A., et al. (1992). Duration of urinary excretion of leptospires by cattle naturally or experimentally infected with *Leptospira interrogans* serovar. *hardjo. Vet Rec, 121,* 435–439.

Levy, M. G., Clabaugh, G., & Ristic, M. (1982). Age resistance in bovine babesiosis: role of blood factors in resistance to Babesia bovis. *Infect Immun, 37,* 1127–1131.

Lewin, H. A., & Bernoco, D. (1986). Evidence for bovine lymphocyte antigen-linked resistance and susceptibility to subclinical progression of bovine leukaemia virus infection. *Anim Genet, 17,* 197–207.

Lincoln, S. D., Zaugg, J. L., & Maas, J. (1987). Bovine anaplasmosis: susceptibility of seronegative cows from an infected herd to experimental infection with Anaplasma marginale. *J Am Vet Med Assoc, 190,* 171–173.

Lischer, C. J., Leutenegger, C. M., Braun, U., et al. (2000). Diagnosis of Lyme disease in two cows by the detection of Borrelia burgdorferi DNA. *Vet Rec, 146,* 497–499.

Long, M. T. (2014). West Nile virus and equine encephalitis viruses: new perspectives. *Vet Clin North Am Equine Pract, 30,* 523–542.

Lopes, C. W., de Sa, W. F., & Botelho, G. G. (2005). Lesions in crossbreed pregnant cows, experimentally infected with *Sarcocystis cruzi* (Hasselmann, 1923) Wenyon, 1926 (Apicomplexa: Sarcocytidae). *Rev Bras Parasitol Vet, 14,* 79–83.

MAF Biosecurity New Zealand. (2009). *Import risk analysis: cattle germplasm from all countries.* New Zealand Ministry of Agriculture, 134–135.

Magnarelli, L. A., Bushmich, S. L., Sherman, B. A., et al. (2004). A comparison of serologic tests for the detection of serum antibodies to whole-cell and recombinant Borrelia burgdorferi antigens in cattle. *Can Vet J, 45,* 667–673.

Magonigle, R. A., & Newby, T. J. (1984). Response of cattle upon reexposure to *Anaplasma marginale* after elimination of chronic carrier infections. *Am J Vet Res, 45,* 695–697.

Magonigle, R. A., Simpson, J. E., & Frank, F. W. (1978). Efficacy of a new oxytetracycline formulation against clinical anaplasmosis. *Am J Vet Res, 39,* 1407–1420.

Maurin, M., & Raoult, D. Q. (1999). Q fever. *Clin Microbiol Rev, 12,* 518–553.

McConnell, S., Livingston, C., Calisher, C. H., et al. (1987). Isolations of Cache Valley virus in Texas, 1981. *Vet Microbiol, 13,* 11–18.

McGee, E. D., Littleton, C. H., Mapp, J. B., et al. (1992). Eastern equine encephalomyelitis in an adult cow. *Vet Pathol, 29,* 361–363.

McNab, W. B., Jacobs, R. M., & Smith, H. E. (1994). A serological survey for bovine immunodeficiency-like virus in Ontario dairy cattle and associations between test results, production records and management practices. *Can J Vet Res, 58,* 36–41.

McQuiston, J. H., & Childs, J. E. (2002). Q fever in humans and animals in the United States. *Vector Borne Zoonotic Dis, 2,* 179–191.

Meas, S., Usui, T., Ohashi, K., et al. (2002). Vertical transmission of bovine leukemia virus and bovine immunodeficiency virus in dairy cattle herds. *Vet Microbiol, 84,* 275–282.

Moeller R. Heartwater, PowerPoint presentation, Veterinary Laboratory Diagnostic Course, Dec 9, 2015.

Monke, D. R. (1986). Noninfectivity of semen from bulls infected with bovine leukosis virus. *J Am Vet Med Assoc, 188,* 823–826.

Monke, D. R., Rohde, R. F., Hueston, W. D., et al. (1992). Estimation of the sensitivity and specificity of the agar gel immunodiffusion test for bovine leukemia virus, 1296 cases 1982–1989. *J Am Vet Med Assoc, 200,* 2001–2004.

Moosawi, M., Ardehaii, M., Farzan, A., et al. (1999). Isolation and identification of Clostridium strains from cattle malignant edema cases. *Arch Razi Institute, 50,* 65–70.

Muller, J., Gwozdz, J., Hodgeman, R., et al. (2015). Diagnostic performance characteristics of a rapid field test for anthrax in cattle. *Prev Vet Med, 120,* 277–282.

National Research Council. (1994). *Livestock disease eradication.* Washington, DC: National Research Council.

Newby, T. J., & Magonigle, R. A. (1983). Long-acting oxytetracycline injectable for the elimination of chronic bovine anaplasmosis under field conditions. *Agri-Practice, 4,* 5–7.

Nicoletti, P., Milward, F. W., Hoffmann, E., et al. (1985). Efficacy of long-acting oxytetracycline alone or combined with streptomycin in the treatment of bovine brucellosis. *J Am Vet Med Assoc, 187,* 493–495.

Nicoletti, P. (2002). A short history of brucellosis. *Vet Microbiol, 90,* 5–9.

Nicoletti, P. (1980). The epidemiology of bovine brucellosis. *Adv Vet Sci Comp Med, 24,* 69–98.

O'Brien, D. J., Schmitt, S. M., Fitzgerald, S. D., et al. (2006). Managing the wildlife reservoir of *Mycobacterium bovis*: the Michigan, USA, experience. *Vet Microbiol, 112,* 313–323.

Onuma, M., Hodatsu, T., Yamamoto, S., et al. (1984). Protection by vaccination against bovine leukemia virus infection in sheep. *Am J Vet Res, 45,* 1212–1215.

Onuma, M., Aida, Y., Okada, K., et al. (1985). Usefulness of monoclonal antibodies for detection of enzootic bovine leukemia cells. *Jpn J Cancer Res, 76,* 959–966.

Orr, K. A., O'Reilly, K. L., & Scholl, D. T. (2003). Estimation of sensitivity and specificity of two diagnostic tests for bovine immunodeficiency virus using Bayesian techniques. *Prev Vet Med, 61,* 79–89.

Ott, S. L., Johnson, R., & Wells, S. J. (2003). Association between bovine-leukosis virus seroprevalence and herd-level productivity on US dairy farms. *Prev Vet Med, 61,* 249–262.

Palmer, G. H., & Lincoln, S. D. (2002). Diseases associated with increased erythrocyte destruction—anaplasmosis. In B. P. Smith (Ed.), *Large animal internal medicine*. St. Louis: Mosby.

Palmer, M. V., & Waters, W. R. (2006). Advances in bovine tuberculosis diagnosis and pathogenesis: what policy makers need to know. *Vet Microbiol, 112*, 181–190.

Parker, J. L., & White, K. K. (1992). Lyme borreliosis in cattle and horses: a review of the literature. *Cornell Vet, 82*, 253–274.

Parma, A. E., Santisteban, G., & Margin, R. A. (1984). Analysis and in vivo assay of *Brucella abortus* agglutinating and non-agglutinating antibodies. *Vet Microbiol, 9*, 391–398.

Parodi, A. L., DaCosta, B., Djilali, S., et al. (1989). Preliminary report of familial thymic lymphosarcoma in Holstein calves. *Vet Rec, 125*, 350–352.

Pelzer, K. D., & Sprecher, D. J. (1993). Controlling BLV infection on dairy operations. *Vet Med, 88*, 275–281.

Piper, C. E., Ferrer, J. F., Abt, D. A., et al. (1979). Postnatal and prenatal transmission of the bovine leukemia virus under natural conditions. *J Natl Cancer Inst, 62*, 165–168.

Pollock, J. M., Rodgers, J. D., Welsh, M. D., et al. (2006). Pathogenesis of bovine tuberculosis: the role of experimental models of infection. *Vet Microbiol, 112*, 141–150.

Potgieter, F. T. (2004). Eperythrozoonosis. *Infect Dis Livestock, 1*, 573–580.

Pursell, A. R., Mitchell, F. E., & Seibold, H. R. (1976). Naturally occurring and experimentally induced Eastern encephalomyelitis in calves. *J Am Vet Med Assoc, 169*, 1101–1103.

Quinn, P. J., Markey, B. K., Carter, M. E., et al. (2002). *Veterinary microbiology and microbial disease*. Oxford: Blackwell Science Ltd.

Radostits, O. M., Gay, C. C., Blood, D. C., et al. (2007). *Veterinary medicine. A textbook of the diseases of cattle, sheep, pigs, goats and horses* (10th ed.). London: WB Saunders Co Ltd.

Ragan, V. E. (2002). The Animal and Plant Health Inspection Service (APHIS) brucellosis eradication program in the United States. *Vet Microbiol, 90*, 11–18.

Ray, W. C., Brown, R. R., Stringfellow, D. A., et al. (1988). Bovine brucellosis: an investigation of latency in progeny of culture-positive cows. *J Am Vet Med Assoc, 192*, 182–186.

Reinbold, J., Coetzee, J., Hollis, L. C., et al. (2010). The efficacy of three chlortetracycline regimens in the treatment of persistent Anaplasma marginale infection. *Vet Microbiol, 145*, 69–75.

Rhodes, J. K., Pelzer, K. D., & Johnson, Y. J. (2003). Economic implications of bovine leukemia virus infection in mid-Atlantic dairy herds. *J Am Vet Med Assoc, 223*, 346–352.

Rhodes, J. K., Pelzer, K. D., Johnson, Y. J., et al. (2003). Comparison of culling rates among dairy cows grouped on the basis of serologic status for bovine leukemia virus. *J Am Vet Med Assoc, 223*, 229–231.

Rhyan, J. C., Nol, P., Quance, C., et al. (2013). Transmission of brucellosis from elk to cattle and bison, Greater Yellowstone area, USA 2002-2012. *Emerg Infect Dis, 19*, 1992–1995.

Richtzenhain, L. J., Cortez, A., Heinemann, M. B., et al. (2002). A multiplex PCR for the detection of Brucella spp. and Leptospira spp. DNA from aborted bovine fetuses. *Vet Microbiol, 87*, 139–147.

Roberts, D. M., Carlyon, J. A., Theisen, M., et al. (2000). The bdr gene families of the Lyme disease and relapsing fever spirochetes: potential influence on biology, pathogenesis, and evolution. *Emerg Infect Dis, 6*, 110–122.

Roby, T. O., Amerault, T. E., Mazzola, V., et al. (1974). Immunity to bovine anaplasmosis after elimination of *Anaplasma marginale* infections with imidocarb. *Am J Vet Res, 35*, 993–995.

Roby, T. O., & Mazzola, V. (1972). Elimination of the carrier state of bovine anaplasmosis with imidocarb. *Am J Vet Res, 33*, 1931–1933.

Ruppanner, R., Jessup, D. A., Ohishi, I., et al. (1983). A strategy for control of bovine leukemia virus infection: test and corrective management. *Can Vet J, 24*, 192–195.

Schiller, I., Oesch, B., Vordermeier, H. M., et al. (2010). Bovine tuberculosis: a review of current and emerging diagnostic techniques in view of their relevance for disease control and eradication. *Transbound Emerg Dis, 57*, 205–220.

Schmidtmann, E. T., Schlater, J. L., Maupin, G. O., et al. (1998). Vegetational association of host-seeking adult blacklegged ticks, Ixodes scapularis Say (Acari: Ixodidae), on dairy farms in northwestern Wisconsin. *J Dairy Sci, 81*, 718–721.

Schmitt, S. M., O'Brien, D. J., Bruning-Fann, C. S., et al. (2002). Bovine tuberculosis in Michigan wildlife and livestock. *Ann N Y Acad Sci, 969*, 262–268.

Schurig, G. G., Sriranganathan, N., & Corbel, M. J. (2002). Brucellosis vaccines: past, present and future. *Vet Microbiol, 90*, 479–496.

Schurig, G. G., Roop, R. M., 2nd, Bagchi, T., et al. (1991). Biological properties of RB51: a stable rough strain of Brucella abortus. *Vet Microbiol, 28*, 171–188.

Schurr, E., Malo, D., Radzioch, D., et al. (1991). Genetic control of innate resistance to mycobacterial infections. *Immunol Today, 12*, A42–A45.

Shettigara, P. T., Samagh, B. S., & Lobinowich, E. M. (1989). Control of bovine leukemia virus infection in dairy herds by agar gel immunodiffusion test and segregation of reactors. *Can J Vet Res, 53*, 108–110.

Shulaw, W., & Zhang, Y. (2008). *EHD in Ohio cattle in 2007: clinical signs and serological findings, USAHA Annual Conference, Extension Veterinarians Meeting*.

Smith, C. R., Corney, B. G., McGowan, M. R., et al. (1997). Amoxycillin as an alternative to dihydrostreptomycin sulphate for treating cattle infected with *Leptospira borgpetersenii* serovar hardjo. *Aust Vet J, 75*, 818–821.

Smith, J. A., Thrall, M. A., Smith, J. L., et al. (1990). *Eperythrozoon wenyonii* infection in dairy cattle. *J Am Vet Med Assoc, 196*, 1244–1250.

Smith, M. O., & George, L. W. (2009). Diseases of the nervous system. In B. P. Smith (Ed.), *Large animal internal medicine*. St. Louis: Mosby.

Snyder, J. H., & Snyder, S. P. (2002). Bacillary hemoglobinuria. In B. P. Smith (Ed.), *Large animal internal medicine*. St. Louis: Mosby.

Stalheim, H. V., Fayer, R., & Hubbert, W. T. (1980). Update on bovine toxoplasmosis and sarcocystosis, with emphasis on their role in bovine abortions. *J Am Vet Med Assoc, 176*, 299–302.

Staples, C. R., & Thatcher, W. W. (2003). Heat stress in dairy cattle. In H. Roginski, J. W. Fuquay, & P. F. Fox (Eds.), *Encyclopedia of dairy sciences*. Boston: Academic Press.

Stevens, G., McClusky, B., King, A., et al. (2012). Review of the 2012 Epizootic Hemorrhagic Disease outbreak in domestic ruminants in the United States. *PLoS One, 10*, e0133359 5.

Surujballi, O., & Mallory, M. (2004). An indirect enzyme linked immunosorbent assay for the detection of bovine antibodies to multiple Leptospira serovars. *Can J Vet Res, 68*, 1–6.

Sweeney, R., Divers, T. J., Ziemer, E., et al. (1986). Intracranial lymphosarcoma in a Holstein bull. *J Am Vet Med Assoc, 189*, 555–556.

Tanner, W. B., Potter, M. E., Teclaw, R. F., et al. (1978). Public health aspects of anthrax vaccination of dairy cattle. *J Am Vet Med Assoc, 173*, 1465–1466.

Thurmond, M. C., Carter, R. L., Puhr, D. M., et al. (1983). An epidemiological study of natural in utero infection with bovine leukemia virus. *Can J Comp Med, 47*, 316–319.

Tripathy, D. N., Hanson, L. E., Mansfield, M. E., et al. (1985). Experimental infection of lactating goats with *Leptospira interrogans* serovars *pomona* and hardjo. *Am J Vet Res, 46*, 2512–2514.

Udall, D. H. (1954). *The practice of veterinary medicine* (6th ed.). Ithaca, NY: Published by the author.

Uilenberg, G., Thiaucourt, F., & Jongejan, F. (2004). On molecular taxonomy: what is in a name? *Exp Appl Acarol, 32*, 301–312.

Van Der Maaten, M. J., Miller, J. B., & Schmerr, M. J. (1981). Effect of colostral antibody on bovine leukemia virus infection of neonatal calves. *Am J Vet Res, 42*, 1498–1500.

Wagenaar, J., Zuerner, R. L., Alt, D., et al. (2000). Comparison of polymerase chain reaction assays with bacteriologic culture, immunofluorescence, and nucleic acid hybridization for detection of *Leptospira borgpetersenii* serovar hardjo in urine of cattle. *Am J Vet Res, 61*, 316–320.

Waters, W. R., & Palmer, M. V. (2015). Mycobacterium bovis infection of cattle and white-tailed deer: translational research of relevance to human tuberculosis. *Inst Lab Anim Res, 56*, 26–43.

Wells, S. J., Trent, A. M., Robinson, R. A., et al. (1993). Association between clinical lameness and *Borrelia-burgdorferi* antibody in dairy cows. *Am J Vet Res, 54*, 398–405.

Williams, B. M. (1977). Clostridial myositis in cattle: bacteriology and gross pathology. *Vet Rec, 100*, 90–91.

Wojnarowicz, C., Ngeleka, M., Sawtell, S. S., et al. (2004). Saskatchewan: unusual winter outbreak of anthrax. *Can Vet J, 45*, 516–517.

Yaeger, M., & Holler, L. D. (1997). Bacterial causes of infertility and abortion. In R. S. Youngquist (Ed.), *Current therapy in large animal theriogenology*. Philadelphia: WB Saunders.

Yeruham, I., Elad, D., Friedman, S., et al. (2003). *Corynebacterium pseudotuberculosis* infection in Israeli dairy cattle. *Epidemiol Infect, 131*, 947–955.

Yeruham, I., Friedman, S., Perl, S., et al. (2004). A herd level analysis of Corynebacterium pseudotuberculosis outbreak in a dairy cattle herd. *Vet Dermatol, 15*, 315–320.

Young, D. B., Mehlert, A., Bal, V., et al. (1988). Stress proteins and the immune response to mycobacteria antigens as virulence factors. *Antonie van Leeuwenhoek, 54*, 431–439.

Yuill, T. M., Gochenour, W. S., Lucas, F. R., et al. (1970). Cache Valley virus in the Del Mar VA Peninsula. *Am J Trop Med Hyg, 19*, 506–512.

Zaugg, J. L. (2002). Babesiosis. In B. P. Smith (Ed.), *Large animal internal medicine* (3rd ed.). St. Louis: Mosby.

17

Toxicities, Poisonings, and Deficiencies

BELINDA S. THOMPSON AND ERIN L. GOODRICH

TABLE 17.1 *Toxicities, Poisonings and Deficiencies*

Agent	Usual Source	Signs	Diagnosis	Treatment
Environmental Toxicities				
Ammoniated forage toxicosis ("bovine bonkers")	Ammoniated feeds	Hyperexcitability, blinking, pupillary dilatation, altered vision, twitching, trembling, frothing, bellowing, charging	History of feeding ammoniated feeds Blood and rumen *ammonia levels normal;* toxic effects caused by pyrazines and imidazoles are implicated	Change diet Proper mixing Gradual adaptation to NPN sources Do not feed to cows that are nursing calves
Nonprotein nitrogen (NPN)–induced ammonia toxicosis (urea toxicosis)	Urea, ammoniated feed, ammonium salts	Rapid onset (maybe sudden death) Colic, bloat, excitement, bellowing, neurologic signs, collapse, salivation	History of consumption Determine NPN in ration Rumen pH >8.0 (in live patients or very fresh postmortem) Blood or vitreous ammonia >1.0 mg/dL	Remove source Administer 2–6 L vinegar and 20–30 L cold water through stomach tube Do not feed more than one third of nitrogen in diet as NPN Do not feed more than 1% of total ration as urea unless animals' diet is gradually increased to higher levels
Anhydrous ammonia	Agricultural liquid fertilizer (theft for methamphetamine laboratories can result in accidental spills near livestock facilities)	Sudden deaths, corneal ulceration, necrosis of the upper respiratory and bronchial mucosa	Detection of ammonia or history of anhydrous ammonia spill	Supportive
Nitrogen dioxide toxicity	Toxic gas that can form during silage fermentation	Dyspnea, methemoglobinemia (brown blood); death	History of exposure; presence of yellow-brown haze from ensiled feed with a strong bleach-like smell	1% Methylene blue solution 4–15 mg/kg IV; not approved in food animals; tissue staining may occur for months after administration
Carbon monoxide toxicity	Toxic gas from engine exhaust, space heater, or furnace; also from house or barn fires (smoke inhalation)	Anorexia, ataxia, weakness, increased respiratory rate, dyspnea, death	Cherry red appearance to blood, tissues appear pink, history of exposure to exhaust or smoke	Supportive, supplemental oxygen
Hydrogen sulfide toxicity	Toxic gas that builds up in manure during anaerobic decomposition and is released upon agitation of the manure slurry	Ocular and respiratory inflammation, recumbency, seizures, death	Based on history, clinical signs and histologic lesions of brain (cerebral laminar necrosis)	Remove source, supportive

TABLE 17.1   *Toxicities, Poisonings and Deficiencies—**cont'd***

Agent	Usual Source	Signs	Diagnosis	Treatment
Dicoumarol or Coumarin toxicities	Rodenticides such as warfarin or second-generation anticoagulants such as brodifacoum Also moldy sweet clover hay or silage Sweet vernal hay (*Anthoxanthum*)	Bleeding caused by vitamin K antagonism leading to decreased production of clotting factors in the liver Resultant hypoprothrombinemia and inability to convert prothrombin to thrombin occurs Hematomas, hemarthrosis, GI bleeding, epistaxis, bleeding from insect bites, ecchymoses, anemia, and abortions	Evidence of hemorrhage Prolonged clotting time Prolonged prothrombin time—always Prolonged activated partial thromboplastin time—sometimes Platelet numbers and FDP values normal	Vitamin K_1 0.5–2.5 mg/kg body weight IM or SC several times (second-generation rodenticides may require therapy for weeks) Fresh whole blood or plasma transfusion. Whole blood if life-threatening anemia is present
Monensin/lasalocid toxicity	Ionophores fed in excess or improperly mixed, especially in young calves! Simultaneous feeding of macrolide antibiotic increases risk of monensin toxicity	Acute: anorexia, pica, diarrhea, depression, dyspnea, CNS signs (especially calves with lasalocid), and acute death Subacute or chronic: heart failure, dyspnea, weakness, diarrhea	Hemorrhage and necrosis in cardiac and skeletal muscle Hydrothorax, ascites, edema, enlarged firm, bluish liver (may occur days to months after ingestion) Feed analysis Elevated serum troponin	Supportive, parenteral selenium and vitamin E
Selenium poisoning	Selenium converter plants in selenium-rich soils (e.g., *Astragalus* spp.), causing dietary intake of 5–40 ppm Se Overdosage of parenteral selenium products; supplement formulation errors	Acute—respiratory distress, heart failure, diarrhea, death Chronic—dullness, weight loss, lameness, poor hair coat, rat tail, deformed hooves "blind staggers"	Hair Se levels >5 ppm Blood Se levels >1.5 ppm Liver Se levels >1.25 ppm wet weight	Remove source Selenium deficiency is a more widespread problem; see section on white muscle disease
Nitrate and nitrite poisoning	Nitrate-accumulating plants—sorghum, Sudan grass, pigweed stems, cereal grains Round bales of hay Fertilizer-contaminated water Nitrate converted to nitrite by rumen; nitrite is usually the toxic ion	Methemoglobinemia (brown blood), >30% of total Hb Dyspnea, weakness Abortion or infertility caused by fetal anoxia	Acute poisoning may be caused by forage nitrate levels >10,000 ppm or water nitrate levels >1500 ppm National Academy of Science cautions that drinking water should not have more than 440 mg nitrates/L or 33 mg nitrites/L Aqueous humor of eye levels >40 μg/mL nitrate confirms diagnosis (40 ppm or 40 mg/L) Field tests using 1% diphenylamine for plant or aqueous nitrate levels	1% Methylene blue solution 4–15 mg/kg IV; not approved in food animals. IV fluids Tissue staining may occur for months after administration Feeds should contain <0.6% nitrate
Plant-Associated Toxicities				
Cyanogenic plants	Sorghum, Sudan grass (usually fresh cut rather than stored forage), *Prunus* spp. trees, Johnson grass	Polypnea, anxiety, progressive weakness and dyspnea followed by death Bright red color to venous blood	Confirmed exposure to cyanogenic plants and signs	0.5 g/kg body weight sodium thiosulfate as a 30–40% solution IV converts cyanide to thiocyanate Also administer orally

Continued

TABLE 17.1 *Toxicities, Poisonings and Deficiencies—cont'd*

Agent	Usual Source	Signs	Diagnosis	Treatment
Gossypol	Cottonseed, cottonseed meal	Cardiac failure caused by alterations in potassium levels (acute) or cardiomyopathy (chronic) Hemoglobinuria Liver necrosis Reproductive failure (chronic)	History of feeding cottonseed or meal to young cattle, 100 ppm in diet support toxicity In adult cattle, 1000–2000 ppm free gossypol in diet is toxic	Change diet; decrease amount fed in hot weather especially
Citrus pulp	Citrus pulp in total mixed ration has been associated with multiple deaths in dairy cattle; it is unknown why this occurs	Skin lesions, hemorrhage, heart failure, and systemic granulomatous disease that is similar to vetch poisoning *(Vicia);* suggested type IV hypersensitivity	Clinical signs and history of citrus pulp feeding	Citrus pulp is often fed with no problems, so there may be a specific toxin that occurs under specific but unknown conditions
Bracken fern	Pasture consumption or bracken in hay	May be delayed after long-term ingestion (1–3 mo) Bleeding and aplastic anemia Enzootic hematuria and bladder neoplasms	Thrombocytopenia Leukopenia Anemia (nonregenerative) Hematuria and bladder carcinomas are rare in United States	None practical other than avoidance and whole blood transfusions
Oak or acorn poisoning	Oak leaves or acorns Oak buds in spring and acorns in the fall	Anorexia, rumen stasis, hemorrhagic enteritis, subcutaneous edema, renal failure	Characteristic signs and history Laboratory confirmation of renal disease by testing serum and urine Necropsy findings of enlarged kidneys, perirenal edema and hemorrhage, GI lesions, oak or acorns in rumen	High volume IV fluid therapy Rumenotomy
Oxalate poisoning	*Rumex* spp. plants (sorrels and docks); rhubarb leaves	Renal failure, hypocalcemia, often with hyperphosphatemia, hyperkalemia, and hypernatremia	Confirm renal disease with oxalate crystals in urinary tract Find plant in rumen	High volume IV fluid therapy Rumenotomy
Redroot pigweed poisoning	*Amaranthus retroflexus*— leafy portions of plants, especially during drought conditions A common source of nitrates and oxalates	SC edema, hypoproteinemia, renal failure	Confirmation of renal failure and ingestion of the plant (in rumen) Cattle rarely eat pigweed although it may be abundant in pastures	High-volume IV fluid therapy Rumenotomy
Yews *(Taxus)*	Discarded trimmings from shrubs or overgrown shrubs	Sudden death common or cardiac dysrhythmias and death several days later	History and finding plant in rumen, in mouth, or around body	None

TABLE 17.1 Toxicities, Poisonings and Deficiencies—cont'd

Agent	Usual Source	Signs	Diagnosis	Treatment
Blue-green algae (*Cyanobacteria*)	Farm ponds, neglected livestock water tanks midsummer to early autumn when warm sunny weather and wind combine to propel toxic algae to pond shore	Hepatotoxicosis Neurotoxicosis Bloody diarrhea Signs depend on specific toxins produced by different species	Identification and culture of various toxic species	Activated charcoal, support; add $CuSO_4$ to pond water to attain a concentration of 0.2–0.4 ppm
Pyrrolizidine alkaloid poisoning	Pasture or hay containing *Senecio* spp., *Crotalaria* sp., *Heliotropium* spp., *Amsinckia* spp., *Cynoglossum officinale*	Hepatic failure, icterus, tenesmus, rectal prolapses, hepatic encephalopathy, GI signs, photosensitization possible	History, signs, hepatic failure based on serum chemistry, typical histopathology findings in liver (megakaryocytosis)	Pasture management to control causative plant species, supportive care for liver dysfunction
Sporodesmin poisoning	Pasture and dead pasture litter containing *Pithomyces chartarum* (mycotoxin), on *Tribulus terrestris*, *Panicum* spp., *Agave lecegilla,* or *Nolina texana* pastures	Biliary obstruction; may lead to icterus, photosensitization, hepatic encephalopathy, anorexia, death	History of exposure, serum blood chemistry, hepatic histopathology	Zinc salts can be protective (oral administration at time of exposure or before exposure)
Kochia scoparia poisoning	Pasture exposure	Photosensitization secondary to toxic hepatic damage Polioencephalomalacia leading to cerebral dysfunction, including blindness, seizures	History, signs, confirmation of hepatic disease by serum chemistry, biopsy, or necropsy	Pasture management to control plant
Locoweed poisoning *Astragalus* spp. *Oxytropis* spp.	Pasture, pod stage of plants containing swainsonine	Tremors, ataxia, anorexia, behavior changes; signs of congestive heart failure if at high altitude	Vacuoles in blood lymphocytes, neurons, and epithelial cells	Remove from pasture
Amanitin toxicosis	Amanitin containing mushrooms	Acute panlobular hepatic necrosis, sudden death	Confirmation of amanitin in rumen contents, liver or urine	Reported cases have been fatal
Cassia spp. (e.g., sicklepod, coffee senna)	Chopped forage containing high levels of plants or pasture exposure, seeds are most toxic, plant stays green in fall	Myopathy, weakness, recumbency, myoglobinuria	Elevated CK and AST Myoglobinuria Rule out selenium deficiency and exertional myopathy	Avoidance or removal of contaminated feed, rumenotomy and IV fluid therapy
White snake root (*Eupatorium rugosum*)	Pasture plant in the northeastern states	Muscle tremors, weakness, ataxia caused by the effects of tremetone	Detection of the plant, signs of muscle tremors, myopathy	Pasture management to control plant
Cocklebur (*Xanthium* spp.)	Pastures containing two leafed seedlings are toxic	Weakness, depression, dyspnea, neurologic signs including convulsions	History, typical GI, hepatic, and renal lesions	Pasture management to control plant

Continued

TABLE 17.1 *Toxicities, Poisonings and Deficiencies—**cont'd***

Agent	Usual Source	Signs	Diagnosis	Treatment
Perilla mint (*Perilla frutescens*) 3-methylindole toxicity (high tryptophan grasses) 4-ipomeanol (moldy sweet potato)	Cattle grazing forest land may be exposed Introduced to new lush pasture 4–14 days before signs Sweet potato infected with *Fusarium solani*	Acute respiratory distress with expiratory grunt, pulmonary edema and emphysema	History, clinical signs, ruling out infectious causes; pulmonary edema and emphysema of lungs on necropsy	Remove from pasture, supportive (diuretics, anti-inflammatories) Ionophores in feed may be preventive before exposure
Brassica spp. (turnips, rape, kale)	Pasturing on turnips or other *Brassica* spp.	Several possible syndromes, including polioencephalomalacia, goiter and other signs of iodine deficiency, acute bovine pulmonary emphysema and edema, bloat, hemolytic anemia Signs of liver disease; photosensitivity	History, clinical signs	Avoidance or limitation of access Replace with roughage
Larkspurs (*Delphinium* spp.)	Pastures	Curare-like neuromuscular blockade Dose-dependent signs of anxiety, excitability, stiffness, base-wide stance, collapse, bloat, vomiting, constipation	History, signs	Physostigmine 0.08 mg/kg body weight IV *or* Neostigmine 0.01 to 0.02 mg/kg body weight IM
Hairy vetch (*Vicia villosa*)	Pastures, hay, silage	Sudden death Acute nervous signs and death after seed ingestion Subcutaneous swelling of head, neck, body with respiratory signs (purulent nasal discharge, cough) Dermatitis, pruritus, alopecia, conjunctivitis, diarrhea Suggested type IV hypersensitivity	History, signs, gross and histopathologic findings (enlarged organs with gray-yellow firm areas of infiltration; multinucleated giant cells)	Remove source, supportive
Oleander	Pasture, hay, or trimmings	Cardiotoxic glycosides Sudden death Cardiac arrhythmia	History, signs, detection of oleandrin in rumen contents by thin layer chromatography	Atropine for arrhythmias, rumenotomy for removal, supportive
Onion (*Allium* sp.)	Wild onions in spring pasture	Onion odor, hemoglobinuria	History of exposure and Heinz bodies in red blood cells on blood smear	Supportive, antioxidants; treatment often not required
Rye grass	Annual ryegrass pasture or hay	Staggers, tremors (lolitrem toxicity), hemoglobinuria possible	Clinical signs, presence of plant; lolitrem B presence in hay detected by HPLC	Removal from source usually results in full recovery within 7–15 days

TABLE 17.1   *Toxicities, Poisonings and Deficiencies—cont'd*

Agent	Usual Source	Signs	Diagnosis	Treatment
Marijuana poisoning (*Cannabis sativa*)	Illegally grown marijuana planted among corn or other feed crops	Muscle tremors, hypersalivation, mydriasis, reluctance to move, incoordination	History of exposure; laboratory assays for detection of THC in GI contents to indicate exposure	Rumenotomy, intraruminal instillation of activated charcoal, cathartics, supportive care
Nicotine toxicosis	*Nicotiana glauca* (wild tree tobacco), *Nicotiana tabacum*	Nicotinic neurologic signs, sudden death, congenital abnormalities (including skeletal deformities in fetus) if pregnant during exposure	History of exposure, remnants of these plants present in rumen contents, analysis of tissues, urine or ingesta for anabasine (an alkaloid in *Nicotiana* spp.)	Supportive
Zygophallaceous plant toxicosis	*Peganum harmala* (African rue*), P. mexicanum* (Mexican rue), *Tribulus terrestris* (cat head), *T. micrococcus* (yellow vine), *Kallstroemia hirsutissima* (hairy caltrop), *K. parviflora* (warty caltrop)	Motor neuron disease, including ataxia, weakness and paresis	History of exposure	Remove from pasture, supportive
Goat's rue toxicosis	*Galega officinalis* (in harvested forages)	Neurologic signs, edema of skin, sudden death, seizures, trembling, tremor	History of exposure, identification of plant in hay being fed or rumen contents	Supportive
Insect Associated Toxicities				
Cantharidin toxicity	Consumption of blister beetles in alfalfa hay or a mixed ration	Agalactia, anorexia, ataxia, diarrhea, oral ulceration, excessive salivation, polyuria, death	GC/LC-MS of urine or rumen contents to detect cantharidin	Rumenotomy, activated charcoal, supportive
Tick paralysis (in North America, *Dermacentor andersoni* most often implicated, but many others are capable of causing disease)	Salivary neurotoxin produced while female tick feeds; impairs acetylcholine release at neuromuscular junction	Pelvic limb weakness, ataxia, lethargy, recumbency, muscle flaccidity of all four limbs, diminished or absent spinal reflexes, absent or diminished withdrawal from noxious stimulus, diminished PLR and menace response, opisthotonus, and seizures	Based on rapid progression of signs, demonstration of appropriate species of tick, and response to tick removal	Removal of all ticks from the animal (most improve within 4 hr of removal and recover in 12–72 hr)
Sawfly (*Lophyrotoma interrupta*) larval toxicity	Larvae of sawflies (*Lophyrotoma interrupta* in Australia, *Arge pullata* in Denmark, and *Perreyia flavipes* in Uruguay) fall out of trees in large numbers and are toxic when ingested (cattle develop a craving for them)	Acute hepatic necrosis leading to apathy, recumbency, tremors, paddling, and death in 24–48 hr; in protracted cases: aggressiveness, icterus, photodermatitis, other neurologic signs consistent with hepatic encephalopathy	Ascites, petechiae and ecchymoses of serosal surfaces with enlarged liver and accentuated lobular pattern on gross necropsy; sawfly larval body fragments found in forestomachs and possibly abomasum; hepatic necrosis on histopathology	Removal of cattle from exposure to larvae; supportive

Continued

TABLE 17.1 *Toxicities, Poisonings and Deficiencies—cont'd*

Agent	Usual Source	Signs	Diagnosis	Treatment
Hyalomma toxicity (sweating sickness)	Epitheliotropic toxin produced by female *Hyalomma truncatum* ticks in Africa	Fever, hyperemia of mucous membranes, salivation, necrosis of oral mucosa, lacrimation, moist dermatitis develops at base of ears, axilla, inguinal region, perineum and later extends over whole body, hyperesthesia, foul odor, later skin may slough, death may occur	Presence of the vector coincident with moist dermatitis and desquamation of the skin	Tick control and removal, supportive, antibiotics and antiinflammatories for secondary infections and pain; immune serum in endemic areas
Miscellaneous Industrial Compound Toxicities				
Pentachlorophenol (PCP or Penta)	Wood preservative	Local irritation (salivation, inflamed oral mucosa, skin lesions) Systemic absorption through skin and lungs may cause acute (neurologic) or chronic (wasting) signs Prolonged residues	Whole blood analysis for PCP	Do not use treated wood for housing or fencing
Polycyclic aromatic hydrocarbons (e.g., cresols, phenols)	Clay pigeons or coal tar pitch Products from distillation of coal tar	Ataxia, bloat, tetraparesis, death	History of exposure and necropsy findings (hepatic damage)	Supportive
Crude oil, petroleum products (kerosene, naphtha, gasoline), lubricating distillates, drilling fluids, diesel fuel	Contamination of water sources or accidental exposure, oil-well drilling fluids, muds and additives, discarded petroleum products (including fuels, greases, and oils), sometimes associated with water deprivation	Enteric—bloat, regurgitation caused by vaporization and expansion of volatile hydrocarbons Pneumonia caused by aspiration of volatile products into the lungs or aspiration during eructation Neurologic signs possible	Confirmation of volatile hydrocarbons in gut contents, feces, or lungs Mix rumen contents with water and look for oil Submit rumen contents for confirmation Petroleum smell on breath	Rumenotomy and supportive therapy
Methyl alcohol, methanol	Antifreeze used in the oil industry	Agalactia, dullness, inability to stand, death	History of exposure, analysis of rumen contents	Supportive
Vanadium, barium, bromide, acrylamide, N-methylolacrylamide	Vanadium mined primarily in Russia and South Africa Barium from lead, silver, and zinc mines Bromide from chemical dump sites N-methylolacrylamide from chemical grouting agents	Weakness, ataxia, tremors, other neurologic signs, excessive salivation, bloody diarrhea, straining, conjunctival injection, periorbital swelling; N-methylolacrylamide can cause blindness	History of exposure, tissue and environmental testing	Supportive

TABLE 17.1 *Toxicities, Poisonings and Deficiencies—cont'd*

Agent	Usual Source	Signs	Diagnosis	Treatment
Halogenated cyclic hydrocarbons (PCB, PBB) poisoning	Residual environmental contamination by compounds no longer produced or transformer accidents	Wasting, skin lesions, hyperkeratosis, immunosuppression, reproductive problems, liver and kidney lesions	Tissue levels (accumulates in fat), milk levels assessed by qualified laboratories; fat deposition *Prolonged residues*	None Culling may be required, but beware of residues
Miscellaneous Insecticide, Pesticide, Rodenticide and Fertilizer Toxicities				
Organophosphate toxicosis	Access or accidental exposure to organophosphate insecticides or lubricants containing triaryl phosphates (e.g., industrial solvents, automotive brake fluids)	Ingestion of insecticides—signs within a few hours Usually salivation, miosis, tremors, weakness, dyspnea, colic dehydration Diarrhea typical, but chlorpyrifos in bulls also causes profound rumen stasis Signs may vary depending on specific toxin and variable muscarinic or nicotinic effects Dermal—signs may be delayed 1 to 7 days or more Ingestion of triaryl phosphates—slowly progressive neurologic signs, 10 days to a few months after exposure; posterior paresis is a predominant sign with this form	Reduced cholinesterase activity in blood, brain, retina, and other tissues Samples should be delivered to laboratory chilled in less than 24 hr; frozen samples may be acceptable for several days Cholinesterase levels decreased over 50% compared to controls are diagnostic Blood samples; serum or heparinized plasma Apparent potentiation with testosterone, therefore bulls may be uniquely affected during a herd exposure For triaryl phosphates—histologic detection of axonopathy in peripheral nerves	Atropine: 0.25–0.50 mg/kg body weight; repeat only if necessary Oral dose of 1–2 lb activated charcoal 2-PAM*: 20–50 mg/kg IM; best given during first 24–48 hr For dermal exposure, gently wash with water and detergent
Carbamate toxicosis	Access or accidental exposure to carbamates	Same as organophosphates	Same as organophosphates, except cholinesterase levels may return to baseline within hours of exposure while patient is still symptomatic and thus may not be diagnostic	Similar to organophosphates but 2-PAM not used for carbamate toxicosis
Boron	Boron fertilizer	Neurologic; weak, depressed, fasciculations, seizures Diarrhea	Colorimetric assay on ashed tissue Minimum lethal dose, 200–600 mg/kg	Supportive
4-Aminopyridine toxicosis	Avicide (starlingcide with limited permitted use in the United States)	Neurologic; aggression, ataxia, salivation, seizures, sudden death	History of exposure; toxicologic assay of GI contents	Supportive
Diquat toxicosis	Pesticides containing diquat (1,1′-ethylene-2,2′-dipyridylium dibromide)	Anorexia, agalactia, ataxia, dysmetria, recumbency, mydriasis, trembling, death, skin lesions in those surviving dermal exposure	History of exposure, detection of diquat in tissues (such as kidney)	Supportive

Continued

TABLE 17.1	Toxicities, Poisonings and Deficiencies—cont'd			
Agent	Usual Source	Signs	Diagnosis	Treatment
Metaldehyde toxicosis	Metaldehyde slug and snail baits	CNS stimulation: salivation, excitement, head pressing, nystagmus, seizures, tetany, tremor, ataxia, fever, cyanosis, blindness, death	Detection of metaldehyde in rumen content or tissues	Supportive
Zinc phosphide or aluminum phosphide rodenticides	Phosphine gas released when rodenticides contact water or stomach contents	Abdominal distention, excitation, cyanosis, salivation, seizures, tremors, tachycardia, dyspnea, tachypnea, hepatic failure, sudden death	History of exposure; phosphine gas odor of decaying fish (garlic-like) when performing postmortem examination; GI contents and tissues should be frozen and packed in air tight container for toxicologic analysis	Supportive
Phosphatic fertilizer toxicosis	Superphosphate fertilizers	Nephritis, PU/PD, hemoglobinuria, anorexia, agalactia, colic, dehydration, abortion, hypocalcemia	Clinical signs and history of exposure; some signs resemble hypocalcemia, but there is no response to calcium administration	None
Sodium fluoroacetate, 1080	Used by professional exterminators in the United States; found in a variety of plants in Australia, Brazil, and Africa	Neurologic; blindness, seizures, hyperesthesia, aimless propulsion, death	Sodium fluoroacetate assay on plasma, tissue, or rumen contents	None
Strychnine toxicosis	Malicious poisoning or rodenticides	Excitement, seizures, CNS stimulation	History and detection in rumen contents	General anesthesia or sedation; removal via rumenotomy or via cathartics
Fluoride poisoning (fluorosis)	Acute poisoning from weed treatment and wood preservative Chronic poisoning from plants and soils downwind from manufacturing plants that process fluoride-containing substances	Acute—gastroenteritis, renal failure, and neurologic Chronic (more common)—lameness caused by exostoses and other bone lesions Dental abnormalities—excessive wear and discoloration	Acute—urine, tissue, and rumen contents >5500 ppm fluoride in compact bone >7000 ppm fluoride in cancellous bone	None
Arsenic toxicosis	Wood preservatives Burn piles Outdated insecticides Rodenticides Herbicides Dirt where these products have concentrated Slag from previous mining Poultry and swine feed additives	Gastroenteritis and diarrhea (sometimes hemorrhagic) Some nervous signs Teeth grinding Possible renal lesions Skin necrosis if topical	>3 ppm arsenic (wet weight) in liver and kidney	Thioctic acid 20% solution 50 mg/kg IM thrice daily or sodium thiosulfate 30 g orally once daily for 4 days Fluid therapy and intestinal protectants

TABLE 17.1   *Toxicities, Poisonings and Deficiencies—cont'd*

Agent	Usual Source	Signs	Diagnosis	Treatment
Lead toxicosis (See Chapter 13)	Old paints, batteries, drained motor oil (when leaded fuel is used), lead shot in feed or pasture; lead solder in pipes especially with low pH water source, industrial waste contamination	Cortical blindness, hyperesthesia, ataxia, tremors, seizures, grinding teeth, rumen atony, and occasionally diarrhea	Signs, possible exposure, look for oil in rumen sample, blood lead concentration >0.35 ppm Liver or kidney >10 ppm Radiography to demonstrate lead in rumen	Thiamine 1 g IV daily; calcium EDTA 35 mg/kg IV every 12 hr for at least 3–5 days Rumenotomy Mg sulfate orally
Mercury toxicosis	Organic mercurial fungicides, ash residues, industrial mercury	Acute gastroenteritis; melena, rumen atony, dysphagia, CNS signs; paresis, recumbency, propulsion, tremors, seizures, blindness, death	Detection of mercury in blood or tissues or rumen contents	None
Mycotoxicoses				
Ergot	Grains or fescue grasses contaminated with sclerotia of *Claviceps purpurea*	Dry gangrene of one or more distal extremities, lameness	Diets containing 0.3–1.0% ergot	Removal of contaminated feed
Fescue toxicosis ("summer syndrome") Fescue foot (usually fall; mostly calves) Fescue fat necrosis	Fescue grass contaminated with *Acremonium coenophialum*	Poor growth, salivation, dyspnea, nervousness, poor heat tolerance Reduced pregnancy rates Lameness, sloughing of extremities Reduced weight gain Abdominal fat necrosis (often in Channel Island breeds)	Endophyte identification in fescue Measure ergopeptide levels in fescue grass	Symptomatic Overseed with legumes and supplement with grain Use low endophyte seed varieties
Tremorogenic toxins	Dallis grass infected with *Claviceps paspali* Bermuda grass (fall) tremors *Phalaris* spp. staggers Perennial ryegrass staggers—contaminated with *Acremonium loliae* Annual ryegrass (corynetoxins) Tremorogenic mycotoxins caused by various *Penicillium* and *Aspergillus* spp. molds; Penitrem is one such toxin White snake root, rayless goldenrod, Jimmy fern, mountain laurel	Tremors accentuated by exercise, hyperexcitability, ataxia, hypermetria, tetany, collapse followed by relaxation White snake root excreted in milk, toxic to calves or people drinking milk from exposed cows	Identify plant and appropriate time of year	Remove from exposure, alternative feed source Recovery often follows removal from exposure
Pithomyces chartarum (see Sporodesmin poisoning)				

Continued

TABLE 17.1	Toxicities, Poisonings and Deficiencies—**cont'd**			
Agent	**Usual Source**	**Signs**	**Diagnosis**	**Treatment**
Zearalenone (F-2)	Usually stored corn contaminated with *Fusarium* as a result of warm moist conditions followed by cold weather	Hyperestrogenism—premature udder development, swollen vulvas, prolapses, abortion, infertility	Feed analysis for zearalenone—usually ≥5 ppm to cause signs	Removal of contaminated feed
Trichothecenes (T-2, DON (Vomitoxin), DAS)	Forages harvested late because of wet weather Corn, wheat, barley, and other grains	Feed refusal or decreased dry matter intake—most common! Necrotic oral mucosal lesions Coagulopathies possible Immunosuppression Reproductive failure Fever, diarrhea	T-2 and DAS levels >10 ppm are toxic	Removal of contaminated feed
Slaframine (slobber factor)	Legumes (often red clover) contaminated with *Rhizoctonia leguminicola*	Salivation that increases over 24 hr followed by anorexia, frequent urination, diarrhea	Clinical signs and identification of specific fungus in forage	Removal of contaminated feed Atropine in severe cases (0.25 mg/kg)
Aflatoxins (B$_1$ most toxic)	Seed grains (especially corn) having excess moisture content	Reduced productivity Hepatotoxicity (central lobular) Immunosuppression	Dietary concentrations ≥20 ppb Milk concentrations should be <0.5 ppb	Removal of contaminated feed Supportive care for liver dysfunction
Mineral and Vitamin Toxicities				
Iron toxicosis	Hematinic preparations	Icterus, nervous signs	History of administration, increased liver enzymes	Supportive, blood removal
Copper poisoning	Accidental or intended ingestion—cattle may be poisoned by intake of greater than 200 mg/kg CuSO$_4$ Normal Cu + low Mo in diet Hepatotoxic plants (pyrrolizidine alkaloids) that cause excessive Cu retention in liver	Acute—severe GI signs and death Chronic—methemoglobinemia, brown mucous membranes, anemia, dyspnea, hemoglobinuria	Elevated blood, liver, and kidney copper levels Normal blood Cu = 0.7–1.3 ppm—blood may not reflect body tissue levels! Normal liver Cu = 30.0–140.0 ppm (wet weight) Normal kidney Cu ≥15.0 ppm (wet weight) Postmortem: blue-black kidneys, hemoglobinuria, icterus, enlarged liver	Remove source Reduce copper or add molybdenum to diet to reduce Cu/Mo ratio 3 g sodium molybdate and 5 g sodium thiosulfate can be added to diet/head/day for 2 weeks and then tapered
Sulfate poisoning	High sulfate-containing plants or water (or both) Distiller grains and other coproducts of ethanol production	Acute; blindness, recumbency, seizures, death Subacute; visual impairment, ataxia, twitching of ears and facial muscles	Polioencephalomalacia High hydrogen sulfide levels in rumen gas; rations >0.4% total sulfur on a dry matter basis. Note; not all animals consuming >0.4% sulfur are affected by clinical disease. Note; considerable sulfur intake may occur via water and must be considered as part of sulfur calculated in ration	Supportive Thiamine treatment Glucocorticoid therapy Removal of affected animals from high-sulfur sources and provision of low-sulfur rations

TABLE 17.1   *Toxicities, Poisonings and Deficiencies—**cont'd***

Agent	Usual Source	Signs	Diagnosis	Treatment
Molybdenum poisoning	Cu:Mo dietary ration <2:1 or dietary Mo >10 ppm Peat bog forages	Chronic—severe diarrhea, poor condition, anemia, lameness, and faded coat with depigmentation around the eyes— same as Cu deficiency Acute—kidney and liver necrosis	Cu:Mo dietary ratios Blood Mo >0.10 mg/kg	Reduce Mo or add Cu as 1%–2% $CuSO_4$ to diet
Salt toxicity	Prolonged water deprivation or from iatrogenic oral administration of abnormally concentrated electrolyte supplements to calves as treatment for diarrhea; commonly occurs if calves are fed high-salt/osmolality milk replacers without free water access	Blindness, seizure, coma	Plasma sodium >160 mEq/L	Slowly correct the hypernatremia with sodium-containing fluids and administer thiamine
Zinc toxicosis	Milk replacer (veal calves) Contaminated water (adult cattle)	Pneumonia, exophthalmos, chemosis, diarrhea, anorexia, bloat, cardiac arrhythmia, convulsions, PU/PD Constipation and reduced milk yield in adults	Preruminant diets containing more than 100 µg/g Zn	Removal of source or add roughage to diet
Vitamin D_3 toxicosis (can be replicated by overzealous and prolonged parenteral calcium administration or ingestion of cholecalciferol-containing rodenticides)	Large parenteral doses to cattle; most commonly young calves or preparturient cows; Jerseys seem more susceptible	Tachycardia, weakness, signs of heart failure, weight loss, stiffness, anorexia	Hypercalcemia and hyperphosphatemia, calcification of heart and greater vessels	Steroids, magnesium, diuresis, and supportive care
†Other byproducts fed to cattle	Food oils, pretzels, and so on may sporadically cause acute or subacute toxicosis in cattle	Variable but may include ruminal atony, diarrhea, neurologic signs in addition to renal or hepatic failure in some cases	A specific toxin is usually not identified, and in many outbreaks. similar byproducts have been fed without prior problems	Symptomatic plus removal of unusual feed source, especially carbohydrates
Iatrogenic Toxicities				
Potassium toxicosis (most cases occur in animals with impaired renal function and in calves with diarrhea and subsequent metabolic acidosis)	Excessive IV supplementation or large doses orally to calves	Cardiotoxic; bradycardia, arrhythmia, syncope or seizures, excitement, trembling, sudden death or collapse	History of administration and elevated potassium on blood chemistry or other fluid analyses (aqueous, CSF)	Correct dehydration in calves by administering IV fluids with glucose and then gradually include potassium in fluid supplementation; to correct cardiac arrhythmia more rapidly due to hyperkalemia, give calcium IV or dextrose and if needed regular insulin IV or SC (0.1 U/kg) with a CRI of 5% glucose (2.2–4.4 mL/kg/hr)

Continued

TABLE 17.1 *Toxicities, Poisonings and Deficiencies—cont'd*

Agent	Usual Source	Signs	Diagnosis	Treatment
Iodine toxicosis	Excessive supplementation or therapeutic administration in diet or repeated parenteral use therapeutically	Respiratory tract disease—cough Naso-ocular discharge Dry scaly coats Immune suppression Decreased production, growth, and fertility	Iodine intake far exceeding 12 mg/head/day Serum iodide or milk iodide ≥20 µg/dL	Maximum of 0.60 ppm in diet for adults Maximum of 0.25 ppm in diet for young stock Discontinue use until signs abate
Magnesium sulfate, oxide or hydroxide toxicosis	Excessive amount or frequency of administration	Anorexia, cold skin, weak, hypothermic, recumbent	History of administration and elevated magnesium on blood chemistry and elevated rumen pH	Calcium borogluconate slowly IV in crystalloids
Propylene glycol toxicosis	Can occur if >12 oz orally BID is given to adult cattle	Anorexia, abdominal distention, dyspnea, abnormal breath odor, increased or decreased borborygmi, foul odor to feces, diarrhea, ataxia, salivation, tachypnea, recumbency, seizures	History of administration, decreased rumen pH with appropriate clinical signs	Supportive care, including transfaunation
Poloxamer toxicosis	Bloat drench containing pluronic-type detergent, e.g., Poloxalene, Phibro Animal Health, Teaneck, NJ, 07664	In calves only; ruminal tympany, vocalization, tachypnea, recumbency, seizures, death	History of administration, clinical signs and concentrations of poloxamer present in abomasal and rumenal contents obtained postmortem	Supportive
Lidocaine toxicity	When given IV for intestinal ileus in young calves or other inadvertent overdose	Tremors and seizures	History of administration and age of calf	Diazepam and supportive fluids; recovery likely
Cobalt toxicosis	Oversupplementation, error in formulation of mineral supplementation	Anorexia, agalactia, colic, diarrhea, weight loss, PU/PD, rough coat, seizures, trembling, death	Blood cobalt analysis	None
Miscellaneous Deficiencies				
Selenium deficiency	Forages and feeds (total diet <0.3 ppm selenium on dry matter basis), inadequate supplementation (deficiency of selenium), vitamin E may play only minor role in white muscle disease	Weakness or stiffness of any striated muscles, including the heart; recumbency; congestive heart failure; death; aspiration pneumonia associated with poor suckling and swallowing; muscle atrophy (seen more in affected adults)	Profoundly elevated CK values, elevated serum troponin, myoglobinuria, whole blood selenium <5.0 µg/dL associated with white muscle disease, glutathione peroxidase less than 20 U/g Hb, CK values >1000–10,000 IU/L, histologic confirmation of lesions typical of Zenker's necrosis	Supplementation by injection and orally in feed Vitamin E and selenium are concentrated in colostrum; supplementation of dams can help prevent disease in calves In selenium-deficient areas, administration of selenium to newborn calves

TABLE 17.1	*Toxicities, Poisonings and Deficiencies—cont'd*			
Agent	**Usual Source**	**Signs**	**Diagnosis**	**Treatment**
Zinc deficiency	Forages from low zinc soils, especially if soil is alkaline and is fertilized heavily with nitrogen and phosphorus Hereditary form reported in Black Pied Danish cattle Idiopathic zinc responsive dermatosis also reported rarely	Parakeratosis and alopecia of head, neck, tail head, and limb flexion sites Poor condition and growth Lameness	Serum zinc levels much lower than normal (80–120 µg/dL) Response to treatment	Add zinc to ration. Minimum daily requirement is 40 ppm (dry matter basis)
Copper deficiency	Primary—forage grown on deficient soils and diet not supplemented adequately Secondary—high molybdenum or low Cu/Mo ratio (peat bog/teart pastures) High zinc, iron, lead, calcium carbonate or inorganic sulfates may also potentiate effect of Mo on copper	Calves—Poor growth, rough, faded or bleached hair coat, diarrhea, musculoskeletal abnormalities Adults—Loss of condition and production, anemia, bleached rough hair coat, chronic diarrhea (usually in secondary Cu deficiency), falling disease (myocardial degeneration)	Pasture having <3 mg Cu/kg dry matter Blood and liver copper levels vary greatly, and overlap occurs between deficient, marginal, and normal values; therefore, response to copper supplementation may provide clinical confirmation of suspected deficient state Plasma copper: 19–57 µg/dL = marginal, <19 µg/dL = low Liver copper: >100 mg/kg (100 ppm) dry weight = normal <30 mg/kg dry weight = low Clinical signs Dietary levels of Cu, Mb, and sulfates	Oral $CuSO_4$: Calves = 4 g/day for 3–5 wk Cows = 8–10 g/day for 3–5 wk Diet should contain 10 mg copper/kg dry matter for prevention Supplementing mineral and salt content of diet to 3%–5% copper sulfate
Iron deficiency	Total milk diet, chronic blood loss	Weakness, tachycardia, pallor	History; clinical signs; microcytic, microchromic, nonregenerative anemia with hematocrit often <12%; serum iron extremely low; iron-binding capacity normal or high	Blood transfusion Parenteral iron
Manganese deficiency	Forages from low Mn soils or alkaline soils with marginal Mn levels	Infertility, calves with congenital limb deformities and knuckling at fetlocks	Blood and tissue levels variable	40 ppm Mn in diet
Magnesium deficiency; less common in dairy cattle than beef cattle; see metabolic diseases	Low magnesium diets, high potassium for ages predisposed to hypomagnesemia Magnesium absorption from milk decreases with age in calves such that 3-month-old calves are most susceptible	Recumbency, tetany, seizures, aggression When tetany is present calcium will also be low Poor growth and poor hair coats Tremors in calves	Serum magnesium levels <1.2 mg/dL in affected cattle Relatively no magnesium in urine (low fractional excretion); vitreous humor Mg <1.2 mg/dL at postmortem	Prevention; magnesium fertilizers spread on pastures, reduced use of potassium fertilizers, balancing the diet Treatment; IV and/or oral supplementation with magnesium chloride or sulfate

Continued

TABLE 17.1   *Toxicities, Poisonings and Deficiencies—cont'd*

Agent	Usual Source	Signs	Diagnosis	Treatment
Sodium chloride deficiency	Lack of supplementation or availability	PU/PD; pica; drinking urine; salt hunger; and loss of appetite, weight, and production	Salivary sodium normal =140–150 mEq/L Deficient = 70–100 mEq/L	Salt fed at 0.5% of diet
Iodine deficiency	Iodine-deficient soils High intake of calcium Diets high in *Brassica* spp.	Enlarged thyroid and weakness in newborn calves Stillbirths, often with fetal goiter	Assess blood and forage for iodine	Lactating and dry cows; 0.6–0.8 mg/kg dry weight feed Calves; 0.1–0.3 mg/kg dry weight feed
Cobalt deficiency	Pastures or diets deficient in cobalt Cobalt deficiency impairs vitamin B_{12} production and prevents propionic acid metabolism	Progressive loss of appetite, weight, and production Anemia, weakness, pica	Liver vitamin B_{12} levels; normal >0.3 mg/kg liver Cobalt deficient <0.1 mg/kg liver	To prevent; 0.11 mg cobalt/kg (dry matter basis) To treat; vitamin B_{12} injection IM or SC, 1 mg cobalt orally, once daily
Vitamin D, calcium, or phosphorus imbalance or deficiency	Lack of sunlight, feeds formulated without appropriate calcium, phosphorus or vitamin D	Rickets—abnormal bone growth, osteoporosis and associated fractures, epiphysitis Urolithiasis in males	Dietary investigation, feed analysis, serum vitamin D analysis	Correction of the diet

*Protopam chloride, Ayerst Labs, New York, NY.
†See http://shaverlab.dysci.wisc.edu/wp-content/uploads/sites/87/2015/04/byproductfeedsrevised2008.pdf
AST, Aspartate transaminase; *BID,* twice a day; *CK,* creatine kinase; *CNS,* central nervous system; *CRI,* constant-rate infusion; *CSF,* cerebrospinal fluid; *DAS,* diacetoxyscirpenol; *DON,* deoxynivalenol; *EDTA,* ethylenediaminetetraacetic acid; *FDP,* fibrin degradation product; *GI,* gastrointestinal; *GC/LC-MS,* gas chromatography/liquid chromatography mass spectrometry; *Hb,* hemoglobin; *HPLC,* high-performance liquid chromatography; *IM,* intramuscular; *IV,* intravenous; *PBB,* polybrominated biphenyl; *PCB,* polychlorinated biphenyl; *PD,* polydipsia; *PLR,* pupillary light reflex; *PU,* polyuria; *SC,* subcutaneous; *THC,* tetrahydrocannabinol.

TABLE 17.2   **Diagnostic Sample Submission Checklist for Suspected Toxicities**

Alive	Dead
CBC Chemistry Coagulation profile (blue tube) Save EDTA and heparin whole-blood samples as well as EDTA and heparinized plasma samples (separated from cells) Serum sample Special tubes for mineral analysis Urine Feed sample; one refrigerated and one frozen in airtight container Water sample: same as feed Rumen contents (if possible) and feces: 100 g in leak-proof container, refrigerated Suspect materials (e.g., pasture, chemicals)	Aqueous humor, 2 mL Heart blood: Save EDTA and heparinized whole blood samples as well as EDTA and heparinized plasma samples (separated from cells) Urine 1 kg rumen contents: frozen, check pH when fresh 100 g of colon contents; frozen Liver and kidney; 100 g frozen Brain; frozen Fat (omental or abdominal); 100 g frozen Complete set of tissues in formalin (include brain, spinal cord, skeletal muscle, all major organs, and any detected gross lesions)

CBC, Complete blood count; *EDTA,* ethylenediaminetetraacetic acid;

Suggested Readings

Bischoff, K., & Smith, M. (2011). Toxic plants of the northeastern United States. *Vet Clin North Am Food Anim Pract, 27*(2), 459–480.

Burrows, G. E. (Ed.). (1989). *Clinical toxicology, Vet Clin North Am Food Anim Pract* (Vol. 5). Philadelphia: Saunders.

Committee on Minerals and Toxic Substances in Diets and Water for Animals, Board on Agriculture and Natural Resources, Division on Earth and Life Studies, National Research Council of the National Academies: Mineral tolerance of animals. (2005). Washington, DC: National Academy Press.

Cowan, V., & Blakley, B. (2016). Characterizing 1341 cases of veterinary toxicosis confirmed in western Canada: a 16-year retrospective study. *Can Vet J, 57*(1), 53–58.

Gabor, L. J., & Downing, G. M. (2003). Monensin toxicity in preruminant dairy heifers. *Aust Vet J, 81*, 476–478.

Gonzalez, M., Barkema, H. W., & Keefe, G. P. (2005). Monensin toxicosis in a dairy herd. *Can Vet J, 46*, 910–912.

Gunes, V. 1, Ozcan, K., Citil, M., et al. (2010). Detection of myocardial degeneration with point-of-care cardiac troponin assays and histopathology in lambs with white muscle disease. *Vet J, 184*(3), 376–378.

Hooser, S. B., Van Alstine, W., Kiupel, M., et al. (2000). Acute pit gas (hydrogen sulfide) poisoning in confinement cattle. *J Vet Diagn Invest, 12*(3), 272–275.

Iizuka, A., Haritani, M., Shiono, M., et al. (2005). An outbreak of systemic granulomatous disease in cows with high milk yields. *J Vet Med Sci, 67*, 693–699.

Kaur, R., Sharma, S., & Rampal, S. (2003). Effect of sub-chronic selenium toxicosis on lipid peroxidation, glutathione redox cycle and antioxidant enzymes in calves. *Vet Hum Toxicol, 45*, 190–192.

Knight, A. P. (2001). *A guide to plant poisoning of animals in North America.* Jackson, WY: Teton New Media.

Lardy, G., & Anderson, V. (2014). Feeding Coproducts of the Ethanol Industry to Beef Cattle. *NDSU Extension Service,* AS1242.

Lopez-Alonso, M., Crespo, A., Miranda, M., et al. (2006). Assessment of some blood parameters as potential markers of hepatic copper accumulation in cattle. *J Vet Diagn Invest, 18*, 71–75.

Machen, M., Montgomery, T., Holland, R., et al. (1996). Bovine hereditary zinc deficiency: lethal trait A 46. *J Vet Diagn Invest, 8*, 219–227.

Mostrom, M. S., & Jacobsen, B. J. (2011). Ruminant mycotoxicosis. *Vet Clin North Am Food Anim Prac, 27*, 315–344.

Nicholson, S. S. (1981). Suspected 4-aminopyridine toxicosis in cattle. *J Am Vet Med Assoc, 178*, 1277–1278.

Osweiler, G. D. (1999). Physical and chemical diseases. In J. L. Howard, & R. A. Smith (Eds.), *Current veterinary therapy 4: food animal practice* (4th ed.). Philadelphia: Saunders.

Osweiler, G. D., & Galey, F. D. (Eds.). (2000). *Toxicology, Vet Clin North Am Food Anim Pract* (Vol. 16). Philadelphia: Saunders.

Pinto, C., Santos, V. M., Dinis, J., et al. (2005). Pithomycotoxicosis (facial eczema) in ruminants in the Azores, Portugal. *Vet Rec, 157*(25), 805–810.

Plumlee, K. H., Holstege, D. M., Blanchard, P. C., et al. (1993). Nicotiana glauca toxicosis of cattle. *J Vet Diagn Invest, 5*(3), 498–499.

Poppenga, R. H. (2011). Commercial and industrial chemical hazards for ruminants. *Vet Clin North Am Food Anim Pract, 27*, 373–387.

Puls, R. (1994). *Mineral levels in animal health* (2nd ed.).

Radostits, O. M., Gay, C. C., Blood, D. C., et al. (2000 and 2006). *Veterinary medicine. A textbook of the diseases of cattle, sheep, pigs, goats and horses* (eds 9 and 10.). Philadelphia: Saunders.

Riet-Correa, F., Rivero, R., Odriozola, E., et al. (2013). Mycotoxicoses of ruminants and horses. *J Vet Diagn Invest, 25*, 692–708.

Santos, J. E., Villasenor, M., Robinson, P. H., et al. (2003). Type of cottonseed and level of gossypol in diets of lactating dairy cows: plasma gossypol, health, and reproductive performance. *J Dairy Sci, 86*, 892–905.

Saunders, G. K., Blodgett, D. J., Hutchins, T. A., et al. (2000). Suspected citrus pulp toxicosis in dairy cattle. *J Vet Diagn Invest, 12*, 269–271.

Smith, B. P. (2002). *Large animal internal medicine* (3rd ed.). St. Louis: Mosby.

Spickett, A. M., Burger, D. B., Crause, J. C., et al. (1991). Sweating sickness: relative curative effect of hyperimmune serum and a precipitated immunoglobulin suspension and immunoblot identification of proposed immunodominant tick salivary gland proteins. *Onderstepoort J Vet Res, 58*(3), 223–226.

Subcommittee on Dairy Cattle Nutrition. (2001). *Committee on Animal Nutrition, Board on Agriculture and Natural Resources, National Research Council of the National Academies: Nutrient requirements of dairy cattle* (7th ed.). Washington, DC: National Academy Press.

Sweeney, R. W. (1999). Treatment of potassium balance disorders. *Vet Clin North Am Food Anim Pract, 15*, 609–617.

Tessele, B., Brum, J. S., Schild, A. L., et al. (2012). Sawfly larval poisoning in cattle: report on new outbreaks and brief review of the literature. *Pesq Vet Bras, 32*(11), 1095–1102.

Velasquez-Pereira, J., Risco, C. A., McDowell, L. R., et al. (1999). Long-term effects of feeding gossypol and vitamin E to dairy calves. *J Dairy Sci, 82*, 1240–1251.

Verhoeff, J., Counotte, G., & Hamhuis, D. (2007). Nitrogen dioxide (silo gas) poisoning in dairy cattle. Tijdschrift Voor Diergeneeskunde, *132*, 780–782.

18

Diagnostic Laboratory Sample Submission

ERIN L. GOODRICH AND BELINDA S. THOMPSON

TABLE 18.1	Diagnostic Laboratory Sample Submission For a Reproductive Failure Disease Investigation		
Condition or Problem[#]	**Sample(s)**	**Test(s)**	**Sample Submission Notes**
Abortion—fetal testing*	Fixed tissue (placenta, liver, lung, brain, adrenal gland, heart, thymus, small intestine, kidney, and any other tissue with a lesion)	Histopathology (with immunohisto-chemical staining as appropriate)	0.5- to 1.0-cm-thick tissue sections fixed in 10% formalin, 10:1 formalin-to-tissue ratio, room temperature
	Placenta	Aerobic bacterial culture	Chilled or frozen[‡]
		Campylobacter fetus FA, PCR, or culture	Chilled or frozen[‡]
		Leptospira PCR or FA	Chilled or frozen[‡]
	Abomasal contents	Aerobic bacterial culture	Chilled or frozen[‡]
	Lung	Aerobic bacterial culture	Chilled or frozen[‡]
	Kidney	*Leptospira* PCR or FA	Chilled or frozen[‡]
	Fresh tissue (placenta, liver, lung, brain, adrenal gland, heart, thymus, small intestine, kidney)	Virus isolation or viral PCRs	Chilled or frozen[‡]
		BVDV FA (more sensitive for detection of acute infection with BVDV than for PI detection)	Chilled or frozen[‡]
		IBR or BHV-1 FA or PCR	Chilled or frozen[‡]
	Skin (ear notch)	BVDV ACE or IHC[†] (will only detect PI fetuses reliably)	Chilled or frozen[‡]; not fixed for ACE Fixed for IHC
	Heart blood (serum) or pleural or peritoneal fluid	*Neospora* IFA	Chilled
		BVDV SN	

[#]Laboratory requirements for sample handling can vary. Please contact your laboratory prior to submission to discuss the preferred sample handling techniques.
*Additional serology (serum antibody detection) or polymerase chain reaction (PCR) (whole-blood pathogen nucleic acid detection) testing may be indicated in the face of other potential aborting or teratogenic infectious agents, including potential transboundary disease outbreaks. These could include Cache Valley fever virus, bluetongue virus, epizootic hemorrhagic disease virus, Schmallenberg virus, foot and mouth disease virus, Akabane virus, or Rift Valley fever.
[‡]Avoid freeze–thaw cycles.
[†]Distinguishing between acute and persistent infection is important when determining appropriate herd detection and control measures for bovine viral diarrhea virus (BVDV) because the timing of exposure can be better predicted. Therefore these two tests are useful even when BVDV is detected by isolation or PCR test.
ACE, antigen-capture enzyme-linked immunosorbent assay; *BHV,* bovine herpesvirus; *FA,* fluorescent antibody; *IBR,* infectious bovine rhinotracheitis; *IFA,* indirect fluorescent antibody assay; *IHC,* immunohistochemistry; *PI,* persistently infected; *SN,* serum neutralization assay.

Condition or Problem	Sample(s)	Test(s)	Sample Submission Notes
Abortion—maternal testing*	Maternal serum (acute and then convalescent collected 14–21 days later)	BVDV SN	Chilled or frozen‡
		Brucella abortus card agglutination test	Chilled or frozen‡
		IBR ELISA or SN	Chilled or frozen‡
		Leptospira MAT, 5 standard serovars	Chilled or frozen‡
		Neospora IFA or ELISA	Chilled or frozen‡
		Salmonella Dublin ELISA†	Chilled or frozen‡
	Maternal EDTA whole blood (acute only)	Selenium analysis	Chilled

*Additional serology (serum antibody detection) or polymerase chain reaction (PCR) (whole-blood pathogen nucleic acid detection) testing may be indicated in the face of other potential aborting or teratogenic infectious agents, including potential transboundary disease outbreaks. These could include Cache Valley fever virus, bluetongue virus, epizootic hemorrhagic disease virus, Schmallenberg virus, foot and mouth disease virus, Akabane virus, or Rift Valley fever.

†*Salmonella* Dublin seroconversion may require 7 weeks for detection; if acute serology results are negative, retest in 7 weeks.

‡Avoid freeze–thaw cycles.

BVDV, bovine viral diarrhea virus; *EDTA,* ethylenediaminetetraacetic acid; *ELISA,* enzyme-linked immunosorbent assay; *IBR,* infectious bovine rhinotracheitis; *IFA,* indirect fluorescent antibody; *MAT,* microscopic agglutination test; *SN,* serum neutralization assay.

TABLE 18.2   Diagnostic Laboratory Sample Submission For Gastrointestinal Disease Investigation

Condition or Problem#	Sample(s)	Test(s)	Sample Submission Notes
Diarrhea (adult—antemortem)	Feces	Quantitative fecal examination (parasites)	Chilled; *not* frozen
		Johne's (paratuberculosis) fecal PCR	Chilled or frozen*
		Salmonella culture	Chilled or frozen*
		Bovine coronavirus PCR	Chilled or frozen*
	EDTA whole blood	BVDV PCR (will detect both acute and persistent infections)	Chilled
	Serum	BVDV ACE (will only detect persistent infections reliably)	Chilled or frozen*
Diarrhea (adult—postmortem)	Fixed tissues (include a segment from every section of the GI tract, all major organs)	Histopathology (with IHC staining as appropriate)	0.5- to 1.0-cm-thick tissue sections fixed in 10% formalin, 10:1 formalin-to-tissue ratio, room temperature
	Colon contents	Quantitative fecal examination (parasites)	Chilled; *not* frozen
		Johne's (paratuberculosis) fecal PCR	Chilled or frozen*
	Colon or affected bowel	*Salmonella* culture	Chilled or frozen*
	Colon	Bovine coronavirus PCR	Chilled or frozen*
	GI tissue (Peyer's patch or affected bowel or mesenteric lymph node)	BVDV PCR or virus isolation	Chilled or frozen*
	Skin (ear notch)	BVDV ACE or IHC† (will only detect persistent infections reliably)	Chilled or frozen*; not fixed for ACE. Fixed for IHC

#Laboratory requirements for sample handling can vary. Please contact your laboratory prior to submission to discuss the preferred sample handling techniques.

*Avoid freeze–thaw cycles.

†Distinguishing between acute and persistent infection is important when determining appropriate herd detection and control measures for bovine viral diarrhea virus (BVDV) because the timing of exposure can be better predicted. Therefore including this test is useful even when BVDV is detected by polymerase chain reaction (PCR) or isolation.

ACE, antigen-capture enzyme-linked immunosorbent assay; *EDTA,* ethylenediaminetetraacetic acid; *GI,* gastrointestinal; *IHC,* immunohistochemistry.

Condition or Problem	Sample(s)	Test(s)	Sample Submission Notes
Diarrhea (calf—antemortem)*	Feces	Quantitative fecal examination (parasites) or other quantitative parasite detection assays for *Giardia* spp., *Cryptosporidium parvum,* and others depending on age (e.g., *Eimeria, Ostertagia, Haemonchus, Strongyloides*)	Chilled; *not* frozen
		Aerobic bacterial culture (only if younger than 14 days of age or if bloody diarrhea)[†]	Chilled or frozen[‡]
		Salmonella culture	Chilled or frozen[‡]
		Bovine coronavirus PCR or antigen detection assay	Chilled or frozen[‡]
		Rotavirus antigen detection assay	Chilled or frozen[‡]
		Clostridium perfringens Enterotoxin detection assay	Preferably *frozen*[‡] or chilled and arriving at laboratory in <24 hr
		Gram stain	Chilled or frozen[‡]; or air-dried thin fecal smear slides
	Fecal swab in anaerobic transport media	Anaerobic culture[§]	Maintain at room temperature; *do not chill*
	EDTA whole blood	BVDV PCR (will detect both acute and persistent infections)	Chilled
	Serum	BVDV ACE (will only detect persistent infections)	Chilled or frozen[‡]
Diarrhea (calf—postmortem)*	Fixed tissues (include a segment from every section of the GI tract, all major organs)	Histopathology (with IHC staining as appropriate)	0.5- to 1.0-cm-thick tissue sections fixed in 10% formalin, 10:1 formalin-to-tissue ratio, room temperature
	Colon contents	Quantitative fecal examination (parasites)	Chilled; *not* frozen
	Tied-off loop of bowel	Anaerobic culture[§]	Preferably *frozen,*[‡] or chilled and arriving at laboratory in <24 hours
	Tied-off loop of bowel	Aerobic bacterial culture (only if younger than 14 days of age or if bloody diarrhea)[†]	Chilled or frozen[‡]
		Salmonella culture	Chilled or frozen[‡]
		BVDV PCR or virus isolation	Chilled or frozen[‡]
	Tied-off loop of small intestine (fresh or frozen)	Rotavirus FA or antigen detection assay	Chilled or frozen[‡]
	Tied-off loop of ileum or colon (fresh or frozen)	Coronavirus FA or antigen detection assay	Chilled or frozen[‡]
	Skin (ear notch)	BVDV ACE or IHC	Chilled or frozen[‡]
	Heart blood (serum) (if calf <7 days old and failure of passive transfer is suspected)	Bovine IgG assay	Chilled
	Liver	Selenium[¶]	Chilled or frozen[‡]

*See also Diarrhea—calf management assessment.

[†]Detection of *Escherichia coli* in aerobic cultures is most valuable if accompanied by genotyping polymerase chain reaction (PCR) for pathogenicity genes and potentially evaluated in multiple animals in an outbreak.

[‡]Avoid freeze–thaw cycles.

[§]Detection of *Clostridium perfringens* is most valuable if accompanied by detection of Enterotoxin in feces or colon contents or by genotyping for toxin-producing genes.

[¶]Especially for situations when nutritional management of pregnant cattle is a concern.

ACE, antigen-capture enzyme-linked immunosorbent assay; *BVDV,* bovine viral diarrhea virus; *EDTA,* ethylenediaminetetraacetic acid; *FA,* fluorescent antibody; *GI,* gastrointestinal; *IgG,* immunoglobulin G; *IHC,* immunohistochemistry.

Condition or Problem	Sample(s)	Test(s)	Sample Submission Notes
Diarrhea—(calf management assessment)	EDTA whole blood (10 calves <7 days old)	Total plasma protein (laboratory assay or refractometer)	Chilled
	5 mL of milk replacer (mixed, as fed)	Osmolality	Chilled
	5 mL of electrolyte supplement (mixed, as fed)	Osmolality	Chilled
	5 mL of colostrum* (ready to feed, collected from feeding utensil)	Modified bacterial counts	Chilled
	Additional colostrum samples, as appropriate*	Modified bacterial counts	Chilled
	5 mL of milk replacer or whole milk† (ready to feed, collected from feeding utensil)	Modified bacterial counts	Chilled
	Additional whole milk samples, as appropriate†	Modified bacterial counts	Chilled
	Bedding (clean stalls and pens, ready to occupy)	Modified bacterial counts	Chilled
	Bedding (stalls and pens with calves)	Modified bacterial counts	Chilled

*"As fed" colostrum bacterial counts can be compared with "as collected" or "pre-" and "post-" heat treatment samples as most appropriate to the management situation.
†"As fed" whole milk bacterial counts can be compared with "pre-" and "post-" pasteurization or acidification samples as most appropriate to the management situation.

TABLE 18.3 Diagnostic Laboratory Sample Submission for Neurologic Disease Investigation

Condition or Problem#	Sample(s)	Test(s)	Sample Submission Notes
Neurologic (postmortem)	Brainstem (complete cross-section) and one-third of the cerebellum (including obex, left, right, and central vermes)	Rabies DFA Public Health Laboratory (rabies-negative samples should be tested for BSE if age appropriate)	Chilled or frozen*; do not fix
	Fixed tissues (cerebrum, cerebellum, brainstem, spinal cord, all major organs, and any other tissue with a lesion)	Histopathology (with IHC staining as appropriate)	0.5- to 1.0-cm-thick tissue sections fixed in 10% formalin, 10:1 formalin-to-tissue ratio, room temperature
	CSF or swab inoculated with CSF or swab of meninges before contamination	Aerobic bacterial culture (including *Listeria* culture or PCR on CSF if available)	CSF in red-top tube; swabs in bacterial transport media; chilled or frozen*
	Fresh brain (brainstem preferred)	Aerobic bacterial culture (including *Listeria* culture)	Chilled or frozen*
	EDTA or heparinized whole blood or fresh liver	Lead analysis	Chilled (liver can be frozen*)
	Fresh brain or CSF (if salt toxicity is considered)	Sodium analysis	CSF in red-top tube; chilled or frozen*
	Fresh brain or CSF (may include additional fresh tissues if systemic viremia suspected)	Virus isolation†	Chilled or frozen* (submit CSF in plain red-top tube)
	Other fresh tissues if systemic bacteremia or focal infection is suspected (list each tissue for specific culture)	Other bacterial cultures (indicate specific tissue and culture desired)	Chilled or frozen*
	Set of fresh tissues, including brain, eye or ocular fluid, liver, kidney, fat, heart blood (heparinized and clotted), urine, stomach contents, colon contents	Assay for specific toxin or class of toxins suspected (e.g., GC/MS for organophosphates, *Clostridium botulinum* culture, toxin gene PCR, or toxin detection by GC/MS)	Chilled or frozen* (can freeze in individual containers and await histopathology results to determine if toxin testing is warranted)
	Spleen or lymph node	MCF PCR	Chilled or frozen*
	Heart blood (serum)	WNV SN; EEE VN; MCF IPT	Chilled

#Laboratory requirements for sample handling can vary. Please contact your laboratory prior to submission to discuss the preferred sample handling techniques.
*Avoid freeze–thaw cycles.
†Most laboratories, other than public health laboratories, will not attempt to isolate rabies virus. Occasionally, neurologic signs may be an early sign of malignant catarrhal fever (MCF). In cattle, the encephalitic form of MCF does not usually occur in multiple animals simultaneously.
BSE, bovine spongiform encephalopathy; CSF, cerebrospinal fluid; DFA, direct fluorescent antibody; EDTA, ethylenediaminetetraacetic acid; EEE, eastern equine encephalitis; GC/MS, gas chromatography–mass spectrometry; IHC, immunohistochemistry; IPT, immunoperoxidase test; PCR, polymerase chain reaction; SN, serum neutralization assay; VN, virus neutralization assay; WNV, West Nile virus.

TABLE 18.4 Diagnostic Laboratory Sample Submission For Respiratory Disease Investigation

Condition or Problem#	Sample(s)	Test(s)	Sample Submission Notes
Respiratory (antemortem)	Nasal or nasopharyngeal swab	Virus isolation	In red-top tube or viral transport media, chilled or frozen*
		Bovine coronavirus PCR	In red-top tube or viral transport media, chilled or frozen*
		BRSV PCR	In red-top tube or viral transport media, chilled or frozen*
		Aerobic culture†	In bacterial transport media, chilled or frozen*
		Mycoplasma culture or PCR†	In bacterial transport media without charcoal (culture); in plain red-top tube or viral transport media (PCR), chilled or frozen*
	Or (preferred) TTW or BAL	Cytology	In purple-top tube (chilled, *not* frozen) and air dried, unstained slides (room temperature)
		Viral FAs or PCRs (BVDV, IBR, BRSV, coronavirus)	In red-top tube, chilled or frozen*
		Virus isolation	In red-top tube, chilled or frozen*
		Aerobic culture	In red-top tube or swab in bacterial transport media, chilled or frozen*
		Mycoplasma culture or PCR	In red-top tube (culture or PCR) or swab in bacterial transport media without charcoal (culture only), chilled or frozen*
	Feces (may be warranted, depending on season and herd presentation)	Fecal examination for evidence of lungworms	Chilled; *not* frozen
	Serum (*acute* and then *convalescent* collected 14–21 days later)	BVDV SN, BRSV SN, IBR kELISA or SN; coronavirus IFA; PI3 SN	Chilled or frozen*
Respiratory (postmortem)	Fixed tissues (lung, heart, liver, diaphragm, skeletal muscle, tongue, and any other tissue with a lesion)	Histopathology (with IHC staining as appropriate)	Maintain at room temperature, 0.5- to 1.0-cm-thick tissue sections fixed in 10% formalin, 10:1 formalin-to-tissue ratio
	Fresh lung tissue	Aerobic culture	Chilled or frozen*
		Mycoplasma culture	Chilled or frozen*
		Bovine coronavirus or PCR	Chilled or frozen*
		Viral FAs, PCRs or virus isolation (BVDV, IBR, BRSV)	Chilled or frozen*
	Heart blood (serum) (especially if illness is chronic and if there is no history of vaccination)	BVDV SN, IBR kELISA BRSV SN	In red-top tube; chilled, *not* frozen
	Feces (only if gross inspection of airways for lungworms is negative and lungworms are still suspected)	Quantitative fecal	Chilled; *not* frozen
	EDTA whole blood or liver	Selenium analysis (especially neonatal calf pneumonia)	Chilled (liver can be frozen*)

#Laboratory requirements for sample handling can vary. Please contact your laboratory prior to submission to discuss the preferred sample handling techniques.
*Avoid freeze–thaw cycles.
†Bacterial respiratory pathogens involved in bovine respiratory disease complex such as *Pasteurella multocida, Mannheimia haemolytica,* and *Mycoplasma bovis* may be part of the commensal nasopharyngeal flora. Isolation from nasal or deep nasopharyngeal swabs may not reflect their involvement in pneumonia.
BAL, bronchoalveolar lavage; *BRSV,* bovine respiratory syncytial virus; *BVDV,* bovine viral diarrhea virus; *EDTA,* ethylenediaminetetraacetic acid; *ELISA,* enzyme-linked immunosorbent assay; *FA,* fluorescent antibody; *IBR,* infectious bovine rhinotracheitis; *IFA,* indirect fluorescent antibody; *IHC,* immunohistochemistry; *kELISA,* kinetic enzyme-linked immunosorbent assay; *PCR,* polymerase chain reaction; *PI3,* parainfluenza 3 virus; *SN,* serum neutralization assay; *TTW,* transtracheal wash.

TABLE 18.5　Diagnostic Laboratory Sample Submission for Ophthalmologic Disease Investigation

Condition or Problem#	Sample(s)	Test(s)	Sample Submission Notes
Conjunctivitis or uveitis	Conjunctival swab*	Aerobic bacterial culture (including *Listeria* culture)	In aerobic bacterial transport media, chilled or frozen†
		Mycoplasma culture	In aerobic bacterial transport media without charcoal, chilled or frozen†
	Conjunctival scraping on glass slide*	IBR FA (BHV-1)	Maintain at room temperature (air dried, unstained)
	Conjunctival swab*	Virus isolation	In red-top tube with 0.5 mL sterile saline or in virus transport media, chilled or frozen†
	EDTA whole blood‡	MCF PCR	Chilled
	Serum‡	MCF IPT	Chilled or frozen†

#Laboratory requirements for sample handling can vary. Please contact your laboratory prior to submission to discuss the preferred sample handling techniques.
*Collect samples from multiple, acutely affected animals.
†Avoid freeze–thaw cycles.
‡Severe uveitis may be an early sign of malignant catarrhal fever (MCF). In cattle, the encephalitic form of MCF does not usually occur in multiple animals simultaneously.
BHV1, bovine herpesvirus 1; EDTA, ethylenediaminetetraacetic acid; FA, fluorescent antibody; IBR, infectious bovine rhinotracheitis; IPT, immunoperoxidase test; PCR, polymerase chain reaction.

TABLE 18.6　Diagnostic Laboratory Sample Submission for Venereal Disease Investigation

Condition or Problem#	Sample(s)	Test(s)	Sample Submission Notes
Venereal disease—bulls	Preputial sample	*Trichomonas fetus* PCR or culture	In the InPouch TF culture system (Biomed Diagnostics, White City, OR, 97503), maintained at room temperature; *do not chill*
	Preputial sample	*Campylobacter fetus* culture, FA, or PCR	In laboratory-recommended transport media, chilled
	Preputial washings	Aerobic culture	In sterile container or swab in bacterial transport media without charcoal, chilled
		Mycoplasma culture	In sterile container or swab in bacterial transport media without charcoal, chilled
		Ureaplasma culture	In sterile container or swab in bacterial transport media without charcoal, chilled
	Serum	*Brucella abortus* card agglutination test	Chilled or frozen*
Venereal disease—cows	Cervical mucus	*Trichomonas fetus* PCR or culture	In the InPouch TF culture system, maintained at room temperature; *do not chill*
	Cervical mucus or vaginal washings	*Campylobacter fetus* culture, FA, or PCR	In laboratory-recommended transport media, chilled
	Uterine or cervical guarded swab	Aerobic culture	In bacterial transport media without charcoal, chilled
		Mycoplasma culture	In bacterial transport media without charcoal, chilled
		Ureaplasma culture	In bacterial transport media without charcoal, chilled
	Serum	*Brucella abortus* card agglutination test	Chilled or frozen*

#Laboratory requirements for sample handling can vary. Please contact your laboratory prior to submission to discuss the preferred sample handling techniques.
*Avoid freeze–thaw cycles.
FA, fluorescent antibody; PCR, polymerase chain reaction; TF, Trichomonas fetus.

TABLE 18.7	**Diagnostic Laboratory Sample Submission for Dermatologic Disease Investigation**		
Condition or Problem[#]	**Sample(s)**	**Test(s)**	**Sample Submission Notes**
Dermatitis—deep lesion	Fresh skin biopsy or deep swab from within tissue	Aerobic culture	Biopsy in red-top tube with 0.5 mL of sterile saline, swab in aerobic transport media; chilled
	Fresh skin biopsy	Parasite examination	In red-top tube with 0.5 mL of sterile saline, chilled
	Fresh skin biopsy or deep swab from within tissue	Fungal culture	Biopsy in red-top tube with 0.5 mL of sterile saline, swab in aerobic transport media; chilled
	Fresh skin biopsies	Gram stain	In red-top tube with 0.5 mL of sterile saline, chilled
	Formalin-fixed skin biopsies	Histopathology (with IHC staining as appropriate)	0.5- to 1.0-cm-thick tissue sections fixed in 10% formalin, 10:1 formalin-to-tissue ratio, room temperature
Dermatitis—superficial lesion	Skin scraping	Ectoparasite identification	In an escape-proof, nonporous container; chilled
	Hair and skin scraping	Fungal culture	In a sealable paper envelope, chilled
	Hair and skin scraping	Gram stain	In a sealable paper envelope, chilled
	Formalin-fixed skin biopsies	Histopathology (with IHC staining as appropriate)	0.5- to 1.0-cm-thick tissue sections fixed in 10% formalin, 10:1 formalin-to-tissue ratio, room temperature
	Impression smears Skin scrapings Fluid aspirates	Cytology	Maintain slides at room temperature (*do not chill*); submit aspirate in a EDTA whole blood tube, chilled

[#]Laboratory requirements for sample handling can vary. Please contact your laboratory prior to submission to discuss the preferred sample handling techniques.
EDTA, ethylenediaminetetracetic acid; *IHC,* immunohistochemistry.

TABLE 18.8	**Diagnostic Laboratory Sample Submission for Investigation of Fever of Unknown Origin**		
Condition or Problem[#]	**Sample(s)**	**Test(s)**	**Sample Submission Notes**
Fever of unknown origin	EDTA whole blood with two blood smears	Hemogram, with manual differential and examination for hemotropic pathogens	Chilled whole blood, slides maintained at room temperature (air dried and unstained)
		Fibrinogen (plasma)	Chilled
		Virus isolation	Chilled
	Serum	Large animal chemistry analysis	Chilled or frozen*
	Three inoculated blood culture media vials (aerobic)	Aerobic or fungal blood cultures	Maintained at room temperature; *do not chill*
	Three inoculated blood culture media vials (anaerobic)	Anaerobic blood cultures	Maintained at room temperature; *do not chill*
	Nasal swab	Virus isolation	In red-top tube with 0.5 mL of sterile saline or in virus transport media, chilled or frozen*
	EDTA whole blood[†]	MCF PCR	Chilled
	Serum[†]	MCF IPT	Chilled or frozen*

[#]Laboratory requirements for sample handling can vary. Please contact your laboratory prior to submission to discuss the preferred sample handling techniques.
*Avoid freeze–thaw cycles.
[†]A fever of unknown origin may be an early sign of malignant catarrhal fever (MCF). In cattle, the encephalitic form of MCF does not usually occur in multiple animals simultaneously.
EDTA, ethylenediaminetetraacetic acid; *IPT,* immunoperoxidase test; *PCR,* polymerase chain reaction.

Legends for Video Clips

To view videos go to: http://dairydiseases.vet.cornell.edu/

Video clip 2.1   A 1-day-old Holstein heifer became distressed with pronounced salivation after feeding of colostrum through an esophageal feeder. When the feeder tube was removed from the calf's mouth, it was noted that a large part of the tube was missing.

Endoscopic findings: Endoscopic retrieval of the broken esophageal feeder lodged in the esophagus of the calf. This feeder had been used for several months on numerous calves with bleach disinfection between use before breaking and becoming trapped in the esophagus of this calf.

Diagnosis: Esophageal obstruction with broken esophageal feeder.

Video clip 2.2   Demonstration of collection of cerebrospinal fluid from the lumbosacral space in cattle.

Video clip 3.1   An adult Holstein cow with persistent fever and weight loss.

Technique for establishing true retrograde filling of the jugular vein associated with right heart failure: The vessel is held off close to the ramus of the mandible, "emptied" by running two fingers down the vein toward the thoracic inlet, and then allowed to "backfill" from the brisket. Ensure that the head is in a neutral position and not held lower than the base of the heart. The animal in this video had severe vegetative endocarditis involving the right atrioventricular valve.

Diagnosis: Vegetative endocarditis and right heart failure.

Video clip 3.2   A 5-year-old Holstein cow with anorexia, tachycardia, and irregular rhythm of the heart noted during auscultation.

Note the rapid "hosepipe"-like filling of the jugular vein from the thoracic inlet to the mandible with the head held in a neutral position. Persistent jugular distension is also evident, as is the arrhythmic nature of the pulse waves. This demonstrates true jugular pulsation associated with right sided heart failure.

Diagnosis: Cardiac lymphosarcoma involving the right atrium.

Video clip 3.3   A 7-day-old calf with increased respiratory and heart rates.

Echocardiographic findings: Doppler flow echocardiogram of 7-day-old Holstein calf with a ventricular septal defect, demonstrating flow across the defect high in the interventricular septum, a classic location for this congenital abnormality.

(Courtesy of Dr. Heidi Kellihan.)

Diagnosis: Ventricular septal defect.

Video clip 3.4   A 14-day-old calf with decreased vigor.

Echocardiographic findings: Doppler flow echocardiogram demonstrating flow across the atria.

(Courtesy of Dr. Rebecca Stepien.)

Diagnosis: Atrial septal defect.

Video clip 3.5   A 4-year-old Holstein cow with anorexia, decreased milk production for the past 3 days, "bottle jaw", enlarged (pipelike) jugular veins, muffled heart sounds, and severe tachycardia (140 beats/min).

Pericardiocentesis: Pericardial effusion was noted on ultrasound examination, and a right-sided pericardiocentesis was performed; 3 L of hemorrhagic fluid was removed. Cytologic examination of the fluid revealed 3,700 white blood cells/µL with 21% neutrophils, 32% macrophages, 36% lymphocytes, and 6% eosinophils. There were large numbers of red blood cells in the fluid, evidence of macrophage erythrophagia, and the total protein was 5.5 g/dL. No neoplastic cells were seen, and the cow was bovine leukemia virus negative. The cow was anemic (hematocrit; 21%) before the procedure, and the hematocrit increased to 32% 5 days later. The cow also had a mild thrombocytopenia (120,000/µL) before pericardiocentesis which increased to greater than 400,000/µL 48 hours after the procedure. The cow's clinical signs resolved within 36 hours. After pericardial drainage, her milk production increased, and she was still healthy 2 years later.

Diagnosis: Idiopathic hemorrhagic and inflammatory pericarditis.

Video clip 3.6   A 3-year-old cow with a 5-day history of poor appetite, decreased rumen contractions, and a sudden drop in milk production. Fever was intermittently present.

Pericardiotomy: Left-sided pericardiotomy being performed in a 3-year-old cow with septic pericarditis caused by "hardware." After incising the pericardium, fetid-smelling yellow fluid was discharged in a projectile manner from the pericardium. The prognosis for similarly affected cattle is poor.

Diagnosis: Traumatic reticulopericarditis; septic pericarditis.

Video clip 3.7   A 5-year-old Holstein cow with fever, decreased production, and muffled heart sounds.

Echocardiographic findings: Note the large volume of anechoic pericardial fluid in which the heart "floats" and the fibrin fronds attached to the epicardial surface. The effusion was reported to be non-neoplastic at the time these images were obtained but transitioned to a lymphoblastic effusion over a 9-month period.

Diagnosis: Idiopathic hemorrhagic pericardial effusion initially.

Final diagnosis: Lymphosarcoma (pericardial).

Video clip 4.1   A 9-month-old Holstein heifer was examined because of stertorous breathing since birth. The difficulty in breathing was accentuated by increased environmental temperature. The heifer was otherwise healthy.

Endoscopy findings: The initial part of the video shows the normally large nasopharyngeal septum, but in the distance, a normal size opening to the nasopharynx cannot be seen. The larynx appears normal, but as the scope is withdrawn away from the larynx or advanced toward the larynx, a collapse of the pharyngeal wall is noted. A diagnosis of functional pharyngeal collapse was made. The heifer's respiratory signs have remained unchanged, but she calved normally 1 year later. The owner reported she is smaller than other 2-year-olds on the farm, and she moves slower than the other cows in the summer months.

Diagnosis: Pharyngeal collapse.

Video clip 4.2   A 2-month-old Holstein bull calf with a 3-week history of progressive dyspnea and upper respiratory stridor.

Endoscopy findings: Swelling of arytenoid cartilages and exudate draining from the left arytenoid area can be seen. A tracheostomy was performed followed by surgical exploration under general anesthesia. The dorsal portion of the left arytenoid cartilage was necrotic and draining pus. The necrotic area was curetted (not shown in video), and the calf was treated with penicillin. The calf had a complete recovery.

Diagnosis: Necrotic laryngitis.

Video clip 4.3   A 2-month-old Holstein heifer was examined because of a 1-month history of progressive respiratory distress with stridor. Tilmicosin, dexamethasone, and flunixin meglumine had been used as treatments but had not been effective.

Endoscopy findings: There is evidence of laryngitis, severe edema of the trachea and larynx, and deformity of the right arytenoid cartilage. A tracheostomy was performed as an emergency procedure and surgery was recommended. The owners declined, and the calf was euthanized.

Diagnosis (necropsy): Chronic necrosuppurative laryngitis, tracheitis, and pneumonia.

Video clip 4.4   An adult Holstein cow with a 5-day history of upper respiratory stridor. There had been some transient improvement in the clinical signs after a combination of corticosteroid and antimicrobial therapy.

Endoscopy findings: (Pre-operative) An inflamed larynx with little movement of the arytenoid cartilages can be noted. A mass can be seen caudal and dorsal to the cartilages. After a tracheostomy, the abscess and the diseased arytenoid cartilage were surgically removed. Three days later on recheck, endoscopy (Post-operative) revealed significant improvement in laryngeal function. The cow was treated with penicillin for 2 weeks and received a single dose of dexamethasone immediately after surgery. The cow recovered and was healthy at a 6-month follow-up.

Diagnosis: *Trueperella pyogenes* arytenoid abscess.

Video clip 4.5   A 9-year-old Brown Swiss cow with a 2-week history of fever and coughing with sudden progression to respiratory distress with stridor.

Endoscopy findings: Evidence of arytenoid chondritis that nearly obstructs the airways. A tracheostomy was performed, and, under local anesthetic, the necrotic left arytenoid was grasped and removed. The cow was treated with ceftiofur, penicillin, and flunixin and was doing well at 6-month follow-up.

Diagnosis: Necrotic arytenoid chondritis.

Video clip 4.6   A 2-year-old Holstein cow that had made an audible upper respiratory noise since shortly after birth. The noise had become louder over time and was beginning to cause some respiratory distress.

Endoscopy findings: A mass is observed on the right ventricle of the larynx. This mass was incised (last segment of the video), and thick mucus material was drained. A biopsy and histopathology of the wall of the mass suggested this was a branchial cyst. After general anesthesia, the lining of the cyst was removed by laser surgery. The cow recovered and has remained normal without any respiratory noise.

Diagnosis: Laryngeal cyst.

Video clip 4.7A   A 7-week-old Holstein heifer with a temporary tracheostomy in place for relief of severe upper respiratory stridor caused by necrotic laryngitis. Video was obtained within 4 hours of the procedure, and the marked difference in comfort and respiratory rate and effort was evident. Medical treatment was only partially successful, and the calf eventually underwent a permanent tracheolaryngotomy.

Diagnosis: Necrotic laryngitis.

Video clip 4.7B   A 4-month-old Holstein calf with progressive respiratory noise and cough that presented in respiratory distress. A tracheostomy had to be performed because of the severity of the airway obstruction. A laryngotomy and partial arytenoidectomy were performed 2 days later, and the calf made a complete recovery.

Diagnosis: Necrotic laryngitis.

Video clip 4.8   A 1-month-old calf with chronic cough, increased respiratory rate, and nasal discharge.

Ultrasound findings: Toward the end of the clip, note the "hepatized" appearance to the lung indicative of lobar consolidation.

Diagnosis: Chronic bronchopneumonia.

Video clip 4.9   A, A 3-month-old Holstein heifer with severe pneumonia and respiratory distress. The calf had been treated on the farm for 2 weeks with various macrolide antibiotics, enrofloxacin, and ceftiofur with no clinical response. B, The same calf as in A after 2 weeks of hospitalization, intranasal oxygen therapy, nebulization for a week, and daily administration of oxytetracycline intravenously every 12 hours and procaine penicillin subcutaneously every 12 hours.

Diagnosis: Bronchopneumonia; marked improvement.

Video clip 4.10   An 8-year-old Holstein cow with recurrent fevers and cough after calving 1 week earlier.

Ultrasound findings: A vector 4- to 1-MHz scan head is used. Ventral is to the left side of the image. The pleural space contains large abscesses; these are the two compartments of fluid with waving tags of fibrin, 5 cm and 18 cm in diameter, with distinct 1-cm thick capsules. The lung is poorly visualized as the dorsal (right side of the image), triangular, hyperechoic structure at 5 to 10 cm depth. The lung is adhered to the pleural abscesses.

Diagnosis: Pleuropneumonia, pleural abscess. *Trueperella pyogenes* and *Clostridium perfringens* were cultured.

Video clip 4.11   Holstein bull calf with respiratory distress. The animal was intolerant of almost any movement without becoming severely distressed and would stand as shown with an extended neck, grunting with each respiratory cycle. Radiographs (see Fig. 4.55 in text) demonstrated severe interstitial pneumonia with bullae formation.

Diagnosis: Severe interstitial pneumonia; bovine respiratory syncytial virus infection.

Video clip 4.12   A 5-week-old calf with chronic cough.

Ultrasound findings: Toward the end of the clip, note the disruption in normal reverberation artifact at the pleural surface.

Diagnosis: Mild lobular consolidation of the lung; pneumonia.

Video clip 4.13   An 8-week-old healthy calf.

Ultrasonographic appearance of normal bovine lung: Note parallel reverberation artifacts created at the pleural surface and hyperechoic appearance to the lung surface.

Diagnosis: Normal pleural ultrasound.

Video clip 4.14   An adult Holstein cow with weight loss, decreased milk production, fever, and subjective increase in size of the mammary veins.

Ultrasonography of the liver: Ultrasonographic appearance of the liver from a mature Holstein cow with caudal vena caval thrombosis syndrome. Note the enlargement of the intrahepatic vasculature and caudal vena cava. A large hepatic abscess is also visible toward the left side of the image at several points in the video clip.

Diagnosis: Hepatic abscess, thrombosis, and obstruction of the caudal vena cava.

Video clip 4.15   A 4-year-old Jersey cow with acute onset of increased respiratory effort and cough after an epidural.

When performing the epidural, air could be heard flowing into the needle, and students were asked to listen to the sound indicating correct placement of the needle. We have noted these respiratory signs in other cows after epidurals when a prolonged "sucking air" sound was reported. We believe air goes from the epidural space into the mediastinum, causing the acute onset of these signs. Affected cattle can also appear distressed and have elevated heart rates, but so far all have recovered with no treatment within 45 minutes.

Diagnosis: Suspected pneumomediastinum.

Video clip 5.1   An adult Holstein cow presented for acute and progressive onset of ruminal bloat with progressive respiratory distress.

The history of rapid progression of ruminal bloat leading to respiratory distress and inability to relieve the bloat by passing a Kingman tube led to the diagnosis of frothy bloat. An emergency rumenotomy was performed and the rumen emptied. The cow made a quick and uneventful recovery. The cause of the frothy bloat could not be determined in this case.

Diagnosis: Frothy bloat.

Video clip 5.2   An adult Holstein cow with acute anorexia, fever, and a dramatic decrease in milk production.

Ultrasonographic examination of the abdomen: Sonogram of cranial ventral abdomen of an adult cow with hardware. The reticulum with can be seen to the bottom right of the image with fluid between it and the diaphragm and fibrin coating its serosal surface. There is also a small amount of free fluid within the thoracic cavity, and the lung can be seen moving in and out of the image.

Diagnosis: Peritonitis—hardware.

Video clip 5.3   A 4-year-old Holstein with weight loss, decreased appetite, and abdominal distension.

Ultrasonographic examination of the abdomen: Sonogram video (first segment) of the cranioventral abdomen of a 4-year-old female Holstein cow with lymphosarcoma. A convex 5- to 2-MHz scan head is used; cranial is to the left side of the image. Viscera are viewed in the following order: first abomasum, then rumen, reticulum,

liver, and again reticulum. The lymphosarcoma is the peritoneal mass, 6.5 × 8 cm, hypoechoic, irregularly interdigitating with abnormally hyperechoic fat and blending with the wall of the reticulum and, to a lesser extent, the wall of the abomasum. The sonographic appearance of lymphosarcoma may resemble abomasitis, reticulitis, and peritonitis. In this case, the diagnosis of lymphosarcoma was confirmed by fine-needle aspirate cytology.

Static sonogram demonstrates first the lymphosarcoma and then the right side of the liver made with a vector 4- to 1-MHz scan head. Ventral is to the left side of the image. In the liver is a 4 × 7 cm hypoechoic mass, most likely lymphosarcoma.

Sonogram video (second segment) of normal left craniodorsal abdomen of a 4-year-old female Holstein. A vector 4- to 1-MHz scan head is placed dorsally in a caudal intercostal space and travels ventrally. Ventral is to the left side of the image. Seen first is a very hyperechoic interface oriented parallel to the body wall and casting reverberation artifact—the normal air-filled lung. Ventral to this is a triangular hyperechoic homogenous soft tissue structure, height about 13 cm, containing a vein in cross-section; the normal spleen. Ventral to the spleen is a curved, very hyperechoic structure casting a hypoechoic shadow—the lumen contents of the normal rumen. Note that the wall of the rumen is thin (≈1–2 mm) and difficult to detect. This sequence repeats twice.

Sonogram video (third segment) of normal small intestines of a 4-year-old female Holstein. A vector 4- to 1-MHz scan head is placed caudal to the costal arch on the right side. Ventral is to the left side of the image. The small intestines are the circular structures with normal motility. The intestine diameter is normal (2.2–4.0 cm), the intestinal walls are normal (thin), and the lumen contains normal granular hyperechoic ingesta.

Diagnosis: Lymphosarcoma (first segment and static image). Normal adult bovine abdomen (second and third segments).

Video clip 5.4   A 6-year-old Holstein cow with fever, inappetence, decreased production, decreased rumination, and a hunched posture since freshening 1 month earlier.

Ultrasound examination of the right abdomen: A vector 4- to 1- MHz scan head is used. The sonogram begins dorsally in the 11th intercostal space and travels ventrally. Ventral is to the left side of the image. At the beginning of the study (first segment), the air-filled right caudal lung lobe, anechoic pleural fluid (abnormal), and normal liver are shown. At times, in the lower left region of the image the aorta and caudal vena cava are seen (1.5 cm in diameter).

The scan head travels farther ventrally (second segment) and is centered on the right kidney. In the center of the kidney are a few 1- to 2-cm, intensely hyperechoic foci that cast faint acoustic shadows. These are calculi. Otherwise, the kidney is normal with normal size (height and width are about 9 cm), lobulated contour, hypoechoic medulla clearly distinguished from the cortex, and the cortex about 1 cm thick.

The normal right adrenal gland (4.5 × 1.5 cm) is visible between the right kidney and caudal vena cava and aorta (third segment). The rumen is the deepest viscus in the image (16 cm deep). Ventral to right kidney is more liver (fourth segment). Ventrally between the liver and rumen are the portal vein, pancreas (3 cm thick), and lymph nodes (2 cm thick). The lymph nodes might be slightly large. When the probe is tipped cranially, the portal vein is larger (2.5 cm diameter). In many adult bovines, the right adrenal gland, pancreas, and periportal lymph nodes are not visible. In this case, conditions were favorable for detecting smaller deeper viscera because the cow was thin, the bowel was relatively empty because of anorexia, and the cow was not pregnant.

Sonogram video (fifth segment) of the right cranioventral abdomen showing focal peritonitis. A convex 5- to 3-MHz scan head is used. Medial is to the left side of the image. The abomasum is between the body wall and rumen. It is small (6 cm in height) because the lumen is nearly empty. Its wall is normal with layer echogenicity, rugal folds, and it is about 0.5 cm thick between folds. In the peritoneal cavity lateral to the abomasum is focal peritonitis; a large (12-cm) irregularly margined region of compartmentalized peritoneal fluid.

Sonogram video (sixth segment) of the left cranioventral abdomen showing a peritoneal abscess. A convex 5- to 3-MHz scan head is used. Cranial is to the left side of the image. The sonogram starts at a 12-cm abscess with hypoechoic fluid surrounded by a distinct capsule and a dorsal gas cap. Next, the scan head travels cranially to the normal reticulum (note the characteristic convex shape of the reticulum), returns to the abscess, and then travels caudally to abnormal hyperechoic fat near the abomasum and then more caudally to show the rumen and peritoneal (or omental) fluid and fibrin.

Diagnosis: Focal peritonitis from a perforated abomasal ulcer.

Video clip 5.5   A 3-year-old Holstein with acute onset of anorexia and decreased production.

Ultrasonographic examination of the abdomen: The convex 5- to 3-MHz scan head is oriented in the transverse plane at the midabdomen. The video begins at ventral midline and progresses dorsally through the right side of the midabdomen.

The distended (8-cm) omental bursa is seen as a distinct fluid compartment located between the body wall and the peritoneal cavity. Deep to the omental bursa, the peritoneal cavity is seen to contain a triangle of anechoic fluid between the rumen ventrally and the small intestine dorsally. The fluid within the omental bursa contains irregular webs of fibrin, in this case indicating inflammation.

Diagnosis: Peritonitis (omental bursitis).

Video clip 6.1   A 10-week-old Holstein heifer with chronic ill thrift, diarrhea and respiratory disease.

Transabdominal ultrasound findings: Using a mid to high frequency probe (suitable for reproductive or thoracic ultrasound examination on-farm), an enlarged abdominal lymph node is visible as an oval-shaped homogeneous structure in the near field (≈2 cm in diameter and 5 cm in length, proximal to a loop of motile intestine). Postmortem examination demonstrated profound mesenteric lymphadenopathy (see Fig. 6.11), and diagnostics confirmed infection with *Salmonella* Dublin.

Diagnosis: *Salmonella* Dublin- associated chronic mesenteric lymphadenopathy.

Video clip 6.2   A 4-year-old Holstein, fresh 5 weeks, with intermittently poor appetite and decreased production for 10 days.

Hepatic ultrasound findings: Sonogram video (first segment) and static image of the liver demonstrating five choleliths in a hepatic duct. The convex 5- to 2-MHz scan head is located within a right intercostal space. Ventral is to the left side of the image. The choleliths are the five, less than 1-cm, well-margined, oval, very hyperechoic structures that cast acoustic shadows. These are located in a hepatic duct as evidenced by their linear distribution and location immediately adjacent and parallel to a portal vein. Normal rumen is deep to the liver.

Sonogram video of the liver within a right intercostal space using a vector 4- to 1- MHz scan head demonstrating that deeper portions of the liver contain multifocal choleliths (second segment). These are in hepatic ducts, which are the many hyperechoic branching linear structures parallel to portal veins.

Additionally, the liver has abnormal increased attenuation of sound, resulting in poor penetration and therefore poor visualization of the deepest portions of the liver. This is a typical but not exclusive finding for lipidosis.

Diagnosis: Hepatic lipidosis, cholelithiasis.

Video clip 6.3   A 6-year-old Holstein with anorexia, lethargy, decreased production, and jaundice for 3 days.

Hepatic ultrasound findings: Sonogram of the liver and gallbladder; a convex 4- to 2-MHz scan head is used. Dorsal is to the left side of the image (first segment). The liver contains many anechoic, branching, tubular structures, some of which are enlarged hepatic ducts. Normally, hepatic ducts are too small to easily detect. The gallbladder is also enlarged (13-cm diameter) (second segment). Extrahepatic bile duct obstruction was suspected.

Enlarged hepatic ducts (third segment) can be distinguished from enlarged hepatic veins because hepatic ducts are largest (in this case, 4.5 cm) at the porta hepatis, and enlarged hepatic ducts frequently have a tortuous shape. Congested hepatic veins are largest near the caudal vena cava (not demonstrated in this study) and are typically not tortuous. Histologically, liver biopsy showed chronic cholangiohepatitis.

Diagnosis: Cholangiohepatitis. *Fusobacterium necrophorum* and *Streptococcus* spp. group D were cultured from the liver biopsy.

Video clip 8.1   Ultrasound examination of the normal udder: Longitudinal sonogram of the normal left hind quarter of the udder at the junction of the gland and teat cisterns. These are patent and filled with hypoechoic milk. The gland cistern has a normal full diameter (2.7 cm), and the lactiferous ducts are also full.

Video clip 8.2   Ultrasound examination of normal teat: Transverse sonogram of normal left hind teat beginning at the udder and moving distally to the teat sphincter. Distal is to the left side of the image. A linear 12- to 5-MHz probe is used. The teat cistern is patent and filled with hypoechoic milk. Note the ring of blood vessels around the teat cistern. The teat sphincter appears as a centrally located hyperechoic dot, 1 mm in size.

Video clip 8.3   A 2-year-old Holstein heifer, recently fresh, with minimal production from the right rear quarter.

Ultrasound examination of teat and gland cistern: Transverse sonogram of right hind teat beginning at the udder and moving to the teat sphincter (distal is to the left of the image). A linear 12- to 5-MHz probe is used. The proximal portion of the teat cistern is obstructed by many soft tissue webs. Distally, the teat cistern is patent, having a normal diameter lumen (8 mm) and containing hypoechoic fluid (milk). At the tip of the teat, the sphincter is normal, appearing as a centrally located hyperechoic dot, 1 mm in size.

Diagnosis: Proximal teat cistern obstruction.

Video clip 8.4   A 2-year-old Holstein heifer in which it was difficult to milk out the right rear quarter.

Ultrasound examination of the teat and gland cisterns: Longitudinal sonogram of the obstructed right hind teat beginning at the teat sphincter and moving toward the udder. Distal is to the left of the image. A linear 12- to 5-MHz probe is used. The length of the teat is 3.6 cm. The teat sphincter is normal and appears as a 9-mm length × 1.5-mm thick hyperechoic stripe at the tip of the teat. The distal third of the teat cistern has a normal 9-mm-wide lumen filled with hypoechoic fluid (milk). The proximal two thirds of the teat cistern is obstructed by many soft tissue webs. These extend into the gland cistern.

Diagnosis: Webbed teat obstruction.

Video clip 8.5   **A 2-year-old Holstein heifer, recently fresh, but in which milk cannot be obtained from one quarter.**
Ultrasound examination findings: Longitudinal sonogram of the abnormal right rear quarter at the gland cistern. Distal is to the left of the image. A convex 8- to 5-MHz probe is used. The teat and gland cisterns are obstructed because the lumen contains many soft tissue webs. The gland cistern is also small in diameter (1.9 cm). The udder parenchyma is normal (hyperechoic background tissue), and lactiferous ducts are normal hypoechoic branching structures full of milk (1-cm lumen diameter).
Diagnosis: Teat and gland cistern obstruction.

Video clip 11.1   **A 2½-month-old Holstein calf with poor growth and dribbling urine since birth.**
Ultrasound examination of the right kidney: Transverse image of right kidney made with a convex 5- to 3-MHz scan head. The kidney is large (10 cm diameter) because all of the calyces and the pelvis are enlarged (2–4 cm). These contain anechoic fluid and round hypoechoic material that could be caseated pus, necrotic debris, or blood clots. The renal cortex is very thin (<5 mm). Right nephrectomy was performed.
Diagnosis: Pyelonephritis; suspect ectopic right ureter.

Video clip 11.2   **A 5-year-old Holstein cow with decreased appetite and milk production and appearance of white crystals in the urine.**
Ultrasound findings: Sonogram of the right kidney. A vector 4- to 1- MHz scan head is used. The center of the kidney contains many oval discrete hyperechoic structures that cast a strong (dark) acoustic shadow (first segment). These calculi have variable diameters with some as large as 2.7 cm. Also in the center of the kidney are five to ten 2-cm anechoic fluid cavities. There are enlarged calyces and an enlarged renal pelvis. The calculi are located dependently within these. Kidney shape (lobulated contour) and corticomedullary definition are normal. Kidney size is normal (11 × 17 cm). The calyces and pelvis are enlarged probably because of obstruction of the right ureter by calculi. The right ureter cannot be seen in the sonograms because it is obscured by acoustic shadowing by renal calculi.

At necropsy, the right renal parenchyma was atrophied, and the right ureter and pelvis were enlarged (8 cm wide) and contained hundreds of calculi (0.1–2 cm). The wall of the pelvis was thick and fibrotic.

Sonogram (second segment) of the left kidney of the same 5-year-old female Holstein with renal failure and calculi. A 4- to 1- MHz vector scan head is used. The left kidney is difficult to visualize, partly because it is so large (≈20 × 30 cm) that its margin extends beyond the equipment's maximum field of view (26.3 cm deep). The left kidney is also difficult to visualize because portions of the renal capsule are poorly defined and portions of the kidney have poor corticomedullary definition. Several 2-cm renal calculi and multiple fluid cavities, some as large as 2 cm in diameter, are detected. Some of these are centrally located and represent enlarged calyces or the renal pelvis. Other fluid cavities are peripheral, and it is uncertain whether these are parenchymal or capsular. These may represent necrosis, abscesses, or hematomas.

At necropsy, the left renal capsule contained a large hematoma. The renal parenchyma had two infarcts (4 and 9 cm). The kidney was enlarged. The pelvis and ureter contained hundreds of calculi (0.1–2 cm).
Diagnosis: Chronic pyelonephritis—renal calculi.

Video clip 11.3   **A 4-month-old Holstein heifer calf with a 2-week history of frequent and painful urination and an enlarged umbilicus. Urinalysis performed on a voided urine sample found a large number of white blood cells with intracellular bacteria and some red blood cells.**

In the video clip the calf can be seen demonstrating agitation, tail switching, flank watching and repeated kicking at the abdomen, consistent with stranguria/dysuria. Ultrasound examination (not shown) revealed an enlarged (3 cm) right umbilical artery with gas echoes seen in the thickened artery. Urine culture had 10^5 CFU *Trueperella pyogenes* and 10^4 CFU *Escherichia coli*. Surgery was performed, and both the infected umbilical artery and the associated diseased part of the bladder were removed. The clinical signs were improved the following day, and by day 3 after surgery, the calf was urinating normally. She was also treated with ampicillin for 7 days.
Diagnosis: Bacterial cystitis associated with umbilical remnant infection.

Video clip 11.4   **A 2-year-old Holstein cow with a 1-week history of hematuria and progressive inappetence. The urinalysis revealed degenerative neutrophils and large numbers of bacteria.**
Endoscopy findings: Endoscopy revealed an edematous and inflamed-appearing bladder with exudate and blood clots on the floor of the bladder. There is also an ulcerative lesion on the ventral bladder mucosa. A biopsy of this confirmed necrotic cystitis. The cow was treated with penicillin and improved, but long-term follow-up was not available.
Diagnosis: Necrotic cystitis caused by *Corynebacterium renale*.

Video clip 11.5   **An 11-year-old Holstein cow with a 6-month history of hematuria and stranguria. The cow was in good body condition, and all other examination findings were normal.**
Endoscopy findings: Endoscopy reveals a large proliferative mass on the ventral floor of the bladder. In the middle of the video, the apex of the bladder can be seen when the scope is retroflexed (causing the image to be upside down). The ureters can be seen traversing through the dorsal bladder wall and opening, with urine flow at the trigone.
Diagnosis: A biopsy confirmed a transitional cell carcinoma.

Video clip 11.6   **A 2½-month-old Holstein with poor growth and an umbilical mass.**
Umbilical ultrasound findings: The umbilical mass is displayed in longitudinal plane (first segment) where cranial is to the left side of the image and transverse (second segment) planes. The sector 5- to 3-MHz scan head is placed on the ventral aspect of the umbilical mass. The umbilical mass has findings typical of an abscess. It is a large (15 cm) single compartment containing echoic fluid and surrounded by a distinct capsule. In real time, it has no motility. The abscess extends caudally in the peritoneal cavity and has a tubular shape, indicating involvement of the urachus or an umbilical artery. The peritoneal cavity is deep in the image, beginning at the calipers.

Sonogram video (third segment) of the umbilical abscess and the normal peritoneal cavity cranial to the abscess demonstrating that the abscess does not involve the abomasum. The convex 8- to 5-MHz scan head is oriented in the transverse plane and begins on the ventral aspect of the umbilical mass and proceeds cranially. The umbilical mass is an abscess with a thick capsule containing echoic fluid. When the scan head reaches the peritoneal cavity, the abscess is no longer detected, and the image changes to show normal abomasum, which has a thin wall (1.2 mm) with layers, thin rugal folds, and normal ingesta that is of much greater echogenicity than the abscess fluid.

Sonogram video (fourth segment) of urachus or umbilical artery abscess demonstrating that the abscess contains gas. The convex 8- to 5-MHz scan head is oriented in the transverse plane in the caudoventral abdomen. The video begins at the apex of the urinary bladder, which contains anechoic urine and has a mildly thick wall (9 mm).

The video proceeds caudally to show an 8-cm-diameter abscess in the peritoneal cavity immediately cranial to the urinary bladder. In addition to the distinct thick capsule and echoic fluid, the abscess has a dorsal gas cap forming a straight, smooth, very echoic, linear interface that casts acoustic shadows at the deep edge of the fluid.

Sonogram of the urachus or umbilical artery abscess and urinary bladder in the longitudinal plane (cranial is to the left side of the image) using a convex 8- to 5-MHz scan head (static image, fifth segment). The capsule of the abscess is continuous with, and distorts, the cranial aspect of the urinary bladder.

Diagnosis: Urachal and umbilical artery abscess.

Video clip 12.1   Adult Holstein cow acutely lame and non-weight bearing on right hind leg.

Caudoventral dislocation of the right coxofemoral joint (into obturator foramen) being reduced under general anesthesia in a mature Holstein cow. This clip shows, by use of mechanical devices, including a calf jack, the profound difficulty faced in lengthening and abducting the femur to bring the femoral head lateral to the pelvis and back cranially toward the acetabulum. This is often impossible in a conscious or even merely sedated individual because of the pain and resistance to such marked tension on the injured limb.

Diagnosis: Coxofemoral luxation.

Video clip 12.2   Adult Holstein cow acutely lame and non-weight bearing on right hind leg.

Continued manipulation of the right hind limb of the cow shown in Video clip 12.1. After limb lengthening and radiographic confirmation that the femoral head had been brought close to the acetabulum, persistent multiple-person pressure is being applied over the region of the greater trochanter and proximal femur while limb lengthening attempts are still ongoing in an attempt to relocate the femoral head into the acetabulum.

Diagnosis: Coxofemoral luxation, attempted manual repair.

Video clip 12.3   Adult Holstein cow acutely lame and non-weight bearing on right hind leg.

Persistence with the cow from Video clips 12.1 and 12.2 was associated with successful relocation of the femoral head into the acetabulum; at about the 45 second mark, it is clear that continued efforts with pressure over the greater trochanter have been successful at reducing the dislocation.

Diagnosis: Coxofemoral luxation, successful repair.

> **Bovine Neurology Videos:** Signalment and history (**H**) are given first followed by
> **AD** = Anatomic diagnosis (neuroanatomical location of dysfunction)
> **CD** = Clinical (or pathologic) diagnosis

Video clip 13.1   A 3-week-old Holstein calf.
H: Abnormal gait since birth with no change in the signs.
AD: Cerebellum.
CD: Necropsy diagnosis of cerebellar hypoplasia and atrophy. Presumptive in utero bovine viral diarrhea virus infection.

Video clip 13.2   Three Holstein calves born to different dams on one farm in a 10-day period.
H: All unable to stand since birth.
AD: Cerebellum.
CD: Necropsy diagnosis of cerebellar hypoplasia and atrophy. Presumptive in utero bovine viral diarrhea virus infection.

Video clip 13.3   Two Holstein calves, 1 and 2 weeks old, respectively.
H: Both unable to stand since birth.
AD: Cerebellum.
CD: The first calf had no lesions at necropsy and is an example of a presumptive congenital functional cerebellar disorder. The second calf had lesions of a presumptive in utero bovine viral diarrhea virus infection. There are no obvious clinical differences.

Video clip 13.4   A 4-day-old Holstein calf.
H: Born unable to get up with diffuse tremors associated with any muscle activity. When recumbent and totally relaxed, the tremors disappear.
AD: Diffuse central nervous system.
CD: Necropsy diagnosis of hypomyelinogenesis. Presumptive in utero bovine viral diarrhea virus infection.

Video clip 13.5   A 5-day-old Holstein calf.
H: Since birth, action-related tremors have been present primarily in the pelvic limb and trunk muscles. When recumbent and totally relaxed, the tremors disappear.
AD: Diffuse central nervous system (CNS). Whole-body tremors require a diffuse disturbance of CNS neurons or their myelin.
CD: Necropsy diagnosis of diffuse axonopathy most pronounced in the spinal cord. Presumptive inherited disorder.

Video clip 13.6   Two, 2-day-old Polled Hereford calves.
H: Unable to stand since birth. Diffuse tremors are associated with any muscle activity. When recumbent and totally relaxed, the tremors disappear.
AD: Diffuse central nervous system (CNS).
CD: Necropsy diagnosis of diffuse CNS edema ("cerebral edema"), a form of spongiform degeneration, which is an inherited autosomal recessive metabolic disorder of Polled Herefords.

Video clip 13.7   A 10-day-old Brown Swiss calf.
H: The calf developed fever and depression on day 3 of life. The calf's plasma protein concentration was 5.2 g/dL, so failure of passive transfer of antibodies was suspected as a predisposing cause for sepsis. The calf was treated with ceftiofur, intravenously administered crystalloids and plasma in additional to nutritional support, and appeared to be responding well until day 10. On day 10 of life, the calf had an acute onset of tremors, and ataxia and fever recurred. Cerebrospinal fluid (CSF) collected from the lumbosacral site was grossly discolored and suppurative. The calf was euthanized, and the brain is shown in Fig. 13.9. *Escherichia coli* was cultured from both the CSF and from a blood culture that had been collected on hospital admission. This organism demonstrated in vitro resistance to ceftiofur and all other antibiotics on the panel except for amikacin.
AD: Prosencephalon, caudal brainstem, cerebellum.
CD: Suppurative meningitis.

Video clip 13.8   A 4-week-old Angus calf.
H: Two weeks of progressive depression and ataxia. Recumbent for 3 days.
AD: Cerebellum, pons, and midbrain; opisthotonus can occur with disorders of these anatomic sites.
CD: Cerebrospinal fluid contained elevated levels of protein and degenerate neutrophils. Necropsy diagnosis of suppurative meningitis.

Video clip 13.9   A 6-month-old Holstein calf.
H: One week of depression, excessive recumbency, sialosis, and tongue protrusion.
AD: Cranial nerves II through XII, caudal brain stem for the mild ataxia or paresis (upper motor neuron/general proprioception systems); more likely parenchymal lesion.
CD: Necropsy diagnosis of probable pituitary abscess that ruptured and extended caudally along the ventral surface of the brain stem.

Video clip 13.10   An 18-month-old Holstein calf.
H: Depression progressing over 48 hours to obtundation and reluctance to move.
AD: Diencephalon based on the severe obtundation from interference with the ascending reticular activating system in an animal that is still able to walk.
CD: Necropsy diagnosis of a large focal pituitary abscess.

Video clip 13.11   A 3-year-old Holstein cow.
H: Six days of intermittent circling to the right and inability to eat normally.
AD: Cranial nerves III through XII—left pons and medulla. This cow had vision but could not close the eyelids because of bilateral facial paralysis. The extensive cranial nerve dysfunction with the mild gait disorder suggested an extramedullary lesion, which turned out to be incorrect in this cow.
CD: Lumbosacral cerebrospinal fluid contained 26 white blood cells/µL with 60% macrophages. Necropsy diagnosis of listeriosis with extensive involvement of cranial nerve nuclei.

Video clip 13.12   A 2-year-old Hereford cow.
H: Ten days of progressive depression and dysphagia.
AD: Pons and medulla.
CD: Necropsy diagnosis of listeriosis.

Video clip 13.13   An 18-month-old Holstein heifer.
H: Acute onset of propulsive circling to the left when stimulated. Intravenous potassium penicillin and supportive therapy led to a full recovery. The heifer was pregnant at the time and maintained the pregnancy to term. This heifer also demonstrated persistent medial strabismus (see Fig. 13.16).
AD: Extrapyramidal system (there was no evidence of vestibular dysfunction) and brainstem (trochlear nerve).
CD: Suspected listeriosis.

Video clip 13.14   A 5-year-old Holstein cow.
H: Five days of progressive difficulty using the pelvic limbs associated with overflexed tarsi and buckled fetlocks. She was recumbent at hospitalization and unable to urinate, and on rectal examination, she had a large bladder. Loss of tail movement and anal reflex developed within the first 6 hours after hospital admission. She became quite agitated and acted in discomfort.
AD: Lumbosacrocaudal spinal cord segments or spinal nerves. Unusual "stringhalt-like" flexor reflex action in the paretic pelvic limbs, which probably reflected disturbed inhibition in the lumbosacral grey matter. Lumbosacral cerebrospinal fluid contained 9 white blood cells/µL (lymphocytes and macrophages) and 97 mg protein/dL.
CD: Necropsy diagnosis of rabies viral myelitis.

Video clip 13.15   A 6-month-old Holstein calf.
H: Acute onset of lethargy, loss of vision, and ataxia. Progressed to recumbency in 24 hours. Improved after therapy.
AD: Prosencephalon. Note depression and loss of vision but the ability to walk. The pupils were small and still reactive to light. The initial signs reflected a diffuse brain lesion that had recovered to just the prosencephalic signs seen on the video.
CD: Presumptive thiamine-deficient polioencephalomalacia.

Video clip 13.16   A 6-month-old Holstein calf.
H: Acute onset of lethargy, loss of vision, and shuffling gait. Became recumbent in 24 hours.
AD: Prosencephalon.
CD: Necropsy diagnosis of polioencephalomalacia. Presumptive thiamine deficiency but beware of sulfur and lead toxicity that cause the same lesions.

Video clip 13.17A   A 2-month-old Holstein calf.
H: One week of a "swaying" gait and progressive depression with loss of vision.
AD: Cerebrocortical disorder.
CD: Blood ammonia was greater than 600 µmol/L (normal, <40 µmol/L). At necropsy, a portocaval shunt was found and a diffuse encephalomyelopathy. On rare occasions, spinal cord signs without obvious cerebral deficits have been observed in other calves with portosystemic shunts (see Fig. 13.31 and Video clip 13.17B).

Video clip 13.17B   A 2-month-old Holstein calf.
H: One week of abnormal gait.
AD: C1 to C5 spinal cord segments, focal or diffuse.
CD: Either discospondylitis or an abscess was suspected. Radiographs were normal. At necropsy, a portocaval shunt was found with a diffuse hepatic form of encephalomyelopathy. No cerebral signs were reported or observed. Similar spinal cord signs have been observed in other calves with portosystemic shunts.

Video clip 13.18A   An 18-month-old Holstein heifer.
H: Escaped from barn 2 days earlier; now demonstrating blindness, hyperesthesia, and ataxia.
AD: Prosencephalon (limbic system) and diffuse brain.
CD: Elevated blood lead concentrations (from licking an old battery). Clinical signs are consistent with lead poisoning.

Video clip 13.18B   A yearling Brown Swiss heifer.
H: This heifer had 2 days of depression and anorexia. On hospital examination, it was noted that the heifer had both a decreased menace and vision but normal pupillary light responses. One day later, the heifer was noted to be grinding her teeth, as can be heard in the video, and abnormally high blood lead levels were found. The heifer was treated with calcium disodium ethylenediaminetetraacetic acid and thiamine intravenously and administered magnesium sulfate orally. She began to improve after 3 days of treatments and had a complete clinical recovery. The owners were instructed by oral communication and letter that follow-up testing for milk lead levels would be required if she were to enter the milking herd. The source of the lead poisoning in this case was unknown.
AD: Cerebral cortex bilateral.
CD: Lead poisoning.

Video clip 13.19   A 10-day-old Brown Swiss heifer.
H: The heifer developed acute and persistent facial twitching with chewing "bubble gum" type seizures. Serum chemistry testing found a profound hypernatremia (serum sodium, 188 mEq/L). Despite attempts at gradual sodium reduction using hypertonic fluids, the neurologic status deteriorated, and the animal was euthanized.
AD: Prosencephalon.
CD: Salt poisoning.

Video clip 13.20   A 3-year-old Jersey cow.
H: Two weeks postpartum, acute depression, decreased milk production, and abnormal behavior. Video shows the maniacal chewing, neck extension, and closed palpebral fissures all observed on hospital admission.
AD: Prosencephalon (limbic system).
CD: Strong elevation of urine ketones, decreased bicarbonate, and increased anion gap diagnosed as ketoacidosis. The clinical signs of nervous ketosis resolved with dextrose therapy.

Video clip 13.21   A 2-year-old Holstein heifer, fresh for 2 weeks.
H: This heifer had an acute onset of circling to the right and propulsively and frequently sticking her tongue out in a dramatic fashion. The cow was strongly ketotic based on urine testing and was sedated (20 mg xylazine) and treated for nervous ketosis with intravenous dextrose and orally administered propylene glycol in addition to transfaunation and forced feeding. The heifer was improved the following day and appeared normal 2 days after treatment was begun.
AD: Prosencephalon—limbic system.
CD: Nervous ketosis.

Video clip 13.22   A 2-week-old Holstein calf.
H: Since birth, unable to stand and walk with the pelvic limbs.
AD: T3 to L3 spinal cord segments, focal or diffuse. The simultaneous use of the pelvic limbs, referred to as "bunny hopping," is a very reliable sign for some form of myelodysplasia. This simultaneous activity is also observed on testing the flexor reflex. Spinal cord malformations are often accompanied by vertebral column malformations. The latter was palpated at L2 and L3 in this calf.
CD: Radiographs and computed tomography (CT) images diagnosed an L2 to L3 malformation. The CT demonstrated segmental spinal cord hypoplasia at this level. Necropsy diagnosis of thoracolumbar myelodysplasia with segmental hypoplasia of the L2 and L3 segments and sacral segment diplomyelia.

Video clip 13.23   A 2-day-old Simmental cross calf.
H: Recumbent since birth.
AD: T10 to T11 focal transverse lesion. This was based on the paraplegia and the T13 line of analgesia. The simultaneous pelvic limb movements were all uninhibited reflex actions similar to spinal walking. There were no vertebrae palpated from T13 to L2.
CD: Myelodysplasia and vertebral malformation were confirmed at necropsy. There were no vertebral arches between T13 and L2, and there were no spinal cord segments from T13 through L3. There was myelodysplasia in the caudal thoracic segments and from L4 through the caudal segments. The extreme pelvic limb hyperreflexia seen here was caused by the complete absence of any brainstem inhibition of the lumbosacral grey matter.

Video clip 13.24   A 1-week-old Holstein calf.
H: Abnormal use of the pelvic limbs since birth.
AD: T3 to L3 spinal cord segments, focal or diffuse. The scoliosis indicates a vertebral malformation, and the congenital simultaneous pelvic limb action indicates a myelodysplasia.
CD: Necropsy diagnosis of multiple thoracolumbar spinal cord segment myelodysplasia.

Video clip 13.25   A 1-month-old Holstein calf.
H: Rapid progression of inability to stand and walk with the pelvic limbs.
AD: T3 to L3 spinal cord segments-focal or diffuse. This is based on the spastic paresis (upper motor neuron dysfunction) and pelvic limb ataxia (general proprioception dysfunction) with retained spinal reflexes and nociception.
CD: Radiographic diagnosis of discospondylitis at the T13 to L1 articulation with a compression fracture of T13.

Video clip 13.26   A 7-year-old Holstein cow with progressive weakness and an abnormal gait.
AD: Tetra-ataxia and paresis, which could be caused by a C1 to C5 lesion or diffuse or multifocal spinal cord disease.
CD: Spinal lymphosarcoma located epidurally in the caudal thoracic and cranial lumbar spine. Although the predominant neoplastic lesion was noted grossly in a more caudal location, there was histologic evidence of infiltration around the cervical cord, explaining the clinical evidence of tetraparesis.

Video clip 13.27   A 1-year-old Holstein heifer.
H: Found at pasture with an abnormal gait.
AD: Cranial thoracic spinal cord segments. Spastic paraparesis and pelvic limb ataxia with lower motor neuron signs of short strides in the thoracic limbs suggest a C5 to T2 spinal cord segment anatomic diagnosis, but note the strength shown by this heifer in her thoracic limbs when she stumbles and is able to get back up. This suggests that the upper motor neuron/general proprioception lesion is in the cranial thoracic spinal cord segments, and there is loss of thoracolumbar axial muscle function.
CD: Necropsy diagnosis of a fracture of T4 with displacement into the vertebral foramen. The cause of the fracture was unknown. There were no lesions of any vertebral body infection.

Video clip 13.28   A 2-year-old Holstein heifer with a dorsal arch in her back since birth.
AD: Note kyphosis in the region of the malformation and hind limb paresis and ataxia consistent with a thoracic cord compression.
CD: Congenital vertebral malformation at T9 to T10 (see Fig. 13.48).

Video clip 13.29   An 8-month-old Holstein bull with chronic stumbling in the rear legs.
AD: T2 to L4 spinal cord disease. Note the bilateral hind limb ataxia and paresis.
CD: Congenital vertebral malformation between T1 and T4 (see Fig. 13.49).

Video clip 13.30   A 5-month-old Holstein calf.
H: One month of a progressively abnormal gait in the left pelvic limb.
AD: Sciatic-tibial nerve or S1, S2 spinal cord segment, gamma efferent dysfunction.

CD: These signs of extreme hyperextension of the tarsus when attempts are made to protract the limb are typical of the functional disorder referred to as spastic paresis or "Elso heel." There are no microscopic lesions. The hyperactive gastrocnemius muscle activity is caused by uninhibited gamma efferents in the sacral spinal cord segments. This is an inherited disorder in many breeds of cattle.

Video clip 13.31   A 3-month-old Hereford calf.
H: Abnormal use of the right pelvic limb since birth with no change in the clinical signs.
AD: Right femoral nerve, L4 to L5 spinal cord segments, or spinal nerve roots. Note the inability to support weight when the left pelvic limb is advanced.
CD: Presumptive dystocia with overextension of the hip during calving and injury to the femoral nerve as it emerges from the iliopsoas muscle or avulsion of its nerve roots. At necropsy, the latter was found in this calf.

Video clip 13.32   A 3-day-old Holstein calf.
H: Abnormal use of the pelvic limbs since birth.
AD: Bilateral femoral nerve, L4 to L5 spinal cord segments, or spinal nerve roots. The lack of pelvic limb support is most severe in the left pelvic limb. Note the intact nociception on the medial side of the left crus, which is innervated by the saphenous nerve, a branch of the femoral nerve. This suggests a better prognosis.
CD: Presumed femoral nerve injury secondary to a dystocia. This calf recovered in a few weeks.

Video clip 13.33   A 4-year-old Holstein.
H: Two months of progressive gait abnormality in both pelvic limbs that began in the right pelvic limb.
AD: Bilateral tibial nerve, S1 and S2 spinal cord segments, or spinal nerves. The latter is least likely with the normal tail, anus, and perineum. Note the overflexion of the tarsus typical of a tibial nerve dysfunction. The buckling dorsally of the fetlock is a unique sign of tibial nerve dysfunction seen only in cattle.
CD: On rectal examination, a bony defect was palpated on the ventral surface of the sacrum. At necropsy, there was a healed displaced fracture of S2 with fibrosis of the intervertebral foramina entrapping the S1 and S2 spinal nerves. The fracture was presumed to be caused by the cow having been ridden by another cow or bull.

Video clip 13.34   A 2-year-old Holstein.
H: Rapidly progressive abnormal gait in both pelvic limbs.
AD: Bilateral L6, sacral, and caudal nerves or spinal cord segments. Compared with the case in Video clip 13.33, note the loss of tail tone and severe hypalgesia of the sacrocaudal dermatomes in this animal.
CD: Necropsy diagnosis of extensive L6 to S1 discospondylitis, with suppurative inflammation involving multiple lumbosacral spinal nerves.

Video clip 13.35   Two Holstein calves, 2- and 4-months-old respectively.
H: Ten days of progressive ataxia, head tilt, and ear droop.
AD: Two-month-old calf: right cranial nerves VII and VIII.
AD: Four-month-old calf: left cranial nerve VII, pons, and medulla. Note the depression, the need for assistance to stand, and the neck extension.

CD: Two-month-old calf; radiographic diagnosis of otitis media/interna. This is a very common cause of facial nerve or vestibulocochlear nerve dysfunction in calves.
CD: Four-month-old calf; necropsy diagnosis of suppurative otitis media/interna, with meningitis and abscess formation in the left side of the pons and medulla.

Video clip 13.36   A 1-month-old Holstein calf.
H: Bilateral ear droop developed over a few days.
AD: Bilateral facial nerve.
CD: Bilateral otitis media diagnosed on computed tomography imaging.

Video clip 13.37   A 12-year-old Holstein cow.
H: Two months before the videotaping, the owner of this cow treated her for "milk fever" with calcium gluconate presumably administered intravenously in the right external jugular vein. A large mass slowly developed at the injection site. The farmer noted that on cold mornings, there was less mist emerging from the cow's right naris during expiration.
AD: Right sympathetic innervation of the head. The right side of the muzzle is dry; the right ear is warmer than the left. There is a smaller right palpebral fissure. Miosis and third eyelid protrusion were minimal. Loss of vasoconstriction in the right nasal cavity would explain the decreased air flow and less mist seen on expiration on a cold morning.
CD: Presumptive dysfunction of the right cervical sympathetic trunk due to the granuloma on the right side of the neck caused by the extravascular injection of calcium gluconate; Horner's syndrome.

Video clip 13.38   A 1-week-old Holstein calf.
H: Since birth, this calf was inactive, walked with short strides, and preferred to remain recumbent.
AD: Diffuse neuromuscular.
CD: A positive response to intravenous Tensilon suggested congenital myasthenia gravis. Over the next few weeks, this calf improved to normal. A delay in the development of normal neuromuscular receptors was presumed.

Video clip 13.39   A 1-month-old Holstein calf.
H: This calf developed a stiff gait and became recumbent over a few days.
AD: Diffuse spinal cord ventral grey columns and brainstem nuclei. Note the typical facial expression with the ears held caudally and the tight lips.
CD: Tetanus caused by infection with *Clostridium tetani*. This calf died from respiratory depression 2 days later.

Video clip 13.40   A 6-week-old Polled Hereford calf.
H: Since birth, this calf had been recumbent and unable to stand and exhibited extensor rigidity.
AD: Diffuse spinal cord ventral grey columns. The clinical signs observed are tetany. Note the prolonged extensor muscle activity when stimulated with mild relaxation between stimuli, and not attempting to move.
CD: This is a hereditary tetany of Polled Herefords caused by an autosomal recessive gene, which results in the abnormal formation of glycine receptors on motor neuronal cell membranes.

Video clip 14.1   An adult Holstein cow.
H: This cow was presented for a displaced abomasum, and the rapid horizontal movement of both eyes was noted. This movement has almost certainly been present since birth but likely went unnoticed.
Diagnosis: Pendular nystagmus in a 5-year-old Holstein cow.

Video clip 15.1   A 2-year-old first lactation cow with acute onset of tremors most pronounced around the head.
(Courtesy of Dr. Matthew Chuff.)

H: A serum sample was submitted for electrolyte measurements; the magnesium level was 0.4 mg/dL, and the total calcium level was less than 4 mg/dL.
AD: Neuromuscular disease.
CD: Hypomagnesemic tetany.

Index

Note: Page numbers followed by *f* indicate figures, *t* indicate tables, and *b* indicate boxes.